P9-CQA-647

EMERGENCY
telephone numbers

Paramedics 911 or __________

Doctor __________

Doctor __________

Doctor __________

Poison control center __________

Hospital emergency room __________

Fire department __________

Police department __________

Parents at work __________

Parents at work __________

Pharmacy __________

Electric company __________

Gas company __________

Neighbor __________

Relative __________

THE AMERICAN MEDICAL ASSOCIATION

FAMILY MEDICAL GUIDE

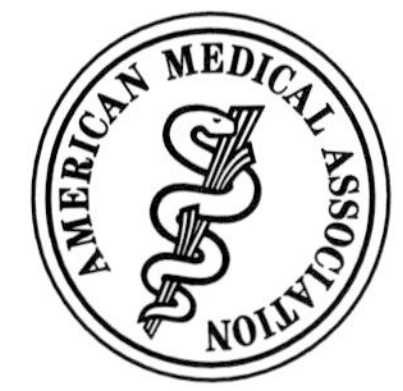

Revised and updated

Third edition

Medical editor
Charles B. Clayman, MD

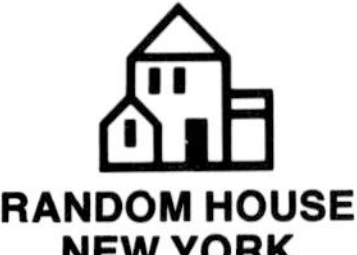

RANDOM HOUSE
NEW YORK

Published in the United States by Random House, Inc., New York.

The recommendations and information in this book are appropriate in most cases; however, they are not a substitute for medical diagnosis. For specific information concerning your personal medical condition, the AMA suggests that you consult a physician. The names of organizations appearing in the book are given for informational purposes only. Their inclusion does not imply AMA endorsement, nor does the omission of any organization, product, or alternative therapy indicate AMA disapproval.

Library of Congress Cataloging-in-Publication Data

American Medical Association family medical guide/
Charles B. Clayman, medical editor.—3rd ed.
p. cm.
Includes index.
ISBN 0-679-41290-5
1. Medicine, Popular. I. Clayman, Charles B. II. Title: Family medical guide.
RC81.A543 1994
616—dc20 94-2116

Manufactured in the United States of America
2 4 6 8 9 7 5 3

American Medical Association

Physicians dedicated to the health of America

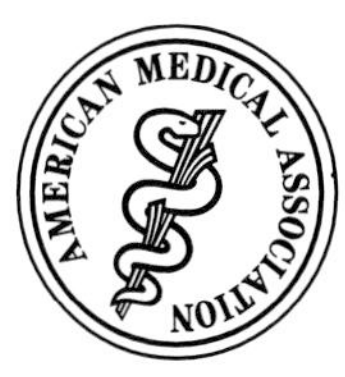

Foreword

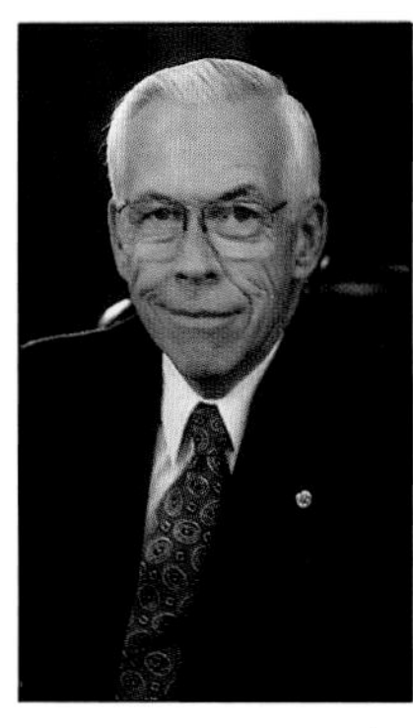

Americans are by definition a highly diverse group of people with many and varied interests and concerns. Today, however, most of us share an active and serious interest in achieving and maintaining good health.

The physicians of the American Medical Association think it is our responsibility to provide you and your family with high-quality, timely, and useful medical information that is geared to your needs and that will help you find the best way to prevent disease and stay healthy.

This newly revised and updated third edition of *The American Medical Association Family Medical Guide* has been edited with some very specific goals; we have worked to make it even more comprehensive and easier to understand. Every article has been reviewed by specialists who work closely with the AMA's team of nonphysician editors to make the best medical information understandable and useful to you. Readers have told us in response to earlier editions that they appreciate this "user-friendly" tone and very clear language.

To make this book even more helpful we have added a new, expanded section in full color, *Your healthy body*, which provides state-of-the-art disease prevention techniques and ways in which you can change your lifestyle to improve your health.

We hope this volume will encourage you and your physician to form a partnership and work together toward a common goal: many years of good health for you and your loved ones.

James S. Todd, MD
Executive Vice President
American Medical Association

The American Medical Association

	James S. Todd, MD	*Executive Vice President*
	Larry E. Joyce	*Senior Vice President, Publishing*
	Steven V. Seekins	*Vice President, Corporate and Consumer Affairs*
	Heidi Hough	*Publisher, Consumer Publishing*
EDITORIAL STAFF	Charles B. Clayman, MD	*Medical Editor*
	Patricia Dragisic	*Managing Editor*
	Steven Michaels	*Senior Editor*
	Mark Ingebretsen	*Contributing Editor*
	Robin Fitzpatrick Husayko	*Editor*
	Daniel Knight	*Copy Editor*
	Barbara Scotese	*Copy Editor*
	Katie Sharp	*Copy Editor*
	Kitty D. Williams	*Editorial Assistant*
	Dorothy A. Johnson	*Administrative Assistant*
	Debra A. Smith	*Production Secretary*
ACKNOWLEDGMENTS	B. J. Anderson, JD	
	Wayne G. Hoppe, JD	
	George Kruto	
	Anne White Michalski	
	William Smith, JD	
	Neil Sutherland	
	Lorri A. Zipperer	
	American Academy of Dermatology	
	American Dietetic Association	
	American Psychiatric Association	
	Mallinckrodt Institute of Radiology	
DORLING KINDERSLEY LIMITED	Jackie Douglas	*Editorial Director*
	Peter Luff	*Art Director*
	Ruth Midgley	*Senior Managing Editor*
	Philip Gilderdale	*Managing Art Editor*
	Christine Murdock	*Editor*
	Ellen Woodward	*Designer*

Medical Consultants		
	Bruce Berkson, MD	*Urology*
	Steven N. Blair, PED	*Epidemiology/Fitness*
	Melvin D. Cheitlin, MD	*Cardiology*
	Priscilla M. Clarkson, PhD	*Physiology*
	Bruce Cohen, MD	*Neurology*
	David Cugell, MD	*Pulmonary Medicine*
	Arthur W. Curtis, MD	*Otolaryngology*
	Kimberly A. Douglass, RN	*Clinical Nurse Specialist*
	Jerome Garden, MD	*Dermatology*
	Richard M. Gore, MD	*Radiology*
	Jourdan Gottlieb, MD	*Plastic and Reconstructive Surgery*
	Steven Gryll, PhD	*Psychology*
	Donald F. Heiman, MD	*Infectious Diseases*
	Linda Hughey Holt, MD	*Obstetrics and Gynecology*
	Allen Horwitz, MD	*Genetics*
	Frederic C. Kass, MD	*Oncology*
	Robert J. Kelsey, Jr., MD	*Obstetrics and Gynecology*
	Gary S. Lissner, MD	*Ophthalmology*
	Kenneth R. Margules, MD	*Rheumatology*
	Arline McDonald, PhD	*Nutrition*
	Ronald M. Meyer, MD	*Anesthesiology*
	Bruce Naughton, MD	*Geriatrics*
	Tom E. Nesbitt, Sr., MD	*Urology*
	Robert V. Rege, MD	*General Surgery*
	Domeena C. Renshaw, MD	*Psychiatry/Sexual Dysfunction*
	Gary A. Rodgers, DDS	*Dentistry*
	Andrew T. Saltzman, MD	*Orthopedics*
	Michael W. T. Shwayder, MD	*Nephrology*
	Tor Shwayder, MD	*Pediatrics*
	Irwin M. Siegel, MD	*Orthopedics*
	Emanuel M. Steindler, PhD	*Addiction Medicine*
	Mark Stolar, MD	*Endocrinology*
	Howard Traisman, MD	*Pediatrics*
	Ronald J. Vasu, MD	*Psychiatry*
	William J. Weigel, MD	*Pharmacology*
	Stanley M. Zydlo, MD	*Emergency Medicine*

Contents

PART ONE *Your healthy body*

PART TWO *Symptoms and self-diagnosis*

PART THREE *Diseases, disorders, and other problems*

How to use this book

A wealth of information on health and disease is at your fingertips in this third edition of *The American Medical Association Family Medical Guide*. Take some time to familiarize yourself with the book to get the most out of it—in terms of specific health questions and general information.

When looking up a topic, start with the index. Note that the index contains many cross-references to other terms (for example, "Botulism, *see* Food poisoning") to help you find the information you need.

Also, scan the contents on pp.8-9 for an overview of how the book is organized.

Your healthy body

Part One begins with a completely revised, expanded full-color section, *Your healthy body*, which contains up-to-date information on preventive medicine. Families today want accurate, clear information on fitness, mental health, diet and nutrition, how to quit smoking, child safety, and environmental health, and all are explored here. *Atlas of the body* is a handy reference for locating bones, muscles, and other parts of the body.

Symptoms and self-diagnosis

Part Two begins with the charts in *Symptoms and self-diagnosis*. By checking out your own and your family's symptoms in these charts (completely revised and updated by medical specialists for this edition), you can get a better idea of when to call your physician about a problem, when to go straight to your hospital emergency department, and what to expect when you get there. As you become familiar with the symptom charts, you may notice that using them is like solving a puzzle; you just need to follow the clues. For example, if you have a headache, do you also have a fever? Where does the pain come from? Answering yes or no to these questions helps you pinpoint the cause of your headache and tells how to get help.

The symptom charts contain many cross-references to articles in Part Three, *Diseases, disorders, and other problems*. To make best use of the symptom charts, follow the cross-references to the disease articles.

Visual aids to diagnosis complements the symptom charts with full-color photos of sores, rashes, and other symptoms, along with a brief description of the disorder or condition they might be linked with. If your symptoms indicate that you need further tests, *Diagnostic imaging techniques*—an all-new section—helps bring you up-to-date on the types of scans your physician might suggest (for example, ultrasound) and which disorders they might help to diagnose.

Diseases, disorders, and other problems

Part Three is the heart of the book, with articles on the most common diseases and conditions arranged by areas of the body and/or by function (for example, *Disorders of the respiratory system*).

The editors have used a standard format for these articles to help answer your most common questions about a disease: What is it? What are the symptoms? What are the risks? What should be done? What is the treatment? When you have certain diseases or conditions, self-care measures are important, so facts about self-care are included in this book whenever appropriate.

Again, to make the most of this book, follow the cross-references to other parts of the book and use the index if you are in doubt about where to look. In addition to articles on disease that apply to most age groups, Part Three features special chapters on health and disease in infants and children, adolescents, and older people.

Caring for the sick

Part Four focuses on additional aspects of health care. *The American health care system* provides useful information about health care delivery in the US. *Caregiving at home* gives you some highly practical ideas on how to take care of a sick person in your home, whether you are taking care of a child who has measles for a week or modifying your home to take care of an older family member who has had surgery or who has dementia.

Dying and death guides you through the grief process on two levels. Included is information on what to tell a dying person and how to deal with your own grief. Practical matters such as organ donation, autopsies, and living wills are also discussed.

The *Drug glossary* and *Glossary* contain useful information to supplement your reading in this book and answer your general questions about health care.

A final section, *Injuries and emergencies*, is a guide with accurate advice on how to handle crises including choking, bleeding, heatstroke, and emergency childbirth.

PART ONE

Your healthy body

Your healthy body

Introduction

Americans are living longer today than at any time in the past. Many of us will remain mentally and physically healthy well into our 80s.

Some people, however, will become ill or die before others of a similar age. To some extent this is a matter of chance, environment, and heredity. But there are some very important factors in determining how healthy you are now—and how healthy you'll be in your later years—that are under your control.

You can stay healthier throughout your life by making positive lifestyle changes and by having regular checkups, so that any disease that develops can be detected and treated early.

Of course, prevention does not mean simply "disease prevention." You can risk illness, injury, and even early death in many other ways. For example, young people in the US are more likely to become disabled or die as a result of motor vehicle and work injuries and violent assaults involving alcohol and illegal drugs than as a result of disease. Because of AIDS, sexual behavior also has become a significant factor in determining both health and survival.

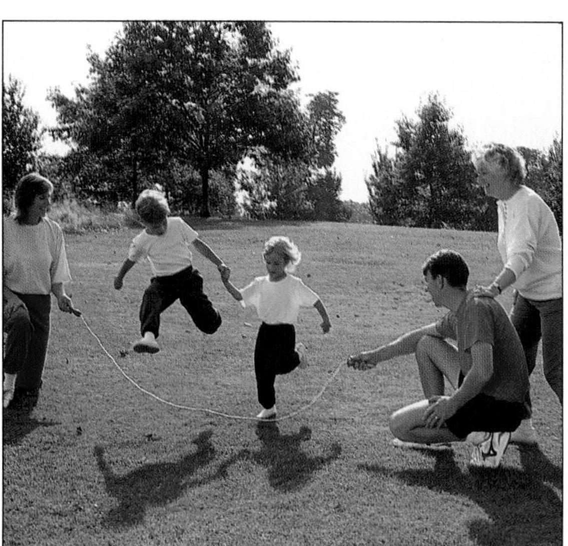

Living a healthy lifestyle is one of the most important things you can do to prevent disease.

Adopting a healthy lifestyle does not mean that you have to stop enjoying life. It does, however, mean taking responsibility for your actions. If you smoke, stop now. Smoking is the leading cause of death before age 65 in the US. You can find suggestions on how to quit smoking on page 51. A healthy diet means eating a wide variety of naturally occurring foods and maintaining your weight at a desirable level. Regular moderate exercise, such as walking, can lead to a gradual, but significant, improvement in your physical condition as well as improved mental energy and alertness. This section of the book will help guide you to a healthier lifestyle.

Medical research performed during the past 20 years clearly shows how a healthy lifestyle can help prevent a variety of diseases that cause most deaths before age 65. For example, heart disease (see Coronary artery disease, p.400) and cancers (see p.16) are major causes of premature death, but you can take steps to prevent some of these diseases.

If disease develops and is detected at any early stage, treatment often is more effective. Detecting and treating conditions that cause no symptoms, such as high blood pressure, have saved millions of lives, and tests have been developed to detect heart and lung disorders and many types of cancer. Evaluating vision and hearing problems is another important part of the regular checkups that are essential to a healthy lifestyle. On pages 14 and 15 you will find a guide to screening tests and checkups that physicians generally recommend for American adults.

The recommendations made in this section of the book are based on scientific research. Six basic rules for healthy living are described in the box on the next page. They sound simple—and they are—but they are valuable guidelines to positive steps that you can take to improve your health both now and in the future.

Six basic rules for healthy living

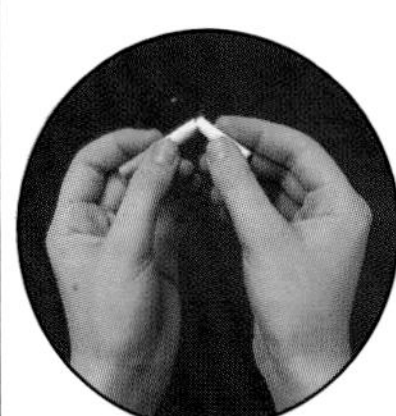

If you smoke, quit now. Smoking is a leading cause of death in the US; it is a major factor in coronary heart disease and in cancers of the lung, mouth, esophagus, throat, bladder, and cervix. Also, smoking accelerates aging of the skin, bones, and lungs.

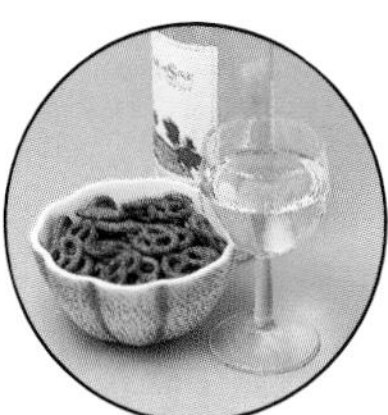

If you drink alcohol, drink only in moderation. Do not drink any alcohol if you are pregnant or if you are driving or operating machinery. If you think you have a problem with alcohol, call Alcoholics Anonymous, your physician, or, your local hospital for assistance.

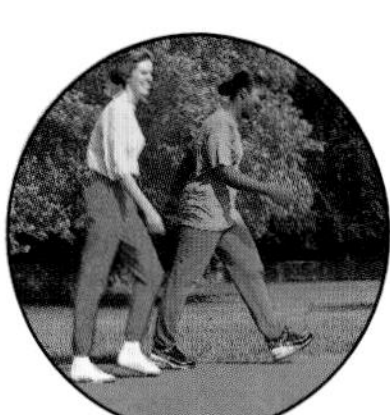

Find some exercise that you enjoy, such as walking or swimming, and do it at least five times per week for a total of at least 30 minutes each day. The 30 minutes can be divided into 10- or 15-minute segments if these are easier to fit into your day.

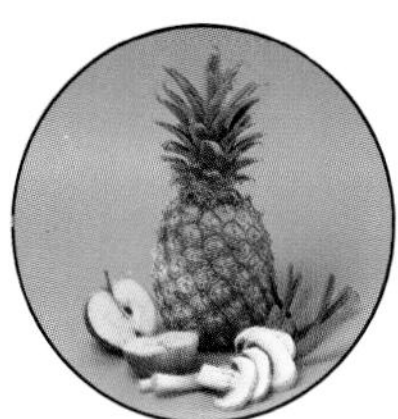

Eat a wide variety of naturally occurring foods, including plenty of whole grains, fresh fruits, and fresh vegetables. Use moderation in your consumption of foods that contain fat. Look at the food pyramid (p.28) for ideas on how to eat for health.

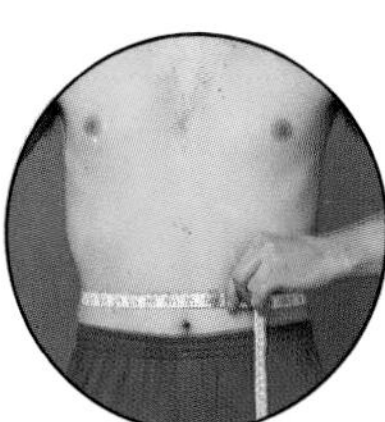

Keep your body trim. Do not let yourself, or your children, become overweight. Obesity (p.530) is linked with many serious disorders such as heart disease and diabetes mellitus. If you are overweight, try hard to make permanent changes in your eating and exercise habits.

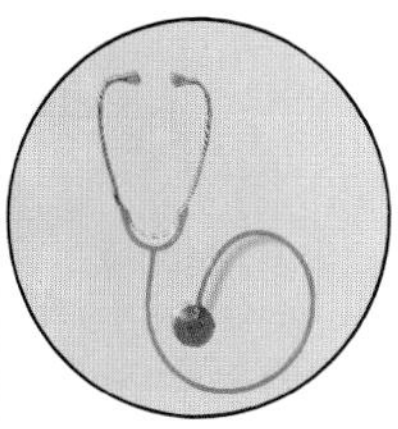

Have regular medical checkups (see pp.14-15). Screening tests can detect many diseases in their early stages, when they may be more successfully treated. Your physician can answer any questions you may have about how often a test should be performed.

The health questionnaire

- Are you within the optimum weight limits for your height (see the Weight charts, p.35)?
- Do you climb at least 40 stairs on most days?
- Do you exercise moderately for a total of 30 minutes at least five times per week?
- Do you walk at least a few blocks every day?
- Do you usually sleep soundly and wake up feeling energetic and ready for the day ahead?
- At the end of a working day do you usually feel energetic enough to go out and enjoy a social evening?
- If you drink alcohol, do you keep your intake low?
- Are you and have you been for at least the last 15 years a nonsmoker?
- Can you walk up three flights of stairs (each flight including about 15 to 20 steps) without having to pause to recover and catch your breath?
- Do you drive carefully and always wear a seat belt?
- Are you happy with your life, and do you generally have a positive outlook?
- Do you have regular medical checkups?
- Is the amount of fat in your diet below 30 percent of your total intake of calories (see p.31)?
- When you are driving, do you always refrain from drinking alcohol or taking any other drugs that affect your coordination?
- Do you not use any type of drug that affects your mood or ability to think?
- If you are not in a monogamous relationship, do you use a latex condom every time you have sex?
- Have you and your family learned essential life-saving first-aid procedures such as the Heimlich maneuver and cardiopulmonary resuscitation (CPR)?

Evaluation

If you can answer YES to all of the above questions, you are maximizing your chances of staying healthy. The more NO answers, the more you need to think about making some changes in your lifestyle.

Tests and screening

Two key components of prevention are adopting a healthy lifestyle and having regular checkups to detect any disease at an early, curable stage. Regular checkups by your physician should include the appropriate tests for your age, background, and health history; these checkups also provide an opportunity for you to ask your physician for advice on such subjects as stress, alcohol consumption, smoking, and your weight.

Physicians test all their patients for common disorders such as high blood pressure, which is found in people of all backgrounds. Other disorders, however, occur more frequently among certain racial or occupational groups, so only those at risk are tested. For example, the genetic blood disorder thalassemia affects many people of southern European and of Middle Eastern descent but not people of northern European descent (see also Genetic counseling, p.664).

If your work regularly exposes you to hazardous chemicals, you may need to be tested regularly to see if your health is being affected by the chemicals. People who have worked with asbestos over a long period of time, for example, should undergo tests periodically for asbestosis or lung cancer. Some types of cancer and heart disease run in families, so tests are performed earlier and more frequently in people who have a family history of a particular disease.

Ask your physician how accurate a particular test might be. An ideal screening test detects virtually everyone who has the disease and does not mistakenly detect the disease in people who do not have it.

Over the years physicians have agreed on the use of selected tests that are of proven value in detecting various diseases. These tests are performed in addition to regular checkups. You generally need more tests as you age, because disorders such as coronary heart disease and cancer are more common in older people. The recommended tests are shown in the chart at right.

Self-examination

In addition to screening tests performed by your physician and dentist, there are several self-examinations designed to identify early signs of cancer that you should perform regularly. Cancer of the breast, skin, or testicle is usually detected first by individuals at home during a self-examination. Since you are most familiar with your body, you are likely to notice any abnormal changes. Because early detection improves the chances of successful treatment, regular self-examination gives you the best chance of detecting a small, early tumor at a stage when a cure may still be possible.

Breast examination

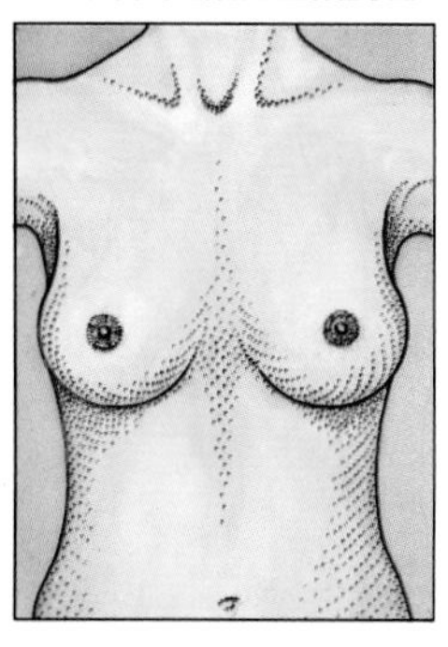

Perform this examination to check for any lump or change in the shape or feel of your breasts. These may be early signs of cancer (see Box, How to examine your breasts, p.630).

All women should do this, but especially women who have a family history of breast cancer.

Start examining your breasts at puberty and repeat every month at the same stage of your menstrual cycle.

Skin examination

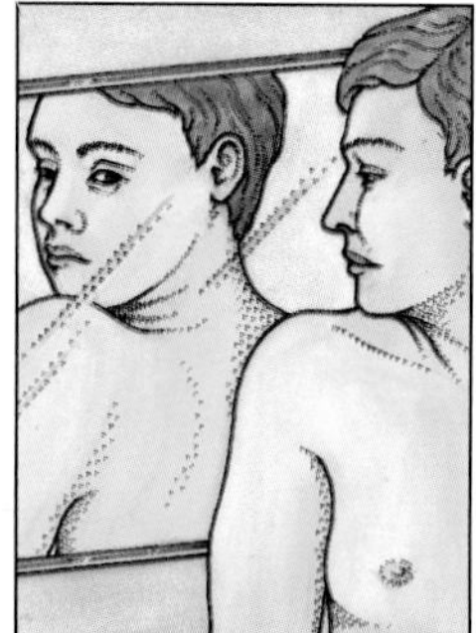

Perform this examination to check for any new mole, or any mole that changes (starts to bleed, itch, or grow), which may be a sign of skin cancer (see also Visual aids to diagnosis, p.251).

Everyone should check his or her skin, but people who have had frequent, prolonged exposure to the sun should check their skin regularly and carefully.

All adults over age 20 should examine their skin regularly.

Testicle examination

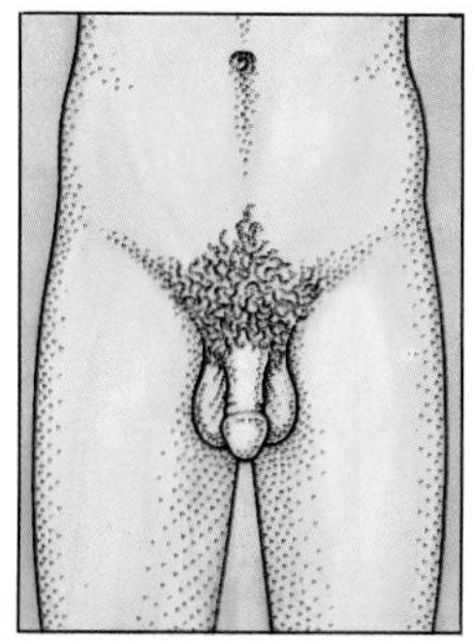

Perform this examination to check for any change in your testicles that may be an early sign of cancer (see Box, Self-examination of the testicles, p.612).

All men should do this.

Start examining your testicles at puberty and repeat the examination once a month, preferably after a warm bath or shower.

Health checkups by medical professionals

Your age and health history determine how often you need specific screening tests. Ask your physician for advice.

● Eye examination
To check for any visual problems or eye muscle disorders and to look for any signs of disease development.
At high risk People who have diabetes or high blood pressure or who have a family history of glaucoma.

● Dental examination
To check the health of your teeth, gums, tongue, and mouth and to look for oral cancer.
At high risk Smokers and tobacco chewers.

● Cervical (Pap) smear—women only
To check for abnormal cells in the lining of the cervix that could develop into cancer.
At high risk Women who have herpes or genital warts.

● Blood pressure measurement
To detect high blood pressure at an early stage, before complications develop.
At high risk People with a family history of high blood pressure, heart or kidney disease, or stroke; people who have diabetes, are overweight, or are taking an oral contraceptive.

● Cholesterol test
To detect a high risk of coronary heart disease.
At high risk People with a family history of early-onset coronary heart disease.

● Mammogram (Breast X ray)—women only
To detect breast cancer early, before it can be detected by physical examination.
At high risk Women with a close relative who has had breast cancer.

● Rectum and colon examination
To check for cancer of the rectum and colon. There are three tests—a) digital rectal examination, b) tests for hidden blood in the stool, and c) flexible sigmoidoscopy.
At high risk People with an immediate family member who has had cancer of the colon or rectum, polyps of the colon, or long-standing, extensive ulcerative colitis.

● Complete physical examination
To determine your current health status and to maintain a relationship with your physician.

	Test	People not at high risk	People at high risk
Adolescents to age 30	Eye	Every 2 years if you have problems with your vision	At least once a year
	Dental	Every 6 months until age 21, then at least once a year	As your dentist recommends
	Cervical (Pap) smear	Annually for women over 18 and all sexually active women, or as your physician recommends	Annually
	Blood pressure	Begin at age 20; after 20, at 3- to 5-year intervals	Annually
	Cholesterol	At the time of your first physical examination	If abnormal, follow your physician's advice
	Rectum/ colon	Usually not necessary	a) Annually after age 20
	Physical	Twice in your 20s	Twice in your 20s
Adults 30 to 50	Eye	Every 2 years; if you have good vision start eye exams at 40	Annually
	Dental	At least once a year	As your dentist recommends
	Cervical (Pap) smear	Every 1 to 3 years	Annually
	Blood pressure	Every 3 to 5 years	Annually
	Cholesterol	Depends on results of last test; if normal, repeat in 5 years	If abnormal, follow your physician's advice
	Breast	Begin at age 40; then every 1 to 2 years to age 50	As your physician recommends
	Rectum/ colon	Annually after 40	a) Annually b) Annually c) Every 3 to 5 years
	Physical	Every 1 to 5 years as your physician recommends	Every 1 to 2 years as your physician recommends
Adults 50 and over	Eye	Every 2 years	At least once a year
	Dental	Every 1 to 2 years	As your dentist recommends
	Cervical (Pap) smear	Every 3 to 5 years	Annually
	Blood pressure	Annually	As your physician recommends
	Cholesterol	Depends on results of last test; if normal, repeat in 3 to 5 years	If abnormal, follow your physician's advice
	Breast	Annually	Annually
	Rectum/ colon	a) Annually b) Annually c) Every 3 to 5 years	a) Annually b) Annually c) Every 3 to 5 years
	Physical	Every 1 to 2 years to age 65; annually after 65	Every 1 to 2 years to age 65; annually after 65

Facts about cancer

Cancer is the second most common cause of death in the US (the first is heart disease), representing about one in five deaths. Cancer has become more common during the twentieth century, not because of pollution or radiation, but because cancer is more common in older people. As the number of older people in the population has increased, so has the frequency of cancer. The disease is very rare in people in their 20s, but the risk of developing cancer roughly doubles between ages 30 and 40 and doubles again with each succeeding decade. This means that people in their 70s have twice the risk of cancer that people in their 60s have, and 16 times the risk of people in their 30s. However, great advances have been made in the diagnosis and treatment of cancer.

What is cancer?

Cancer is the unregulated growth and spread of cells. Cancer is not a single disease; it is a group of diseases in which a breakdown occurs in the normal processes that control the multiplication of cells. Almost all our cells need to be replaced regularly; some cells (such as those that line the intestine) divide every few hours and are shed after living for only a few days; other cells live for years. The processes of cell division and growth are controlled by genes that start and stop the growth process. Some of these growth-controlling genes may undergo changes (mutations) that cause them to malfunction. Cell growth is then uncontrolled; the cell divides, forming more cells with the same mutated genes. Simple overgrowth of cells may lead to a relatively harmless, benign (not likely to spread) tumor such as a wart or polyp, but two or three (or more) genes within a single cell may undergo changes that cause a growth that becomes malignant (likely to spread) and invades and damages blood vessels, nerves, and other body tissues. Invasion of healthy tissues by the growth of malignant tumor cells is called metastasis. It usually takes 10 years or more for a malignant tumor to grow large enough to cause symptoms. Malignant tumor cells may be carried by the bloodstream or spread through the lymphatic system to all parts of the body, where they form other tumors. Once a cancer has metastasized (spread) it is usually incurable. However, treatment can prolong and improve the quality of life.

What causes cancer?

The three major causes of changes in growth-controlling cells include viruses, chemicals, and radiation. Several human viruses have been shown to cause cancer. For example, the hepatitis B virus causes a type of liver cancer, some papillomaviruses are closely linked with cancer of the cervix, and another virus is responsible for a rare type of leukemia. The most significant chemical cause of cancer is tobacco; smoking is the cause of most lung cancers and is an

Warning signs of cancer

Here are some common signs and symptoms that may be caused by undetected cancer in its early stages. Although all of these warning signs can have other causes, you should see your physician immediately if you notice any of them. He or she can then examine you and provide appropriate treatment. Remember that early detection and treatment give you the best chances for a cure.

- A scab, sore, or ulcer that does not heal within 3 weeks.

- A skin blemish or mole that enlarges, bleeds, or itches.

- A lump or swelling beneath the skin.

- Recurrent indigestion or difficulty swallowing.

- Hoarseness that lasts for more than a week.

- A persistent cough or coughing up blood.

- Any change in bowel or bladder habits.

- Blood in the stools or urine.

- Vaginal bleeding in the interval between regular periods or after menopause.

How do I avoid getting cancer?

Although some of the causes of cancer remain unknown, and some are beyond a person's control, you can use the information already available to significantly reduce your chances of getting cancer.

Preventing cancer has two aspects: a healthy lifestyle and effective cancer detection.

Effective cancer detection requires regular medical checkups; follow the schedule on p.15. You should also learn the basic skills of self-examination (see p.14) so you can check for skin cancer, breast cancer, and cancer of the testicle. Watch for the early warning signs of cancer (see Box, previous page). Also, if you are exposed to any chemicals at work, ask your employer or your local office of OSHA (Occupational Safety and Health Administration) if you need to wear any protective clothing and whether you should be screened regularly for possible job-related cancers.

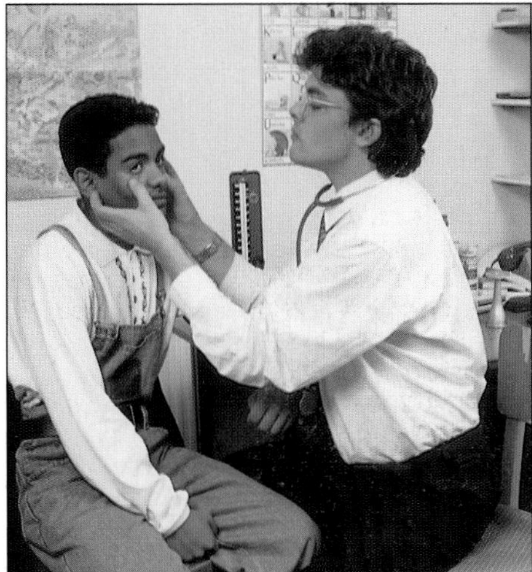

Regular checkups
Be sure to see your physician regularly for physical examinations.

Here are six steps you can take to avoid getting cancer:

1 Do not smoke or chew tobacco. If you do, quit now—it is never too late to quit.

2 Eat a low-fat, low-salt, balanced diet of naturally occurring foods, with plenty of fruit and vegetables and very little smoked meat or fish (see Box, next page).

3 Keep your weight within the normal range for your height and build (see p.35).

4 If you drink alcohol, drink only in moderation (see p.45).

5 Do not expose your skin repeatedly to excessive amounts of direct sunlight.

6 Practice "safer" sex (see Box, p.466) to avoid sexually transmitted diseases.

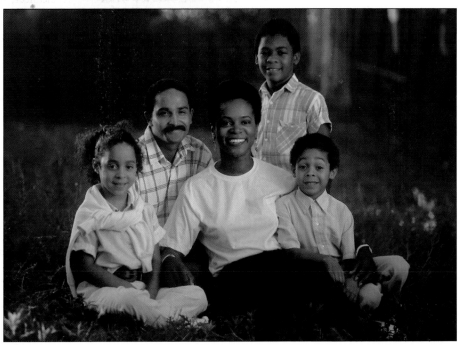

Health by example
Set a good example for your children by taking steps to avoid getting cancer.

Continued from page 16

important factor in cancers of the tongue, larynx, esophagus, cervix, and bladder. Chewing tobacco can cause mouth and tongue cancer. Workers who are exposed to chemicals such as benzene, coal tar, rubber, and some plastics can develop cancers of the blood cells, kidneys, bladder, and liver. Radiation from radioactive isotopes, X rays, and nuclear waste can cause cancer, especially some types of leukemia. The main radiation hazard is sunlight, which causes most skin cancers. People with fair skin that is repeatedly exposed to excessive amounts of direct sunlight have an increased risk of developing skin cancer.

These factors do not, however, always cause cancer in everyone who is exposed to the risk; for example, only a minority of people who have ever smoked cigarettes get lung cancer (although many others die prematurely of chronic illnesses such as heart disease and emphysema). In part, this is because some people are genetically more or less susceptible to a particular risk. Other variables in resisting development of cancer include the amount of alcohol that you drink and the ability of your body's immune system to detect and destroy cancer cells at an early stage.

A diet to help reduce the risk of cancer

Research groups such as the National Cancer Institute have published guidelines that can help you choose a diet that is nutritious and that will help lower your risk of getting cancer.

Reduce the amount of fat you eat. Many Americans get 40 percent of their calories from fats; make an effort to reduce your fat intake to no more than 30 percent of total calories.

Eat more fruits, vegetables, and whole-grain products. This will increase your intake of vitamins A, C, and E. It will also increase your intake of fiber, which shortens the length of time food takes to pass through your intestines, thereby helping eliminate body wastes.

Drink alcohol only in moderation. Excessive alcohol consumption increases your risk of cancers of the mouth, larynx, esophagus, and liver.

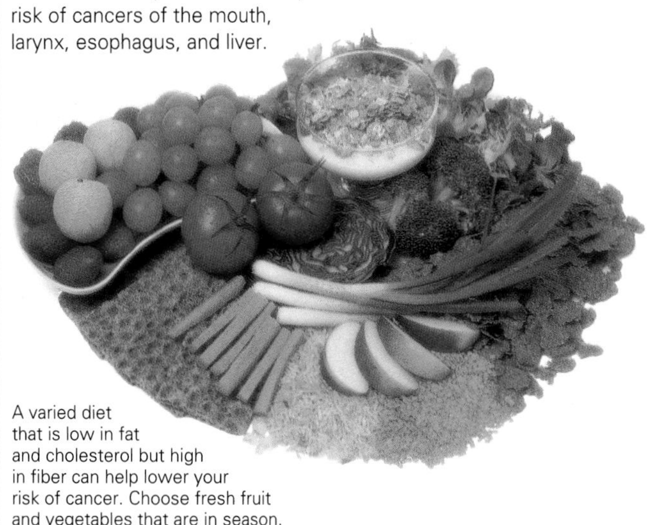

A varied diet that is low in fat and cholesterol but high in fiber can help lower your risk of cancer. Choose fresh fruit and vegetables that are in season.

What are the chances for a cure?

The key to curing some types of cancer is early diagnosis and treatment. Successful treatment is far less likely once malignant cells have spread from the original tumor to form cancers in other parts of the body.

Tests currently used to detect cancer are designed to achieve early diagnosis. Mammography, for example, detects possible breast tumors in women when such tumors are still too small to be found by physical examination of the breasts. Research has shown that the cure rate is more than 80 percent when a breast tumor is under half an inch in diameter at diagnosis.

Regular Pap smears (see p.641) in women detect precancerous changes in the cervix at an early stage when treatment is simple and effective. The death rate from cancer of the cervix has fallen dramatically in recent years in communities where most women have regular Pap smears.

There is evidence that regular examination of the large intestine (colon) in people over age 50 improves survival from cancers of the rectum and colon.

When cancer is suspected, imaging techniques (see p.257) reveal accurate details of tumors, increasing the chances of successful treatment; these techniques include CT scans, MRI scans, and radionuclide scans including PET scans. Also, many internal organs can now be examined directly by endoscopy (examination with a viewing tube).

Advances have been made in treatment as well as in diagnosis of cancer. Drugs may be injected directly into the arteries that supply blood to a tumor, thereby allowing a more targeted destruction of the tumor. In addition, reconstructive plastic surgery offers the possibility of restoring a person's appearance after major surgery on the breast, head, or neck.

Some forms of chemotherapy and treatment with hormones are more effective and less difficult for the patient than treatments used in the past. For example, tamoxifen, the drug used most commonly to treat breast cancer, has few major side effects in most women. Radiation therapy, too, has become more precise and therefore is more effective and causes fewer side effects.

How to strengthen your back

Exercises that strengthen your abdominal muscles can help prevent back injury. They are also important because they help keep your back muscles flexible. For best results, do these exercises at least three times per week. If the exercises cause you any pain or if you have pain and are stiff the next day, check with your physician—you may be overdoing it, performing the exercises incorrectly, or simply out of shape. Repeat each exercise 2 or 3 times and gradually work up to 10 repetitions of each over several days or weeks.

Flexion (bending) exercises

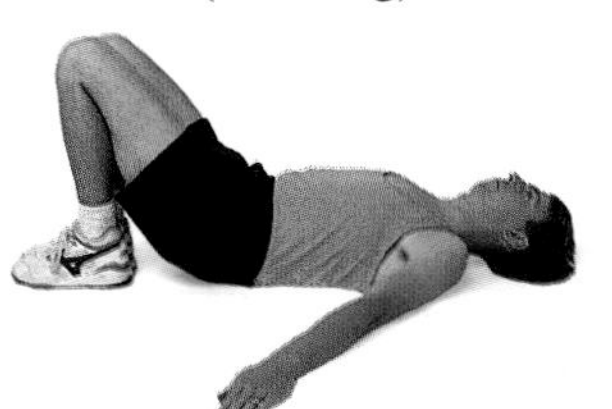

1 Lie on your back with your knees bent. Pull in your abdomen and roll your pelvis to flatten your lower back to the floor. Hold for a count of 5. Relax.

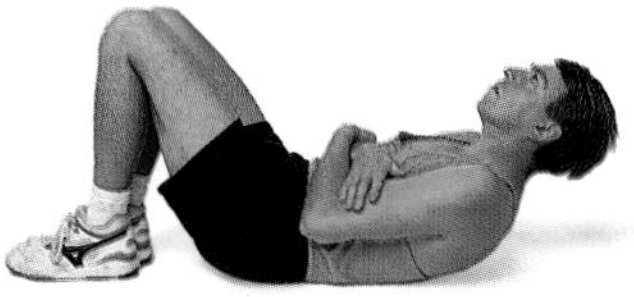

2 Starting in the same position, but with your arms folded across your chest, lift your head and shoulders off the floor up to an angle of 45 degrees. Hold for a count of 5. Relax.

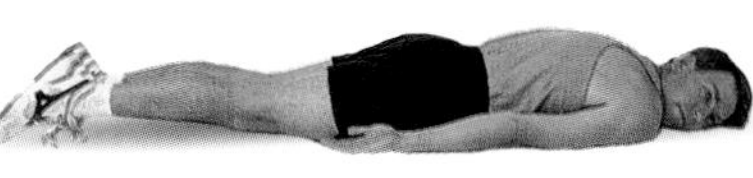

3 Lie on your back with one knee bent. Hold one knee against your chest, and bend your foot toward your head. Then straighten your leg. Hold for a count of 5. Relax; repeat with your other leg.

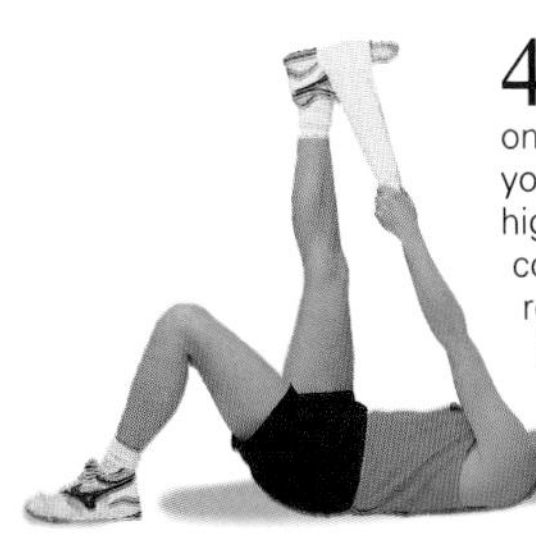

4 Lie on your back with your knees bent and straighten one leg. Bend your foot toward your head and lift your leg as high as you can. Hold for a count of 5 and then slowly return to the starting position. Repeat with your other leg. You can vary your routine by holding a towel around your foot and then pressing against the towel to stretch the muscles at the back of your thigh.

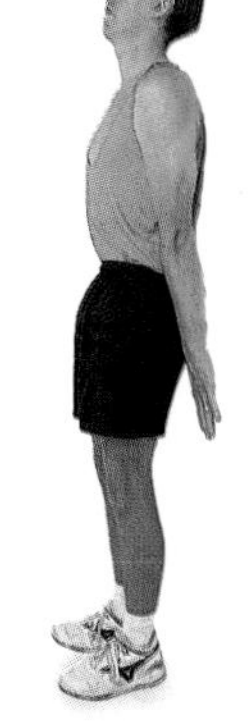

5 Stand against a wall with your heels 4 inches away from it. Then do the same exercise as in 1, pushing against the wall instead of the floor.

Extension (straightening) exercises

6 Lie on your abdomen with your hands at your sides. Tighten your buttocks hard for a count of 5. Relax.

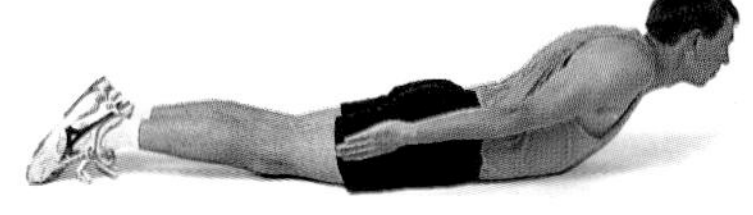

7 Lying on your abdomen with your hands at your sides, squeeze your shoulders together toward your back and raise your head and chest. Hold for a count of 5. Relax.

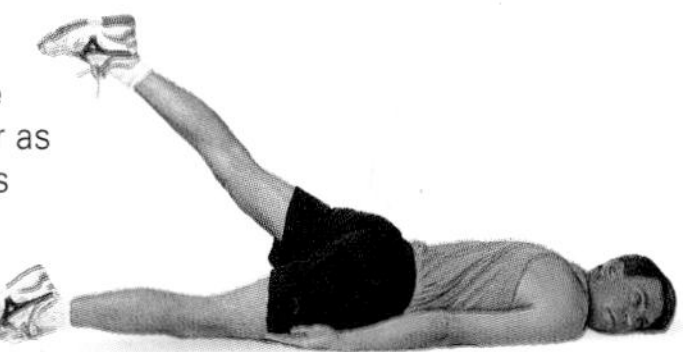

8 From the same position slowly raise one leg into the air as far as possible; do not hold this position but slowly return your leg to the floor. Repeat with each leg.

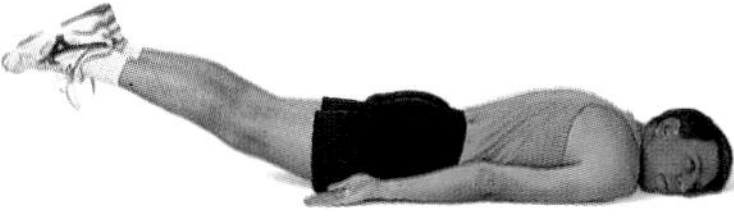

9 Perform the same procedure as exercise 8 but with both legs raised together.

10 Lie on your abdomen with one arm raised above your head. Raise that arm and the opposite leg as high as you can without bending either. Do not hold the position but slowly return your arm and leg to the floor. Repeat with your other arm and leg.

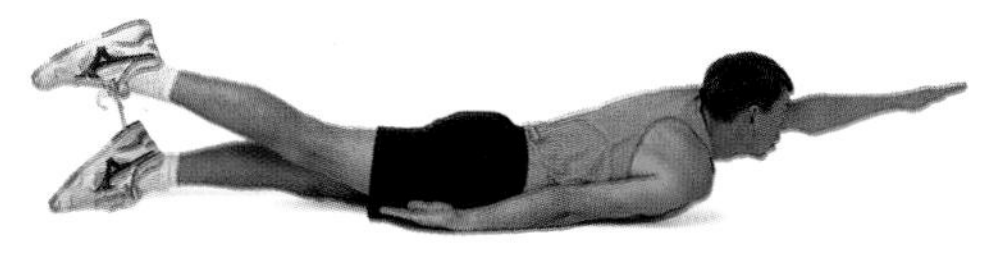

Why exercise is good for you

People who exercise are stronger and have greater endurance than people who do not. Exercise has other health benefits, too. Research has shown that exercise protects against coronary heart disease. Part of this protection comes from improvement in the heart's pumping action; a person who is physically fit pumps more blood with each heart beat and is able to sustain demanding physical exertion at a lower heart rate than someone who is out of shape.

Regular, moderate exercise improves your capacity for endurance, meaning you will be able to walk (or swim or bike) farther as you continue to work out. Exercise lowers the blood pressure—a clear benefit since high blood pressure is associated with both heart disease and stroke. Exercise also burns up fat, controls weight, lowers your harmful cholesterol level, and raises your good cholesterol level (see Fats and cholesterol, p.32). Research has also shown that people who are physically active are less susceptible to the type of diabetes that develops in adulthood (type II diabetes).

Anyone who has been confined to bed for more than a few days knows that his or her muscles and bones became weak. This occurs because the minerals in the bones are excreted by the kidneys in large quantities during long periods of immobility. Exercise, however, builds up the strength of bones by stimulating bone-building cells to create new bone. Research has shown that exercise at all ages improves bone strength. This is especially important for women after they reach menopause, when a lack of the hormone estrogen may lead to osteoporosis (thinning and weakening of bone). Exercise will help build up the bones to help protect against fractures in the future.

Finally, exercise makes people feel good. People who exercise regularly feel healthy and are less likely to become depressed.

The benefits of exercise

Sports

Gymnastics combines strength, endurance, and flexibility, resulting in a high level of physical fitness. Other sports such as running require simply endurance.

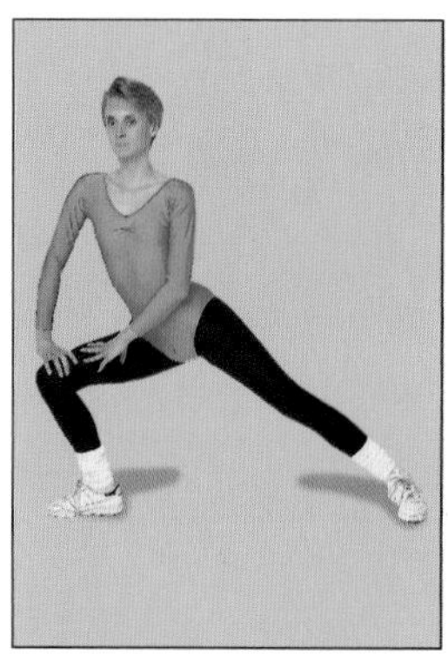

Joints

Joints that are exercised regularly stay flexible and healthy. And regular exercise will benefit the muscles that work the joints and the ligaments that support the joints. Brisk walking and swimming are good exercises to help keep your joints moving smoothly.

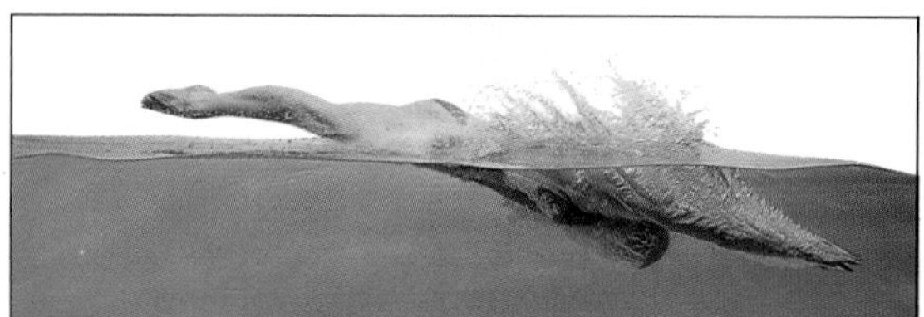

Heart, lungs, and arteries

Regular, moderate exercise will make your heart and lungs stronger and more resilient. Although exercise may not decrease the amount of fat deposits laid down in arteries, it may increase HDL cholesterol (the good cholesterol), widen the arteries, and make complete blockage, such as that from a clot, less likely.

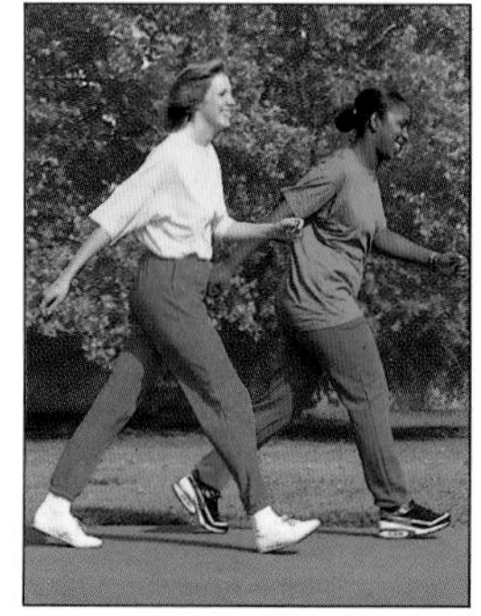

Muscles

Because the muscles that move the legs are among the largest muscles in the body, activities that exercise your legs, such as brisk walking, bicycling, and aerobic dancing, are excellent ways to place healthy demands on your heart and lungs and help improve fitness.

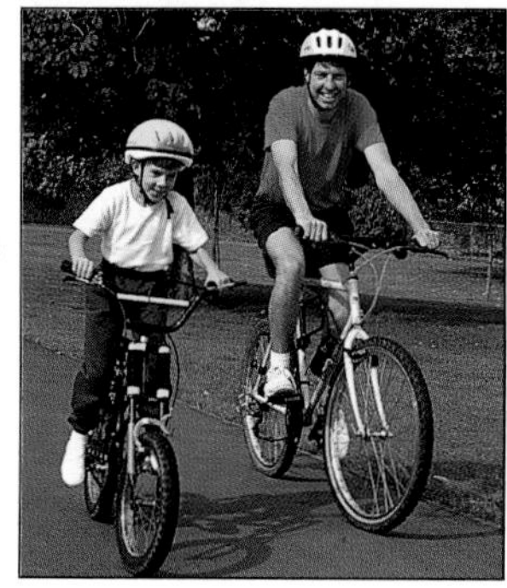

Choosing a good exercise program

The best exercise for you is exercise that you will enjoy and will do regularly. The following recommendations are based on guidelines that apply to most people.

1 Exercise throughout the day for a total of 30 minutes at least 5 days every week. You do not need to do the exercise in one session. Exercise moderately. If you begin to get dizzy or nauseated, or if you feel any pain, stop what you are doing. These are signs that you are overdoing it. Always do warm-up, stretching exercises (see next page) before the main exercise session and cool-down, stretching exercises (see p.23) at the end.

2 Choose types of exercise that you enjoy and that you can fit into your schedule. If you dislike competitive sports then consider brisk walking, bicycling, or swimming. Energetic gardening or do-it-yourself work around the house can also be good ways to exercise. Many people find that bicycling or brisk walking to and from work, or walking up stairs instead of taking the elevator, fits nicely into their everyday routines. The goal is to develop a habit of integrating physical activity into your life, so that you look forward to your chosen activity.

3 Do not attempt to get into shape too rapidly. Start slowly, exercising just hard enough to become aware that you feel mild strain, and increase your efforts gradually over the first 4 weeks. If you are out of condition and start a new sport, avoid vigorous sports that can demand unhealthy sudden bursts of strength and energy.

Before you exercise

Healthy people of any age can generally increase their routine physical activity with very little risk. An increase in an activity you normally do, such as walking, does not require a medical examination. If you belong to one of the following groups, however, it may be wise to call your physician for advice before you begin an exercise program:

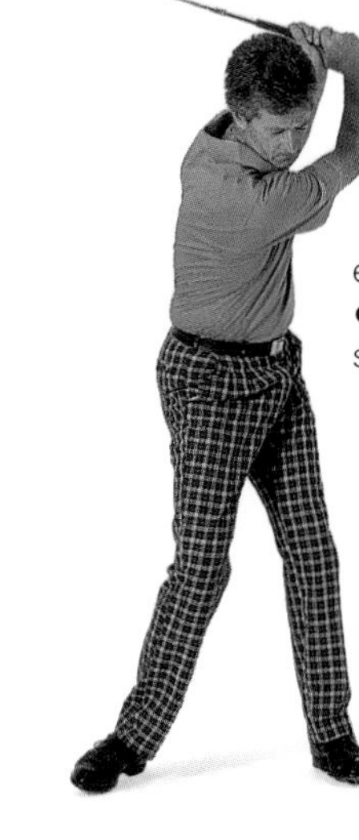

- People over 50 years of age, or those over 40 who have had little or no exercise since early adulthood.
- Heavy smokers (those who smoke more than 20 cigarettes per day).
- People who are overweight (see Weight charts, p.35).
- People under medical treatment or supervision for a long-term health problem such as high blood pressure; heart, lung, or kidney disease; or diabetes.

Aerobic exercise

Aerobic is a term used in exercise physiology. Muscles working at a steady, sustained pace get their energy by combining oxygen with glucose and fats to produce and release energy (along with carbon dioxide). This process is called aerobic metabolism. Regular sessions of moderate aerobic exercise are important for maintaining good health; aerobic exercise benefits your bones and muscles and is especially good for both your heart and your lungs.

Try to find an aerobic activity that you enjoy, and make it a part of your regular exercise program. Exercise at least 5 days per week for a total of 30 minutes per day. Ideally, all your muscles should work at a comfortable pace. This is achieved most easily by activities such as brisk walking, swimming, and bicycling.

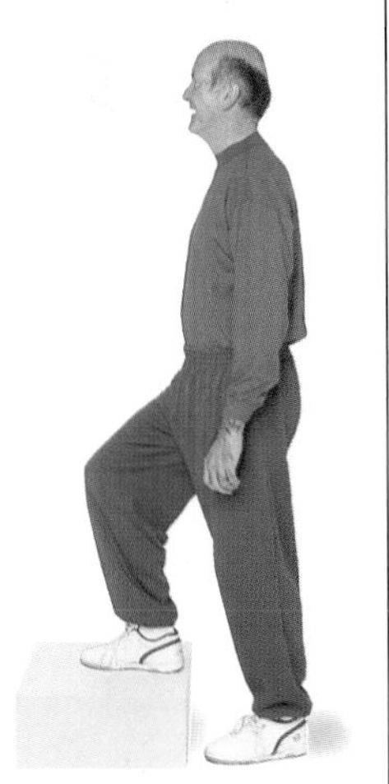

Warm-up exercises

It is important to warm up for at least 10 minutes immediately before exercising. Slowly stretching your muscles helps increase blood flow and can help prevent injury to your muscles, tendons, and ligaments. Try to stretch all the major muscle groups (your chest, abdomen, shoulders, arms, and legs) before starting your exercise. Begin your warm-up gradually, stretching slowly and carefully. Notice how your body feels, being careful not to overstretch. Never bounce or jerk your body while warming up. If your activity is walking, start slowly and gradually accelerate to your preferred pace. Work in some stretching after you have been walking for several minutes. Stretching will improve your flexibility. After exercising, be sure to cool down (see Box, Cooling down, p.23).

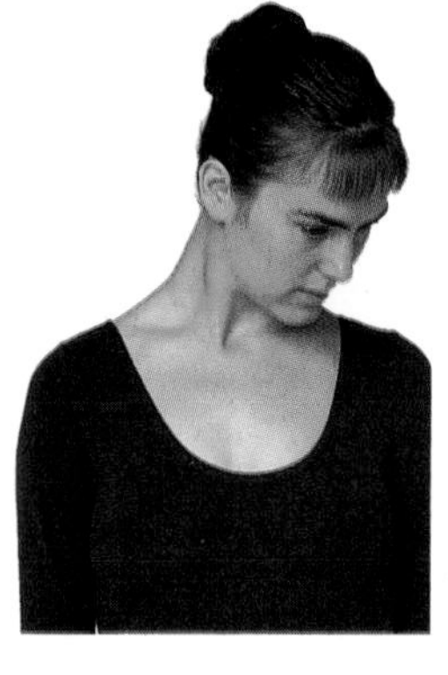

1 Head and neck Roll your head slowly around in a full circle, flexing your neck so that you face up at the back of the circle, and down at the front. Repeat 5 to 10 times.

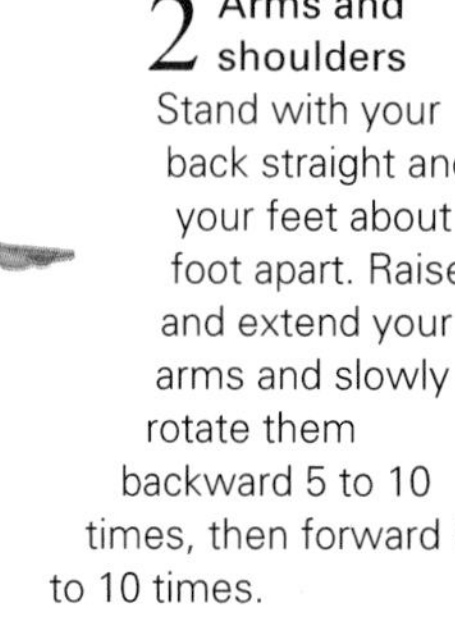

2 Arms and shoulders Stand with your back straight and your feet about 1 foot apart. Raise and extend your arms and slowly rotate them backward 5 to 10 times, then forward 5 to 10 times.

4 Trunk Stand with your back straight and your feet about $1\frac{1}{2}$ feet apart. Bend to the right at the waist, sliding your right hand down your leg to just below the knee. Straighten, then do a similar bend to the left. Repeat 5 to 10 times.

5 Hips and trunk Stand with your back straight, bend forward at the waist, and bring one leg up to touch your face with your knee; then straighten. Do the same with your other leg. Repeat 5 to 10 times.

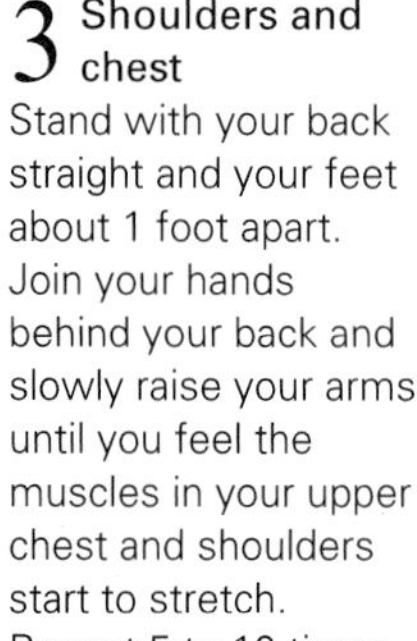

3 Shoulders and chest Stand with your back straight and your feet about 1 foot apart. Join your hands behind your back and slowly raise your arms until you feel the muscles in your upper chest and shoulders start to stretch. Repeat 5 to 10 times.

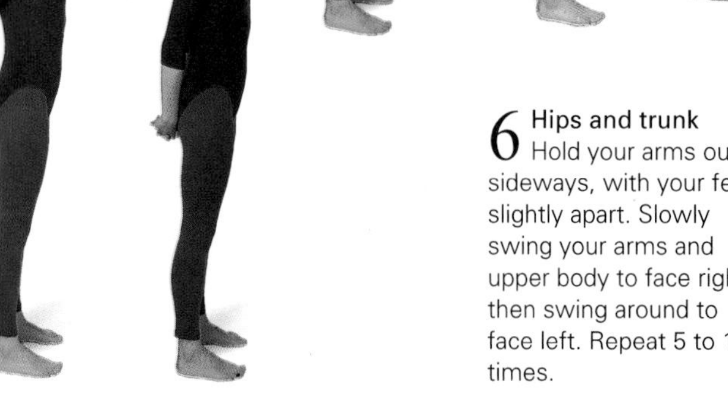

6 Hips and trunk Hold your arms out sideways, with your feet slightly apart. Slowly swing your arms and upper body to face right, then swing around to face left. Repeat 5 to 10 times.

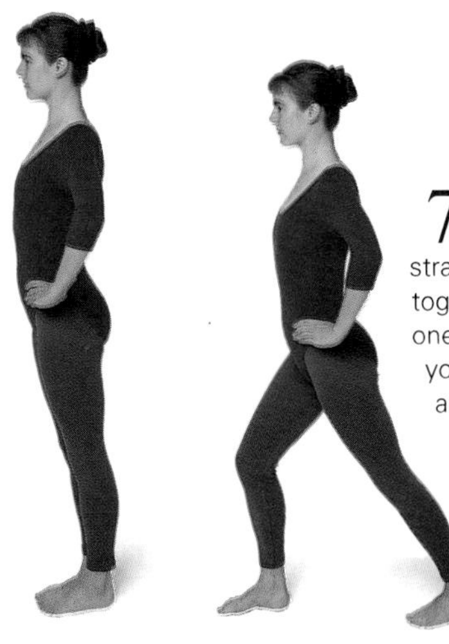

7 Knees and calves Stand with your back straight and your feet together. Carefully move one leg forward, putting your weight on that leg, and bending your knee. Do the same with your other leg. Repeat 5 to 10 times.

Cooling down

Cooling down is just as important as warming up because it helps prevent muscle cramps and muscle injury, and it helps blood return to the heart. Always stop exercising slowly and gradually; never stop exercising suddenly. After a long run, for example, gradually slow down to a walk, and continue walking for several minutes. Massaging your muscles after cooling down will help your blood circulate.

8 Hamstrings Stand with your back straight and your feet together. Slowly raise one leg, bending your knee. Grasp the front of your leg with both hands, and gently pull it up toward your chest. Lower your leg and then do the same with your other leg. Repeat 5 to 10 times.

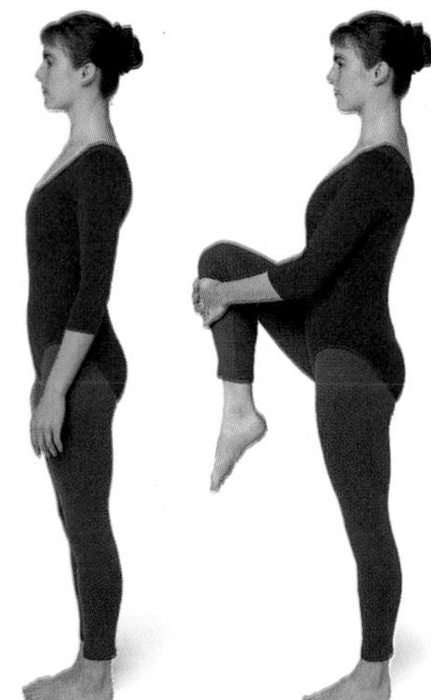

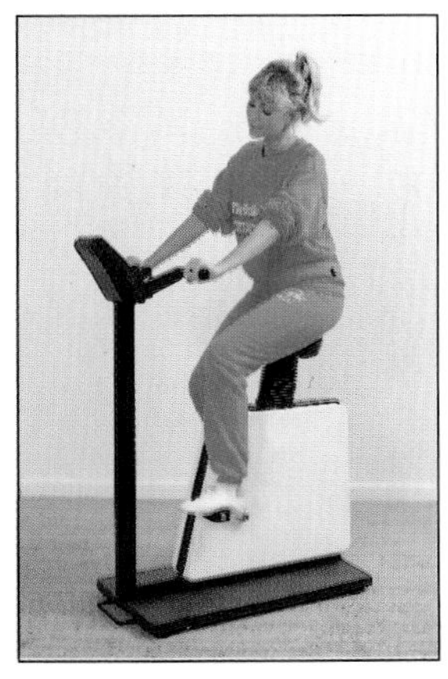

Exercise bicycle
A stationary exercise bicycle is useful fitness equipment in all weather. Measure each day's performance against your previous performance, and aim for a steady, week-by-week improvement. Also, adjust the tension mechanism on the bicycle as you gradually increase your fitness level.

Brisk walking
Walking briskly is an easy way to add aerobic exercise to your daily routine. Start slowly at first, gradually walking greater distances for a longer period of time. Brisk walking helps improve your endurance, your circulation, and the condition of your heart.

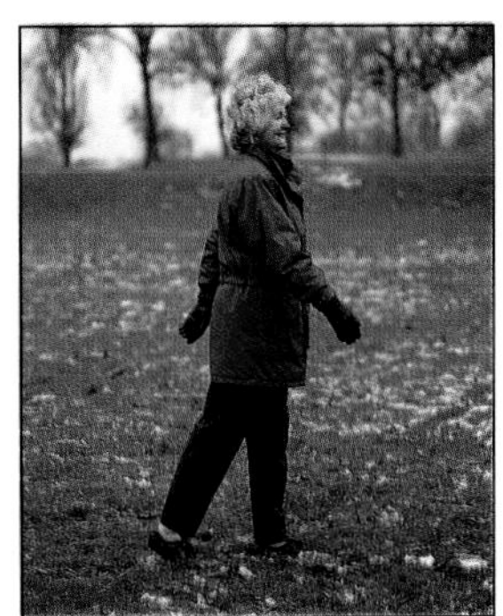

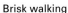

When to stop exercising

No matter how physically fit you are, or how long you may have been playing a particular sport, never ignore certain warning symptoms of overexercise. The following warning symptoms are potentially serious, and might mean you are having a heart attack or some other medical emergency. If you injure yourself, stop what you are doing. Do not continue with the exercise. You won't "work through" the pain; you can make the damage worse. For example, if during a tennis game you feel a tear or strain in your shoulder, don't continue the game. If after a few days of rest and following the RICE routine (see Box, p.574) the injury is still painful, or if you think the injury might be serious, call your physician for advice.

Stop exercising right away if you have any of these symptoms:

- chest pain or chest pressure
- pain in your neck, jaw, or running down your left arm
- heart palpitations
- dizziness or light-headedness
- nausea
- blurred vision
- severe breathlessness
- feeling faint or fainting

Preventing osteoporosis

Bones thinned by osteoporosis (see p.581) break more easily. In the US each year about 1.3 million fractures are attributed to osteoporosis; half a million of these are fractures of the spine and another 250,000 are fractures of the hip and wrist. Hip and spine fractures in older people whose general health is frail can be fatal, so it is vital to try to prevent them.

Osteoporosis is not simply a lack of calcium in the bones. In osteoporosis the protein framework of the bones becomes thinned so

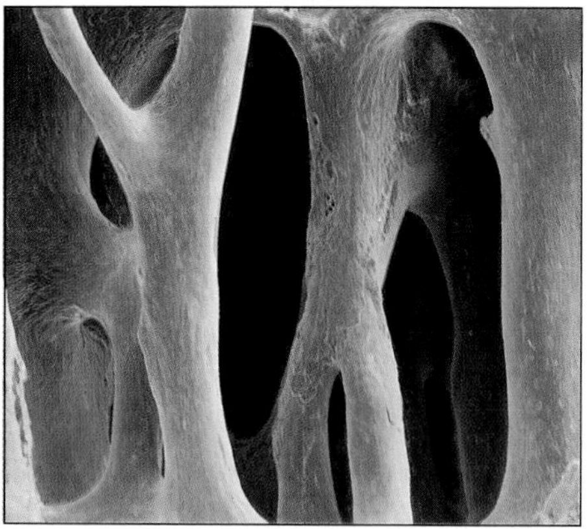

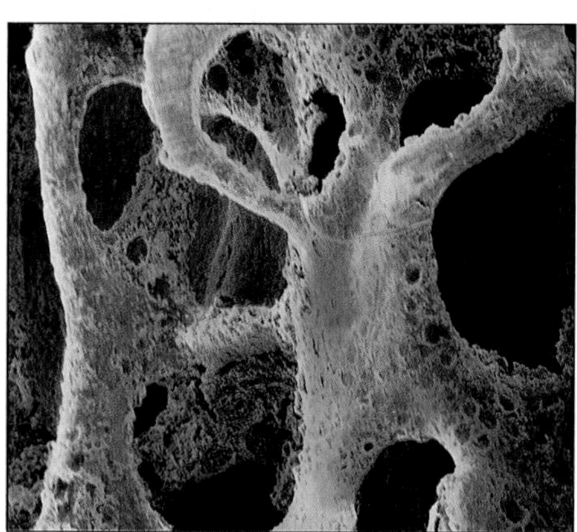

Changes in bone
Healthy bone (right) appears dense. In osteoporosis, the protein framework becomes thinned, calcium does not attach itself to the framework, and bones become less dense (far right) and fracture more easily.

Steps you can take to prevent osteoporosis

You may be able to slow the rate at which your bones become thinned by taking some preventive steps. Ideally, women should start prevention in their teens, which is the time when healthy bones reach their maximum density.

During the teenage years and their 20s and 30s, women should eat foods containing plenty of calcium and vitamin D, especially low-fat dairy products, green leafy vegetables, whole grains, citrus fruits, and beans. This type of diet is also good for your general health and should be followed throughout life, but your bones benefit most from a healthy diet in your youth. Your skin will produce vitamin D from sunlight if you spend time outdoors.

You should begin exercising as a child and continue throughout life. Women who have been physically active have stronger bones and have fewer fractures than women who have lived inactive lives. Almost any weight-bearing exercise seems to increase the density of bones, so it is a good idea to choose one, such as brisk walking, jogging, or stair-climbing, that will also benefit your heart and lungs. At the very least try to climb three flights of stairs every day and take a brisk walk. Women who exercise regularly benefit by having stronger bones.

Do not smoke, and cut down on alcohol. Alcohol consumption and smoking increase the risk of osteoporosis and bone fractures.

Women approaching menopause should consider the advantages and disadvantages of hormone replacement therapy (see Box, next page). This treatment has been shown to slow the decline in bone density that normally occurs after menopause, helping the bones to keep more of their strength.

Not everyone develops osteoporosis, but certain factors are associated with an increased risk of the disorder. The most important factor is gender; women are at much greater risk than men. This is because formation of protein in bones is heavily dependent on the sex hormones. And although men continue to produce some testosterone until well into old age, women produce very little estrogen after menopause. Osteoporosis tends to occur much earlier and more severely in women than in men.

Other known risk factors are:

- Lack of exercise. Regular exercise stimulates bones to stay strong.
- Early menopause. The earlier a woman's ovaries stop producing estrogen, the earlier her bones begin to lose protein and calcium.
- Cigarette smoking.
- Alcohol consumption.
- Being underweight.
- Not having children.
- White or Asian descent.
- Low calcium intake or vitamin D deficiency.
- Long-term treatment with corticosteroid drugs.
- Metabolic disorders such as an overactive thyroid gland.
- A strong family history of osteoporosis.

that less calcium is able to bind to the framework. This makes the bones lighter, less dense, weaker, and thus more susceptible to fracture with an injury.

The protein framework of the bones is built up partly as a result of stimulation from male and female sex hormones in childhood, adolescence, and through early adulthood. It is strengthened by deposits of calcium phosphate and other minerals. Bone is a living tissue, and throughout life its cells are constantly replaced and its shape changing. This growth process is controlled by hormones and vitamins and is also influenced by factors such as physical activity. Like other tissues, such as muscle, bone is also affected by how often it is used. Lack of use encourages wasting of bones. Skin, muscles, and bones are also vulnerable to the aging process, which causes bone to become less dense, in part because it is used less. Some degree of osteoporosis is a natural and inevitable part of aging. The decline in bone density that occurs with age may progress faster or slower depending on individual factors (see Box, facing page).

Hormone replacement therapy

At menopause, a woman's ovaries stop producing estrogen, the female sex hormone, and her estrogen level gradually falls to about 20 percent of its premenopause level. Some symptoms of menopause, such as hot flashes, night sweats, and vaginal dryness, are the result of this lower estrogen level. Also, lack of estrogen is a factor in osteoporosis (thinning of the bones; see p.581).

Hormone replacement therapy is a controversial treatment that gives replacement estrogen, with a form of progesterone (another hormone), to prevent or treat problems caused by a lowered estrogen level. Hormone replacement therapy includes synthetic progesterone because treatment with estrogen alone (estrogen replacement therapy) increases a woman's risk of endometrial cancer (cancer of the lining of the uterus). Estrogen replacement therapy without progesterone may be recommended for women who have had a hysterectomy.

Treatment with hormone replacement therapy for severe symptoms of menopause usually lasts for about 1 year. Symptoms may return in a few months; if they do, treatment is resumed. To help reduce the effects of osteoporosis, your physician may recommend treatment with replacement hormones for at least 5 to 10 years, or indefinitely. Estrogen protects women against heart disease and atherosclerosis (see p.398), but there is some evidence that progesterone may limit this protection. If you decide to take hormone replacement therapy, be sure to have regular checkups, including blood pressure checks, mammograms, pelvic examinations, Pap smears, and uterine biopsies. In a biopsy, your physician removes a small sample of tissue from the uterus for examination under a microscope.

Some possible side effects of hormone replacement therapy are headache, nausea, bloating, breast tenderness, weight gain, jaundice, and depression. If any of these occur, talk to your physician; he or she will probably lower your dosage or may stop the medication.

Some physicians may not recommend hormone replacement therapy unless a woman's symptoms are severe; others may recommend it for most women to help prevent osteoporosis. Hormone replacement therapy is usually not recommended for women who have been treated for endometrial cancer or breast cancer, or those who have some blood disorders. Also, this treatment may not be recommended for women who are obese or who smoke heavily because complications are more likely.

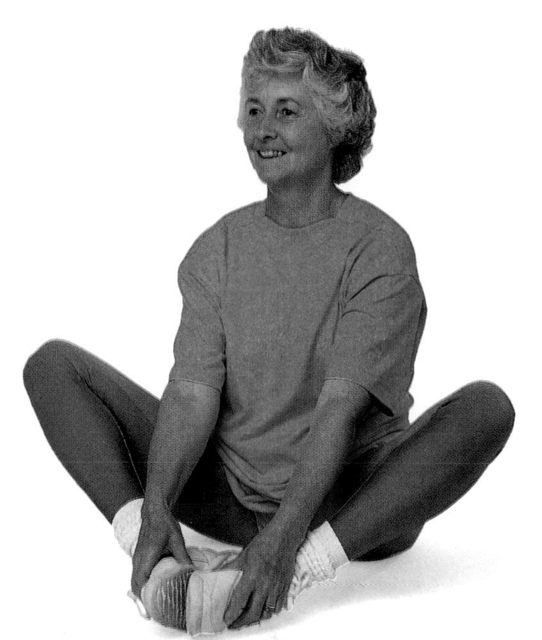

Estrogen replacement can help slow down bone loss, but exercise and diet are equally important for middle-aged women.

Hormone replacement therapy is available in many forms. You may take estrogen orally, by injection, through a skin patch, or in creams and suppositories. You may take progesterone orally or by injection.

Although hormone replacement therapy has improved the health of many women, and possibly extended their lives, its long-term effects regarding cancer are still unknown. Before you decide to take this treatment, talk to your physician and to women who have had the treatment, read about hormone replacement therapy, and then carefully weigh the risks and benefits.

Your diet and health

Probably the biggest problem with the average American's diet is that we eat too much for the amount of energy we use. Generally we are too sedentary. The result is that many of us are overweight, and many others try to maintain their weight only by repeated periods of dieting. Maintaining an adequate level of physical activity is essential to maintaining your weight. A healthy diet does more than match your energy intake to energy output. It provides all the elements required for good health.

Eating and drinking sensibly

If you eat a balanced diet—the widest possible selection of naturally occurring foods, as opposed to packaged processed foods—you are following the first rule of sensible eating. Many people, however, tend to disregard the second rule, which is eating only what you need. Eating a balanced, adequate diet helps promote good health in many ways. More and more people are taking a major interest in eating for health, while still enjoying the food they select.

The components of a healthy diet

A healthy diet contains adequate quantities of six groups of essential substances: proteins, carbohydrates, and fats, all of which contain calories (that is, they are nutrients that produce energy); and fiber, vitamins, and minerals, which, although they are essential to a healthy diet, do not contain any calories. In addition, you need plenty of water, without which life is impossible. A human being deprived of both food and drink usually can survive for only 4 or 5 days, but can live for as long as 2 months on liquids alone.

Proteins

Proteins are the chemical compounds that form the basis of living matter. You need a regular daily intake of protein for the repair, replacement, growth, and function of the body. Animal proteins (meat, fish, eggs, and cheese) can provide essential protein in the form your body needs, but it is vital to limit your intake of fats—meats and cheeses can be high in fat. A wide variety of vegetable proteins is also available. These are found most abundantly in peas, beans, and other legumes, but also are present in grains. If you eat more protein than your body needs, the extra protein is converted to glucose and provides energy or is converted to fat and stored by your body.

The Dietary Guidelines for Americans

The Dietary Guidelines for Americans, developed through research by the US Department of Health and Human Services and the US Department of Agriculture, can help you choose a healthy diet. The guidelines apply to Americans who are age 2 and older. Following these guidelines will help you improve your overall health and will help lower your risk of developing such diseases as high blood pressure, heart disease, stroke, diabetes mellitus, and possibly some types of cancer.

- Eat a variety of foods.
- Maintain a healthy weight (see Weight charts, p.35).
- Choose a diet low in total fat, saturated fat, and cholesterol (see p.32).
- Choose a diet with plenty of vegetables, fruits, and grain products.
- Use sugar only in moderation.
- Use salt (sodium) only in moderation.
- If you drink alcohol, do so in moderation (see Alcohol problems, p.42).

Water

Your body is made up of about 65 to 70 percent water. You lose 4 pints (about 2 liters) every day in breathed-out moisture, urine, stools, and sweat. The lost fluid must be replaced. To replace fluids, drink 6 to 8 glasses of water every day.

Carbohydrates

These are chemicals that contain carbon, hydrogen, and oxygen. All the foods that we think of as being either "starchy" or "sugary" contain a high proportion of carbohydrates. Some examples are sugar, bread, pasta, rice, potatoes, and cereals. These foods are our main source of energy, and some of them contribute other essential elements of a balanced diet, such as vitamins and minerals. For example, potatoes and whole-grain bread contain fiber, cereals contain protein, and whole-grain bread is a good source of iron.

Fiber

The human digestive tract is unable to digest fiber, which is plant material such as

Caffeine

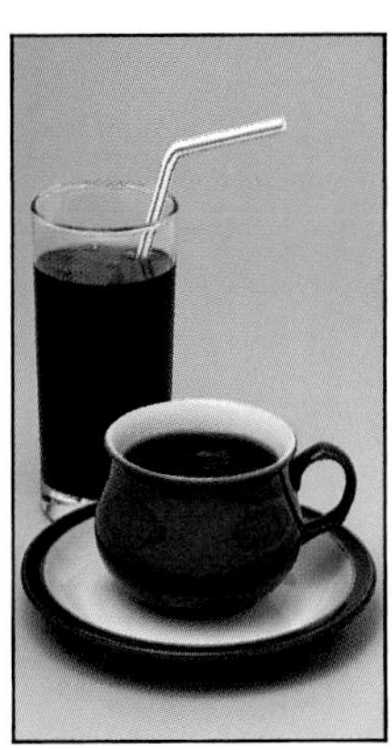

Caffeine, a drug found in coffee, tea, cocoa, and some soft drinks, stimulates your central nervous system and makes you feel more energetic. It also increases blood flow through the kidneys, which in turn produces more urine. Although the effects of caffeine vary from person to person, one or two cups of either tea or coffee are generally enough to act as a stimulant.

Very large doses of caffeine—1,000 mg (about the amount in 10 cups of strong coffee) or more—can lead to restlessness, trembling, sleeplessness, palpitations, and diarrhea. An average-sized cup of coffee contains about 100 mg of caffeine. Weak coffee contains less caffeine. There is much less caffeine in tea and cocoa, and even less in most caffeine-containing beverages. Try to keep your average consumption below three cups of coffee daily, especially if you notice that caffeine makes you feel jittery. Or drink decaffeinated coffee as a general rule.

Tea, coffee, or cola drinkers may become psychologically dependent on the drug, and addiction (physical dependence on the drug, with withdrawal symptoms when it is not available) does occur. Remember also that there are no vitamins or minerals in coffee, tea, or cola. Fruit juice and water are better alternatives when you are thirsty.

cellulose and pectin that is found in unrefined cereals, fruit, vegetables, and legumes. Fiber is very important because it provides bulk to help the large intestine efficiently carry away body wastes. Also, fiber may help prevent diverticular disease (see p.515) and cancer of the large intestine (see p.518).

Fats

Fats are found in plant foods such as olives and peanuts as well as in animal products. Fats provide energy, and minute quantities are also used for growth and repair. In addition, they make food more palatable and filling. Excess fat is stored in the body as fatty tissue. Fat can cause serious health problems (see Obesity, p.530).

Depending on chemical composition, fats are either saturated or unsaturated—a distinction that matters primarily because eating saturated fats is thought to increase the amount of cholesterol (see p.32) in the blood. Animal fats, especially those in milk, butter, cheese, and meat, are mostly saturated and may be partly responsible for the development of atherosclerosis (see p.398). The fat in fish and some vegetable oils is largely unsaturated (see illustration on p.33). In chicken and turkey most of the fat is in the skin. From the standpoint of health, the better fats are polyunsaturated and monounsaturated. However, all forms of fat contain the same number of calories—a substantial 135 calories per tablespoon.

Vitamins

Vitamins are chemicals. Your body can make small amounts of some vitamins, such as vitamin D, which is made in the skin when it is exposed to sunlight, but most vitamins can be obtained only from food or supplements. Anyone who eats a varied diet of fresh fruits and vegetables, grains, dairy products, fish, and meat generally gets enough vitamins. There is, however, some evidence that the average American diet does not contain enough vitamin A and C year-round or enough vitamin D in the winter months. The best solution is not, however, to take vitamin supplements. Instead, you should change your diet so that you eat more fresh, vitamin-rich foods. If you eat additional fresh fruits and vegetables, your diet will provide enough vitamins A, C, and E to avoid osteoporosis and possibly cancer. Also, fruits and vegetables contain valuable fiber and reduce your appetite for the less-healthy fats and sugars.

Minerals

You need to include at least 20 minerals in your diet, but only iron, calcium, iodine, and sodium are of major nutritional importance. An apparently reasonable diet may be deficient in iron, calcium, or iodine. Foods such as bread, however, may be fortified with added iron and calcium. And in parts of the world where the soil is deficient in iodine, it is often added to salt. A well-balanced diet usually provides enough iron, calcium, and iodine.

Many people eat too much sodium (salt), and this is known to increase the risk of heart disease for people who already have high blood pressure. Many people add salt to food in cooking and at the table out of habit. Taste your food before salting it, and you will discover that your food tastes better without added salt.

The Food Guide Pyramid

The Food Guide Pyramid is a simple, general plan for eating sensibly every day. It is based on the Dietary Guidelines for Americans listed in the Box on page 26. You can use the pyramid to choose the right amounts of all of the foods that are essential to a well-balanced diet. Following these recommendations will help ensure that you get enough protein, carbohydrates, vitamins, minerals, and fiber every day, while also limiting your intake of fats, cholesterol, sugar, and salt (sodium). Note that one serving is not necessarily the same as your usual helping.

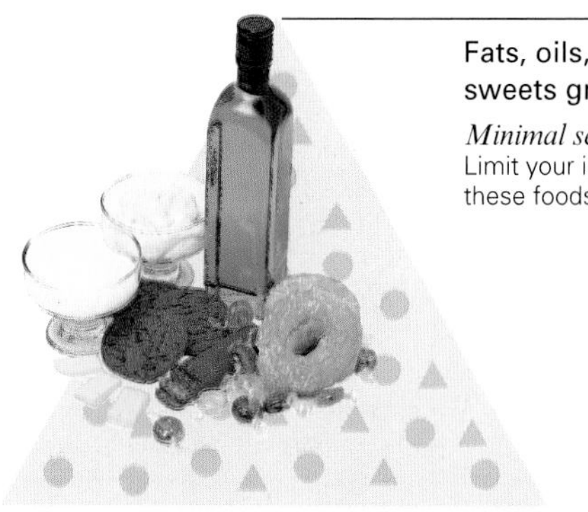

Fats, oils, and sweets group

Minimal servings
Limit your intake of these foods

Milk, yogurt, and cheese group

2-3 servings per day
- 1 cup of milk
- 1 cup of yogurt
- 1½ oz of natural cheese
- 2 oz of processed cheese

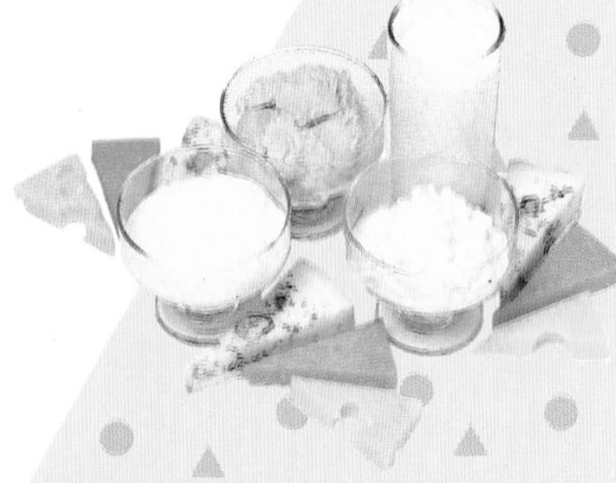

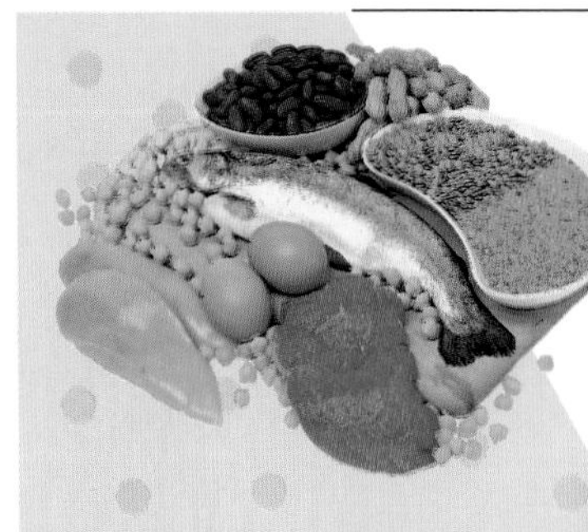

Vegetable group

3-5 servings per day
- 1 cup of raw leafy vegetables
- ½ cup of other vegetables (raw or cooked)
- ¾ cup of vegetable juice

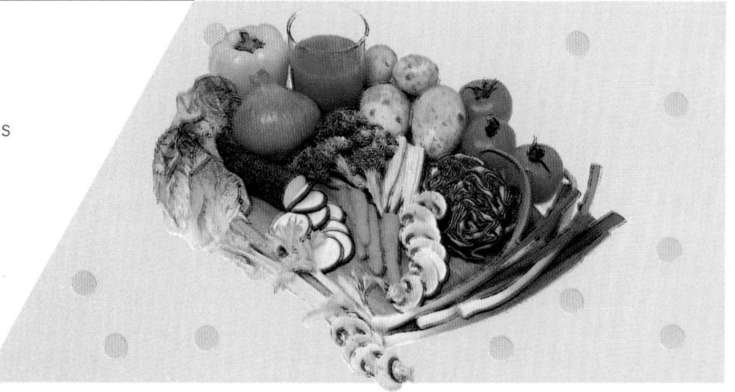

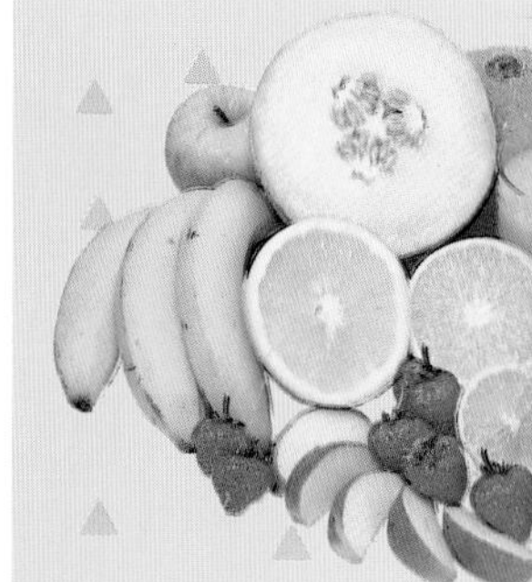

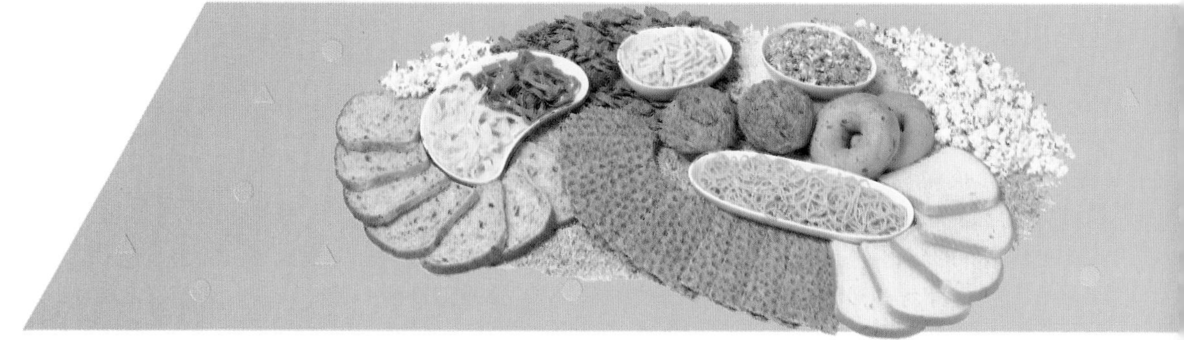

What are the food groups?

Bread, cereal, rice, and pasta group
Foods from this group provide carbohydrates, vitamins, minerals, and fiber. Choose whole-grain products; read package labels to check amounts of added fat, sugar, and salt (sodium), especially in ready-to-eat cereals; and watch out for added fats, cholesterol, and sugar in spreads and toppings.

Vegetable group
Foods from this group are low in fat and provide vitamins such as A and C, minerals such as iron, and fiber. Choose plenty of dark green, leafy vegetables, deep yellow vegetables, and legumes (peas and beans). Use low-fat or nonfat dressings and toppings to limit added fats and cholesterol.

Fruit group
Foods from this group are low in fat and sodium and provide vitamins such as A and C, minerals such as potassium, and fiber. Choose fresh, whole fruits whenever possible. Choose only canned fruit packed in its own juice, and read package labels to check for added sugar in canned fruits and canned or bottled juices.

Milk, yogurt, and cheese group
Foods from this group provide calcium, protein, vitamins, and minerals. Choose skim, low-fat, or nonfat milk and dairy products.

Meat, poultry, fish, dry beans, eggs, and nuts group
Foods from this group provide protein, B vitamins, and minerals such as iron. Choose lean cuts of red meat and trim all visible fat. Remove skin from poultry. Bake, broil, or roast meat, fish, and poultry. Limit yourself to three or four eggs per week to cut down on cholesterol. Go easy on nuts; they are high in fat.

Fats, oils, and sweets group
Foods from this group include butter, margarine, vegetable oils, salad dressings, soft drinks, and candy. They are generally high in calories and low in nutritional value. Fats should account for no more than 30 percent of your total daily intake of calories. On the diagram note that sugars and fats can show up in all food groups.

Key
- ◆ One serving
- ■ One third of a serving
- Sugars
- Fats

Meat, poultry, fish, dry beans, eggs, and nuts group

2-3 servings per day
- ◆ 2-3 oz of meat, fish, or poultry
- ■ 1/2 cup of cooked dry beans
- ■ 1 egg
- ■ 2 Tbsp of peanut butter

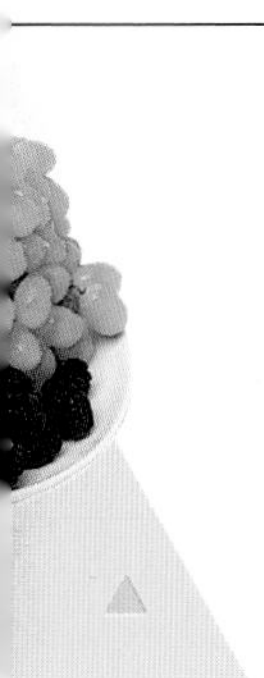

Fruit group

2-4 servings per day
- ◆ 1 medium-sized piece of fresh fruit
- ◆ 1/2 cup of cooked, chopped, or canned fruit
- ◆ 1/4 cup of dried fruit
- ◆ 3/4 cup of 100 percent fruit juice

Bread, cereal, rice, and pasta group

6-11 servings per day
- ◆ 1 slice of bread
- ◆ 1 oz of ready-to-eat cereal
- ◆ 1/2 cup of cooked cereal, rice, or pasta

How many servings do I need?

Try to eat at least the lowest number of servings shown at left in each group every day. And do not confuse a "serving" with a "helping"; a larger portion provides more than one serving.

Recommended number of servings each day from the five major food groups

Food group	1,600 calories per day	2,200 calories per day	2,800 calories per day
Bread	6	9	11
Vegetables	3	4	5
Fruit	2	3	4
Milk	2-3*	2-3*	2-3*
Meat	2 (5 oz, total)	2 (6 oz, total)	3 (7 oz, total)

* Teenagers, young adults through age 24, and women who are pregnant or breast-feeding need at least 3 servings of milk and other dairy products each day.

To summarize
In general, to maintain a healthy weight, sedentary women and older people need to take in about 1,600 calories per day; children, teenage girls, active women, and sedentary men need to take in about 2,200 calories per day; and teenage boys, active men, and very active women need to take in about 2,800 calories per day. If you are not sure about how many calories you need per day, talk to your physician.

Healthy diet options

Today, many families do not have enough time to eat all of their meals at home together. We tend to eat many of our meals at work, at school, or in restaurants, which can make it difficult to stick to a well-balanced diet. Although there are plenty of healthy food options available to us, we often choose to eat fast foods, many of which contain large amounts of fat, cholesterol, sugar, and salt (sodium). Because our eating habits affect our health, it is important for all of us to understand the health benefits of eating sensibly every day. (For information on healthy eating see The Food Guide Pyramid on pages 28 and 29.)

Breakfast

Try not to skip breakfast. It is an important meal that provides energy for starting your day. However, it is a good idea to avoid eating traditional high-fat, high-cholesterol breakfast foods such as bacon, sausage, eggs, and hash browns. Instead, choose healthy options such as fresh fruit, high-fiber cereal such as bran flakes served with skim milk, and whole-grain toast.

Lunch

Many of us eat lunch away from home, and we often eat it in a hurry. Because of this, it often seems convenient to choose high-fat fast foods such as hot dogs, hamburgers, and french fries. However, a more nutritious and equally satisfying meal includes salad, whole-grain bread, and fresh fruit. You can bring a lunch like this with you from home or purchase it at your favorite salad bar.

Snacks

For a well balanced diet, avoid eating snacks that are high in fat or calories. However, if you become hungry or need an energy boost between meals, choose a healthy alternative such as fresh fruit, plain popcorn, or a bagel. Although snacks such as donuts and potato chips may taste good, they provide mostly empty calories, and snacking on them can lead to obesity and tooth decay.

Dinner

For most people, dinner is the main meal of the day; it should ideally include sensible choices from each of the food groups that make up the Food Guide Pyramid. Large servings of fatty red meat, once a significant part of our diet, should be replaced by smaller portions of lean red meat, chicken, or fish, served with large helpings of fresh vegetables. Fresh fruit or low-fat frozen yogurt is a healthier choice for dessert than high-fat options such as ice cream.

Traditional options

Bacon, eggs, hash browns, and white bread

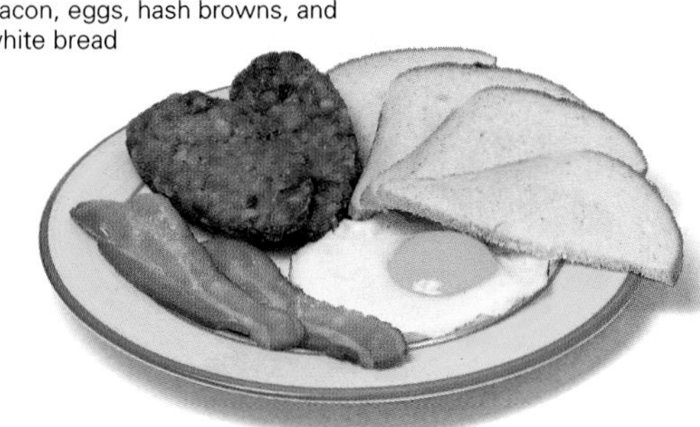

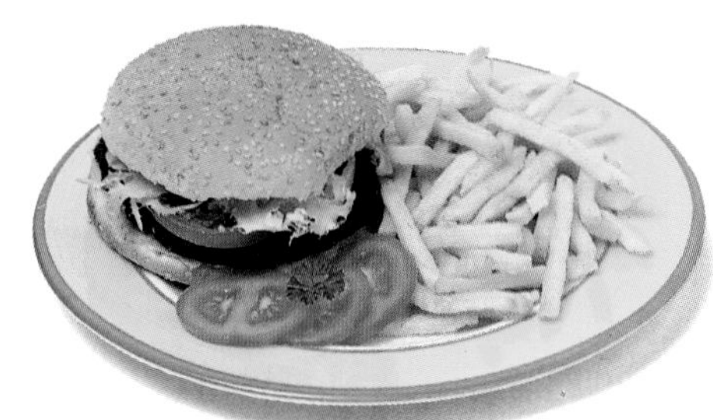

Hamburger and french fries

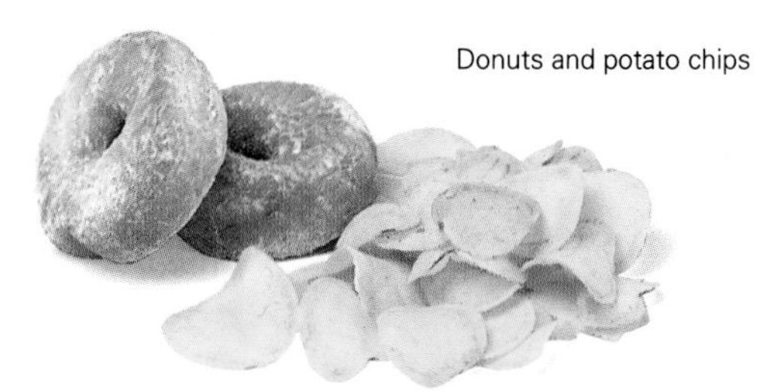

Donuts and potato chips

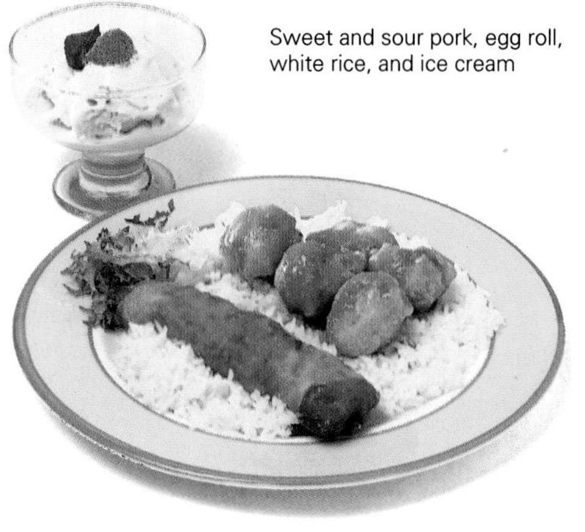

Sweet and sour pork, egg roll, white rice, and ice cream

Healthy options

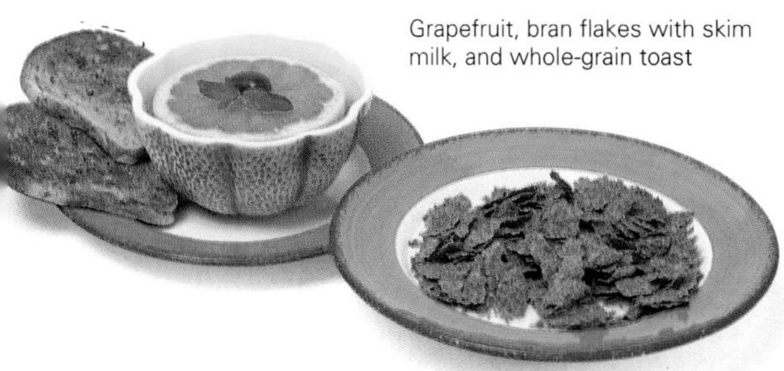

Grapefruit, bran flakes with skim milk, and whole-grain toast

Mixed salad in pita bread

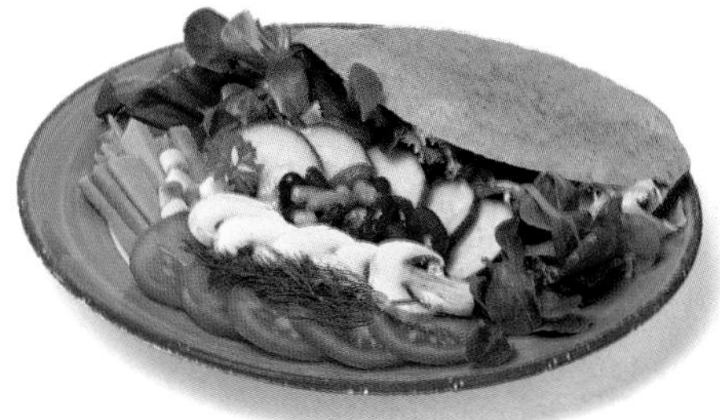

Apple, bagel, and unbuttered, unsalted, low-fat popcorn

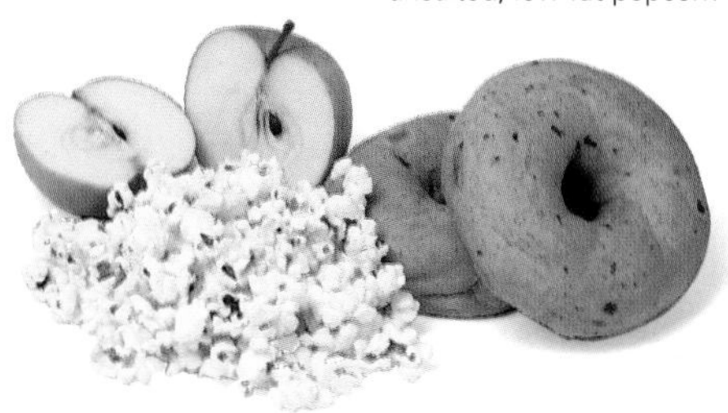

Broiled chicken, baked potato, ratatouille, whole-grain roll, fresh fruit salad with low-fat yogurt topping

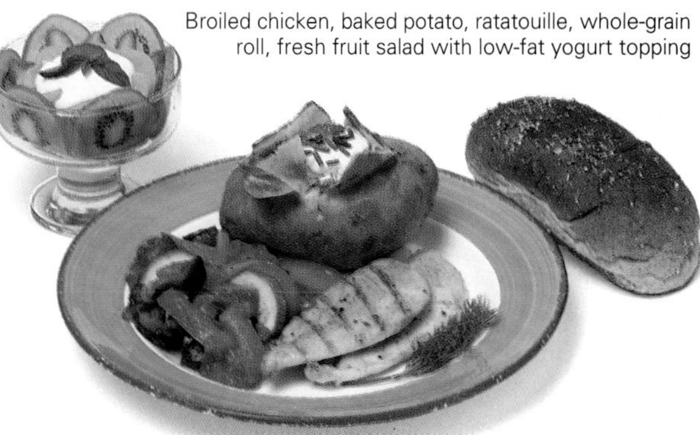

Healthy drink options

Drinking plenty of fluids is an essential part of a healthy diet. Always try to choose one of the healthy drink options shown below.

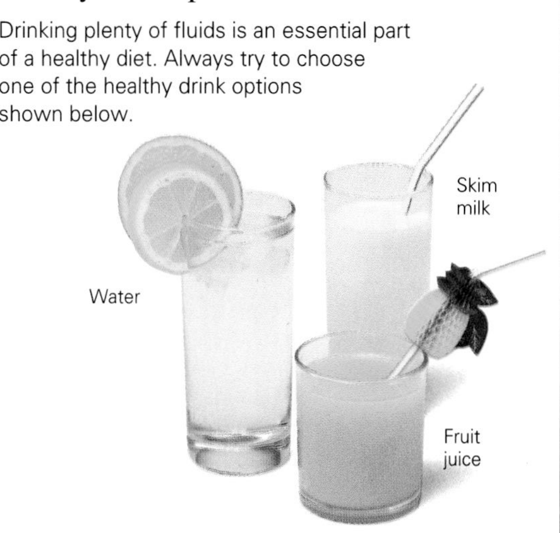

Counting calories

A calorie is a measurement of energy. If you burn a piece of coal, you can measure the resultant energy (released as heat) in calories. Similarly, your body burns a given quantity of food to release a certain number of calories. The three basic dietary components—proteins, carbohydrates, and fats—produce different amounts of energy. Ounce for ounce, high-protein and high-carbohydrate foods have fewer calories than the same amount of fat.

The number of calories you need depends largely on how physically active you are (see Obesity, p.530). For example, sedentary women need, on average, 1,600 calories per day; active women, about 2,200 calories per day; and women who are very active, about 2,800 calories per day. On average, sedentary men need 2,200 calories per day and active men need 2,800 calories per day. Teenage girls need about 2,200 calories per day and teenage boys need about 2,800 calories per day. Talk to your physician about what daily intake of calories is right for you. You gain weight if you consume a few hundred calories more than you need each day, unless you get more exercise. If you are in the later stages of pregnancy or are breast-feeding, you may need up to 800 extra calories each day. As you get older, you may find that it becomes harder to keep your weight down even when your daily calorie intake has not increased. This may occur in part because as you get older, you may become less active, but you do not reduce your intake of calories. Your body stores these extra calories as body fat. Starting a regular program of moderate exercise, such as brisk walking or swimming, will help keep your weight in check.

Fats and cholesterol

Health-conscious Americans are aware that high levels of cholesterol in their blood increase their risk of heart disease. However, many of us are not sure what cholesterol is or what it does, or how to control cholesterol levels.

Cholesterol is not a fat but it is closely related to fats. It is a chemical that is an essential component in the structure of cells and is also involved in the formation of important hormones. If your diet contained no cholesterol, your liver would still produce all the cholesterol you need.

High levels of cholesterol can contribute to atherosclerosis (see p.398), in which the blood vessels are narrowed by deposits of a fatty tissue called atheroma, which are made up largely of cholesterol. Narrowing of the heart's coronary arteries by patches of atheroma causes angina (see p.403) when you exercise and the artery has become narrowed enough to deprive the heart muscle of needed blood. This also increases the risk of an artery becoming blocked by a blood clot. In most instances, the more cholesterol there is in your blood, the higher your risk of heart disease (see Box on cholesterol levels, next page). High cholesterol levels in your bloodstream generally lead to more cholesterol being deposited in patches of atheroma. As a rule, the more cholesterol there is in the bloodstream, the greater the risk of severe atherosclerosis.

The amount of cholesterol you have in your bloodstream depends on several factors, including your genes, your diet, and your lifestyle.

The genetic factor is very important. Some families have an inherited tendency to high cholesterol levels, and members of these families may have heart attacks at an early age. One cause of this tendency is a genetic disorder called hyperlipoproteinemia (see p.538), but there are a number of other genetic conditions that are associated with high cholesterol levels.

Whatever your background, the amount of fat you eat affects your cholesterol level. However, there are good fats and bad fats, just as there are good cholesterols (HDL cholesterol) and bad cholesterols (LDL cholesterol). Fats that raise the cholesterol level most dramatically are called saturated. They are found in meat and high-fat dairy products and are easily recognized because they are always solid at room temperature. Unsaturated fats are found in plant oils, which are liquid at room temperature, and are less likely to elevate your cholesterol level. Too much unsaturated fat in your diet also has disadvantages, however. The overall fat content of your diet should be low (no more than 30 percent of your daily intake of calories) and it should consist largely of unsaturated fats. There are some simple guidelines that will help you choose a diet that keeps your cholesterol level low, thereby reducing your risk of heart disease (see The Food Guide Pyramid, pp.28-29).

A diet for a healthy heart

Is your diet a healthy one? Study the illustration of the food pyramid (pp.28-29) to understand the ideal proportions of various foods in your diet. Get most of your calories from complex carbohydrates, especially whole grains, beans, fruits, and vegetables. The fat in your diet should provide 30 percent or less of the total intake of calories. Avoid foods rich in saturated fat. These are animal fats found in meat, butter, whipped cream, sour cream, cheese, and whole milk. When you eat meat, choose skinless (or remove the skin from) poultry or lean cuts of beef and pork, and trim off all the fat you can see. Limit yourself to small portions of meat, too (about 3 oz, which is approximately the size of a deck of cards).

Whenever possible, choose foods that have a low fat content or that contain unsaturated fats. Eat more fish and less red meat. Eat more fruits and vegetables, cook in as little vegetable oil as possible, and drink skim milk rather than whole milk.

For a healthy diet, choose the widest possible variety of naturally occurring foods, including fruits, vegetables, and whole grains.

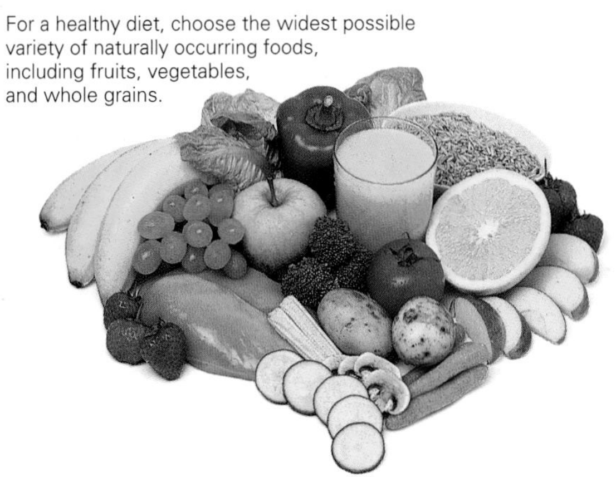

Limit foods that contain large amounts of cholesterol. Eat no more than three or four eggs a week and limit your intake of shellfish, such as shrimp, and liver.

The third factor that determines your cholesterol level is your lifestyle; the more you exercise the higher your HDL and the lower your LDL cholesterol levels are likely to be. An inactive lifestyle appears to lead to high LDL cholesterol levels, which are a factor in the development of atherosclerosis and heart disease.

What types of fat are you eating?

Fats should provide no more than 30 percent of your total intake of calories each day, and most of the fat you eat should be unsaturated. While most plant oils are high in unsaturated fat, others are high in saturated fat.

The relative percentages of types of fat contained in the most common plant oils used in cooking are shown in this table.

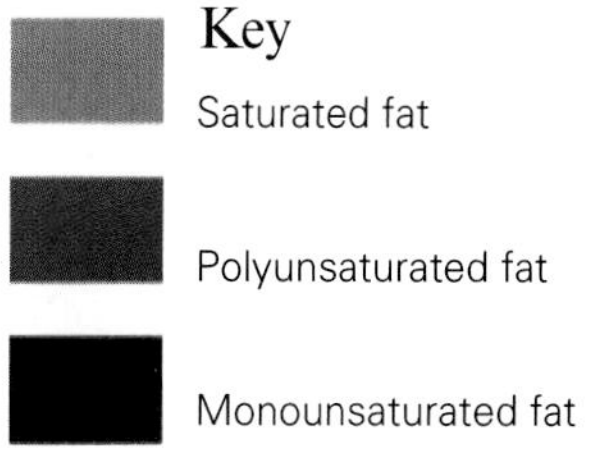

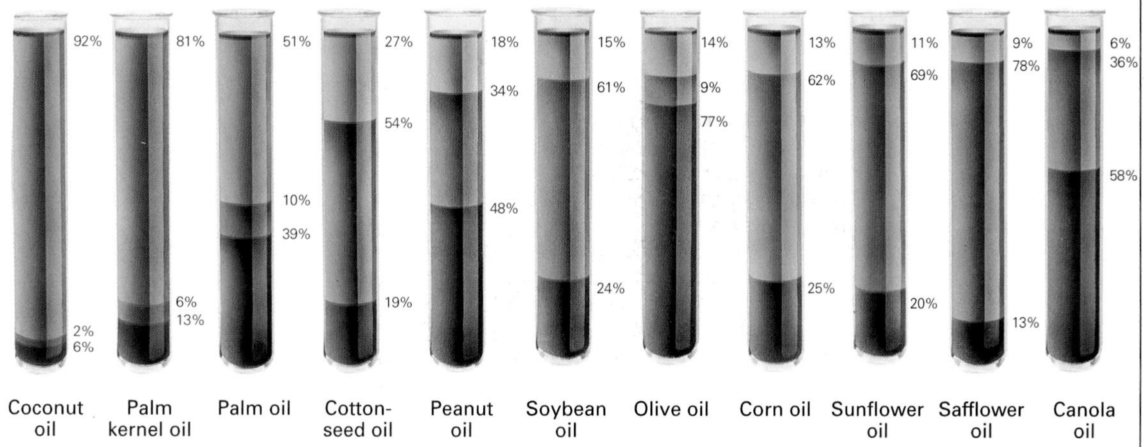

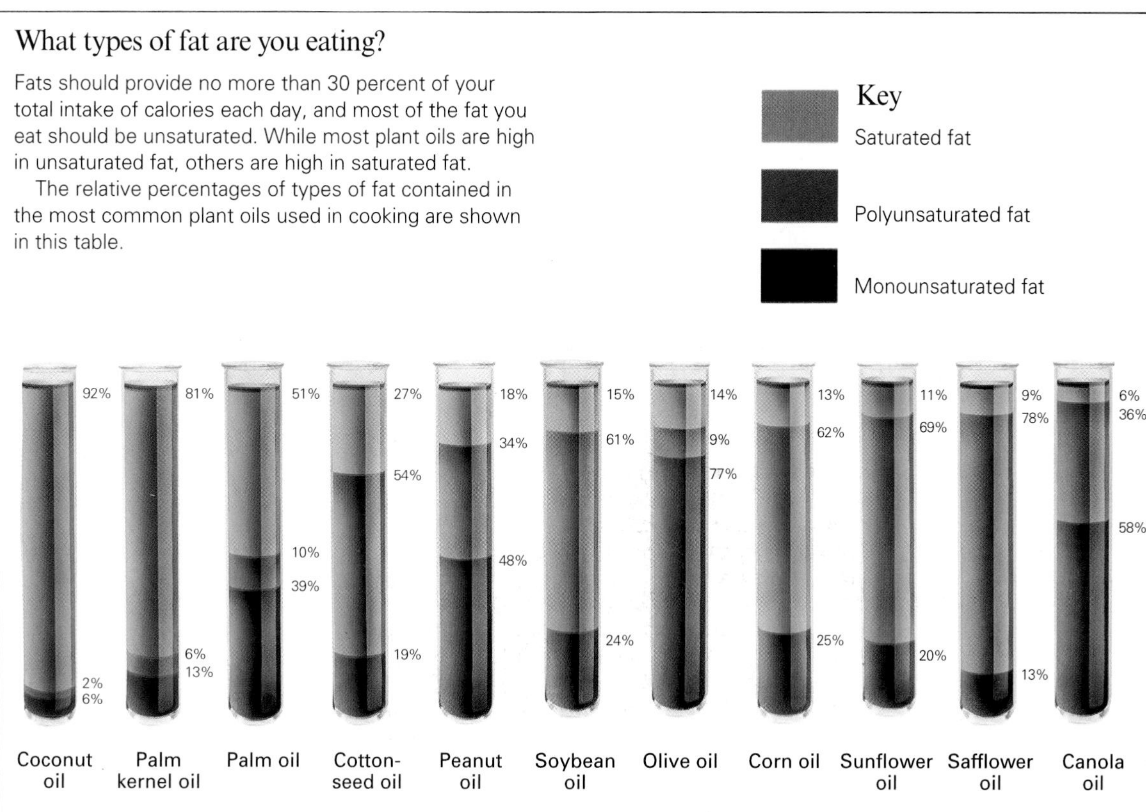

Know your cholesterol levels

Have your blood cholesterol measured when you are in your 20s. If the result is within the normal range, the test should be repeated every 5 to 10 years (see Health checkups by medical professionals, p.15). If the result is abnormal, your physician will probably recommend that you change your diet and exercise habits. You will then need to have your cholesterol level checked more often to monitor your response to treatment.

If your cholesterol level is below 200 milligrams per deciliter (mg/dL), you need not be concerned. If your cholesterol level is between 200 and 239 mg/dL, your physician will evaluate your health and your lifestyle. Your physician may recommend changes in your diet as the only treatment if your weight and blood pressure are normal, you do not have diabetes, you do not smoke, you exercise regularly, and there is no history of heart disease in persons younger than 50 to 55 in your family. But if you have two or more of these risk factors or if your cholesterol level is over 240 mg/dL, your physician will perform additional tests.

These tests are necessary to evaluate more precisely your risk of heart disease. Fats and fatty substances such as cholesterol are not soluble in water, and to carry them in the bloodstream the body incorporates them into units called lipoproteins, which are made up of fats, cholesterol, and proteins. There are several different types of lipoproteins. The most important are low-density lipoprotein (LDL cholesterol, the bad cholesterol) and high-density lipoprotein (HDL cholesterol, the good cholesterol). If your cholesterol level is elevated, your physician will probably arrange for tests that involve a detailed analysis of the lipoproteins and fats in your blood. If the tests reveal high levels of low-density lipoproteins (which carry the harmful LDL cholesterol), that is additional evidence of a cholesterol problem. These test results will be the basis for evaluating your risk of heart disease. A single elevated cholesterol level reading is almost impossible to interpret without further tests, but a single lower cholesterol level reading is a good indicator of improvement.

Losing weight

If you are overweight (see Weight charts, next page), you are at increased risk of heart disease, stroke, diabetes, cancer, and other disorders. The more overweight you are, the greater the risk (see Obesity, p.530).

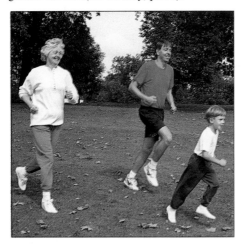

Regular moderate exercise that you enjoy is a vital factor in keeping your weight at a healthy level.

Losing weight safely and permanently means that you will need to modify your lifestyle by changing both your eating and your exercising habits. You must eat less and exercise more.

Choose from a wide variety of naturally occurring foods to make sure that your diet is well-balanced (see p.28). At the same time, begin an exercise program that is suited to your needs and abilities. Your goal should be to lose no more than 1 or 2 pounds per week. Read the information on exercise (p.20) and try to include a variety of exercises in your daily routine. Walk to the train, take stairs instead of the elevator, or ride your bike to the store. Exercising every day will help you keep off the weight you lose through dieting.

It is a good idea to talk to your physician before starting any weight-loss or exercise program, especially if you have a medical problem, are severely overweight, or have been out of shape for some time.

Tips for dieters

Here are some useful ideas that will help you stick to your diet.

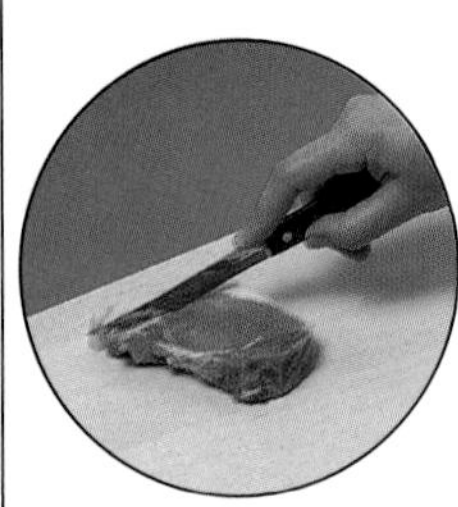

Cooking

- Bake, broil, roast, steam, or microwave your food.
- If you fry food, use a small amount of vegetable oil or a nonstick cooking spray. Do not use butter or margarine.
- Choose lean cuts of red meat and remove all visible fat before cooking. Remove skin from poultry before cooking to avoid hidden fat.
- Season your food with herbs, spices, and lemon juice. Go easy on salt.

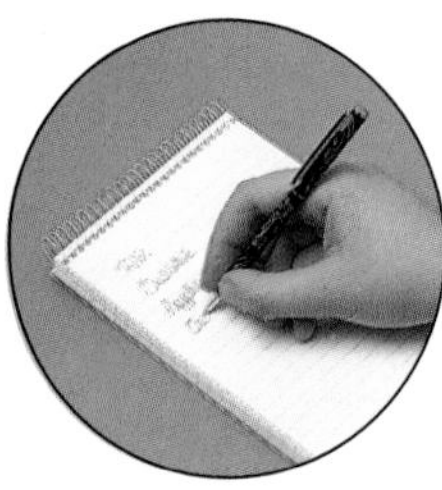

Shopping

- Never shop for food when you are hungry.
- Make a grocery list and stick to it. Do not buy on impulse.

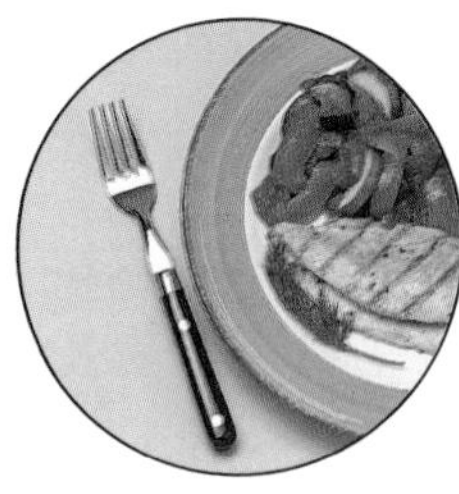

Eating

- Plan your meals in advance. It may be helpful to eat five or six small, well-balanced meals rather than three large meals each day.
- Eat only when you are hungry.
- Never skip a meal; this can lead to excessive hunger and binge eating.
- Take a bite, put down your fork, and chew slowly and thoroughly before swallowing. Then pick up your fork and take another bite.
- Try to eat at the same time every day. Eat sitting down and use a knife and fork.
- Make a habit of eating fresh fruit for dessert.

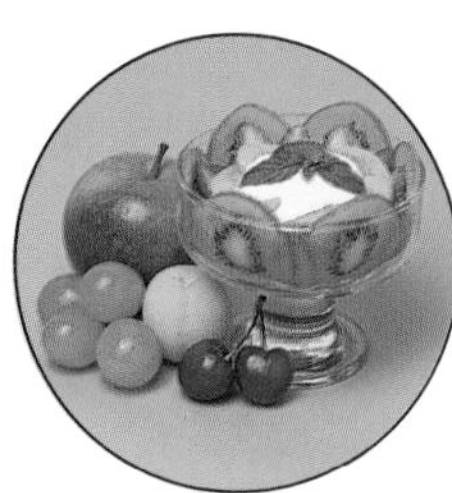

Weight charts

Statistics show that people who are significantly underweight or overweight are less healthy than people who are close to the average weight for their sex, height, and build. People who are overweight are more susceptible to heart disease, diabetes, rheumatoid arthritis, and many other disorders. People who are underweight are more susceptible to respiratory and other disorders. Your ideal weight for your height depends on your build (or "frame"). Some people have broader bones than others, which is apparent from the thickness of the bones at the wrist, elbow, knee, and ankle.

To check your actual weight against the desirable weight range for you, try to assess your build honestly. Then find your height under your gender on the chart and look at the range for your build. If you are unsure of your desirable weight range, ask your physician for his or her advice when you have your next checkup.

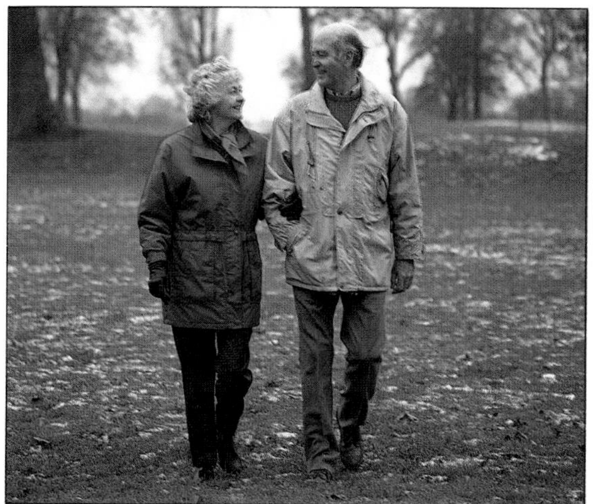

Regular exercise and a healthy diet should keep you trim.

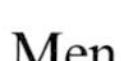

Men

Desirable weight range

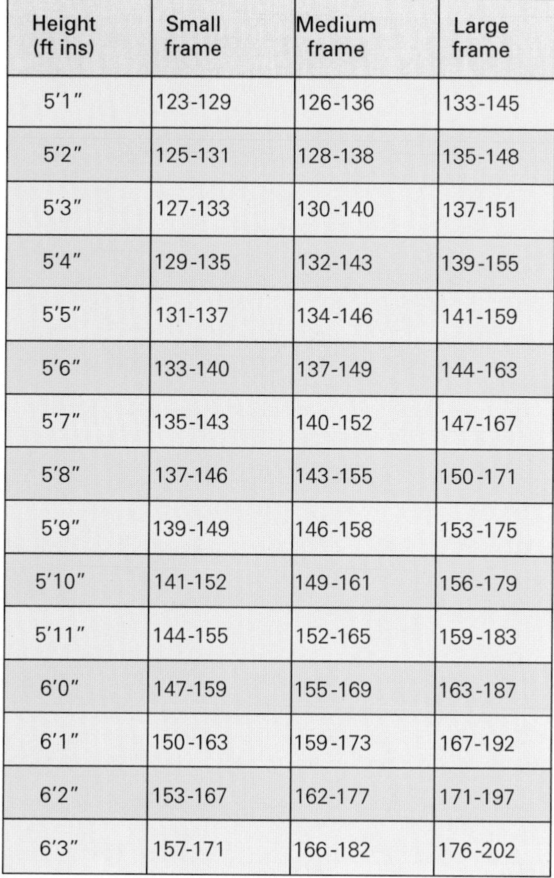

Height (ft ins)	Small frame	Medium frame	Large frame
5'1"	123-129	126-136	133-145
5'2"	125-131	128-138	135-148
5'3"	127-133	130-140	137-151
5'4"	129-135	132-143	139-155
5'5"	131-137	134-146	141-159
5'6"	133-140	137-149	144-163
5'7"	135-143	140-152	147-167
5'8"	137-146	143-155	150-171
5'9"	139-149	146-158	153-175
5'10"	141-152	149-161	156-179
5'11"	144-155	152-165	159-183
6'0"	147-159	155-169	163-187
6'1"	150-163	159-173	167-192
6'2"	153-167	162-177	171-197
6'3"	157-171	166-182	176-202

Women

Desirable weight range

Height (ft ins)	Small frame	Medium frame	Large frame
4'9"	99-108	106-118	115-128
4'10"	100-110	108-120	117-131
4'11"	101-112	110-123	119-134
5'0"	103-115	112-126	121-137
5'1"	105-118	115-129	125-140
5'2"	108-121	118-132	128-144
5'3"	111-124	121-135	131-148
5'4"	114-127	124-138	134-152
5'5"	117-130	127-141	137-156
5'6"	120-133	130-144	140-160
5'7"	123-136	133-147	143-164
5'8"	126-139	136-150	146-167
5'9"	129-142	139-153	149-170
5'10"	132-145	142-156	152-173
5'11"	135-148	145-159	155-176

Sex and health

Sex is a normal, natural part of a healthy lifestyle; a satisfying sex life contributes to the overall physical and emotional well-being of both men and women. Sex can enhance a loving relationship by providing intimacy and pleasure. However, a good sex life does not happen by chance, and it is not realistic to expect your sex life always to be perfect. Like any other significant aspect of a close, caring relationship, it requires thought and effort from both partners. Keep in mind that your partner has his or her own expectations, needs, and desires. Through open, honest communication and with mutual respect and consideration, you can work together to achieve and maintain a healthy, satisfying sexual relationship.

No one outgrows the need for sexual intimacy and affection.

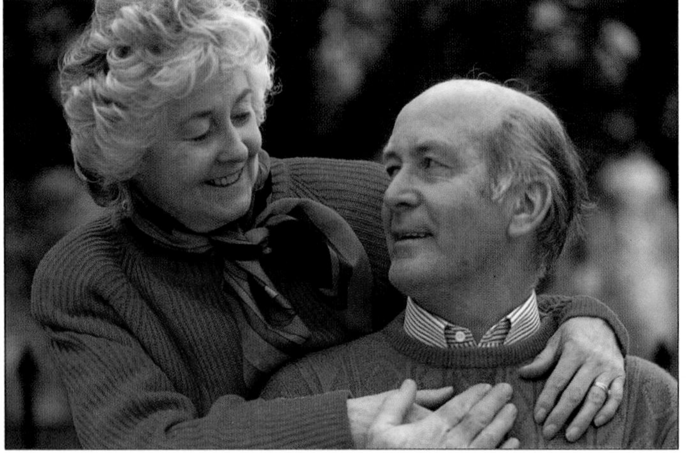

Experimenting with sex and relationships is part of growing up (see Adolescent sexuality, p.764). Research suggests that most American teenagers today become sexually active at an earlier age than their parents did. Because of this, it is important for parents to be aware of their children's sexuality and, more importantly, to take the time to talk to them about sex. Explain the risks and responsibilities associated with sexual activity: teenage boys and girls alike need accurate information about topics such as pregnancy (see p.662), contraception (see p.650), sexually transmitted diseases (see p.654), "safer" sex (see Box, p.466), and sexual orientation (see p.660).

Based on your values, begin to educate your children about sex as soon as it is practical, and continue that process throughout their adolescence and young adulthood. Open communication with your children is essential to establish trust. Be honest and direct, and answer their questions to the best of your ability. And if you do not know the answer, talk to your physician. He or she can answer your questions or guide you to the best sources of information on sex education. Talking about sex does not mean you are encouraging your children or giving them permission to be sexually active. Rather, you are providing your children with the information, values, support, and education they need to make responsible, informed decisions about sex, both now and in the future.

Balancing life's pressures

If you and your partner are both employed outside the home, you probably devote a large amount of your time to your jobs and job-related activities. If your lifestyle is hectic and stressful, sexual activity could easily become a casualty. Even if one of you works at home, especially if you are raising a family, there may often seem to be no time for intimacy. Young children in particular demand a great deal of their parents' attention, and there are frequently problems with finding privacy. You may be too rushed or too tired or both, and you may wonder how you could ever fit sex into your hectic schedule. Think about scheduling time with your partner to nurture your relationship. Planning ahead does not mean that there can never be spontaneity in your sex life; it simply ensures that you will not place your sex life in the deep freeze while other events take up most of your time.

For some couples, there may be more privacy and more time for sexual activity in midlife, after their children have left home. However, many couples in this so-called "sandwich generation" must care for aging parents while they are still raising a family, or divorced children with children of their own may return home. There may seem to be no time for intimacy and sex. And in some cases, fatigue, stress, and anxiety contribute to loss of interest in sex (see Boxes, Loss of sexual desire in men, p.658, and Loss of sexual desire in women, p.659) and other sexual problems such as impotence (see p.657). That is why, if you find yourself neglecting your relationship, it is important that you and your partner watch for potential problems, discuss your feelings openly and honestly, and make every effort to spend time together on a regular basis. Agree to make your overall goal the enrichment of a caring relationship that includes an active sex life.

Seniors and sex

Sex is not just for younger people; the need for intimacy and sex does not diminish as you get older. Research shows that both men and women can have satisfying sex lives well into their 70s, 80s, and even 90s. There is no reason for you to give up your sex life (or settle for an unsatisfactory one) because you think you are too old for sex or because you are having a sexual problem. Sex is for everyone, and virtually all sexual problems can be treated. Remember that intercourse is only one aspect of sexuality; kissing, hugging, and petting all show that you care for each other.

Physical changes related to aging need not interfere with your sex life if you are open-minded and willing to adjust to predictable changes. In fact, some changes that many of us experience may actually increase your enjoyment of sex. For example, after a woman reaches menopause (see p.624), both partners often find sex more enjoyable because they are no longer concerned about contraception and pregnancy. Also, the delay that some older men experience in getting an erection can provide more time for foreplay and intercourse, giving greater pleasure to both partners. (For information about impotence, which is the inability to have an erection, see p.657.) Focus on quality instead of quantity, and work together to improve your sexual abilities, range of positions, and playfulness; you can make sex more satisfying than ever before.

If you need help

If you are having problems with sex, talk to your physician, who will examine you to determine whether the problem is physical, psychological, or a combination of both. He or she will then treat your problem or may refer you to another professional such as a counselor, a psychiatrist, or a sex therapist. Treatment often involves both partners, so both will benefit.

If you want to learn more about sex, read the section on Sexuality (see p.648). Many other good sources of information about sex are also available. For example, your family physician can answer questions about sex. And if you are a teenager, talk to your parents, other family members whom you trust, your physician, or your school nurse. Another excellent resource is your local public library; ask your librarian to recommend some sources of information about sex. You can also get assistance from support groups, as well as telephone helplines and hotlines. Ask your physician about groups in your area.

HIV infection and AIDS

HIV (human immunodeficiency virus) is the virus that causes AIDS (acquired immune deficiency syndrome; see p.465). HIV infection progressively weakens the body's natural defenses. HIV is usually spread by having unprotected sex (sex without using condoms) with an infected person or sharing HIV-contaminated needles when injecting drugs. The virus can be transmitted from an HIV-infected woman to her baby and through a transfusion with blood from an infected donor.

When HIV infection reaches its advanced stage and the person's immune system is no longer able to resist certain diseases, the person has AIDS.

There are several steps you can take to help prevent HIV infection (see Box, "Safer" sex, p.466):

- When you have sex, always use latex condoms and a water-based spermicidal lubricant containing nonoxynol-9
- Have a sex partner who has only you as a partner
- Never use intravenous drugs
- Never mix sex with alcohol or other drugs

If you think you may be infected with HIV, talk to your physician or call your local health department. You can schedule a blood test to find out if you have been infected. And knowing whether you are infected with HIV will allow you to start medical treatment early.

The effects of stress

Any significant change in your routine, whether it is positive or negative, can be stressful. As stresses accumulate, an individual becomes increasingly susceptible to physical illness, behavioral and emotional problems, and injuries. The illustration below shows some important ways in which stress affects various parts of your body, although the precise cause-and-effect relationship is often unclear.

Brain
Many behavioral and emotional problems, such as anxiety and depression, can be triggered by stress.

Hair
Some forms of baldness, such as alopecia areata, have been linked to high levels of stress.

Heart
Periodic angina and disturbances of heart rate and rhythm often occur during or shortly after a period of stress.

Digestive tract
Diseases of the digestive tract may be caused or aggravated by stress. They include nervous indigestion, dyspepsia, stomach and duodenal ulcers, and irritable colon.

Bladder
The bladder may react to stress by becoming "irritable," causing an urgent sense that you need to urinate.

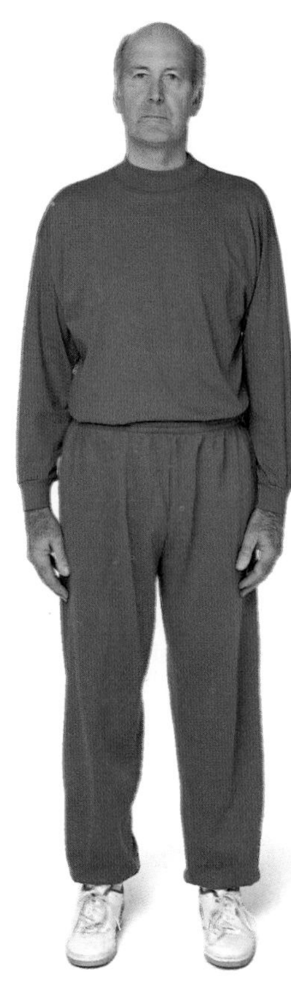

Mouth
Certain mouth problems such as bruxism (grinding of teeth) and mouth ulcers often seem to occur during times of stress.

Skin
Some people have outbreaks of skin problems such as eczema and psoriasis when they are under stress.

Lungs
People with asthma often find that their condition worsens when they are under stress.

Reproductive organs
Stress-related problems include menstrual disorders such as absence of periods in women, and impotence and premature ejaculation in men.

Muscles
Various minor muscular twitches and tics become more noticeable, particularly on the face and hands, when an individual is under stress.

Are you under too much stress?

Here are examples of some common stressful situations. If you are trying to cope with one or more of these or similar situations, you may be at increased risk of stress-related illness. It is important to recognize that positive changes (for example, getting married or having a baby) can produce stress just as negative changes do. (For suggestions on reducing stress, see How to cope with stress, next page).

- Has someone close to you died?
- Have you been divorced or separated from your partner?
- Have you or a family member been hospitalized because of injury or illness?
- Have you married or reconciled after a separation?
- Have you lost your job or retired?
- Are you having any sexual problems?
- Is there a new baby at home?
- Have your finances gotten significantly better or worse?
- Have you changed jobs?
- Have any of your children left or returned home?
- Have you had a significant personal success, such as a promotion at work?
- Have you moved or are you remodeling your house?
- Are there problems at work (for example, with the financial health of your employer) that may be putting your job at risk?
- Have you taken on a substantial debt, such as a mortgage?

What should I do about stress?

Moving can be a stressful time for a family, even if they are eager to move.

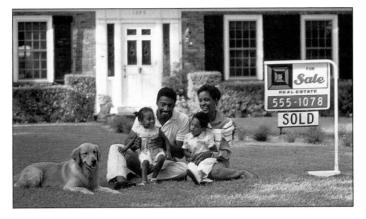

An occasional period of stress is usually distinct from behavioral and emotional problems (see p.318), which may require treatment. Death in the family or among friends, financial difficulties, illness, and worry are all part of life, but it is often when several of these events occur together that severe stress occurs. Although these times of excessive stress may not cause a mental or physical illness, they affect your quality of life and may make you more susceptible to illness (see Are you under too much stress?, previous page).

Since you cannot always avoid stress, review the following pages for ideas on how you can protect your mental and physical health. If you are having difficulty dealing with stressful situations, the Box below may be particularly helpful.

In order to cope successfully with the tensions of difficult experiences in life, everyone should have a healthy attitude and a healthy body. However, if you feel that you cannot cope with the stress in your life, talk to your physician, who will help you or refer you to a qualified therapist.

How to cope with stress

No matter how healthy you are, you will probably have occasional difficulty coping with stress throughout your life. However, there are a number of steps you can take to minimize the impact of stressful situations. If you are under stress, the best way to cope is to make an effort to adopt the following attitudes and behavior:

1 Concentrate on the present. Do not brood about the past. Think about the future in terms of changes you can make. Do not worry about a future that you cannot control.

2 Consider your problems one at a time. Sometimes lumping them together can make them seem overwhelming, but if you look at each of your problems individually it may be easier to see that each one is not as serious as you thought it was. Then you can begin to look for solutions.

3 Do not complain about your problems. Instead, talk things over with your family and friends; seek positive feedback and listen to their opinions.

4 Once you have decided what you want to do about a problem that you can do something about, act quickly and firmly. Positive action is usually helpful.

5 Occupy yourself and your mind as much as possible. Social activities such as sports, volunteer work, discussion groups, or outings with friends are often better than being alone during a time of stress.

6 Do not hold grudges or blame other people for your problems. Even if you have been treated badly, a constant sense of frustrated hostility will accomplish nothing and can only make you feel worse.

7 Make a point of devoting some time every day to physical relaxation that takes your mind off your problems. If you go for a walk, concentrate on what you see around you instead of thinking about your problems.

8 Be more sociable and more physically active than usual and stick as closely as you can to your daily routine. At times of stress a familiar pattern of regular meals and activities at the usual hours can encourage a sense of security by providing an orderly environment.

9 To avoid taking your problems to bed with you, try not to think about them late at night. You will probably sleep better if you can relax for a few hours before going to bed. For additional suggestions on how to deal with problems sleeping, see next page.

10 If you need help coping with stress, talk to your physician as soon as possible, contact your local health department, or go to a community mental health agency. You may be able to get help from an agency that specializes in dealing with certain problems such as alcoholism, child abuse, or Alzheimer's disease. Sometimes you may benefit from joining a support group for people with similar problems; for example, Reach for Recovery is a support group for women who have had breast cancer.

Stress-related problems

Prevention is usually the best strategy for stress-related illness. If you feel stressed (see Are you under too much stress?, p.38) take steps that will help you cope. First, try to manage the sources of stress in your life. For example, you may need to agree with your spouse to visit a marriage counselor, or possibly ask your employer to hire additional staff to ease your workload (see Box, How to cope with stress, previous page).

Do you feel tense? Do you have difficulty sleeping? Have you gained or lost a significant amount of weight? Have you been socially withdrawn or involved in frantic social activity? Do you work too much or not at all? Do you have no personal life outside of work? Do you worry a lot, or drink too much, or smoke? Are you easily upset? If so, you are probably under too much stress and should consider talking to someone about it.

Help is available from three main sources:

- Your physician
- A psychiatrist, psychologist, psychotherapist, or counselor
- Self-help groups

See your physician first when you are under stress, especially if you are feeling anxious or depressed. He or she will talk to you about the sources of stress in your life and the effects they are having on your health. Your physician will then advise you about possible counseling options, with or without medication. If your physician thinks that counseling would be helpful, he or she may then refer you to a psychiatrist or psychotherapist. And if you have developed a stress-related physical illness such as eczema or a peptic ulcer, your physician will provide appropriate treatment.

Counseling consists of talking things over with a counselor or therapist and trying to

How to get a good night's sleep

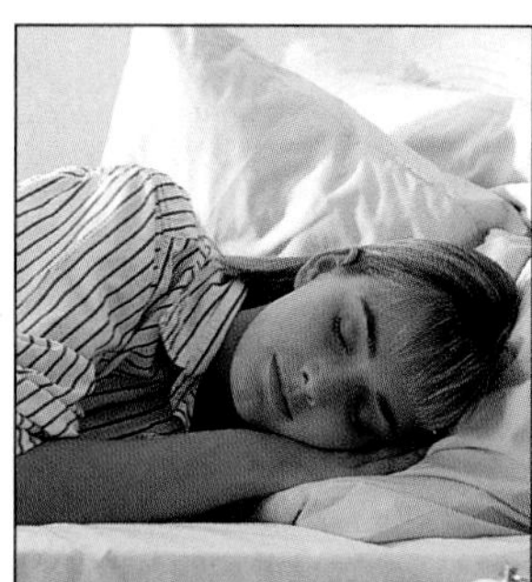

Most people get between 7 and 8 hours of sleep, but sleep requirements differ widely. If you always wake up after only 5 or 6 hours and find it impossible to fall asleep again, do not worry; this is probably as much sleep as you need. And there is generally no cause for concern if you usually wake up once or twice during the night. Many people not only overestimate their need for sleep but also underestimate the amount they get during a restless night. Research into sleep-time behavior and electrical brain waves indicates that most people who think they get little sleep really get more sleep during a restless night than they realize.

A few days of very little sleep will not harm you as long as you remain energetic and alert during waking hours. If, however, you feel overtired or too tense to relax and sleep when you go to bed, try some of the suggestions listed here. If you continue to have difficulty sleeping and it appears to be affecting your daily routine, consult your physician. Although prolonged periods of sleeplessness may not damage your health, insomnia is sometimes a warning symptom of an emotional problem such as anxiety (see p.324) or depression (see p.321). For other possible causes of difficulty sleeping, see the Self-diagnosis symptom chart on page 84.

1 Do not take work-related reading material to bed with you. If you like to read in bed, do some light reading that is not filled with suspense or vivid descriptions of other people's problems.

2 Exercise moderately during the day so that you are tired and ready to rest at bedtime. If you do not get enough exercise, try taking a brisk walk before bedtime. Also, read Why exercise is good for you (p.20) to learn about other benefits of exercise.

3 A warm glass of milk and a warm bath, not a brisk shower, just before bedtime may help you relax.

4 Sexual intercourse at bedtime may have a relaxing effect. However, other strenuous exercise or arguments just before going to bed are likely to interfere with sleep.

5 Make sure that your bed is comfortable and that you are neither too hot nor too cold. Most people sleep best in a room temperature of 60 to 65°F (16 to 18°C); adjust the thermostat before you go to bed.

6 If all else fails, rather than trying to sleep and turning and tossing restlessly in bed, get out of bed, drink a glass of warm milk, and stay up reading or doing a simple chore or two until you are tired. Then go to bed and let yourself fall asleep. Be sure to get up at your normal time and try to make it through the day without falling asleep. Take a very short nap only if you must do so to keep going. Do not let your days and nights get turned around.

understand what is causing your stress, how you are reacting to the stress, and helping you resolve the problem. You may prefer individual counseling, or you may benefit from group therapy involving discussions with several people who have similar emotional problems.

Your physician may recommend medications such as tranquilizers and antidepressants. Medication is sometimes useful in treating stress but is most effective when used in conjunction with one-on-one counseling or psychotherapy.

In many cases, however, the main source of stress may remain. The source, for example, may be the care you must provide for an older relative with Alzheimer's disease, your anxiety about one of your children, or external stress that has resulted in underlying emotional conflicts that cannot be quickly resolved without achieving understanding through psychotherapy.

Also, there are many self-help organizations available to help you by providing information and support regarding a wide variety of stress-related problems. Ask your physician for the name of an appropriate organization in your area.

If the sources of your stress cannot be easily managed, or if you think you might have an emotional disorder (see p.318) as opposed to stress that is caused by situations in your life, then you should quickly seek professional help. Asking for help is not a sign of weakness; it is the intelligent thing to do to protect your health.

Breathing exercises

Deep breathing helps to keep your heart and lungs working efficiently, and making a habit of breathing deeply can help to reduce tension. Get into the habit of breathing deeply by sitting or lying in a comfortable position, and breathing deeply and slowly, timing the breaths so that you take about half as many as usual in the course of 1 minute. Continue for 5 minutes, but stop if you begin to feel dizzy. Whenever you begin to feel tense, make a point of breathing slowly and deeply for a few minutes. This should help relieve tension.

Perform breathing exercises just before you go to bed, or first thing in the morning. It is a good idea to lie on your back with your hands on your ribs as shown.

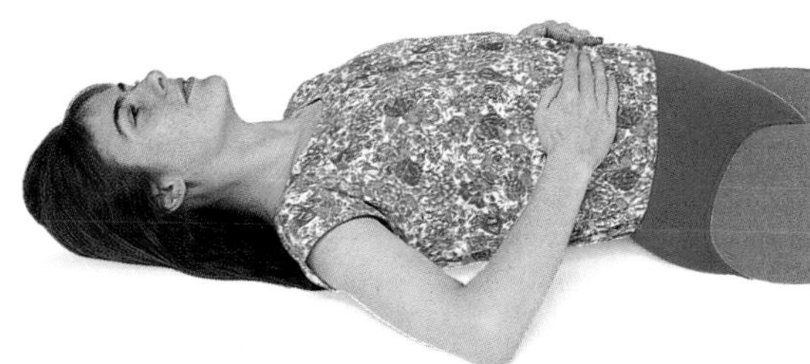

For maximum benefit, breathe deeply, drawing air deep into your lungs. As you breathe in, you will feel your rib cage moving upward and outward.

Take time out every day to breathe deeply.

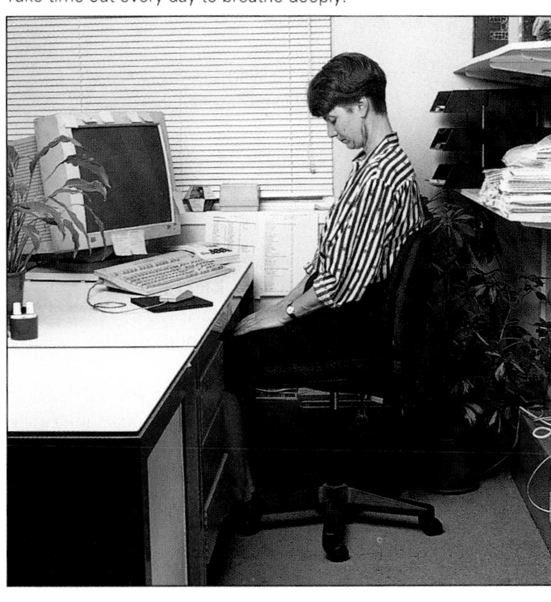

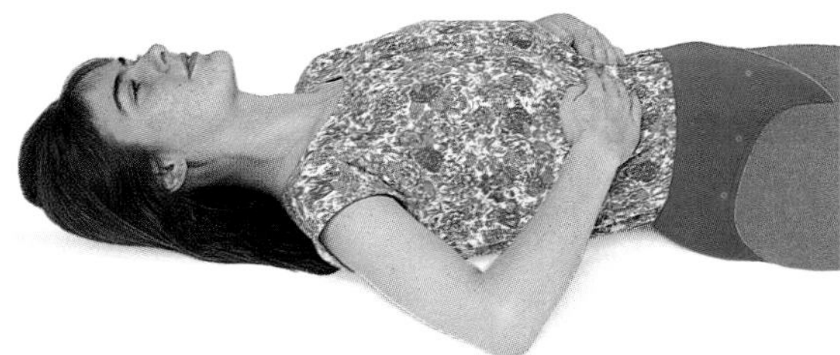

When you breathe out, exhale as much air as possible to make room for your next breath. As you breathe out, you will feel your rib cage moving downward and inward.

Alcohol problems

The most serious and widespread form of drug abuse in the US is alcohol abuse. Millions of people drink alcohol regularly and many, mistakenly, do not regard themselves as alcoholics. In reality, however, regular drinking can gradually evolve into heavier alcohol consumption and the inability to stop voluntarily. A person who drinks regularly may never become "drunk" or have problems at home or at work but may still be damaging his or her health. The heart, brain, nervous system, stomach, and liver can all be damaged by alcohol. Drinking also substantially increases the risk of cancers of the mouth, throat, larynx, and esophagus. The next few pages discuss the damage that excessive consumption of alcohol can cause. For more information on alcohol addiction, read the article on Alcohol abuse (see p.329).

Regular alcohol consumption can damage all your internal organs even if it does not appear to cause drunkenness. Several serious diseases occur much more frequently in regular drinkers than in the rest of the population. Some possible effects of alcohol on various parts of the body are summarized in the Box below.

Parts of the body affected by alcohol

Heart
Heavy drinkers are at risk for a condition called cardiomyopathy, in which the heart muscle becomes weak and damaged.

Liver
Prolonged, heavy intake of alcohol usually causes liver damage, which in some cases leads to cirrhosis of the liver. A diseased liver can no longer process nutrients from digestion or break down drugs. Symptoms of cirrhosis include edema (fluid retention and swelling), jaundice (yellowing of the skin and the whites of the eyes), ascites (swollen abdomen), and hematemesis (vomiting blood).

Skin
Alcohol is a vasodilator; it widens blood vessels at the surface of the body. Besides making you look flushed, this can allow excessive heat loss from body tissues, which may lead to chilling (hypothermia) and pneumonia in cold temperatures.

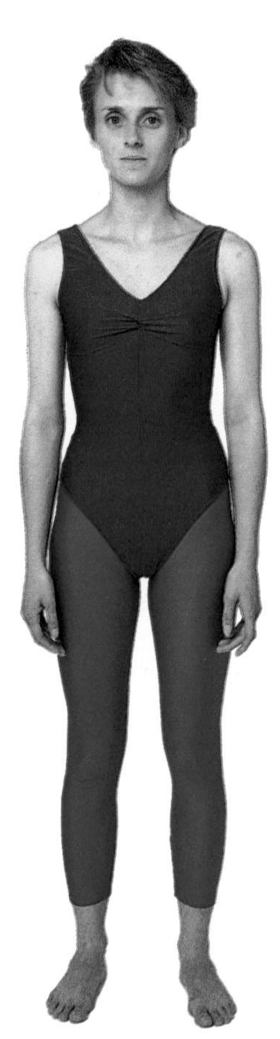

Brain
Some people believe that a small amount of alcohol makes you feel more stimulated, alert, and attentive, but tests have shown that this is not true. Alcohol has a depressant effect. Taken in higher doses it may cause serious problems with memory, concentration, judgment, coordination, and emotional reactions. Speech becomes slurred, vision is blurred, and balance is lost.

Stomach
A single heavy drinking session may give you the unpleasant symptoms of acute gastritis (inflammation of the stomach lining), which can lead to hemorrhagic (bleeding) gastritis.

Reproductive organs
In men, alcohol can produce impotence. In pregnant women, alcohol can increase the risk of damage to the fetus. The infant could be born physically deformed and/or mentally retarded. If a pregnant woman drinks even small amounts of alcohol, it can have adverse effects on the fetus and, later, on the child's emotional and mental development.

How much is too much?

The real question is, how much is too much for you? If you are a pregnant woman, any amount is too much because of potential harm to the fetus. If you are planning to drive, any amount is too much because even one drink can impair your reaction time, coordination, and judgment. If you are taking medication, any amount can be too much because alcohol can increase or diminish the effects of medications. If you are under age 21, any amount is too much because it is illegal for you to drink.

The effect that alcohol has on the body and mind depends on its concentration in the blood. Alcohol is absorbed into the blood from the digestive system and remains in the blood until it is broken down by the liver and exhaled by the lungs or excreted in urine. The rate at which the alcohol level in the blood falls is fairly constant. Whatever the circumstances and however long it may take for you to be affected, once you have reached a certain blood alcohol level it takes the alcohol about the same time to leave your system as it takes to leave the system of someone who is affected more slowly or more quickly than you. However, the rate at which the alcohol level in the blood rises is variable, depending on the circumstances.

Body size

Because a large person has more blood in his or her body than a small person does, the concentration of alcohol in a larger person's blood tends to rise more slowly and to reach lower levels overall when identical amounts of alcohol are consumed.

You can enjoy yourself without drinking alcohol.

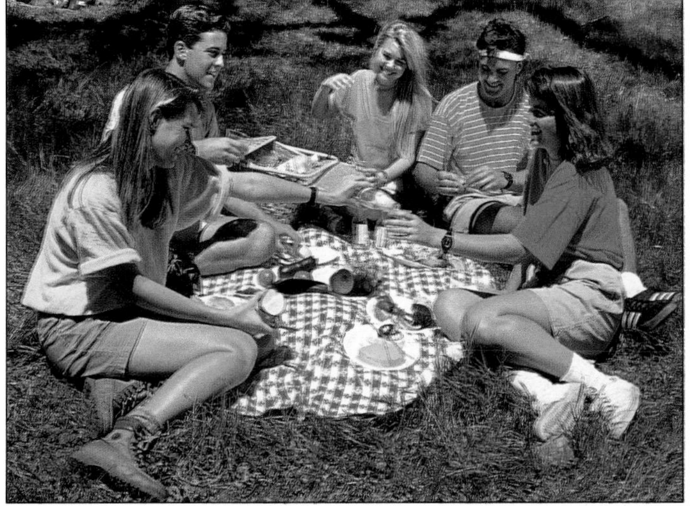

Eating while drinking

Food in the stomach and intestines slows the rate at which alcohol is absorbed in the bloodstream. If you eat before or while drinking, you temporarily slow down the absorption of alcohol.

Type of drink and speed of drinking

The more slowly you drink, the less drastic the effects. If you drink liquor straight, the high alcohol content produces a high concentration of alcohol in your blood more quickly than does a similar amount of wine or beer. If you gulp a shot of liquor, the alcohol is quickly absorbed into your system, especially on an empty stomach.

Physical tolerance

Regular intake of alcohol causes an individual to gradually tolerate a substantial quantity in the blood. The brain gets used to alcohol. As a result, if you have drunk heavily for years, you may be able to look and behave normally even though your blood level would produce drunkenness in a person with a lower tolerance for alcohol. Heavy drinkers who have built up a physical tolerance to alcohol may talk coherently, but their ability to drive a car is still impaired and progressive damage to the brain, liver, and other organs will still occur.

A negative result of increased tolerance is that you become dependent on having a concentration of alcohol in your blood. You gradually need to drink greater amounts to give you whatever effects you expect from drinking. This dependence degenerates into addiction (see p.329), and the greater levels of alcohol further damage the organs of your body including the brain.

Women and alcohol

Alcohol can affect men and women in different ways. Because of this, women who are heavy drinkers are at greater risk of liver disease than men.

A single drink briefly raises the alcohol concentration in a woman's blood to a higher level than in a man's blood. This is partly because a difference in the amount of enzymes in the stomach lining causes women to absorb more rapidly a greater proportion of the alcohol from a drink than men; because women are generally smaller than men; and because women have a higher proportion of fat in their body weight—fat tissue does not absorb alcohol.

The dangers of alcohol

What we usually call social drinking is a habit in which millions of people indulge. Moderate drinking of beer, wine, or mixed drinks is not generally harmful to adults, but it can gradually develop into a serious problem. Remember that alcohol is a drug, and any drug consumed in excess, or at the wrong time, can be dangerous. The following pages describe the harm that alcohol can cause. For information on various aspects of alcohol dependence, read the article on Alcohol abuse (see p. 329).

How much alcohol is in your drink?

Pure alcohol is a colorless liquid too strong for the mouth and stomach to tolerate undiluted. There are many types of alcohol, but the type that is present in varying proportions in alcoholic drinks is known as ethyl alcohol or ethanol (grain alcohol). Shown below is a summary of the approximate alcohol content of selected popular drinks. This will give you a rough guide to use in estimating your actual intake of alcohol. For example, although beer is weaker than whiskey, keep in mind that the alcohol adds up quickly if you drink several beers.

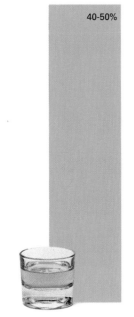

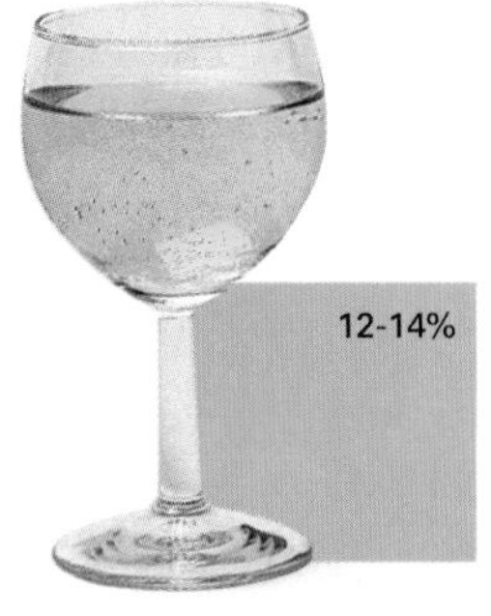

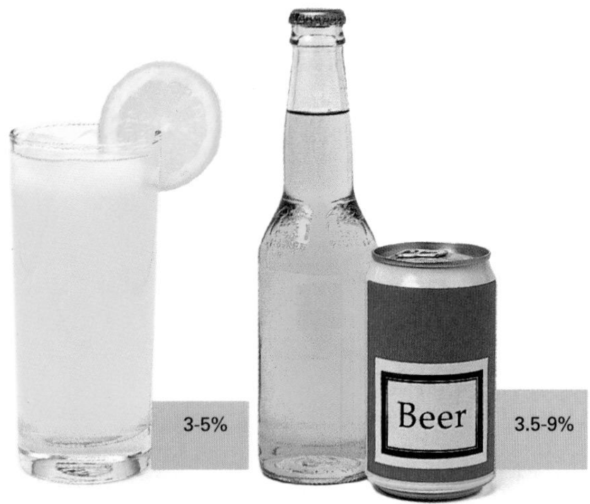

Liquor
Whiskey, gin, vodka, brandy, and other "hard" liquors, including most liqueurs, contain from 40 to 50 percent alcohol by volume.

Wine
Typical table wines contain about 12 to 14 percent alcohol by volume. The alcohol content of a wine is not necessarily related to its taste or bouquet; a "powerful, full-bodied" vintage may contain less alcohol than a "light, fragrant" wine.

Wine cooler
A wine cooler is a blend of wine, sparkling water, and fruit juice. Although they have the flavor and appearance of a soft drink, wine coolers contain 3 to 5 percent alcohol by volume—as much alcohol as beer.

Beer
Most types of beer contain about 5 percent alcohol by volume. "Light" beer usually contains 3.5 percent alcohol by volume. Some malt liquors are stronger and can contain up to 8 or 9 percent alcohol by volume.

Equivalent sizes

The size of the container in which a drink is usually served determines the quantity of alcohol found in that drink. So although there is a smaller proportion of alcohol in beer than there is in wine, a single can of beer is ordinarily a few times the size of a single glass of wine. The equivalents shown above are based on typical sizes of drinks.

The alcohol content of 12 ounces of beer is about the same as the alcohol content of 4 ounces of wine, 12 ounces of wine cooler, or one shot of liquor. Fortified wines such as sherry contain up to 20 percent alcohol by volume. It is important for you to understand that whatever drink you choose, your intake of alcohol will be about the same.

Teenagers, drinking, and other drugs

Adolescent problems with alcohol and other drugs are occurring at an earlier age than ever before. Children today commonly have their first alcohol drinking experience at age 12, in contrast to age 13 to 14 in previous generations. Each year an estimated 4.6 million adolescents age 14 through 17 have alcohol-related problems such as poor school performance, trouble with their parents, or criminal behavior and arrests.

According to the US surgeon general, beer is now the drug of choice for teenagers. Alcohol damages the health of teenagers as well as disturbing their behavior. Drinking and the aftereffects of drinking impair concentration, learning, and performance at skilled tasks, and induce irritability, hostility, and aggression.

A person who begins to use alcohol or other drugs at an early age is very likely to become seriously dependent on them. Alcohol abuse is a major problem for teenagers as a group, including the added possibility of moving on to other drugs such as cocaine and heroin. Young people who drink heavily or use other drugs soon find that they are part of a drug culture in which their friends all share the same habits, reinforcing one another's beliefs and problems through peer pressure that makes it extremely difficult to quit.

Along with dangers to personal health, abuse of alcohol and other drugs contributes to a substantial number of serious injuries every year in the US: about half of all adolescent drivers who are involved in traffic accidents have been drinking alcohol. Also, deaths caused by falls and drowning and diving injuries are more common among teenagers who have been drinking. Alcohol and other drugs are also involved in a large portion of teenage crimes.

Many teenagers experiment with alcohol and other drugs. Parents should not ignore such experimentation in the hope that their teenager will somehow learn about risks involved or outgrow his or her drug-related behavior. Parents should talk to their children about the risks of alcohol and other drug abuse, emphasizing the very serious dangers of drinking and driving and the health hazards involved (see p.42). Teenagers should understand the danger of being in a car driven by someone who has been drinking or using other drugs. Parents should also set a good example for their teenagers.

Set reasonable limits for yourself

Decide to limit the number of drinks you will have, and stick to your decision. If you are not dependent on alcohol, no more than two beers or one mixed drink per day is a reasonable limit. If you are already an alcoholic, however, do not delude yourself that one or two drinks are acceptable for you. Attend an Alcoholics Anonymous meeting and get information and help on quitting.

Learn to say no

Many people have another drink because others in their group are having one or because someone puts pressure on them. When you reach the sensible limit you have set for yourself, politely but firmly refuse to exceed it. Drink a glass of water or juice.

Drink slowly

Never gulp down a drink. Choose your drinks for their flavor, and sip them slowly.

If you prefer a mixed drink, dilute it with a large amount of mixer such as tonic, water, juice, or soda in a tall glass. That way, you can enjoy drinking, but it will take longer to finish your drink. Also, you can make your two-drink limit last all evening or switch to drinking the mixer by itself.

Do not drink alone

Drink only at social gatherings. It is sometimes hard to resist the urge to pour yourself a drink when you are alone at the end of a hard day, but many drinkers have found that a cup of tea, water, juice, or a soft drink satisfies the urge just as well as alcohol can. What may help you unwind without a drink is a comfortable chair, loose clothing, and some soothing music or a good book.

Where to get help

If you think you, your teenager, or anyone else in your family may have a problem with alcohol or another drug, talk to your physician as soon as possible, or contact one of these organizations:

- The local chapter of Alcoholics Anonymous
- The National Council on Alcoholism
- The local chapter of Narcotics Anonymous

Alcohol and driving

This could be your car if you drink and drive, even if you have had only one drink.

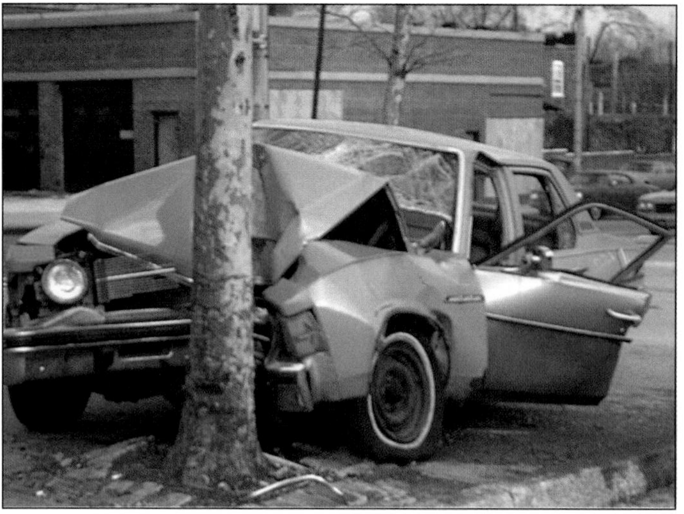

In addition to concerns about an individual's health, alcohol consumption causes many problems related to public health and safety. Because even small amounts of alcohol affect judgment, reaction time, and physical coordination, there is no safe limit for anyone driving a car, school bus, or other vehicle, or for pilots, operators of boats, and heavy equipment operators such as construction workers.

Never mix drinking and driving. Alcohol use is responsible for many severe, disabling injuries and fatal traffic accidents each year in the US. And even if you may not be technically or legally intoxicated (that is, with a blood alcohol concentration of 0.10 percent or greater), you may still be alcohol-impaired. Even one drink will affect your reflexes, coordination, and judgment. If you are going with a group to an event or party where drinking will take place, choose a designated driver who will agree to abstain from alcohol for the evening.

If you have teenagers in the family, discuss with them clearly and often the dangers of drinking and driving. Also, advise them never to get into a car driven by someone who has been drinking; assure your children you will pick them up if they are stranded in such a situation. Further, be sure you are setting a good example for them. Currently all states have a minimum drinking age of 21 years, and studies have shown that the highest rates of driving while intoxicated are found in drivers in their early 20s.

Alcohol and pregnancy

Fetal alcohol syndrome refers to birth defects caused by consumption of alcohol during pregnancy. The condition occurs most often in the children of women who are binge drinkers or consistent drinkers, but there is no safe level for alcohol drinking in pregnancy. Even small amounts of alcohol may produce a lower-than-average birth weight and less obvious adverse effects, as well as increase the risk of birth defects and miscarriage. If you are pregnant, do not drink any alcohol.

A baby who has fetal alcohol syndrome will have some or all of the following symptoms or signs:

- Lower-than-average birth weight
- Facial abnormalities, including a cleft lip and cleft palate, small eyes, and a small jaw
- Small brain
- Heart defects
- Abnormal arm and leg development
- Poor sucking reflex
- Irritability
- Short stature
- Difficulty sleeping
- Lower-than-average intelligence

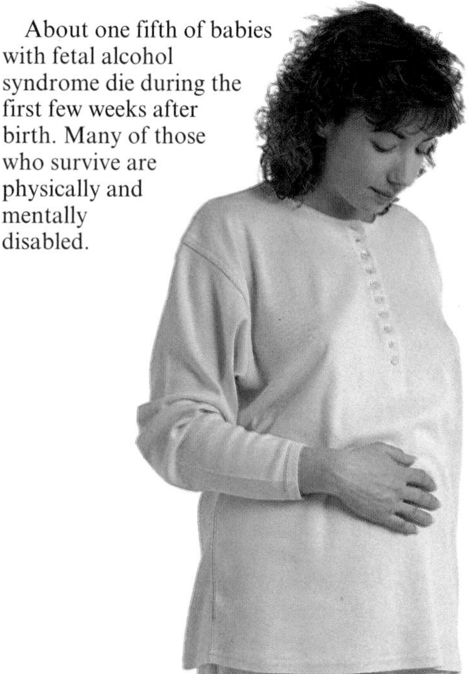

About one fifth of babies with fetal alcohol syndrome die during the first few weeks after birth. Many of those who survive are physically and mentally disabled.

Other drug abuse and drug dependence

Throughout history people have taken drugs for their mind-altering effects. But any drug—whether it is cocaine, marijuana, nicotine, or alcohol—eventually leads to dependence in people who take it. There are two forms of dependence: psychological and physical. You are psychologically dependent on a drug if you experience a profound craving and severe emotional distress when the drug is not available. In physical dependence this emotional feeling of need is accompanied by physical symptoms such as cramps and sweating, which are caused by withdrawal of the drug.

Most drugs of abuse have such powerful effects on the brain that a person who is dependent on them is not able to function, think, and coordinate normally. He or she cannot safely work, drive a car, or care for a family. (Similar problems may occur in people who abuse prescription drugs such as sleeping pills or tranquilizers.) For more information on drugs, see Drugs of abuse and their effects, p.331.

People who use illegal drugs may also rationalize that using these drugs offers little threat to health when it takes the form of occasionally smoking marijuana or using cocaine. All such use of drugs, however, definitely damages health. For example, studies show that marijuana is just as harmful to the lungs as tobacco.

Hazards of illegal drugs

A person who becomes dependent on a drug exposes himself or herself to multiple risks. First, dependence is associated with increased use of the drug so that eventually it has to be taken many times every day; and since most of these drugs may, at least for a time, substantially impair performance of activities such as working or attending school, the drug user may soon find himself or herself outside the mainstream of society.

Second, illegal drugs are obtainable only through illegal sources and are therefore expensive. Regular drug users often turn to crime or prostitution (which has its own serious health risks) to finance their habits.

Third, and most important, a person who is dependent on illegal drugs endangers his or her health. Illegal drugs are of variable quality and purity, and poisonings and overdoses are common and often fatal. Drug dealers often dilute a drug with a hazardous substance to increase profits. If the drugs are injected intravenously, the drug user risks bacterial or viral infection of the lungs, heart, brain, kidneys, and other organs if he or she uses or shares contaminated needles and syringes. This puts the drug user at high risk of hepatitis and infection with HIV (human immunodeficiency virus, which causes AIDS). Even if precautions are taken to avoid sharing contaminated needles and syringes, repeated use of illegal drugs often leads to loss of appetite, malnutrition, and a progressive decline in health.

Finally, many psychoactive drugs of abuse, such as amphetamines or lysergic acid diethylamide (LSD), produce visual and auditory hallucinations, which may lead to irreversible psychoses in the user.

Hazards of drug abuse

There are potentially serious health risks involved in the misuse of any drug, no matter how harmless that drug might seem to be. For example, alcohol, nicotine, and caffeine, although commonly used, are drugs that often lead to some level of dependence. To learn how these drugs can damage your health, see the Boxes, Parts of the body affected by alcohol, p.42, How smoking damages your health, p.49, and Caffeine, p.27.

Use of amphetamines (stimulants once widely used for weight loss) and opiates (painkillers such as morphine and codeine) has frequently led to dependence on them. And drugs such as marijuana and cocaine, which have only limited medical use, are widely abused because of their mood-altering effects. For more information on misuse of these and other drugs, see the Box, Drugs of abuse and their effects, p.331.

Anabolic steroid drugs (see Sex hormones, p.818), commonly called "steroids," are synthetic hormones that imitate the actions of the male sex hormone testosterone. These drugs, which increase muscle bulk and muscle strength, have been abused by athletes who want quick improvement in their overall athletic performance. However, abuse of anabolic steroids involves many serious potential health risks, including fluid retention, hardening of the arteries, damage to the adrenal glands, infertility, impotence, damage to the testicles, liver damage, some types of cancer, and even death. Also, teenage males who abuse anabolic steroids risk problems with bone and muscle development that may cause their growth to be stunted.

Use of anabolic steroids by athletes is widely criticized by physicians and prohibited by athletic organizations worldwide.

The dangers of tobacco

Smoking is the leading preventable cause of death in the US. If you are a regular smoker, you are probably losing about 5½ minutes of life expectancy for each cigarette you smoke. Up to age 65, people who smoke 20 or more cigarettes per day die at almost twice the rate for nonsmokers in the same age group. Cigarette smoking is a major cause of lung cancer (see p.392). Yet, despite the vast medical evidence supporting such statistics, and the publicity given to them, most heavy smokers continue to smoke. While many smokers have stopped smoking, thousands of adolescents every year begin to smoke, often to appear more mature, or because of peer pressure. Research indicates that about 85 percent of adolescent smokers continue to smoke as adults.

The following pages outline the health problems associated with smoking, discuss the dangerous substances contained in tobacco, and suggest ways that you can begin the difficult work of breaking this life-threatening habit.

Smoking during pregnancy

Any couple planning to start a family should be aware of the risks of smoking during pregnancy and after the baby is born; if either partner smokes he or she should quit now. The developing fetus is nourished during pregnancy by the placenta, and research has shown that circulation of blood through the placenta is impaired if a pregnant woman smokes. The most important stages in the development of a fetus are completed by the time a woman is 8 weeks pregnant. Therefore, you should start to think about these risks well before attempting to conceive. Some risks associated with smoking are:

- Smoking reduces fertility, making conception less likely.
- Smoking interferes with the growth of the fetus during pregnancy.
- Smoking increases the risk of complications during pregnancy.
- Smoking increases the risk of miscarriage, premature delivery, and fetal death.
- Smoking increases the risk of low birth weight.
- Smoking increases the risk of respiratory distress syndrome (difficulty breathing after birth due to failure of the lungs to expand).
- Smoking threatens the health of newborns in their critical first days or weeks.
- Smoking increases the risk of sudden infant death syndrome (see p.699).

In addition to the risks listed above, research has shown that babies born to women who smoke during pregnancy develop at a slightly slower pace, both physically and mentally, than those born to nonsmokers. And infants raised in a smoking environment are more likely to require medical treatment for respiratory disorders in the first 2 years of their lives than are infants who are raised in a nonsmoking environment.

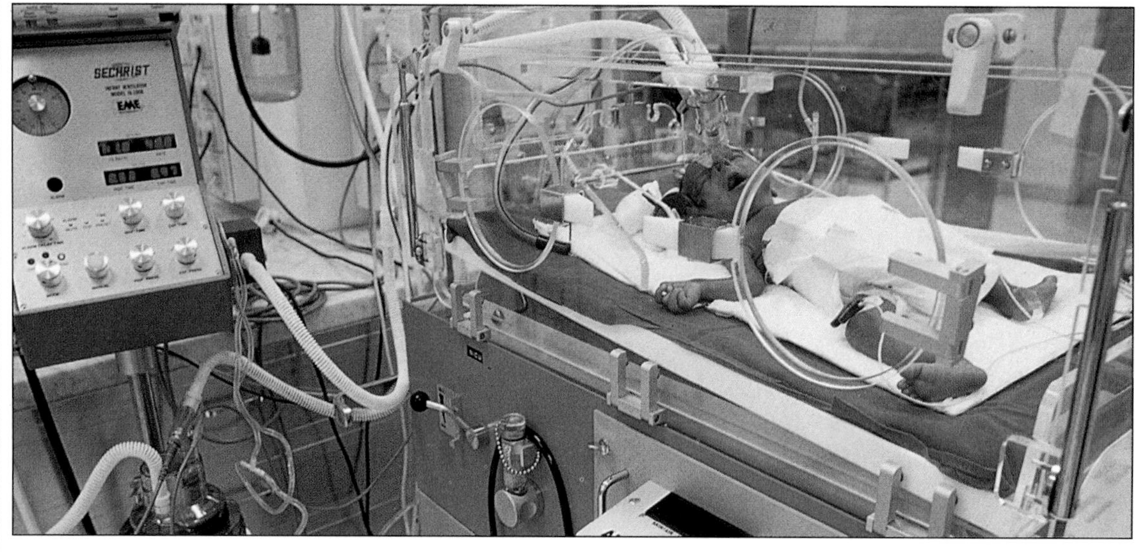

How smoking damages your health

Tobacco smoke contains three principal dangerous chemicals: tar, nicotine, and carbon monoxide. Tar is a mixture of several substances (hydrocarbons) that condense into a sticky substance in the lungs. Nicotine is an addictive drug that is absorbed from the lungs and acts mainly on the nervous and cardiovascular systems. And carbon monoxide decreases the amount of oxygen that red blood cells can carry throughout the body.

Consider the average smoker, a person who smokes 15 to 20 cigarettes per day. Compared with nonsmokers he or she is about 14 times more likely to die from cancer of the lung, throat, or mouth; 4 times more likely to die from cancer of the esophagus; twice as likely to die from cancer of the bladder; and twice as likely to die from a heart attack. Cigarettes are a principal cause of chronic bronchitis and emphysema, and having a chronic lung disease increases the risks of pneumonia and heart failure. The usually minor risks of blood clots from oral contraceptives are much, much greater among women smokers (see p.650), and physicians do not usually prescribe oral contraceptives for smokers over 35 for this reason. Smoking also increases the risk of high blood pressure.

Some brands of cigarettes contain less tar and nicotine than others, but there is no such thing as a safe cigarette. Switching to mild cigarettes does not usually help; habitually heavy smokers usually adapt their smoking habits to the switch by inhaling longer and more deeply and by smoking more cigarettes.

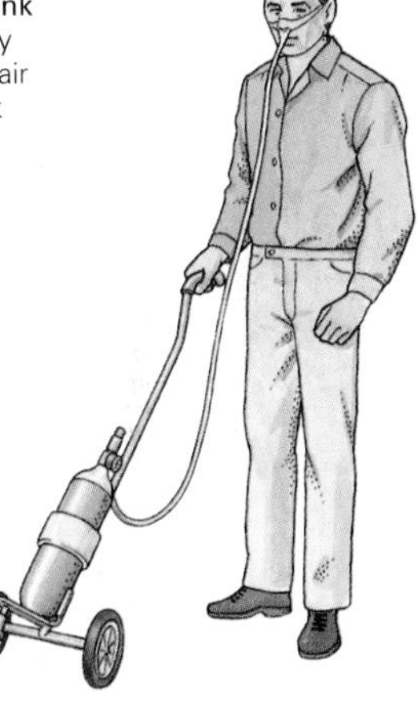

Portable oxygen tank
Breathing in a supply of oxygen-enriched air from a portable tank can improve the mobility and prolong the survival of former smokers with damaged lungs.

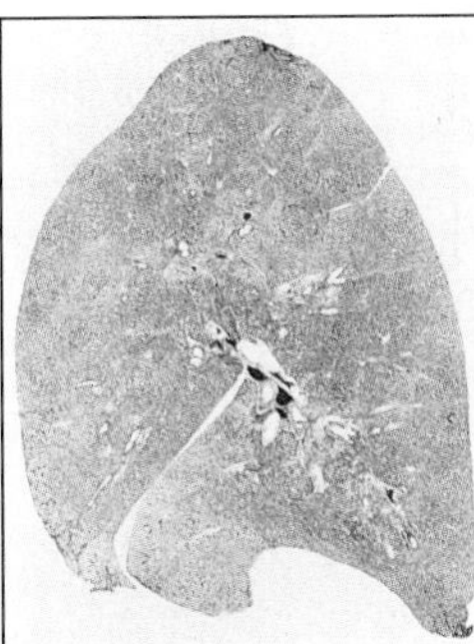

Healthy lung
This photograph shows a slice of healthy tissue from a nonsmoker's lung.

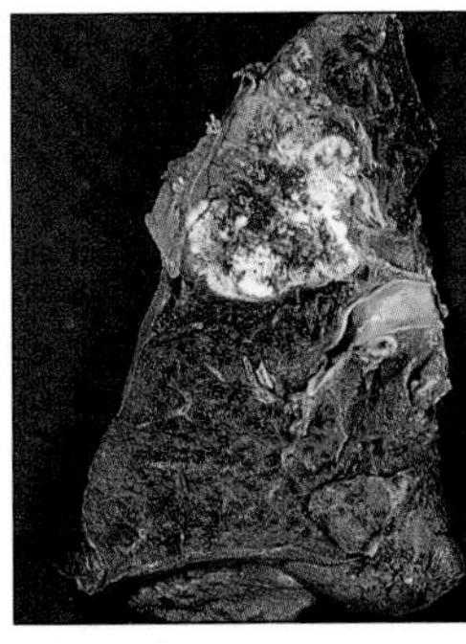

Cancerous lung
This tissue slice from a smoker's lung shows cancerous cell changes.

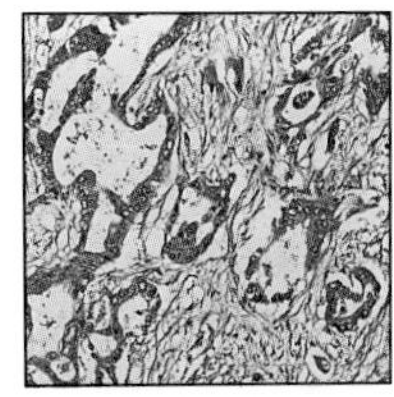

Cancer of the pancreas
Long-term smokers are at high risk of developing cancer of the pancreas. This photograph shows a tissue slice through such a cancer.

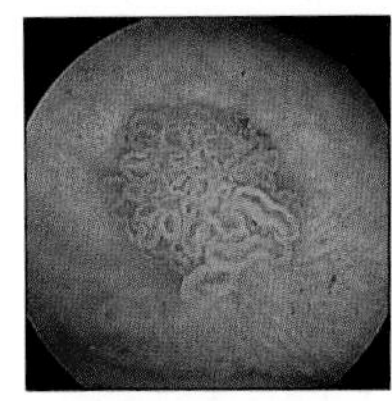

Bladder cancer
Cigarette smoke in the urine can cause cells in the bladder to become cancerous, as shown in this view through a cystoscope (viewing tube).

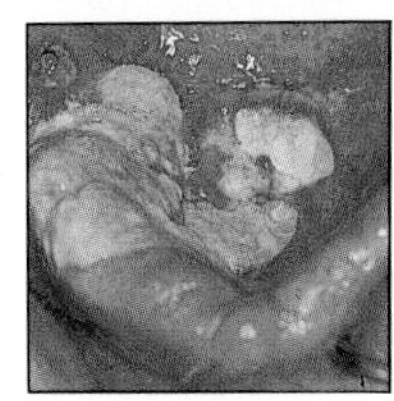

Mouth cancer
Repeated exposure to hot tobacco smoke causes cell changes that can lead to cancer of the mouth, throat, or larynx (voice box).

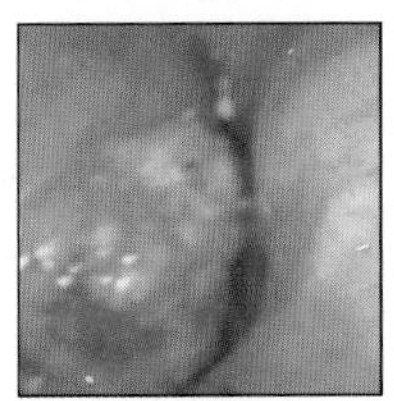

Cancer of the esophagus
This type of cancer occurs more commonly in smokers than it does in nonsmokers.

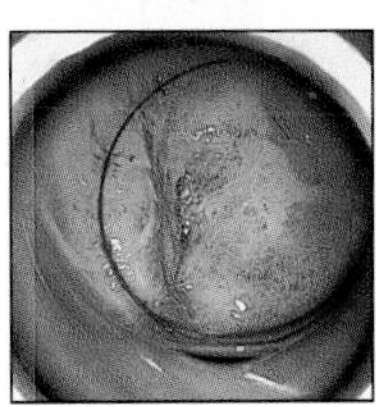

Cervical cancer
The mucus that coats the lining of a smoker's cervix contains substances that can cause precancerous cell changes.

Passive smoking

In the past, nonsmokers came repeatedly into contact with tobacco smoke wherever they went, whether they liked it or not. People once smoked without thinking in restaurants, public buildings, offices, factories, and other people's homes.

Attitudes have changed, however, as evidence has accumulated that nonsmokers may be at risk of contracting serious illnesses from inhaling other people's tobacco smoke. Physicians have discovered that passive smoking—the unavoidable inhaling of tobacco smoke by nonsmokers—increases the risk of lung cancer and coronary heart disease in adults, and the risk of respiratory disorders and sudden infant death syndrome in children. In addition, breathing secondhand smoke often contributes to respiratory problems in people who have asthma, hay fever, and other allergies. Studies have shown that a nonsmoker who lives in the same house as a smoker has almost twice the risk of developing lung cancer as a nonsmoker who lives in a smoke-free environment. Health experts believe that passive smoking by nonsmokers is a factor in nearly 4,000 deaths each year from lung cancer in the US.

How dangerous is tobacco smoke?

Tobacco smoke contains about 4,000 different chemicals, of which at least 200 are known to be poisonous to people. When someone is smoking tobacco, two kinds of smoke are released: mainstream smoke, which has been inhaled by the smoker and is then breathed out, and sidestream smoke, which is released by the burning cigarette, pipe, or cigar. This sidestream smoke actually has higher concentrations of some harmful chemicals than the mainstream smoke, which has already been cleansed in part by the deposit of some of these poisons in the smoker's respiratory tract before it is exhaled.

Studies of smokers have shown that the main health dangers from tobacco—lung cancer, emphysema, chronic bronchitis, and coronary heart disease—are related to how much the person smokes. The more someone smokes, the greater his or her risk of contracting one or more of these diseases. Studies have also shown that there is no safe level of exposure to tobacco; someone who smokes occasionally is still at greater risk of disease than is a nonsmoker. Tobacco smoke is like nuclear radiation; although increased exposure leads to increased risk, any exposure at all carries a threat to your health and your life.

Medical treatment to help you quit smoking

If you have tried conventional methods to quit smoking (see Box, How to quit smoking, opposite page) but have not been successful, you may be able to quit by chewing nicotine gum or by wearing nicotine patches. Both of these methods, available only through your physician, slowly release a small amount of nicotine into your bloodstream. Over time, the amount of gum you chew is reduced or the interval between changing patches is increased, to gradually reduce the amount of nicotine in your body. This will help you to eliminate your physical dependence on the drug. Withdrawal of nicotine is combined with changes in your smoking-related behavior in an attempt also to eliminate your psychological dependence. If you continue to smoke while wearing the patch or chewing the gum, you risk dangerous health complications from nicotine overdose.

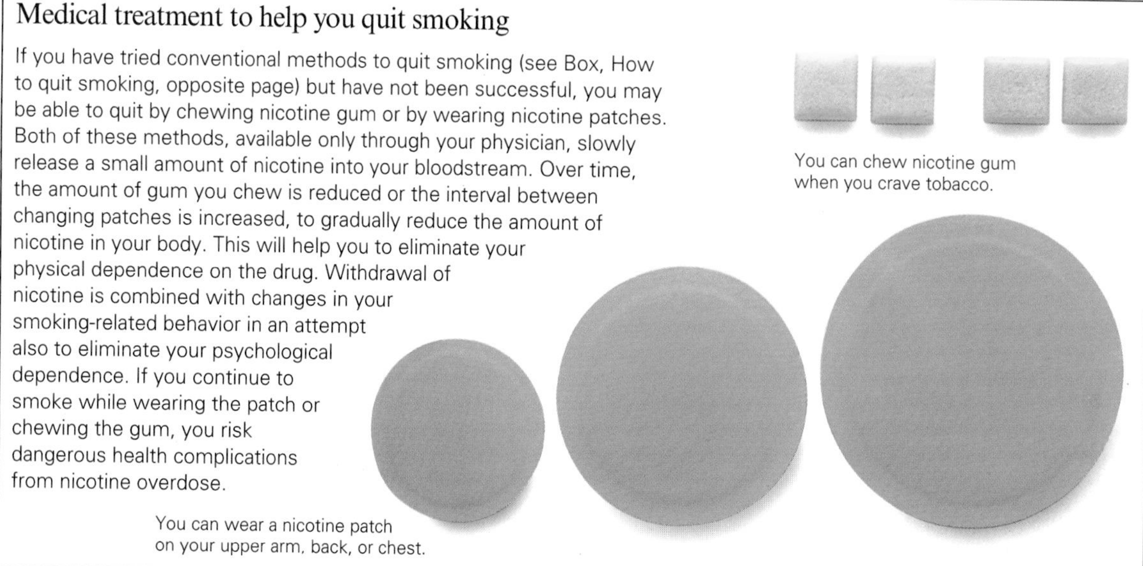

You can chew nicotine gum when you crave tobacco.

You can wear a nicotine patch on your upper arm, back, or chest.

How to quit smoking

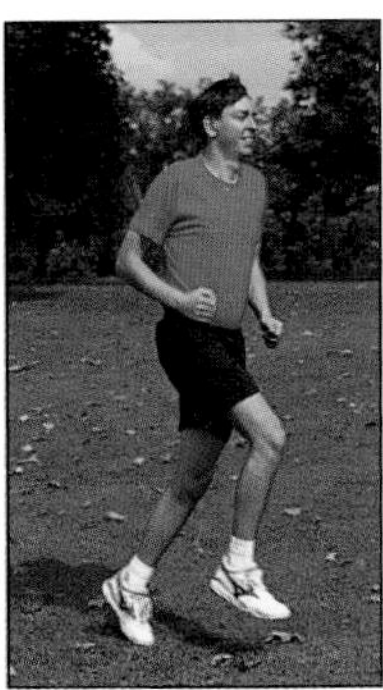

Quit smoking and you will have more energy.

Almost all health risks associated with smoking begin to decrease as soon as you quit, no matter how long you have smoked. Your chances of having a heart attack, for example, drop rapidly. After 1 or more nonsmoking years, the risk of premature death from smoking-related diseases is greatly reduced. After 1 year, for example, the risk of heart disease from smoking is cut in half. After 15 years, smoking-related health risks have almost disappeared.

Research about smoking indicates that while nearly 4 out of 5 smokers want to quit, fewer than 20 percent of those who try manage to do so. Those who try and fail are usually determined to try again, despite the inconvenience, craving, and withdrawal symptoms that quitting smoking almost always involves. Methods such as hypnotism, group therapy, or acupuncture may help ease those symptoms in some people. Using nicotine gum or a nicotine patch (see opposite page), which slowly release small amounts of nicotine into the bloodstream, will prevent the withdrawal symptoms caused by nicotine deprivation. These substitutes, which are available only when prescribed by your physician, should be discontinued gradually over several weeks, during which time the smoker's self-confidence is being restored. Success with nicotine substitution in quitting cigarette smoking is improved when combined with other forms of support or behavior modification. Dangerous complications from excess nicotine can occur in people who chew the gum or wear the patch and continue to smoke. If you want to stop and have been unable to succeed on your own, talk to your physician. He or she may be able to suggest methods to help you stop or refer you to a quit-smoking program.

However, most smokers who have the determination can stop by themselves. The following step-by-step procedure has proved effective for thousands of people who have been able to quit smoking. It is also important to recognize that quitting is very difficult. If you resume smoking, don't be discouraged; try again. You will succeed.

Be sure to drink plenty of water.

Step 1
Analyze your smoking habits. Prepare a chart showing every cigarette you smoke in a 24-hour period, including the times when you almost automatically smoke, such as with every cup of coffee, after every meal, or as you begin work. Give yourself 2 or 3 weeks in which to determine when and why you smoke cigarettes.

Step 2
Make up your mind that there can be no turning back. List all the reasons why you want to quit, including all the benefits. For instance, you will save money, food will taste better, and you may get rid of that morning cough. Convince yourself that the effort is worth making before you start.

Step 3
Choose the day, circle it on your calendar, and quit on that day. It helps if family members or close friends can act together, quitting on the same date and supporting one another through the difficult early days. It may help to choose a time when your usual routine is being changed for another reason (for example, as you leave for vacation). Some smokers have found that it helps to tell as many people as possible. This makes it a matter of pride to keep your resolution to quit.

Step 4
Use any method you can as a cigarette substitute during the difficult early days. It may help to chew sugarless gum or suck on sugarless hard candies. It often helps to give up, at least temporarily, some of the activities that you associate with smoking. For instance, if you usually smoked while having a drink at the neighborhood bar, stay away for a while. Avoid situations that encourage smoking; for example, sit in the nonsmoking section of restaurants.

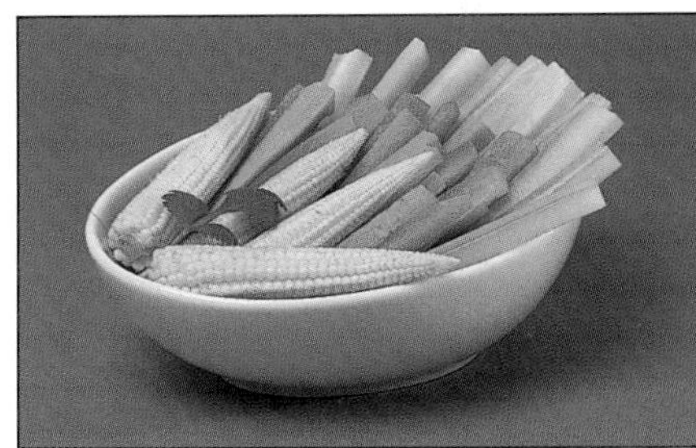

Snack on raw vegetables instead of smoking.

Step 5
Enjoy not smoking! Do not forget that you are saving a lot of money. You can give yourself a positive reward by saving up the unspent money to buy something you would not otherwise purchase.

Step 6
During the first few difficult weeks, eat as much as you want of low-calorie food and drink plenty of water. Your appetite will probably increase, and when you are feeling tense and restless (the natural result of trying to overcome an addictive habit), you may often want to eat something, so you will probably gain a few pounds. To help prevent weight gain, stock up on sugarless candy and gum, as well as low-calorie vegetables such as celery and carrots. Remember that the first 4 weeks are the hardest. You can expect to lose your intense craving for tobacco after about 8 weeks, and you can then return to your usual eating habits.

Safety and environment

Every day you and your family are exposed to many health risks. While some of these risks are fairly obvious, others are less apparent. Where you live, your occupation, your daily routine, and how you spend your leisure time are just a few examples of the wide variety of factors that can affect your health and the overall quality of your life. Factors such as the source of your drinking water, the amount and strength of sunlight you are regularly exposed to, and the kinds of transportation you use all have potential impact on your health and well-being. Some of these factors are within your control; others are not.

To reduce your health risks, it is most practical to deal with factors that you can do something about. For example, if you smoke, you can try to quit; if you drive a car, remember to wear your seat belt at all times. However, for most people, moving to a new home just to ensure a cleaner water supply is not possible or practical. Many people have had an impact on larger health-related risks, such as air and water pollution, by working with environmental or community organizations. You can help to improve your environment by getting involved in such groups.

Injuries account for 5 percent of all deaths each year in the US. However, there are many steps you can take to make the world a safer place for you and your family. By initiating preventive measures in your home, on the road, and at your workplace you can help to protect your family. Read the checklists below to learn about some of the steps that you can take to help reduce the risk of injury.

Are you doing enough to prevent injuries?

Injuries cause a large number of deaths each year in the US (see chart, p.800). How well do you protect yourself and your family from injuries? The following safety guidelines deal with possible risks in and around your house or apartment, preventing injuries that might happen to you or your family while you are on the road, and safety in the workplace. By following these guidelines, you can help reduce your risk of injury.

Basic safety at home

Bathroom safety
In the tub or shower, use a nonskid rubber mat or adhesive safety treads and grab rails to reduce the risk of falling. When getting out of the tub or shower, always step onto a nonskid bath mat.

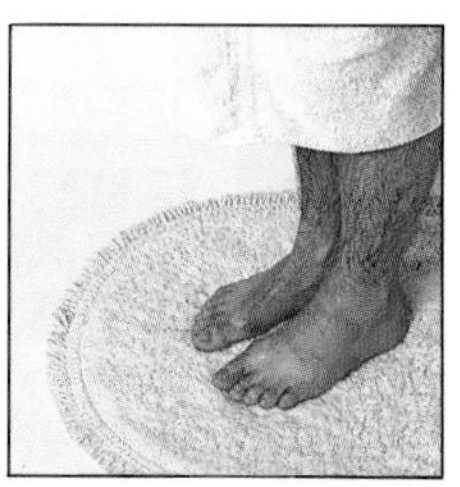

Stair safety
To prevent falls, make sure that all carpet on stairs is held securely in place with bars nailed over the carpet, or gripper rods under the carpet. Nonskid rubber edging can also hold the carpet in place.

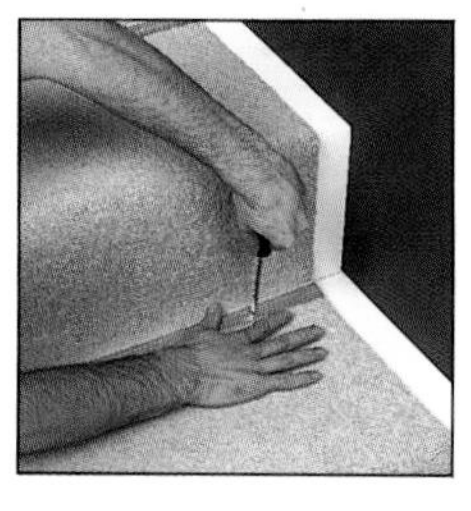

Safety at home

- Never smoke in bed (better yet, don't smoke at all).
- If you have fireplaces, keep screens in front of them.
- When cooking, protect against tipping and burns by positioning pan handles so that they do not extend over the edge of the stove.
- If you own a gun, keep it unloaded, separate from the ammunition, and in a locked place.
- Be sure all carpeting is held down firmly, with no ragged spots or edges, and that loose rugs are placed to minimize the risk of sliding or tripping.
- Be sure all stairways, hallways, and other passages are well lighted.
- Never leave anything on the stairs.
- If you spill or drop something that might be slippery on the floor, clean it up immediately.
- Keep nonskid mats both in and alongside the bathtub and shower.
- When working around the house, wear safety goggles, ear plugs, and protective clothing such as sturdy shoes and gloves when appropriate.
- Make sure you read instructions carefully before using any tools or equipment.
- Never leave safety guards off power tools.

Air and water pollution

Clean air and clean water are the most basic components of a healthy environment. And when we pollute these natural resources we place our own health and survival at risk.

Contamination of the atmosphere by industrial emissions has probably decreased in the second half of the 20th century as a result of laws regulating smokestack emissions and decreasing use of coal. The greatest current source of air pollution is exhaust from motor vehicles, containing carbon monoxide and dioxide, nitrogen oxides, sulfur oxides, decreasing amounts of lead, and particulate hydrocarbons. Stricter government control over vehicle emissions has reduced the amount of pollution released by automobiles, but continuing growth in the number of vehicles, especially in large cities, is forcing up levels of some pollutants.

Although there is no direct evidence, air pollution is considered one possible explanation for the increasing incidence of asthma in young people in the US. Improving the quality of our air and further reducing vehicle emissions should continue to be one of our major environmental goals at the community, state, and national level.

Indoor air pollution has also become a cause for concern as more and more people spend their working days in air-conditioned buildings with windows that don't open. The air inside these buildings is recirculated so that any air pollutants inside the building may gradually accumulate if they are not filtered out. Examples of some indoor air pollutants include resins from construction materials, insulation materials, adhesives used to lay carpets and tiles, cleaning agents, and chemicals from photocopiers and other office equipment. Illnesses caused by air pollution from these sources have been called "sick building syndrome" and

Safety on the road

- Make sure that you and all passengers in your car wear seat belts.
- Always place your children in appropriate car seats or restraints.
- Do not drink any alcohol if you are driving, and never ride with a driver who has been drinking.
- Always drive within the speed limit and drive defensively.
- Keep a safe distance between your car and the one ahead of you—at least 3 feet for each mile-per-hour.
- Avoid driving when you feel ill or unusually tired, or if you are taking medications that cause drowsiness.
- Pull off the road and rest if you get sleepy while driving.
- Have your car fully serviced either every 6,000 miles or at least every 6 months.
- Carry a spare tire and a jack in your trunk at all times, and know how to change a flat tire.
- If your car breaks down, pull as far off the road as possible.
- Check at least once a week to make sure that your car windows, lights, mirrors, and reflectors are clean.
- When walking on streets or open roads at dawn or dusk or in the dark, carry a flashlight and wear light-colored or reflective clothing.

Safety at work

- Make sure that you understand and follow all safety rules at all times.
- Wear protective clothing, including a helmet, goggles, and boots when your work exposes you to hazards.
- Wear gloves, a mask, and safety goggles when handling dangerous chemicals.
- Wear a mask to protect your lungs from inhaled fumes or particles if you work in a dusty environment.
- Check any machinery you operate to make sure that the required guards and shields are in place.
- Make sure that equipment like ladders and scaffold towers is checked regularly, and replaced when necessary.
- Have all electrical equipment serviced regularly, and make routine checks of cables, plugs, and sockets.
- Make sure that operators of dangerous machinery do not become overtired.
- Train employees in first aid, and make sure that every employee knows who to contact in an emergency.
- Report all injuries immediately to your supervisors.
- Make sure that all staff are familiar with evacuation procedures and escape routes in case of an emergency.
- Take all recommended screening tests to check for early signs of work-related illness.

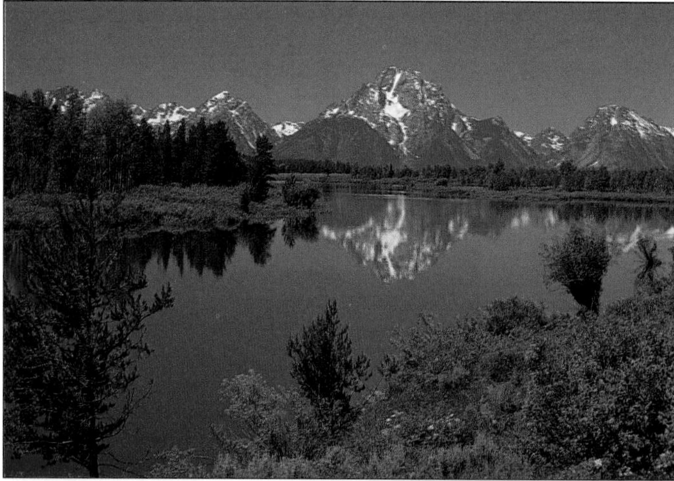

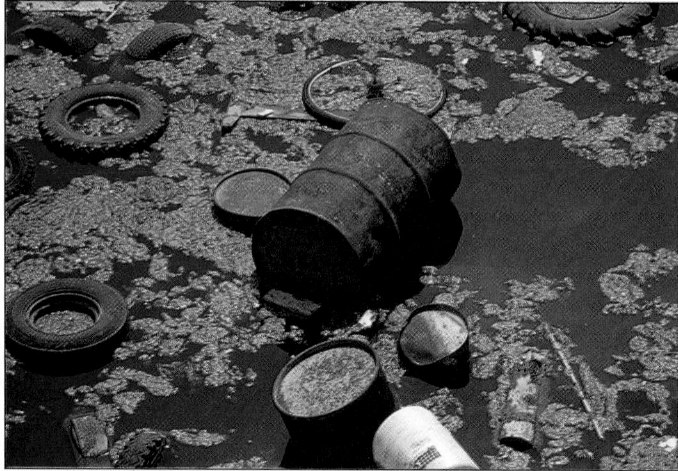

Effects of pollution
Air and water pollution contribute to poor health and destroy the beauty of the landscape. Pollution control should be an important goal for every community.

tentatively linked to a variety of medical problems. Air quality can be and usually is improved in new buildings by increasing the amount of fresh, outside air introduced into the ventilation system by air conditioning and in other ways.

The main concern about our water supply is that the sources from which it is drawn—rivers, lakes, and underground aquifers—are being polluted by runoff that contains fertilizers, pesticides, and herbicides and by acid rain and industrial wastes. Today's water treatment plants were designed to protect against water-borne infectious diseases such as typhoid and dysentery, which can result when the water supply is contaminated with either human or animal wastes. These facilities are not intended to, and in most cases cannot, remove chemical pollutants from water. If you are concerned about the purity of your water supply, have your tap water tested by the designated agency in your state for contamination by microorganisms; or have a reliable, independent laboratory check it for toxic pollutants. If levels of chemical pollutants are found to be high, contact your local public water utility as soon as possible. If the pollution is in your own water source, such as a well, you must attempt to clean it up or abandon it for drinking purposes. Be cautious of bottled water sources too; their purity varies, and the water in most cases is no safer than that from public water supplies.

Lead poisoning

Lead is a powerful poison, and workers who are exposed to high concentrations of the metal may develop damage to their kidneys or nervous systems. But there is no clear evidence that the concentration of air-borne lead is great enough anywhere in the US to damage health. There is, however, a public health problem of lead poisoning, especially of children, from lead-based paint, which is most often found in older homes and apartment buildings, and from lead that leaches from water pipes into tap water.

Occupational and environmental risks

Injuries at work remain a major cause of death and disability, especially those involving motor vehicles. Some occupations—notably in the construction industry, the off-shore oil industry, and deep-sea fishing—are hazardous by their very nature. However, the rate of injuries can be kept lower by closely following all safety standards.

Exposure to chemicals, dusts, vibration, noise, or radioactivity can be hazardous to health. In many cases, legislation and regulation have caused the industries concerned to reduce the risks of exposure. For example, dust control measures have been introduced into coal mines and have lowered the chances of miners developing black lung disease. Also, many industries have occupational health programs; some workers are screened for early signs of disease, since in many cases early detection and treatment can prevent the disease from becoming more serious. Be sure to schedule screenings for yourself at regular intervals.

However, occupational diseases are likely to remain common. Even when they use masks, quarry workers, miners, and other industrial workers are exposed to the hazards of asbestos, silica, and other types of dust (see Pneumoconiosis, p.390). Some agricultural workers may be susceptible to farmer's lung (see p.391), and they always face the risk of injury by machinery or animals. People who work with vibrating machinery may develop Raynaud's disease (see p.440) and possibly occupational hearing loss (see p.364). People who work with asbestos, tar or tar derivatives, certain chemicals, or radioactive compounds are at increased risk of various types of cancer. The health of these workers needs to be monitored regularly throughout their lives, since occupational cancers may develop 30 years or more after the last exposure to the carcinogen (cancer-causing agent).

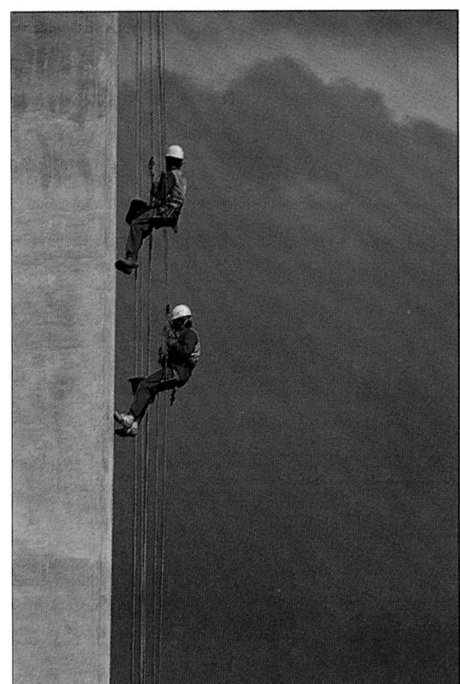

Reducing risks
Always follow the appropriate work safety guidelines, and wear protective equipment if required.

Health hazards exist for office workers also, but research on these risks is in its infancy. People who operate computer and word-processor keyboards are at risk of developing disorders such as headaches and back problems. The possibility of repetitive strain disorder of the wrist is a concern, but medical evidence on this disorder is not conclusive. Concern that working with a video display terminal, or monitor, might increase the risk of miscarriage in early pregnancy has been reduced by several studies showing no excess risk.

Are you at risk?

No list of potential hazards can cover all the possible risks. For one thing, new industries create different types of work, and these jobs may create new risks. Also, unsuspected links between certain jobs and diseases may be discovered in the future. There is evidence, for instance, that workers exposed to certain chemicals used in the industrial manufacture of polyvinyl chloride (PVC) are susceptible to a rare form of cancer of the liver. In fact, virtually every job has its health risks. If you sit at a desk all day, you are more likely than others to develop coronary artery disease; be sure to do exercises regularly after work (including brisk walking). Many white-collar workers have an additional risk of stress.

In general, you are most at risk of a job-related disorder if your occupation:

- exposes your respiratory system to chemicals, dusts, or harmful gases;
- exposes your skin to a chemical (especially in concentrated form);
- exposes your ears to loud noise; or
- exposes you to machinery of any type.

What should be done?

Today most obvious occupational hazards are recognized and publicized, and employers are legally required to take steps to minimize injuries. If your job is even slightly risky, be sure you understand what the hazards are. Also, at times, you may feel pressured to speed up work to a pace that does not seem safe to you. You should talk to your employer or union representative about that. Make sure you take all recommended safety precautions and wear approved protective clothing. Use the ear plugs or protectors provided if you work with noisy machinery, to protect your ears from occupational hearing loss (see p.364). Do not trust your luck instead of wearing a hard hat on a construction site. In short, take advantage of every safety precaution.

If you are concerned about the adequacy of injury prevention measures at your place of work, do not hesitate to bring up the subject. Start by talking to a representative of your employer or union. If you are not satisfied with their response, get in touch with the local or state health department or the nearest branch of the Occupational Safety and Health Administration (OSHA), which is the federal agency that deals with such matters.

Safeguarding your children

Young children must rely on adults to protect them from accident and injury. As children grow and learn, by experience and by example, they will gradually be able to recognize and avoid potential hazards. A child's natural curiosity makes an occasional minor injury unavoidable, but you can reduce the chance of serious injury by making your children's environment as safe as possible. Guide your children toward safe behavior by explaining why something is dangerous. Also, make sure that your children memorize their address and telephone number in case they get lost, and show them how to dial 911 in an emergency.

Choose fireproof clothing.

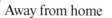

Away from home

- Teach your children how, when, and where to cross the street safely.
- Make sure your children wear highly visible clothing when out after dark.
- Teach your children never to talk to or accept a ride from a stranger.
- Teach your children to swim.
- Make sure your children use the correct equipment and protective gear for activities such as skateboarding and roller blading.
- Make sure that bicycles are in good working order and that your children wear safety helmets whenever they ride.
- Make sure that your car has childproof locks and seat belts and/or car seats appropriate for children—and use them.
- Make sure you know where and with whom your children are playing.

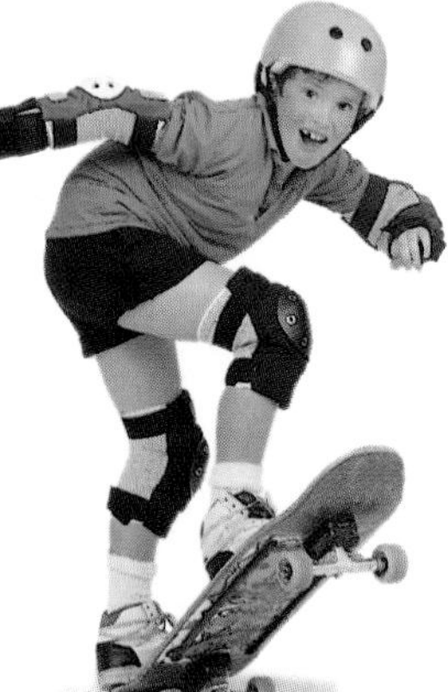

Wear protective gear.

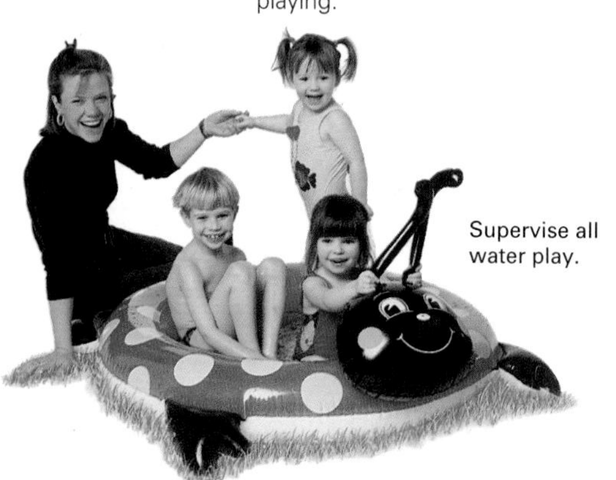

Supervise all water play.

At home

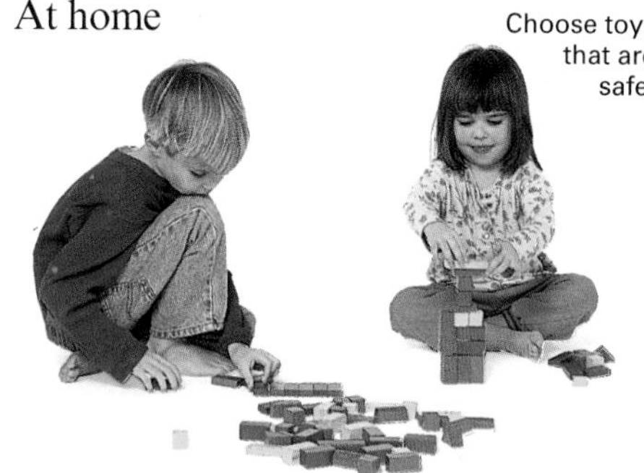

Choose toys that are safe.

- Use safety gates on stairs.
- Put childproof locks on windows and cabinets.
- Never leave a young child unsupervised in the bathroom, kitchen, yard, or pool.
- Cover a fireplace with a screen.
- Teach your children not to touch the stove.
- Keep pot handles turned inward.
- Choose fireproof clothing whenever possible.
- Cover unused electrical outlets.
- Keep all medications, cleaning materials, and other poisonous substances locked out of children's reach.
- Keep the number of your local poison control center near the telephone.
- Keep syrup of ipecac on hand to induce vomiting if your child swallows a poison (see p.843).
- Make sure that toys are safe; for young children, toys should have no parts small enough to swallow or inhale.
- Remove all lead-based paint from surfaces in your home.
- Keep firearms and ammunition locked in separate places.
- Learn first aid.

Turn pot handles inward.

Atlas of the body

Introduction

Until the Middle Ages, medicine was based almost entirely on the teaching of Ancient Greek physicians Hippocrates and Galen. Their methods of treating common illnesses and injuries came from practical experience, but they had little understanding of how the human body is put together and how it works. Medieval medicine was still based on such concepts as the "four humors"—blood, phlegm, yellow bile, and black bile.

The science of medicine began in the 16th century with careful dissection and detailed study of corpses by Italian artist and inventor Leonardo da Vinci. In 1543 Belgian scientist Andreas Vesalius produced the first comprehensive textbook of anatomy, *De humani corporis fabrica* ("The Structure of the Human Body"). Vesalius was able to correct many of the misconceptions in the teachings of the Ancient Greeks, laying the foundation for modern anatomy (structure of the body) and physiology (functioning of the body). The next major achievement came in 1628 when English physician William Harvey accurately described blood circulation.

The study of anatomy and physiology has developed steadily since Harvey. And the pace of discovery has accelerated with development of new techniques for studying the body—including CT scans, ultrasound scans, and MRI scans (see Diagnostic imaging techniques, p.257), and with new understanding of the genetic basis of many diseases (see Genetics, p.752).

This section deals with the anatomy of the body. It illustrates the major divisions of the body's structure and shows how imaging techniques help physicians view the structures of internal organs. (Descriptions of how the various parts and systems of the body function are given in the section introductions in Part III.)

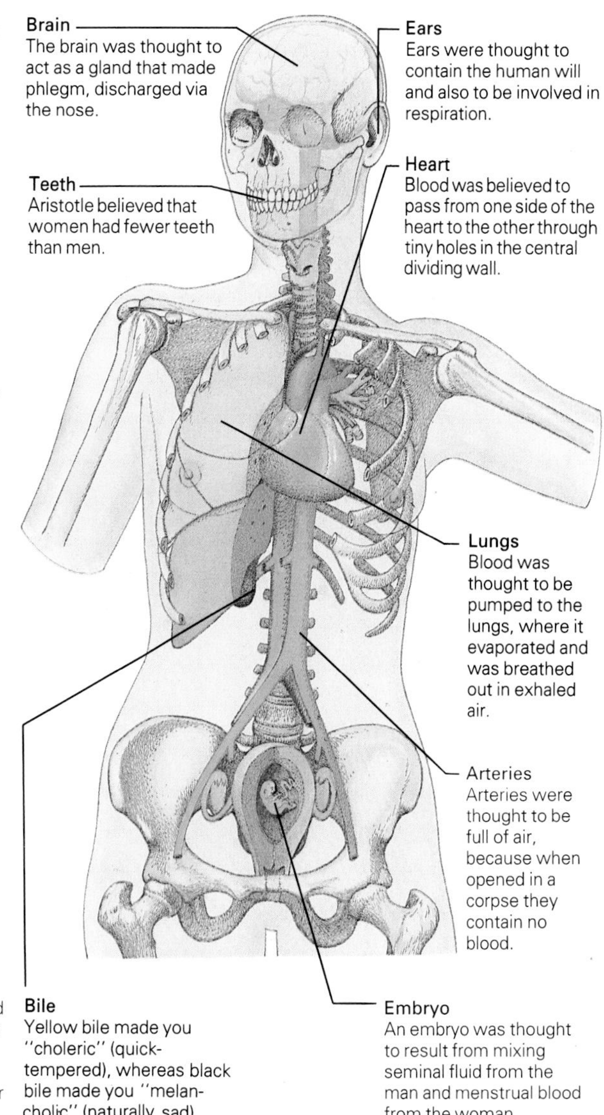

Brain
The brain was thought to act as a gland that made phlegm, discharged via the nose.
Ears
Ears were thought to contain the human will and also to be involved in respiration.
Teeth
Aristotle believed that women had fewer teeth than men.
Heart
Blood was believed to pass from one side of the heart to the other through tiny holes in the central dividing wall.
Lungs
Blood was thought to be pumped to the lungs, where it evaporated and was breathed out in exhaled air.
Arteries
Arteries were thought to be full of air, because when opened in a corpse they contain no blood.
Bile
Yellow bile made you "choleric" (quick-tempered), whereas black bile made you "melancholic" (naturally sad).
Embryo
An embryo was thought to result from mixing seminal fluid from the man and menstrual blood from the woman.

Historical beliefs about the body
Until the 16th century, religious beliefs and other restrictions prevented dissection of corpses to study how the human body is put together. As a result, a number of beliefs developed about anatomy and physiology that we now know are misconceptions. To us, many of these beliefs seem surprising and bizarre; but it is likely that in the future some of our own beliefs will be disproved by scientists.

Skeleton

The average human skeleton consists of 206 bones in most people. There are 32 bones in each arm, 31 in each leg, 29 in the skull, 26 in the spine, and 25 in the chest. In some people the number of bones varies slightly from the norm—for example, about 5 percent of us have an extra pair of ribs, and some of us may have a few extra bones in our hands or feet, or one or more bones may be missing.

The individual bones of the skeleton are connected by joints. There are several types of joints. Fixed joints (sutures) hold the bones firmly together, as in the skull. Partly movable joints allow some flexibility, as in the bones of the spine. And freely movable joints provide variable flexibility, in several planes of movement, as in the jaw, hip, knee, or shoulder.

The skeletons of men and women differ very little. One difference is that men's bones are generally slightly larger and heavier than those of women. Also, the cavity in the male pelvis, surrounded by the hipbones and sacrum, is narrower than the cavity in the female pelvis, through which an infant's head and body pass during childbirth.

Ossification (bone formation)

In the first 6 months before birth, very little of the skeleton contains calcified bone. Most of the bones that eventually form are made of cartilage. After birth, as a child grows, the cartilage turns into calcified bone in a process known as ossification. The areas of ossification appear at predictable times during the growth of a healthy child. On an X ray, the only areas that show up are those formed of bone (cartilage is almost invisible). In long bones such as the femur, the humerus, and the finger bones, growth is greatest in a region known as the epiphysis (where the slender part of the bone, or shaft, joins the wider end of the bone). Such areas of growth can be seen in the X-ray photographs below of the finger and wrist bones of a 2-year-old and a 7-year-old child. The bones of the wrist and fingers are mostly cartilage at age 2 but bone develops as a child grows; in the 15-year-old, bone formation is almost complete.

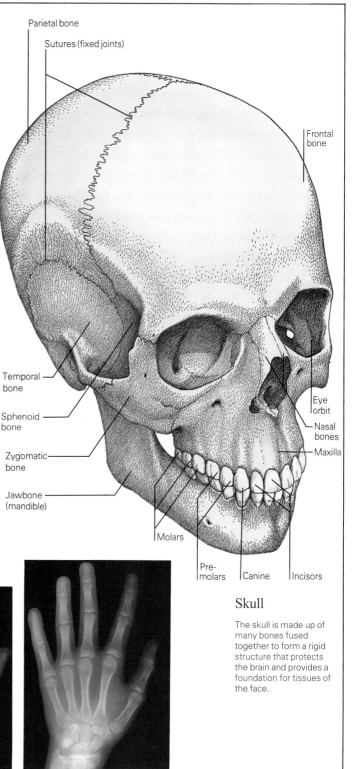

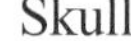

Skull

The skull is made up of many bones fused together to form a rigid structure that protects the brain and provides a foundation for tissues of the face.

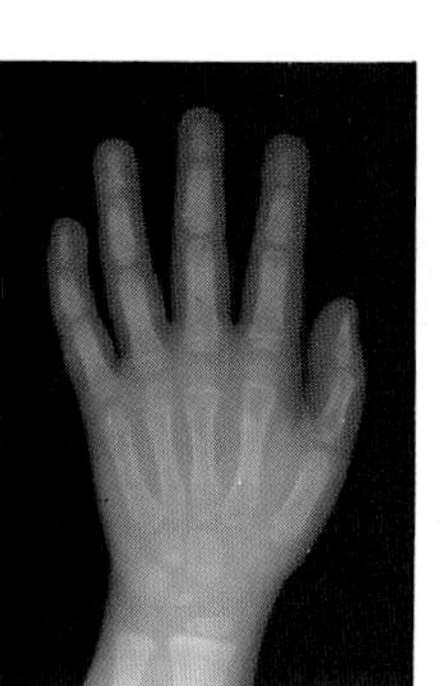

2 years

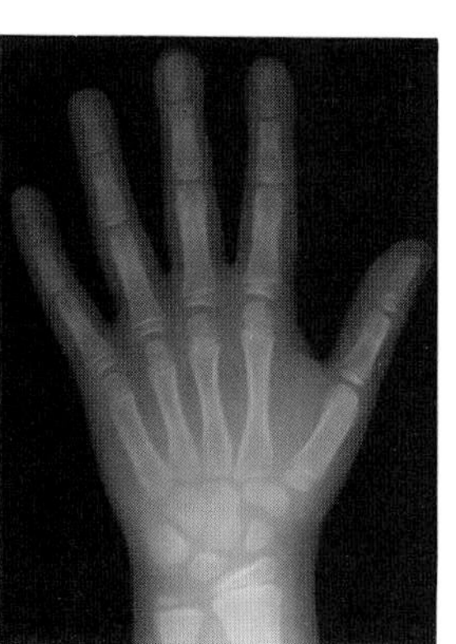

7 years

15 years

Skeleton

Skeletons of men and women differ in the heaviness of the arm and leg bones, the shape of the pelvis, and the angle at the elbow joint, but the skeletons are otherwise identical.

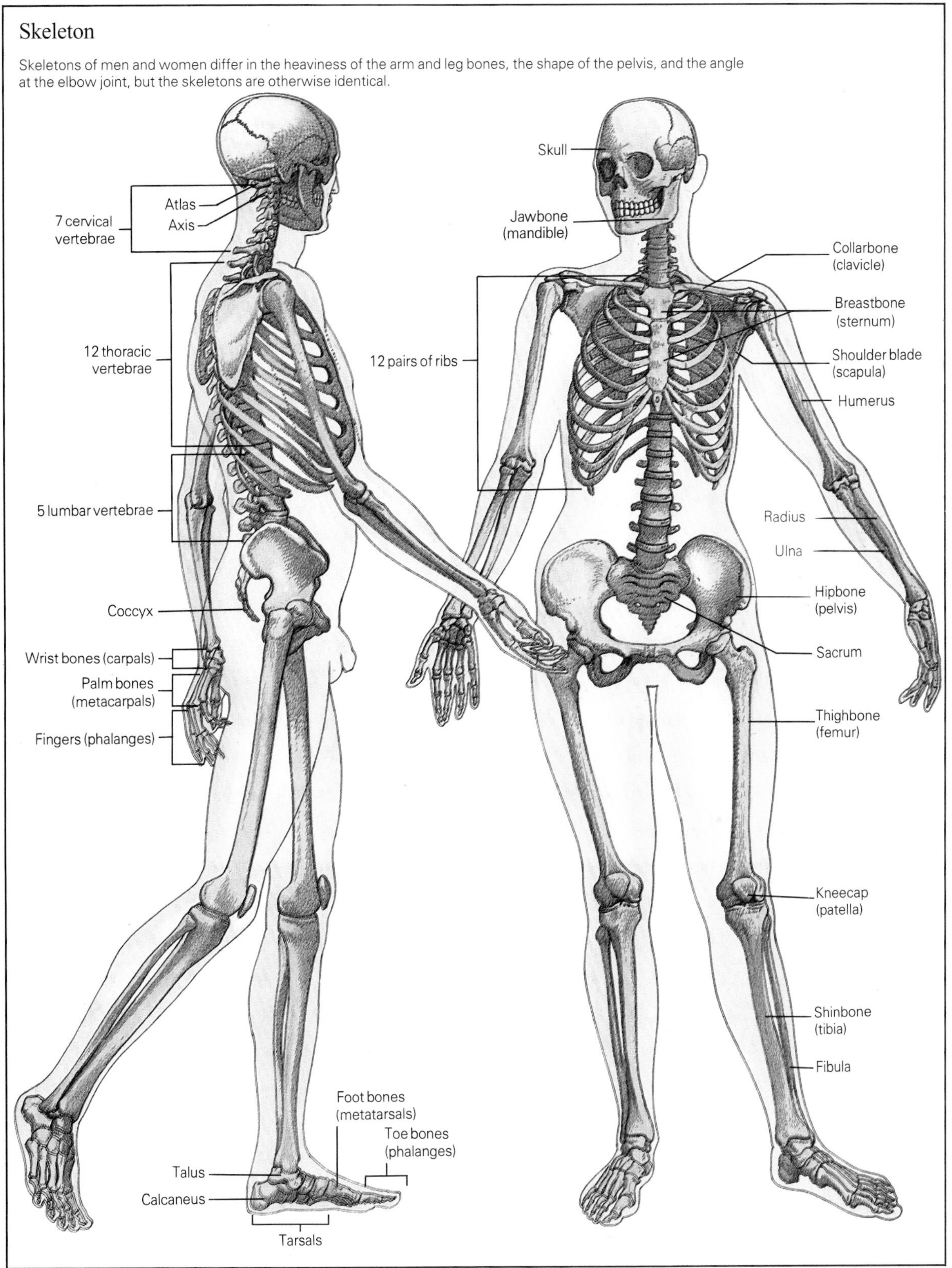

Muscles

There are more than 600 muscles in the human body. Each muscle is made up of bundles of closely interlocking muscle fibers, which vary in length from a fraction of an inch, as in the muscles that move the iris in your eye, to about 1 ft (30 cm), as in your thigh muscles. Some of these muscle fibers contract and relax very quickly; other muscle fibers are designed for the long-term contraction that is required to maintain body posture.

Each end of skeletal muscle is attached to a bone (except for a few muscles in the face, which are attached to skin or other tissue), either directly or by means of a tendon. The tendon may be long and tapering or a flat sheet of tissue. In addition to the skeletal muscles shown here, there are many other muscles in the body; the heart and the digestive-tract walls, for example, contain large quantities of muscular tissue.

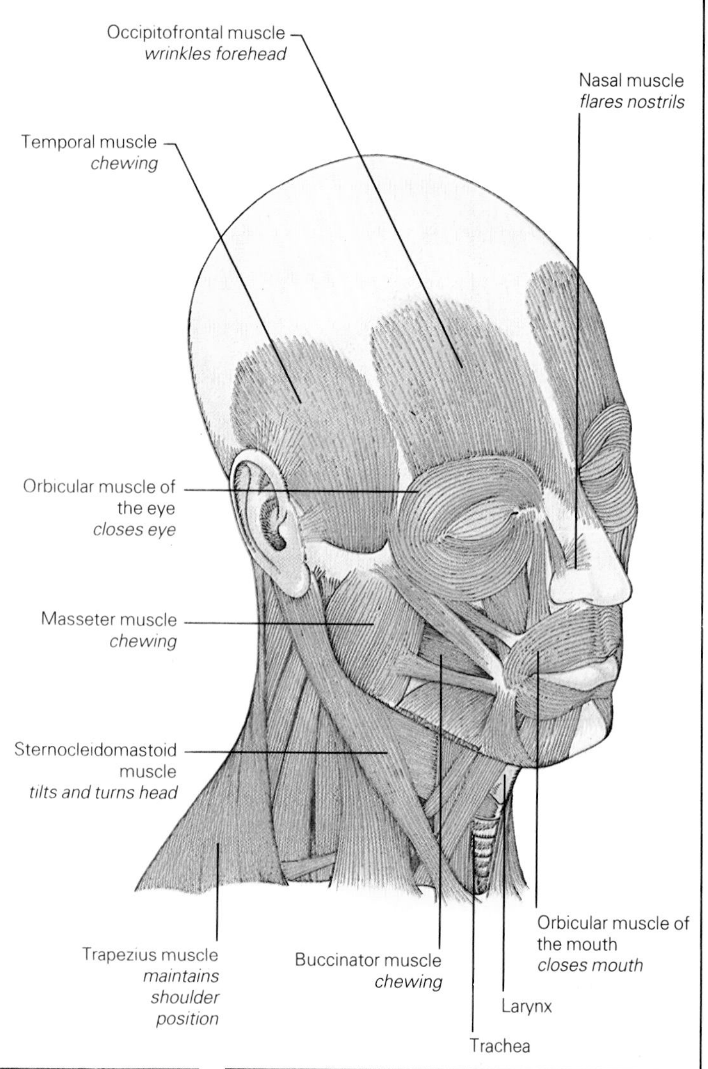

Muscles of the head and neck (right)

These muscles produce the movements associated with eating and with positioning of the head. In addition, they are responsible for the vast range of facial expressions that we use to communicate our moods and emotions to others.

Muscle biopsies
In a muscle biopsy, your physician removes a small sample of muscle tissue for examination under a microscope. These photographs show very thin slices of healthy muscle, magnified 8,000 times. Each fiber is made of many tiny dark stripes (myosin molecules) and light stripes (actin molecules). In a relaxed muscle (right) the stripes overlap only slightly. In a contracted muscle (far right) they slide over each other, shortening the length of the muscle.

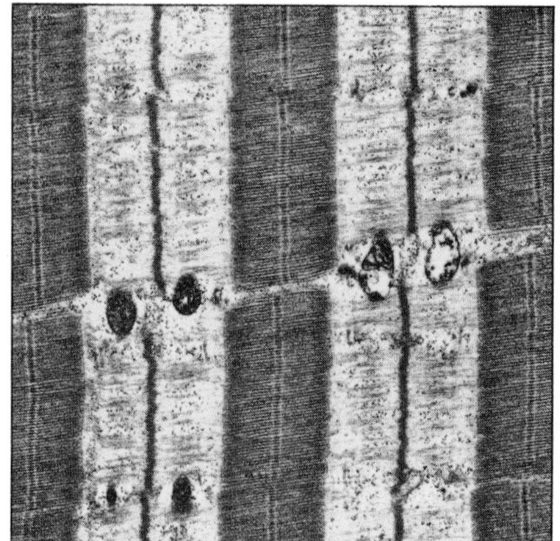

Relaxed muscle fiber

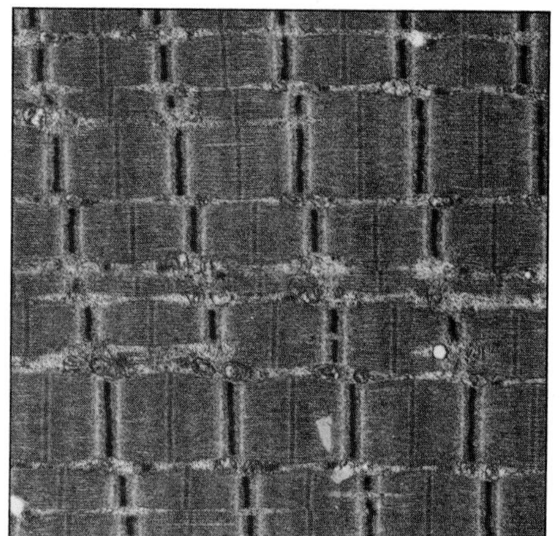

Contracted muscle fiber

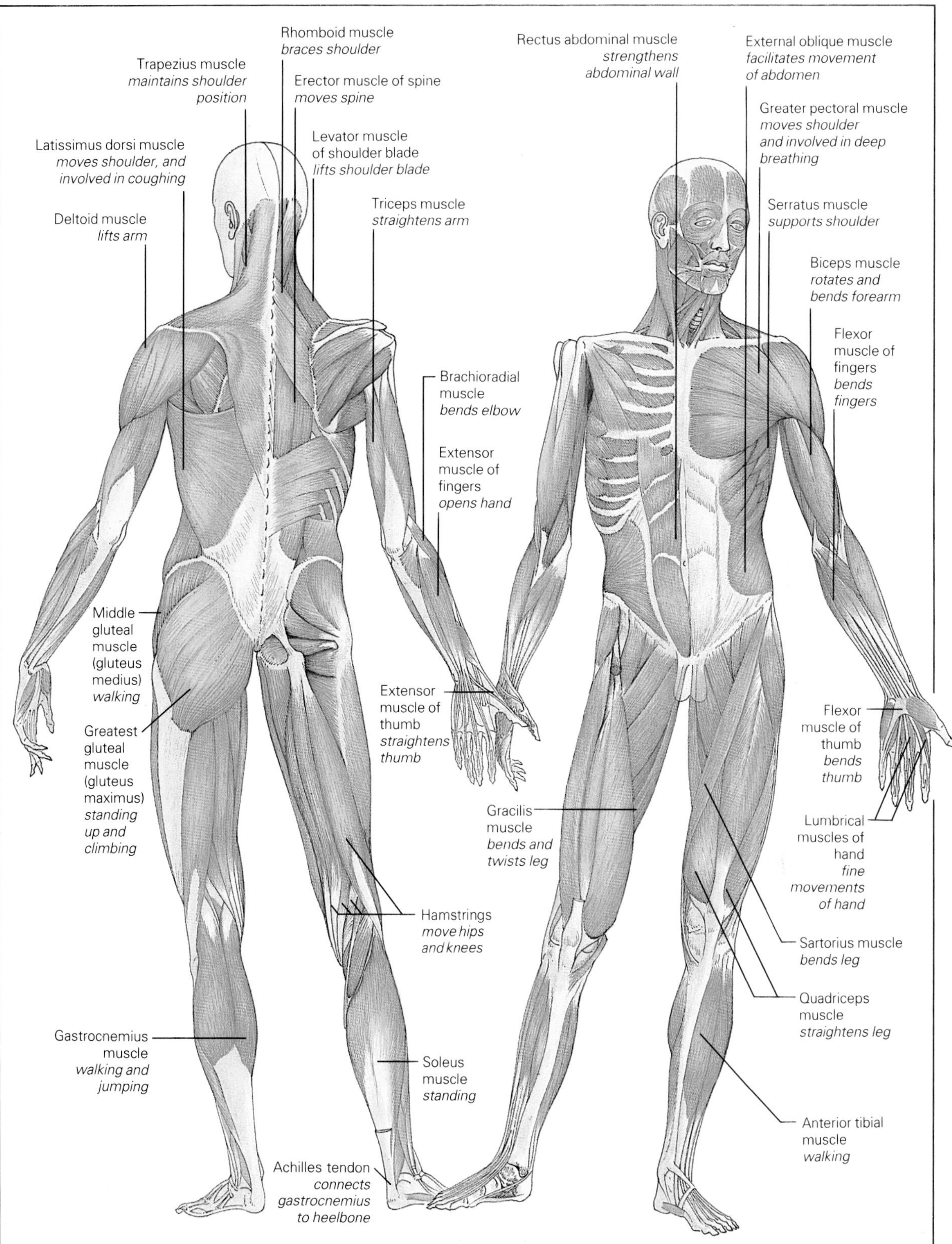
Rhomboid muscle
braces shoulder
Trapezius muscle
maintains shoulder position
Erector muscle of spine
moves spine
Levator muscle of shoulder blade
lifts shoulder blade
Latissimus dorsi muscle
moves shoulder, and involved in coughing
Deltoid muscle
lifts arm
Triceps muscle
straightens arm
Rectus abdominal muscle
strengthens abdominal wall
External oblique muscle
facilitates movement of abdomen
Greater pectoral muscle
moves shoulder and involved in deep breathing
Serratus muscle
supports shoulder
Biceps muscle
rotates and bends forearm
Flexor muscle of fingers
bends fingers
Brachioradial muscle
bends elbow
Extensor muscle of fingers
opens hand
Middle gluteal muscle (gluteus medius)
walking
Greatest gluteal muscle (gluteus maximus)
standing up and climbing
Extensor muscle of thumb
straightens thumb
Flexor muscle of thumb
bends thumb
Lumbrical muscles of hand
fine movements of hand
Gracilis muscle
bends and twists leg
Hamstrings
move hips and knees
Sartorius muscle
bends leg
Quadriceps muscle
straightens leg
Gastrocnemius muscle
walking and jumping
Soleus muscle
standing
Anterior tibial muscle
walking
Achilles tendon
connects gastrocnemius to heelbone

Brain and nerves

Lying well protected within the rigid, bony container formed by the skull bones is the brain. The main components of the brain are the two cerebral hemispheres, the cerebellum, and the brain stem.

The cerebral hemispheres form nearly 90 percent of brain tissue. Each hemisphere is about 6 in (15 cm) from front to back, and together they are about 4½ in (11 cm) across. They are made up of intricate folds of nerve tissue whose total surface area is approximately the same as the area of a large sheet of newspaper.

The cerebellum, which is concerned with muscular coordination, lies beneath the rear of the cerebral hemispheres. The cerebellum also consists of nerve cells and is divided into two hemispheres.

The brain stem, which is about 3 in (75 mm) long, connects the rest of the brain to the spinal cord and contains the nerve centers that control automatic functions.

Inside the brain are four interconnected cavities, called ventricles, filled with a fluid called cerebrospinal fluid. The ventricles are connected to the long, thin cavity that runs down the middle of the spinal cord. This cavity is also filled with cerebrospinal fluid.

Nerve junctions

Shown below are two small parts of the nervous system, the brachial plexus (upper diagram) in the lower neck, and the lumbosacral plexus (lower diagram) in the lower back. These nerve junctions illustrate the tremendous complexity of the nervous system.

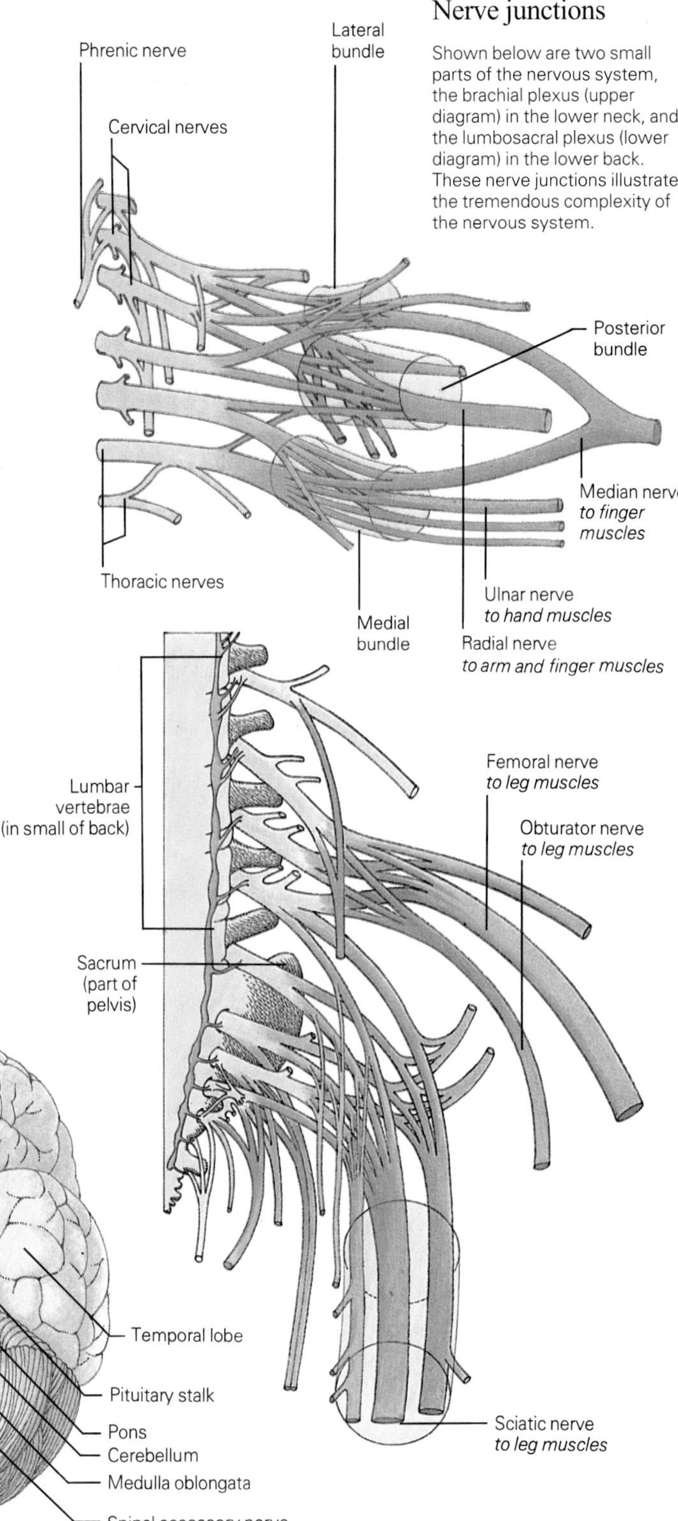

Cranial nerves
There are 12 pairs of cranial nerves (below) that run from the underside of the brain to various organs and body parts. Some of the more important nerves carry information from the main sense organs. For example, the optic nerves transmit visual information from the eyes to the brain, where it is coordinated and interpreted.

Frontal lobe
Olfactory nerve
Optic nerve
Oculomotor nerve
Trochlear nerve
Abducent nerve
Trigeminal nerve
Facial nerve
Auditory nerve
Glossopharyngeal nerve
Vagus nerve
Hypoglossal nerve
Temporal lobe
Pituitary stalk
Pons
Cerebellum
Medulla oblongata
Spinal accessory nerve

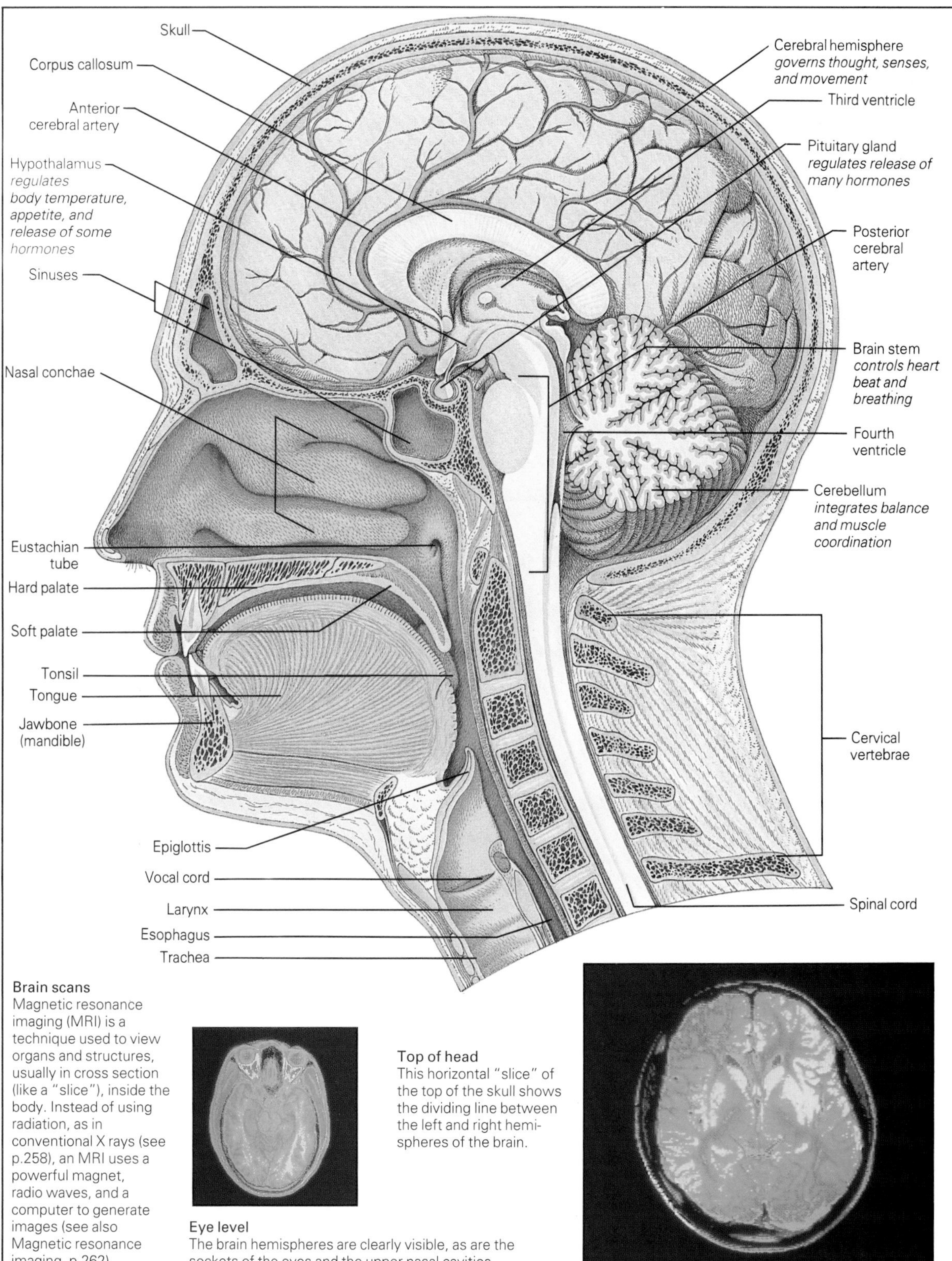

Brain scans
Magnetic resonance imaging (MRI) is a technique used to view organs and structures, usually in cross section (like a "slice"), inside the body. Instead of using radiation, as in conventional X rays (see p.258), an MRI uses a powerful magnet, radio waves, and a computer to generate images (see also Magnetic resonance imaging, p.262).

Eye level
The brain hemispheres are clearly visible, as are the sockets of the eyes and the upper nasal cavities.

Top of head
This horizontal "slice" of the top of the skull shows the dividing line between the left and right hemispheres of the brain.

Heart, lungs, and blood vessels

The heart is made almost entirely of muscle and is about the size of your clenched fist. It lies roughly in the center of the chest. Two thirds of the heart is to the left of the breastbone, the other third to the right.

The lungs lie on either side of the heart. The left lung is slightly smaller than the right one, to accommodate the heart. Between them, the lungs contain about 300 million tiny air sacs (called alveoli), whose combined surface area equals that of a tennis court. The tops of the lungs come right up to the collar line at the base of the neck. When you breathe in deeply, the bases of the lungs extend to the depth of the tenth pair of ribs. When you breathe out, they retract to the level of the eighth pair of ribs.

Magnetic resonance imaging of upper chest
An MRI scan of the chest reveals both lungs (red-tinted areas) with the heart (yellow-tinted area) and great vessels (small blue circles) between them (see also Magnetic resonance imaging, p.262).

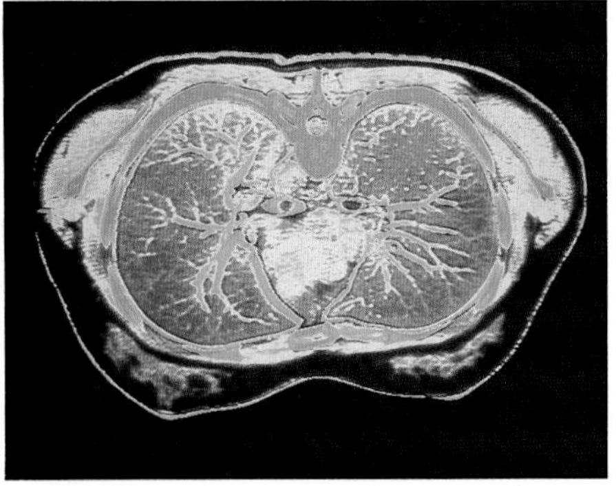

Endoscopic picture of the trachea and bronchi
The inside of the lungs can be viewed directly by a bronchoscope, a type of viewing tube. This picture shows the trachea (windpipe) dividing into the two main airways, or bronchi (see also Endoscopy, p.264).

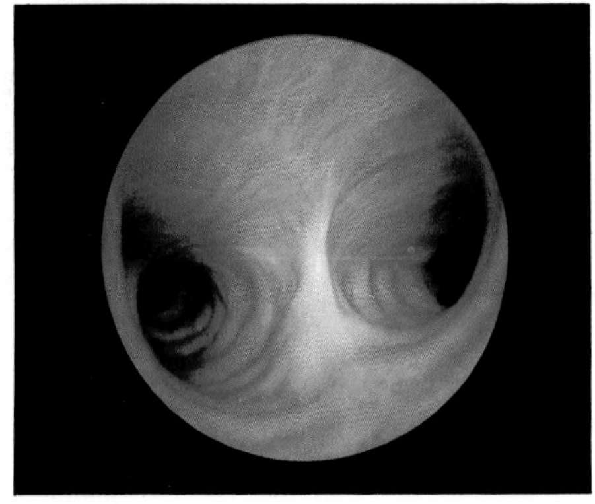

Circulatory system

The circulatory system carries blood to and from every part of the body. Arteries carry blood away from the heart. Veins return blood to the heart.

Internal carotid artery
External carotid artery
Vertebral artery
Subclavian artery
Aorta
Pulmonary artery
Brachial artery
Lower aorta
Celiac trunk
Hepatic artery
Superior mesenteric artery
Radial artery
Ulnar artery
Testicular artery in men
Ovarian artery in women
Femoral artery
Anterior tibial artery
Posterior tibial artery
Peroneal artery
External jugular vein
Internal jugular vein
Subclavian vein
Pulmonary vein
Cephalic vein
Hepatic vein
Basilic vein
Inferior vena cava
Renal vein
Testicular vein in men
Ovarian vein in women
Iliac vein
Femoral vein
Great saphenous vein
Small saphenous vein
Anterior tibial vein

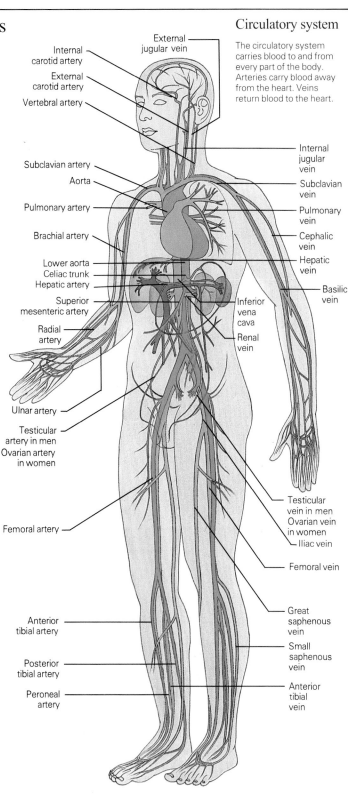

Chest

This illustration of the chest reveals the intimate and complex connections between the lungs (part of the respiratory system) and the heart (part of the circulatory system).

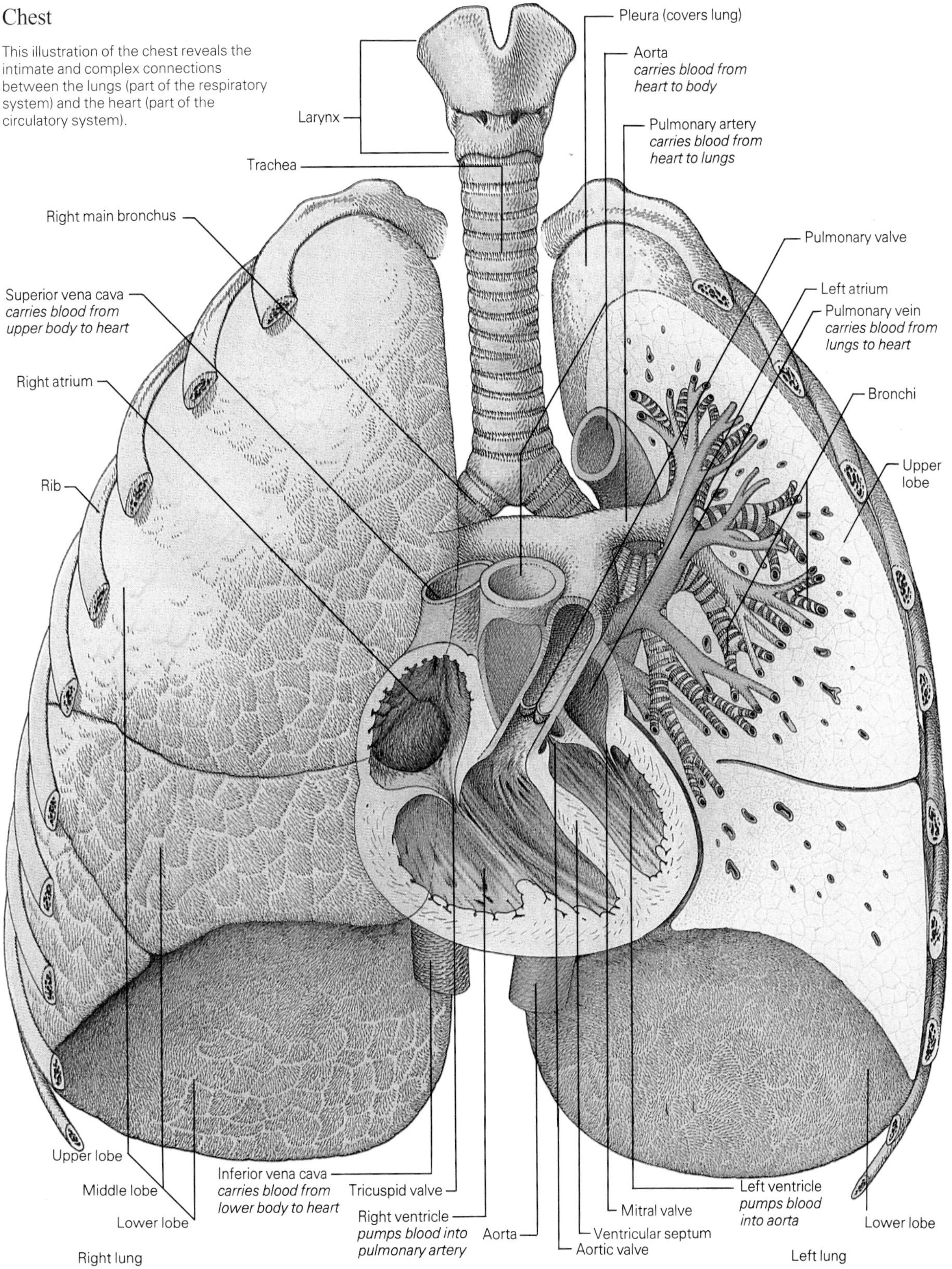

Larynx

Trachea

Right main bronchus

Superior vena cava
carries blood from upper body to heart

Right atrium

Rib

Pleura (covers lung)

Aorta
carries blood from heart to body

Pulmonary artery
carries blood from heart to lungs

Pulmonary valve

Left atrium

Pulmonary vein
carries blood from lungs to heart

Bronchi

Upper lobe

Upper lobe

Middle lobe

Lower lobe

Right lung

Inferior vena cava
carries blood from lower body to heart

Tricuspid valve

Right ventricle
pumps blood into pulmonary artery

Aorta

Mitral valve

Ventricular septum

Aortic valve

Left ventricle
pumps blood into aorta

Lower lobe

Left lung

Torso

The upper part of the torso is the chest, which contains the heart and lungs (see also previous page). The chest is separated from the lower part of the torso—the abdomen—by the diaphragm, a dome-shaped sheet of muscle. The edge of the diaphragm is attached to the bottom of the rib cage. Because of its domed shape, the middle of the diaphragm reaches to only 1 in (25 mm) below the level of the nipples.

Packed into the abdomen are the organs of the digestive and urinary systems. The lower part of the abdomen, cradled within the hipbone, is called the pelvis. In the female, the pelvis contains the reproductive organs.

CT scans of the torso

Pictures of horizontal "slices" through the body can be taken by a CT scanner (see also CT scanning, p.261). The denser the tissue that is scanned, the lighter it will appear on the final image.

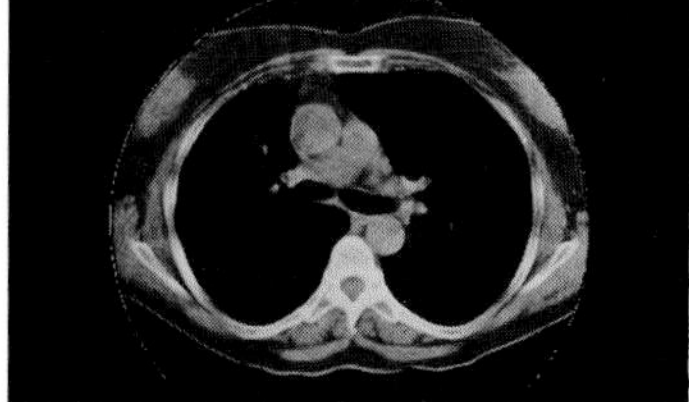

At mid-chest level, the palest areas are the backbone and ribs, the heart appears slightly darker, and the air-filled lungs look black.

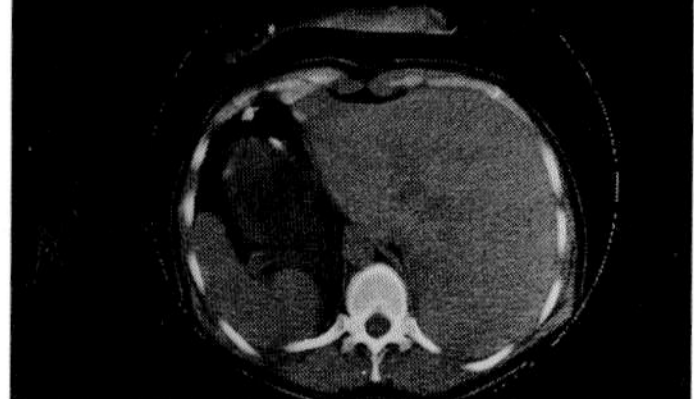

At a level just below the breastbone, the large light area on the right is the liver, and the similar, smaller area to the left is the spleen. The darker patch is the stomach.

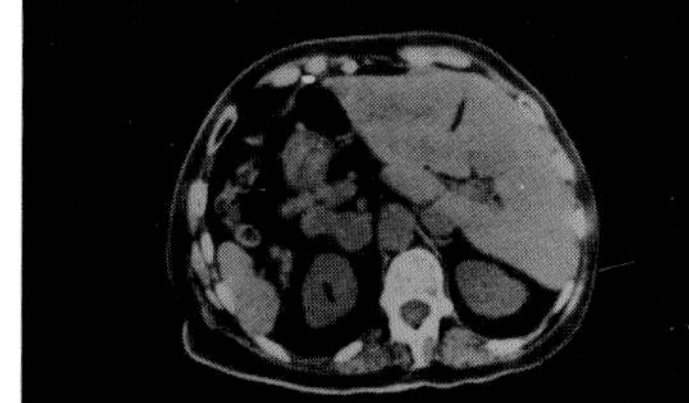

Just above the navel, the liver shows up as a large light area to the right. The light circles on either side of the backbone are the kidneys. The patchy areas toward the left are loops of intestine.

Female torso

The right lung and part of the liver have been omitted to show the heart and abdominal organs. The main blood vessels and nerves in the chest are visible, but those in the abdomen are hidden by the intestines.

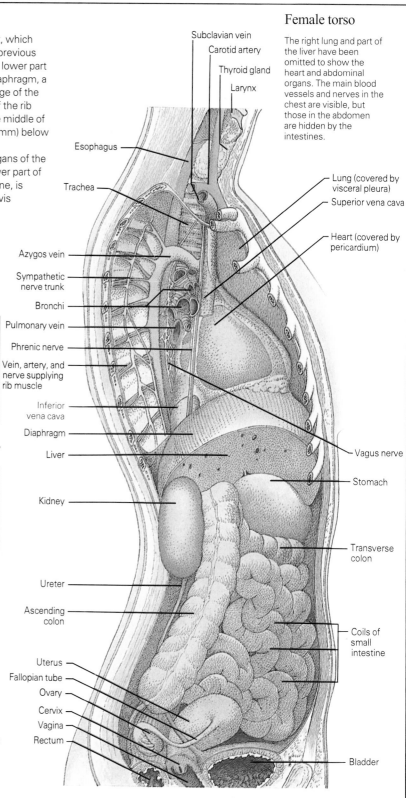

Subclavian vein
Carotid artery
Thyroid gland
Larynx
Esophagus
Trachea
Lung (covered by visceral pleura)
Superior vena cava
Heart (covered by pericardium)
Azygos vein
Sympathetic nerve trunk
Bronchi
Pulmonary vein
Phrenic nerve
Vein, artery, and nerve supplying rib muscle
Inferior vena cava
Diaphragm
Liver
Vagus nerve
Stomach
Kidney
Transverse colon
Ureter
Ascending colon
Coils of small intestine
Uterus
Fallopian tube
Ovary
Cervix
Vagina
Rectum
Bladder

Male torso

A clear view inside the abdomen is shown here by omitting a large flap of tissue, the omentum, which normally extends from the lower edge of the stomach and covers the intestines.

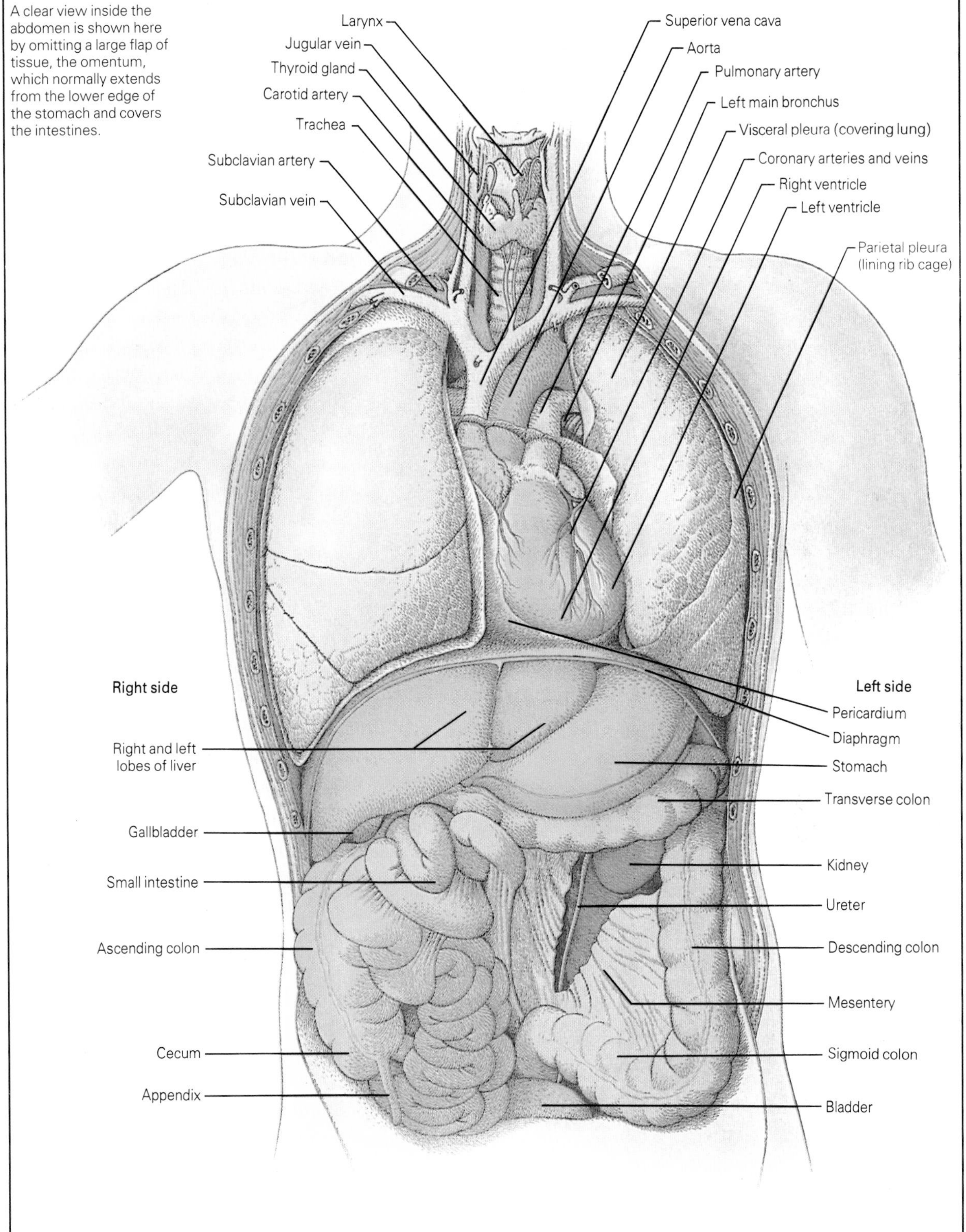

Larynx
Jugular vein
Thyroid gland
Carotid artery
Trachea
Subclavian artery
Subclavian vein
Superior vena cava
Aorta
Pulmonary artery
Left main bronchus
Visceral pleura (covering lung)
Coronary arteries and veins
Right ventricle
Left ventricle
Parietal pleura (lining rib cage)

Right side

Right and left lobes of liver
Gallbladder
Small intestine
Ascending colon
Cecum
Appendix

Left side

Pericardium
Diaphragm
Stomach
Transverse colon
Kidney
Ureter
Descending colon
Mesentery
Sigmoid colon
Bladder

Digestive organs

The digestive tract is basically one long tube extending from the mouth to the anus. Food passes from the mouth down the esophagus, a section of the tube about 10 in (25 cm) long, to the stomach, which holds about 2½ pints (1.5 liters) when nearly full. The section after the stomach is the duodenum, a C-shaped tube about the same length as the esophagus. Small ducts carry digestive juices from the liver and pancreas into the duodenum. The next section of the tract is about 16 ft (about 5 m) of coiled small intestine, followed by about 5 ft (about 1.5 m) of large intestine, which leads into the rectum and, finally, the anus.

The lengths of the various sections of digestive tract vary somewhat from person to person.

Digestive system

The digestive system is composed of the digestive tract—the tube from mouth to anus—plus two other organs, the liver and pancreas, which manufacture digestive fluids.

Tongue
Lip
Pharynx
Epiglottis
Esophagus
Stomach
Liver
Pancreas
Duodenum
Colon
Small intestine
Appendix
Rectum
Anus

Endoscopy

Today's endoscopes (long, flexible tubes that transmit visual images) can reach and view much of the digestive tract. Most regions of the tract are normally flattened and contain murky semi-liquids. So, to obtain a clear view, air is pumped down the endoscope into the tract to hold its wall apart during the examination. Below left is an endoscopic image of the stomach lining with its shiny, ridged surface. Below right is the lining of the duodenum. It has a smooth interior on which an abnormality—such as an ulcer—would be clearly visible (see also Endoscopy, p.264).

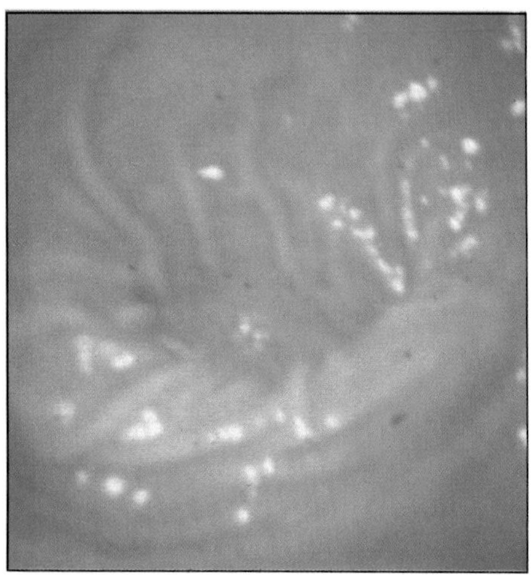

Endoscopic view of stomach

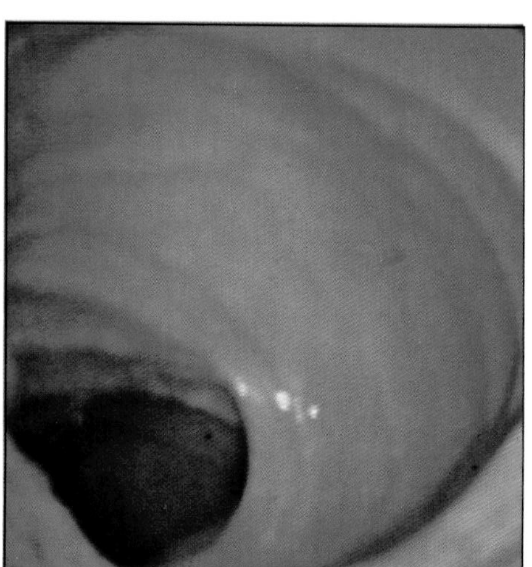

Endoscopic view of duodenum

Abdominal digestive organs

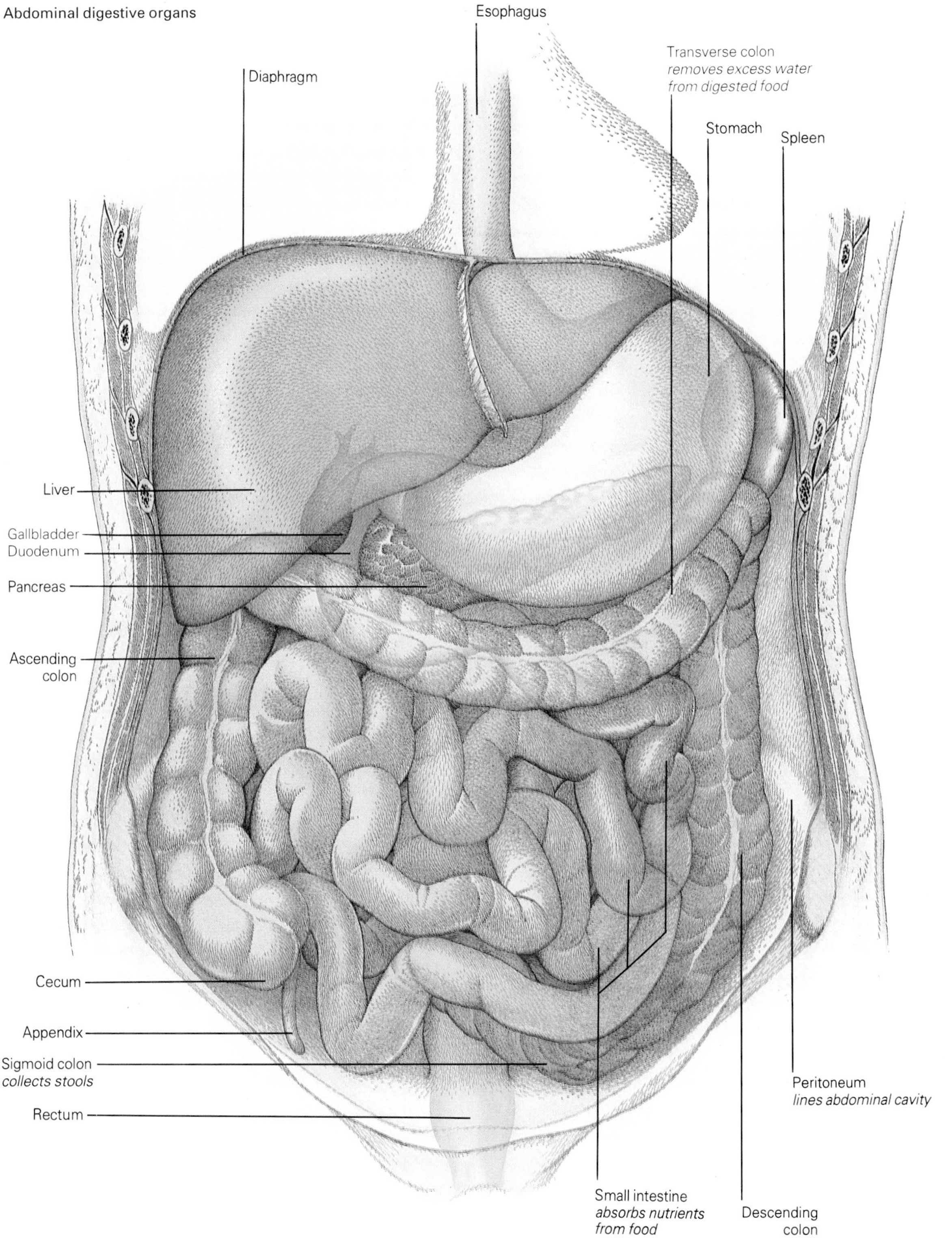

Esophagus

Diaphragm

Transverse colon
removes excess water from digested food

Stomach

Spleen

Liver

Gallbladder

Duodenum

Pancreas

Ascending colon

Cecum

Appendix

Sigmoid colon
collects stools

Rectum

Small intestine
absorbs nutrients from food

Descending colon
collects stools

Peritoneum
lines abdominal cavity

Organs of the lower abdomen

The lower abdominal organs are concerned principally with removal of wastes, in the form of urine and stools, and with reproduction (see below). The bladder, which stores urine from the kidneys, is a muscular sac about 3 in (75 mm) in diameter when full. The urine is passed to the outside via a tube called the urethra, which in a man is about 10 in (25 cm) long but in a woman about 1 in (25 mm) long. The lower abdominal organs are sometimes called the pelvic organs because they are situated within the cup-shaped hipbone, or pelvis.

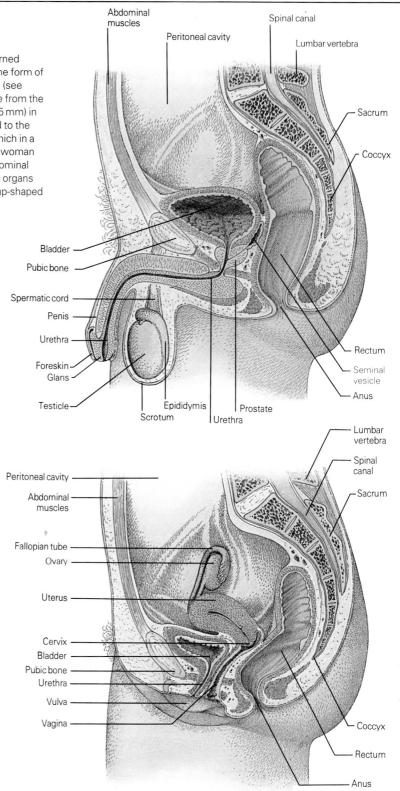

Abdominal muscles
Peritoneal cavity
Spinal canal
Lumbar vertebra
Sacrum
Coccyx
Bladder
Pubic bone
Spermatic cord
Penis
Urethra
Foreskin
Glans
Testicle
Scrotum
Epididymis
Urethra
Prostate
Rectum
Seminal vesicle
Anus

Male reproductive organs

In addition to the visible male genitalia—two testicles in their pouch (the scrotum) and the penis—there are glands and ducts inside the abdomen. These internal organs are the prostate gland, two seminal vesicles, and the two tubes that are called the vas deferens.

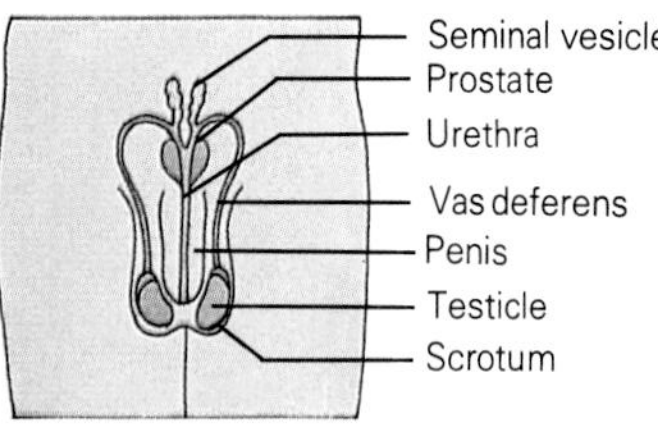

Lumbar vertebra
Spinal canal
Sacrum
Peritoneal cavity
Abdominal muscles
Fallopian tube
Ovary
Uterus
Cervix
Bladder
Pubic bone
Urethra
Vulva
Vagina
Coccyx
Rectum
Anus

Female reproductive organs

The female genitalia are located inside the abdomen, except for the vagina, which leads from the abdominal area to the external genitals, the vulva. Inside the abdomen are two ovaries connected by the two fallopian tubes to the uterus.

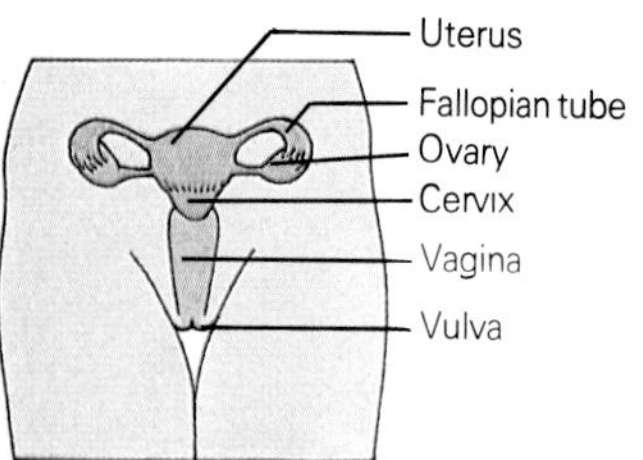

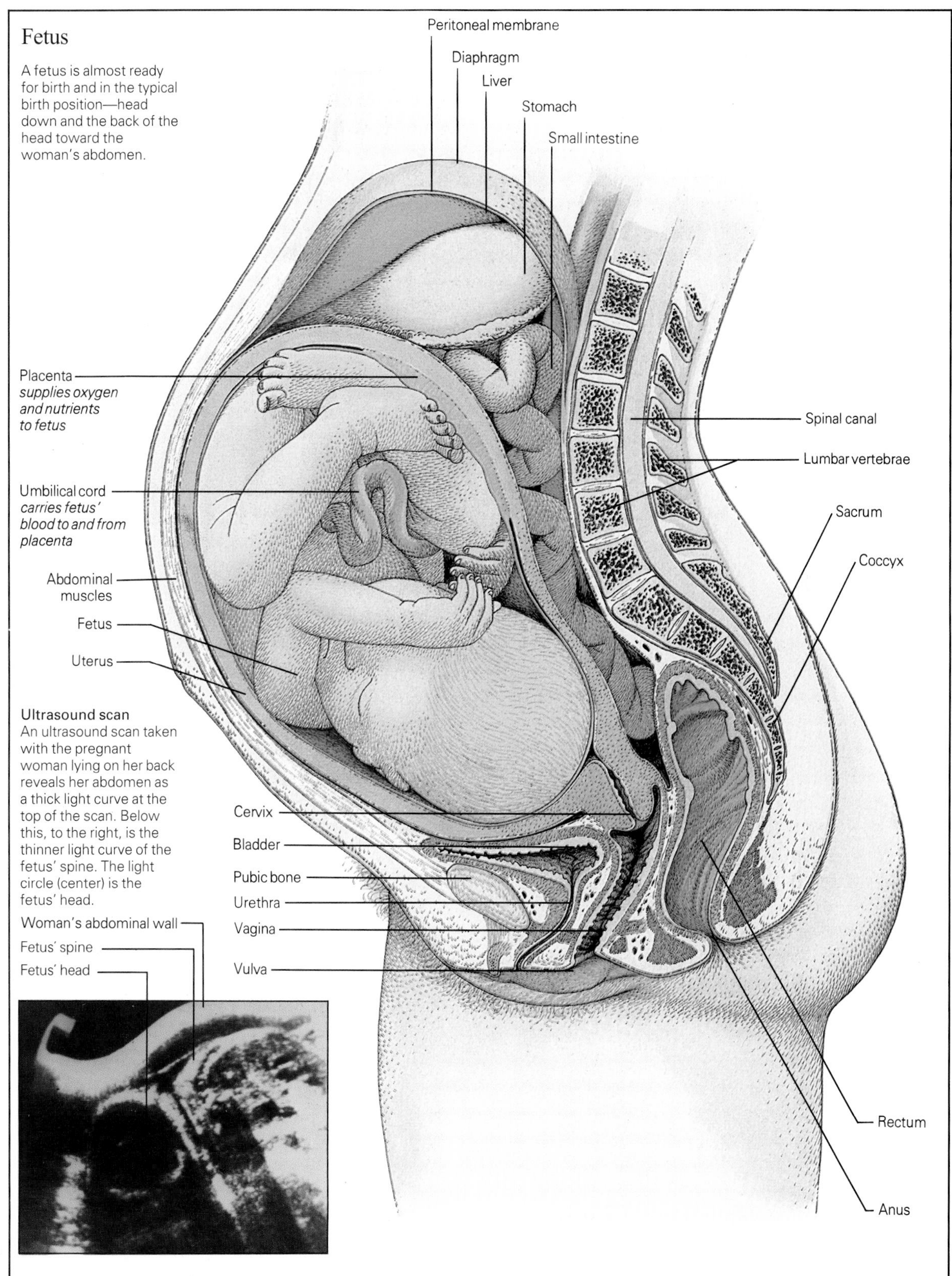
Fetus
A fetus is almost ready for birth and in the typical birth position—head down and the back of the head toward the woman's abdomen.
Peritoneal membrane
Diaphragm
Liver
Stomach
Small intestine
Placenta *supplies oxygen and nutrients to fetus*
Umbilical cord *carries fetus' blood to and from placenta*
Abdominal muscles
Fetus
Uterus
Spinal canal
Lumbar vertebrae
Sacrum
Coccyx
Cervix
Bladder
Pubic bone
Urethra
Vagina
Vulva
Rectum
Anus
Ultrasound scan
An ultrasound scan taken with the pregnant woman lying on her back reveals her abdomen as a thick light curve at the top of the scan. Below this, to the right, is the thinner light curve of the fetus' spine. The light circle (center) is the fetus' head.
Woman's abdominal wall
Fetus' spine
Fetus' head

Sense organs

Two senses that provide most information about the world around us are sight and hearing. Eyes and ears are delicate and sensitive structures of great complexity, but they lie well protected inside cavities in the skull bones. The eye is "directional" in that six separate muscles attached to the eyeball swivel it to look at objects in various locations, and this directional information is passed to the brain. The human ear does not have this ability, although many other animals are able to pinpoint the direction a sound comes from by moving the external ear, or pinna.

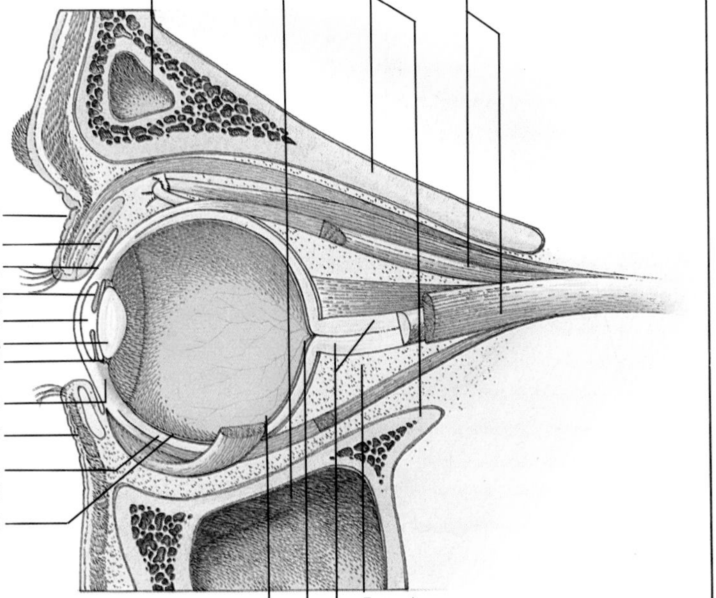

A close-up of the retina
As seen through an ophthalmoscope (viewing instrument), the pale disc is the optic disc, where all the nerves come together and leave the eye on their way to the brain. The blood vessels radiating from the disc are arteries that supply the retina and other structures in the eye with blood.

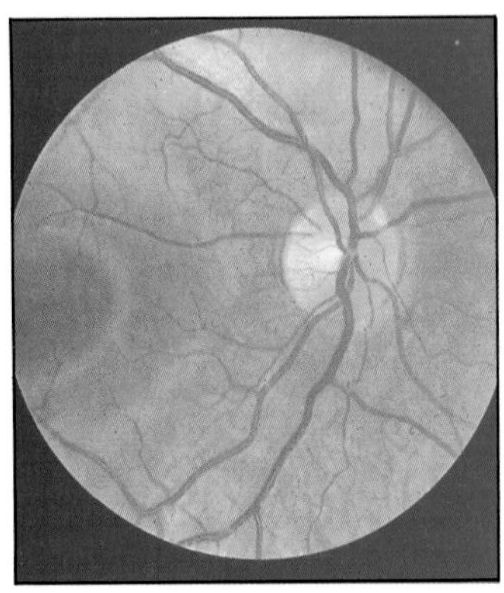

Eye

The eyeball is about 1 in (25 mm) in diameter. The socket for it in the skull bone is larger to allow room for the muscles that control eye movement.

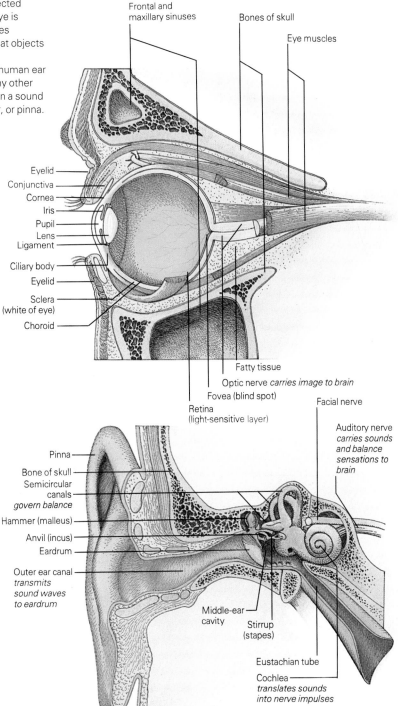

Frontal and maxillary sinuses
Bones of skull
Eye muscles
Eyelid
Conjunctiva
Cornea
Iris
Pupil
Lens
Ligament
Ciliary body
Eyelid
Sclera (white of eye)
Choroid
Fatty tissue
Optic nerve *carries image to brain*
Fovea (blind spot)
Retina (light-sensitive layer)

Ear

The outer ear canal, which is about ¾ in (2 cm) long, leads through the skull bone to the middle and inner ear. Connecting the middle ear to the back of the throat is another tube about 1½ in (about 4 cm) long, the eustachian tube. Besides enabling you to hear, the ear contains the semicircular canals, which help you keep your balance.

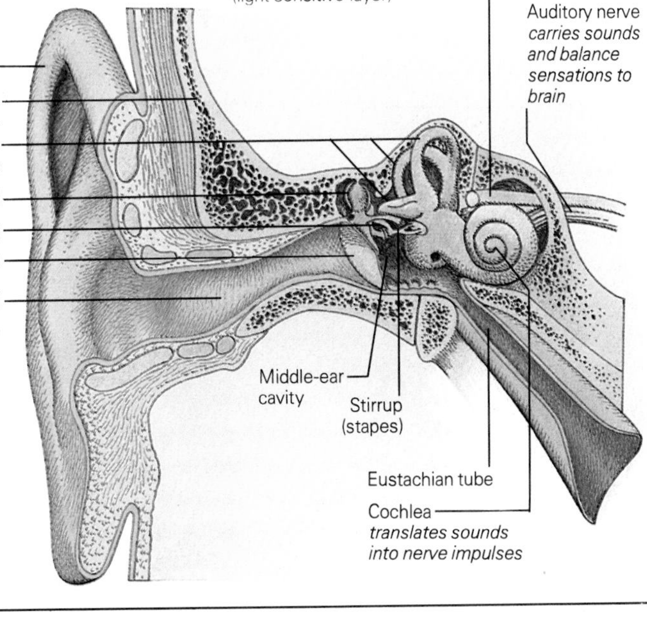

Facial nerve
Auditory nerve *carries sounds and balance sensations to brain*
Pinna
Bone of skull
Semicircular canals *govern balance*
Hammer (malleus)
Anvil (incus)
Eardrum
Outer ear canal *transmits sound waves to eardrum*
Middle-ear cavity
Stirrup (stapes)
Eustachian tube
Cochlea *translates sounds into nerve impulses*

PART TWO

Symptoms and self-diagnosis

Self-diagnosis symptom charts

How to use the charts

Each of the self-diagnosis charts in this section is designed to help you track down the possible significance of a particular symptom, either on its own or combined with other symptoms. Every chart has a common symptom as its starting point, and then you are led by a series of questions and answers to a logical conclusion. The end point you reach will probably refer you to other charts or articles in this book and may also tell you to seek professional help. First find the chart you want by consulting the Chart-finder index (see p.76), which gives you the appropriate chart number. Then, turn to the chart itself, and check whether it is relevant by noting the definition.

As shown on the two samples on these pages, each chart consists of a series of simple YES or NO questions. Begin at the first question, and follow through to the diagnosis that fits your case. Here you will usually find one—or

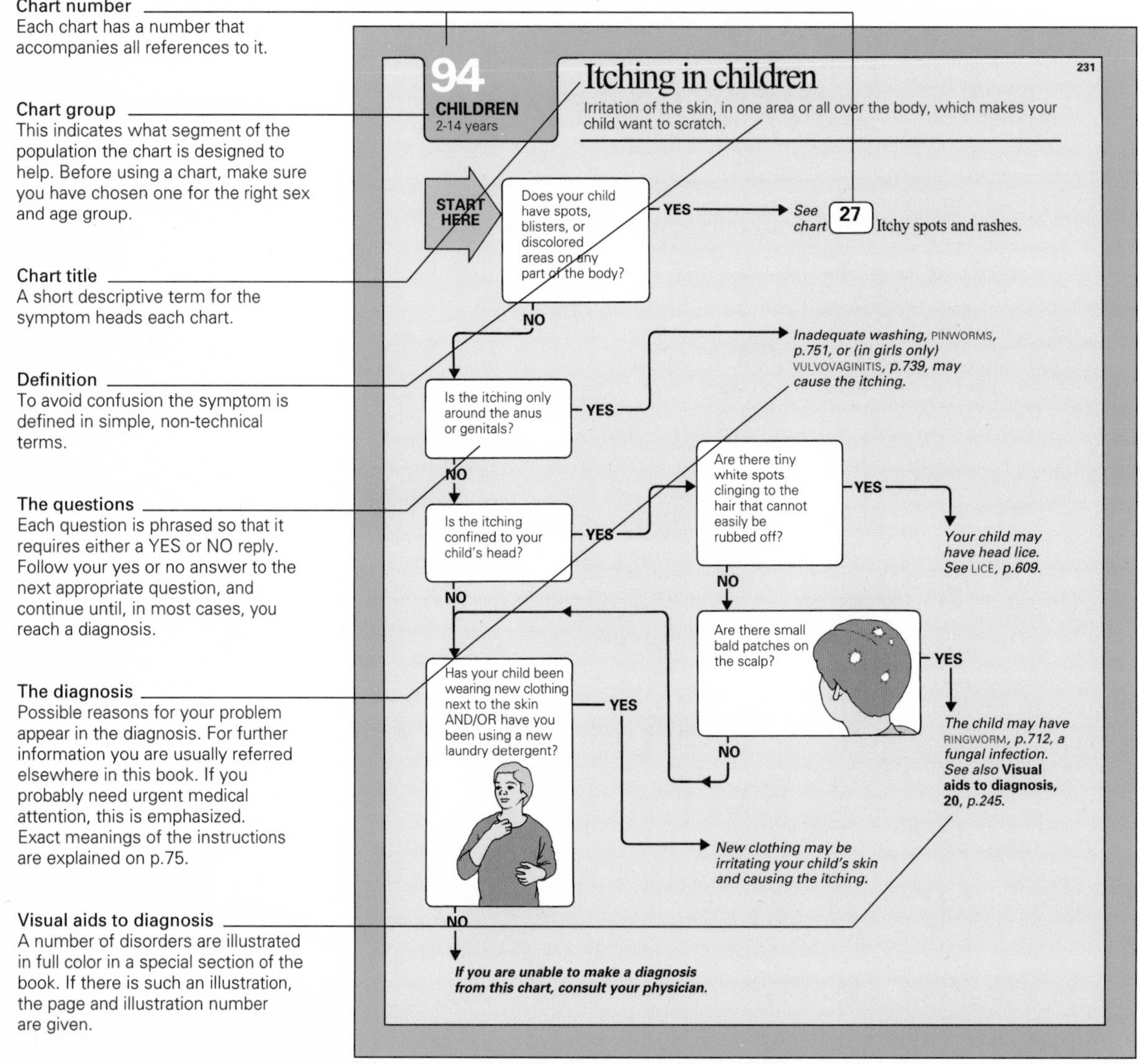

Chart number
Each chart has a number that accompanies all references to it.
Chart group
This indicates what segment of the population the chart is designed to help. Before using a chart, make sure you have chosen one for the right sex and age group.
Chart title
A short descriptive term for the symptom heads each chart.
Definition
To avoid confusion the symptom is defined in simple, non-technical terms.
The questions
Each question is phrased so that it requires either a YES or NO reply. Follow your yes or no answer to the next appropriate question, and continue until, in most cases, you reach a diagnosis.
The diagnosis
Possible reasons for your problem appear in the diagnosis. For further information you are usually referred elsewhere in this book. If you probably need urgent medical attention, this is emphasized. Exact meanings of the instructions are explained on p.75.
Visual aids to diagnosis
A number of disorders are illustrated in full color in a special section of the book. If there is such an illustration, the page and illustration number are given.
94
CHILDREN
2-14 years
Itching in children
231
Irritation of the skin, in one area or all over the body, which makes your child want to scratch.
START HERE
Does your child have spots, blisters, or discolored areas on any part of the body?
YES
See chart 27 Itchy spots and rashes.
NO
Is the itching only around the anus or genitals?
YES
Inadequate washing, PINWORMS, p.751, or (in girls only) VULVOVAGINITIS, p.739, may cause the itching.
NO
Is the itching confined to your child's head?
YES
Are there tiny white spots clinging to the hair that cannot easily be rubbed off?
YES
Your child may have head lice. See LICE, p.609.
NO
Are there small bald patches on the scalp?
YES
The child may have RINGWORM, p.712, a fungal infection. See also Visual aids to diagnosis, 20, p.245.
NO
NO
Has your child been wearing new clothing next to the skin AND/OR have you been using a new laundry detergent?
YES
New clothing may be irritating your child's skin and causing the itching.
NO
If you are unable to make a diagnosis from this chart, consult your physician.

sometimes more than one—likely explanation of your problem, along with instructions on what steps to take. Except in emergency cases, be sure to follow through on all cross-references to get as much information as possible. Important: Remember that the charts help you arrive at a tentative diagnosis. For diagnosis and treatment, consult your physician.

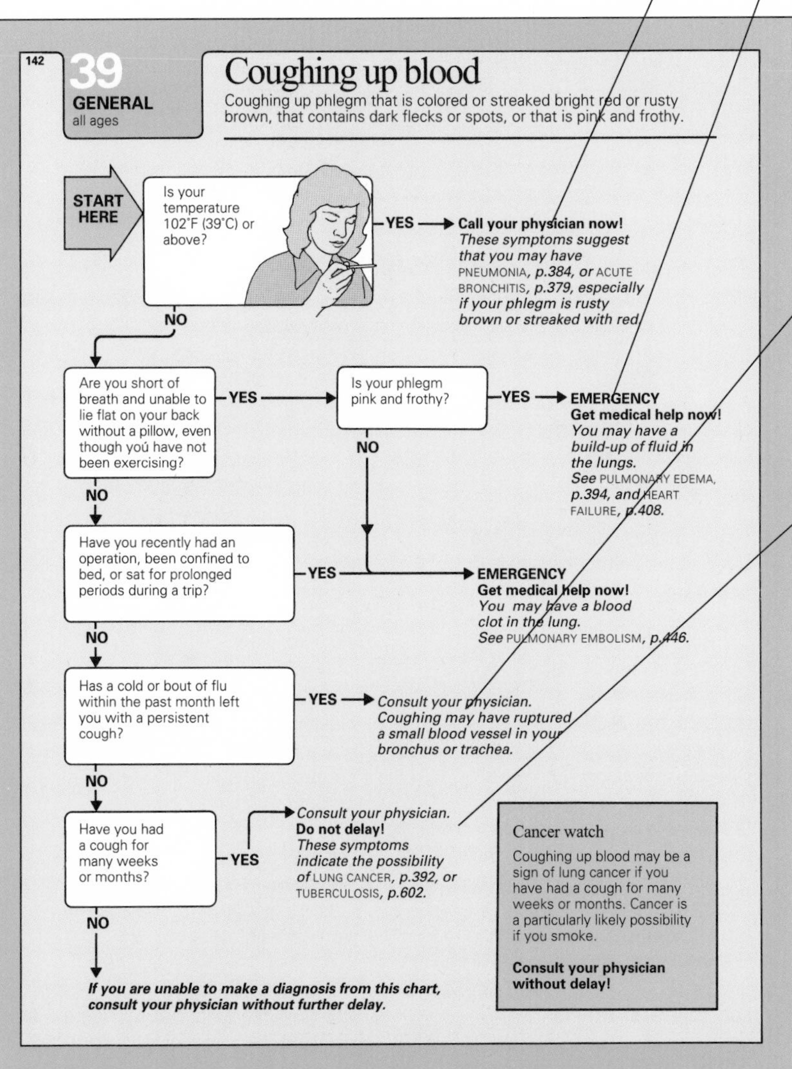

142
39
GENERAL
all ages
Coughing up blood
Coughing up phlegm that is colored or streaked bright red or rusty brown, that contains dark flecks or spots, or that is pink and frothy.
START HERE
Is your temperature 102°F (39°C) or above?
YES
Call your physician now!
These symptoms suggest that you may have PNEUMONIA, p.384, or ACUTE BRONCHITIS, p.379, especially if your phlegm is rusty brown or streaked with red.
NO
Are you short of breath and unable to lie flat on your back without a pillow, even though you have not been exercising?
YES
Is your phlegm pink and frothy?
YES
EMERGENCY
Get medical help now!
You may have a build-up of fluid in the lungs.
See PULMONARY EDEMA, p.394, and HEART FAILURE, p.408.
NO
NO
Have you recently had an operation, been confined to bed, or sat for prolonged periods during a trip?
YES
EMERGENCY
Get medical help now!
You may have a blood clot in the lung.
See PULMONARY EMBOLISM, p.446.
NO
Has a cold or bout of flu within the past month left you with a persistent cough?
YES
Consult your physician.
Coughing may have ruptured a small blood vessel in your bronchus or trachea.
NO
Have you had a cough for many weeks or months?
YES
Consult your physician.
Do not delay!
These symptoms indicate the possibility of LUNG CANCER, p.392, or TUBERCULOSIS, p.602.
NO
If you are unable to make a diagnosis from this chart, consult your physician without further delay.
Cancer watch
Coughing up blood may be a sign of lung cancer if you have had a cough for many weeks or months. Cancer is a particularly likely possibility if you smoke.
Consult your physician without delay!

What the instructions mean

Call your physician now!

Seek medical advice within a few hours at the most. Telephone your physician immediately. If your physician is not available, telephone or go to the nearest hospital emergency room.

EMERGENCY
Get medical help now!

The problem may be life-threatening and needs immediate attention. If you cannot reach your own physician within minutes, call for an ambulance, or take the person to the nearest hospital emergency room if he or she can be moved safely.

Consult your physician.

If your problem is not identified as one requiring immediate attention, you can assume that an urgent consultation is not vital. Turn to the page(s) indicated for further information.

Consult your physician.
Do not delay!

Get medical advice within a day or two. Ask your doctor's receptionist for an appointment or discuss the problem with your physician by telephone.

Boxed information

Some charts contain boxes with important additional information such as self-help advice or, more often, warnings about possibly dangerous symptoms. Generally when there is a possibility of cancer the box is headed Cancer watch.

How to find the chart you need

The Chart-finder index (below) directs you to the number of the chart (rather than a page number) that deals with your problem. To find the chart you want, follow these steps:

1 Single out your major problem. If you have two or more symptoms (such as a high fever, a cough, and a runny nose), select the one that bothers you the most.

2 Find the symptom in the chart-finder index. For your convenience the charts are indexed according to a wide variety of key words. Irregular vaginal bleeding, for instance, is listed in three places, under B, I, and V.

3 If you cannot find your main symptom in the chart-finder index, look for a chart dealing with any additional symptom (if you have one).

4 When you have found the correct chart, turn to the chart number (not the page number) indicated and proceed to answer the questions. For a full explanation of how to use the charts, see p.74.

Chart-finder index

1
GENERAL
all ages

Feeling under the weather

A vague, generalized sense of not being well.

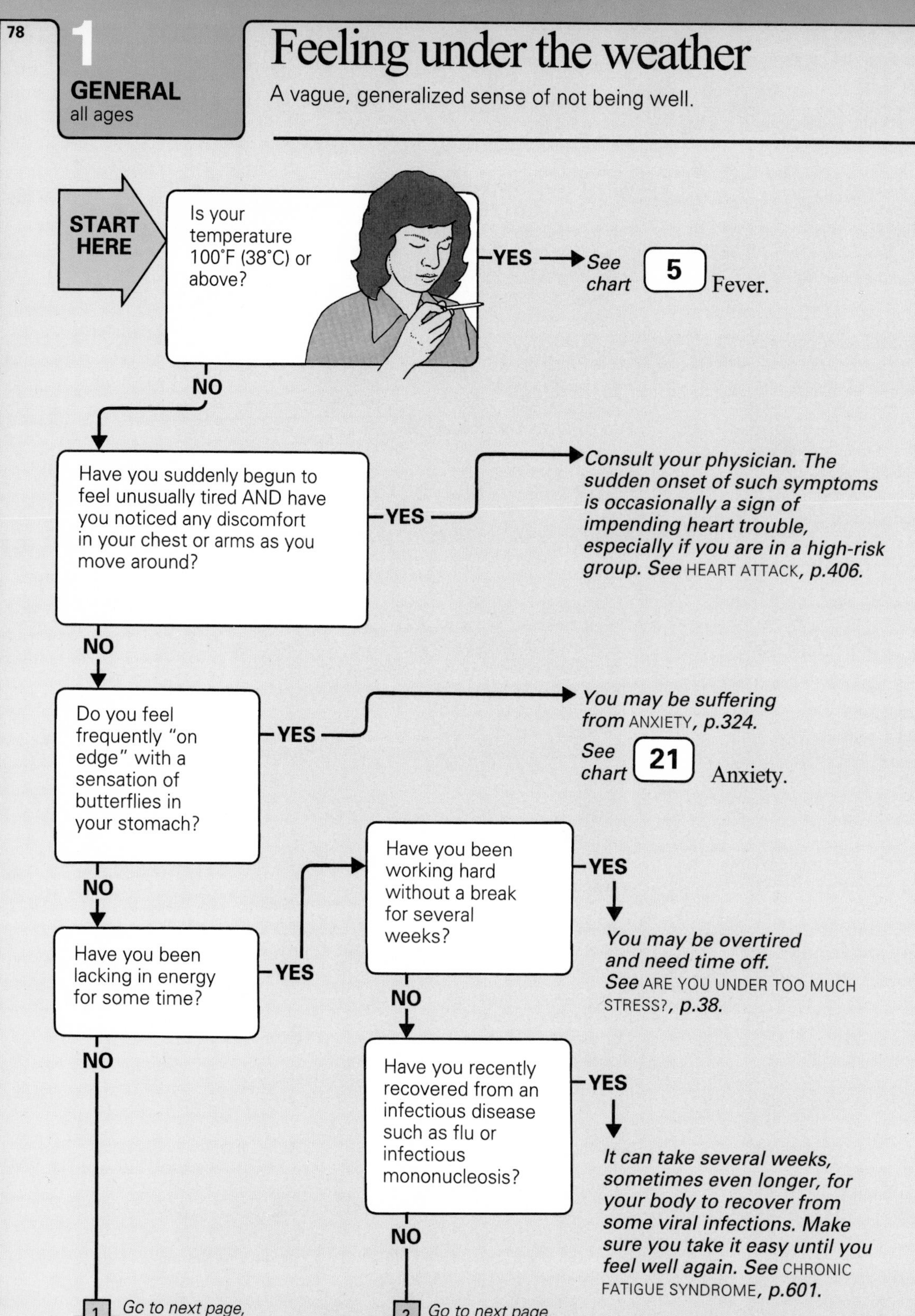

START HERE
Is your temperature 100°F (38°C) or above?
YES → See chart 5 Fever.
NO
Have you suddenly begun to feel unusually tired AND have you noticed any discomfort in your chest or arms as you move around?
YES → Consult your physician. The sudden onset of such symptoms is occasionally a sign of impending heart trouble, especially if you are in a high-risk group. See HEART ATTACK, p.406.
NO
Do you feel frequently "on edge" with a sensation of butterflies in your stomach?
YES → You may be suffering from ANXIETY, p.324.
See chart 21 Anxiety.
NO
Have you been lacking in energy for some time?
YES
Have you been working hard without a break for several weeks?
YES
You may be overtired and need time off.
See ARE YOU UNDER TOO MUCH STRESS?, p.38.
NO
Have you recently recovered from an infectious disease such as flu or infectious mononucleosis?
YES
It can take several weeks, sometimes even longer, for your body to recover from some viral infections. Make sure you take it easy until you feel well again. See CHRONIC FATIGUE SYNDROME, p.601.
NO
2 Go to next page, second column
NO
1 Go to next page, first column

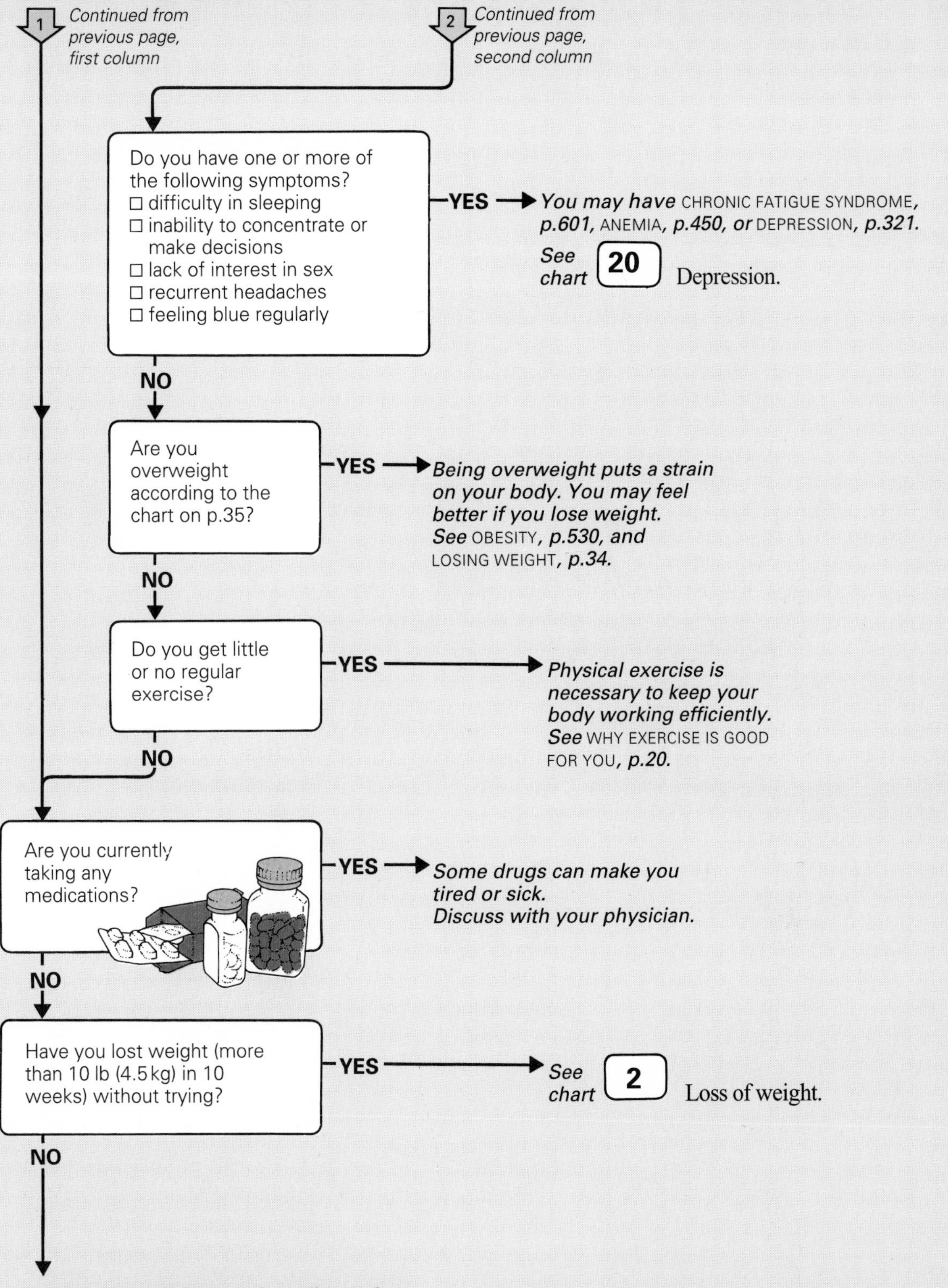

1
Continued from previous page, first column
2
Continued from previous page, second column
Do you have one or more of the following symptoms?
☐ difficulty in sleeping
☐ inability to concentrate or make decisions
☐ lack of interest in sex
☐ recurrent headaches
☐ feeling blue regularly
YES
You may have CHRONIC FATIGUE SYNDROME, p.601, ANEMIA, p.450, or DEPRESSION, p.321.
See chart 20 Depression.
NO
Are you overweight according to the chart on p.35?
YES
Being overweight puts a strain on your body. You may feel better if you lose weight. See OBESITY, p.530, and LOSING WEIGHT, p.34.
NO
Do you get little or no regular exercise?
YES
Physical exercise is necessary to keep your body working efficiently. See WHY EXERCISE IS GOOD FOR YOU, p.20.
NO
Are you currently taking any medications?
YES
Some drugs can make you tired or sick. Discuss with your physician.
NO
Have you lost weight (more than 10 lb (4.5 kg) in 10 weeks) without trying?
YES
See chart 2 Loss of weight.
NO
If you are unable to make a diagnosis from this chart, consult your physician.

Loss of weight

Loss of 10 lb (4.5 kg) or more over a period of 10 weeks or less, without a deliberate change in eating habits.

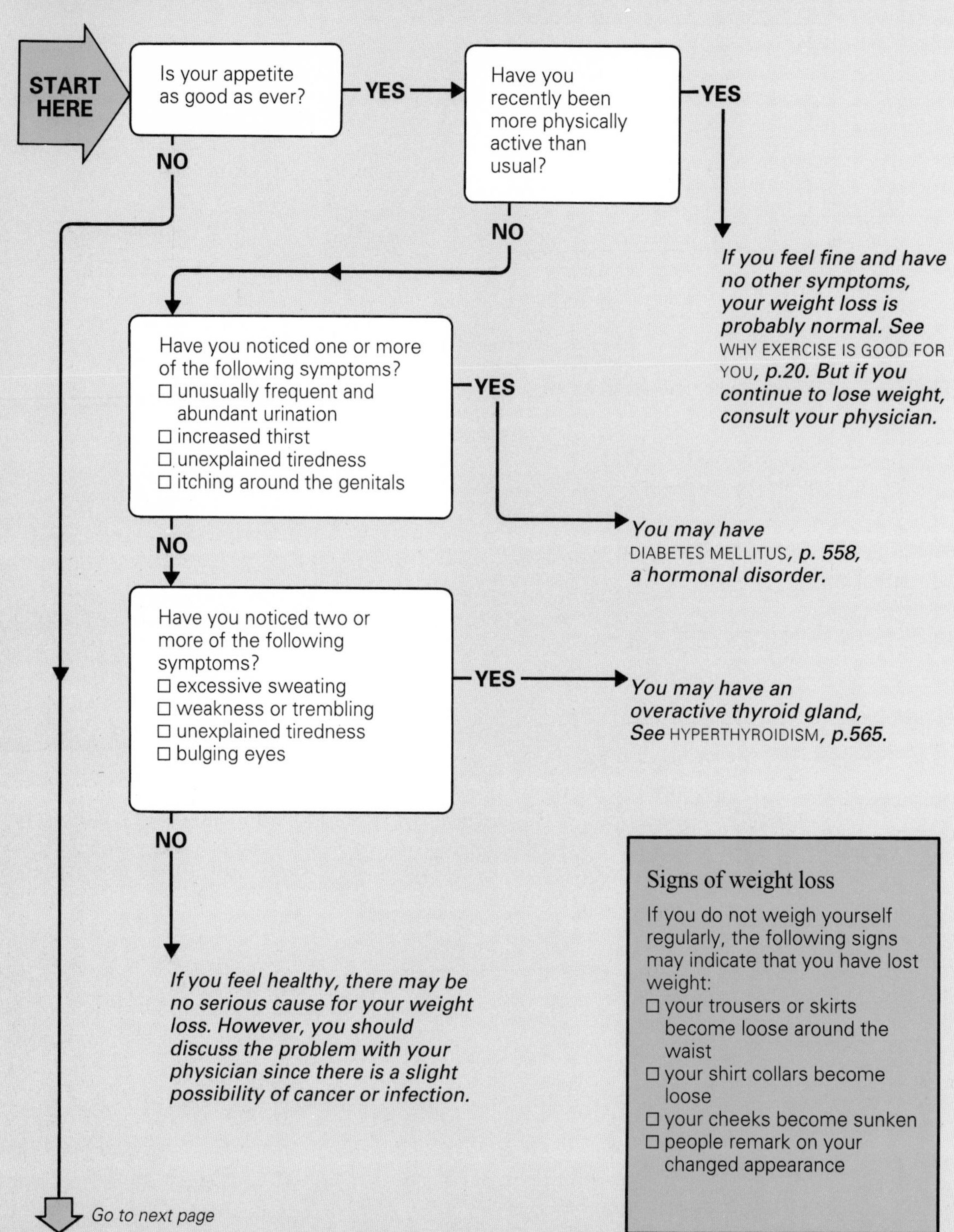

START HERE
Is your appetite as good as ever?
YES
NO
Have you recently been more physically active than usual?
YES
NO
If you feel fine and have no other symptoms, your weight loss is probably normal. See WHY EXERCISE IS GOOD FOR YOU, p.20. But if you continue to lose weight, consult your physician.
Have you noticed one or more of the following symptoms?
☐ unusually frequent and abundant urination
☐ increased thirst
☐ unexplained tiredness
☐ itching around the genitals
YES
You may have DIABETES MELLITUS, p. 558, a hormonal disorder.
NO
Have you noticed two or more of the following symptoms?
☐ excessive sweating
☐ weakness or trembling
☐ unexplained tiredness
☐ bulging eyes
YES
You may have an overactive thyroid gland, See HYPERTHYROIDISM, p.565.
NO
If you feel healthy, there may be no serious cause for your weight loss. However, you should discuss the problem with your physician since there is a slight possibility of cancer or infection.
Signs of weight loss
If you do not weigh yourself regularly, the following signs may indicate that you have lost weight:
☐ your trousers or skirts become loose around the waist
☐ your shirt collars become loose
☐ your cheeks become sunken
☐ people remark on your changed appearance
Go to next page

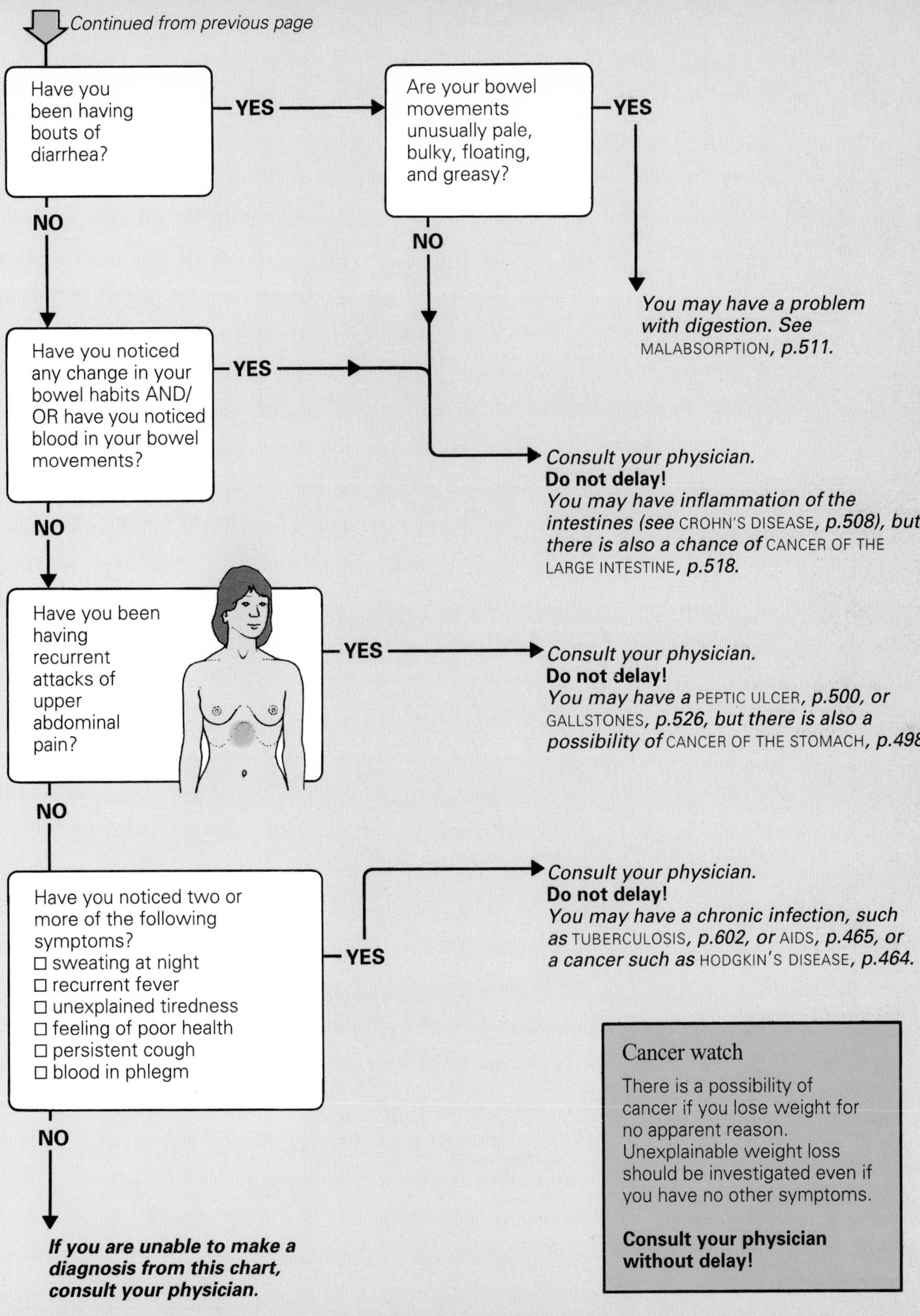

Continued from previous page
Have you been having bouts of diarrhea?
YES
Are your bowel movements unusually pale, bulky, floating, and greasy?
YES
You may have a problem with digestion. See MALABSORPTION, *p.511.*
NO
NO
Have you noticed any change in your bowel habits AND/OR have you noticed blood in your bowel movements?
YES
Consult your physician.
Do not delay!
You may have inflammation of the intestines (see CROHN'S DISEASE, *p.508), but there is also a chance of* CANCER OF THE LARGE INTESTINE, *p.518.*
NO
Have you been having recurrent attacks of upper abdominal pain?
YES
Consult your physician.
Do not delay!
You may have a PEPTIC ULCER, *p.500, or* GALLSTONES, *p.526, but there is also a possibility of* CANCER OF THE STOMACH, *p.498.*
NO
Have you noticed two or more of the following symptoms?
☐ sweating at night
☐ recurrent fever
☐ unexplained tiredness
☐ feeling of poor health
☐ persistent cough
☐ blood in phlegm
YES
Consult your physician.
Do not delay!
You may have a chronic infection, such as TUBERCULOSIS, *p.602, or* AIDS, *p.465, or a cancer such as* HODGKIN'S DISEASE, *p.464.*
NO
If you are unable to make a diagnosis from this chart, consult your physician.
Cancer watch
There is a possibility of cancer if you lose weight for no apparent reason. Unexplainable weight loss should be investigated even if you have no other symptoms.
Consult your physician without delay!

3

GENERAL
all ages

Overweight

If you weigh more than the optimum weight for your height (see p.35), you are overweight and may be endangering your health.

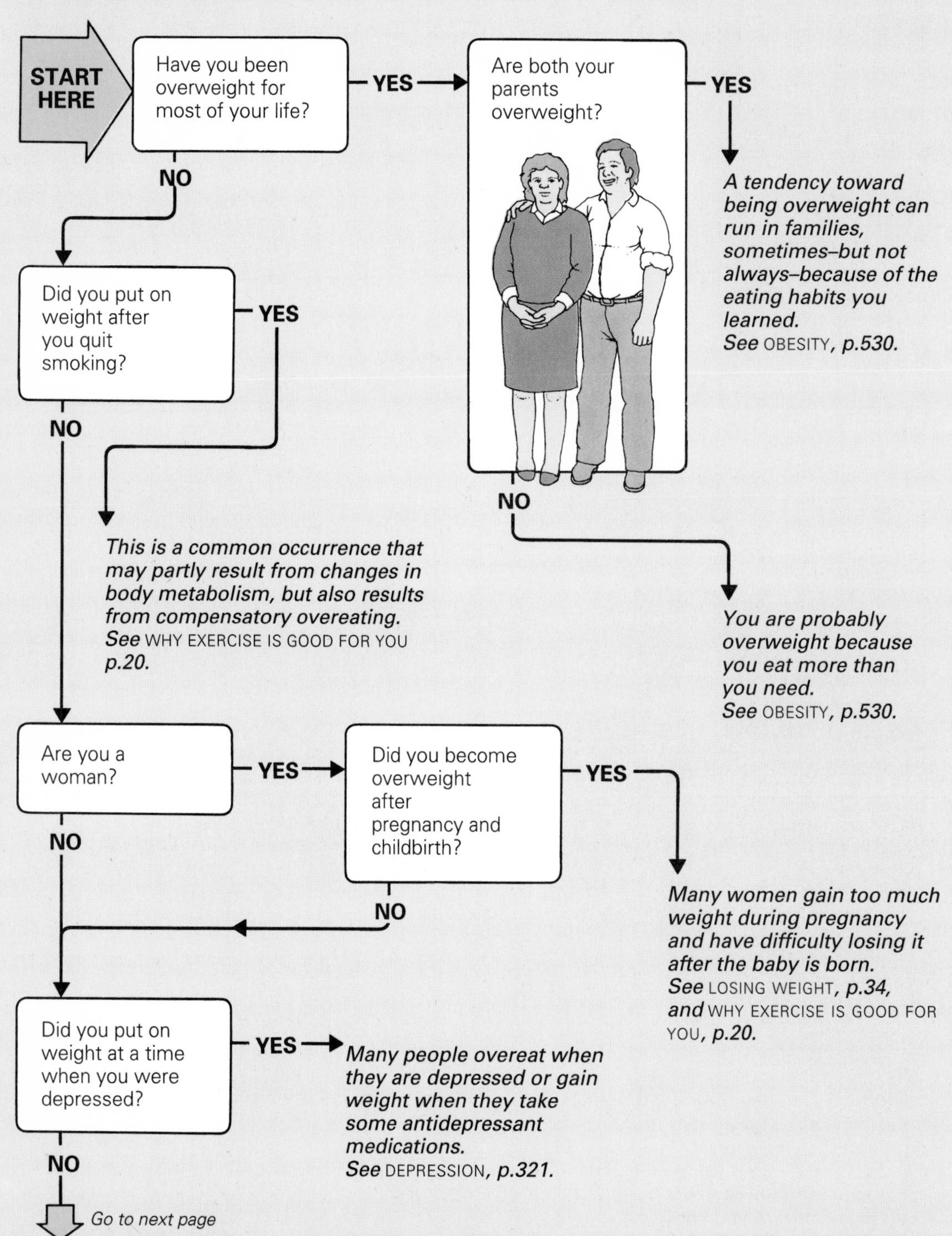

START HERE
Have you been overweight for most of your life?
YES
Are both your parents overweight?
YES
A tendency toward being overweight can run in families, sometimes–but not always–because of the eating habits you learned.
See OBESITY, *p.530.*
NO
You are probably overweight because you eat more than you need.
See OBESITY, *p.530.*
NO
Did you put on weight after you quit smoking?
YES
This is a common occurrence that may partly result from changes in body metabolism, but also results from compensatory overeating.
See WHY EXERCISE IS GOOD FOR YOU *p.20.*
NO
Are you a woman?
YES
Did you become overweight after pregnancy and childbirth?
YES
Many women gain too much weight during pregnancy and have difficulty losing it after the baby is born.
See LOSING WEIGHT, *p.34, and* WHY EXERCISE IS GOOD FOR YOU, *p.20.*
NO
NO
Did you put on weight at a time when you were depressed?
YES
Many people overeat when they are depressed or gain weight when they take some antidepressant medications.
See DEPRESSION, *p.321.*
NO
Go to next page

Continued from previous page

Did the weight gain follow a change from a physically strenuous job to sedentary work?

YES → *In your former job you probably used more calories than you do now. You should therefore eat less and exercise more after work. See* COUNTING CALORIES, *p.31, and* WHY EXERCISE IS GOOD FOR YOU, *p.20.*

NO ↓

Have you noticed any of the following symptoms since you began to put on weight?
- ☐ feeling cold more than you used to
- ☐ thinning or brittle hair
- ☐ dry skin

YES → *You may have an underactive thyroid gland See* HYPOTHYROIDISM, *p.567.*

NO ↓

Have you been taking corticosteroid drugs for a problem such as asthma or rheumatoid arthritis?

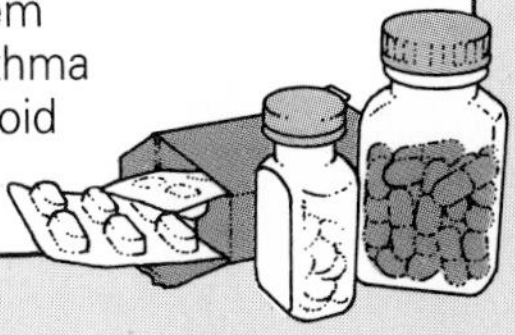

YES → *Such drugs can cause weight gain. Discuss with your physician.*

NO ↓

Are you over 40?

YES → *Weight gain as you grow older may be a result of such factors as a decline in the amount of exercise you get and changes in the rate that your body burns up food.*

NO ↓

If you are unable to make a diagnosis from this chart, your excess weight probably results from overeating and lack of exercise. Follow a balanced weight-loss diet for a month and get more exercise. If you fail to lose weight, consult your physician.

Losing weight

Whatever the cause of your weight gain, follow a balanced diet like the one described on p.31 and exercise. See also WHY EXERCISE IS GOOD FOR YOU, p.20.

4 GENERAL all ages

Difficulty sleeping

Frequent problems in either falling asleep or staying asleep during the night (often called insomnia).

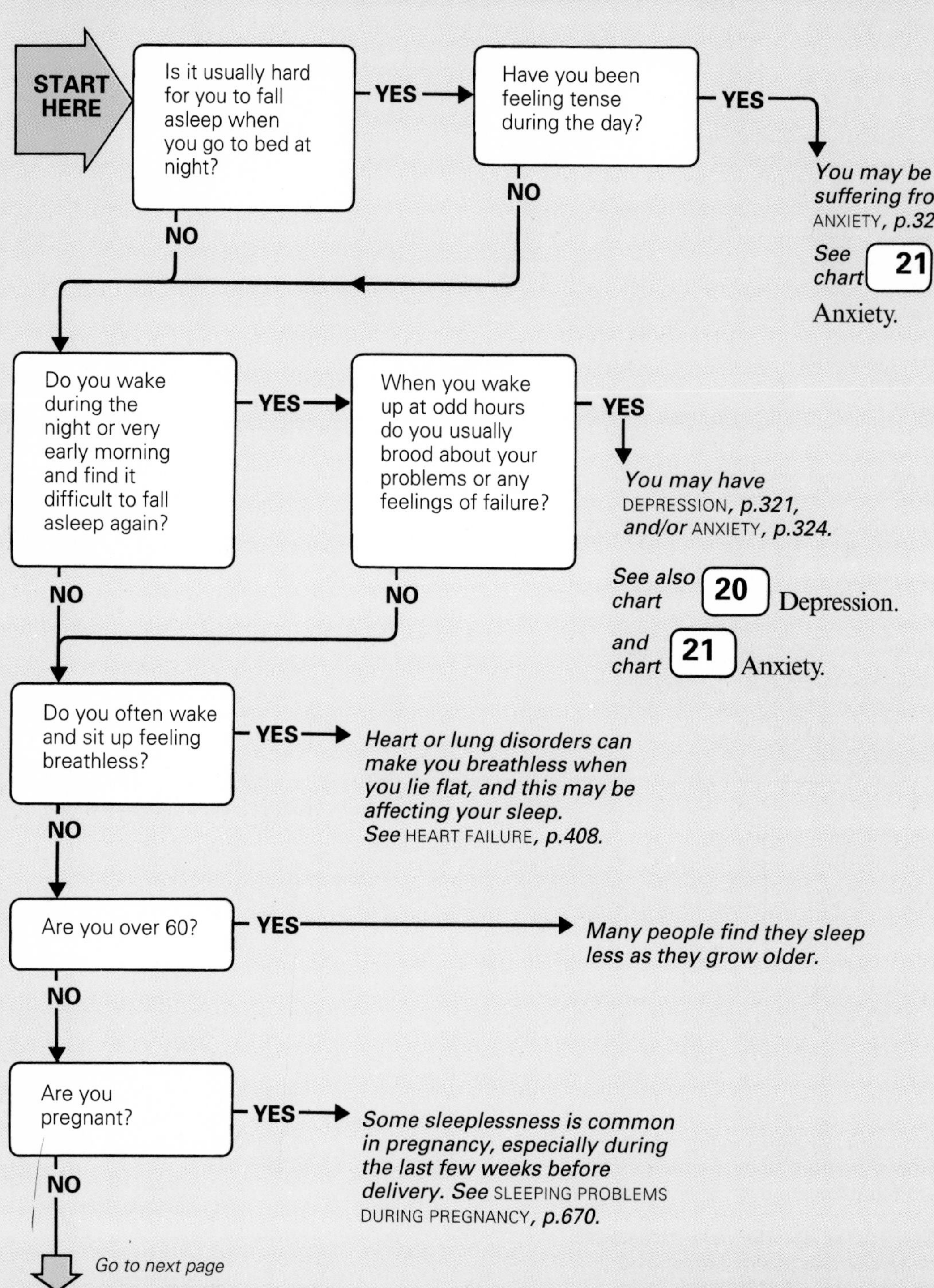
START HERE
Is it usually hard for you to fall asleep when you go to bed at night?
YES
NO
Have you been feeling tense during the day?
YES
NO
You may be suffering from ANXIETY, p.324.
See chart 21 Anxiety.
Do you wake during the night or very early morning and find it difficult to fall asleep again?
YES
NO
When you wake up at odd hours do you usually brood about your problems or any feelings of failure?
YES
NO
You may have DEPRESSION, p.321, and/or ANXIETY, p.324.
See also chart 20 Depression.
and chart 21 Anxiety.
Do you often wake and sit up feeling breathless?
YES
NO
Heart or lung disorders can make you breathless when you lie flat, and this may be affecting your sleep. See HEART FAILURE, p.408.
Are you over 60?
YES
NO
Many people find they sleep less as they grow older.
Are you pregnant?
YES
NO
Some sleeplessness is common in pregnancy, especially during the last few weeks before delivery. See SLEEPING PROBLEMS DURING PREGNANCY, p.670.
Go to next page

Continued from previous page

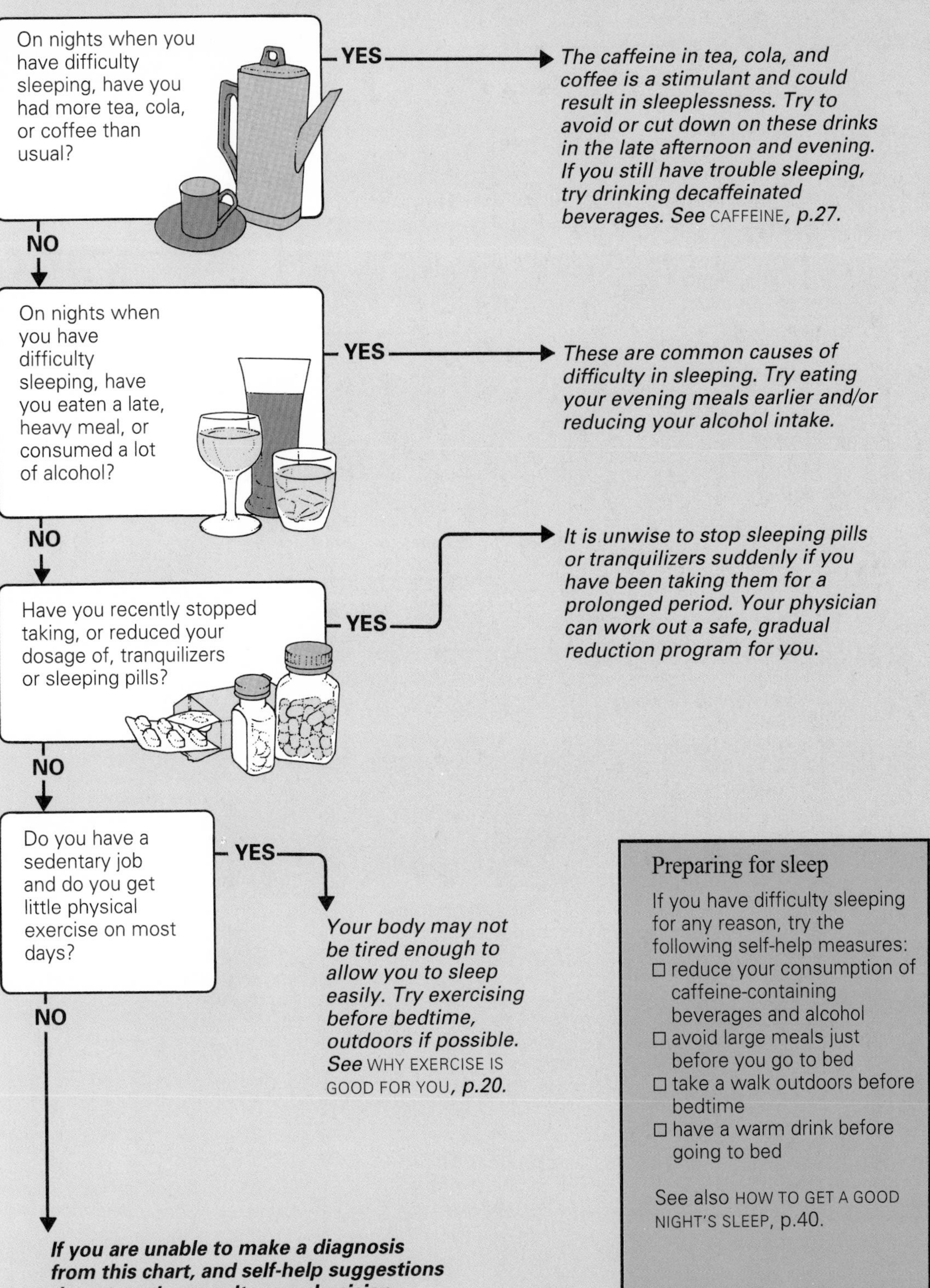

On nights when you have difficulty sleeping, have you had more tea, cola, or coffee than usual?

YES → *The caffeine in tea, cola, and coffee is a stimulant and could result in sleeplessness. Try to avoid or cut down on these drinks in the late afternoon and evening. If you still have trouble sleeping, try drinking decaffeinated beverages. See* CAFFEINE, *p.27.*

NO ↓

On nights when you have difficulty sleeping, have you eaten a late, heavy meal, or consumed a lot of alcohol?

YES → *These are common causes of difficulty in sleeping. Try eating your evening meals earlier and/or reducing your alcohol intake.*

NO ↓

Have you recently stopped taking, or reduced your dosage of, tranquilizers or sleeping pills?

YES → *It is unwise to stop sleeping pills or tranquilizers suddenly if you have been taking them for a prolonged period. Your physician can work out a safe, gradual reduction program for you.*

NO ↓

Do you have a sedentary job and do you get little physical exercise on most days?

YES → ***Your body may not be tired enough to allow you to sleep easily. Try exercising before bedtime, outdoors if possible. See*** WHY EXERCISE IS GOOD FOR YOU, ***p.20.***

NO ↓

If you are unable to make a diagnosis from this chart, and self-help suggestions do not work, consult your physician.

Preparing for sleep

If you have difficulty sleeping for any reason, try the following self-help measures:

- ☐ reduce your consumption of caffeine-containing beverages and alcohol
- ☐ avoid large meals just before you go to bed
- ☐ take a walk outdoors before bedtime
- ☐ have a warm drink before going to bed

See also HOW TO GET A GOOD NIGHT'S SLEEP, p.40.

5 GENERAL over 14 years

Fever

Temperature of about 100°F (38°C) or above. For children see chart 91, **Fever in infants**, or chart 92, **Fever in children.**

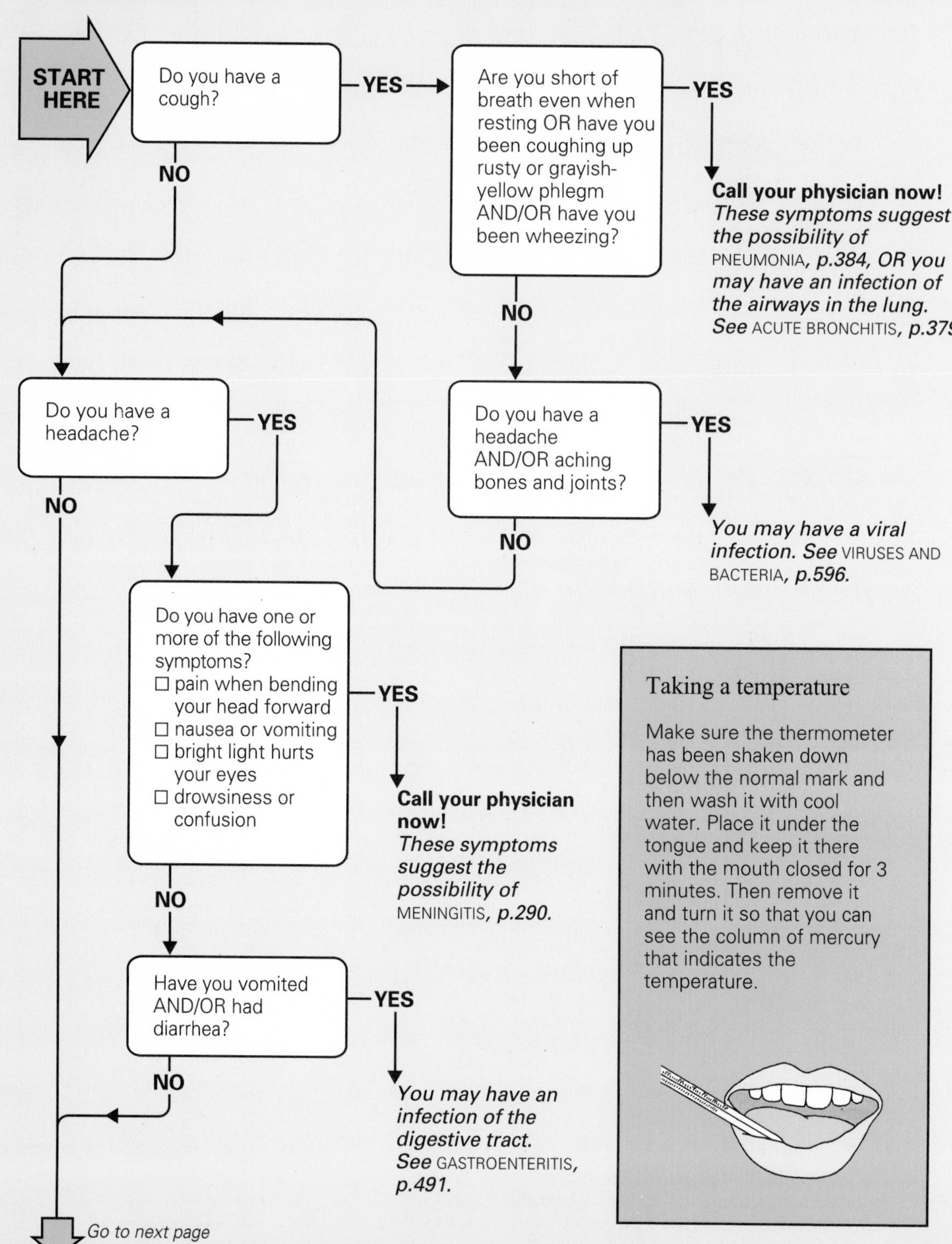

START HERE
Do you have a cough?
YES
Are you short of breath even when resting OR have you been coughing up rusty or grayish-yellow phlegm AND/OR have you been wheezing?
YES
Call your physician now!
These symptoms suggest the possibility of PNEUMONIA*, p.384, OR you may have an infection of the airways in the lung. See* ACUTE BRONCHITIS*, p.379.*
NO
Do you have a headache AND/OR aching bones and joints?
YES
You may have a viral infection. See VIRUSES AND BACTERIA*, p.596.*
NO
NO
Do you have a headache?
YES
Do you have one or more of the following symptoms?
☐ pain when bending your head forward
☐ nausea or vomiting
☐ bright light hurts your eyes
☐ drowsiness or confusion
YES
Call your physician now!
These symptoms suggest the possibility of MENINGITIS*, p.290.*
NO
Have you vomited AND/OR had diarrhea?
YES
You may have an infection of the digestive tract. See GASTROENTERITIS*, p.491.*
NO
NO
Go to next page
Taking a temperature
Make sure the thermometer has been shaken down below the normal mark and then wash it with cool water. Place it under the tongue and keep it there with the mouth closed for 3 minutes. Then remove it and turn it so that you can see the column of mercury that indicates the temperature.

Continued from previous page

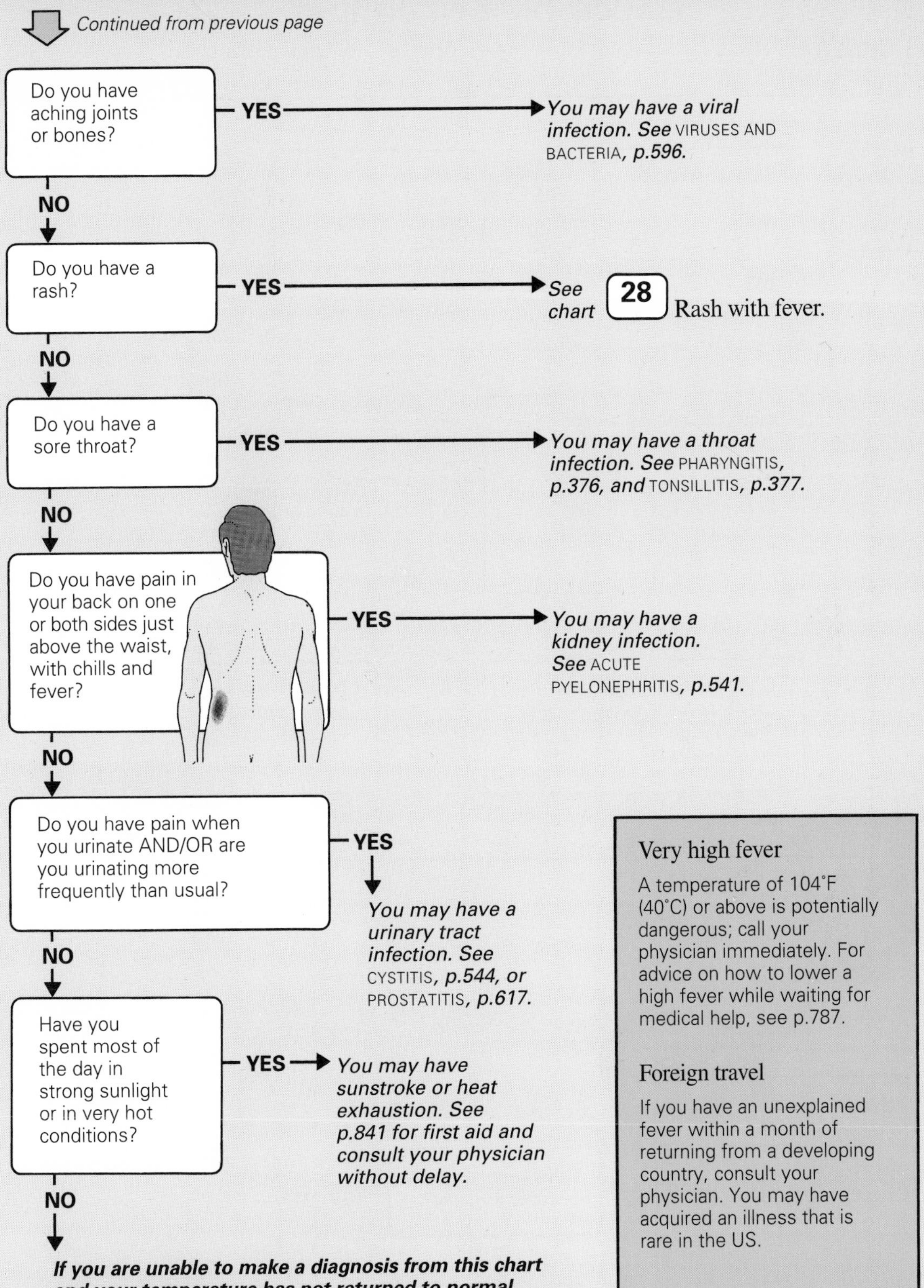

Do you have aching joints or bones?
YES
You may have a viral infection. See VIRUSES AND BACTERIA, p.596.
NO
Do you have a rash?
YES
See chart 28 Rash with fever.
NO
Do you have a sore throat?
YES
You may have a throat infection. See PHARYNGITIS, p.376, and TONSILLITIS, p.377.
NO
Do you have pain in your back on one or both sides just above the waist, with chills and fever?
YES
You may have a kidney infection. See ACUTE PYELONEPHRITIS, p.541.
NO
Do you have pain when you urinate AND/OR are you urinating more frequently than usual?
YES
You may have a urinary tract infection. See CYSTITIS, p.544, or PROSTATITIS, p.617.
NO
Have you spent most of the day in strong sunlight or in very hot conditions?
YES
You may have sunstroke or heat exhaustion. See p.841 for first aid and consult your physician without delay.
NO
If you are unable to make a diagnosis from this chart and your temperature has not returned to normal within 24 hours or rises again, consult your physician.

Very high fever

A temperature of 104°F (40°C) or above is potentially dangerous; call your physician immediately. For advice on how to lower a high fever while waiting for medical help, see p.787.

Foreign travel

If you have an unexplained fever within a month of returning from a developing country, consult your physician. You may have acquired an illness that is rare in the US.

6
GENERAL
all ages

Excessive sweating

Sweating that is not associated with heat or exercise.

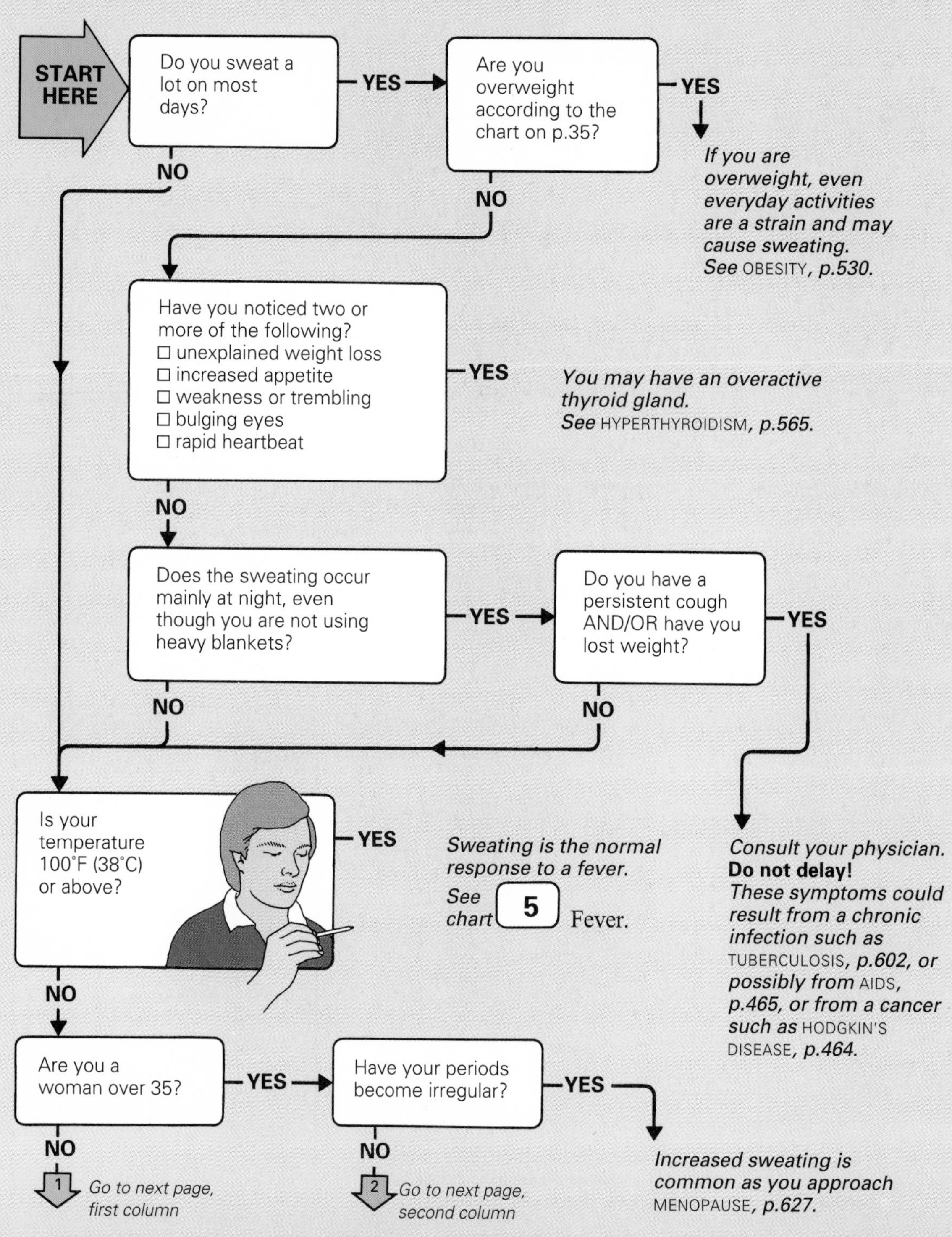

START HERE
Do you sweat a lot on most days?
YES
NO
Are you overweight according to the chart on p.35?
YES
NO
If you are overweight, even everyday activities are a strain and may cause sweating. See OBESITY, *p.530.*
Have you noticed two or more of the following?
☐ unexplained weight loss
☐ increased appetite
☐ weakness or trembling
☐ bulging eyes
☐ rapid heartbeat
YES
NO
You may have an overactive thyroid gland. See HYPERTHYROIDISM, *p.565.*
Does the sweating occur mainly at night, even though you are not using heavy blankets?
YES
NO
Do you have a persistent cough AND/OR have you lost weight?
YES
NO
Consult your physician. **Do not delay!** *These symptoms could result from a chronic infection such as* TUBERCULOSIS, *p.602, or possibly from* AIDS, *p.465, or from a cancer such as* HODGKIN'S DISEASE, *p.464.*
Is your temperature 100°F (38°C) or above?
YES
NO
Sweating is the normal response to a fever. See chart 5 Fever.
Are you a woman over 35?
YES
NO
Have your periods become irregular?
YES
NO
Increased sweating is common as you approach MENOPAUSE, *p.627.*
1 *Go to next page, first column*
2 *Go to next page, second column*

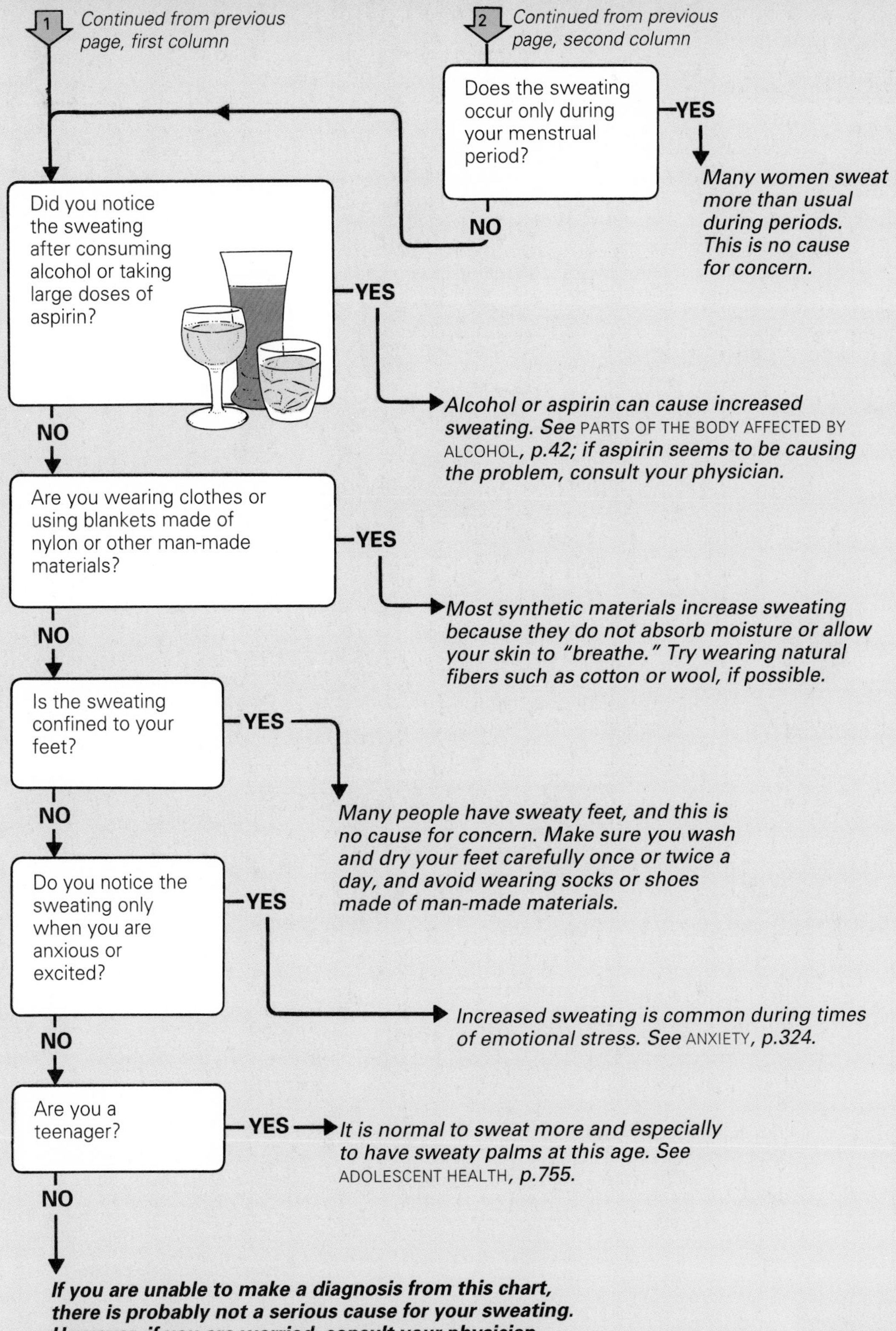

1 Continued from previous page, first column
2 Continued from previous page, second column
Does the sweating occur only during your menstrual period?
YES
Many women sweat more than usual during periods. This is no cause for concern.
NO
Did you notice the sweating after consuming alcohol or taking large doses of aspirin?
YES
Alcohol or aspirin can cause increased sweating. See PARTS OF THE BODY AFFECTED BY ALCOHOL, p.42; if aspirin seems to be causing the problem, consult your physician.
NO
Are you wearing clothes or using blankets made of nylon or other man-made materials?
YES
Most synthetic materials increase sweating because they do not absorb moisture or allow your skin to "breathe." Try wearing natural fibers such as cotton or wool, if possible.
NO
Is the sweating confined to your feet?
YES
Many people have sweaty feet, and this is no cause for concern. Make sure you wash and dry your feet carefully once or twice a day, and avoid wearing socks or shoes made of man-made materials.
NO
Do you notice the sweating only when you are anxious or excited?
YES
Increased sweating is common during times of emotional stress. See ANXIETY, p.324.
NO
Are you a teenager?
YES
It is normal to sweat more and especially to have sweaty palms at this age. See ADOLESCENT HEALTH, p.755.
NO

If you are unable to make a diagnosis from this chart, there is probably not a serious cause for your sweating. However, if you are worried, consult your physician.

7

GENERAL
over 14 years

Swellings under the skin

Any new lump or swollen area that you can see or feel under your skin. For children see chart 96, **Swellings in children**.

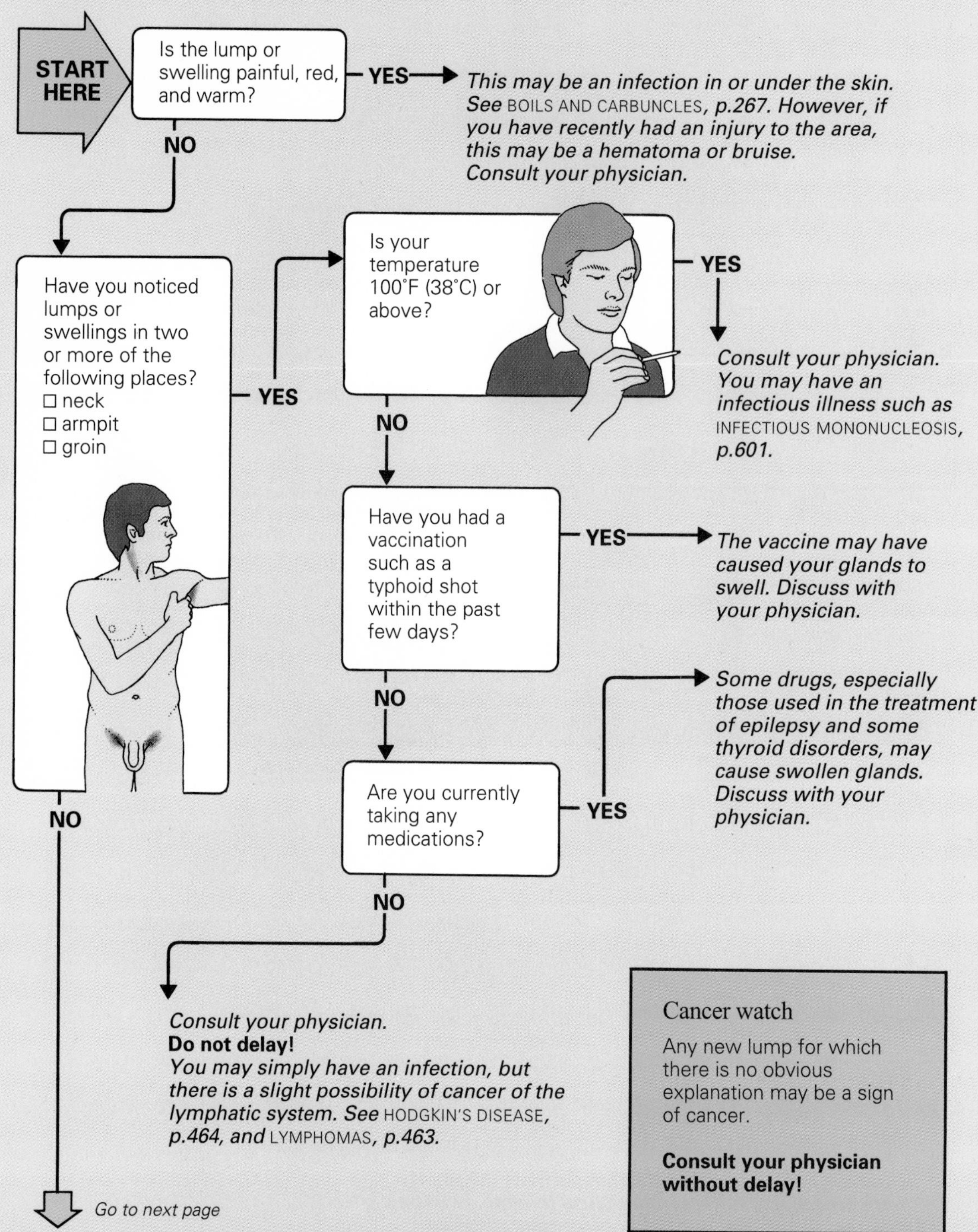

START HERE
Is the lump or swelling painful, red, and warm?
YES
This may be an infection in or under the skin. See BOILS AND CARBUNCLES, p.267. However, if you have recently had an injury to the area, this may be a hematoma or bruise. Consult your physician.
NO
Have you noticed lumps or swellings in two or more of the following places?
☐ neck
☐ armpit
☐ groin
YES
Is your temperature 100°F (38°C) or above?
YES
Consult your physician. You may have an infectious illness such as INFECTIOUS MONONUCLEOSIS, p.601.
NO
Have you had a vaccination such as a typhoid shot within the past few days?
YES
The vaccine may have caused your glands to swell. Discuss with your physician.
NO
Are you currently taking any medications?
YES
Some drugs, especially those used in the treatment of epilepsy and some thyroid disorders, may cause swollen glands. Discuss with your physician.
NO
Consult your physician.
Do not delay!
You may simply have an infection, but there is a slight possibility of cancer of the lymphatic system. See HODGKIN'S DISEASE, p.464, and LYMPHOMAS, p.463.
NO

Go to next page

Cancer watch

Any new lump for which there is no obvious explanation may be a sign of cancer.

Consult your physician without delay!

Continued from previous page

Is the swelling on your face between the ear and the angle of your jaw?

YES → Is the swelling on both sides?

- **YES** → *This may be* MUMPS, *p.748.*
- **NO** → *Consult your physician.*
  Do not delay!
  One-sided swelling of the face may be due to MUMPS, *p.748, a tooth abscess (see* TOOTH ABSCESS, *p.473), or a salivary gland problem such as a* SALIVARY DUCT STONE, *p.486. However, there is a slight chance of a* SALIVARY GLAND TUMOR, *p.486.*

NO → Is there swelling on both sides of the back of your neck?

YES → Do you have a pink rash AND/OR is your temperature 100°F (38°C) or above?

- **YES** → *You may have* GERMAN MEASLES, *p.746, or* INFECTIOUS MONONUCLEOSIS, *p.601.*
- **NO** → Is your throat sore?

NO → Are there swellings on both sides of your neck?

YES → Is your throat sore?

- **YES** → *You may have a throat infection (see* PHARYNGITIS, *p.376, and* TONSILLITIS, *p.377) or* INFECTIOUS MONONUCLEOSIS, *p.601, but there is also a slight possibility of* AIDS, *p.465.*
- **NO** → *Consult your physician.*
  Do not delay!
  You may simply have an infection, but there is a slight possibility of cancer of the lymphatic system (see HODGKIN'S DISEASE, *p.464, and* LYMPHOMAS, *p.463) or of* AIDS, *p.465.*

NO → *Go to next page*

Swellings under the skin

Continued from previous page

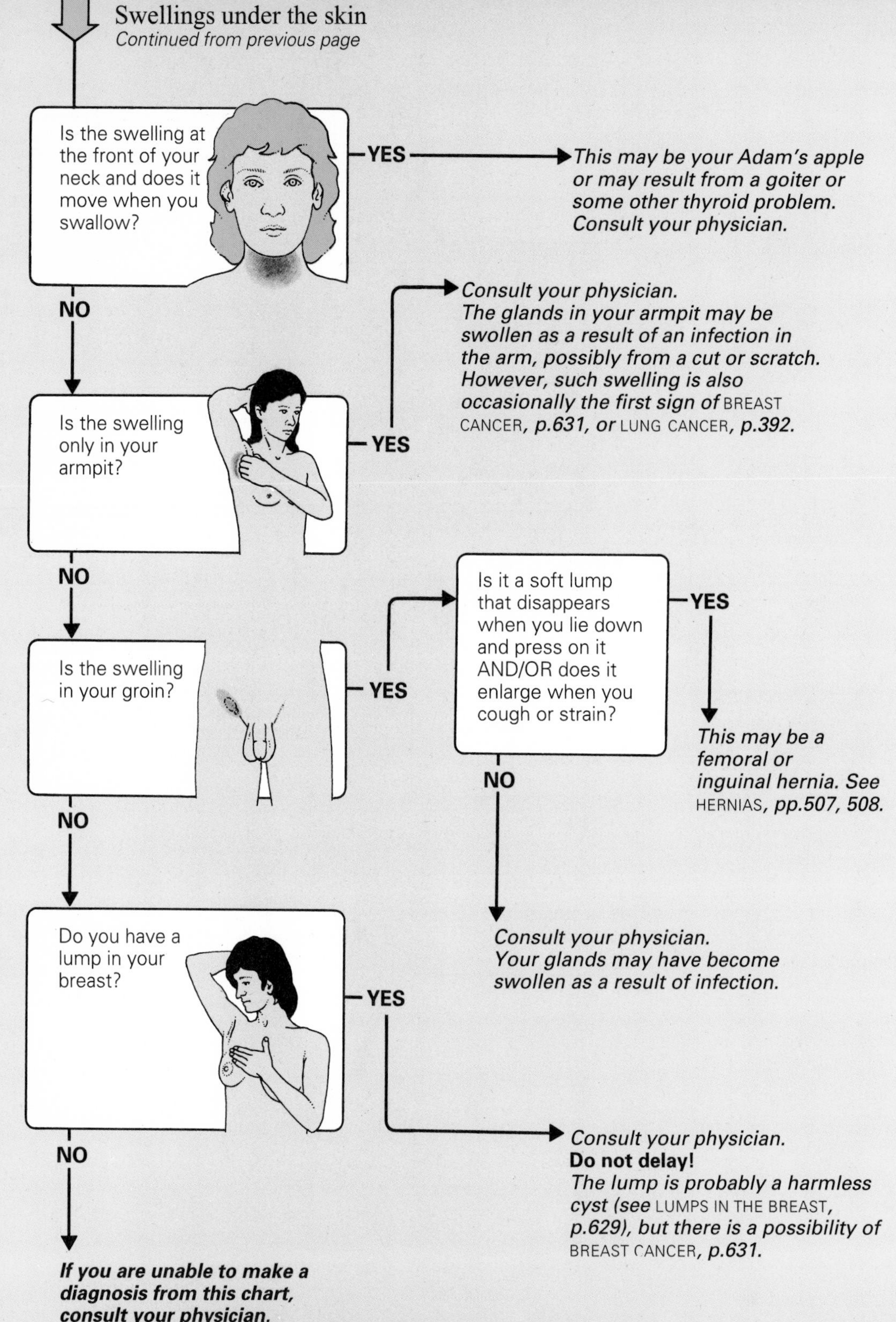

Is the swelling at the front of your neck and does it move when you swallow?
YES
This may be your Adam's apple or may result from a goiter or some other thyroid problem. Consult your physician.
NO
Is the swelling only in your armpit?
YES
Consult your physician. The glands in your armpit may be swollen as a result of an infection in the arm, possibly from a cut or scratch. However, such swelling is also occasionally the first sign of BREAST CANCER, *p.631, or* LUNG CANCER, *p.392.*
NO
Is the swelling in your groin?
YES
Is it a soft lump that disappears when you lie down and press on it AND/OR does it enlarge when you cough or strain?
YES
This may be a femoral or inguinal hernia. See HERNIAS, *pp.507, 508.*
NO
Consult your physician. Your glands may have become swollen as a result of infection.
NO
Do you have a lump in your breast?
YES
Consult your physician. **Do not delay!** *The lump is probably a harmless cyst (see* LUMPS IN THE BREAST, *p.629), but there is a possibility of* BREAST CANCER, *p.631.*
NO
If you are unable to make a diagnosis from this chart, consult your physician.

Itching without a rash

Desire to scratch the skin but no change in its appearance.
For children see chart 94, **Itching in children**.

START HERE

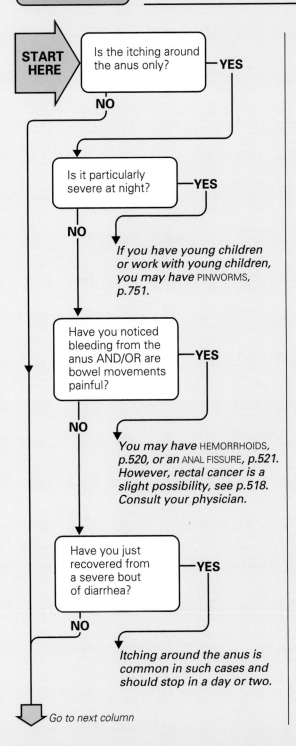

Is the itching around the anus only? — **YES** / **NO**

Is it particularly severe at night? — **YES**

If you have young children or work with young children, you may have PINWORMS, *p.751.*

NO

Have you noticed bleeding from the anus AND/OR are bowel movements painful? — **YES**

You may have HEMORRHOIDS, *p.520, or an* ANAL FISSURE, *p.521. However, rectal cancer is a slight possibility, see p.518. Consult your physician.*

NO

Have you just recovered from a severe bout of diarrhea? — **YES**

Itching around the anus is common in such cases and should stop in a day or two.

NO

Go to next column

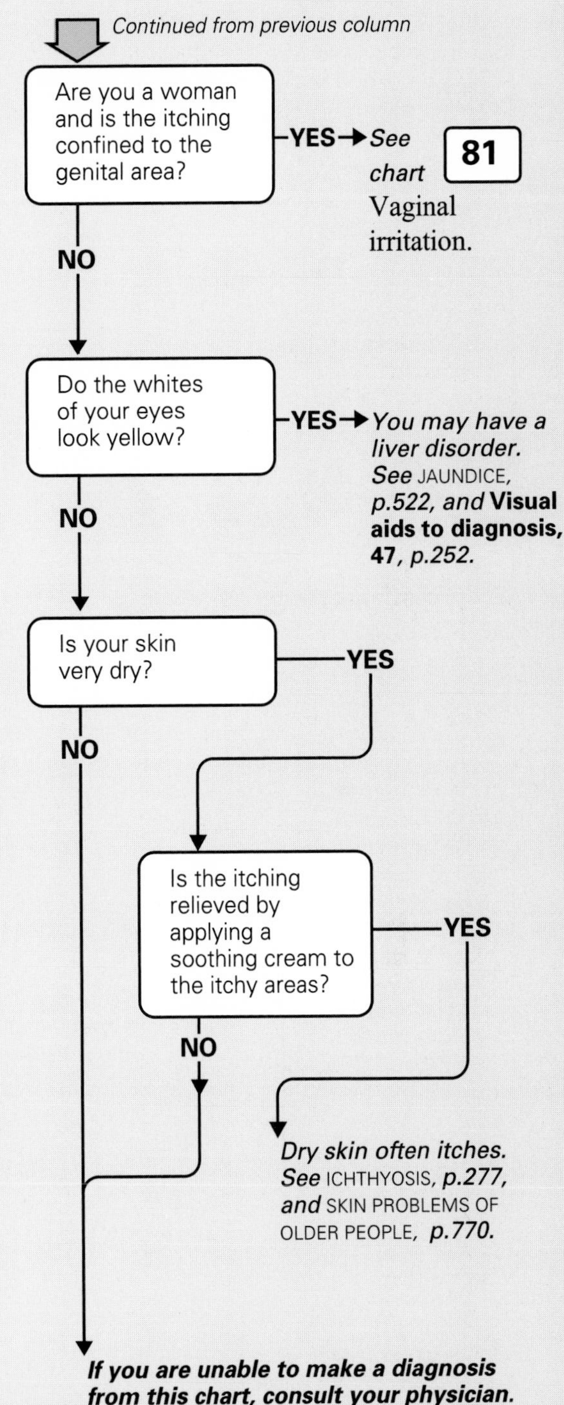

Continued from previous column

Are you a woman and is the itching confined to the genital area? — **YES** → *See chart* **81** Vaginal irritation.

NO

Do the whites of your eyes look yellow? — **YES** → *You may have a liver disorder. See* JAUNDICE, *p.522, and* **Visual aids to diagnosis, 47**, *p.252.*

NO

Is your skin very dry? — **YES** / **NO**

Is the itching relieved by applying a soothing cream to the itchy areas? — **YES**

Dry skin often itches. See ICHTHYOSIS, *p.277, and* SKIN PROBLEMS OF OLDER PEOPLE, *p.770.*

NO

If you are unable to make a diagnosis from this chart, consult your physician.

9

GENERAL

all ages

Feeling faint and fainting

A sudden feeling of weakness and unsteadiness that may result in brief loss of consciousness.

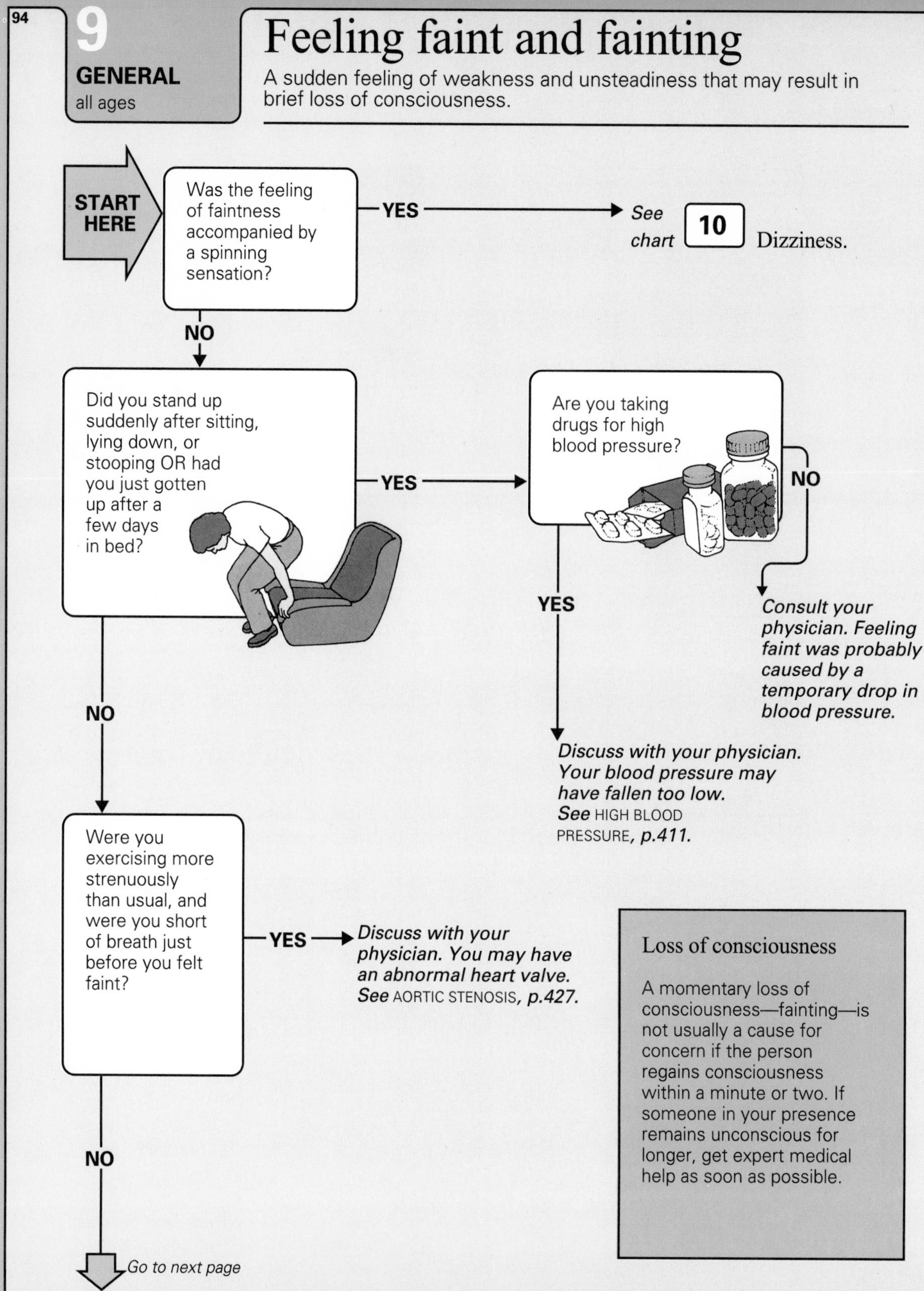

START HERE
Was the feeling of faintness accompanied by a spinning sensation?
YES
See chart 10 Dizziness.
NO
Did you stand up suddenly after sitting, lying down, or stooping OR had you just gotten up after a few days in bed?
YES
Are you taking drugs for high blood pressure?
NO
Consult your physician. Feeling faint was probably caused by a temporary drop in blood pressure.
YES
Discuss with your physician. Your blood pressure may have fallen too low. See HIGH BLOOD PRESSURE, p.411.
NO
Were you exercising more strenuously than usual, and were you short of breath just before you felt faint?
YES
Discuss with your physician. You may have an abnormal heart valve. See AORTIC STENOSIS, p.427.
NO
Go to next page

Loss of consciousness

A momentary loss of consciousness—fainting—is not usually a cause for concern if the person regains consciousness within a minute or two. If someone in your presence remains unconscious for longer, get expert medical help as soon as possible.

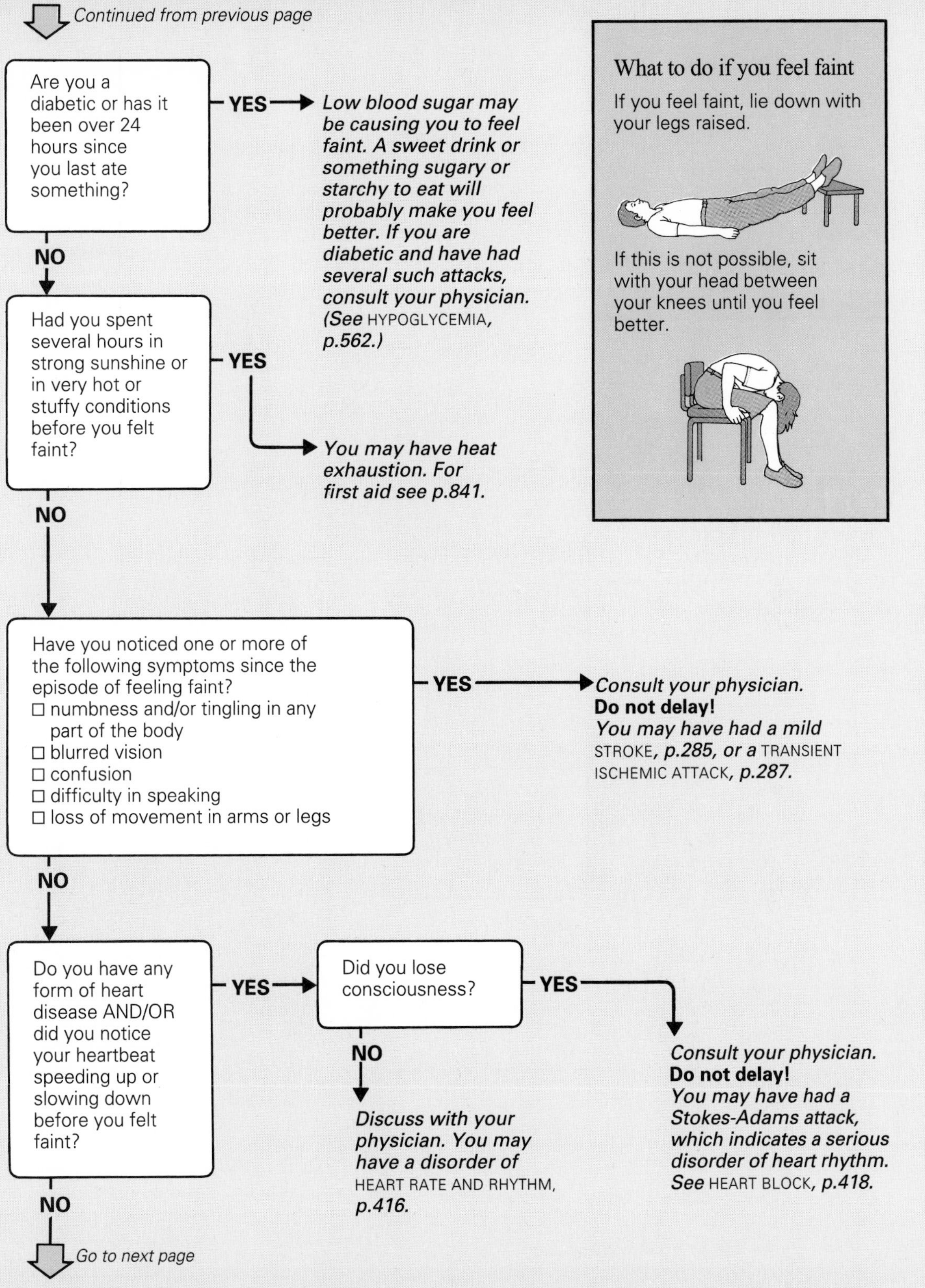

Continued from previous page

Are you a diabetic or has it been over 24 hours since you last ate something?
YES
Low blood sugar may be causing you to feel faint. A sweet drink or something sugary or starchy to eat will probably make you feel better. If you are diabetic and have had several such attacks, consult your physician. (See HYPOGLYCEMIA, *p.562.)*
NO
Had you spent several hours in strong sunshine or in very hot or stuffy conditions before you felt faint?
YES
You may have heat exhaustion. For first aid see p.841.
NO
Have you noticed one or more of the following symptoms since the episode of feeling faint?
☐ numbness and/or tingling in any part of the body
☐ blurred vision
☐ confusion
☐ difficulty in speaking
☐ loss of movement in arms or legs
YES
Consult your physician.
Do not delay!
You may have had a mild STROKE, *p.285, or a* TRANSIENT ISCHEMIC ATTACK, *p.287.*
NO
Do you have any form of heart disease AND/OR did you notice your heartbeat speeding up or slowing down before you felt faint?
YES
Did you lose consciousness?
YES
Consult your physician.
Do not delay!
You may have had a Stokes-Adams attack, which indicates a serious disorder of heart rhythm. See HEART BLOCK, *p.418.*
NO
Discuss with your physician. You may have a disorder of HEART RATE AND RHYTHM, *p.416.*
NO
Go to next page

What to do if you feel faint

If you feel faint, lie down with your legs raised.

If this is not possible, sit with your head between your knees until you feel better.

Feeling faint and fainting

Continued from previous page

Were you breathing very deeply or rapidly before you felt faint?

- **YES** → *Feeling faint was probably caused by hyperventilation or "overbreathing," possibly as a result of anxiety or stress. See* ANXIETY, *p.324.*
- **NO** ↓

Did you feel faint after an emotional shock?

- **YES** → *Emotional upsets can easily affect the nerves that control blood pressure, and this may cause faintness.*
- **NO** ↓

Did you feel faint while you were doing any of the following?
- ☐ coughing
- ☐ urinating
- ☐ stretching
- ☐ holding your breath

- **YES** → *Any of these activities can occasionally affect the supply of oxygen to the brain, causing faintness. This is usually no cause for concern. But if it happens more than once, consult your physician.*
- **NO** ↓

Are you over 50?

- **YES** → **Does raising or turning your head make you feel faint?**
  - **YES** → *This may be a rare symptom of a disorder that involves the nerves and bones in the neck. See* CERVICAL OSTEOARTHRITIS, *p.299.*
  - **NO** ↓
- **NO** ↓

Do you feel inexplicably tired AND/OR are you often short of breath?

- **YES** → *You may have a form of* ANEMIA, *p.450, or* HEART FAILURE, *p.408.*
- **NO** ↓

If you are unable to make a diagnosis from this chart, consult your physician.

10
GENERAL
all ages

Dizziness

A sense of being dazed and unsteady accompanied by a sensation of spinning.

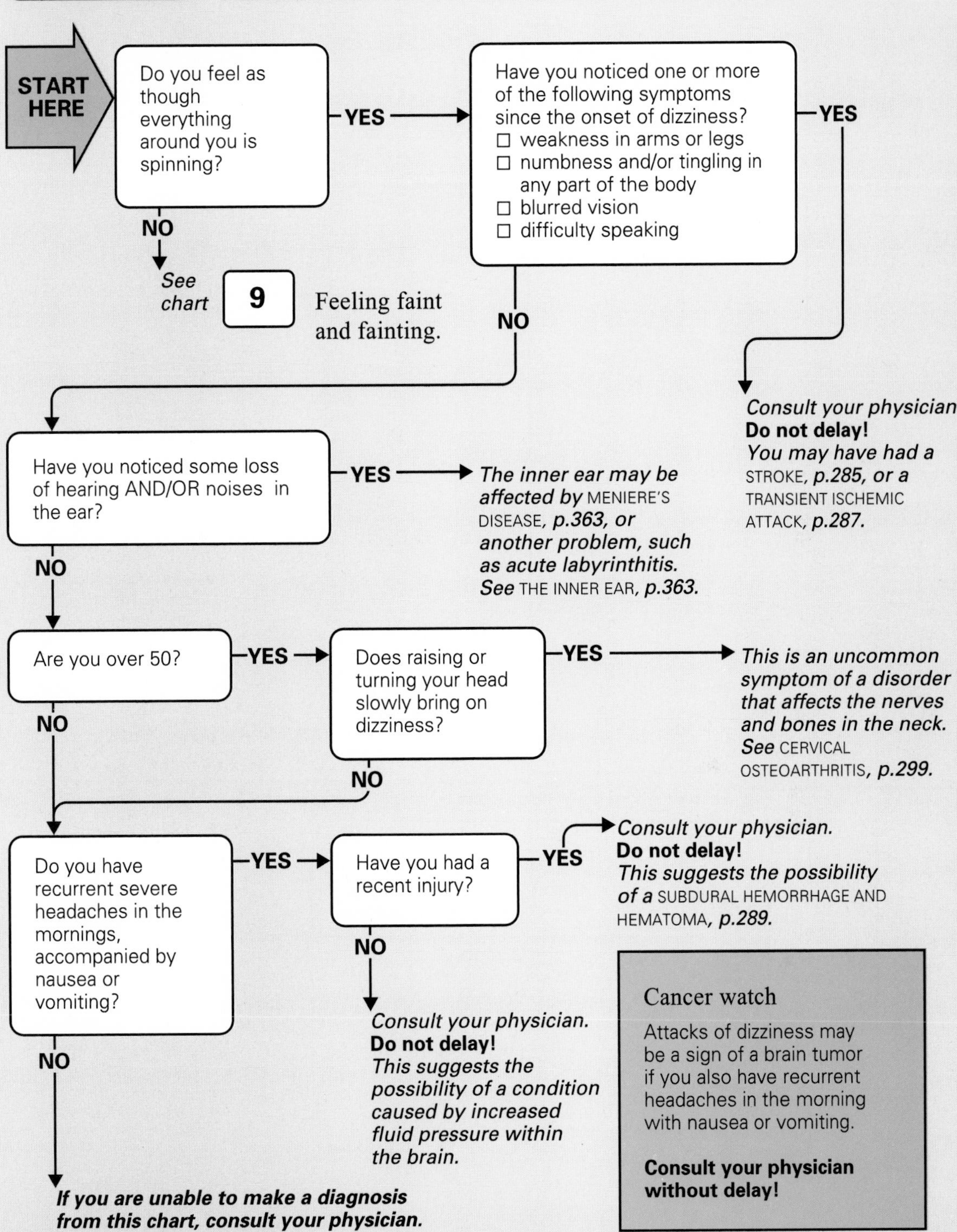

START HERE
Do you feel as though everything around you is spinning?
YES
NO
See chart 9 Feeling faint and fainting.
Have you noticed one or more of the following symptoms since the onset of dizziness?
☐ weakness in arms or legs
☐ numbness and/or tingling in any part of the body
☐ blurred vision
☐ difficulty speaking
YES
NO
Consult your physician. Do not delay! You may have had a STROKE, p.285, or a TRANSIENT ISCHEMIC ATTACK, p.287.
Have you noticed some loss of hearing AND/OR noises in the ear?
YES
NO
The inner ear may be affected by MENIERE'S DISEASE, p.363, or another problem, such as acute labyrinthitis. See THE INNER EAR, p.363.
Are you over 50?
YES
NO
Does raising or turning your head slowly bring on dizziness?
YES
NO
This is an uncommon symptom of a disorder that affects the nerves and bones in the neck. See CERVICAL OSTEOARTHRITIS, p.299.
Do you have recurrent severe headaches in the mornings, accompanied by nausea or vomiting?
YES
NO
Have you had a recent injury?
YES
NO
Consult your physician. Do not delay! This suggests the possibility of a SUBDURAL HEMORRHAGE AND HEMATOMA, p.289.
Consult your physician. Do not delay! This suggests the possibility of a condition caused by increased fluid pressure within the brain.
If you are unable to make a diagnosis from this chart, consult your physician.
Cancer watch
Attacks of dizziness may be a sign of a brain tumor if you also have recurrent headaches in the morning with nausea or vomiting.
Consult your physician without delay!

11
GENERAL
all ages

Headache

Pain in the head that may range from mild to severe and may be incapacitating.

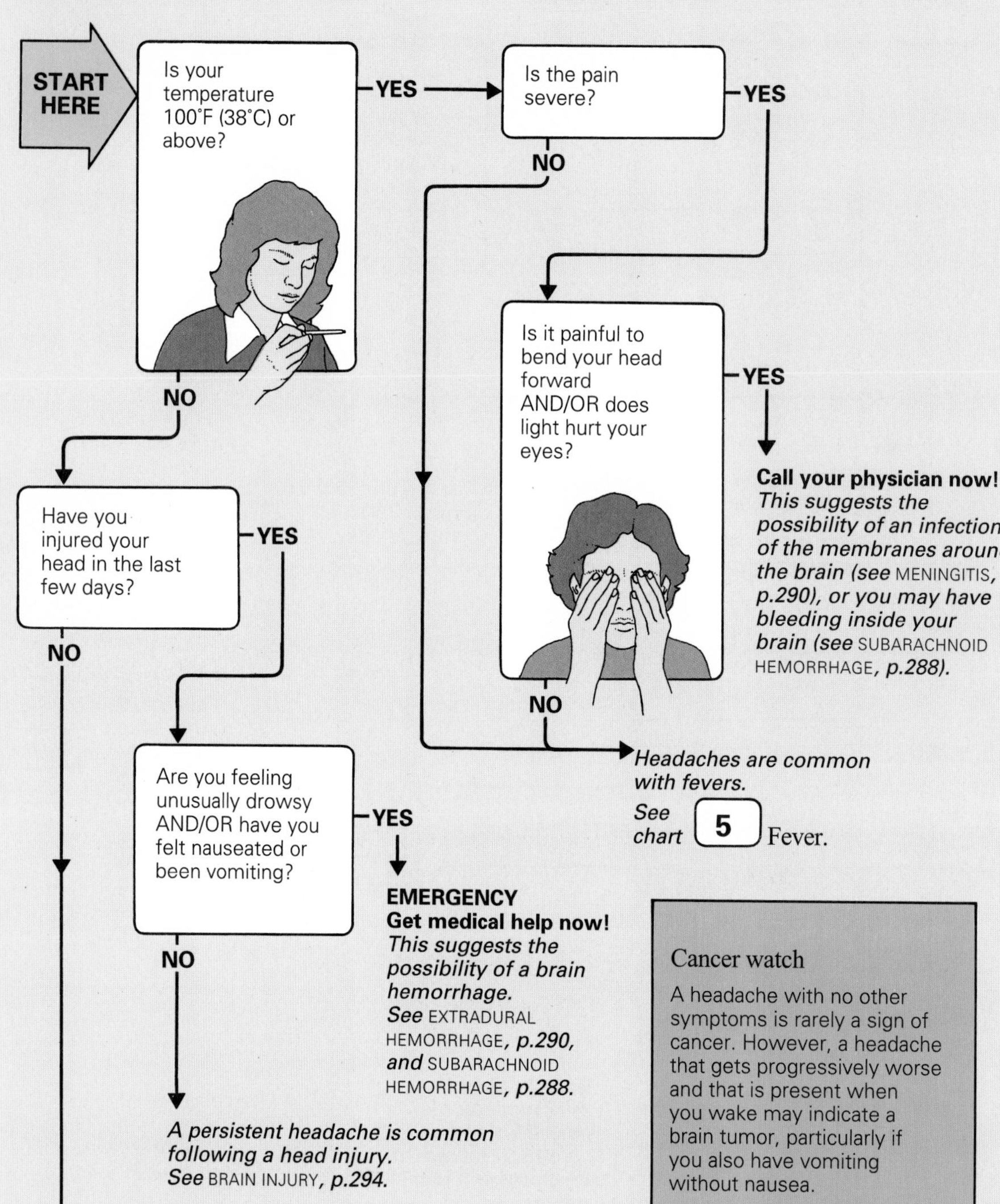

START HERE
Is your temperature 100°F (38°C) or above?
YES
NO
Is the pain severe?
YES
NO
Is it painful to bend your head forward AND/OR does light hurt your eyes?
YES
NO
Call your physician now!
This suggests the possibility of an infection of the membranes around the brain (see MENINGITIS*, p.290), or you may have bleeding inside your brain (see* SUBARACHNOID HEMORRHAGE*, p.288).*
Headaches are common with fevers.
See chart 5 Fever.
Have you injured your head in the last few days?
YES
NO
Are you feeling unusually drowsy AND/OR have you felt nauseated or been vomiting?
YES
NO
EMERGENCY
Get medical help now!
This suggests the possibility of a brain hemorrhage.
See EXTRADURAL HEMORRHAGE*, p.290, and* SUBARACHNOID HEMORRHAGE*, p.288.*
A persistent headache is common following a head injury.
See BRAIN INJURY*, p.294.*
Go to next page

Cancer watch

A headache with no other symptoms is rarely a sign of cancer. However, a headache that gets progressively worse and that is present when you wake may indicate a brain tumor, particularly if you also have vomiting without nausea.

Consult your physician without delay!

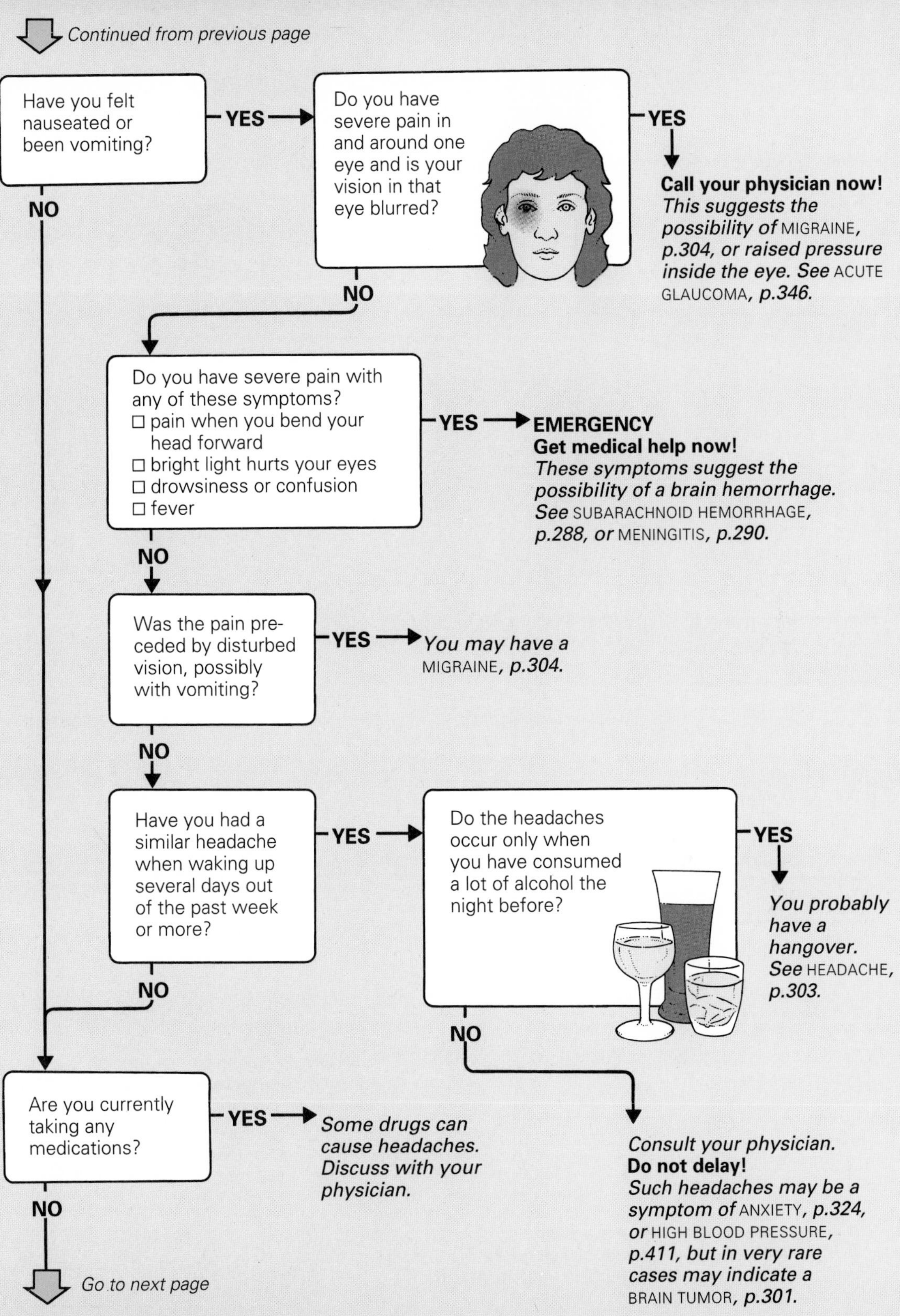
Continued from previous page
Have you felt nauseated or been vomiting?
YES
NO
Do you have severe pain in and around one eye and is your vision in that eye blurred?
YES
NO
Call your physician now!
This suggests the possibility of MIGRAINE, p.304, or raised pressure inside the eye. See ACUTE GLAUCOMA, p.346.
Do you have severe pain with any of these symptoms?
☐ pain when you bend your head forward
☐ bright light hurts your eyes
☐ drowsiness or confusion
☐ fever
YES
NO
EMERGENCY
Get medical help now!
These symptoms suggest the possibility of a brain hemorrhage. See SUBARACHNOID HEMORRHAGE, p.288, or MENINGITIS, p.290.
Was the pain preceded by disturbed vision, possibly with vomiting?
YES
NO
You may have a MIGRAINE, p.304.
Have you had a similar headache when waking up several days out of the past week or more?
YES
NO
Do the headaches occur only when you have consumed a lot of alcohol the night before?
YES
NO
You probably have a hangover. See HEADACHE, p.303.
Are you currently taking any medications?
YES
NO
Some drugs can cause headaches. Discuss with your physician.
Consult your physician.
Do not delay!
Such headaches may be a symptom of ANXIETY, p.324, or HIGH BLOOD PRESSURE, p.411, but in very rare cases may indicate a BRAIN TUMOR, p.301.
Go to next page

Headache

Continued from previous page

Have you recently had or do you now have a runny or stuffy nose?

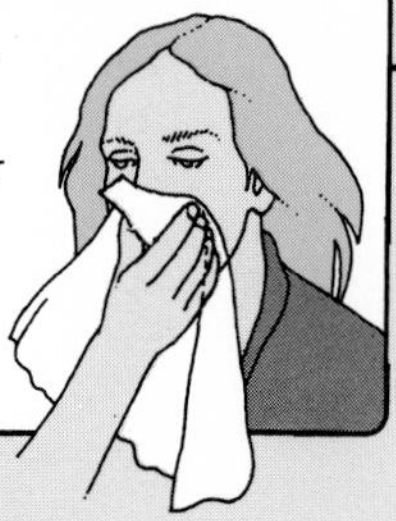

YES → Do you have dull pain and tenderness around the eyes and cheekbones that worsen when you bend forward?

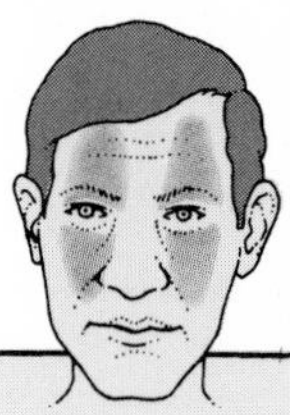

- YES → *You may have an infection of the sinuses. See* SINUSITIS, ***p.373.***
- NO → *Headache is a common symptom of a* COLD, ***p.368.***

NO ↓

Are you feeling tense or under stress AND/OR are you sleeping poorly?

YES → ***Anxiety often causes headaches. See*** ANXIETY, ***p.324, and*** HEADACHE, ***p.303.***

NO ↓

Did the headache occur after you had been reading or doing close work such as sewing?

YES → ***Strain on your neck muscles may have caused the headache. See*** HEADACHE, ***p.303.***

NO ↓

Did any of the following apply in the 12 hours before the headache started?

- ☐ you were exposed to strong sunlight
- ☐ you were in stuffy, smoky, or noisy surroundings
- ☐ you drank more alcohol than usual
- ☐ you missed a meal

YES → ***Headaches are often brought on by such circumstances and are usually no cause for concern. See*** HEADACHE, ***p.303.***

NO ↓

If you are unable to make a diagnosis from this chart and the headache persists overnight or if you develop other symptoms, consult your physician.

Numbness and/or tingling

Loss of feeling and/or a "pins and needles" sensation in any part of the body.

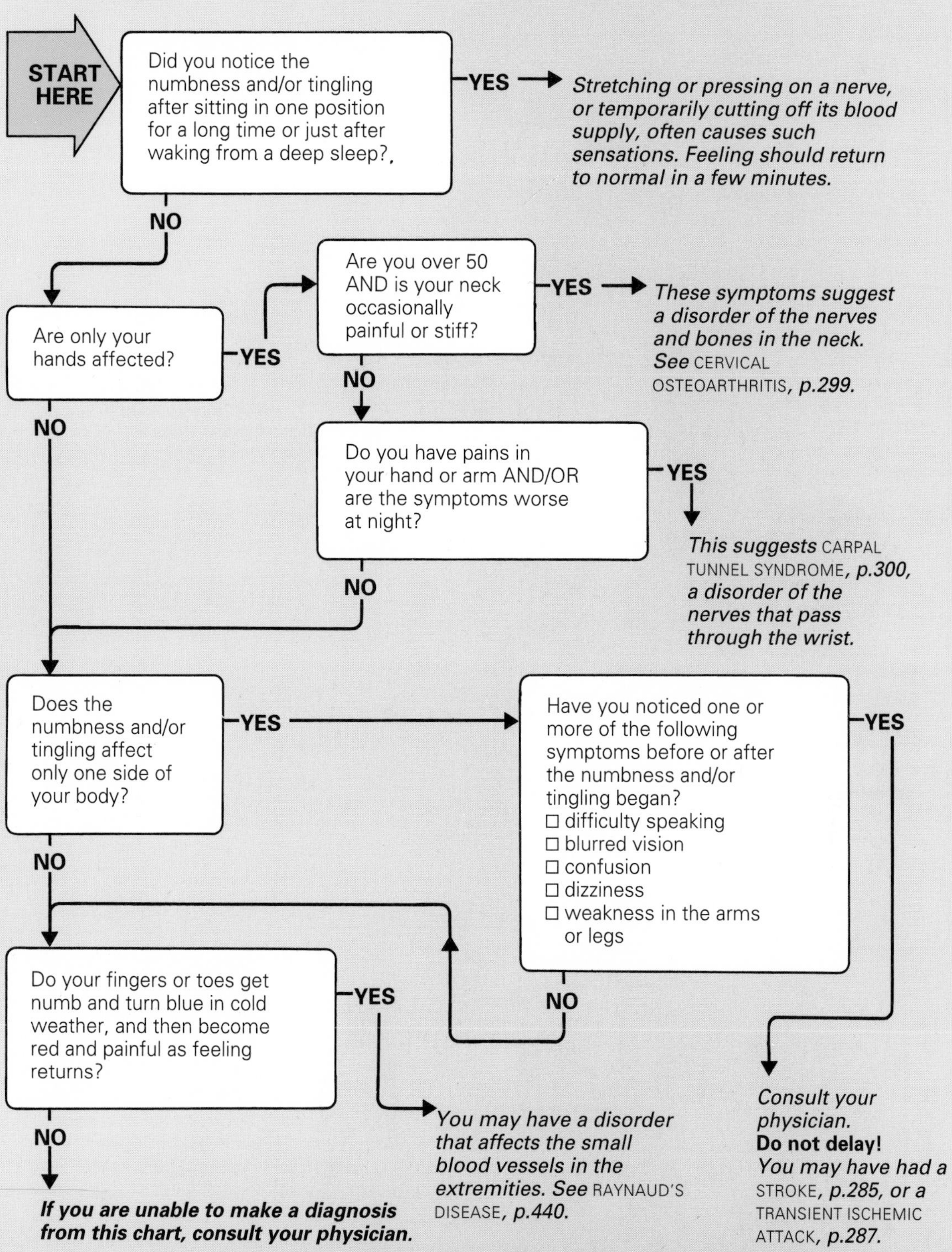

START HERE
Did you notice the numbness and/or tingling after sitting in one position for a long time or just after waking from a deep sleep?
YES
Stretching or pressing on a nerve, or temporarily cutting off its blood supply, often causes such sensations. Feeling should return to normal in a few minutes.
NO
Are only your hands affected?
YES
Are you over 50 AND is your neck occasionally painful or stiff?
YES
These symptoms suggest a disorder of the nerves and bones in the neck. See CERVICAL OSTEOARTHRITIS, p.299.
NO
Do you have pains in your hand or arm AND/OR are the symptoms worse at night?
YES
This suggests CARPAL TUNNEL SYNDROME, p.300, a disorder of the nerves that pass through the wrist.
NO
NO
Does the numbness and/or tingling affect only one side of your body?
YES
Have you noticed one or more of the following symptoms before or after the numbness and/or tingling began?
☐ difficulty speaking
☐ blurred vision
☐ confusion
☐ dizziness
☐ weakness in the arms or legs
YES
Consult your physician.
Do not delay!
You may have had a STROKE, p.285, or a TRANSIENT ISCHEMIC ATTACK, p.287.
NO
NO
Do your fingers or toes get numb and turn blue in cold weather, and then become red and painful as feeling returns?
YES
You may have a disorder that affects the small blood vessels in the extremities. See RAYNAUD'S DISEASE, p.440.
NO
If you are unable to make a diagnosis from this chart, consult your physician.

13

GENERAL
all ages

Twitching and trembling

Any involuntary movements including persistent trembling and shaking or sudden twitching.

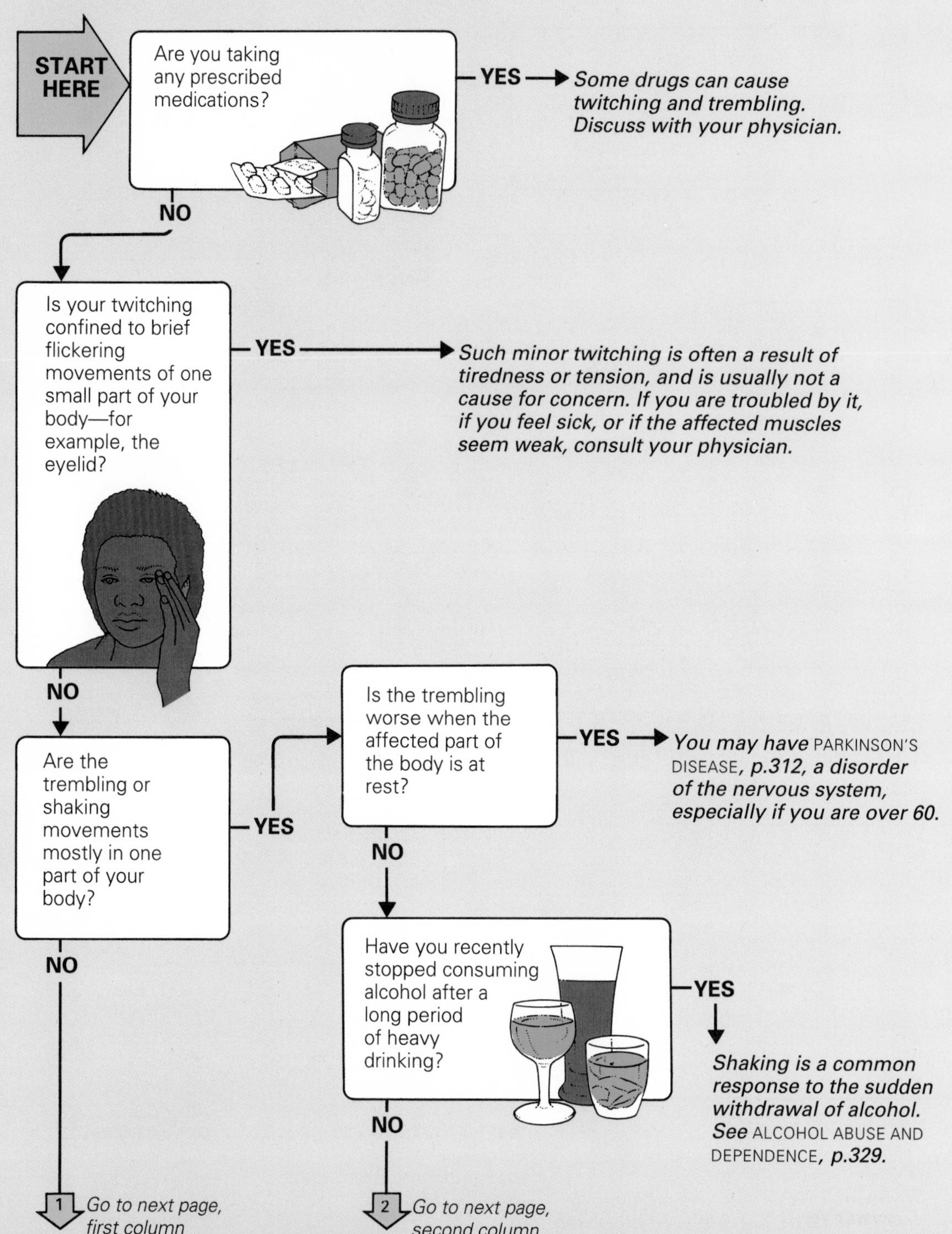

START HERE
Are you taking any prescribed medications?
YES → Some drugs can cause twitching and trembling. Discuss with your physician.
NO
Is your twitching confined to brief flickering movements of one small part of your body—for example, the eyelid?
YES → Such minor twitching is often a result of tiredness or tension, and is usually not a cause for concern. If you are troubled by it, if you feel sick, or if the affected muscles seem weak, consult your physician.
NO
Are the trembling or shaking movements mostly in one part of your body?
YES
Is the trembling worse when the affected part of the body is at rest?
YES → You may have PARKINSON'S DISEASE, p.312, a disorder of the nervous system, especially if you are over 60.
NO
Have you recently stopped consuming alcohol after a long period of heavy drinking?
YES
Shaking is a common response to the sudden withdrawal of alcohol. See ALCOHOL ABUSE AND DEPENDENCE, p.329.
NO
1 Go to next page, first column
NO
2 Go to next page, second column

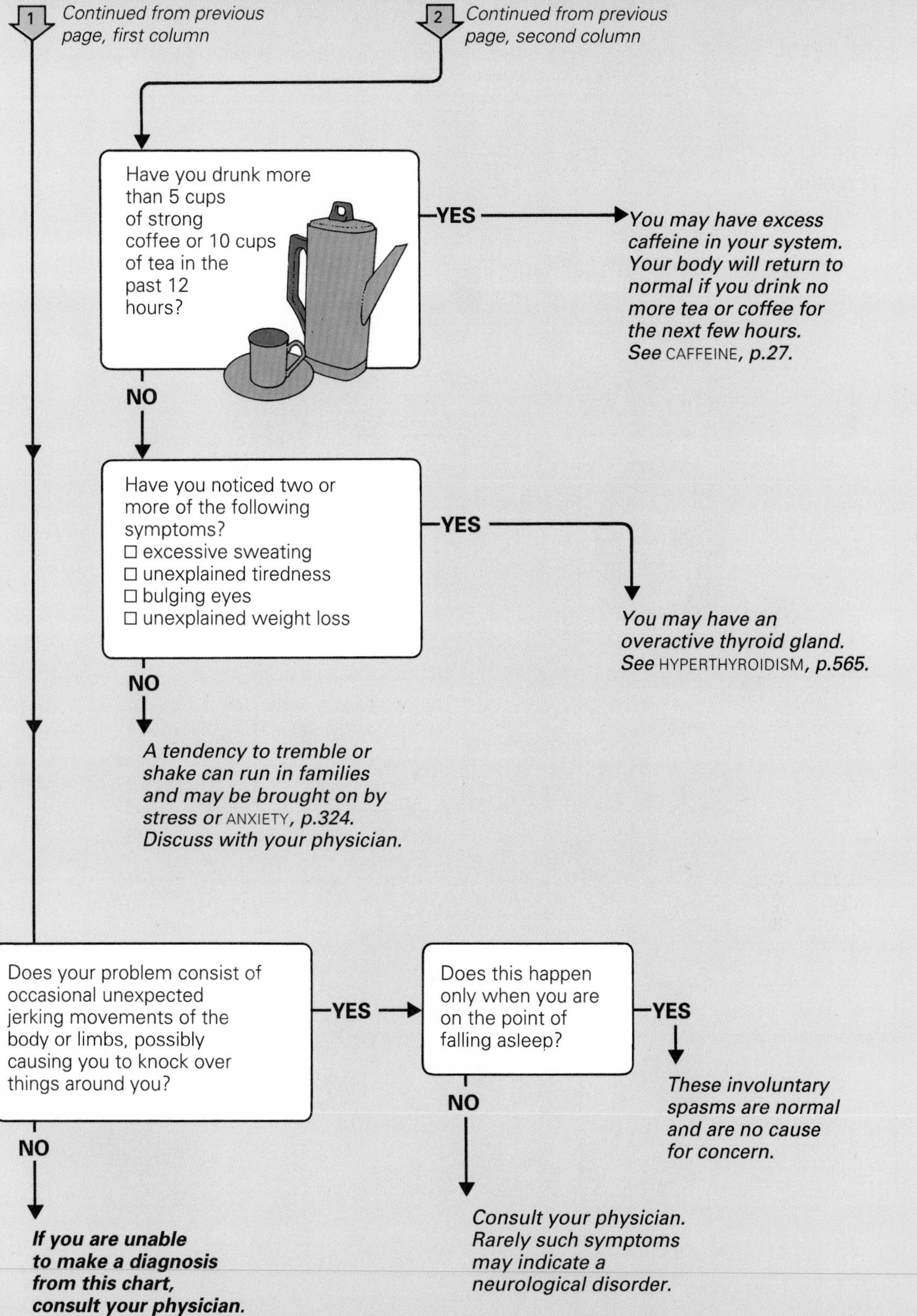
1
Continued from previous page, first column
2
Continued from previous page, second column
Have you drunk more than 5 cups of strong coffee or 10 cups of tea in the past 12 hours?
YES
You may have excess caffeine in your system. Your body will return to normal if you drink no more tea or coffee for the next few hours. See CAFFEINE, p.27.
NO
Have you noticed two or more of the following symptoms?
☐ excessive sweating
☐ unexplained tiredness
☐ bulging eyes
☐ unexplained weight loss
YES
You may have an overactive thyroid gland. See HYPERTHYROIDISM, p.565.
NO
A tendency to tremble or shake can run in families and may be brought on by stress or ANXIETY, p.324. Discuss with your physician.
Does your problem consist of occasional unexpected jerking movements of the body or limbs, possibly causing you to knock over things around you?
YES
Does this happen only when you are on the point of falling asleep?
YES
These involuntary spasms are normal and are no cause for concern.
NO
Consult your physician. Rarely such symptoms may indicate a neurological disorder.
NO
If you are unable to make a diagnosis from this chart, consult your physician.

14
GENERAL
all ages

Pain in the face

Pain in one or both sides of the face or forehead that may be dull and throbbing or intense and stabbing.

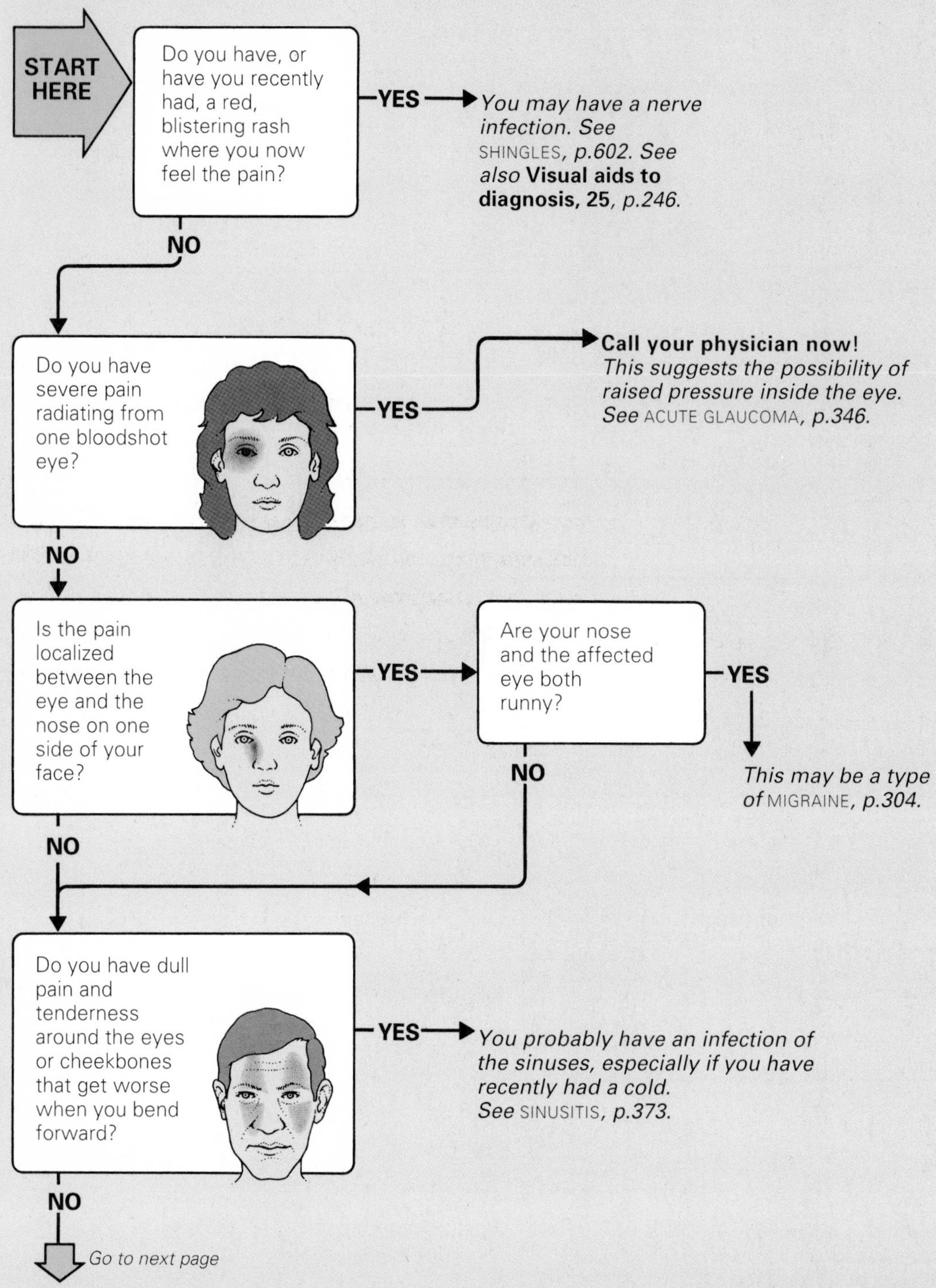

START HERE
Do you have, or have you recently had, a red, blistering rash where you now feel the pain?
YES
You may have a nerve infection. See SHINGLES, *p.602. See also* **Visual aids to diagnosis, 25**, *p.246.*
NO
Do you have severe pain radiating from one bloodshot eye?
YES
Call your physician now!
This suggests the possibility of raised pressure inside the eye. See ACUTE GLAUCOMA, *p.346.*
NO
Is the pain localized between the eye and the nose on one side of your face?
YES
Are your nose and the affected eye both runny?
YES
This may be a type of MIGRAINE, *p.304.*
NO
NO
Do you have dull pain and tenderness around the eyes or cheekbones that get worse when you bend forward?
YES
You probably have an infection of the sinuses, especially if you have recently had a cold. See SINUSITIS, *p.373.*
NO
Go to next page

Continued from previous page

Do you have a continuous, throbbing pain on one side of your face?

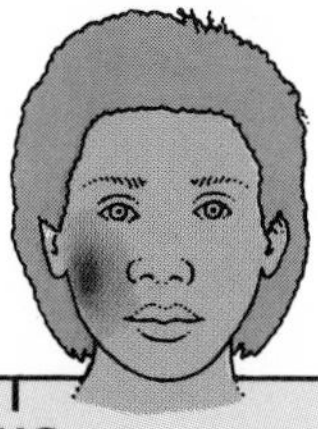

YES → Is the pain worse at night, when you eat, or when you touch a particular tooth?

YES → *Consult your physician or dentist.* **Do not delay!** *You may have a* TOOTH ABSCESS, *p.473.*

NO ↓

Do you have a severe throbbing pain that comes on suddenly in one or both temples?

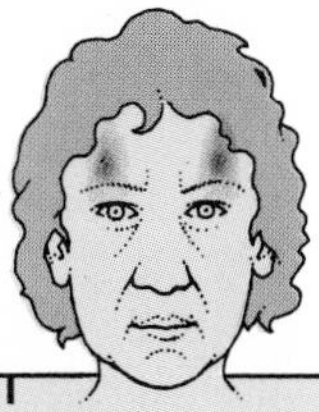

YES → Have you been feeling generally sick AND/OR is your scalp sensitive to touch?

YES → *Consult your physician.* **Do not delay!** *You may have inflammation of the arteries in your head, which can affect your vision. See* TEMPORAL ARTERITIS, *p.439.*

NO ↓

Is there stabbing pain on one side of your face, brought on by any of the following?

- ☐ touching your face
- ☐ chewing
- ☐ breathing cold air
- ☐ drinking cold liquid

YES → *The pain is probably caused by a damaged nerve. See* TRIGEMINAL NEURALGIA, *p.770.*

NO ↓

If you are unable to make a diagnosis from this chart, consult your physician.

15
GENERAL
all ages

Confusion

Confusion may vary from feeling bewildered about times, places, and events, to an alarming loss of contact with reality.

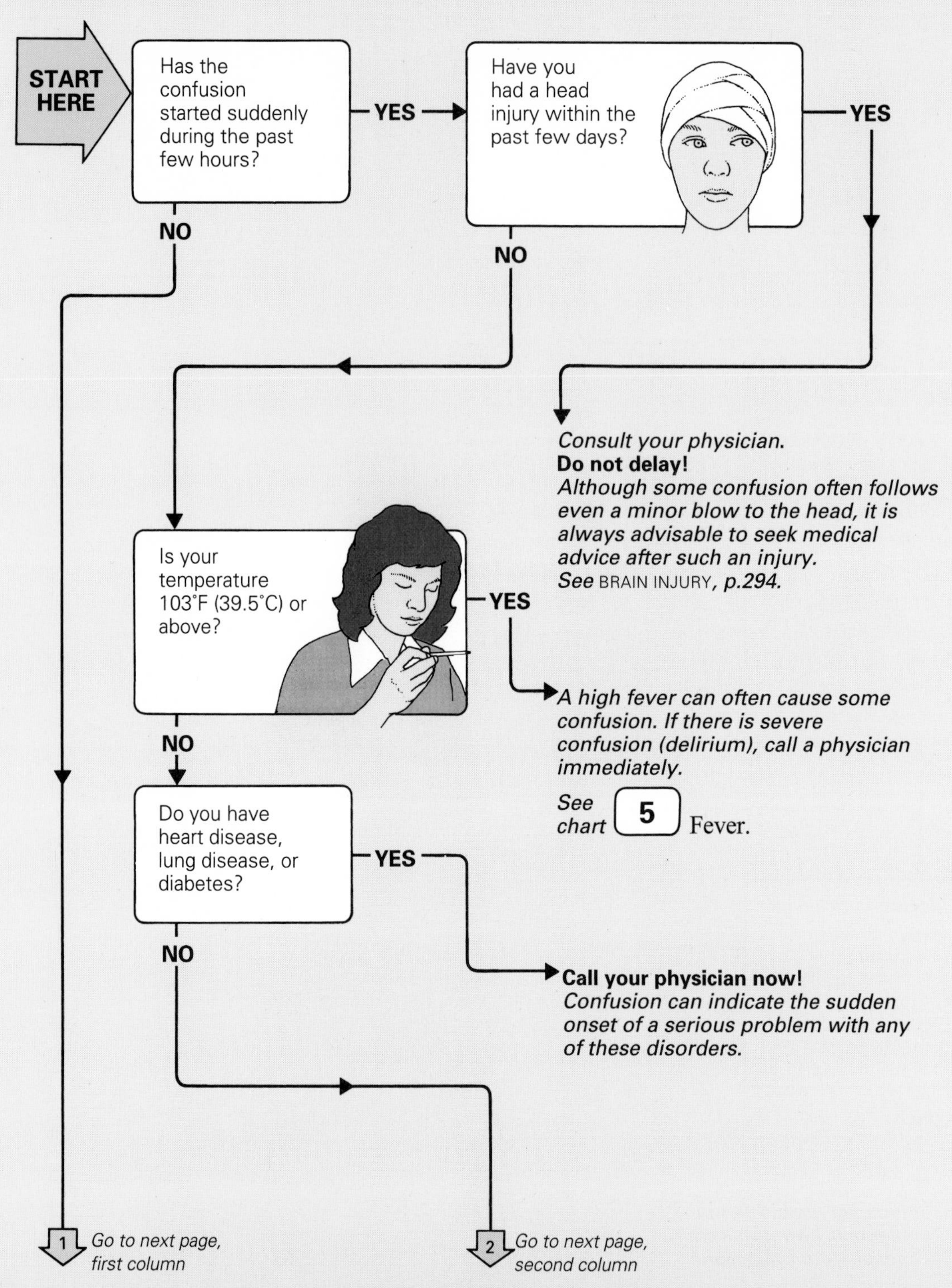

START HERE
Has the confusion started suddenly during the past few hours?
YES
NO
Have you had a head injury within the past few days?
YES
NO
Consult your physician.
Do not delay!
Although some confusion often follows even a minor blow to the head, it is always advisable to seek medical advice after such an injury.
See BRAIN INJURY, *p.294.*
Is your temperature 103°F (39.5°C) or above?
YES
NO
A high fever can often cause some confusion. If there is severe confusion (delirium), call a physician immediately.
See chart 5 Fever.
Do you have heart disease, lung disease, or diabetes?
YES
NO
Call your physician now!
Confusion can indicate the sudden onset of a serious problem with any of these disorders.
1 *Go to next page, first column*
2 *Go to next page, second column*

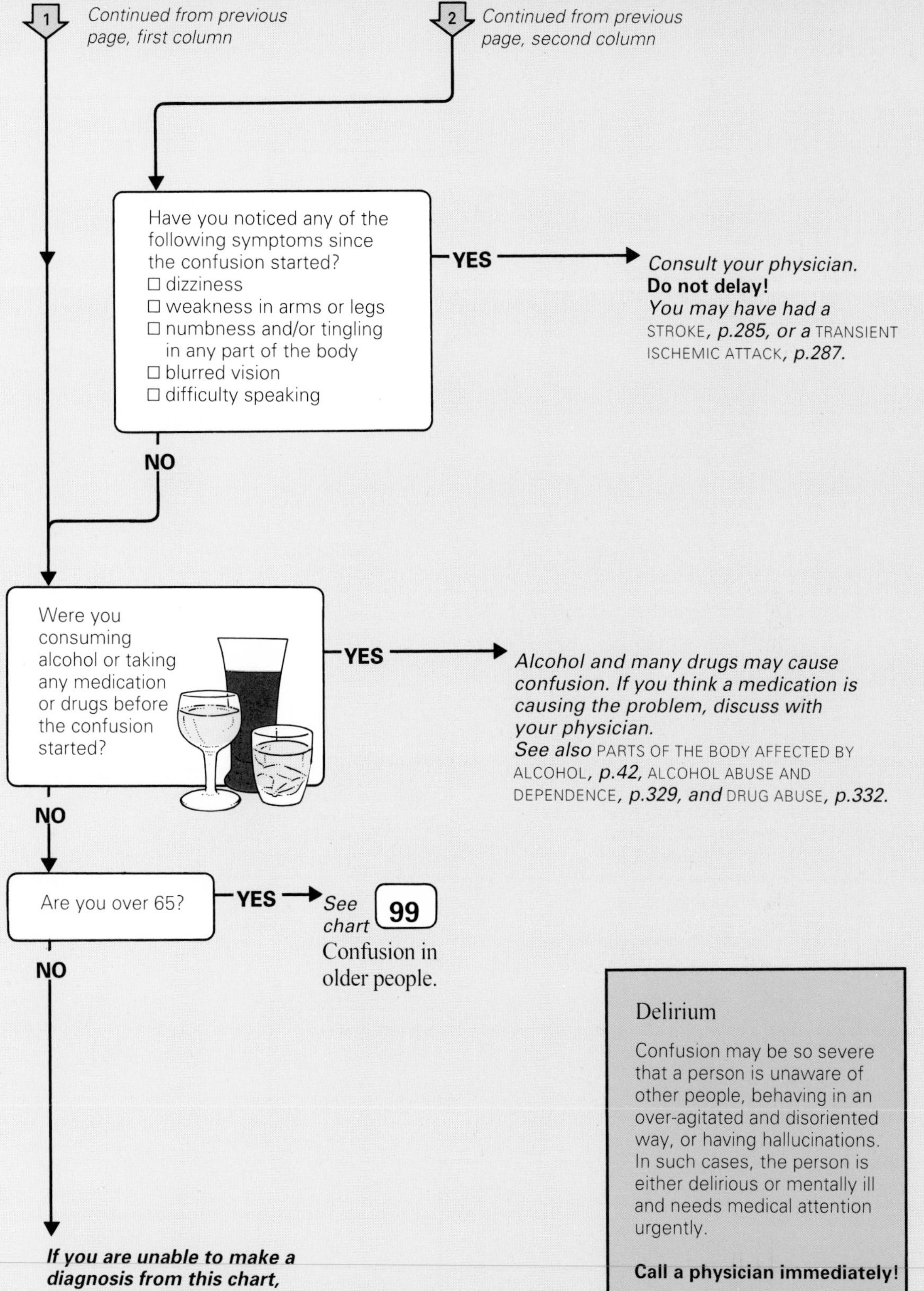

1
Continued from previous page, first column
2
Continued from previous page, second column
Have you noticed any of the following symptoms since the confusion started?
☐ dizziness
☐ weakness in arms or legs
☐ numbness and/or tingling in any part of the body
☐ blurred vision
☐ difficulty speaking
YES
Consult your physician.
Do not delay!
You may have had a STROKE, *p.285, or a* TRANSIENT ISCHEMIC ATTACK, *p.287.*
NO
Were you consuming alcohol or taking any medication or drugs before the confusion started?
YES
Alcohol and many drugs may cause confusion. If you think a medication is causing the problem, discuss with your physician.
See also PARTS OF THE BODY AFFECTED BY ALCOHOL, *p.42,* ALCOHOL ABUSE AND DEPENDENCE, *p.329, and* DRUG ABUSE, *p.332.*
NO
Are you over 65?
YES
See chart **99** Confusion in older people.
NO
If you are unable to make a diagnosis from this chart, consult your physician.

Delirium

Confusion may be so severe that a person is unaware of other people, behaving in an over-agitated and disoriented way, or having hallucinations. In such cases, the person is either delirious or mentally ill and needs medical attention urgently.

Call a physician immediately!

16
GENERAL
all ages

Impaired memory

Difficulty in remembering specific events and facts (often called absent-mindedness) or whole periods of time (amnesia).

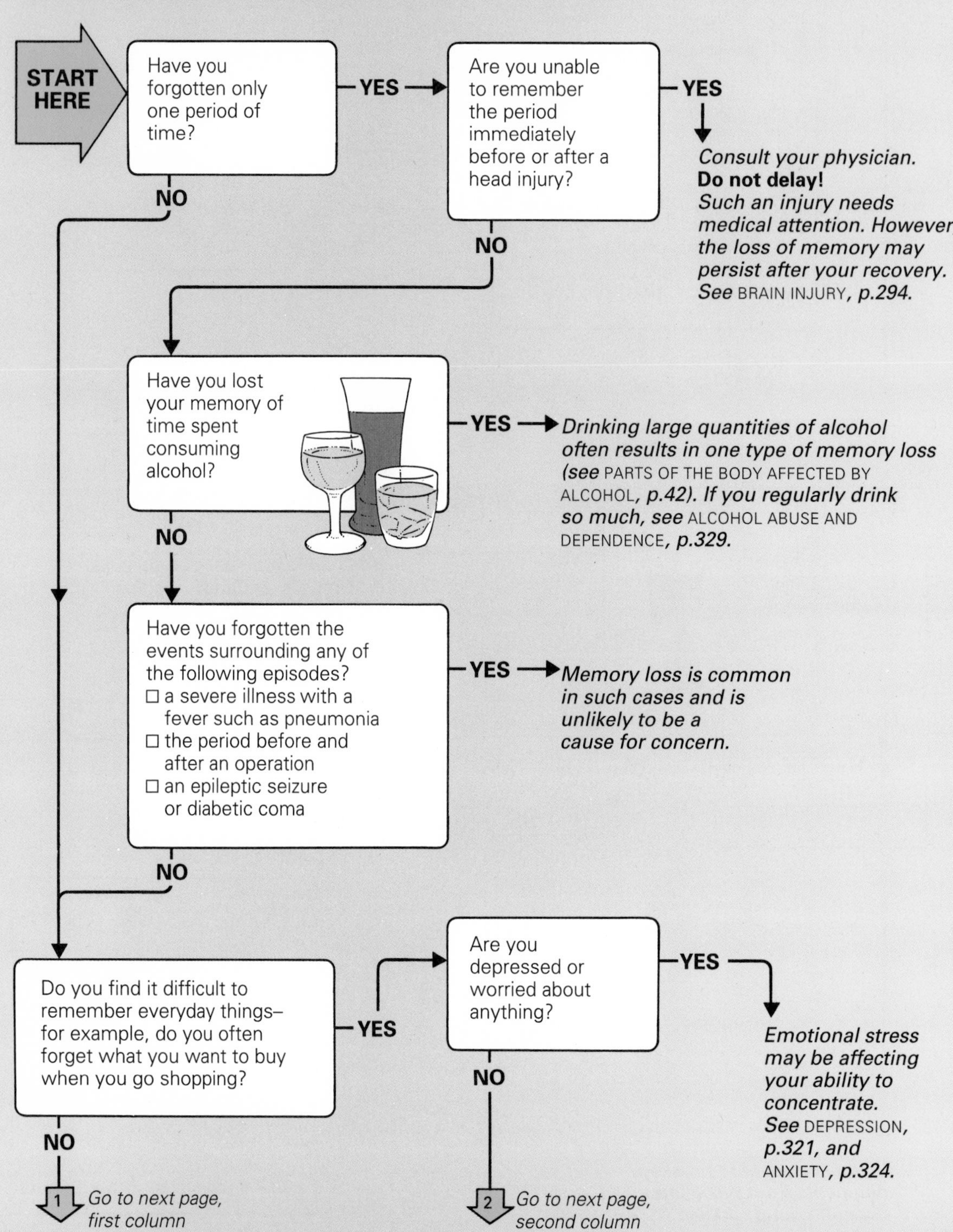

START HERE
Have you forgotten only one period of time?
YES
Are you unable to remember the period immediately before or after a head injury?
YES
Consult your physician.
Do not delay!
Such an injury needs medical attention. However, the loss of memory may persist after your recovery. See BRAIN INJURY, p.294.
NO
NO
Have you lost your memory of time spent consuming alcohol?
YES
Drinking large quantities of alcohol often results in one type of memory loss (see PARTS OF THE BODY AFFECTED BY ALCOHOL, p.42). If you regularly drink so much, see ALCOHOL ABUSE AND DEPENDENCE, p.329.
NO
Have you forgotten the events surrounding any of the following episodes?
☐ a severe illness with a fever such as pneumonia
☐ the period before and after an operation
☐ an epileptic seizure or diabetic coma
YES
Memory loss is common in such cases and is unlikely to be a cause for concern.
NO
Do you find it difficult to remember everyday things– for example, do you often forget what you want to buy when you go shopping?
YES
Are you depressed or worried about anything?
YES
Emotional stress may be affecting your ability to concentrate. See DEPRESSION, p.321, and ANXIETY, p.324.
NO
1 Go to next page, first column
NO
2 Go to next page, second column

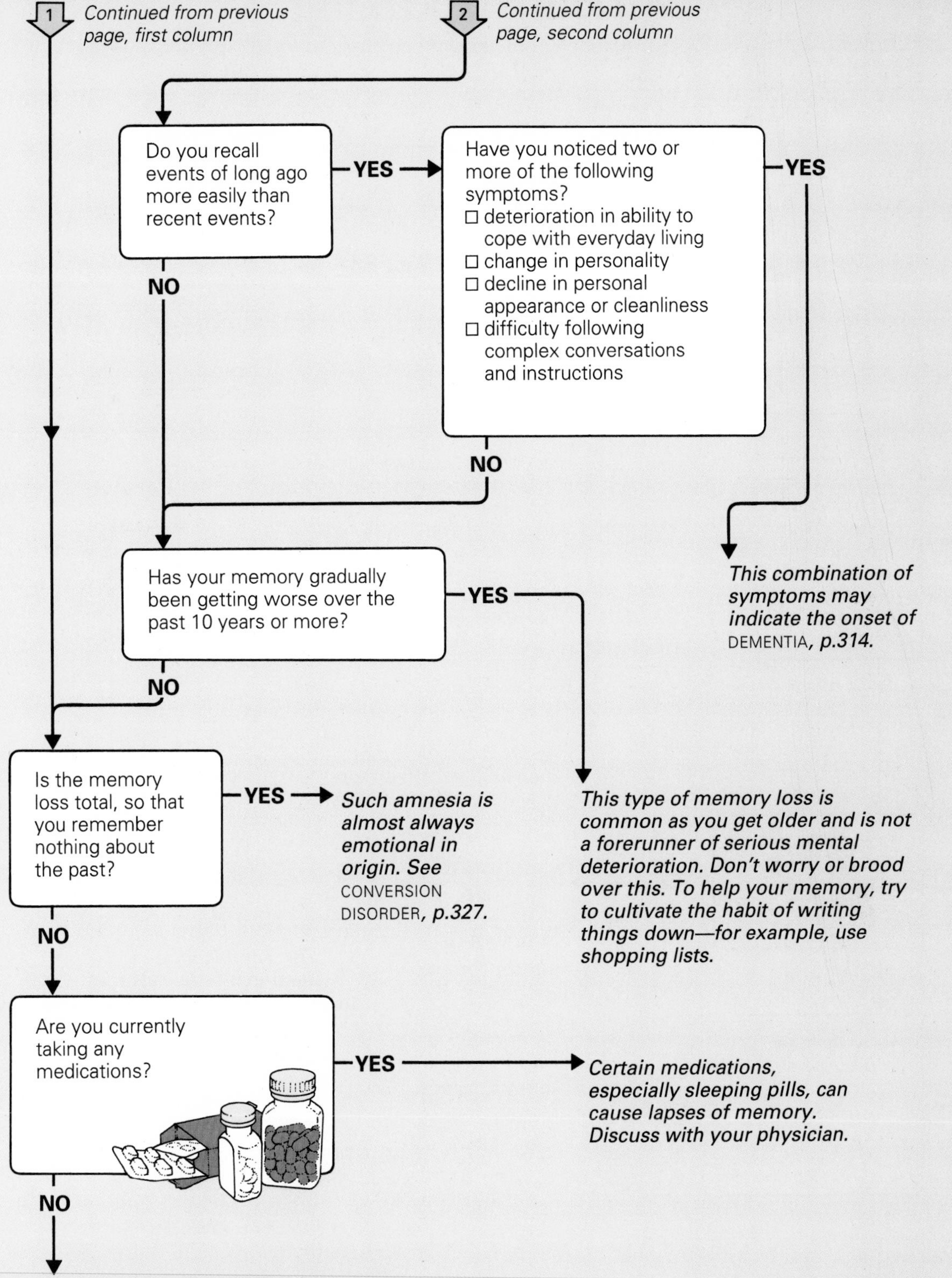

1
Continued from previous page, first column
2
Continued from previous page, second column
Do you recall events of long ago more easily than recent events?
YES
NO
Have you noticed two or more of the following symptoms?
□ deterioration in ability to cope with everyday living
□ change in personality
□ decline in personal appearance or cleanliness
□ difficulty following complex conversations and instructions
YES
NO
This combination of symptoms may indicate the onset of DEMENTIA, p.314.
Has your memory gradually been getting worse over the past 10 years or more?
YES
NO
Is the memory loss total, so that you remember nothing about the past?
YES
Such amnesia is almost always emotional in origin. See CONVERSION DISORDER, p.327.
This type of memory loss is common as you get older and is not a forerunner of serious mental deterioration. Don't worry or brood over this. To help your memory, try to cultivate the habit of writing things down—for example, use shopping lists.
NO
Are you currently taking any medications?
YES
Certain medications, especially sleeping pills, can cause lapses of memory. Discuss with your physician.
NO

If you are unable to make a diagnosis from this chart, consult your physician.

17 GENERAL all ages

Difficulty speaking

A deterioration in the ability to choose, use, or pronounce words.

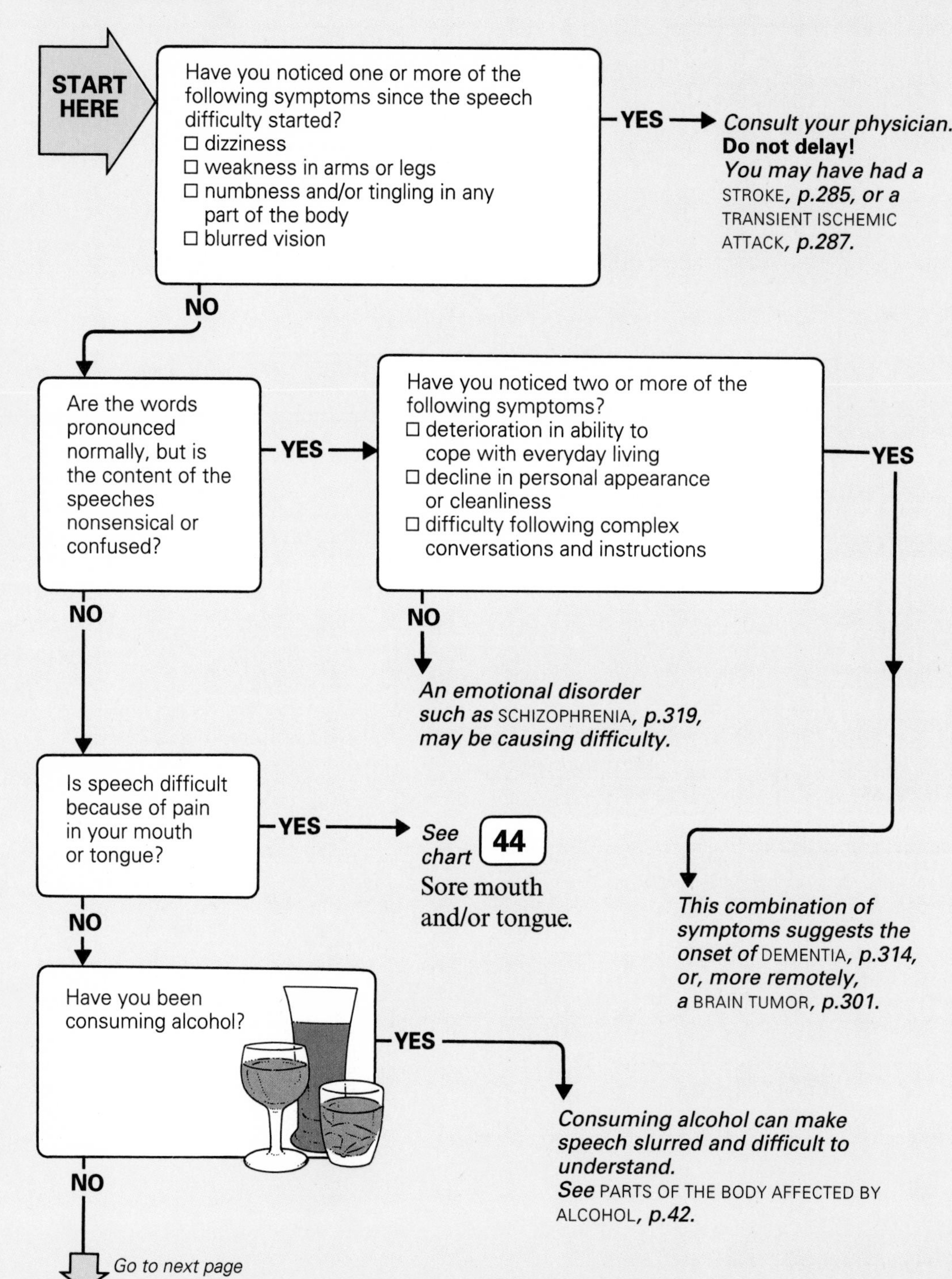

START HERE
Have you noticed one or more of the following symptoms since the speech difficulty started?
☐ dizziness
☐ weakness in arms or legs
☐ numbness and/or tingling in any part of the body
☐ blurred vision
YES
Consult your physician. **Do not delay!** *You may have had a* STROKE, *p.285, or a* TRANSIENT ISCHEMIC ATTACK, *p.287.*
NO
Are the words pronounced normally, but is the content of the speeches nonsensical or confused?
YES
Have you noticed two or more of the following symptoms?
☐ deterioration in ability to cope with everyday living
☐ decline in personal appearance or cleanliness
☐ difficulty following complex conversations and instructions
YES
This combination of symptoms suggests the onset of DEMENTIA, *p.314, or, more remotely, a* BRAIN TUMOR, *p.301.*
NO
An emotional disorder such as SCHIZOPHRENIA, *p.319, may be causing difficulty.*
NO
Is speech difficult because of pain in your mouth or tongue?
YES
See chart 44 Sore mouth and/or tongue.
NO
Have you been consuming alcohol?
YES
Consuming alcohol can make speech slurred and difficult to understand.
See PARTS OF THE BODY AFFECTED BY ALCOHOL, *p.42.*
NO
Go to next page

Continued from previous page

Are you currently taking any medications?

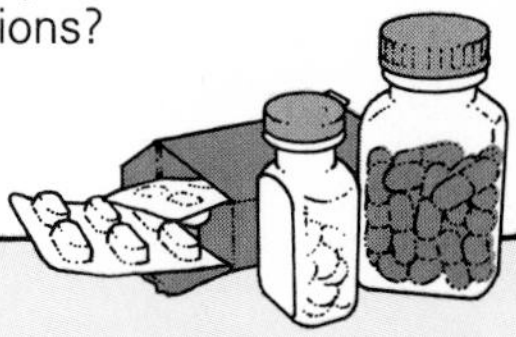

YES → ***Some drugs can affect speech. Discuss with your physician.***

NO ↓

Is speech difficult because you are unable to move the muscles on one side of your face?

YES → ***You may have*** BELL'S PALSY, ***p.298, a disorder of the facial nerves.***

NO ↓

Does your speech lack normal variations in tone and pauses, so that it sounds expressionless?

YES → Do your hands tremble?

YES → ***These symptoms suggest*** PARKINSON'S DISEASE, ***p.312, a disorder of the nervous system.***

NO ↓

NO ↓

Are you sometimes unable to speak even though you know what you want to say AND/OR do you sometimes get stuck at the beginning of a word and find yourself repeating the first consonant for several seconds before you can get the whole word out?

YES → ***Discuss with your physician. This stammering or stuttering often develops in early childhood but—even if it is brought under control in the school years—may recur in an adult under stress.***

NO ↓

If you are unable to make a diagnosis from this chart, consult your physician.

18 GENERAL all ages

Disturbing thoughts and feelings

Any thoughts or feelings that may seem (whether to other people or to you) to be abnormal or unhealthy.

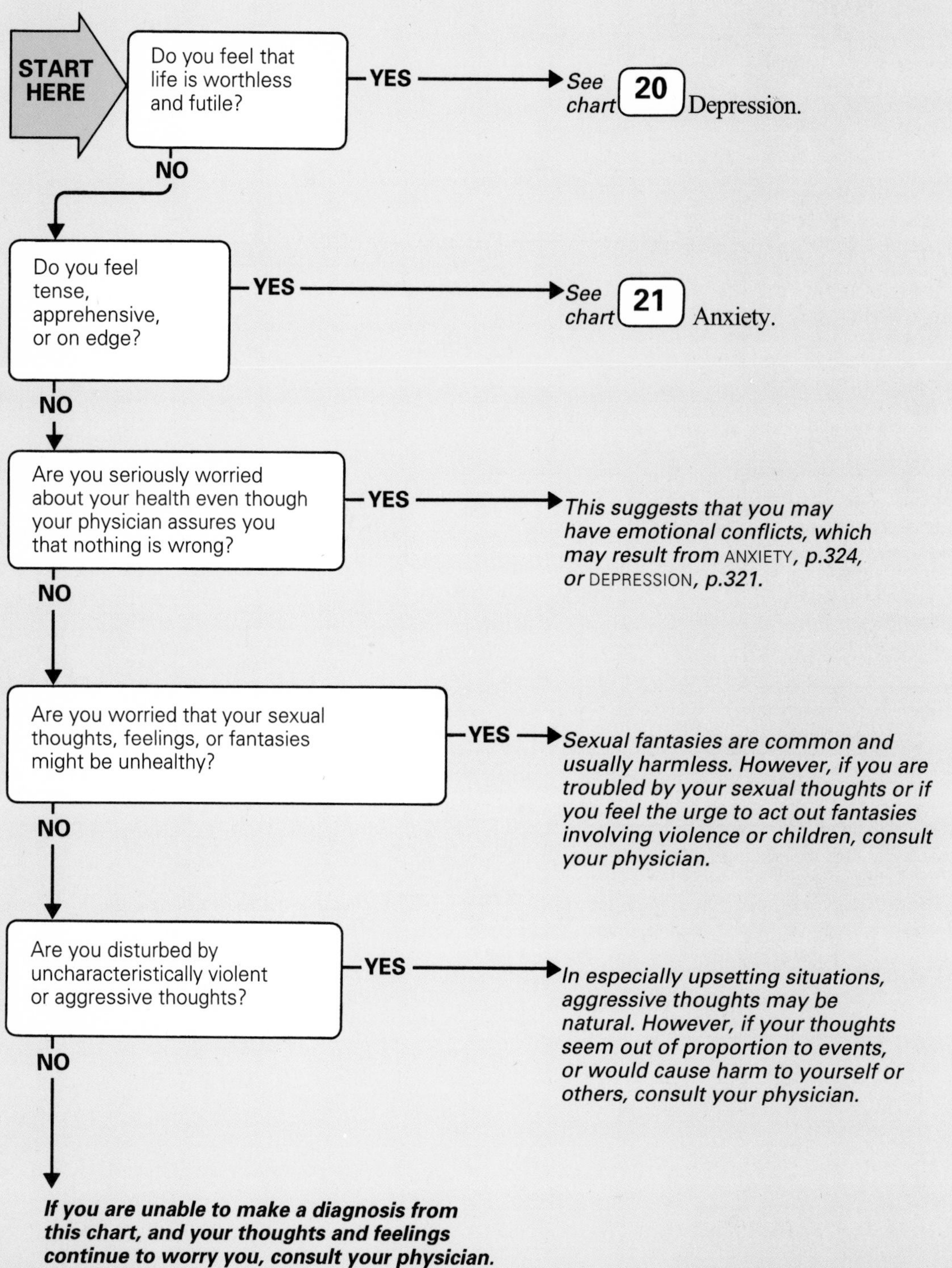

START HERE
Do you feel that life is worthless and futile?
YES
See chart 20 Depression.
NO
Do you feel tense, apprehensive, or on edge?
YES
See chart 21 Anxiety.
NO
Are you seriously worried about your health even though your physician assures you that nothing is wrong?
YES
This suggests that you may have emotional conflicts, which may result from ANXIETY, p.324, or DEPRESSION, p.321.
NO
Are you worried that your sexual thoughts, feelings, or fantasies might be unhealthy?
YES
Sexual fantasies are common and usually harmless. However, if you are troubled by your sexual thoughts or if you feel the urge to act out fantasies involving violence or children, consult your physician.
NO
Are you disturbed by uncharacteristically violent or aggressive thoughts?
YES
In especially upsetting situations, aggressive thoughts may be natural. However, if your thoughts seem out of proportion to events, or would cause harm to yourself or others, consult your physician.
NO
If you are unable to make a diagnosis from this chart, and your thoughts and feelings continue to worry you, consult your physician.

19 **GENERAL** all ages

Strange behavior

Any behavior, whether it develops suddenly or gradually, that seems out of keeping with previous behavior patterns.

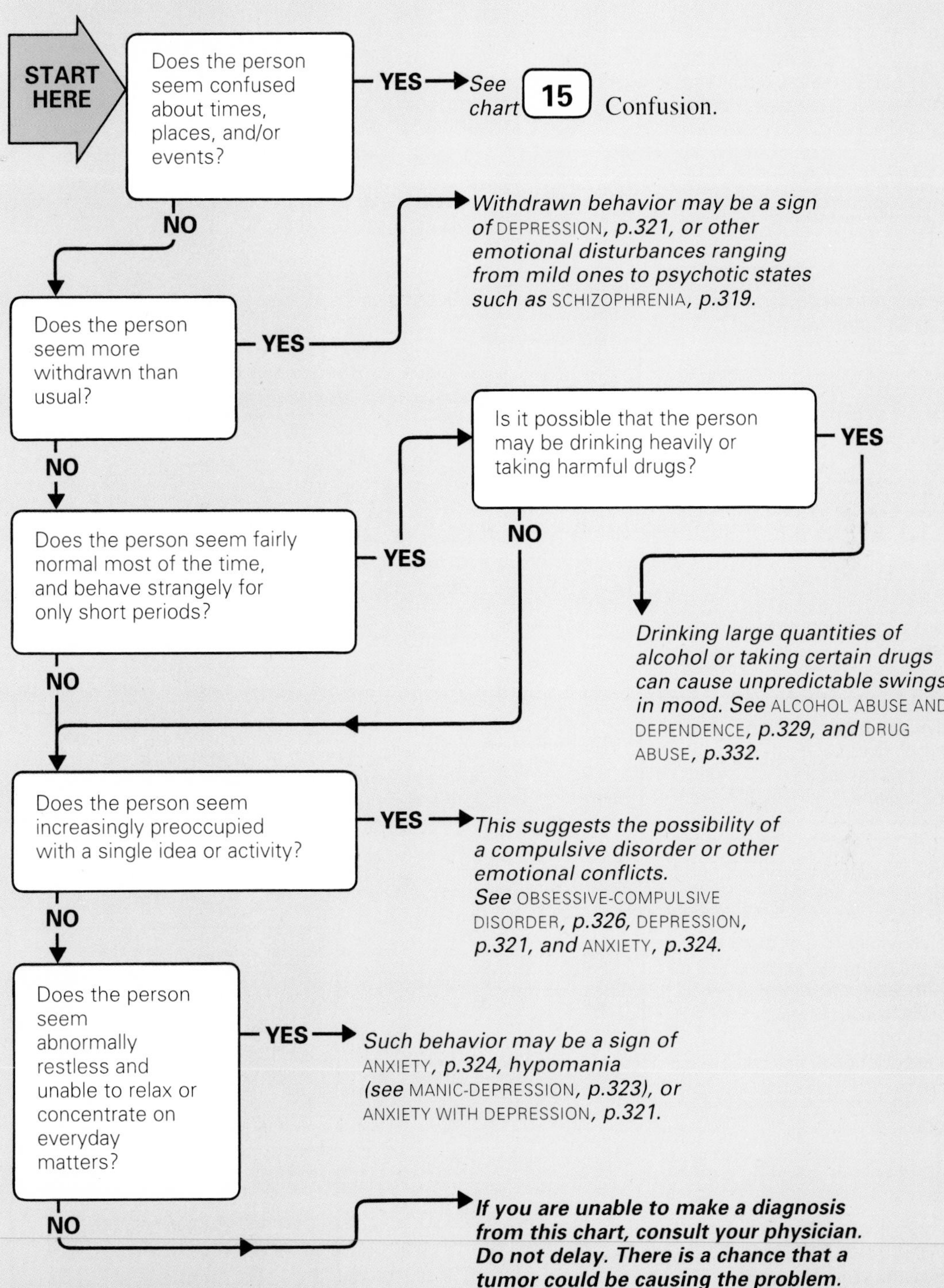

START HERE
Does the person seem confused about times, places, and/or events?
YES → See chart 15 Confusion.
NO
Does the person seem more withdrawn than usual?
YES → *Withdrawn behavior may be a sign of* DEPRESSION, *p.321, or other emotional disturbances ranging from mild ones to psychotic states such as* SCHIZOPHRENIA, *p.319.*
NO
Does the person seem fairly normal most of the time, and behave strangely for only short periods?
YES → Is it possible that the person may be drinking heavily or taking harmful drugs?
YES → *Drinking large quantities of alcohol or taking certain drugs can cause unpredictable swings in mood. See* ALCOHOL ABUSE AND DEPENDENCE, *p.329, and* DRUG ABUSE, *p.332.*
NO
NO
Does the person seem increasingly preoccupied with a single idea or activity?
YES → *This suggests the possibility of a compulsive disorder or other emotional conflicts. See* OBSESSIVE-COMPULSIVE DISORDER, *p.326,* DEPRESSION, *p.321, and* ANXIETY, *p.324.*
NO
Does the person seem abnormally restless and unable to relax or concentrate on everyday matters?
YES → *Such behavior may be a sign of* ANXIETY, *p.324, hypomania (see* MANIC-DEPRESSION, *p.323), or* ANXIETY WITH DEPRESSION, *p.321.*
NO
If you are unable to make a diagnosis from this chart, consult your physician. Do not delay. There is a chance that a tumor could be causing the problem.

20
GENERAL
all ages

Depression

A feeling of sadness, futility, unworthiness, despair, or guilt that may make you unable to cope with normal life.

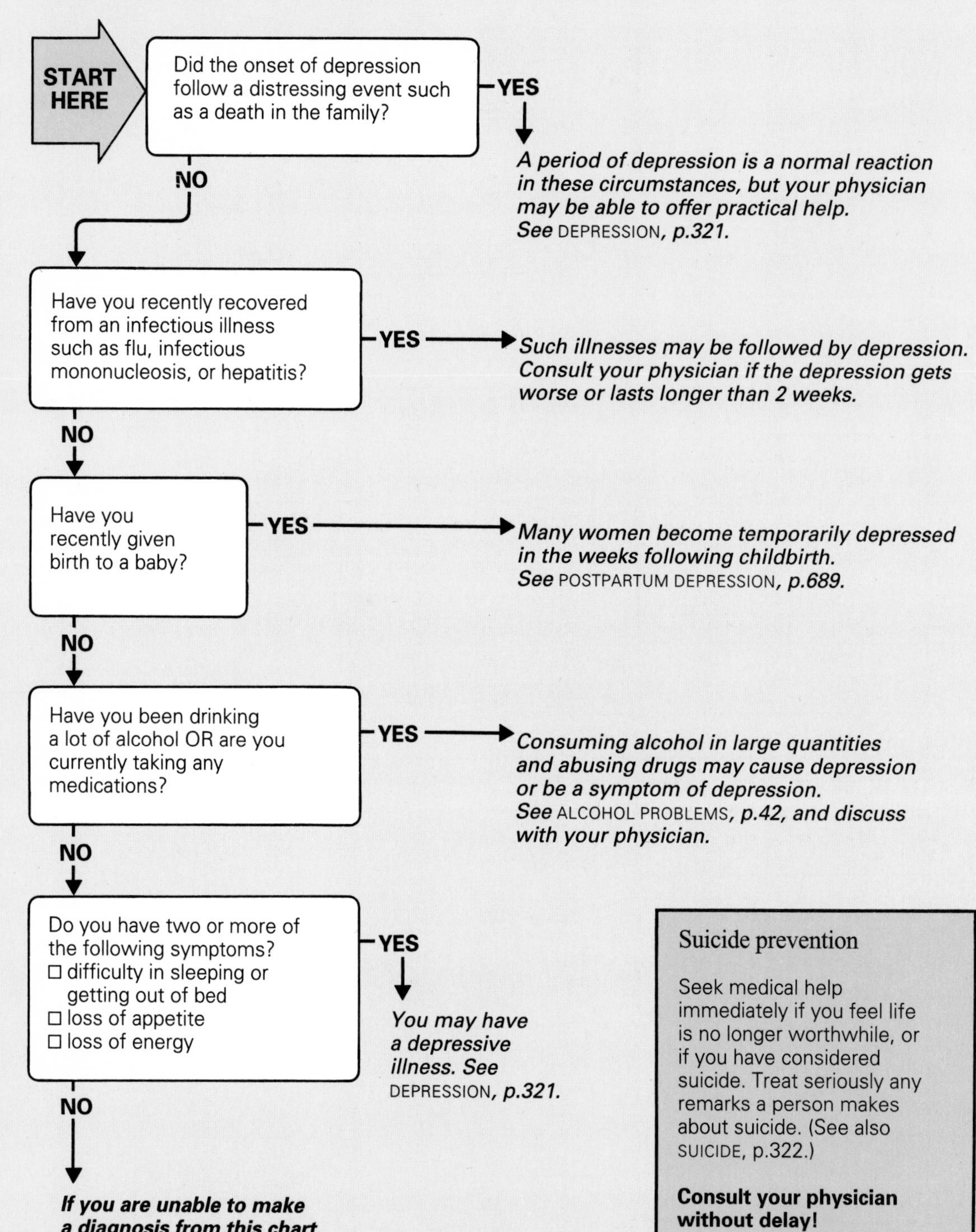

START HERE
Did the onset of depression follow a distressing event such as a death in the family?
YES
A period of depression is a normal reaction in these circumstances, but your physician may be able to offer practical help. See DEPRESSION, p.321.
NO
Have you recently recovered from an infectious illness such as flu, infectious mononucleosis, or hepatitis?
YES
Such illnesses may be followed by depression. Consult your physician if the depression gets worse or lasts longer than 2 weeks.
NO
Have you recently given birth to a baby?
YES
Many women become temporarily depressed in the weeks following childbirth. See POSTPARTUM DEPRESSION, p.689.
NO
Have you been drinking a lot of alcohol OR are you currently taking any medications?
YES
Consuming alcohol in large quantities and abusing drugs may cause depression or be a symptom of depression. See ALCOHOL PROBLEMS, p.42, and discuss with your physician.
NO
Do you have two or more of the following symptoms?
☐ difficulty in sleeping or getting out of bed
☐ loss of appetite
☐ loss of energy
YES
You may have a depressive illness. See DEPRESSION, p.321.
NO
If you are unable to make a diagnosis from this chart, consult your physician.

Suicide prevention

Seek medical help immediately if you feel life is no longer worthwhile, or if you have considered suicide. Treat seriously any remarks a person makes about suicide. (See also SUICIDE, p.322.)

Consult your physician without delay!

21
GENERAL
all ages

Anxiety

A feeling of tenseness, apprehension, or edginess, which may be accompanied by physical symptoms such as palpitations or diarrhea.

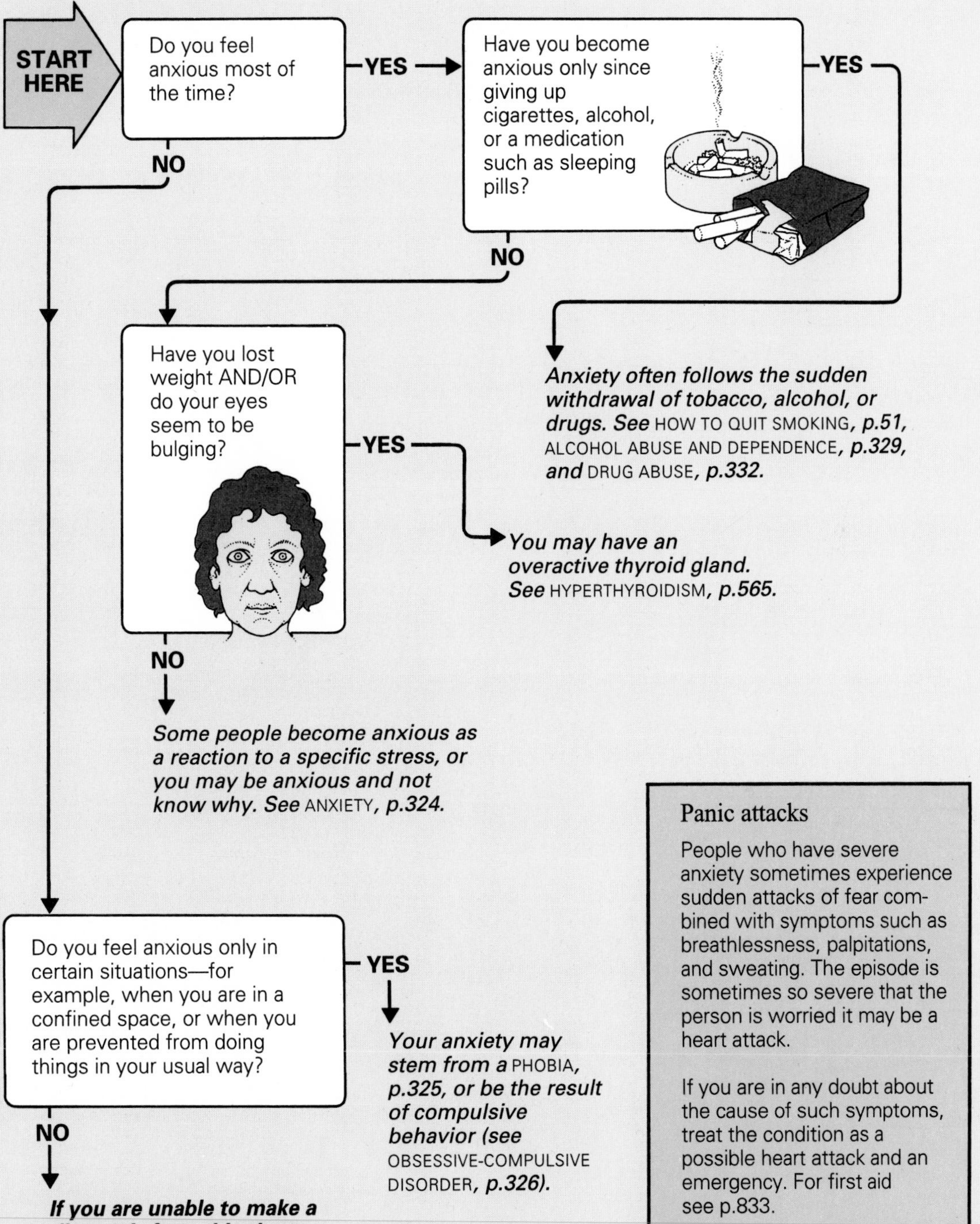

START HERE
Do you feel anxious most of the time?
YES
NO
Have you become anxious only since giving up cigarettes, alcohol, or a medication such as sleeping pills?
YES
NO
Anxiety often follows the sudden withdrawal of tobacco, alcohol, or drugs. See HOW TO QUIT SMOKING, *p.51,* ALCOHOL ABUSE AND DEPENDENCE, *p.329, and* DRUG ABUSE, *p.332.*
Have you lost weight AND/OR do your eyes seem to be bulging?
YES
You may have an overactive thyroid gland. See HYPERTHYROIDISM, *p.565.*
NO
Some people become anxious as a reaction to a specific stress, or you may be anxious and not know why. See ANXIETY, *p.324.*
Do you feel anxious only in certain situations—for example, when you are in a confined space, or when you are prevented from doing things in your usual way?
YES
Your anxiety may stem from a PHOBIA, *p.325, or be the result of compulsive behavior (see* OBSESSIVE-COMPULSIVE DISORDER, *p.326).*
NO
If you are unable to make a diagnosis from this chart, consult your physician.

Panic attacks

People who have severe anxiety sometimes experience sudden attacks of fear combined with symptoms such as breathlessness, palpitations, and sweating. The episode is sometimes so severe that the person is worried it may be a heart attack.

If you are in any doubt about the cause of such symptoms, treat the condition as a possible heart attack and an emergency. For first aid see p.833.

22
GENERAL
all ages

Hallucinations

Mistakenly and repeatedly hearing, feeling, smelling, or seeing things that are not heard, felt, smelled, or seen by other people.

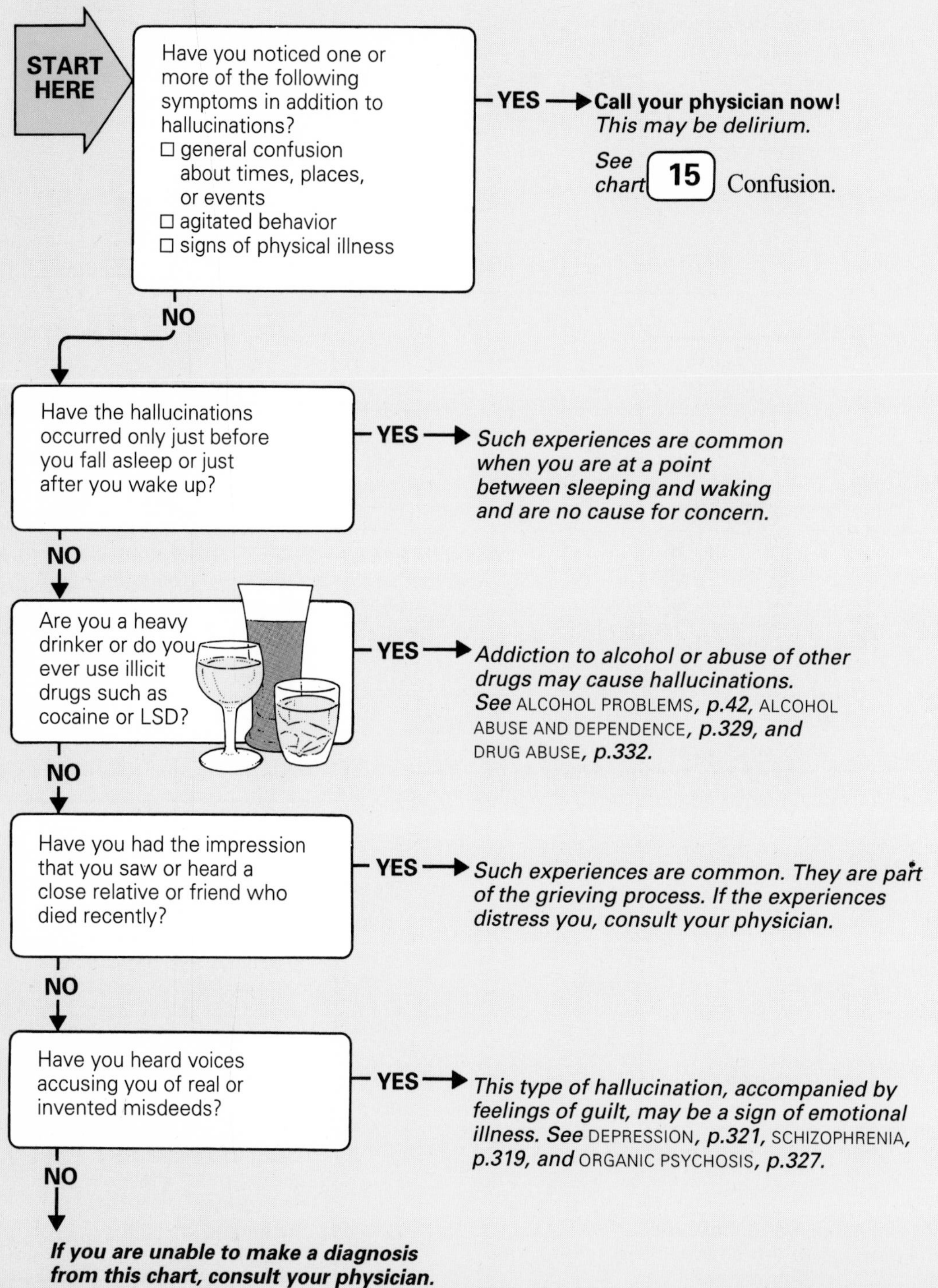

START HERE
Have you noticed one or more of the following symptoms in addition to hallucinations?
☐ general confusion about times, places, or events
☐ agitated behavior
☐ signs of physical illness
YES → Call your physician now! This may be delirium.
See chart 15 Confusion.
NO
Have the hallucinations occurred only just before you fall asleep or just after you wake up?
YES → Such experiences are common when you are at a point between sleeping and waking and are no cause for concern.
NO
Are you a heavy drinker or do you ever use illicit drugs such as cocaine or LSD?
YES → Addiction to alcohol or abuse of other drugs may cause hallucinations. See ALCOHOL PROBLEMS, p.42, ALCOHOL ABUSE AND DEPENDENCE, p.329, and DRUG ABUSE, p.332.
NO
Have you had the impression that you saw or heard a close relative or friend who died recently?
YES → Such experiences are common. They are part of the grieving process. If the experiences distress you, consult your physician.
NO
Have you heard voices accusing you of real or invented misdeeds?
YES → This type of hallucination, accompanied by feelings of guilt, may be a sign of emotional illness. See DEPRESSION, p.321, SCHIZOPHRENIA, p.319, and ORGANIC PSYCHOSIS, p.327.
NO
If you are unable to make a diagnosis from this chart, consult your physician.

23 GENERAL all ages

Nightmares

Frightening dreams that may be disturbing enough to wake you.

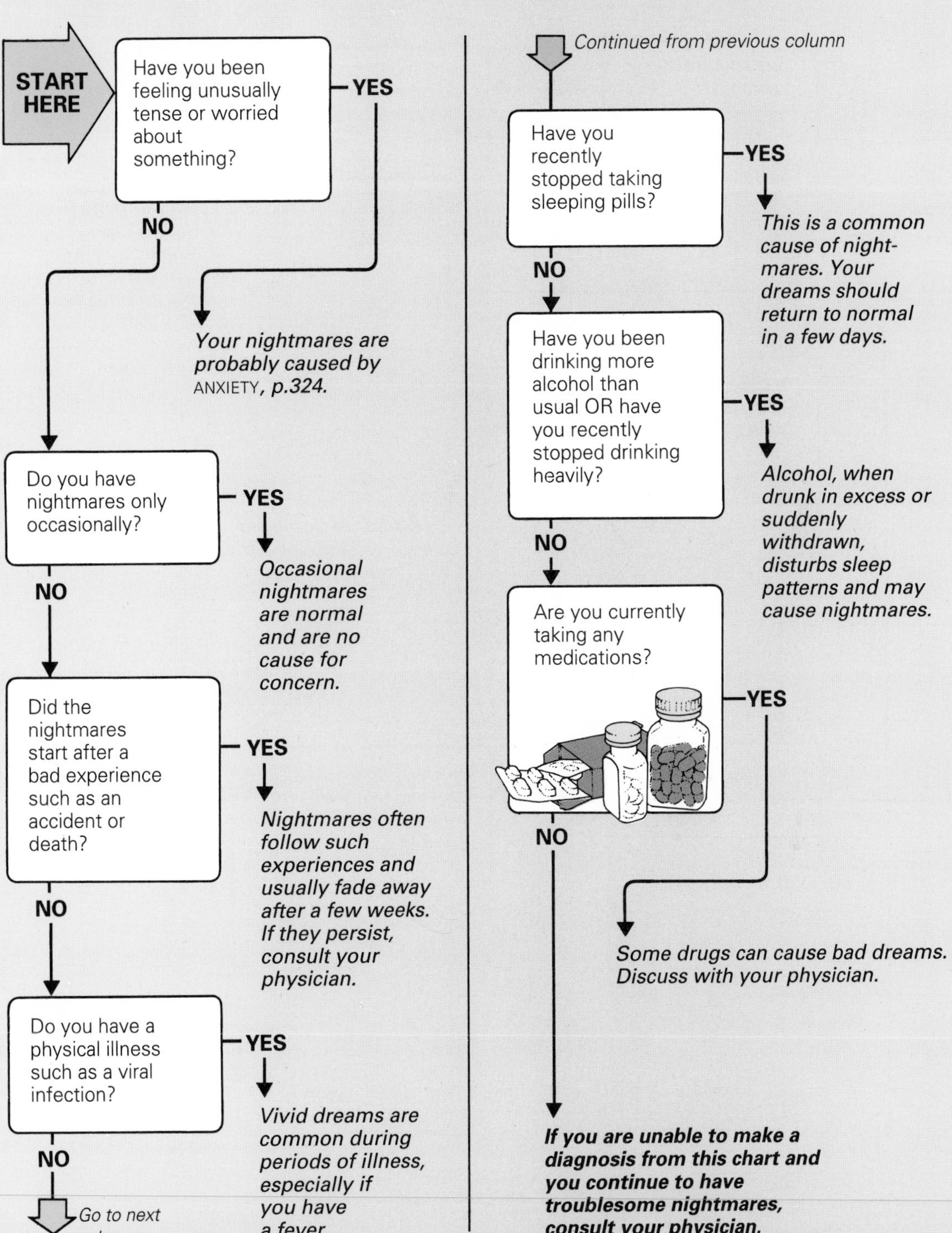

START HERE
Have you been feeling unusually tense or worried about something?
YES
Your nightmares are probably caused by ANXIETY*, p.324.*
NO
Do you have nightmares only occasionally?
YES
Occasional nightmares are normal and are no cause for concern.
NO
Did the nightmares start after a bad experience such as an accident or death?
YES
Nightmares often follow such experiences and usually fade away after a few weeks. If they persist, consult your physician.
NO
Do you have a physical illness such as a viral infection?
YES
Vivid dreams are common during periods of illness, especially if you have a fever.
NO
Go to next column
Continued from previous column
Have you recently stopped taking sleeping pills?
YES
This is a common cause of night-mares. Your dreams should return to normal in a few days.
NO
Have you been drinking more alcohol than usual OR have you recently stopped drinking heavily?
YES
Alcohol, when drunk in excess or suddenly withdrawn, disturbs sleep patterns and may cause nightmares.
NO
Are you currently taking any medications?
YES
Some drugs can cause bad dreams. Discuss with your physician.
NO
If you are unable to make a diagnosis from this chart and you continue to have troublesome nightmares, consult your physician.

24

GENERAL
all ages

Hair loss

Thinning or loss of hair on all or part of the head.

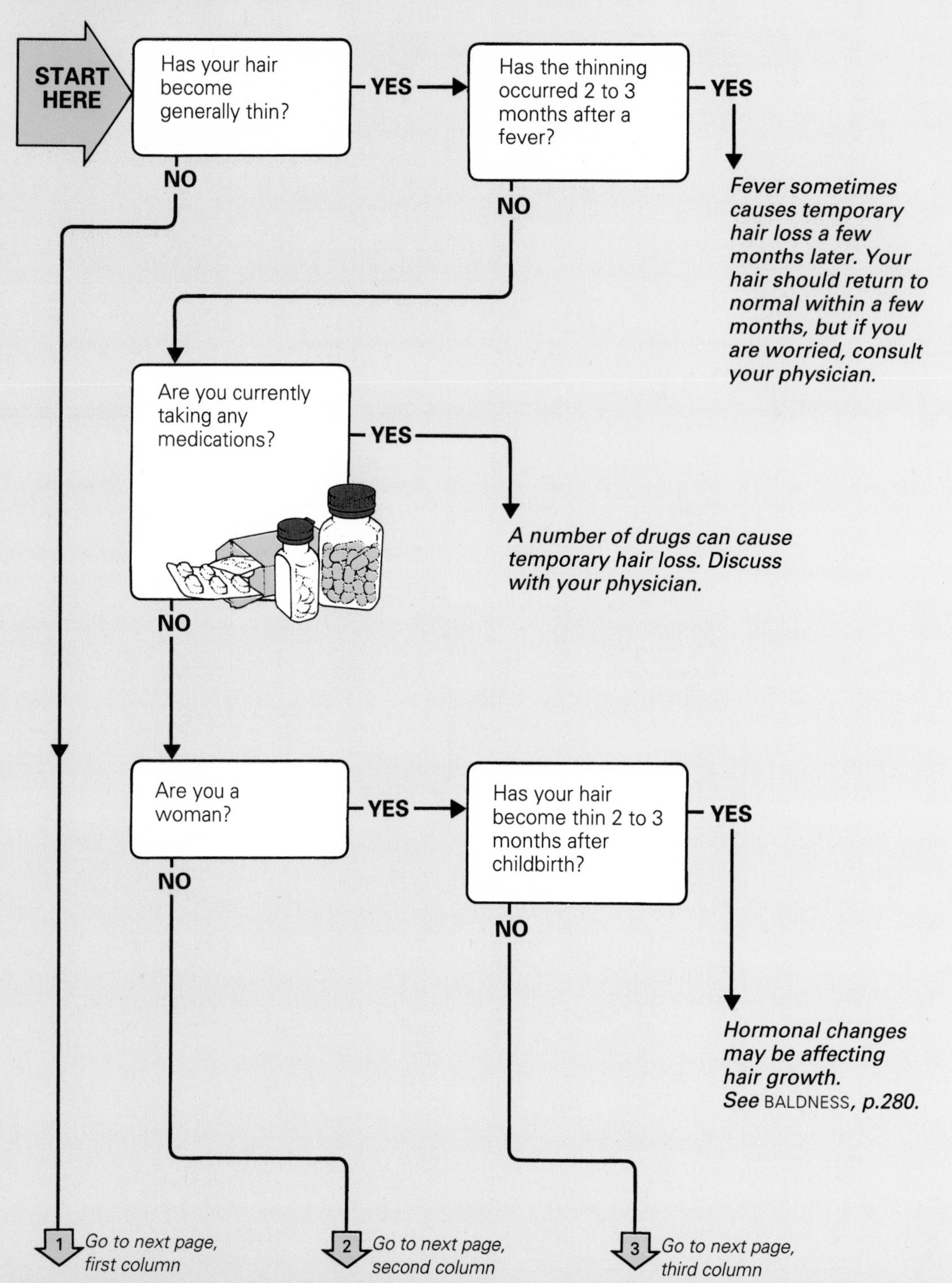
START HERE
Has your hair become generally thin?
YES
Has the thinning occurred 2 to 3 months after a fever?
YES
Fever sometimes causes temporary hair loss a few months later. Your hair should return to normal within a few months, but if you are worried, consult your physician.
NO
NO
Are you currently taking any medications?
YES
A number of drugs can cause temporary hair loss. Discuss with your physician.
NO
Are you a woman?
YES
Has your hair become thin 2 to 3 months after childbirth?
YES
Hormonal changes may be affecting hair growth.
See BALDNESS, *p.280.*
NO
NO
1 *Go to next page, first column*
2 *Go to next page, second column*
3 *Go to next page, third column*

23 **GENERAL** all ages

Nightmares

Frightening dreams that may be disturbing enough to wake you.

START HERE

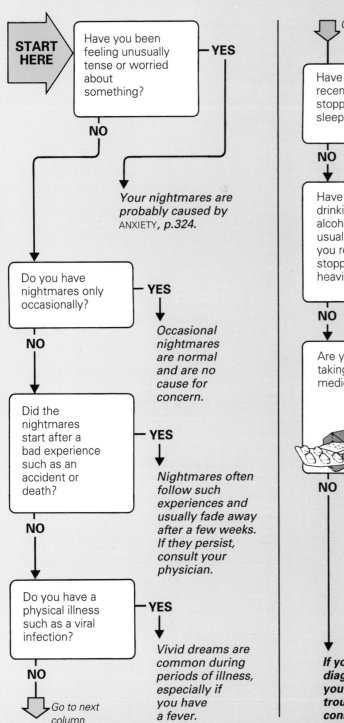

Have you been feeling unusually tense or worried about something?

YES → *Your nightmares are probably caused by* ANXIETY*, p.324.*

NO ↓

Do you have nightmares only occasionally?

YES → *Occasional nightmares are normal and are no cause for concern.*

NO ↓

Did the nightmares start after a bad experience such as an accident or death?

YES → *Nightmares often follow such experiences and usually fade away after a few weeks. If they persist, consult your physician.*

NO ↓

Do you have a physical illness such as a viral infection?

YES → *Vivid dreams are common during periods of illness, especially if you have a fever.*

NO ↓

Go to next column

Continued from previous column

Have you recently stopped taking sleeping pills?

YES → *This is a common cause of night-mares. Your dreams should return to normal in a few days.*

NO ↓

Have you been drinking more alcohol than usual OR have you recently stopped drinking heavily?

YES → *Alcohol, when drunk in excess or suddenly withdrawn, disturbs sleep patterns and may cause nightmares.*

NO ↓

Are you currently taking any medications?

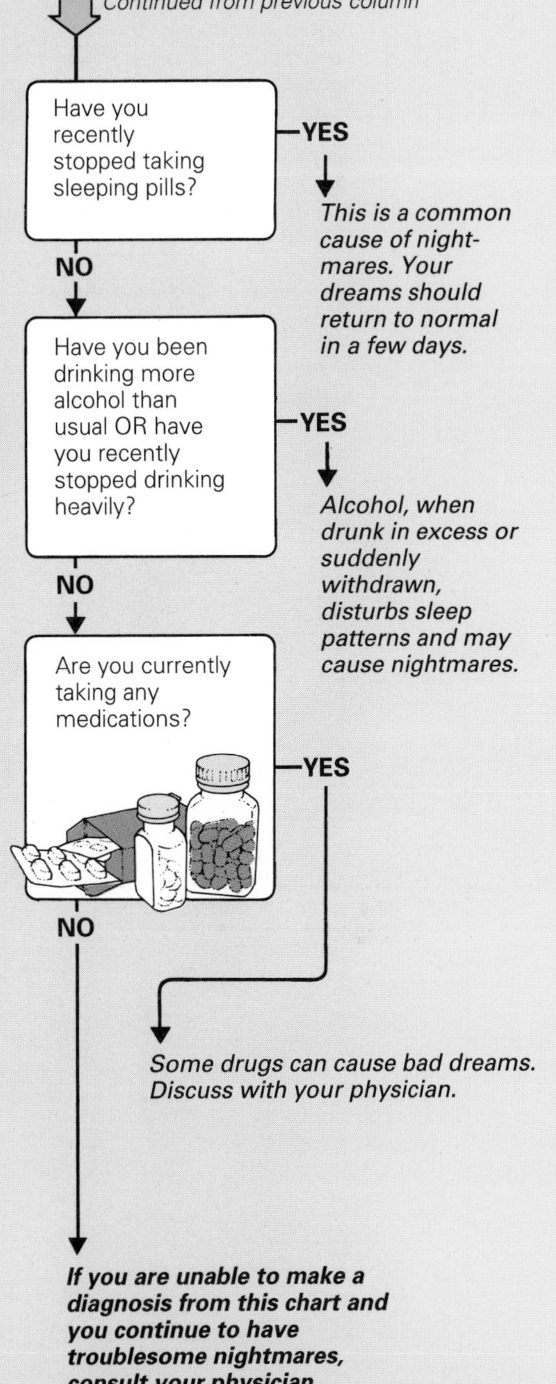

YES → *Some drugs can cause bad dreams. Discuss with your physician.*

NO ↓

If you are unable to make a diagnosis from this chart and you continue to have troublesome nightmares, consult your physician.

24 GENERAL all ages

Hair loss

Thinning or loss of hair on all or part of the head.

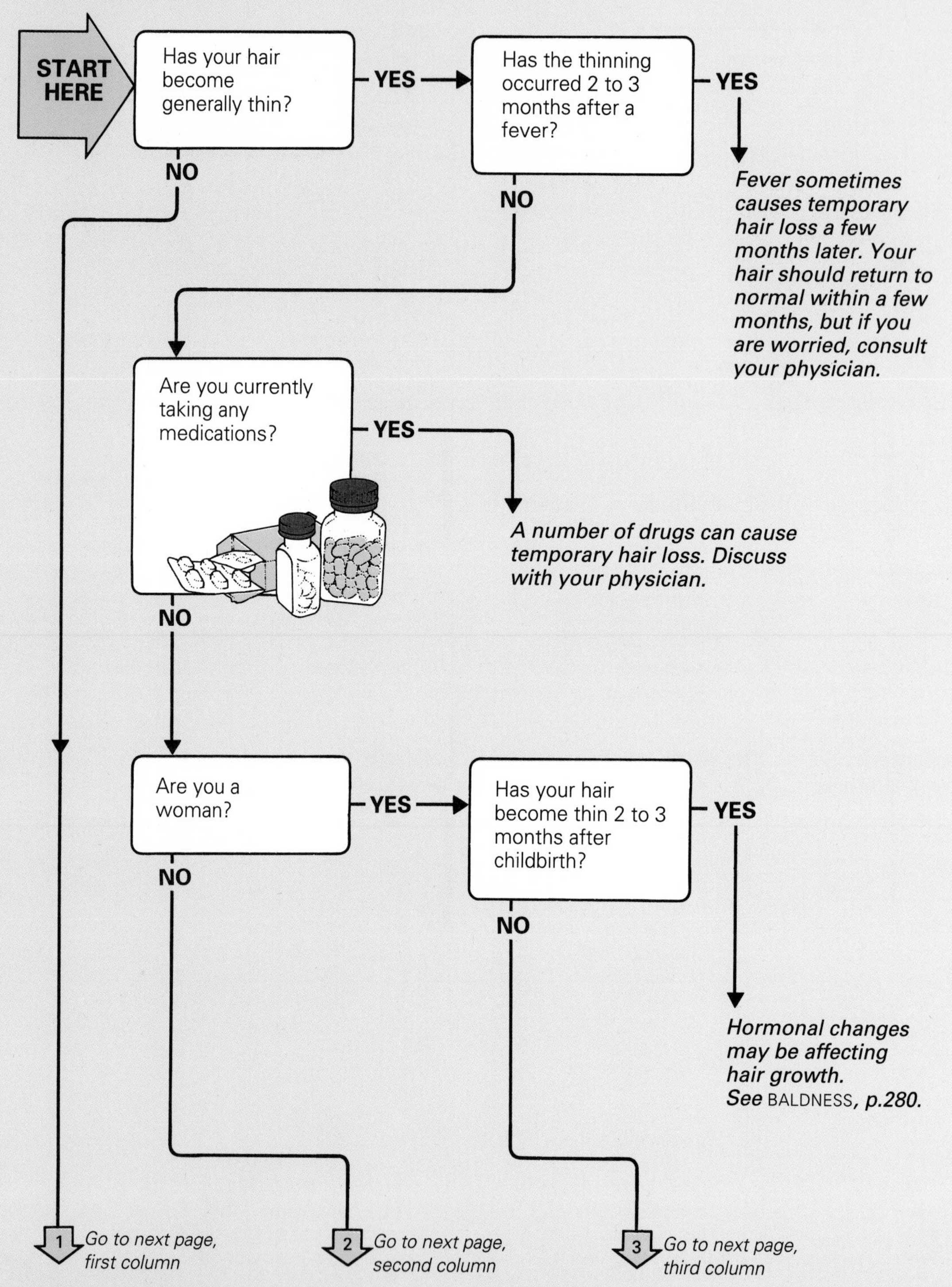
START HERE
Has your hair become generally thin?
YES
NO
Has the thinning occurred 2 to 3 months after a fever?
YES
NO
Fever sometimes causes temporary hair loss a few months later. Your hair should return to normal within a few months, but if you are worried, consult your physician.
Are you currently taking any medications?
YES
NO
A number of drugs can cause temporary hair loss. Discuss with your physician.
Are you a woman?
YES
NO
Has your hair become thin 2 to 3 months after childbirth?
YES
NO
Hormonal changes may be affecting hair growth.
See BALDNESS, p.280.
1 Go to next page, first column
2 Go to next page, second column
3 Go to next page, third column

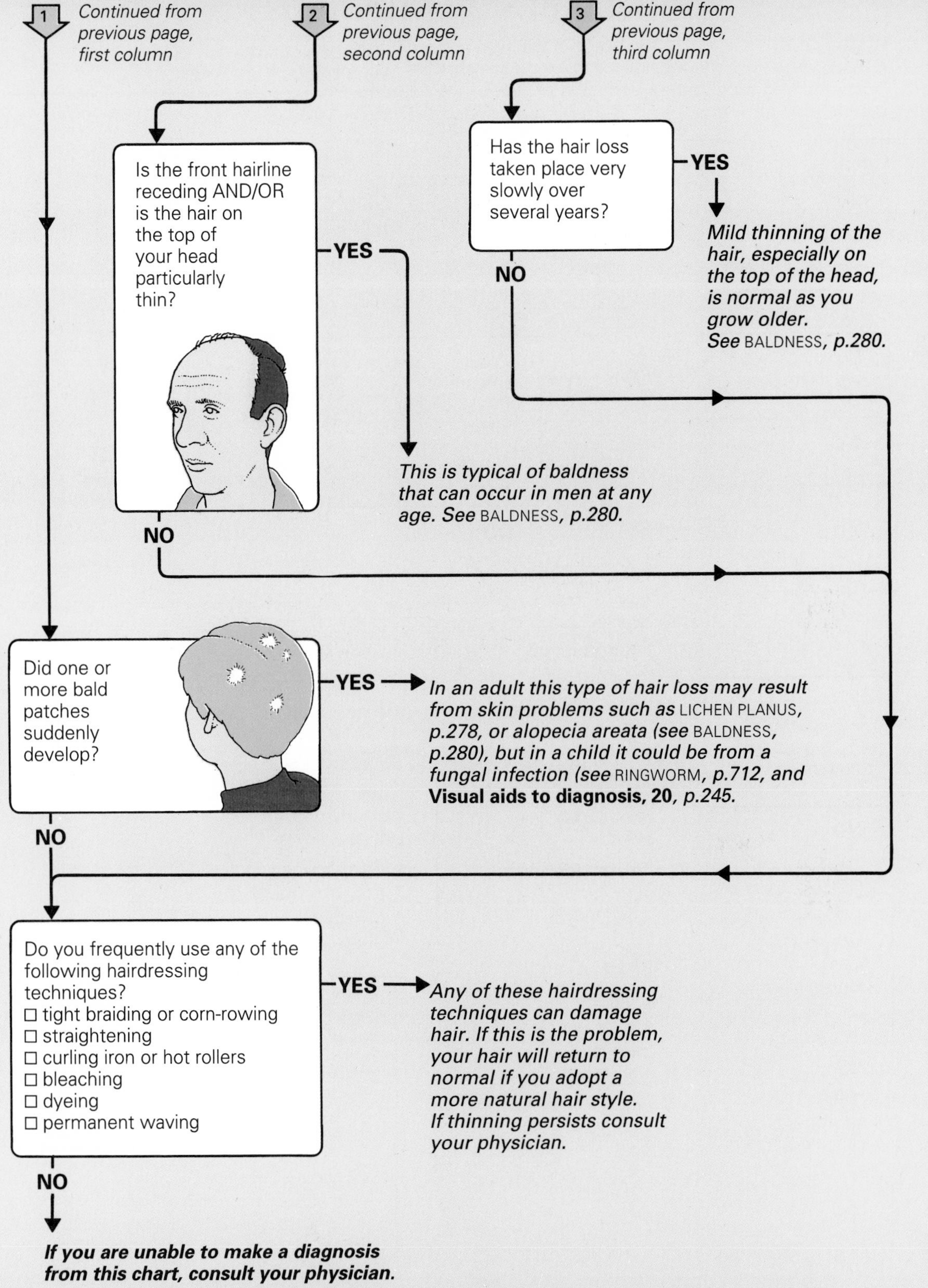
1
Continued from previous page, first column
2
Continued from previous page, second column
3
Continued from previous page, third column
Has the hair loss taken place very slowly over several years?
YES
Mild thinning of the hair, especially on the top of the head, is normal as you grow older. See BALDNESS, *p.280.*
NO
Is the front hairline receding AND/OR is the hair on the top of your head particularly thin?
YES
This is typical of baldness that can occur in men at any age. See BALDNESS, *p.280.*
NO
Did one or more bald patches suddenly develop?
YES
In an adult this type of hair loss may result from skin problems such as LICHEN PLANUS, *p.278, or alopecia areata (see* BALDNESS, *p.280), but in a child it could be from a fungal infection (see* RINGWORM, *p.712, and* **Visual aids to diagnosis, 20**, *p.245.*
NO
Do you frequently use any of the following hairdressing techniques?
☐ tight braiding or corn-rowing
☐ straightening
☐ curling iron or hot rollers
☐ bleaching
☐ dyeing
☐ permanent waving
YES
Any of these hairdressing techniques can damage hair. If this is the problem, your hair will return to normal if you adopt a more natural hair style. If thinning persists consult your physician.
NO
If you are unable to make a diagnosis from this chart, consult your physician.

25
GENERAL
over 2 years

General skin problems

Any change in the skin, including rashes and spots.
For babies under 2 see chart 89, **Skin problems in infants**.

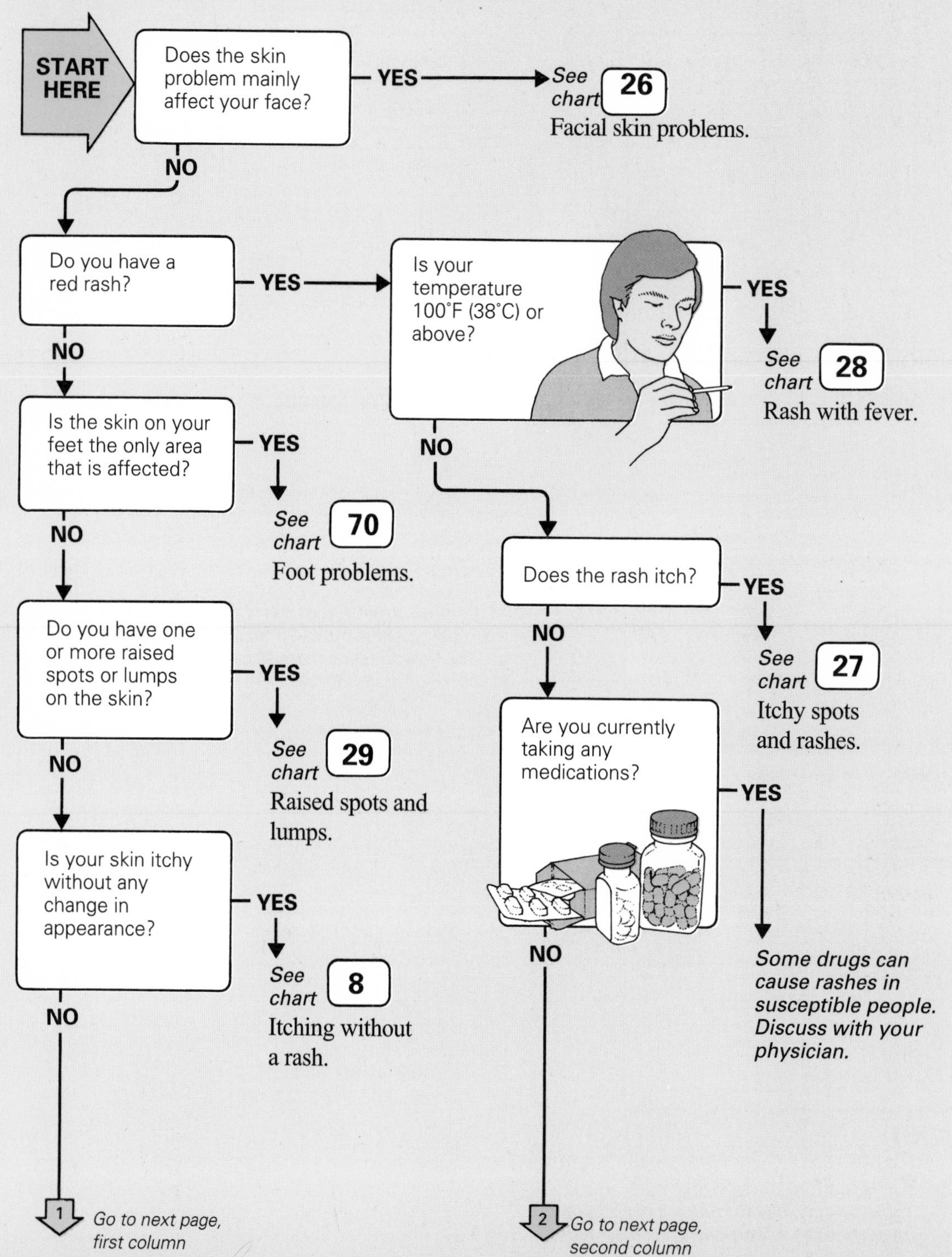

START HERE
Does the skin problem mainly affect your face?
YES
See chart 26
Facial skin problems.
NO
Do you have a red rash?
YES
Is your temperature 100°F (38°C) or above?
YES
See chart 28
Rash with fever.
NO
Does the rash itch?
YES
See chart 27
Itchy spots and rashes.
NO
Are you currently taking any medications?
YES
Some drugs can cause rashes in susceptible people. Discuss with your physician.
NO
2 Go to next page, second column
NO
Is the skin on your feet the only area that is affected?
YES
See chart 70
Foot problems.
NO
Do you have one or more raised spots or lumps on the skin?
YES
See chart 29
Raised spots and lumps.
NO
Is your skin itchy without any change in appearance?
YES
See chart 8
Itching without a rash.
NO
1 Go to next page, first column

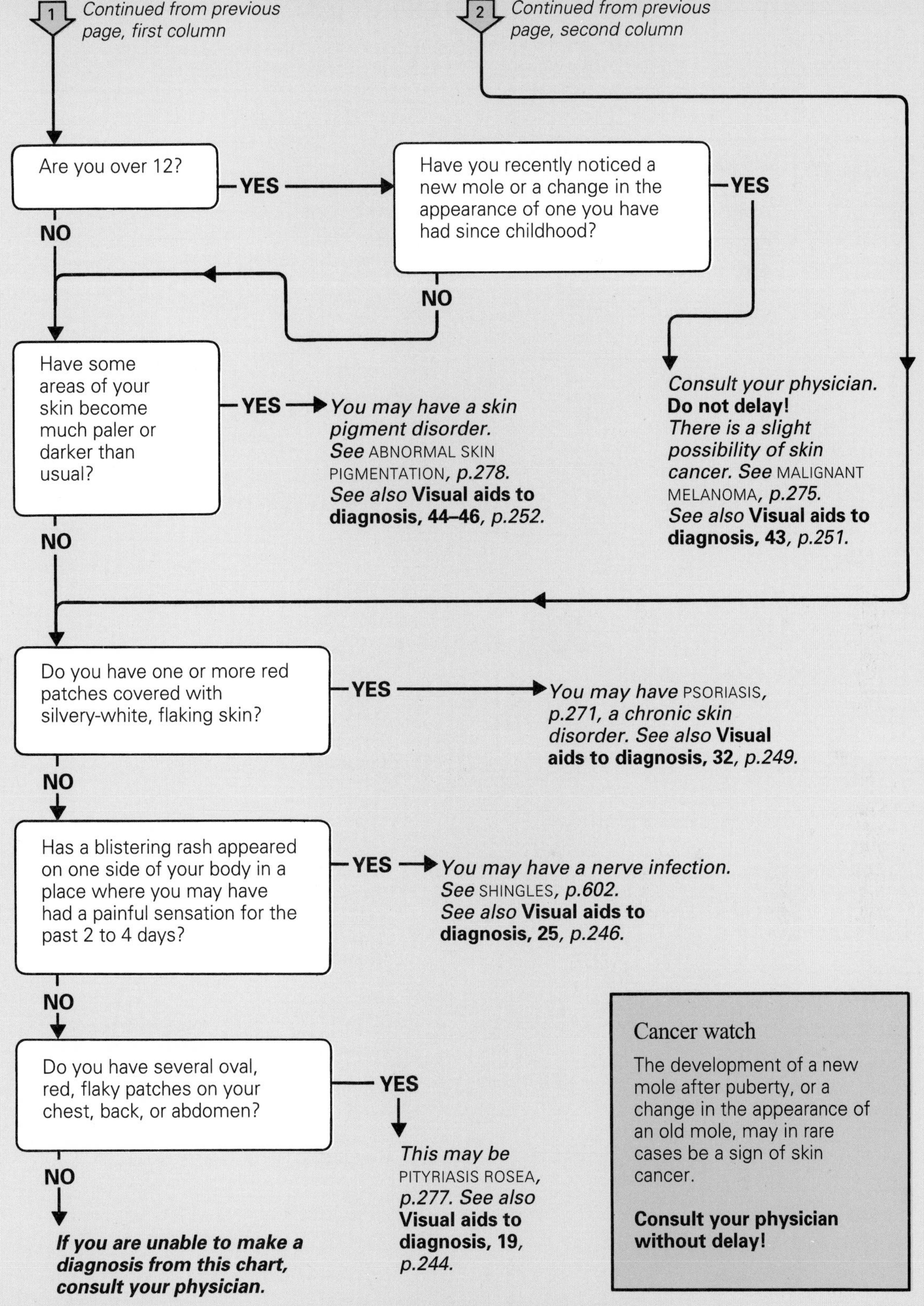
1 Continued from previous page, first column
2 Continued from previous page, second column
Are you over 12?
YES
NO
Have you recently noticed a new mole or a change in the appearance of one you have had since childhood?
YES
NO
Consult your physician. Do not delay! There is a slight possibility of skin cancer. See MALIGNANT MELANOMA, p.275. See also Visual aids to diagnosis, 43, p.251.
Have some areas of your skin become much paler or darker than usual?
YES
You may have a skin pigment disorder. See ABNORMAL SKIN PIGMENTATION, p.278. See also Visual aids to diagnosis, 44–46, p.252.
NO
Do you have one or more red patches covered with silvery-white, flaking skin?
YES
You may have PSORIASIS, p.271, a chronic skin disorder. See also Visual aids to diagnosis, 32, p.249.
NO
Has a blistering rash appeared on one side of your body in a place where you may have had a painful sensation for the past 2 to 4 days?
YES
You may have a nerve infection. See SHINGLES, p.602. See also Visual aids to diagnosis, 25, p.246.
NO
Do you have several oval, red, flaky patches on your chest, back, or abdomen?
YES
This may be PITYRIASIS ROSEA, p.277. See also Visual aids to diagnosis, 19, p.244.
NO
If you are unable to make a diagnosis from this chart, consult your physician.
Cancer watch
The development of a new mole after puberty, or a change in the appearance of an old mole, may in rare cases be a sign of skin cancer.
Consult your physician without delay!

26
GENERAL
over 2 years

Facial skin problems

Any rash, spots, or change in the skin of the face. For babies under 2 years see chart 89, **Skin problems in infants**.

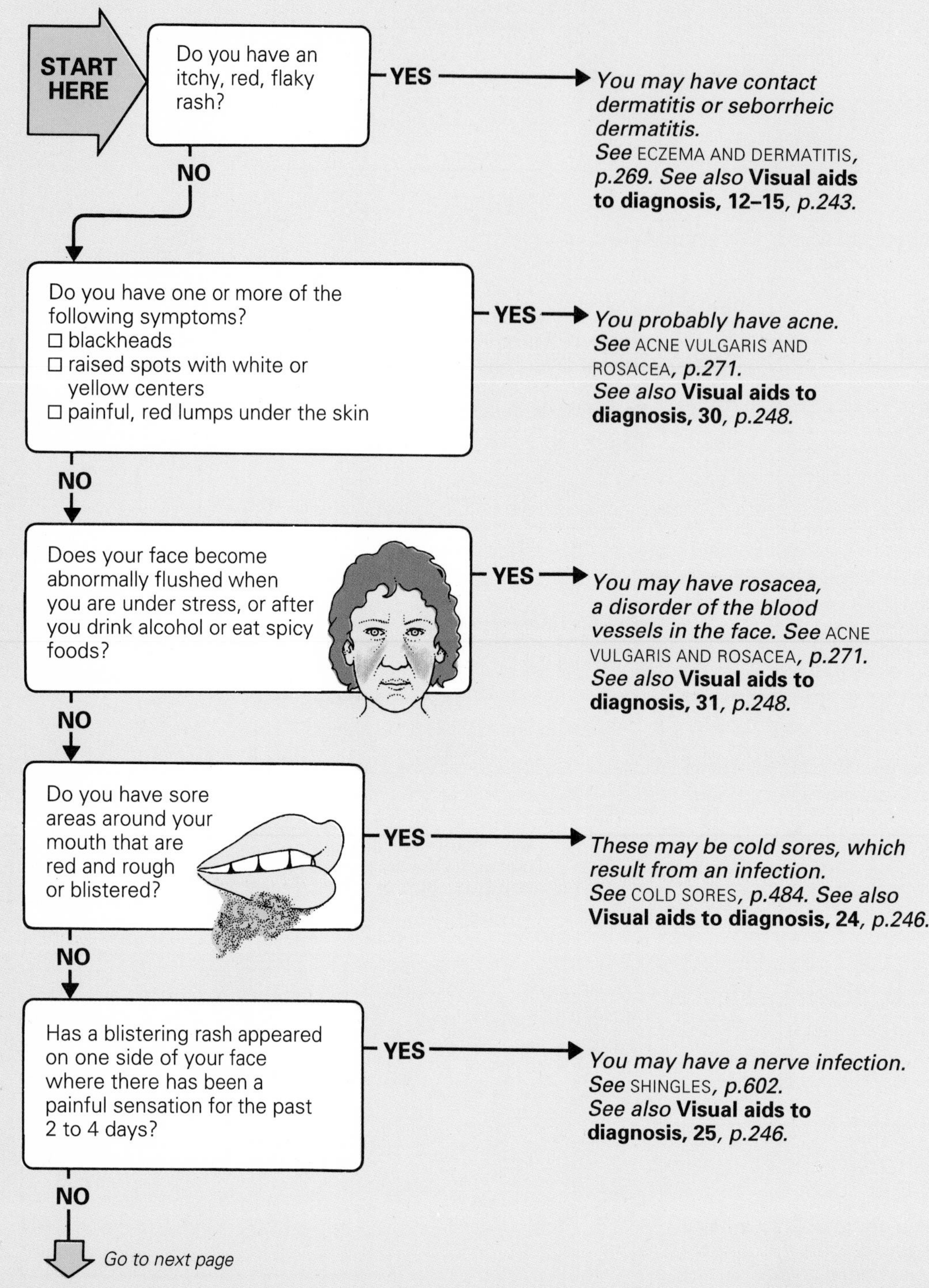

START HERE

Do you have an itchy, red, flaky rash?

YES → *You may have contact dermatitis or seborrheic dermatitis.* *See* ECZEMA AND DERMATITIS, *p.269. See also* **Visual aids to diagnosis, 12–15**, *p.243.*

NO ↓

Do you have one or more of the following symptoms?
- ☐ blackheads
- ☐ raised spots with white or yellow centers
- ☐ painful, red lumps under the skin

YES → *You probably have acne.* *See* ACNE VULGARIS AND ROSACEA, *p.271.* *See also* **Visual aids to diagnosis, 30**, *p.248.*

NO ↓

Does your face become abnormally flushed when you are under stress, or after you drink alcohol or eat spicy foods?

YES → *You may have rosacea, a disorder of the blood vessels in the face. See* ACNE VULGARIS AND ROSACEA, *p.271.* *See also* **Visual aids to diagnosis, 31**, *p.248.*

NO ↓

Do you have sore areas around your mouth that are red and rough or blistered?

YES → *These may be cold sores, which result from an infection.* *See* COLD SORES, *p.484. See also* **Visual aids to diagnosis, 24**, *p.246.*

NO ↓

Has a blistering rash appeared on one side of your face where there has been a painful sensation for the past 2 to 4 days?

YES → *You may have a nerve infection.* *See* SHINGLES, *p.602.* *See also* **Visual aids to diagnosis, 25**, *p.246.*

NO ↓

Go to next page

Continued from previous page

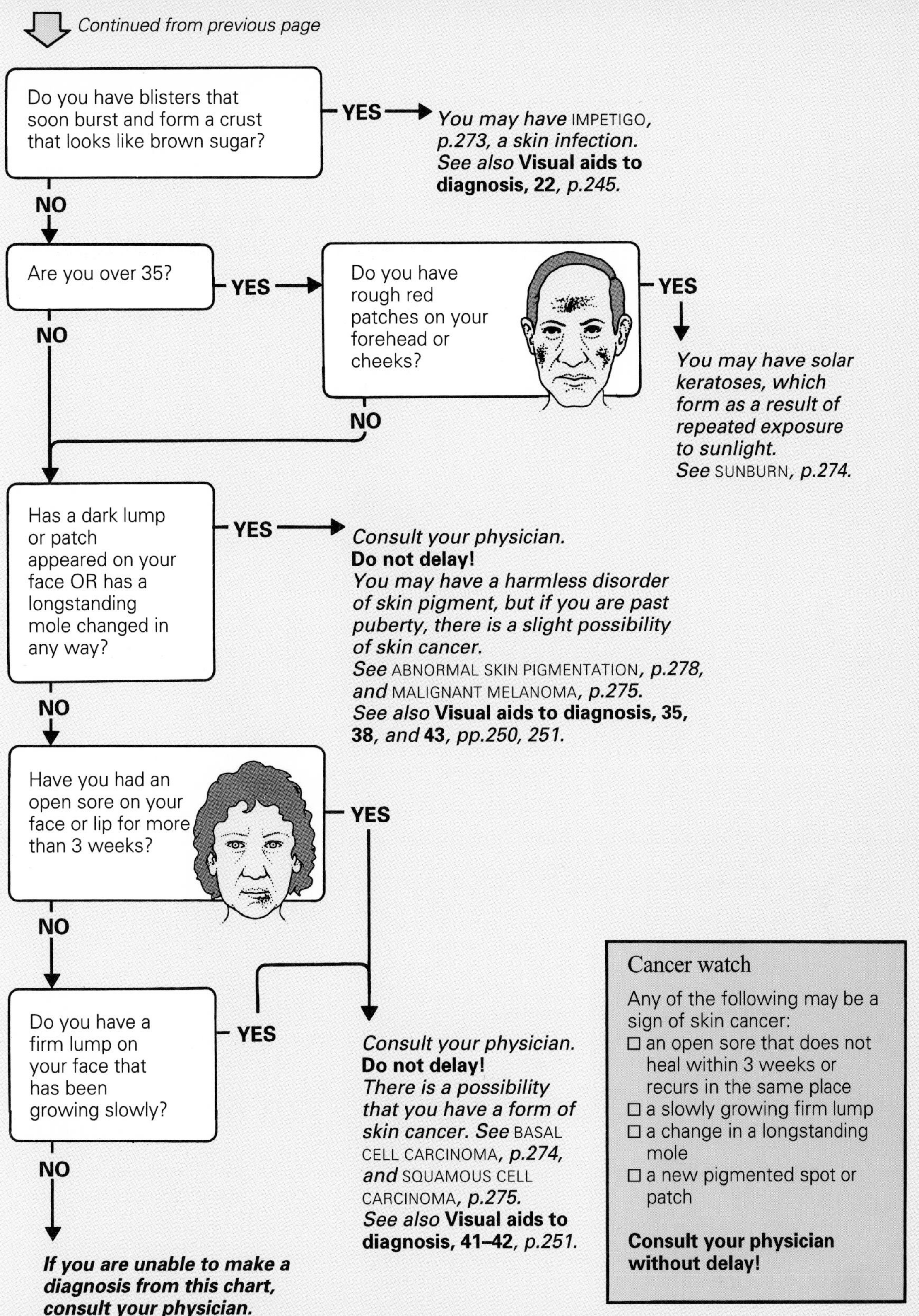

Do you have blisters that soon burst and form a crust that looks like brown sugar?
YES
You may have IMPETIGO, p.273, a skin infection. See also Visual aids to diagnosis, 22, p.245.
NO
Are you over 35?
YES
Do you have rough red patches on your forehead or cheeks?
YES
You may have solar keratoses, which form as a result of repeated exposure to sunlight. See SUNBURN, p.274.
NO
NO
Has a dark lump or patch appeared on your face OR has a longstanding mole changed in any way?
YES
Consult your physician. Do not delay! You may have a harmless disorder of skin pigment, but if you are past puberty, there is a slight possibility of skin cancer. See ABNORMAL SKIN PIGMENTATION, p.278, and MALIGNANT MELANOMA, p.275. See also Visual aids to diagnosis, 35, 38, and 43, pp.250, 251.
NO
Have you had an open sore on your face or lip for more than 3 weeks?
YES
NO
Do you have a firm lump on your face that has been growing slowly?
YES
Consult your physician. Do not delay! There is a possibility that you have a form of skin cancer. See BASAL CELL CARCINOMA, p.274, and SQUAMOUS CELL CARCINOMA, p.275. See also Visual aids to diagnosis, 41–42, p.251.
NO
If you are unable to make a diagnosis from this chart, consult your physician.

Cancer watch

Any of the following may be a sign of skin cancer:

- ☐ an open sore that does not heal within 3 weeks or recurs in the same place
- ☐ a slowly growing firm lump
- ☐ a change in a longstanding mole
- ☐ a new pigmented spot or patch

Consult your physician without delay!

27
GENERAL
over 2 years

Itchy spots and rashes

Discolored and/or raised areas of itchy skin.
For babies under 2 years see chart 89, **Skin problems in infants.**

START HERE

Is your temperature 100°F (38°C) or above?

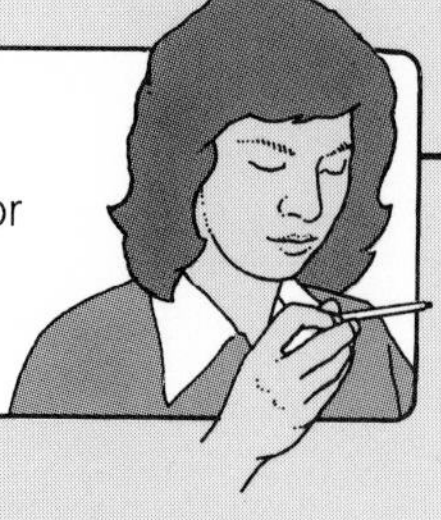

YES → *See chart* **28** Rash with fever.

NO ↓

Do you have a red, flaky, or moist rash that fades away into the surrounding skin?

YES → Is the rash on a part of the body that has come into contact with a new cosmetic or a new item of clothing or jewelry?

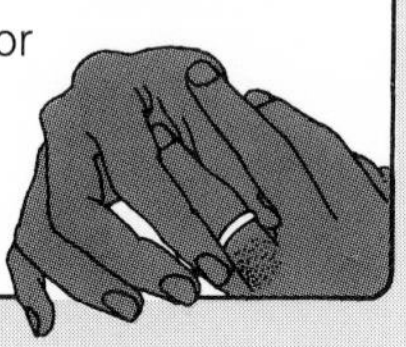

YES → *This may be contact dermatitis, a type of allergic reaction. See* ECZEMA AND DERMATITIS, *p.269. See also* **Visual aids to diagnosis, 13–15,** *p.243.*

NO ↓

Is it possible that you touched a plant to which you may be sensitive, such as poison ivy, poison oak, or poison sumac?

YES → *This may be contact dermatitis, a type of allergic reaction. See* ECZEMA AND DERMATITIS, *p.269. See also* **Visual aids to diagnosis, 13–15,** *p.243.*

NO ↓

Is the rash only on your hands AND have you spent a lot of time working with detergents or other substances that might irritate the skin?

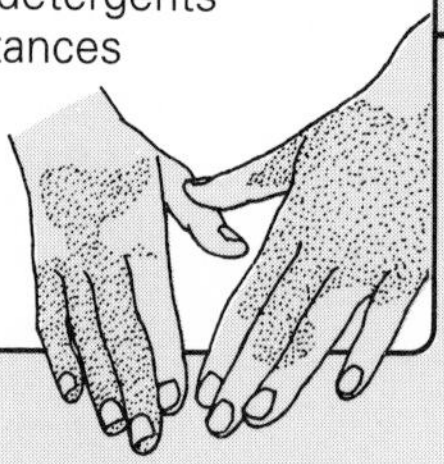

YES → *You may have "dishwashing hand" dermatitis. See* ECZEMA AND DERMATITIS, *p.269. See also* **Visual aids to diagnosis, 8,** *p.243.*

NO → *You may have one of the many types of* ECZEMA AND DERMATITIS, *p.269. See also* **Visual aids to diagnosis, 8–15,** *p.243.*

(From "Do you have a red, flaky, or moist rash…?") **NO** ↓

Do you have a smooth, raised, light-red rash with clearly defined edges?

YES → *This may be* HIVES, *p.272, an allergic rash. See also* **Visual aids to diagnosis, 16,** *p.244.*

NO ↓

Go to next page

Continued from previous page

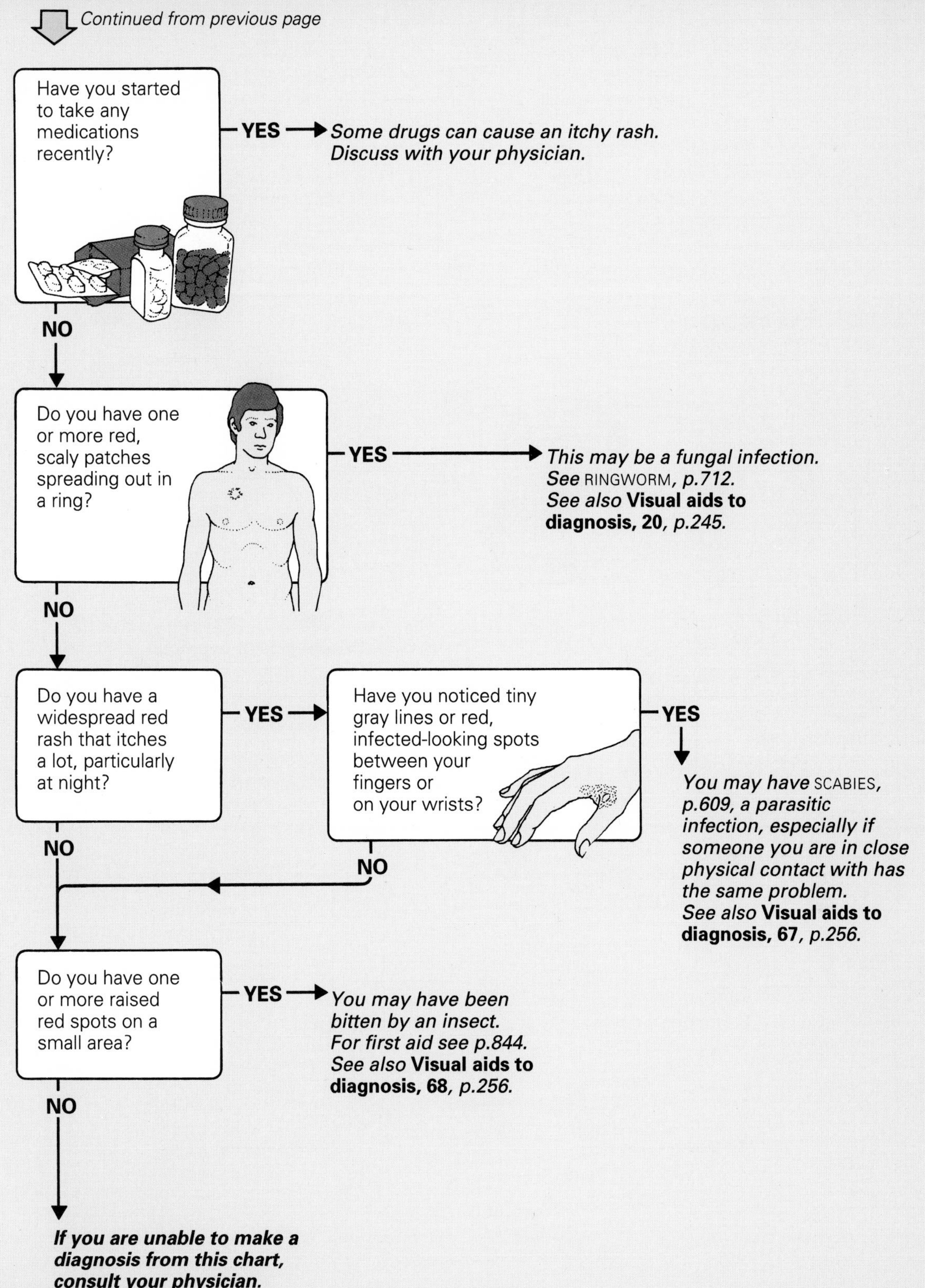

Have you started to take any medications recently?
YES
Some drugs can cause an itchy rash. Discuss with your physician.
NO
Do you have one or more red, scaly patches spreading out in a ring?
YES
This may be a fungal infection. See RINGWORM, *p.712.*
See also **Visual aids to diagnosis, 20**, *p.245.*
NO
Do you have a widespread red rash that itches a lot, particularly at night?
YES
Have you noticed tiny gray lines or red, infected-looking spots between your fingers or on your wrists?
YES
You may have SCABIES, *p.609, a parasitic infection, especially if someone you are in close physical contact with has the same problem.*
See also **Visual aids to diagnosis, 67**, *p.256.*
NO
NO
Do you have one or more raised red spots on a small area?
YES
You may have been bitten by an insect. For first aid see p.844.
See also **Visual aids to diagnosis, 68**, *p.256.*
NO
If you are unable to make a diagnosis from this chart, consult your physician.

28
GENERAL
all ages

Rash with fever

Any spots, discolored areas, or blisters on the skin combined with a temperature of 100°F (38°C) or above.

START HERE

Do you have any red spots or blotches?
- **YES** → Do you have two or more of the following symptoms?
  - ☐ runny nose
  - ☐ sore red eyes
  - ☐ dry cough
  - **YES** → *You may have* MEASLES, *p.745, or a similar viral infection, especially if the rash is mainly on your face or trunk. See also* **Visual aids to diagnosis, 26**, *p.247.*
  - **NO** → Is there an abnormal swelling down the sides of the back of your neck or at the base of your skull? 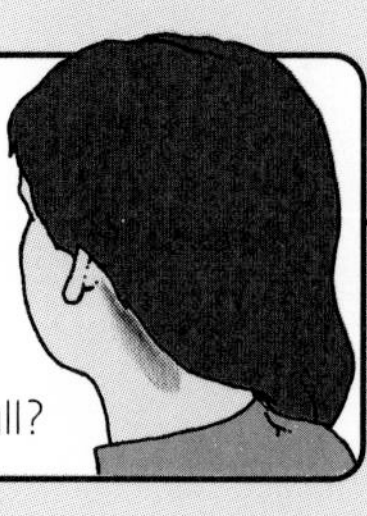
    - **YES** → *You may have* RUBELLA *(German measles), p.746. See also* **Visual aids to diagnosis, 27**, *p.247.*
    - **NO** → go to next question
- **NO** → go to next question

Do you have raised red and itchy spots that turn into blisters?
- **YES** → *This may be* CHICKENPOX, *p.747. See also* **Visual aids to diagnosis, 28**, *p.247.*
- **NO** ↓

Do you have one or more reddish brown spots that expand, leaving a whitish center?
- **YES** → *Consult your physician. If you have been bitten by a tick, this may be* LYME DISEASE, *p.605.*
- **NO** ↓

Do you have a rash of purple spots?
- **YES** → Do you have two or more of the following symptoms?
  - ☐ vomiting
  - ☐ headache
  - ☐ strong light hurts your eyes
  - ☐ pain when you try to bend your head forward
  - **YES** → **EMERGENCY Get medical help now!** *These symptoms suggest the possibility of* MENINGITIS, *p.290.*
  - **NO** → **Call your physician now!** *You may have a serious disorder,* ALLERGIC PURPURA, *p.728.*
- **NO** → ***If you are unable to make a diagnosis from this chart, consult your physician.***

29
GENERAL
all ages

Raised spots and lumps

Any raised areas on the surface of the skin that may be inflamed, dark, or the same color as the surrounding skin.

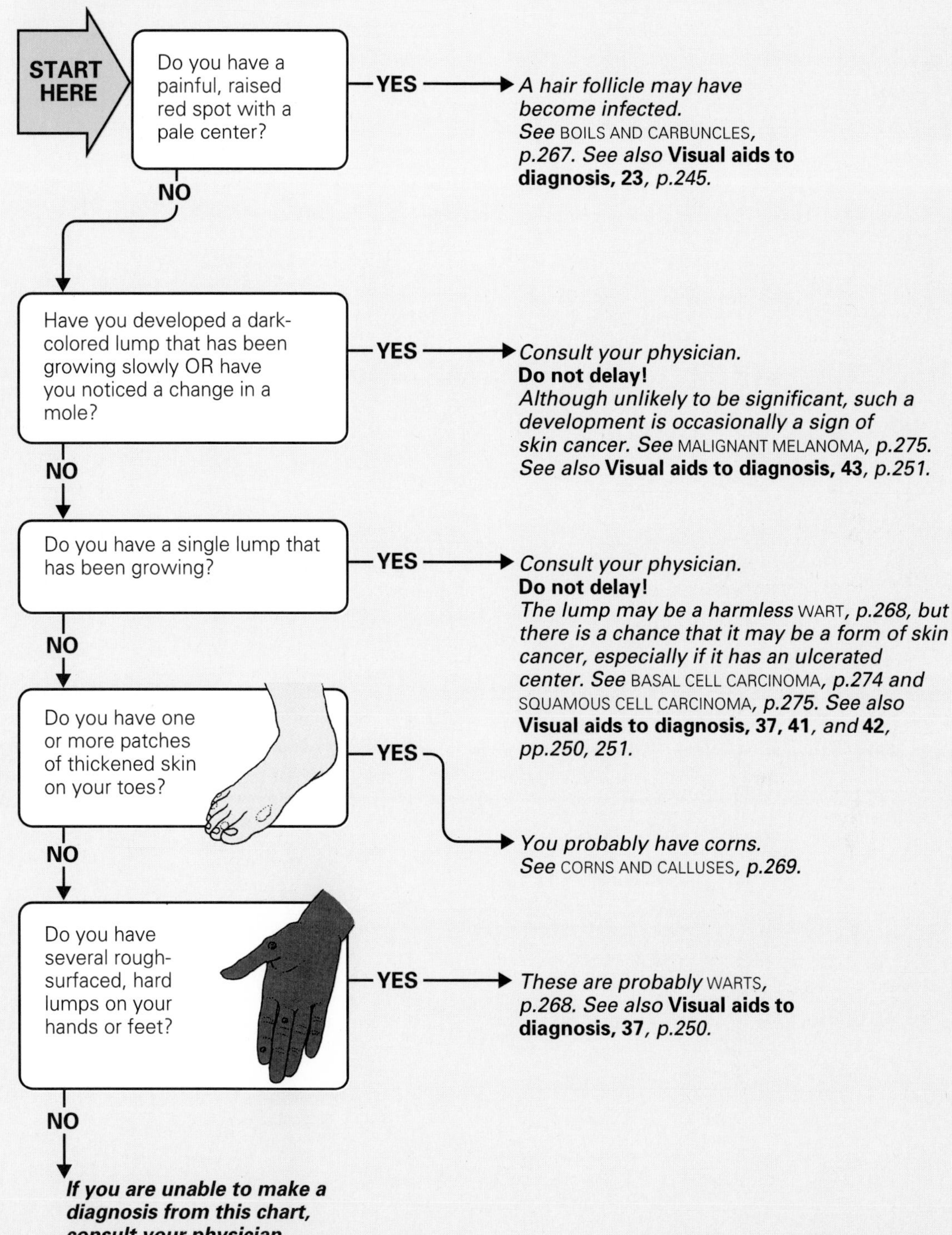

START HERE

Do you have a painful, raised red spot with a pale center?

YES → *A hair follicle may have become infected.* *See* BOILS AND CARBUNCLES, *p.267. See also* **Visual aids to diagnosis, 23**, *p.245.*

NO ↓

Have you developed a dark-colored lump that has been growing slowly OR have you noticed a change in a mole?

YES → *Consult your physician.* **Do not delay!** *Although unlikely to be significant, such a development is occasionally a sign of skin cancer. See* MALIGNANT MELANOMA, *p.275. See also* **Visual aids to diagnosis, 43**, *p.251.*

NO ↓

Do you have a single lump that has been growing?

YES → *Consult your physician.* **Do not delay!** *The lump may be a harmless* WART, *p.268, but there is a chance that it may be a form of skin cancer, especially if it has an ulcerated center. See* BASAL CELL CARCINOMA, *p.274 and* SQUAMOUS CELL CARCINOMA, *p.275. See also* **Visual aids to diagnosis, 37, 41**, *and* **42**, *pp.250, 251.*

NO ↓

Do you have one or more patches of thickened skin on your toes?

YES → *You probably have corns. See* CORNS AND CALLUSES, *p.269.*

NO ↓

Do you have several rough-surfaced, hard lumps on your hands or feet?

YES → *These are probably* WARTS, *p.268. See also* **Visual aids to diagnosis, 37**, *p.250.*

NO ↓

If you are unable to make a diagnosis from this chart, consult your physician.

30
GENERAL
all ages

Painful eye

Pain may be continuous or intermittent and may occur in or around the eye.

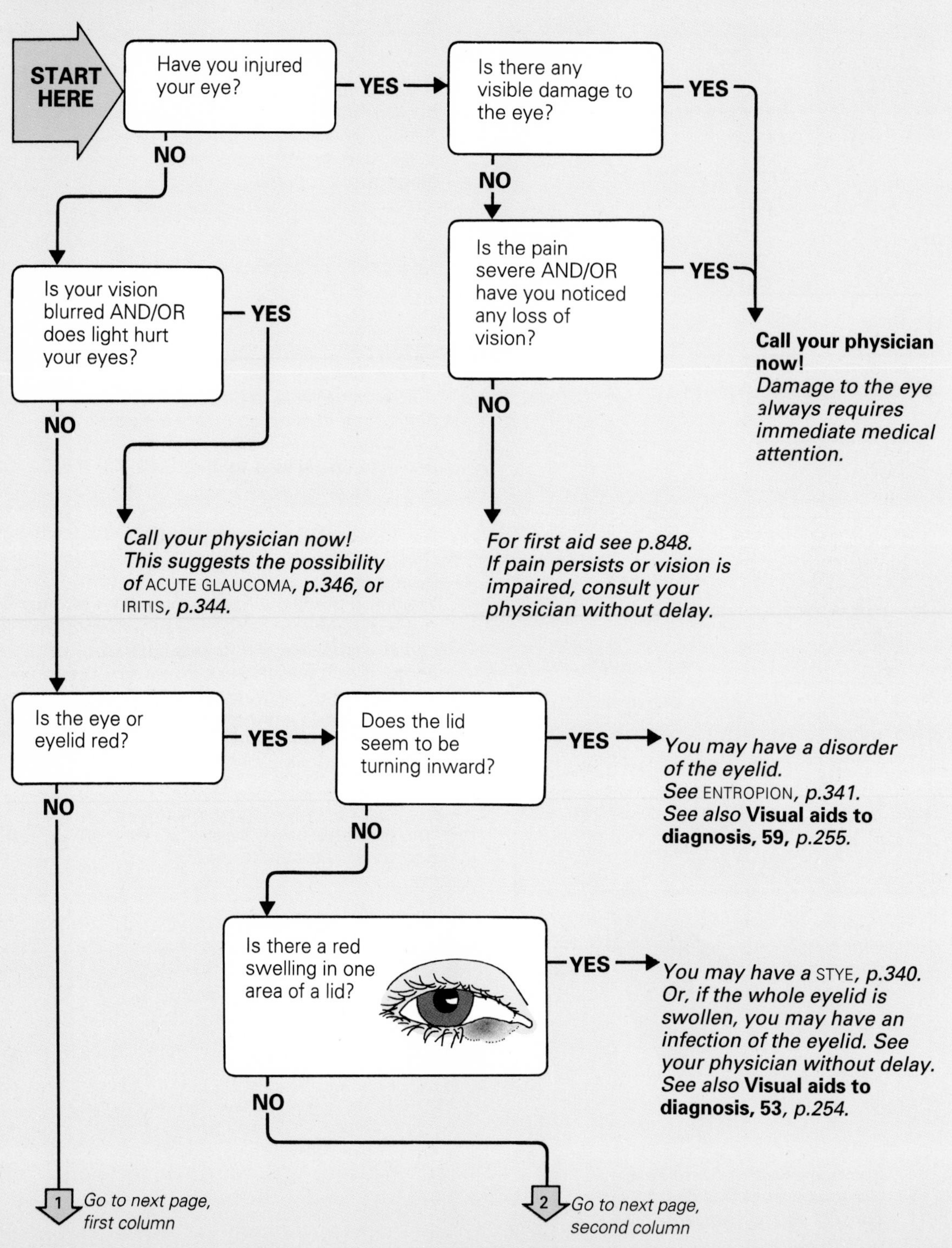

START HERE
Have you injured your eye?
YES
Is there any visible damage to the eye?
YES
NO
Is the pain severe AND/OR have you noticed any loss of vision?
YES
Call your physician now!
Damage to the eye always requires immediate medical attention.
NO
For first aid see p.848.
If pain persists or vision is impaired, consult your physician without delay.
NO
Is your vision blurred AND/OR does light hurt your eyes?
YES
Call your physician now!
This suggests the possibility of ACUTE GLAUCOMA, p.346, or IRITIS, p.344.
NO
Is the eye or eyelid red?
YES
Does the lid seem to be turning inward?
YES
You may have a disorder of the eyelid.
See ENTROPION, p.341.
See also Visual aids to diagnosis, 59, p.255.
NO
Is there a red swelling in one area of a lid?
YES
You may have a STYE, p.340.
Or, if the whole eyelid is swollen, you may have an infection of the eyelid. See your physician without delay.
See also Visual aids to diagnosis, 53, p.254.
NO
2 Go to next page, second column
NO
1 Go to next page, first column

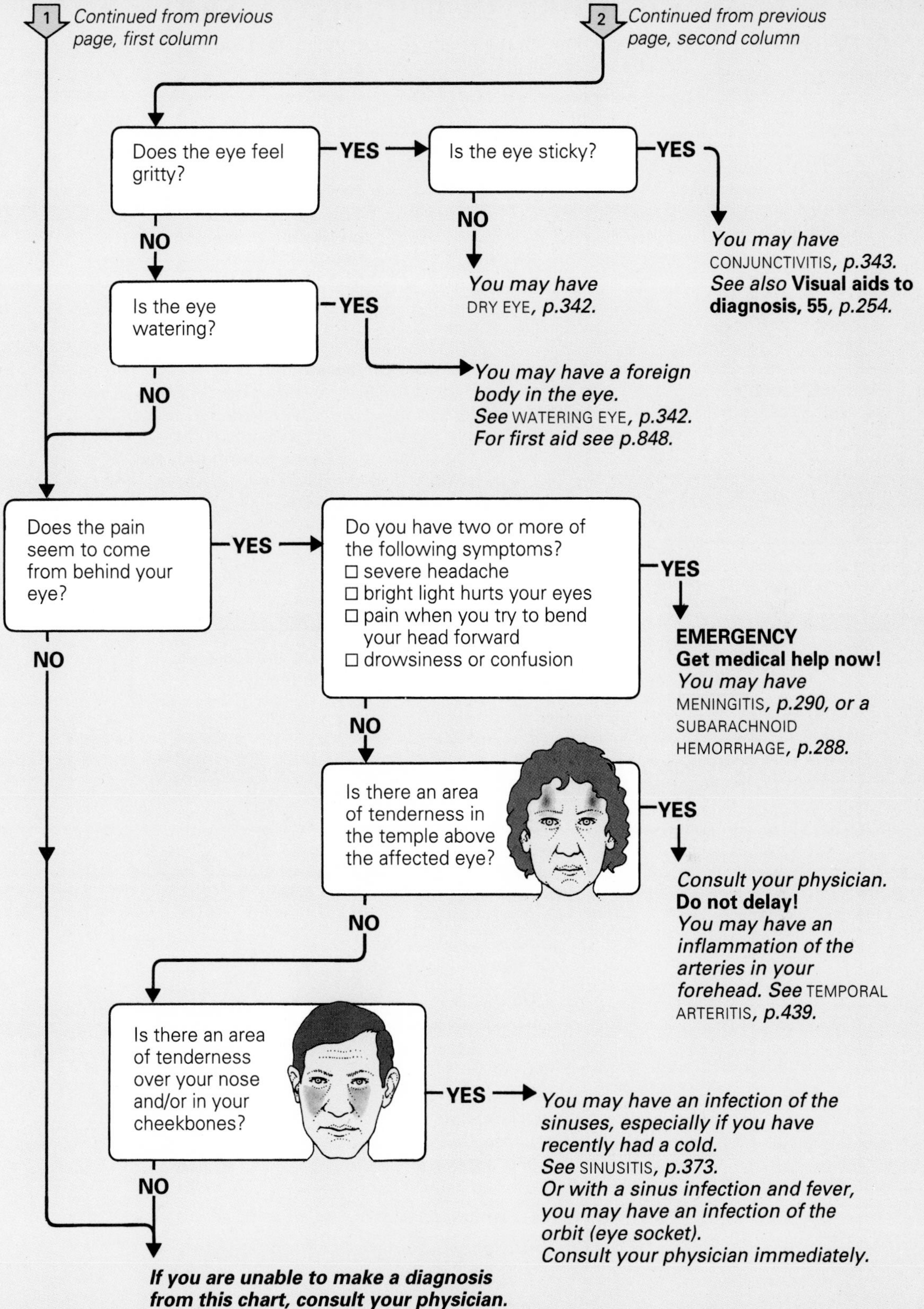

1 Continued from previous page, first column
2 Continued from previous page, second column
Does the eye feel gritty?
YES
Is the eye sticky?
YES
You may have CONJUNCTIVITIS, p.343. See also **Visual aids to diagnosis, 55**, p.254.
NO
You may have DRY EYE, p.342.
NO
Is the eye watering?
YES
You may have a foreign body in the eye. See WATERING EYE, p.342. For first aid see p.848.
NO
Does the pain seem to come from behind your eye?
YES
Do you have two or more of the following symptoms?
☐ severe headache
☐ bright light hurts your eyes
☐ pain when you try to bend your head forward
☐ drowsiness or confusion
YES
EMERGENCY
Get medical help now!
You may have MENINGITIS, p.290, or a SUBARACHNOID HEMORRHAGE, p.288.
NO
Is there an area of tenderness in the temple above the affected eye?
YES
Consult your physician. **Do not delay!** You may have an inflammation of the arteries in your forehead. See TEMPORAL ARTERITIS, p.439.
NO
NO
Is there an area of tenderness over your nose and/or in your cheekbones?
YES
You may have an infection of the sinuses, especially if you have recently had a cold. See SINUSITIS, p.373. Or with a sinus infection and fever, you may have an infection of the orbit (eye socket). Consult your physician immediately.
NO
If you are unable to make a diagnosis from this chart, consult your physician.

31
GENERAL
all ages

Disturbed or impaired vision

Any reduction in your ability to see, including blurring, double vision, and/or seeing flashing lights or floating spots.

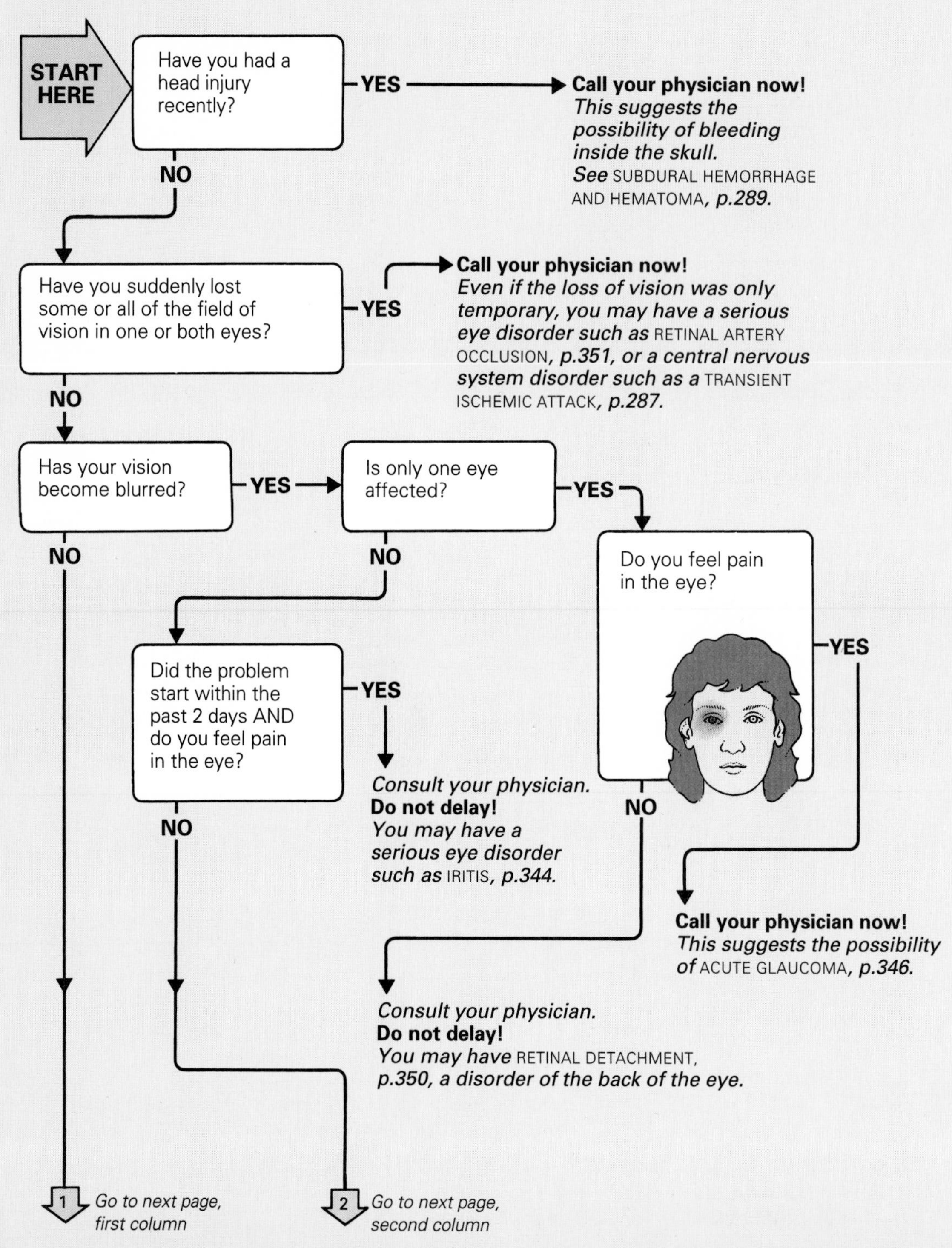

START HERE
Have you had a head injury recently?
YES
Call your physician now!
This suggests the possibility of bleeding inside the skull.
See SUBDURAL HEMORRHAGE AND HEMATOMA, *p.289.*
NO
Have you suddenly lost some or all of the field of vision in one or both eyes?
YES
Call your physician now!
Even if the loss of vision was only temporary, you may have a serious eye disorder such as RETINAL ARTERY OCCLUSION, *p.351, or a central nervous system disorder such as a* TRANSIENT ISCHEMIC ATTACK, *p.287.*
NO
Has your vision become blurred?
YES
Is only one eye affected?
YES
Do you feel pain in the eye?
YES
Call your physician now!
This suggests the possibility of ACUTE GLAUCOMA, *p.346.*
NO
Consult your physician.
Do not delay!
You may have RETINAL DETACHMENT, *p.350, a disorder of the back of the eye.*
NO
Did the problem start within the past 2 days AND do you feel pain in the eye?
YES
Consult your physician.
Do not delay!
You may have a serious eye disorder such as IRITIS, *p.344.*
NO
NO
1 *Go to next page, first column*
2 *Go to next page, second column*

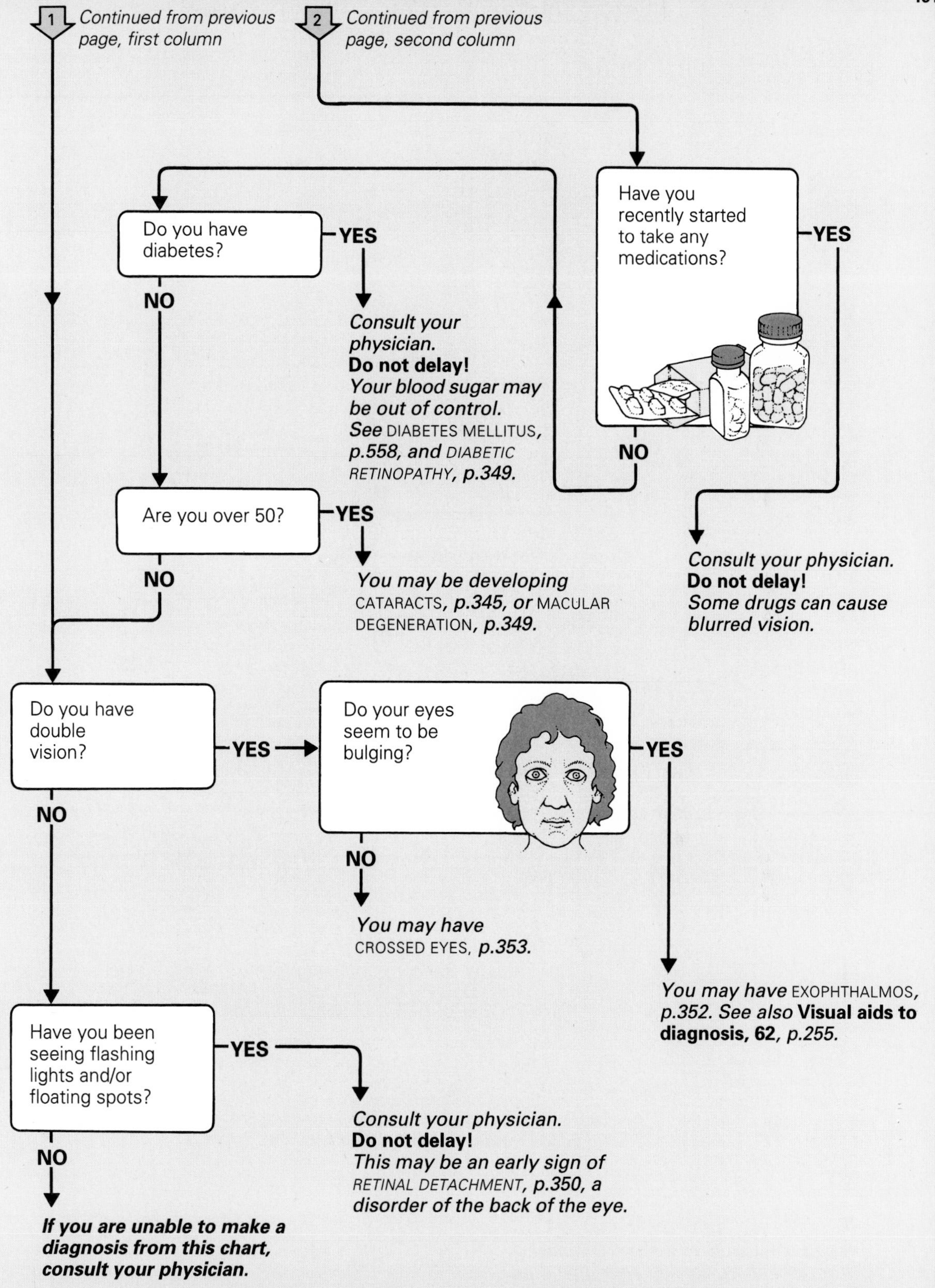
1 Continued from previous page, first column
2 Continued from previous page, second column
Have you recently started to take any medications?
YES
NO
Consult your physician.
Do not delay!
Some drugs can cause blurred vision.
Do you have diabetes?
YES
NO
Consult your physician.
Do not delay!
Your blood sugar may be out of control.
See DIABETES MELLITUS, p.558, and DIABETIC RETINOPATHY, p.349.
Are you over 50?
YES
NO
You may be developing CATARACTS, p.345, or MACULAR DEGENERATION, p.349.
Do you have double vision?
YES
NO
Do your eyes seem to be bulging?
YES
NO
You may have CROSSED EYES, p.353.
You may have EXOPHTHALMOS, p.352. See also Visual aids to diagnosis, 62, p.255.
Have you been seeing flashing lights and/or floating spots?
YES
NO
Consult your physician.
Do not delay!
This may be an early sign of RETINAL DETACHMENT, p.350, a disorder of the back of the eye.
If you are unable to make a diagnosis from this chart, consult your physician.

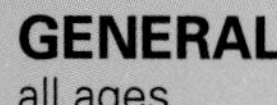

GENERAL
all ages

Earache

Pain in one or both ears, either sharp and stabbing or dull and throbbing.

START HERE

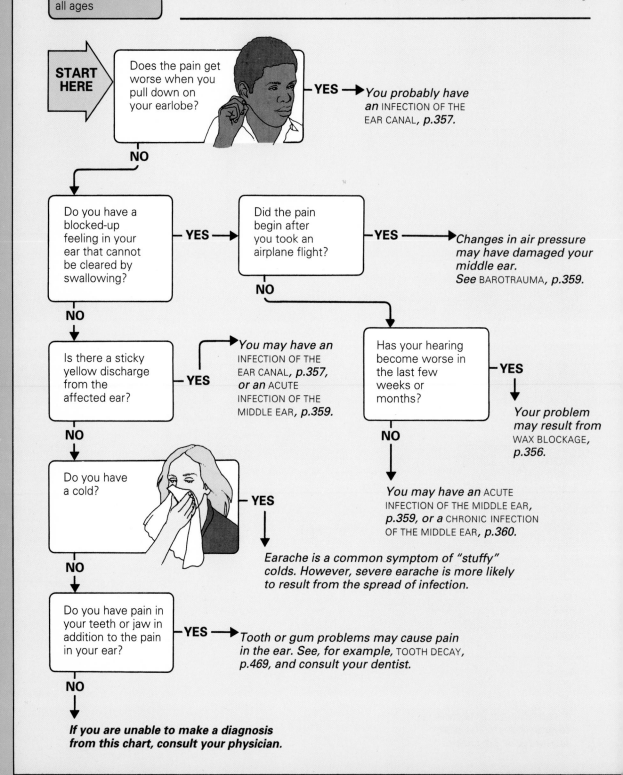

Does the pain get worse when you pull down on your earlobe?

YES → *You probably have an* INFECTION OF THE EAR CANAL, ***p.357.***

NO ↓

Do you have a blocked-up feeling in your ear that cannot be cleared by swallowing?

YES → Did the pain begin after you took an airplane flight?

- **YES** → ***Changes in air pressure may have damaged your middle ear. See*** BAROTRAUMA, ***p.359.***
- **NO** ↓ Has your hearing become worse in the last few weeks or months?
  - **YES** → ***Your problem may result from*** WAX BLOCKAGE, ***p.356.***
  - **NO** → ***You may have an*** ACUTE INFECTION OF THE MIDDLE EAR, ***p.359, or a*** CHRONIC INFECTION OF THE MIDDLE EAR, ***p.360.***

NO ↓

Is there a sticky yellow discharge from the affected ear?

YES → ***You may have an*** INFECTION OF THE EAR CANAL, ***p.357, or an*** ACUTE INFECTION OF THE MIDDLE EAR, ***p.359.***

NO ↓

Do you have a cold?

YES → ***Earache is a common symptom of "stuffy" colds. However, severe earache is more likely to result from the spread of infection.***

NO ↓

Do you have pain in your teeth or jaw in addition to the pain in your ear?

YES → ***Tooth or gum problems may cause pain in the ear. See, for example,*** TOOTH DECAY, ***p.469, and consult your dentist.***

NO ↓

If you are unable to make a diagnosis from this chart, consult your physician.

Noises in the ear

Any ringing, buzzing, or hissing sounds (not including speech or music) that only you can hear.

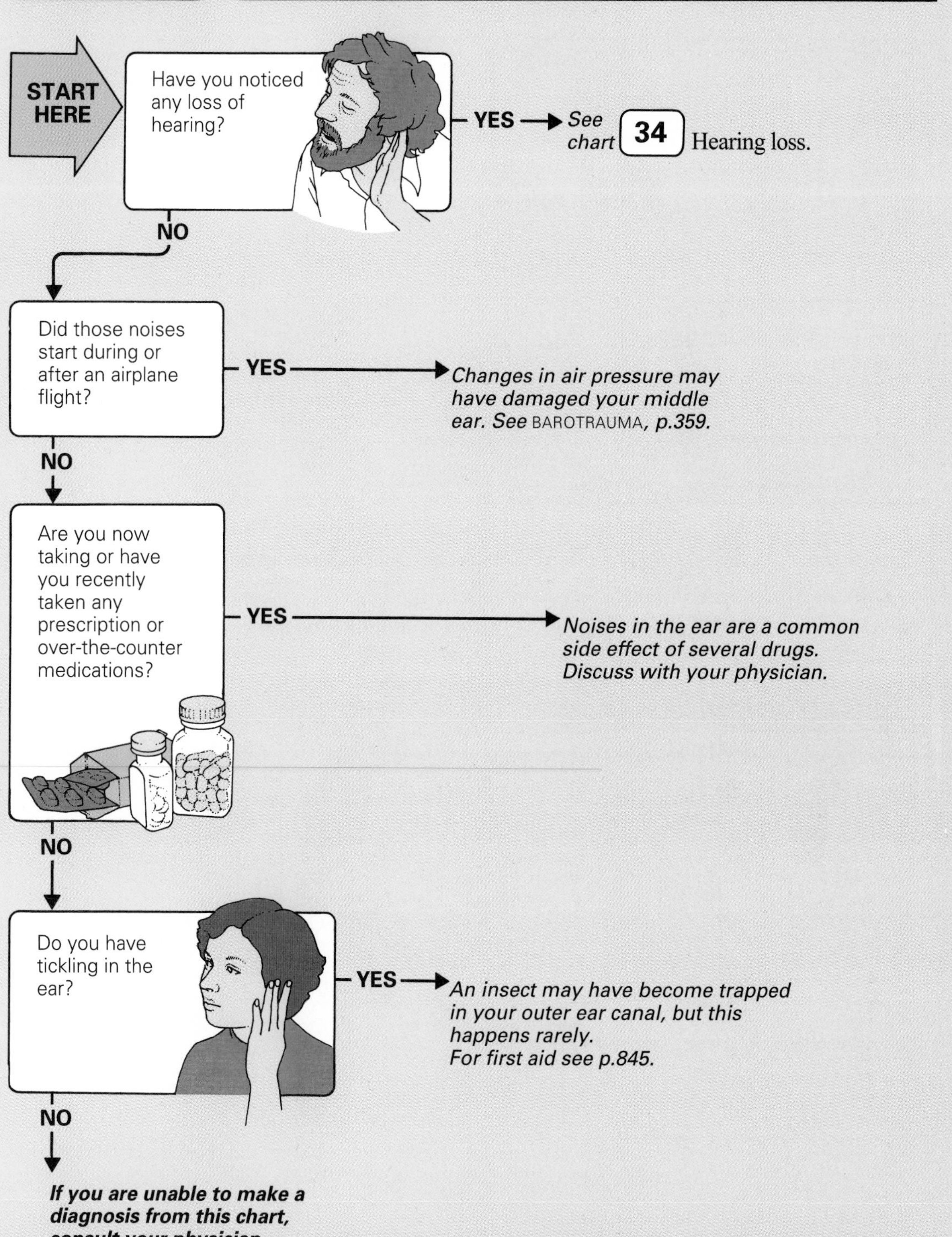

START HERE

Have you noticed any loss of hearing?

YES → *See chart* **34** Hearing loss.

NO

Did those noises start during or after an airplane flight?

YES → *Changes in air pressure may have damaged your middle ear. See* BAROTRAUMA, *p.359.*

NO

Are you now taking or have you recently taken any prescription or over-the-counter medications?

YES → *Noises in the ear are a common side effect of several drugs. Discuss with your physician.*

NO

Do you have tickling in the ear?

YES → *An insect may have become trapped in your outer ear canal, but this happens rarely.*
For first aid see p.845.

NO

If you are unable to make a diagnosis from this chart, consult your physician.

34
GENERAL
all ages

Hearing loss

Reduction in the ability to hear some or all sounds in one or both ears.

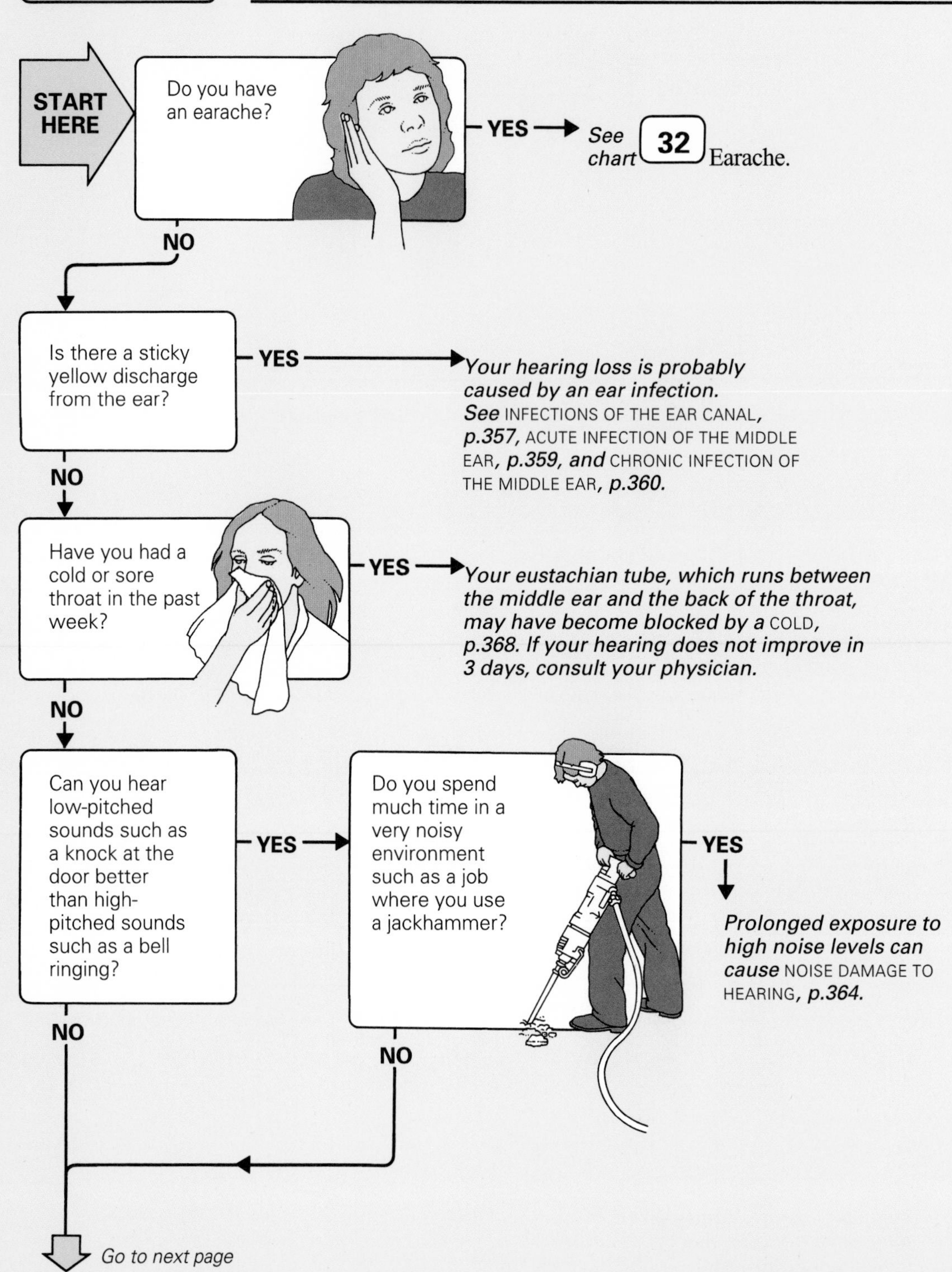

START HERE

Do you have an earache?

YES → See chart **32** Earache.

NO ↓

Is there a sticky yellow discharge from the ear?

YES → *Your hearing loss is probably caused by an ear infection. See* INFECTIONS OF THE EAR CANAL, *p.357,* ACUTE INFECTION OF THE MIDDLE EAR, *p.359, and* CHRONIC INFECTION OF THE MIDDLE EAR, *p.360.*

NO ↓

Have you had a cold or sore throat in the past week?

YES → *Your eustachian tube, which runs between the middle ear and the back of the throat, may have become blocked by a* COLD, *p.368. If your hearing does not improve in 3 days, consult your physician.*

NO ↓

Can you hear low-pitched sounds such as a knock at the door better than high-pitched sounds such as a bell ringing?

YES → Do you spend much time in a very noisy environment such as a job where you use a jackhammer?

YES ↓ *Prolonged exposure to high noise levels can cause* NOISE DAMAGE TO HEARING, *p.364.*

NO ↓

NO ↓

Go to next page

Continued from previous page

Have you recently taken any prescription medications?

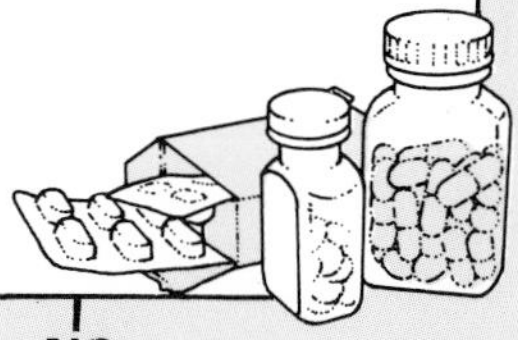

— YES → *Hearing loss is a common side effect of several drugs. Discuss with your physician.*

NO ↓

Do you have occasional attacks of dizziness when everything around you seems to spin?

— YES → *You may have* MENIERE'S DISEASE, ***p.363,*** *which affects the balance mechanism of the inner ear.*

NO ↓

Are you over 60?

— YES → *Some hearing loss is common as you grow older, but it often can be treated. See* AGING AND THE SENSES, ***p.771.***

NO ↓

Has your hearing been getting worse over a period of several weeks or more?

— YES → Have other members of your family had a gradual loss of hearing?

— YES → *You may have* OTOSCLEROSIS, ***p.358,*** *which affects the working of the middle ear.*

NO ↓ *Your problem may result from* WAX BLOCKAGE, ***p.356.***

NO ↓

If you are unable to make a diagnosis from this chart, consult your physician.

Hearing loss in children

Hearing loss is a possibility if your child seems to ignore your questions and/or turns up the volume on the television set. Hearing loss in children often results from fluid in the ear. See THE MIDDLE EAR, p.358. Consult your physician.

35
GENERAL
all ages

Runny nose

Completely or partially blocked nose, with a liquid discharge.

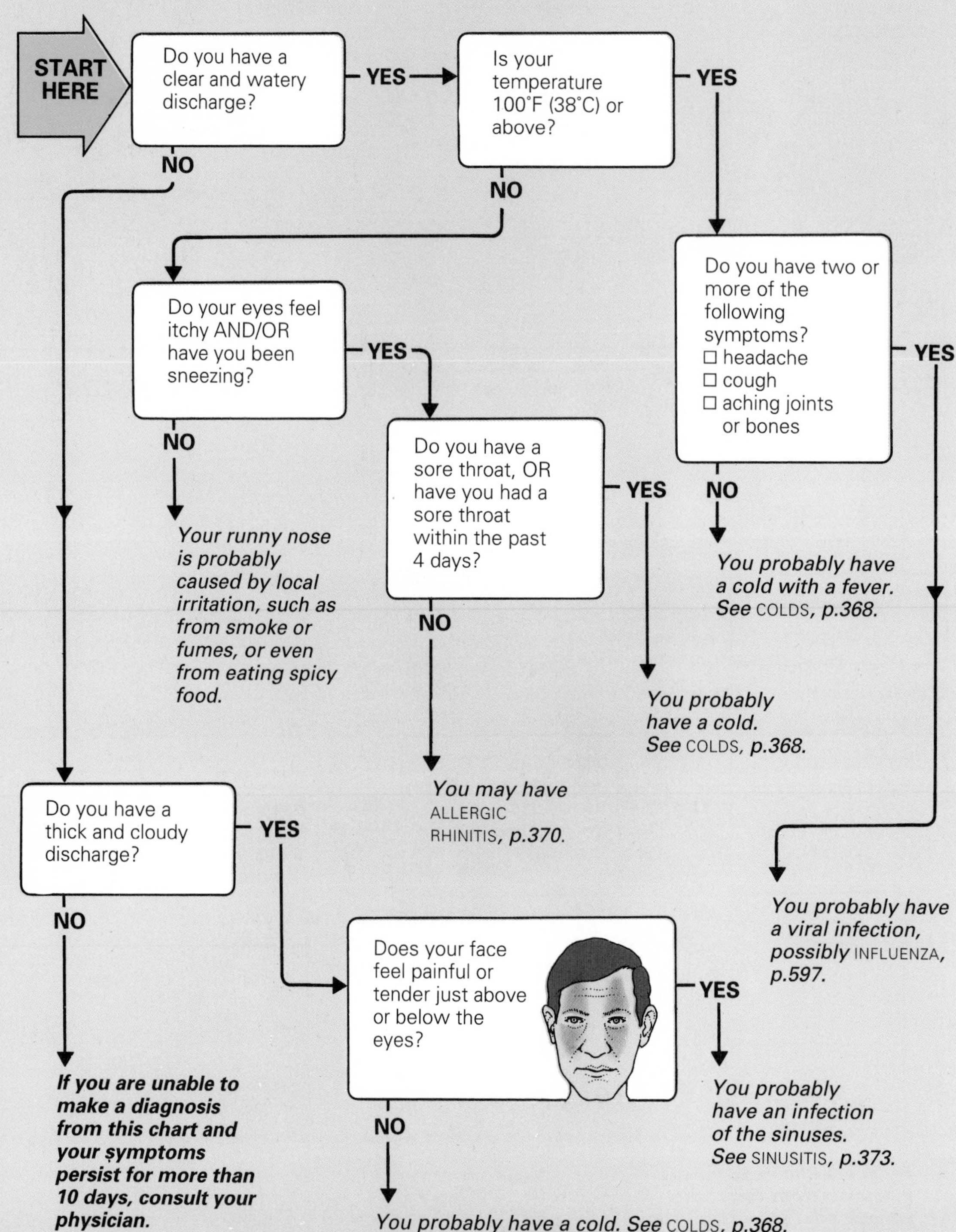

START HERE
Do you have a clear and watery discharge?
YES
NO
Is your temperature 100°F (38°C) or above?
YES
NO
Do you have two or more of the following symptoms?
☐ headache
☐ cough
☐ aching joints or bones
YES
NO
You probably have a cold with a fever. See COLDS, p.368.
You probably have a viral infection, possibly INFLUENZA, p.597.
Do your eyes feel itchy AND/OR have you been sneezing?
YES
NO
Your runny nose is probably caused by local irritation, such as from smoke or fumes, or even from eating spicy food.
Do you have a sore throat, OR have you had a sore throat within the past 4 days?
YES
NO
You probably have a cold. See COLDS, p.368.
You may have ALLERGIC RHINITIS, p.370.
Do you have a thick and cloudy discharge?
YES
NO
If you are unable to make a diagnosis from this chart and your symptoms persist for more than 10 days, consult your physician.
Does your face feel painful or tender just above or below the eyes?
YES
NO
You probably have an infection of the sinuses. See SINUSITIS, p.373.
You probably have a cold. See COLDS, p.368.

36
GENERAL
all ages

Sore throat

Any rough or raw feeling in the back of the throat that causes discomfort, especially when you swallow.

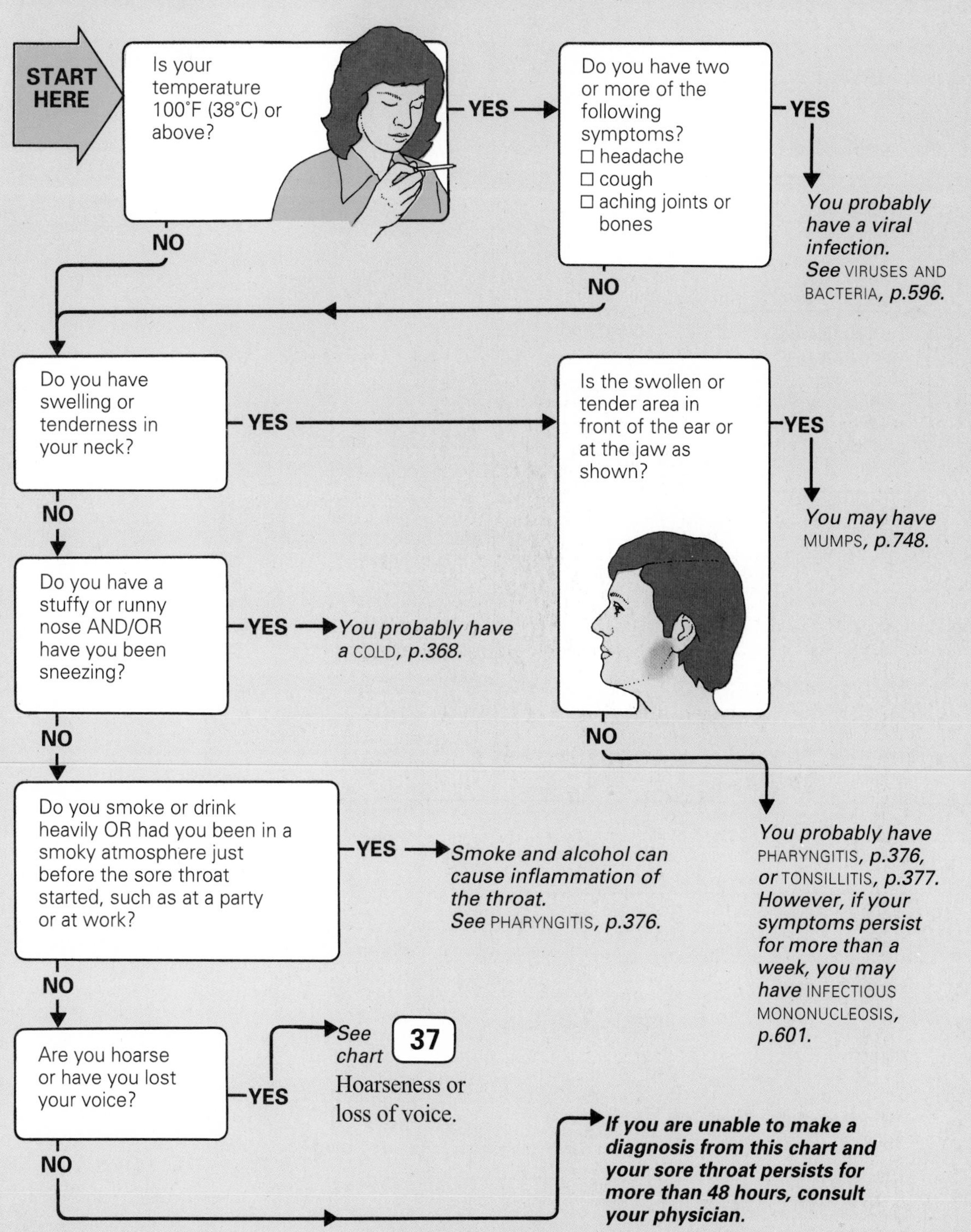

START HERE
Is your temperature 100°F (38°C) or above?
YES
NO
Do you have two or more of the following symptoms?
☐ headache
☐ cough
☐ aching joints or bones
YES
NO
You probably have a viral infection.
See VIRUSES AND BACTERIA, p.596.
Do you have swelling or tenderness in your neck?
YES
NO
Is the swollen or tender area in front of the ear or at the jaw as shown?
YES
NO
You may have MUMPS, p.748.
Do you have a stuffy or runny nose AND/OR have you been sneezing?
YES
NO
You probably have a COLD, p.368.
You probably have PHARYNGITIS, p.376, or TONSILLITIS, p.377. However, if your symptoms persist for more than a week, you may have INFECTIOUS MONONUCLEOSIS, p.601.
Do you smoke or drink heavily OR had you been in a smoky atmosphere just before the sore throat started, such as at a party or at work?
YES
NO
Smoke and alcohol can cause inflammation of the throat.
See PHARYNGITIS, p.376.
Are you hoarse or have you lost your voice?
YES
NO
See chart 37
Hoarseness or loss of voice.
If you are unable to make a diagnosis from this chart and your sore throat persists for more than 48 hours, consult your physician.

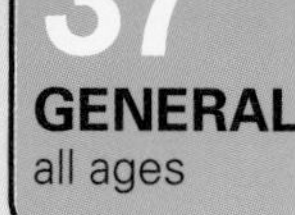

GENERAL
all ages

Hoarseness or loss of voice

Any abnormal huskiness in the voice that may be so severe that you can make little or no sound.

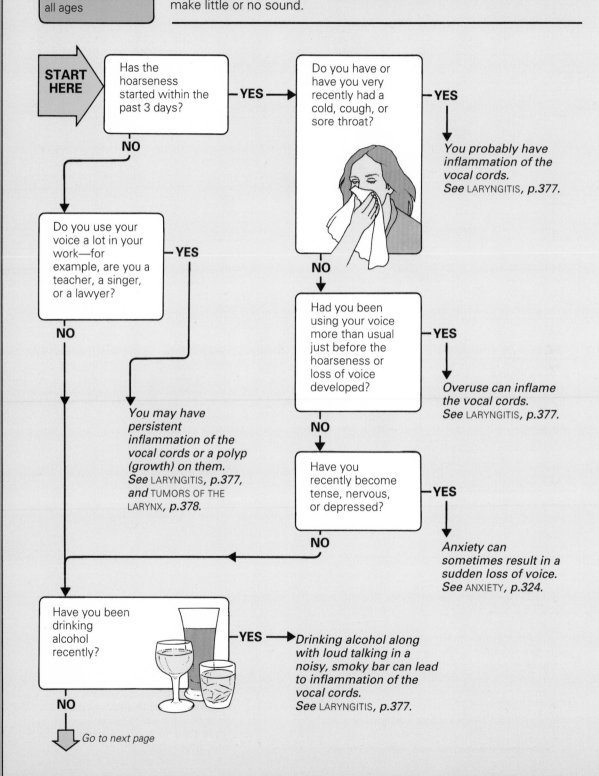

START HERE

Has the hoarseness started within the past 3 days?

- **YES** → Do you have or have you very recently had a cold, cough, or sore throat?
  - **YES** → *You probably have inflammation of the vocal cords. See* LARYNGITIS, *p.377.*
  - **NO** → Had you been using your voice more than usual just before the hoarseness or loss of voice developed?
    - **YES** → *Overuse can inflame the vocal cords. See* LARYNGITIS, *p.377.*
    - **NO** → Have you recently become tense, nervous, or depressed?
      - **YES** → *Anxiety can sometimes result in a sudden loss of voice. See* ANXIETY, *p.324.*
      - **NO** → go to "Have you been drinking alcohol recently?"
- **NO** → Do you use your voice a lot in your work—for example, are you a teacher, a singer, or a lawyer?
  - **YES** → *You may have persistent inflammation of the vocal cords or a polyp (growth) on them. See* LARYNGITIS, *p.377, and* TUMORS OF THE LARYNX, *p.378.*
  - **NO** → Have you been drinking alcohol recently?
    - **YES** → *Drinking alcohol along with loud talking in a noisy, smoky bar can lead to inflammation of the vocal cords. See* LARYNGITIS, *p.377.*
    - **NO** → *Go to next page*

Continued from previous page

Do you smoke?

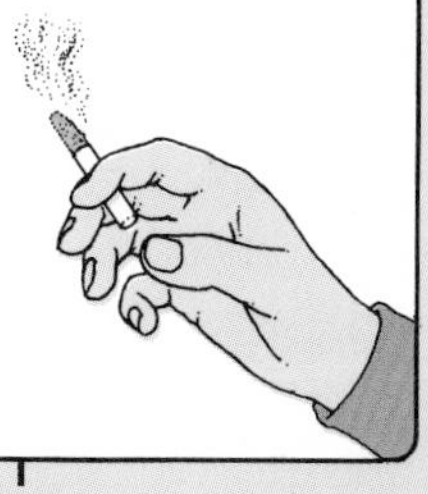

YES → *Smoking can lead to inflammation or cancer of the vocal cords. See* LARYNGITIS, *p.377, and* TUMORS OF THE LARYNX, *p.378.*

NO ↓

Do you have two or more of the following symptoms?

- ☐ feeling more affected by cold weather
- ☐ dry skin or hair
- ☐ weight gain without overeating
- ☐ unexplained tiredness

YES → *You may have an underactive thyroid gland. See* HYPOTHYROIDISM, *p.567.*

NO ↓

Has your hoarseness or loss of voice lasted for more than a week?

YES → *Consult your physician.* **Do not delay!** *Although there is probably a simple explanation for your hoarseness or loss of voice, there is a possibility of a polyp or cancer on the larynx. See* TUMORS OF THE LARYNX, *p.378.*

NO ↓

Have you had several attacks of hoarseness or loss of voice in the last 6 months?

YES → (see "Consult your physician" above)

NO ↓

If you are unable to make a diagnosis from this chart and your hoarseness persists for more than a week, consult your physician.

Cancer watch

Frequent hoarseness or loss of voice or an episode that lasts for more than a week may indicate cancer of the larynx.

Consult your physician without delay!

38
GENERAL
over 14 years

Coughing

A noisy expulsion of air from the lungs that may produce phlegm or be "dry." For children see chart 95, **Coughing in children**.

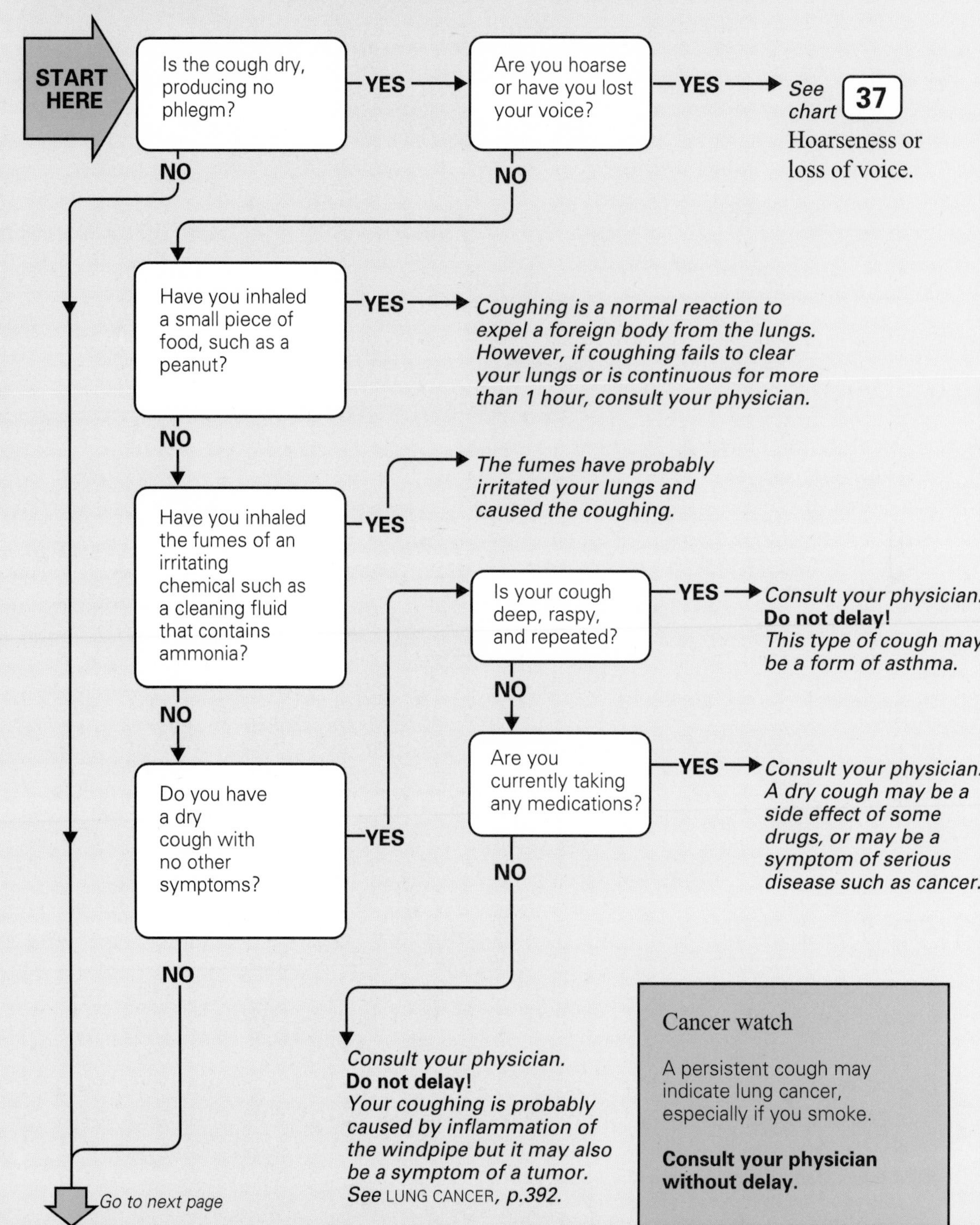

START HERE
Is the cough dry, producing no phlegm?
YES
NO
Are you hoarse or have you lost your voice?
YES
NO
See chart 37
Hoarseness or loss of voice.
Have you inhaled a small piece of food, such as a peanut?
YES
NO
Coughing is a normal reaction to expel a foreign body from the lungs. However, if coughing fails to clear your lungs or is continuous for more than 1 hour, consult your physician.
Have you inhaled the fumes of an irritating chemical such as a cleaning fluid that contains ammonia?
YES
NO
The fumes have probably irritated your lungs and caused the coughing.
Do you have a dry cough with no other symptoms?
YES
NO
Is your cough deep, raspy, and repeated?
YES
NO
Consult your physician.
Do not delay!
This type of cough may be a form of asthma.
Are you currently taking any medications?
YES
NO
Consult your physician. A dry cough may be a side effect of some drugs, or may be a symptom of serious disease such as cancer.
Consult your physician.
Do not delay!
Your coughing is probably caused by inflammation of the windpipe but it may also be a symptom of a tumor. See LUNG CANCER, p.392.
Go to next page

Cancer watch

A persistent cough may indicate lung cancer, especially if you smoke.

Consult your physician without delay.

Continued from previous page

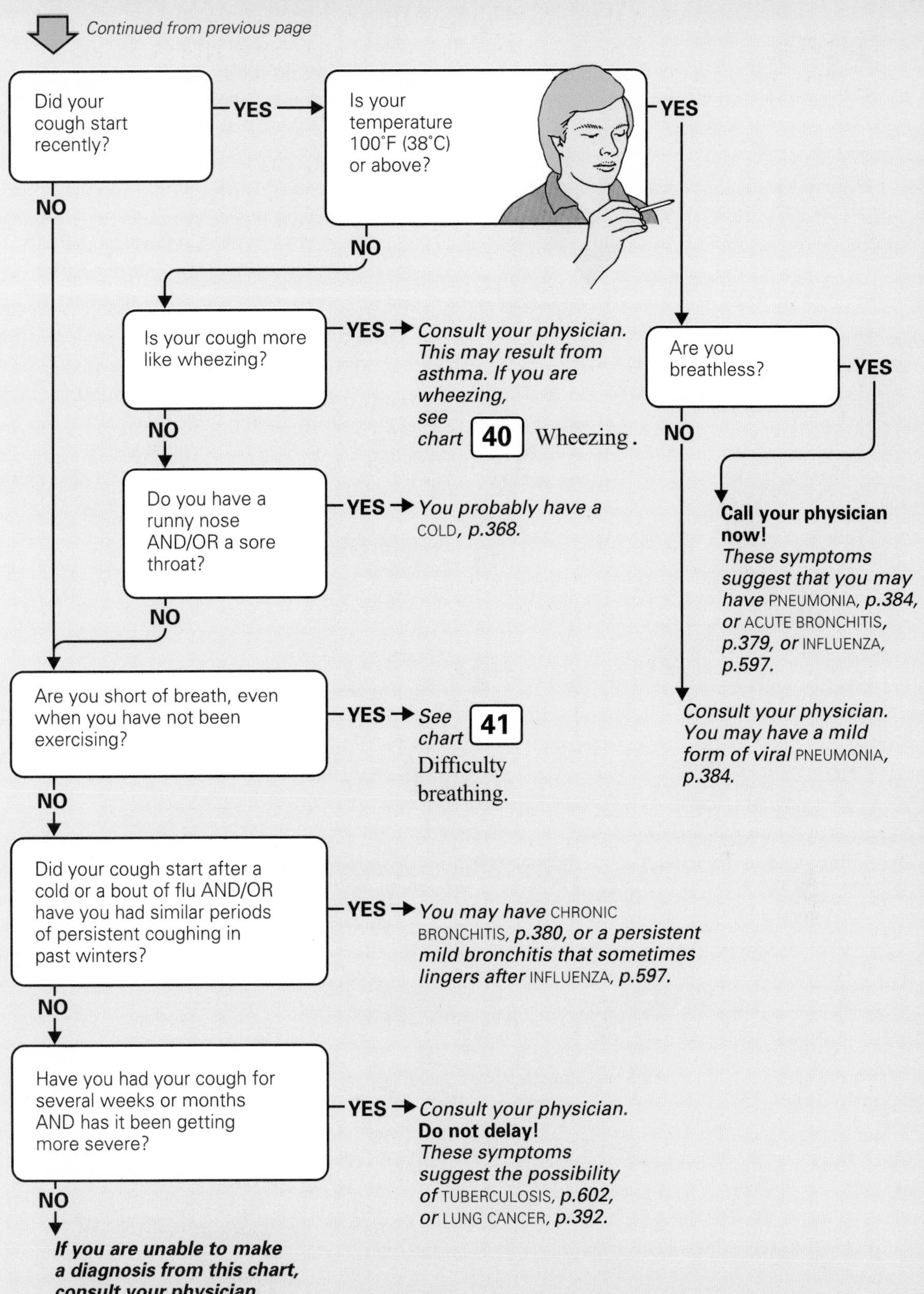

Did your cough start recently?
YES
Is your temperature 100°F (38°C) or above?
YES
Are you breathless?
YES
Call your physician now!
These symptoms suggest that you may have PNEUMONIA, p.384, or ACUTE BRONCHITIS, p.379, or INFLUENZA, p.597.
NO
Consult your physician. You may have a mild form of viral PNEUMONIA, p.384.
NO
Is your cough more like wheezing?
YES
Consult your physician. This may result from asthma. If you are wheezing, see chart 40 Wheezing.
NO
Do you have a runny nose AND/OR a sore throat?
YES
You probably have a COLD, p.368.
NO
NO
Are you short of breath, even when you have not been exercising?
YES
See chart 41 Difficulty breathing.
NO
Did your cough start after a cold or a bout of flu AND/OR have you had similar periods of persistent coughing in past winters?
YES
You may have CHRONIC BRONCHITIS, p.380, or a persistent mild bronchitis that sometimes lingers after INFLUENZA, p.597.
NO
Have you had your cough for several weeks or months AND has it been getting more severe?
YES
Consult your physician. Do not delay! These symptoms suggest the possibility of TUBERCULOSIS, p.602, or LUNG CANCER, p.392.
NO
If you are unable to make a diagnosis from this chart, consult your physician.

39
GENERAL
all ages

Coughing up blood

Coughing up phlegm that is colored or streaked bright red or rusty brown, that contains dark flecks or spots, or that is pink and frothy.

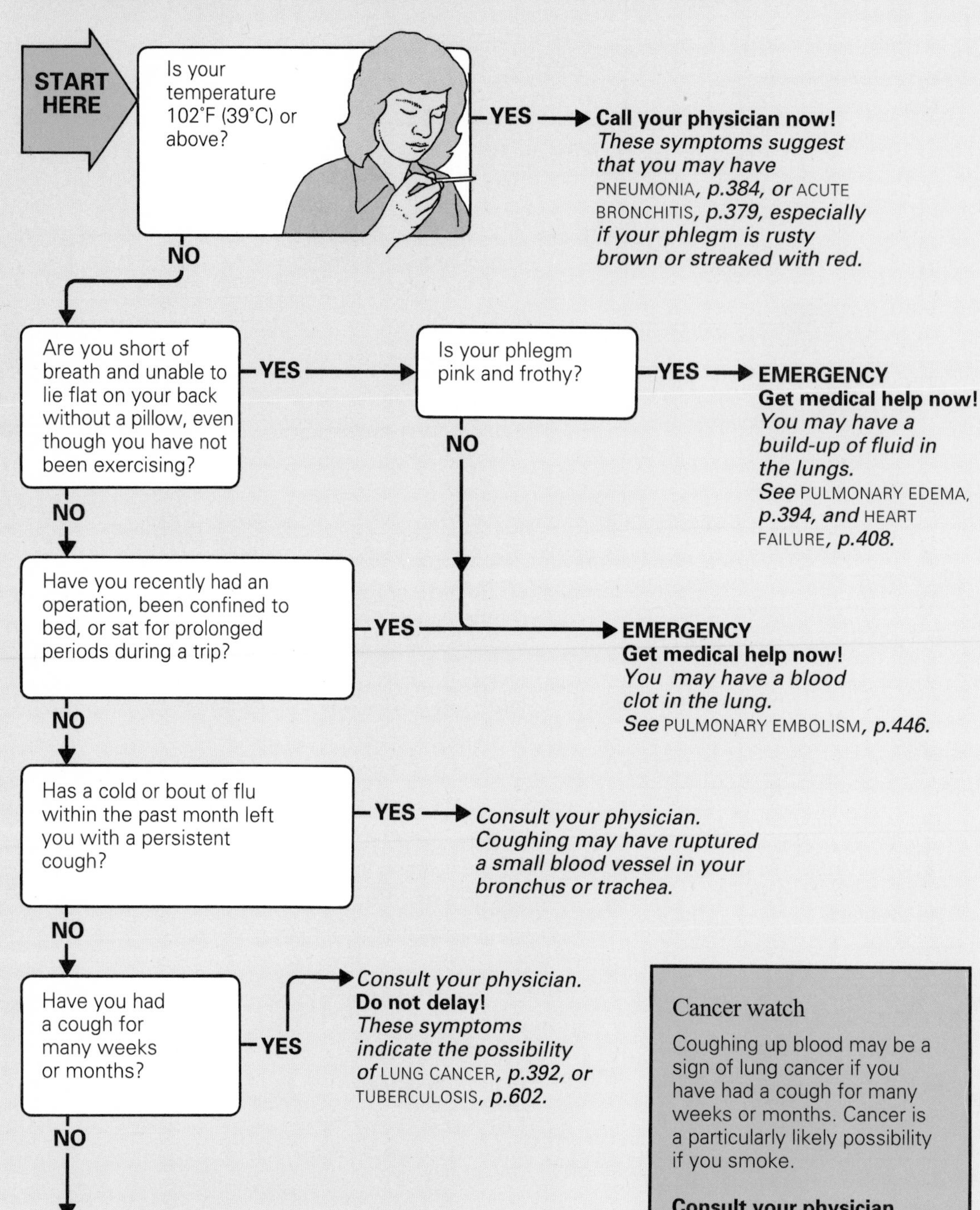

START HERE
Is your temperature 102°F (39°C) or above?
YES → **Call your physician now!** *These symptoms suggest that you may have* PNEUMONIA, *p.384, or* ACUTE BRONCHITIS, *p.379, especially if your phlegm is rusty brown or streaked with red.*
NO
Are you short of breath and unable to lie flat on your back without a pillow, even though you have not been exercising?
YES → Is your phlegm pink and frothy?
YES → **EMERGENCY** **Get medical help now!** *You may have a build-up of fluid in the lungs. See* PULMONARY EDEMA, *p.394, and* HEART FAILURE, *p.408.*
NO
NO
Have you recently had an operation, been confined to bed, or sat for prolonged periods during a trip?
YES → **EMERGENCY** **Get medical help now!** *You may have a blood clot in the lung. See* PULMONARY EMBOLISM, *p.446.*
NO
Has a cold or bout of flu within the past month left you with a persistent cough?
YES → *Consult your physician. Coughing may have ruptured a small blood vessel in your bronchus or trachea.*
NO
Have you had a cough for many weeks or months?
YES → *Consult your physician.* **Do not delay!** *These symptoms indicate the possibility of* LUNG CANCER, *p.392, or* TUBERCULOSIS, *p.602.*
NO
If you are unable to make a diagnosis from this chart, consult your physician without further delay.

Cancer watch

Coughing up blood may be a sign of lung cancer if you have had a cough for many weeks or months. Cancer is a particularly likely possibility if you smoke.

Consult your physician without delay!

40
GENERAL
all ages

Wheezing

Noisy, difficult breathing, when breathing in or breathing out.

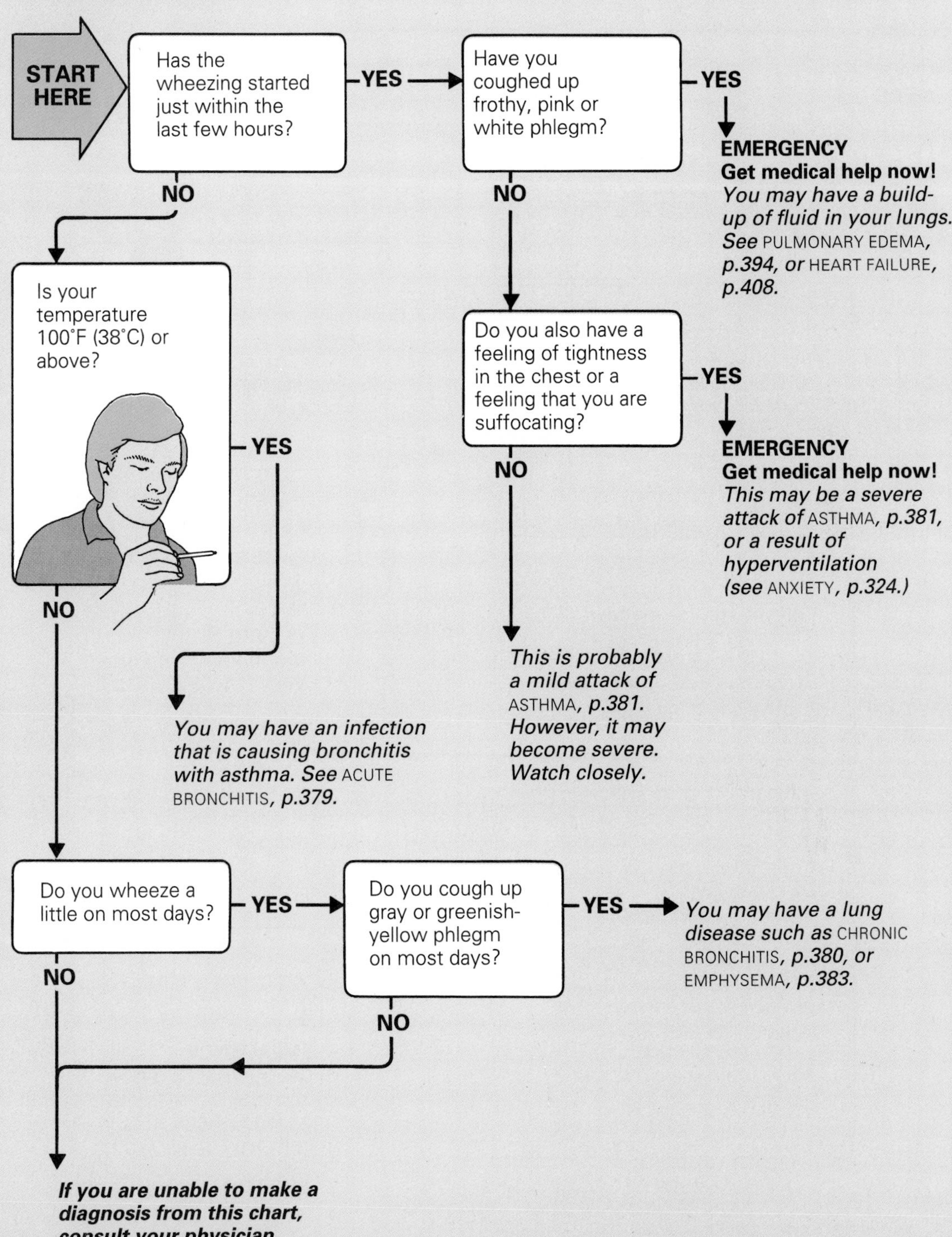

START HERE
Has the wheezing started just within the last few hours?
YES
NO
Have you coughed up frothy, pink or white phlegm?
YES
EMERGENCY
Get medical help now!
You may have a build-up of fluid in your lungs. See PULMONARY EDEMA, p.394, or HEART FAILURE, p.408.
NO
Do you also have a feeling of tightness in the chest or a feeling that you are suffocating?
YES
EMERGENCY
Get medical help now!
This may be a severe attack of ASTHMA, p.381, or a result of hyperventilation (see ANXIETY, p.324.)
NO
This is probably a mild attack of ASTHMA, p.381. However, it may become severe. Watch closely.
Is your temperature 100°F (38°C) or above?
YES
You may have an infection that is causing bronchitis with asthma. See ACUTE BRONCHITIS, p.379.
NO
Do you wheeze a little on most days?
YES
Do you cough up gray or greenish-yellow phlegm on most days?
YES
You may have a lung disease such as CHRONIC BRONCHITIS, p.380, or EMPHYSEMA, p.383.
NO
NO
If you are unable to make a diagnosis from this chart, consult your physician.

41

GENERAL
all ages

Difficulty breathing

Breathlessness or tightness in the chest that makes you aware of your breathing.

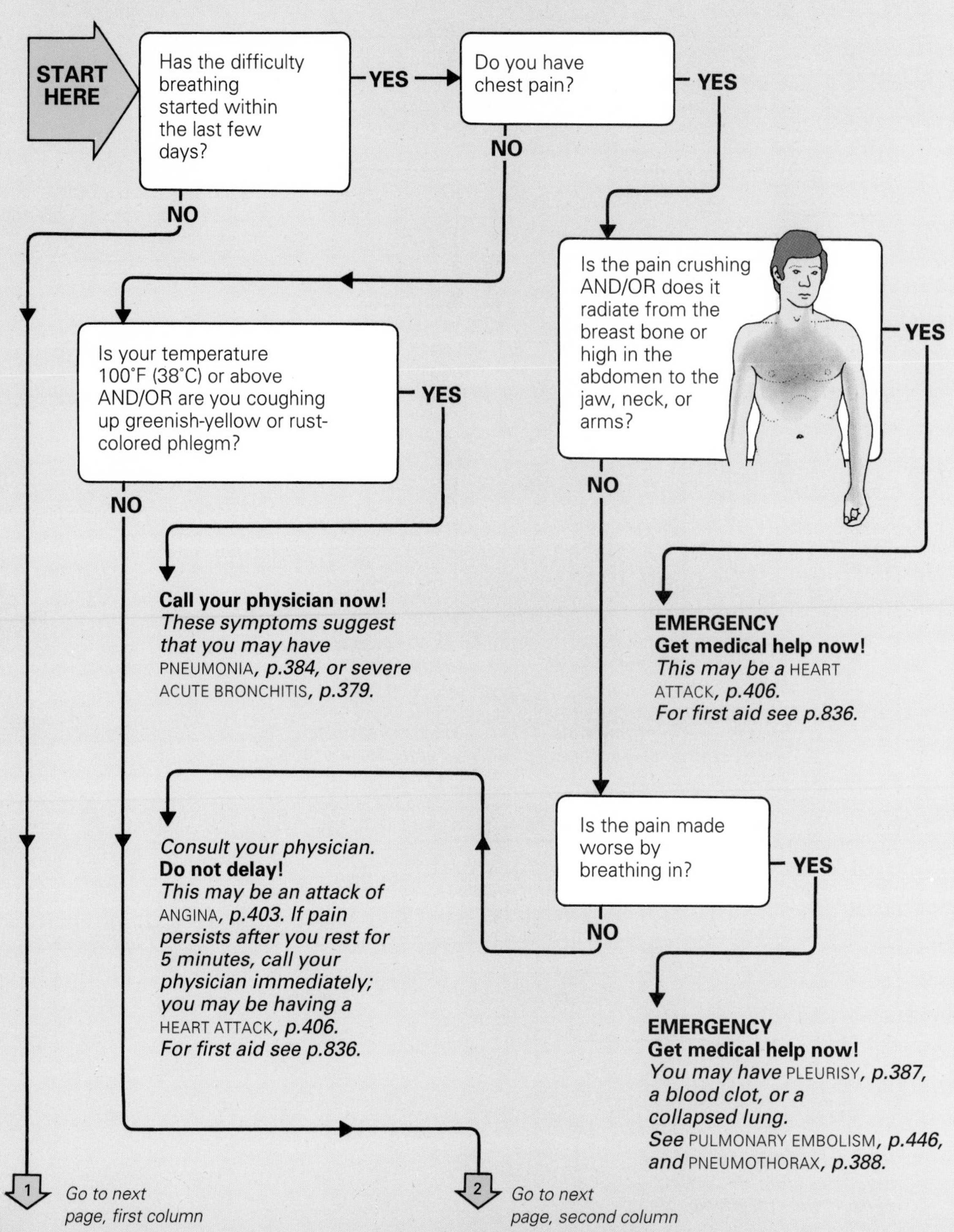

START HERE
Has the difficulty breathing started within the last few days?
YES
NO
Do you have chest pain?
YES
NO
Is the pain crushing AND/OR does it radiate from the breast bone or high in the abdomen to the jaw, neck, or arms?
YES
NO
Is your temperature 100°F (38°C) or above AND/OR are you coughing up greenish-yellow or rust-colored phlegm?
YES
NO
Call your physician now!
These symptoms suggest that you may have PNEUMONIA, p.384, or severe ACUTE BRONCHITIS, p.379.
EMERGENCY
Get medical help now!
This may be a HEART ATTACK, p.406.
For first aid see p.836.
Is the pain made worse by breathing in?
YES
NO
Consult your physician.
Do not delay!
This may be an attack of ANGINA, p.403. If pain persists after you rest for 5 minutes, call your physician immediately; you may be having a HEART ATTACK, p.406.
For first aid see p.836.
EMERGENCY
Get medical help now!
You may have PLEURISY, p.387, a blood clot, or a collapsed lung.
See PULMONARY EMBOLISM, p.446, and PNEUMOTHORAX, p.388.
1
Go to next page, first column
2
Go to next page, second column

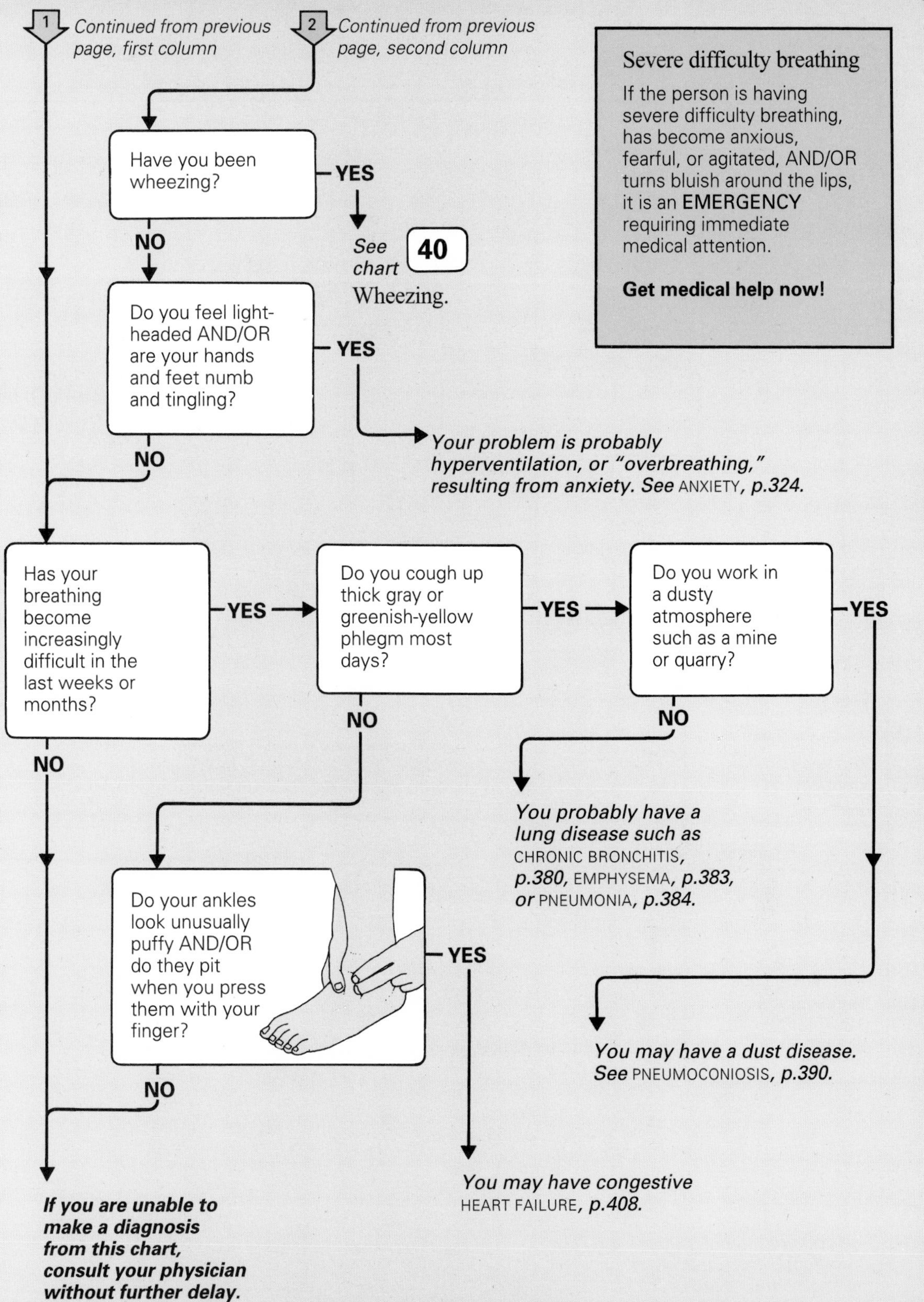
1 Continued from previous page, first column
2 Continued from previous page, second column
Have you been wheezing?
YES
See chart 40 Wheezing.
NO
Do you feel light-headed AND/OR are your hands and feet numb and tingling?
YES
Your problem is probably hyperventilation, or "overbreathing," resulting from anxiety. See ANXIETY, p.324.
NO
Has your breathing become increasingly difficult in the last weeks or months?
YES
Do you cough up thick gray or greenish-yellow phlegm most days?
YES
Do you work in a dusty atmosphere such as a mine or quarry?
YES
You may have a dust disease. See PNEUMOCONIOSIS, p.390.
NO
You probably have a lung disease such as CHRONIC BRONCHITIS, p.380, EMPHYSEMA, p.383, or PNEUMONIA, p.384.
NO
Do your ankles look unusually puffy AND/OR do they pit when you press them with your finger?
YES
You may have congestive HEART FAILURE, p.408.
NO
NO
If you are unable to make a diagnosis from this chart, consult your physician without further delay.
Severe difficulty breathing
If the person is having severe difficulty breathing, has become anxious, fearful, or agitated, AND/OR turns bluish around the lips, it is an EMERGENCY requiring immediate medical attention.
Get medical help now!

42
GENERAL
all ages

Toothache

Pain in one tooth, or in the teeth and gums generally, either in the form of a dull throb or a sharp twinge.

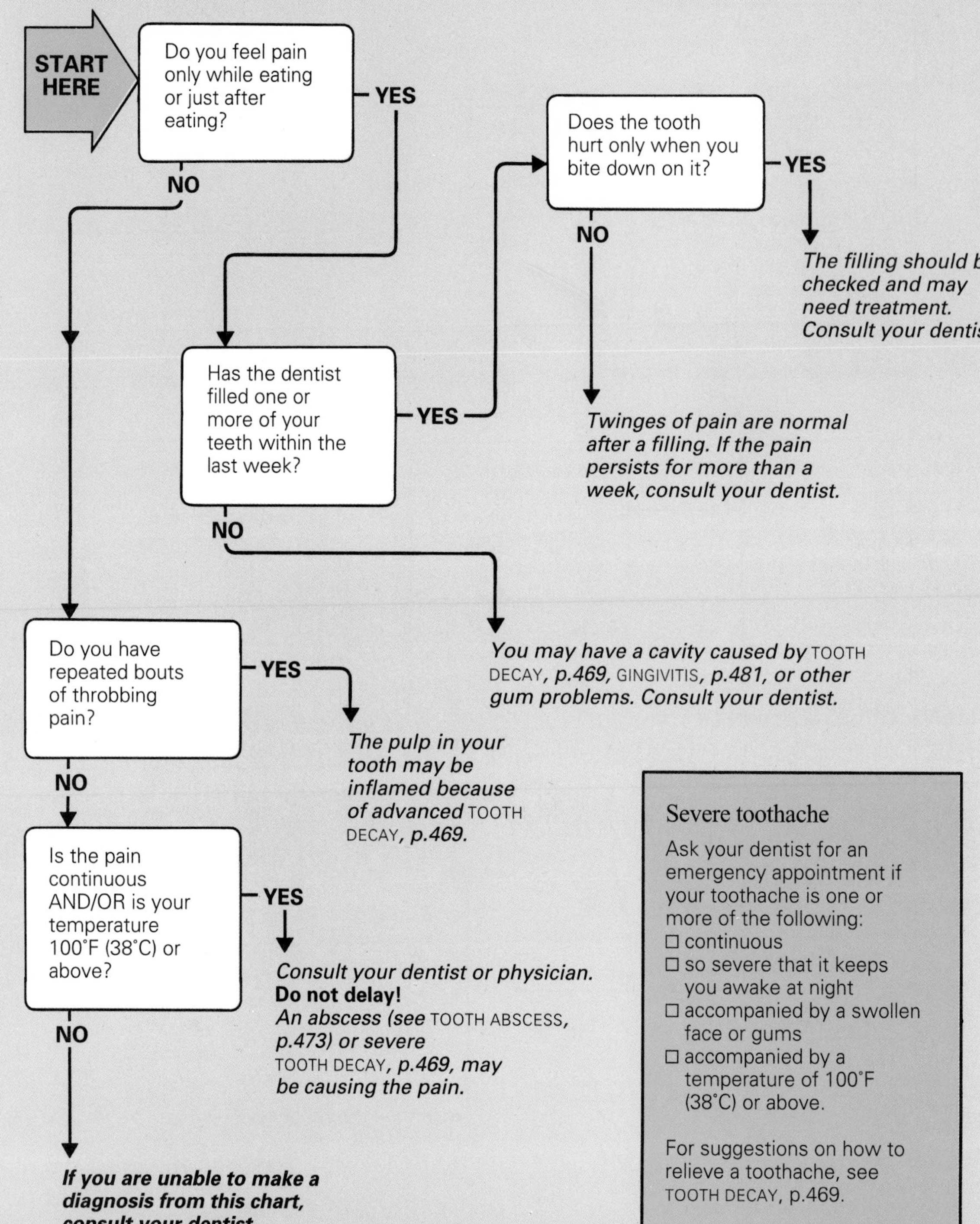

START HERE
Do you feel pain only while eating or just after eating?
YES
NO
Does the tooth hurt only when you bite down on it?
YES
NO
The filling should be checked and may need treatment. Consult your dentist.
Has the dentist filled one or more of your teeth within the last week?
YES
NO
Twinges of pain are normal after a filling. If the pain persists for more than a week, consult your dentist.
Do you have repeated bouts of throbbing pain?
YES
NO
You may have a cavity caused by TOOTH DECAY, p.469, GINGIVITIS, p.481, or other gum problems. Consult your dentist.
The pulp in your tooth may be inflamed because of advanced TOOTH DECAY, p.469.
Is the pain continuous AND/OR is your temperature 100˚F (38˚C) or above?
YES
NO
Consult your dentist or physician. Do not delay! An abscess (see TOOTH ABSCESS, p.473) or severe TOOTH DECAY, p.469, may be causing the pain.
If you are unable to make a diagnosis from this chart, consult your dentist.
Severe toothache
Ask your dentist for an emergency appointment if your toothache is one or more of the following:
☐ continuous
☐ so severe that it keeps you awake at night
☐ accompanied by a swollen face or gums
☐ accompanied by a temperature of 100˚F (38˚C) or above.
For suggestions on how to relieve a toothache, see TOOTH DECAY, p.469.

43
GENERAL
all ages

Difficulty swallowing

Discomfort or pain when swallowing, or difficulty in making food go down at all.

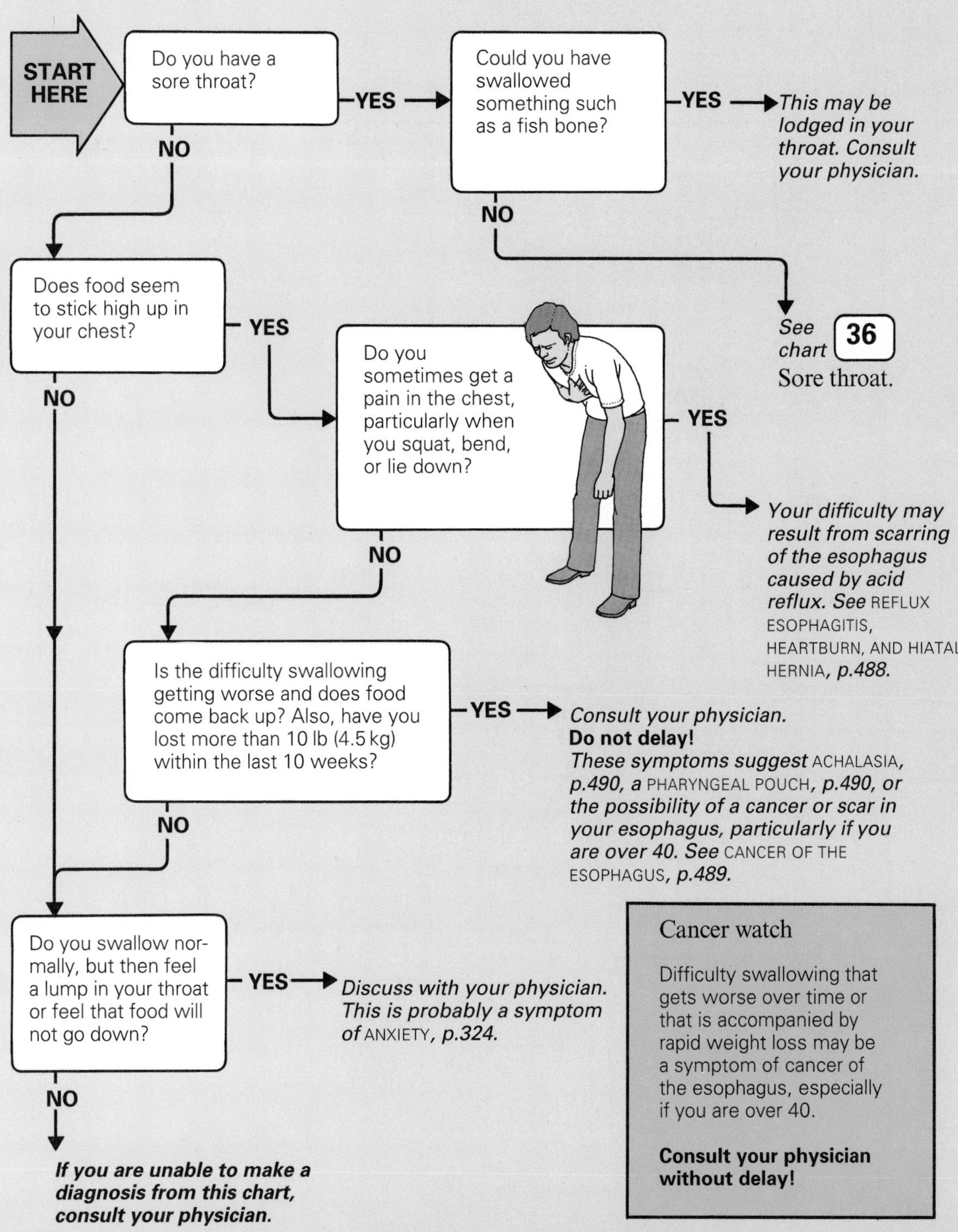

START HERE
Do you have a sore throat?
YES
Could you have swallowed something such as a fish bone?
YES
This may be lodged in your throat. Consult your physician.
NO
See chart 36 Sore throat.
NO
Does food seem to stick high up in your chest?
YES
Do you sometimes get a pain in the chest, particularly when you squat, bend, or lie down?
YES
Your difficulty may result from scarring of the esophagus caused by acid reflux. See REFLUX ESOPHAGITIS, HEARTBURN, AND HIATAL HERNIA*, p.488.*
NO
NO
Is the difficulty swallowing getting worse and does food come back up? Also, have you lost more than 10 lb (4.5 kg) within the last 10 weeks?
YES
Consult your physician.
Do not delay!
These symptoms suggest ACHALASIA*, p.490, a* PHARYNGEAL POUCH*, p.490, or the possibility of a cancer or scar in your esophagus, particularly if you are over 40. See* CANCER OF THE ESOPHAGUS*, p.489.*
NO
Do you swallow normally, but then feel a lump in your throat or feel that food will not go down?
YES
Discuss with your physician. This is probably a symptom of ANXIETY*, p.324.*
NO
If you are unable to make a diagnosis from this chart, consult your physician.
Cancer watch
Difficulty swallowing that gets worse over time or that is accompanied by rapid weight loss may be a symptom of cancer of the esophagus, especially if you are over 40.
Consult your physician without delay!

44

GENERAL
all ages

Sore mouth and/or tongue

Soreness anywhere inside the mouth and/or on or around the tongue and lips.

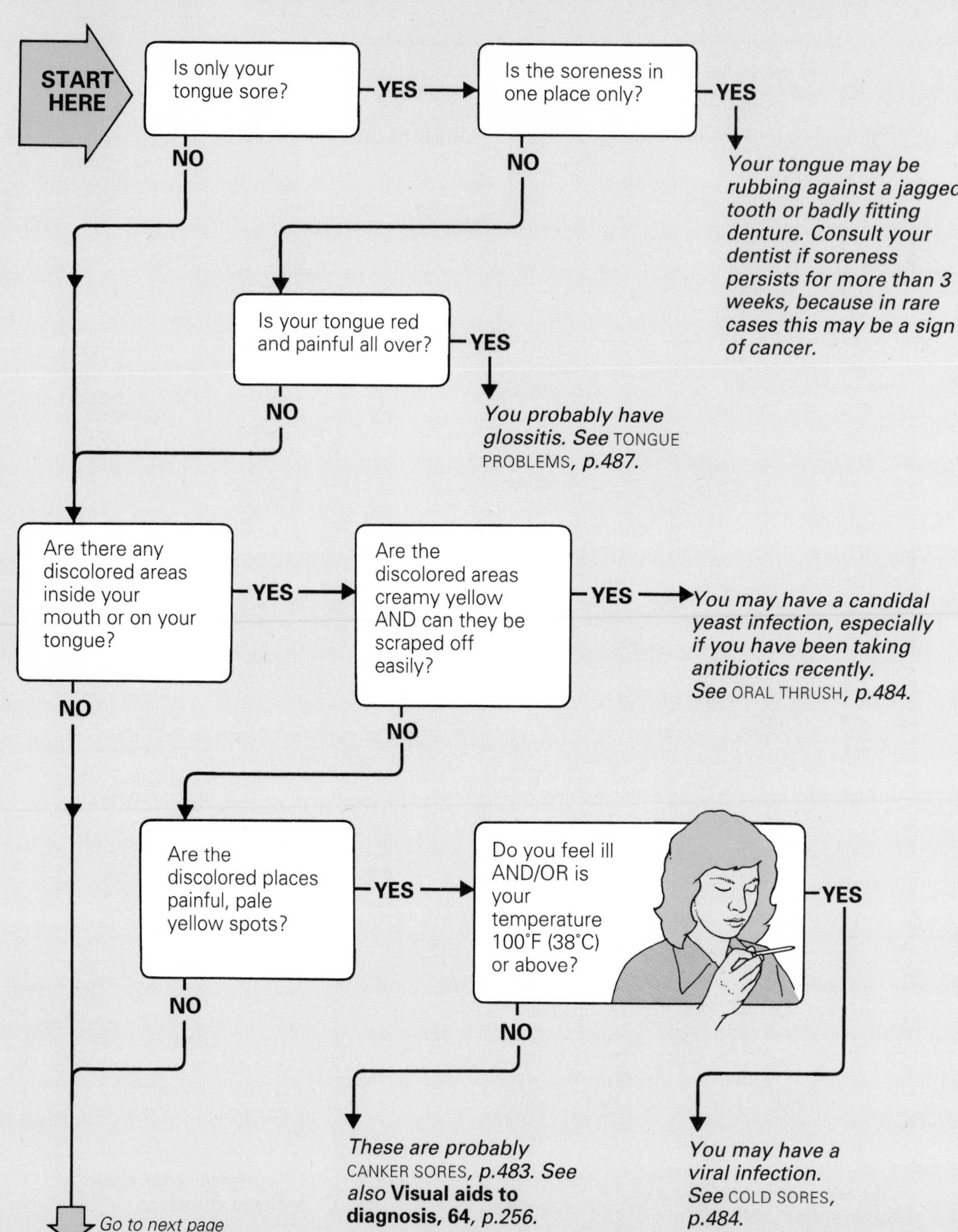

START HERE
Is only your tongue sore?
YES
NO
Is the soreness in one place only?
YES
NO
Your tongue may be rubbing against a jagged tooth or badly fitting denture. Consult your dentist if soreness persists for more than 3 weeks, because in rare cases this may be a sign of cancer.
Is your tongue red and painful all over?
YES
NO
You probably have glossitis. See TONGUE PROBLEMS, p.487.
Are there any discolored areas inside your mouth or on your tongue?
YES
NO
Are the discolored areas creamy yellow AND can they be scraped off easily?
YES
NO
You may have a candidal yeast infection, especially if you have been taking antibiotics recently. See ORAL THRUSH, p.484.
Are the discolored places painful, pale yellow spots?
YES
NO
Do you feel ill AND/OR is your temperature 100°F (38°C) or above?
YES
NO
These are probably CANKER SORES, p.483. See also Visual aids to diagnosis, 64, p.256.
You may have a viral infection. See COLD SORES, p.484.
Go to next page

Continued from previous page

Are your gums painful, red, and swollen?

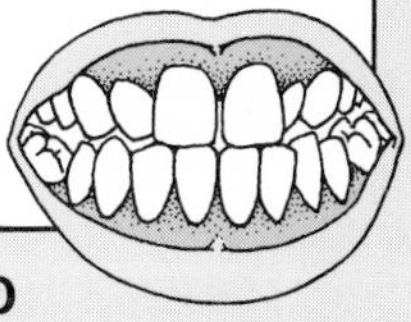

YES → Does your breath smell bad AND/OR do you have a foul taste in your mouth?

YES → *Consult your dentist. You may have* ORAL LICHEN PLANUS, *p.485, an infection of the gums.*

NO → *You may have severe* GINGIVITIS, *p.481, other gum disease, or a viral infection. See* COLD SORES, *p.484.*

NO → Do you have sore places on or around the lips?

YES → Are the sores red, rough, AND/OR blistered?

YES → *You probably have a* COLD SORE, *p.484. See also* **Visual aids to diagnosis, 24**, *p.246.*

NO → Are there cracks at the corners of your mouth?

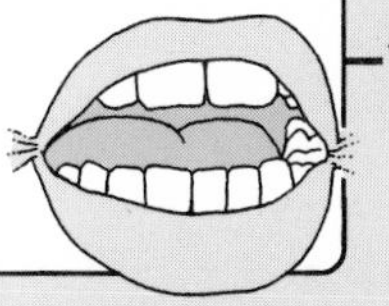

YES → *This soreness may be caused by badly fitting dentures. See* DENTURE PROBLEMS, *p.479. Or you may have a vitamin deficiency, see* VITAMIN AND MINERAL DEFICIENCY, *p.532, or you may have an overbite that causes the cracks in your skin; consult your dentist about applying petroleum jelly to the affected skin.*

NO → Have you recently started to use any new cosmetics or lotions on your lips?

YES → *The soreness may be an allergic reaction to an ingredient in your cosmetics. See* ECZEMA AND DERMATITIS, *p.269.*

NO →

If you are unable to make a diagnosis from this chart, consult your physician.

Cancer watch

Any sore area in the mouth or on the tongue may indicate cancer if it fails to heal within 3 weeks.

Consult your physician or dentist without delay!

45
GENERAL
all ages

Bad breath

An offensive smell from your mouth that you may or may not be aware of until it is mentioned by somebody else.

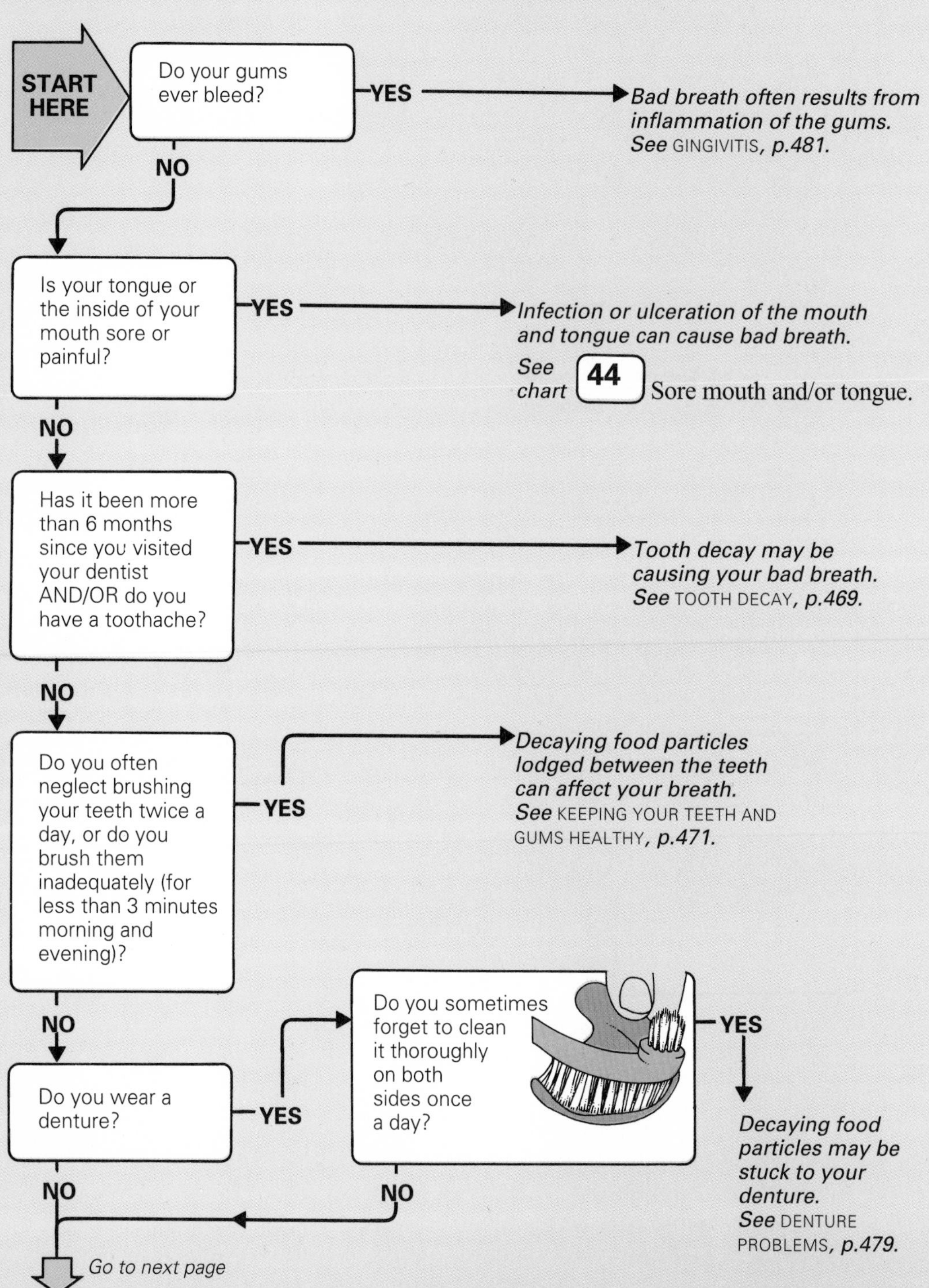

START HERE
Do your gums ever bleed?
YES
Bad breath often results from inflammation of the gums. See GINGIVITIS*, p.481.*
NO
Is your tongue or the inside of your mouth sore or painful?
YES
Infection or ulceration of the mouth and tongue can cause bad breath.
See chart 44 Sore mouth and/or tongue.
NO
Has it been more than 6 months since you visited your dentist AND/OR do you have a toothache?
YES
Tooth decay may be causing your bad breath. See TOOTH DECAY*, p.469.*
NO
Do you often neglect brushing your teeth twice a day, or do you brush them inadequately (for less than 3 minutes morning and evening)?
YES
Decaying food particles lodged between the teeth can affect your breath. See KEEPING YOUR TEETH AND GUMS HEALTHY*, p.471.*
NO
Do you wear a denture?
YES
Do you sometimes forget to clean it thoroughly on both sides once a day?
YES
Decaying food particles may be stuck to your denture. See DENTURE PROBLEMS*, p.479.*
NO
NO
Go to next page

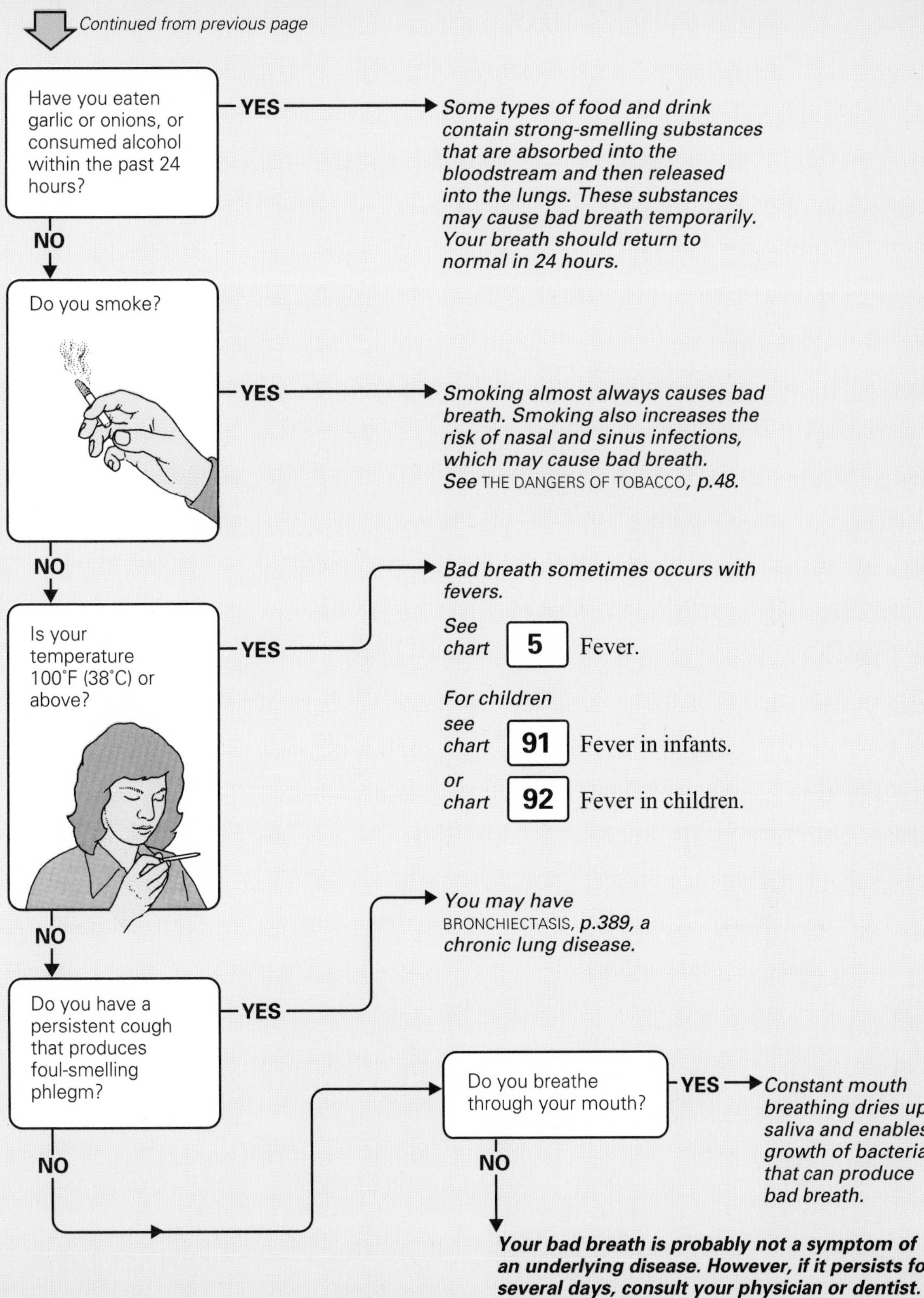
Continued from previous page
Have you eaten garlic or onions, or consumed alcohol within the past 24 hours?
YES
Some types of food and drink contain strong-smelling substances that are absorbed into the bloodstream and then released into the lungs. These substances may cause bad breath temporarily. Your breath should return to normal in 24 hours.
NO
Do you smoke?
YES
Smoking almost always causes bad breath. Smoking also increases the risk of nasal and sinus infections, which may cause bad breath. See THE DANGERS OF TOBACCO, p.48.
NO
Is your temperature 100°F (38°C) or above?
YES
Bad breath sometimes occurs with fevers.
See chart 5 Fever.
For children see chart 91 Fever in infants.
or chart 92 Fever in children.
NO
Do you have a persistent cough that produces foul-smelling phlegm?
YES
You may have BRONCHIECTASIS, p.389, a chronic lung disease.
NO
Do you breathe through your mouth?
YES
Constant mouth breathing dries up saliva and enables growth of bacteria that can produce bad breath.
NO
Your bad breath is probably not a symptom of an underlying disease. However, if it persists for several days, consult your physician or dentist.

46
GENERAL
all ages

Vomiting

Throwing up of stomach contents that may be preceded by nausea. For babies under 6 months see chart 87, **Vomiting in infants**.

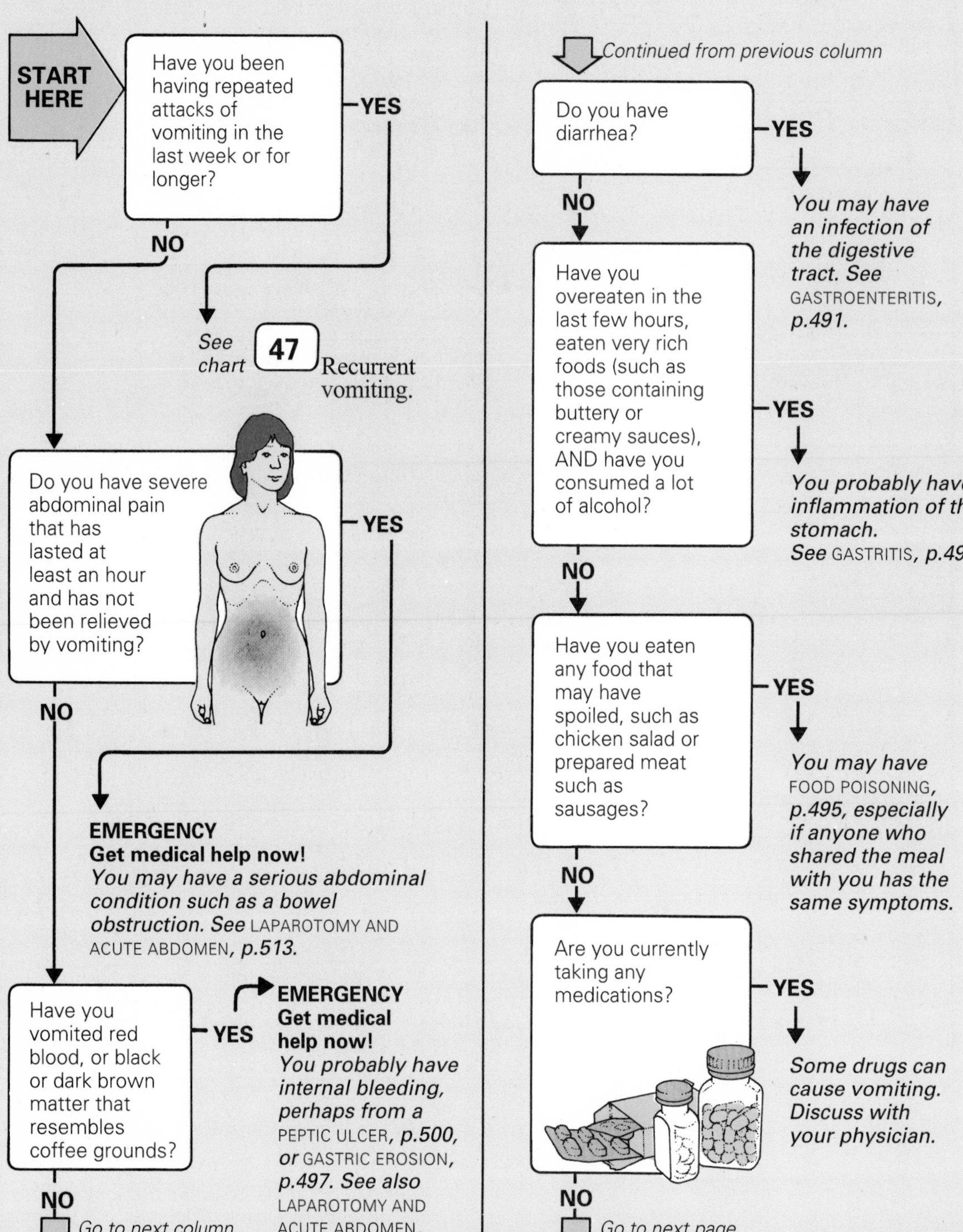

START HERE

Have you been having repeated attacks of vomiting in the last week or for longer?

YES → *See chart* **47** Recurrent vomiting.

NO ↓

Do you have severe abdominal pain that has lasted at least an hour and has not been relieved by vomiting?

YES → **EMERGENCY Get medical help now!** *You may have a serious abdominal condition such as a bowel obstruction. See* LAPAROTOMY AND ACUTE ABDOMEN, *p.513.*

NO ↓

Have you vomited red blood, or black or dark brown matter that resembles coffee grounds?

YES → **EMERGENCY Get medical help now!** *You probably have internal bleeding, perhaps from a* PEPTIC ULCER, *p.500, or* GASTRIC EROSION, *p.497. See also* LAPAROTOMY AND ACUTE ABDOMEN, *p.513.*

NO ↓

Go to next column

Continued from previous column

Do you have diarrhea?

YES → *You may have an infection of the digestive tract. See* GASTROENTERITIS, *p.491.*

NO ↓

Have you overeaten in the last few hours, eaten very rich foods (such as those containing buttery or creamy sauces), AND have you consumed a lot of alcohol?

YES → *You probably have inflammation of the stomach. See* GASTRITIS, *p.497.*

NO ↓

Have you eaten any food that may have spoiled, such as chicken salad or prepared meat such as sausages?

YES → *You may have* FOOD POISONING, *p.495, especially if anyone who shared the meal with you has the same symptoms.*

NO ↓

Are you currently taking any medications?

YES → *Some drugs can cause vomiting. Discuss with your physician.*

NO ↓

Go to next page, first column

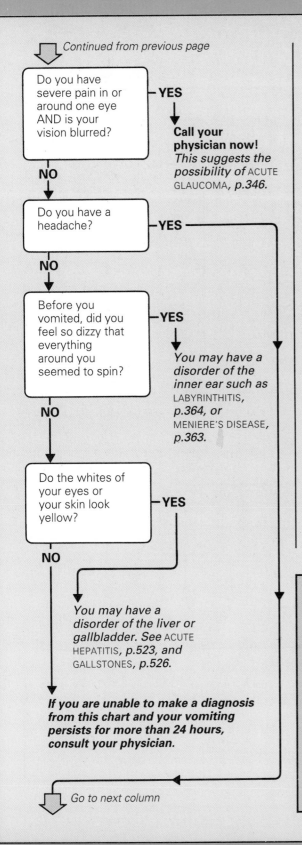

Continued from previous page

Do you have severe pain in or around one eye AND is your vision blurred?

YES → **Call your physician now!** *This suggests the possibility of* ACUTE GLAUCOMA, *p.346.*

NO ↓

Do you have a headache?

YES → Go to next column

NO ↓

Before you vomited, did you feel so dizzy that everything around you seemed to spin?

YES → *You may have a disorder of the inner ear such as* LABYRINTHITIS, *p.364, or* MENIERE'S DISEASE, *p.363.*

NO ↓

Do the whites of your eyes or your skin look yellow?

YES → *You may have a disorder of the liver or gallbladder. See* ACUTE HEPATITIS, *p.523, and* GALLSTONES, *p.526.*

NO ↓

If you are unable to make a diagnosis from this chart and your vomiting persists for more than 24 hours, consult your physician.

Go to next column

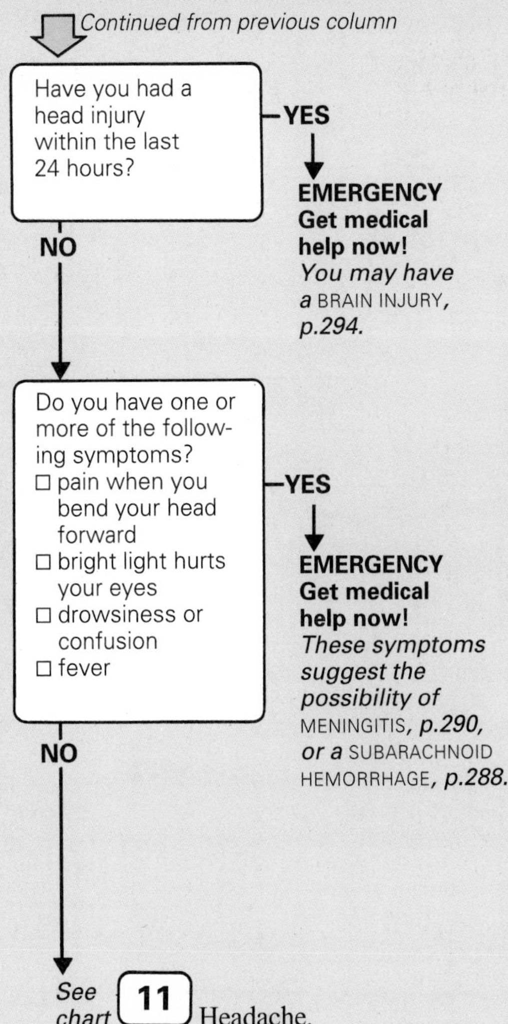

Continued from previous column
Have you had a head injury within the last 24 hours?
YES
EMERGENCY
Get medical help now!
You may have a BRAIN INJURY, p.294.
NO
Do you have one or more of the following symptoms?
☐ pain when you bend your head forward
☐ bright light hurts your eyes
☐ drowsiness or confusion
☐ fever
YES
EMERGENCY
Get medical help now!
These symptoms suggest the possibility of MENINGITIS, p.290, or a SUBARACHNOID HEMORRHAGE, p.288.
NO
See chart 11 Headache.

Persistent vomiting

If you have vomited numerous times in the course of one day, you may have lost a dangerous amount of body fluid.

Consult your physician without delay!

Red or dark blood in vomit

If your vomit contains dark red blood or dark brown matter that resembles coffee grounds (partly digested blood), it is an EMERGENCY that indicates gastrointestinal bleeding.

Get medical help now!

47

GENERAL
over 6 months

Recurrent vomiting

Throwing up of stomach contents several times in a week.
For babies under 6 months see chart 87, **Vomiting in infants**.

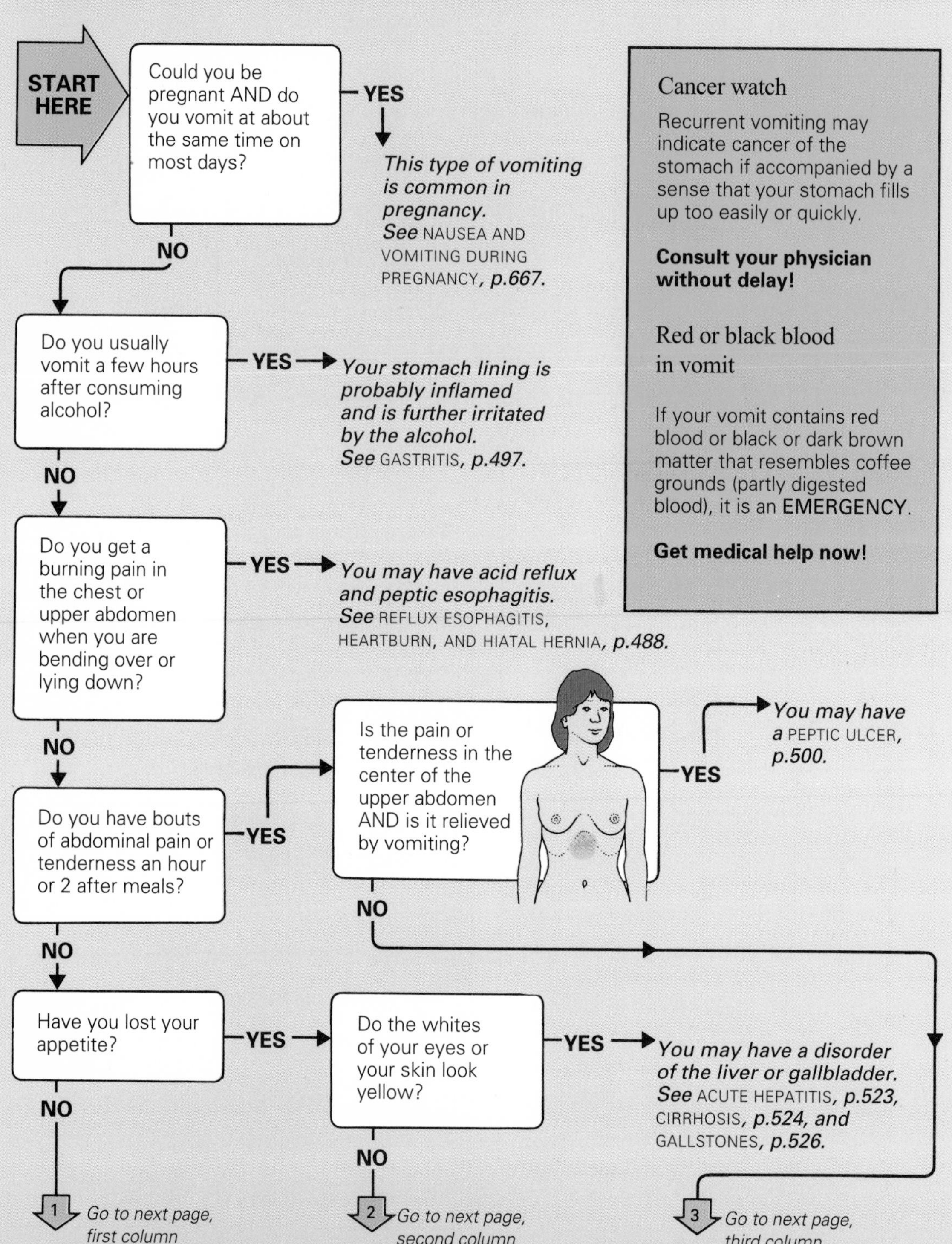

START HERE
Could you be pregnant AND do you vomit at about the same time on most days?
YES
This type of vomiting is common in pregnancy. See NAUSEA AND VOMITING DURING PREGNANCY, *p.667.*
NO
Do you usually vomit a few hours after consuming alcohol?
YES
Your stomach lining is probably inflamed and is further irritated by the alcohol. See GASTRITIS, *p.497.*
NO
Do you get a burning pain in the chest or upper abdomen when you are bending over or lying down?
YES
You may have acid reflux and peptic esophagitis. See REFLUX ESOPHAGITIS, HEARTBURN, AND HIATAL HERNIA, *p.488.*
NO
Do you have bouts of abdominal pain or tenderness an hour or 2 after meals?
YES
Is the pain or tenderness in the center of the upper abdomen AND is it relieved by vomiting?
YES
You may have a PEPTIC ULCER, *p.500.*
NO
NO
Have you lost your appetite?
YES
Do the whites of your eyes or your skin look yellow?
YES
You may have a disorder of the liver or gallbladder. See ACUTE HEPATITIS, *p.523,* CIRRHOSIS, *p.524, and* GALLSTONES, *p.526.*
NO
NO
1 *Go to next page, first column*
2 *Go to next page, second column*
3 *Go to next page, third column*

Cancer watch

Recurrent vomiting may indicate cancer of the stomach if accompanied by a sense that your stomach fills up too easily or quickly.

Consult your physician without delay!

Red or black blood in vomit

If your vomit contains red blood or black or dark brown matter that resembles coffee grounds (partly digested blood), it is an EMERGENCY.

Get medical help now!

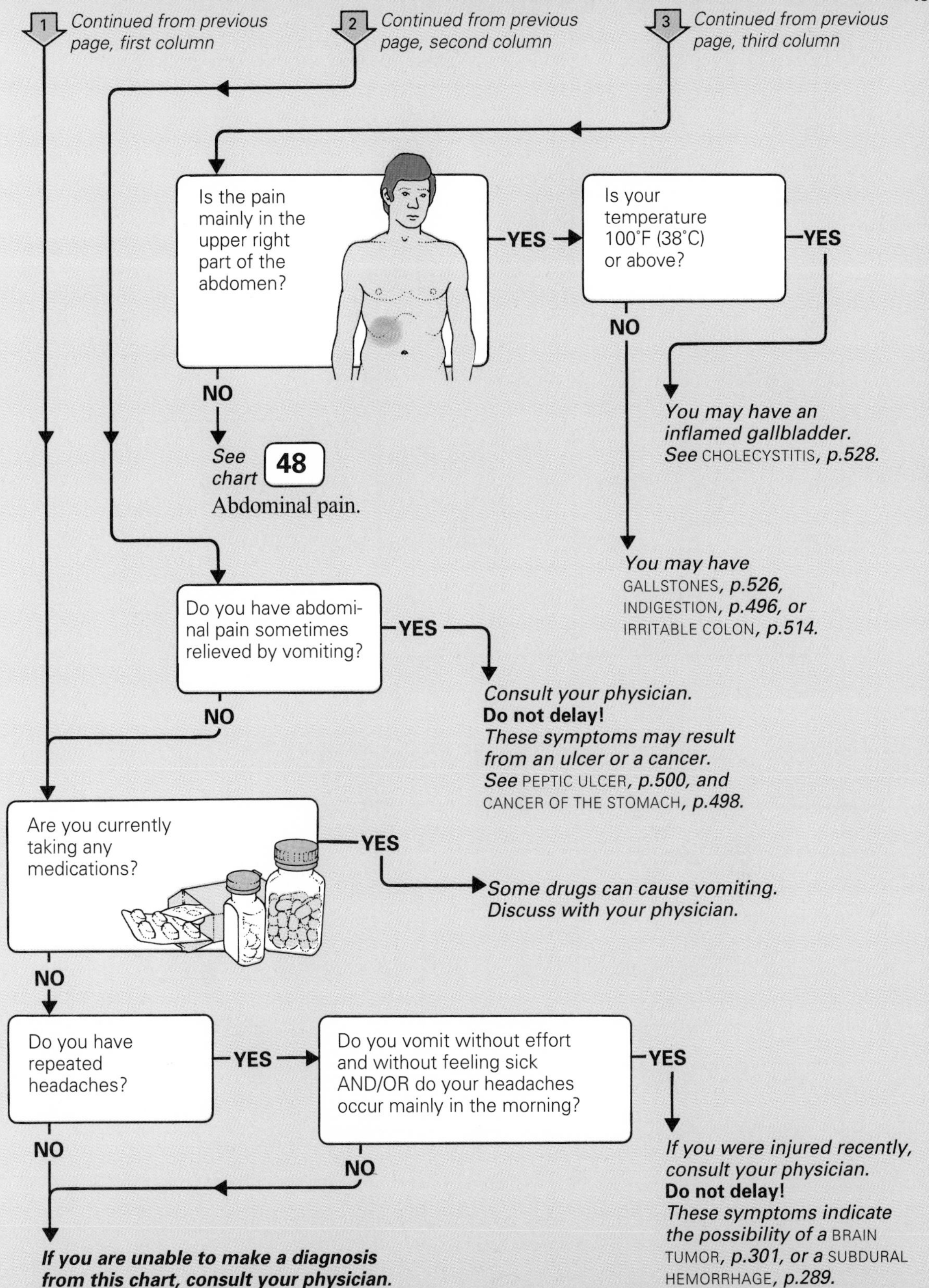
1
Continued from previous page, first column
2
Continued from previous page, second column
3
Continued from previous page, third column
Is the pain mainly in the upper right part of the abdomen?
YES
Is your temperature 100°F (38°C) or above?
YES
NO
You may have an inflamed gallbladder. See CHOLECYSTITIS, p.528.
NO
See chart
48
Abdominal pain.
You may have GALLSTONES, p.526, INDIGESTION, p.496, or IRRITABLE COLON, p.514.
Do you have abdominal pain sometimes relieved by vomiting?
YES
Consult your physician.
Do not delay!
These symptoms may result from an ulcer or a cancer.
See PEPTIC ULCER, p.500, and CANCER OF THE STOMACH, p.498.
NO
Are you currently taking any medications?
YES
Some drugs can cause vomiting. Discuss with your physician.
NO
Do you have repeated headaches?
YES
Do you vomit without effort and without feeling sick AND/OR do your headaches occur mainly in the morning?
YES
If you were injured recently, consult your physician.
Do not delay!
These symptoms indicate the possibility of a BRAIN TUMOR, p.301, or a SUBDURAL HEMORRHAGE, p.289.
NO
NO
If you are unable to make a diagnosis from this chart, consult your physician.

48
GENERAL
over 14 years

Abdominal pain

General or localized pain between the bottom of the rib cage and the groin. For children see chart 93, **Abdominal pain in children**.

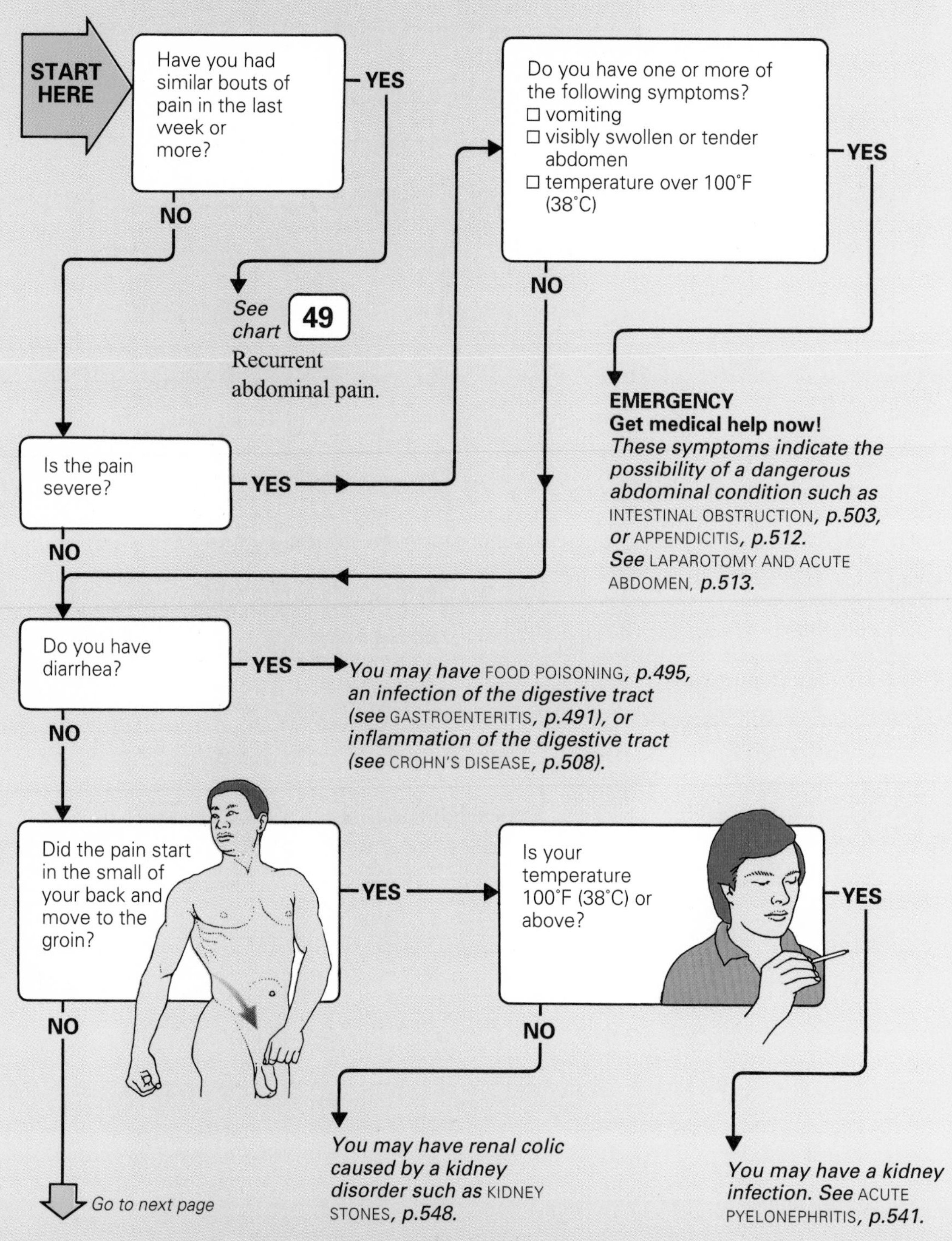

START HERE
Have you had similar bouts of pain in the last week or more?
YES
See chart 49 Recurrent abdominal pain.
NO
Is the pain severe?
YES
Do you have one or more of the following symptoms?
☐ vomiting
☐ visibly swollen or tender abdomen
☐ temperature over 100°F (38°C)
YES
EMERGENCY
Get medical help now!
These symptoms indicate the possibility of a dangerous abdominal condition such as INTESTINAL OBSTRUCTION, p.503, or APPENDICITIS, p.512.
See LAPAROTOMY AND ACUTE ABDOMEN, p.513.
NO
NO
Do you have diarrhea?
YES
You may have FOOD POISONING, p.495, an infection of the digestive tract (see GASTROENTERITIS, p.491), or inflammation of the digestive tract (see CROHN'S DISEASE, p.508).
NO
Did the pain start in the small of your back and move to the groin?
YES
Is your temperature 100°F (38°C) or above?
YES
You may have a kidney infection. See ACUTE PYELONEPHRITIS, p.541.
NO
You may have renal colic caused by a kidney disorder such as KIDNEY STONES, p.548.
NO
Go to next page

Continued from previous page

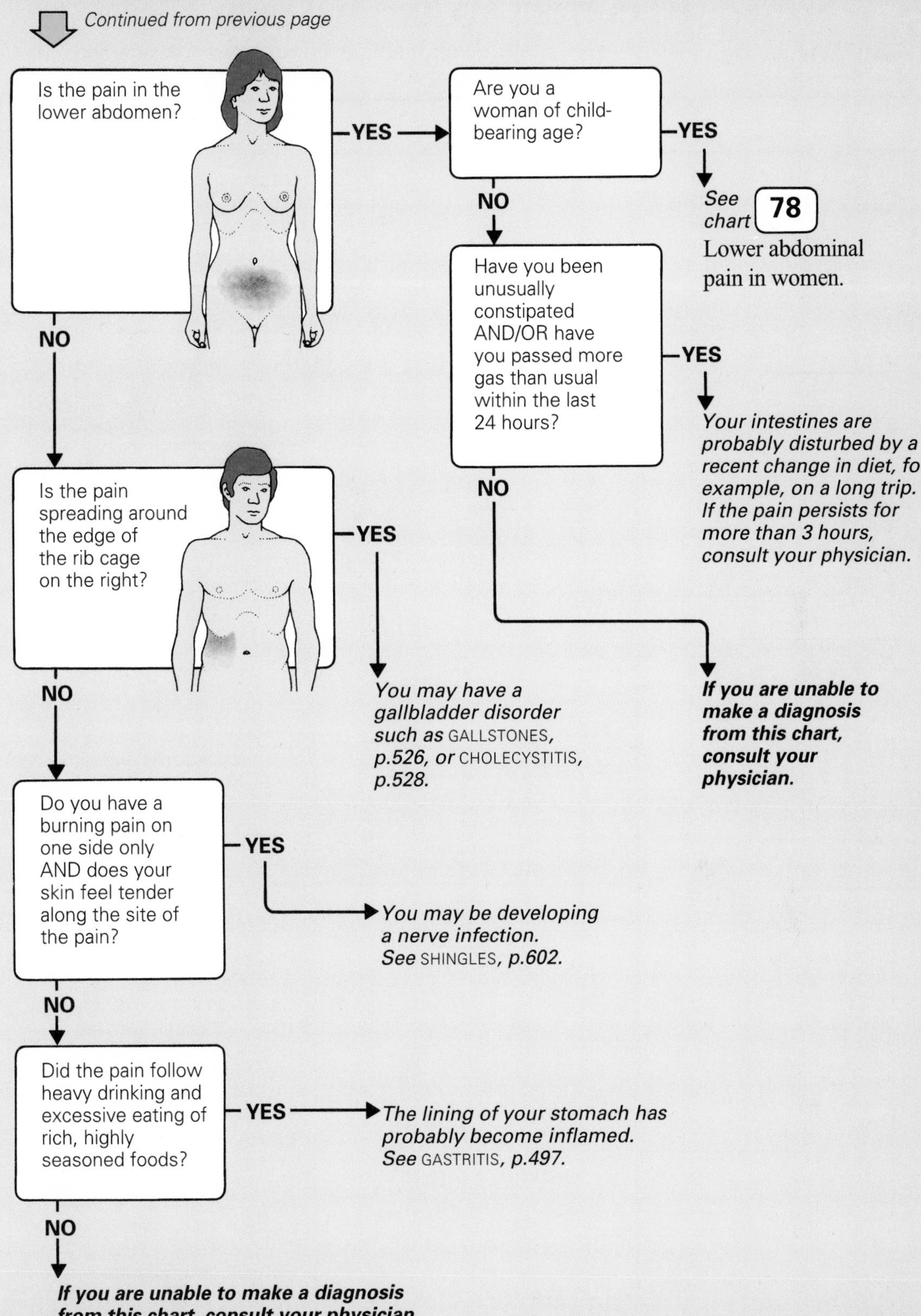

Is the pain in the lower abdomen?
YES
Are you a woman of child-bearing age?
YES
See chart 78
Lower abdominal pain in women.
NO
Have you been unusually constipated AND/OR have you passed more gas than usual within the last 24 hours?
YES
Your intestines are probably disturbed by a recent change in diet, for example, on a long trip. If the pain persists for more than 3 hours, consult your physician.
NO
If you are unable to make a diagnosis from this chart, consult your physician.
NO
Is the pain spreading around the edge of the rib cage on the right?
YES
You may have a gallbladder disorder such as GALLSTONES, p.526, or CHOLECYSTITIS, p.528.
NO
Do you have a burning pain on one side only AND does your skin feel tender along the site of the pain?
YES
You may be developing a nerve infection. See SHINGLES, p.602.
NO
Did the pain follow heavy drinking and excessive eating of rich, highly seasoned foods?
YES
The lining of your stomach has probably become inflamed. See GASTRITIS, p.497.
NO
If you are unable to make a diagnosis from this chart, consult your physician.

49
GENERAL
over 14 years

Recurrent abdominal pain

Abdominal pain that returns on several days over a week or more. For children see chart 93, **Abdominal pain in children**.

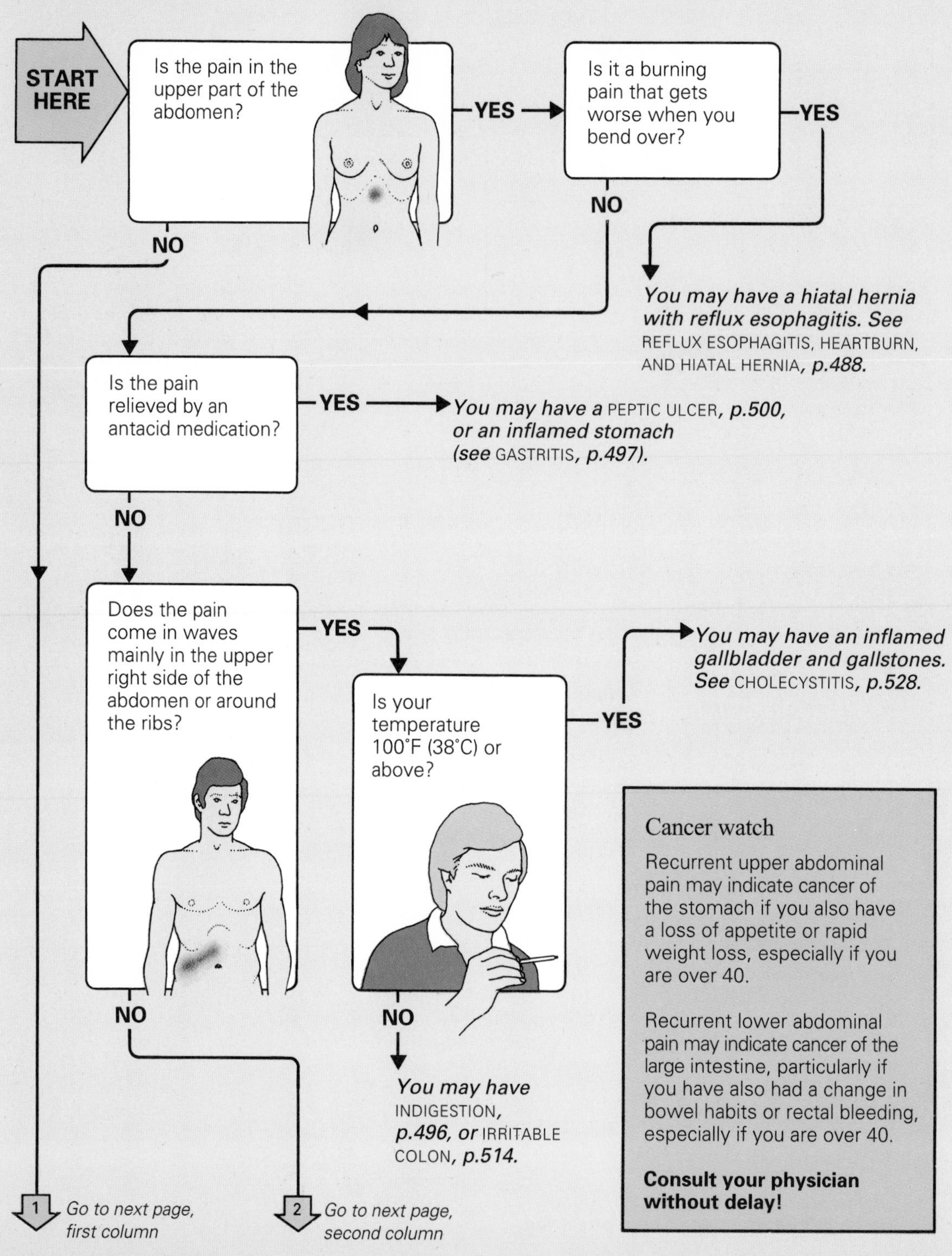

START HERE
Is the pain in the upper part of the abdomen?
YES
Is it a burning pain that gets worse when you bend over?
YES
You may have a hiatal hernia with reflux esophagitis. See REFLUX ESOPHAGITIS, HEARTBURN, AND HIATAL HERNIA, *p.488.*
NO
NO
Is the pain relieved by an antacid medication?
YES
You may have a PEPTIC ULCER, *p.500, or an inflamed stomach (see* GASTRITIS, *p.497).*
NO
Does the pain come in waves mainly in the upper right side of the abdomen or around the ribs?
YES
Is your temperature 100°F (38°C) or above?
YES
You may have an inflamed gallbladder and gallstones. See CHOLECYSTITIS, *p.528.*
NO
NO
You may have INDIGESTION, *p.496, or* IRRITABLE COLON, *p.514.*
1 *Go to next page, first column*
2 *Go to next page, second column*

Cancer watch

Recurrent upper abdominal pain may indicate cancer of the stomach if you also have a loss of appetite or rapid weight loss, especially if you are over 40.

Recurrent lower abdominal pain may indicate cancer of the large intestine, particularly if you have also had a change in bowel habits or rectal bleeding, especially if you are over 40.

Consult your physician without delay!

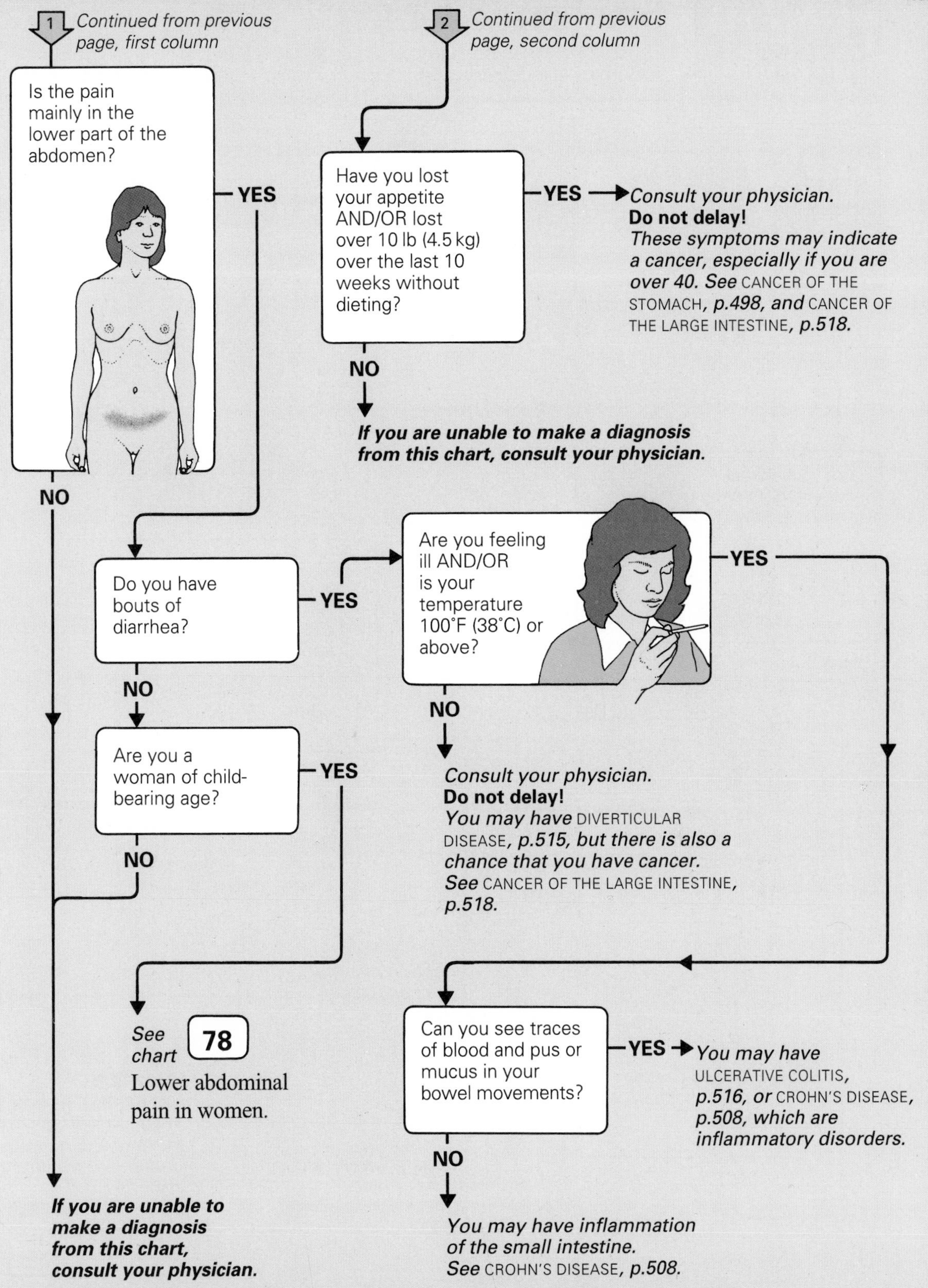

1 Continued from previous page, first column
Is the pain mainly in the lower part of the abdomen?
YES
NO
2 Continued from previous page, second column
Have you lost your appetite AND/OR lost over 10 lb (4.5 kg) over the last 10 weeks without dieting?
YES
Consult your physician.
Do not delay!
These symptoms may indicate a cancer, especially if you are over 40. See CANCER OF THE STOMACH, p.498, and CANCER OF THE LARGE INTESTINE, p.518.
NO
If you are unable to make a diagnosis from this chart, consult your physician.
Do you have bouts of diarrhea?
YES
NO
Are you feeling ill AND/OR is your temperature 100°F (38°C) or above?
YES
NO
Consult your physician.
Do not delay!
You may have DIVERTICULAR DISEASE, p.515, but there is also a chance that you have cancer. See CANCER OF THE LARGE INTESTINE, p.518.
Are you a woman of child-bearing age?
YES
NO
See chart 78
Lower abdominal pain in women.
Can you see traces of blood and pus or mucus in your bowel movements?
YES
You may have ULCERATIVE COLITIS, p.516, or CROHN'S DISEASE, p.508, which are inflammatory disorders.
NO
You may have inflammation of the small intestine. See CROHN'S DISEASE, p.508.
If you are unable to make a diagnosis from this chart, consult your physician.

50

GENERAL
all ages

Swollen abdomen

Generalized swelling over the entire abdomen between the bottom of the rib cage and the groin.

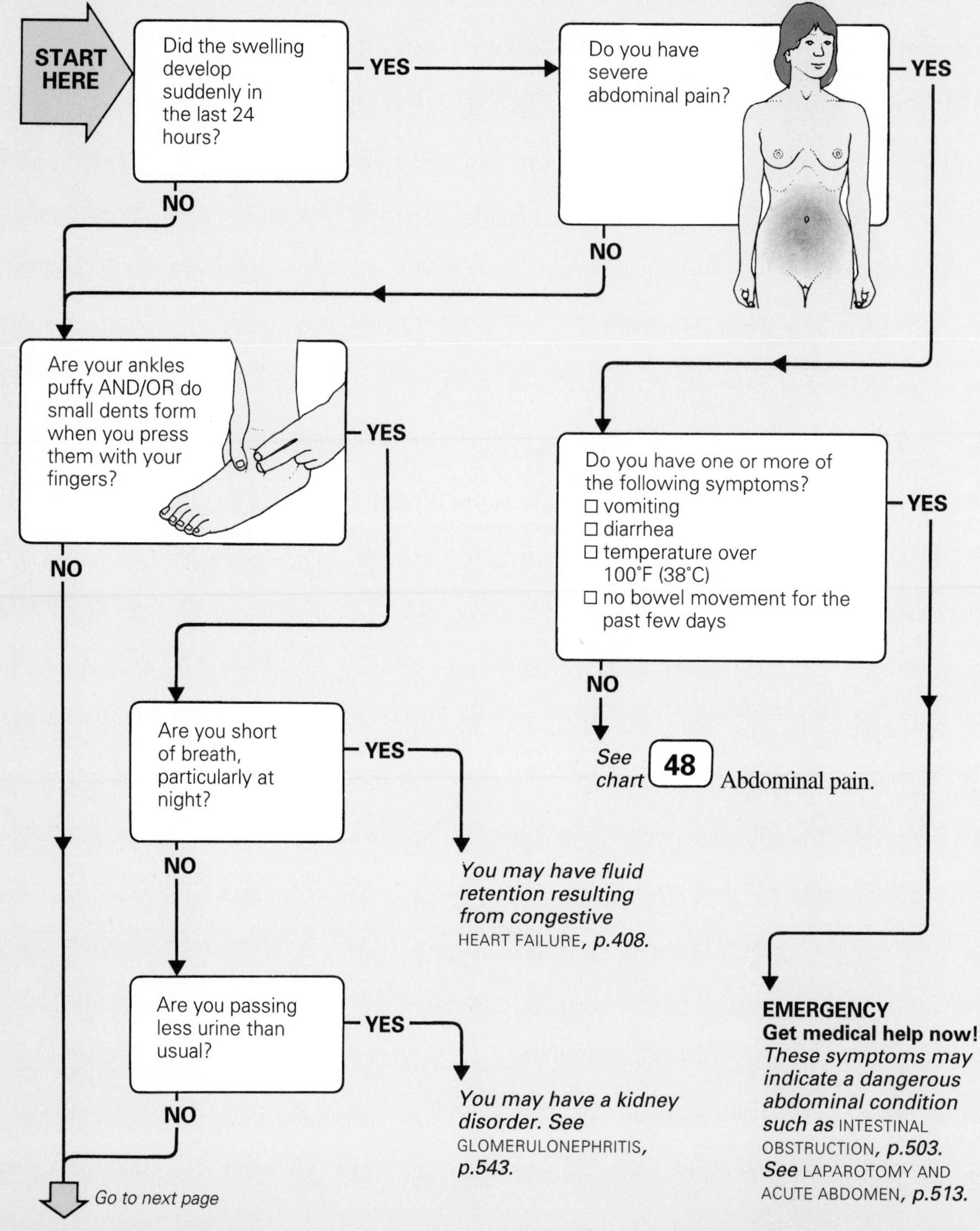

START HERE
Did the swelling develop suddenly in the last 24 hours?
YES
NO
Do you have severe abdominal pain?
YES
NO
Are your ankles puffy AND/OR do small dents form when you press them with your fingers?
YES
NO
Do you have one or more of the following symptoms?
☐ vomiting
☐ diarrhea
☐ temperature over 100°F (38°C)
☐ no bowel movement for the past few days
YES
NO
See chart 48 Abdominal pain.
Are you short of breath, particularly at night?
YES
NO
You may have fluid retention resulting from congestive HEART FAILURE, p.408.
Are you passing less urine than usual?
YES
NO
You may have a kidney disorder. See GLOMERULONEPHRITIS, p.543.
EMERGENCY
Get medical help now!
These symptoms may indicate a dangerous abdominal condition such as INTESTINAL OBSTRUCTION, p.503. See LAPAROTOMY AND ACUTE ABDOMEN, p.513.
Go to next page

Continued from previous page

Do the whites of your eyes or your skin look yellow?

YES → *Consult your physician.* **Do not delay!** *This suggests a liver disorder such as* CIRRHOSIS OF THE LIVER, *p.524.*

NO ↓

Are you a woman of child-bearing age?

YES → Could you be more than 3 months pregnant?

- **YES** → *Perform a home pregnancy test; if it indicates that you are pregnant, consult your physician, who will verify whether you are pregnant. See* GENERAL CONCERNS OF PREGNANCY, *p.666.*
- **NO** → Did the swelling develop just before or during your period?
  - **YES** → *Many women have a swollen abdomen at this time. See* PREMENSTRUAL SYNDROME, *p.627.*
  - **NO** ↓

NO ↓

Do you have persistent constipation?

YES → *Constipation infrequently accompanies a swollen abdomen. See* CONSTIPATION AND DIARRHEA, *p.510.*

NO ↓

Are you over-weight according to the chart on p.35 AND is your navel deeply sunken?

YES → *Your problem is probably* OBESITY, *p.530.*

NO ↓

If you are unable to make a diagnosis from this chart, and your abdomen remains swollen for more than 24 hours, consult your physician.

Painful swollen abdomen

Go to a hospital immediately if you have a swollen abdomen accompanied by severe pain AND one or more of the following symptoms:

- ☐ vomiting
- ☐ temperature over 100°F (38°C)
- ☐ diarrhea

EMERGENCY
Get medical help now!

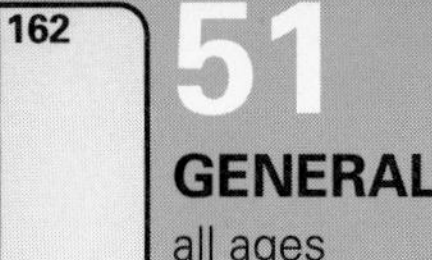

Gas and belching

The expulsion of air from the digestive tract through the mouth or anus (also called flatulence).

START HERE

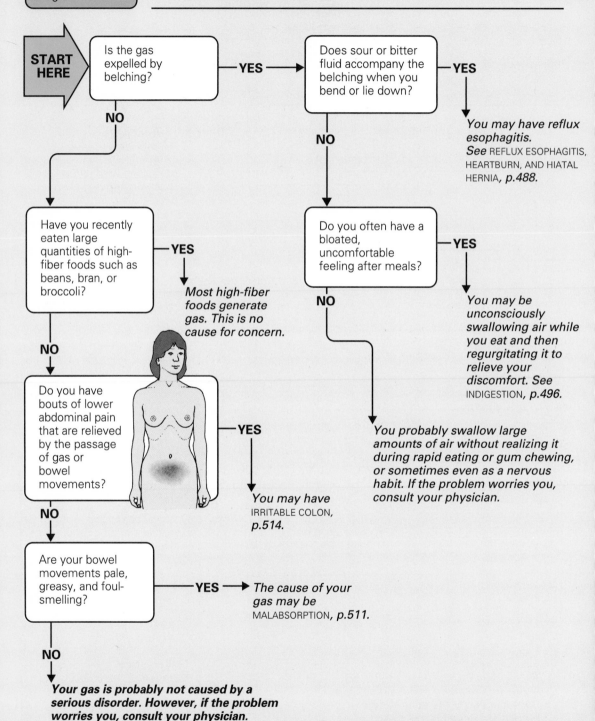

Is the gas expelled by belching?

- **YES** → Does sour or bitter fluid accompany the belching when you bend or lie down?
  - **YES** → *You may have reflux esophagitis. See* REFLUX ESOPHAGITIS, HEARTBURN, AND HIATAL HERNIA, *p.488.*
  - **NO** → Do you often have a bloated, uncomfortable feeling after meals?
    - **YES** → *You may be unconsciously swallowing air while you eat and then regurgitating it to relieve your discomfort. See* INDIGESTION, *p.496.*
    - **NO** → *You probably swallow large amounts of air without realizing it during rapid eating or gum chewing, or sometimes even as a nervous habit. If the problem worries you, consult your physician.*
- **NO** → Have you recently eaten large quantities of high-fiber foods such as beans, bran, or broccoli?
  - **YES** → *Most high-fiber foods generate gas. This is no cause for concern.*
  - **NO** → Do you have bouts of lower abdominal pain that are relieved by the passage of gas or bowel movements?
    - **YES** → *You may have* IRRITABLE COLON, *p.514.*
    - **NO** → Are your bowel movements pale, greasy, and foul-smelling?
      - **YES** → *The cause of your gas may be* MALABSORPTION, *p.511.*
      - **NO** → ***Your gas is probably not caused by a serious disorder. However, if the problem worries you, consult your physician.***

52 GENERAL all ages

Diarrhea

Frequent passing of unusually loose bowel movements.
For babies under 6 months see chart 88, **Diarrhea in infants**.

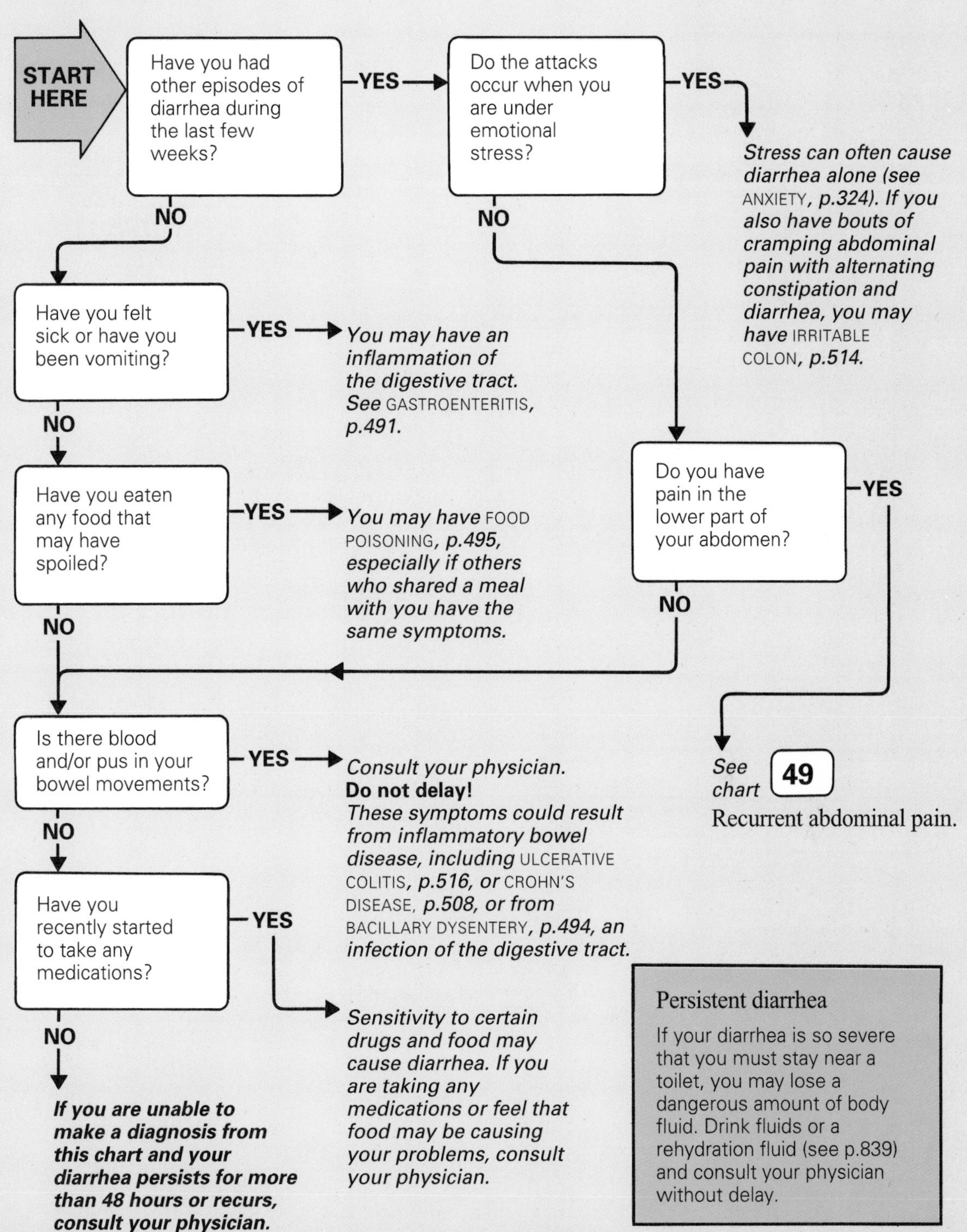

START HERE
Have you had other episodes of diarrhea during the last few weeks?
YES
Do the attacks occur when you are under emotional stress?
YES
Stress can often cause diarrhea alone (see ANXIETY, p.324). If you also have bouts of cramping abdominal pain with alternating constipation and diarrhea, you may have IRRITABLE COLON, p.514.
NO
Do you have pain in the lower part of your abdomen?
YES
See chart 49 Recurrent abdominal pain.
NO
NO
Have you felt sick or have you been vomiting?
YES
You may have an inflammation of the digestive tract. See GASTROENTERITIS, p.491.
NO
Have you eaten any food that may have spoiled?
YES
You may have FOOD POISONING, p.495, especially if others who shared a meal with you have the same symptoms.
NO
Is there blood and/or pus in your bowel movements?
YES
Consult your physician. Do not delay! These symptoms could result from inflammatory bowel disease, including ULCERATIVE COLITIS, p.516, or CROHN'S DISEASE, p.508, or from BACILLARY DYSENTERY, p.494, an infection of the digestive tract.
NO
Have you recently started to take any medications?
YES
Sensitivity to certain drugs and food may cause diarrhea. If you are taking any medications or feel that food may be causing your problems, consult your physician.
NO
If you are unable to make a diagnosis from this chart and your diarrhea persists for more than 48 hours or recurs, consult your physician.

Persistent diarrhea

If your diarrhea is so severe that you must stay near a toilet, you may lose a dangerous amount of body fluid. Drink fluids or a rehydration fluid (see p.839) and consult your physician without delay.

53

GENERAL
all ages

Constipation

Infrequent, difficult passing of hard bowel movements.

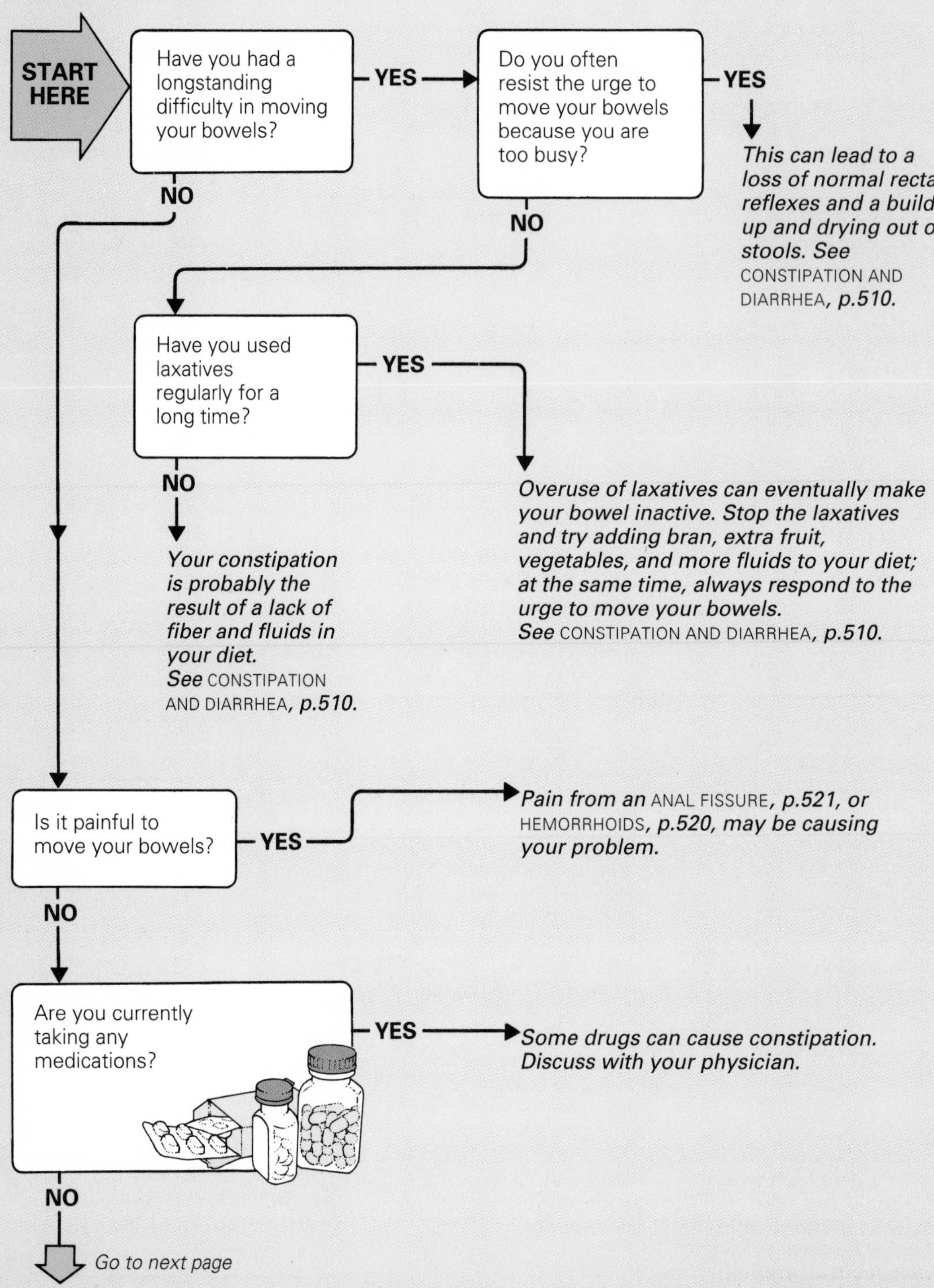

START HERE
Have you had a longstanding difficulty in moving your bowels?
YES
Do you often resist the urge to move your bowels because you are too busy?
YES
This can lead to a loss of normal rectal reflexes and a build-up and drying out of stools. See CONSTIPATION AND DIARRHEA, p.510.
NO
Have you used laxatives regularly for a long time?
YES
Overuse of laxatives can eventually make your bowel inactive. Stop the laxatives and try adding bran, extra fruit, vegetables, and more fluids to your diet; at the same time, always respond to the urge to move your bowels. See CONSTIPATION AND DIARRHEA, p.510.
NO
Your constipation is probably the result of a lack of fiber and fluids in your diet. See CONSTIPATION AND DIARRHEA, p.510.
NO
Is it painful to move your bowels?
YES
Pain from an ANAL FISSURE, p.521, or HEMORRHOIDS, p.520, may be causing your problem.
NO
Are you currently taking any medications?
YES
Some drugs can cause constipation. Discuss with your physician.
NO
Go to next page

Continued from previous page

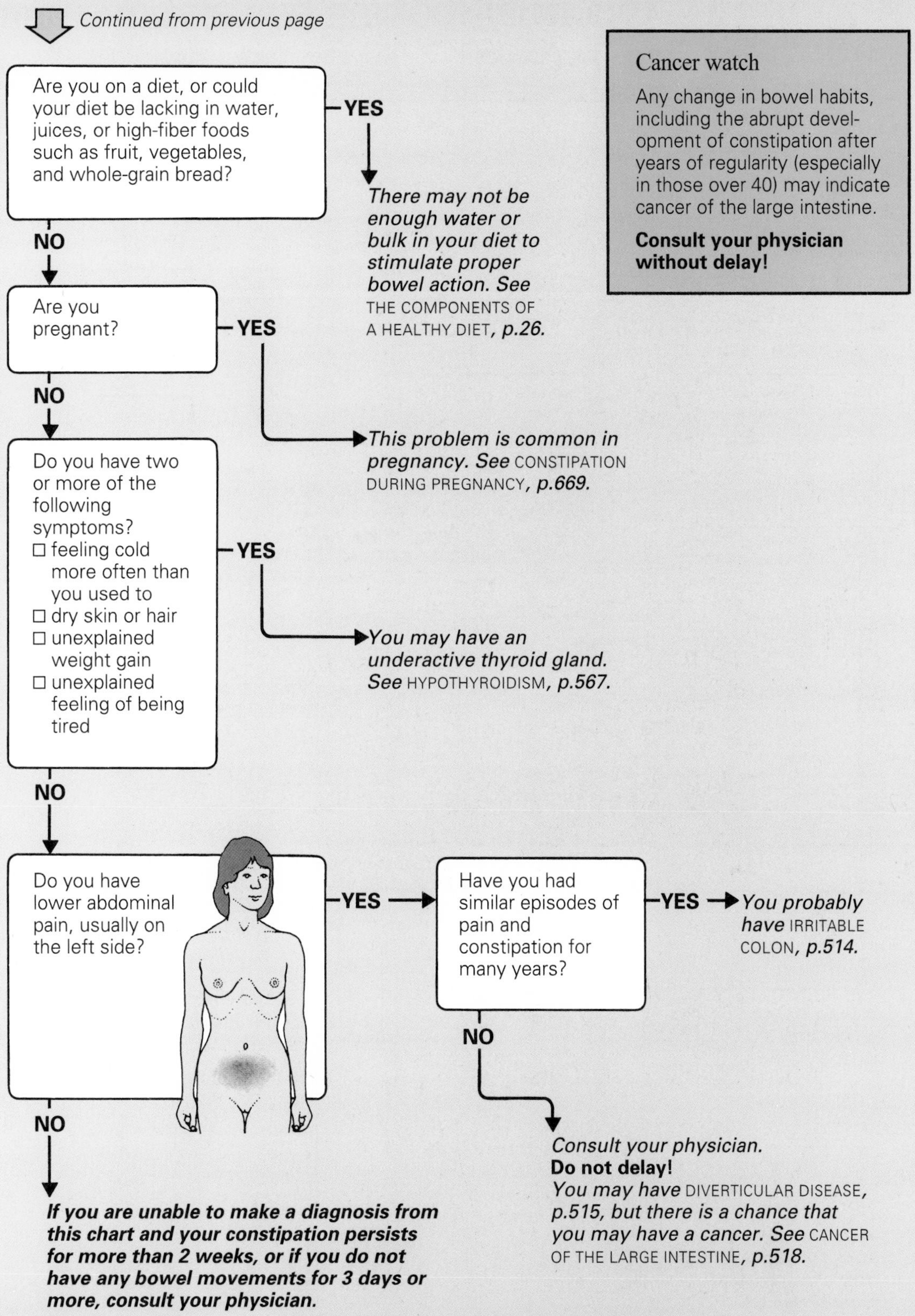

Are you on a diet, or could your diet be lacking in water, juices, or high-fiber foods such as fruit, vegetables, and whole-grain bread?
YES
There may not be enough water or bulk in your diet to stimulate proper bowel action. See THE COMPONENTS OF A HEALTHY DIET, *p.26.*
NO
Are you pregnant?
YES
This problem is common in pregnancy. See CONSTIPATION DURING PREGNANCY, *p.669.*
NO
Do you have two or more of the following symptoms?
☐ feeling cold more often than you used to
☐ dry skin or hair
☐ unexplained weight gain
☐ unexplained feeling of being tired
YES
You may have an underactive thyroid gland. See HYPOTHYROIDISM, *p.567.*
NO
Do you have lower abdominal pain, usually on the left side?
YES
Have you had similar episodes of pain and constipation for many years?
YES
You probably have IRRITABLE COLON, *p.514.*
NO
Consult your physician.
Do not delay!
You may have DIVERTICULAR DISEASE, *p.515, but there is a chance that you may have a cancer. See* CANCER OF THE LARGE INTESTINE, *p.518.*
NO
If you are unable to make a diagnosis from this chart and your constipation persists for more than 2 weeks, or if you do not have any bowel movements for 3 days or more, consult your physician.

Cancer watch

Any change in bowel habits, including the abrupt development of constipation after years of regularity (especially in those over 40) may indicate cancer of the large intestine.

Consult your physician without delay!

54
GENERAL
all ages

Abnormal-looking bowel movements

Passing bowel movements that are not the usual color.

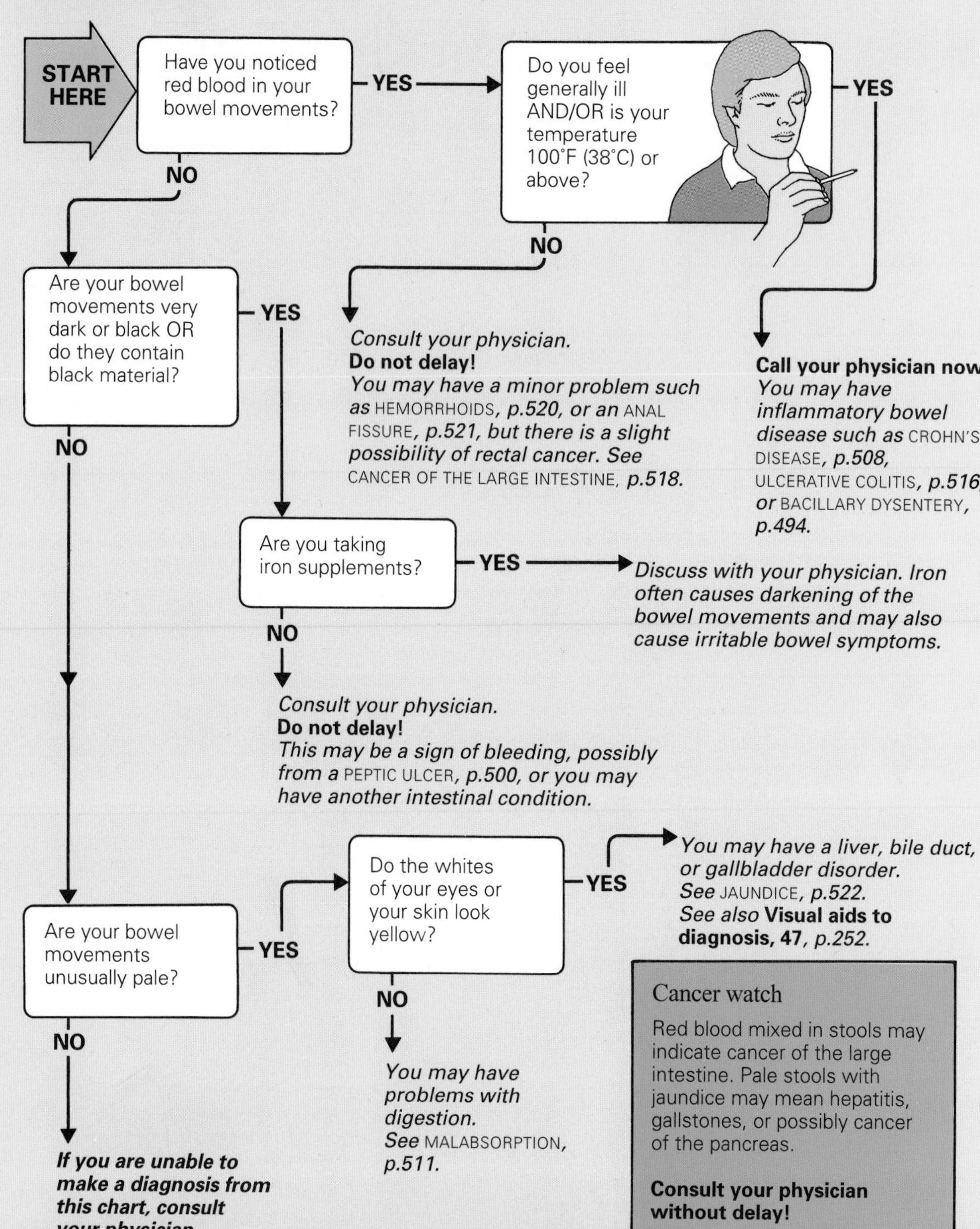

START HERE
Have you noticed red blood in your bowel movements?
YES
Do you feel generally ill AND/OR is your temperature 100°F (38°C) or above?
YES
Call your physician now!
You may have inflammatory bowel disease such as CROHN'S DISEASE, p.508, ULCERATIVE COLITIS, p.516, or BACILLARY DYSENTERY, p.494.
NO
Consult your physician.
Do not delay!
You may have a minor problem such as HEMORRHOIDS, p.520, or an ANAL FISSURE, p.521, but there is a slight possibility of rectal cancer. See CANCER OF THE LARGE INTESTINE, p.518.
NO
Are your bowel movements very dark or black OR do they contain black material?
YES
Are you taking iron supplements?
YES
Discuss with your physician. Iron often causes darkening of the bowel movements and may also cause irritable bowel symptoms.
NO
Consult your physician.
Do not delay!
This may be a sign of bleeding, possibly from a PEPTIC ULCER, p.500, or you may have another intestinal condition.
NO
Are your bowel movements unusually pale?
YES
Do the whites of your eyes or your skin look yellow?
YES
You may have a liver, bile duct, or gallbladder disorder.
See JAUNDICE, p.522.
See also Visual aids to diagnosis, 47, p.252.
NO
You may have problems with digestion.
See MALABSORPTION, p.511.
NO
If you are unable to make a diagnosis from this chart, consult your physician.

Cancer watch

Red blood mixed in stools may indicate cancer of the large intestine. Pale stools with jaundice may mean hepatitis, gallstones, or possibly cancer of the pancreas.

Consult your physician without delay!

55
GENERAL
all ages

Palpitations

A feeling that your heart is beating irregularly, more strongly, or more rapidly than normal.

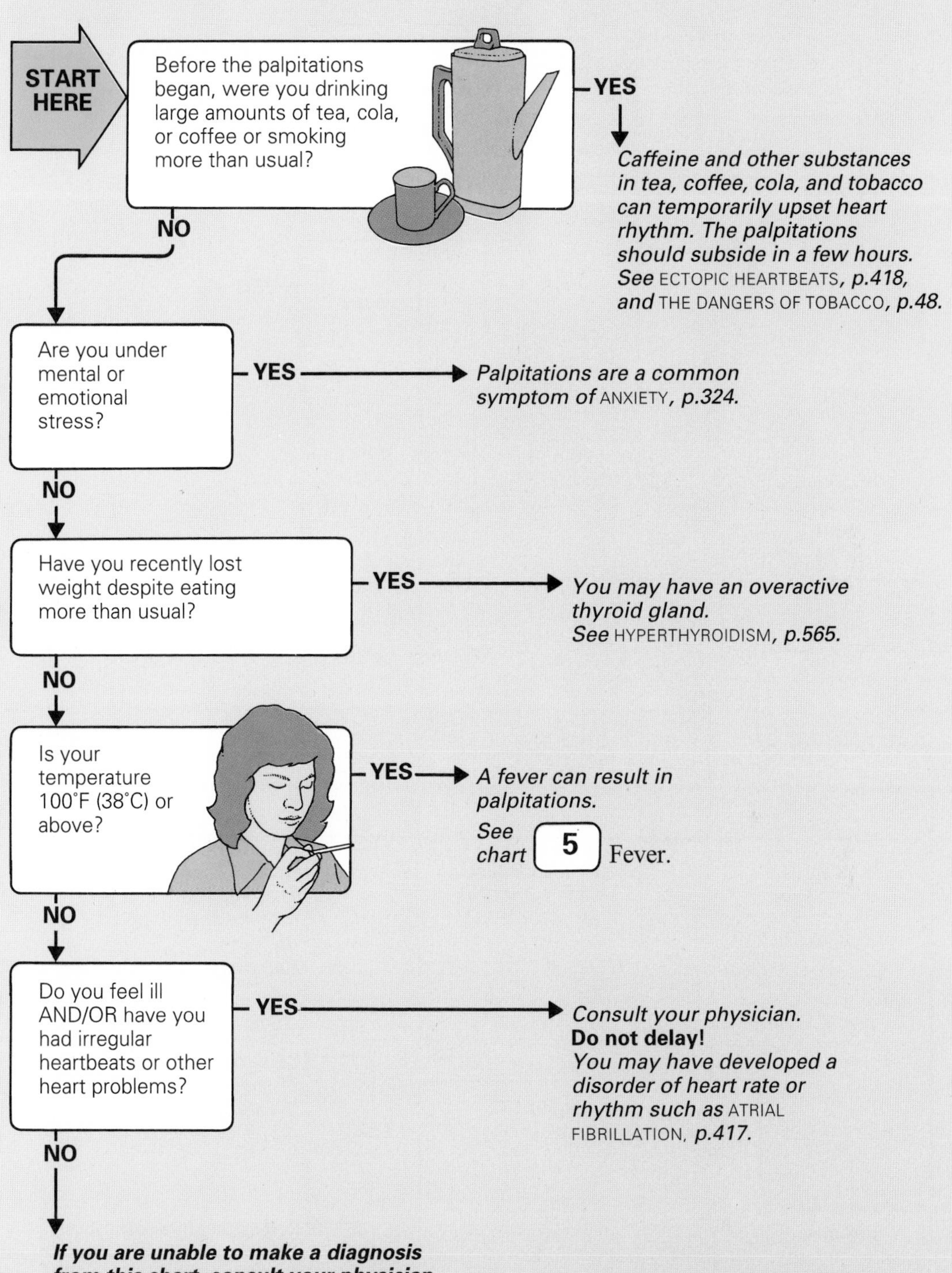

START HERE

Before the palpitations began, were you drinking large amounts of tea, cola, or coffee or smoking more than usual?

YES → *Caffeine and other substances in tea, coffee, cola, and tobacco can temporarily upset heart rhythm. The palpitations should subside in a few hours. See* ECTOPIC HEARTBEATS, *p.418, and* THE DANGERS OF TOBACCO, *p.48.*

NO ↓

Are you under mental or emotional stress?

YES → *Palpitations are a common symptom of* ANXIETY, *p.324.*

NO ↓

Have you recently lost weight despite eating more than usual?

YES → *You may have an overactive thyroid gland. See* HYPERTHYROIDISM, *p.565.*

NO ↓

Is your temperature 100°F (38°C) or above?

YES → *A fever can result in palpitations.* *See chart* 5 Fever.

NO ↓

Do you feel ill AND/OR have you had irregular heartbeats or other heart problems?

YES → *Consult your physician.* **Do not delay!** *You may have developed a disorder of heart rate or rhythm such as* ATRIAL FIBRILLATION, *p.417.*

NO ↓

If you are unable to make a diagnosis from this chart, consult your physician.

56

GENERAL
all ages

Chest pain

Pain anywhere between the neck and the bottom of the rib cage, which may be dull and pressing, aching, stabbing, burning, or crushing.

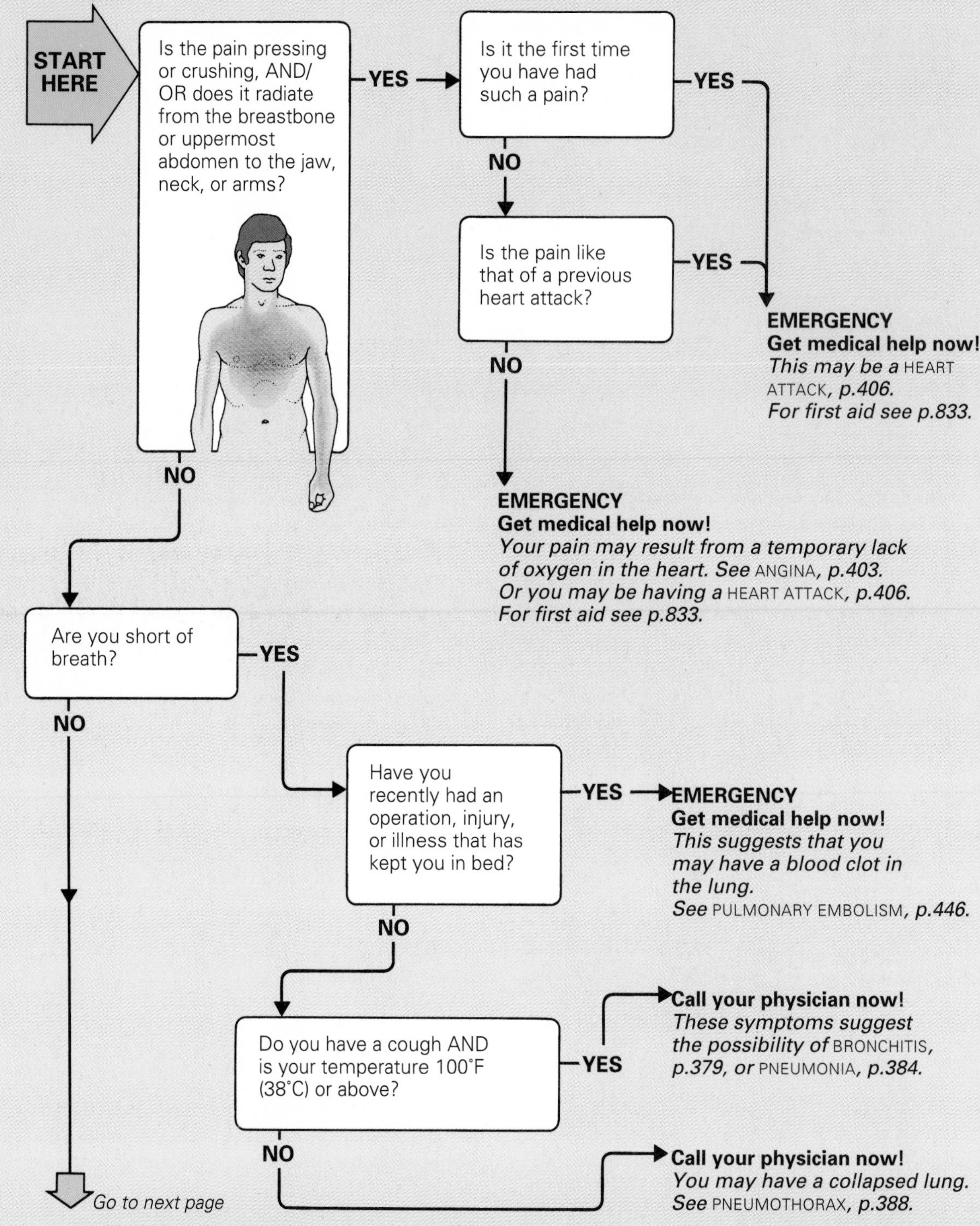

START HERE
Is the pain pressing or crushing, AND/OR does it radiate from the breastbone or uppermost abdomen to the jaw, neck, or arms?
YES
Is it the first time you have had such a pain?
YES
NO
Is the pain like that of a previous heart attack?
YES
EMERGENCY
Get medical help now!
This may be a HEART ATTACK, p.406.
For first aid see p.833.
NO
EMERGENCY
Get medical help now!
Your pain may result from a temporary lack of oxygen in the heart. See ANGINA, p.403.
Or you may be having a HEART ATTACK, p.406.
For first aid see p.833.
NO
Are you short of breath?
YES
Have you recently had an operation, injury, or illness that has kept you in bed?
YES
EMERGENCY
Get medical help now!
This suggests that you may have a blood clot in the lung.
See PULMONARY EMBOLISM, p.446.
NO
Do you have a cough AND is your temperature 100˚F (38˚C) or above?
YES
Call your physician now!
These symptoms suggest the possibility of BRONCHITIS, p.379, or PNEUMONIA, p.384.
NO
Call your physician now!
You may have a collapsed lung.
See PNEUMOTHORAX, p.388.
NO
Go to next page

Continued from previous page

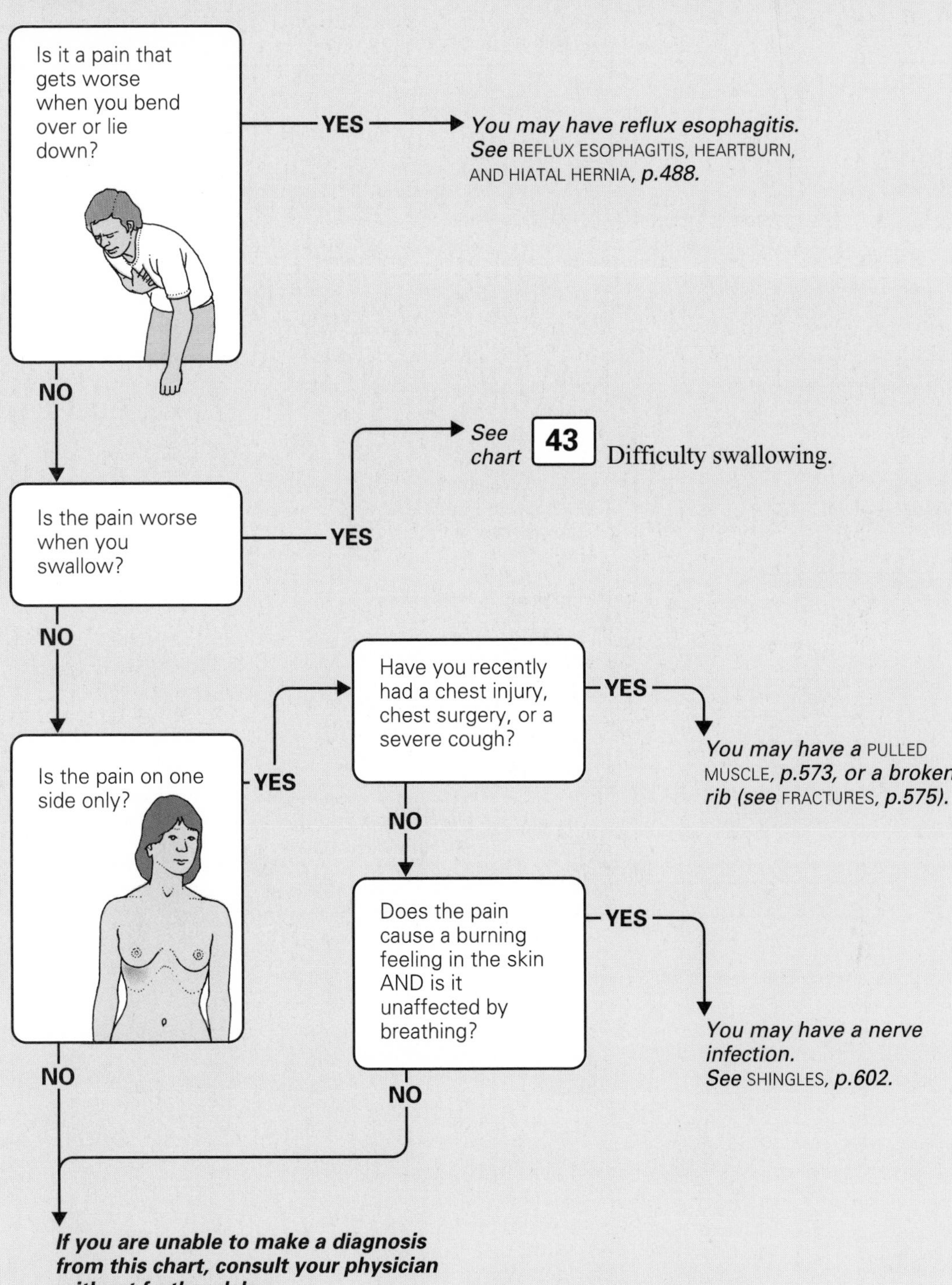
Is it a pain that gets worse when you bend over or lie down?
YES
You may have reflux esophagitis.
See REFLUX ESOPHAGITIS, HEARTBURN, AND HIATAL HERNIA, p.488.
NO
Is the pain worse when you swallow?
YES
See chart 43 Difficulty swallowing.
NO
Is the pain on one side only?
YES
Have you recently had a chest injury, chest surgery, or a severe cough?
YES
You may have a PULLED MUSCLE, p.573, or a broken rib (see FRACTURES, p.575).
NO
Does the pain cause a burning feeling in the skin AND is it unaffected by breathing?
YES
You may have a nerve infection.
See SHINGLES, p.602.
NO
NO

If you are unable to make a diagnosis from this chart, consult your physician without further delay.

57

GENERAL
all ages

Abnormally frequent urination

Feeling the urge to urinate and doing so more often than usual, even though you may be producing little urine.

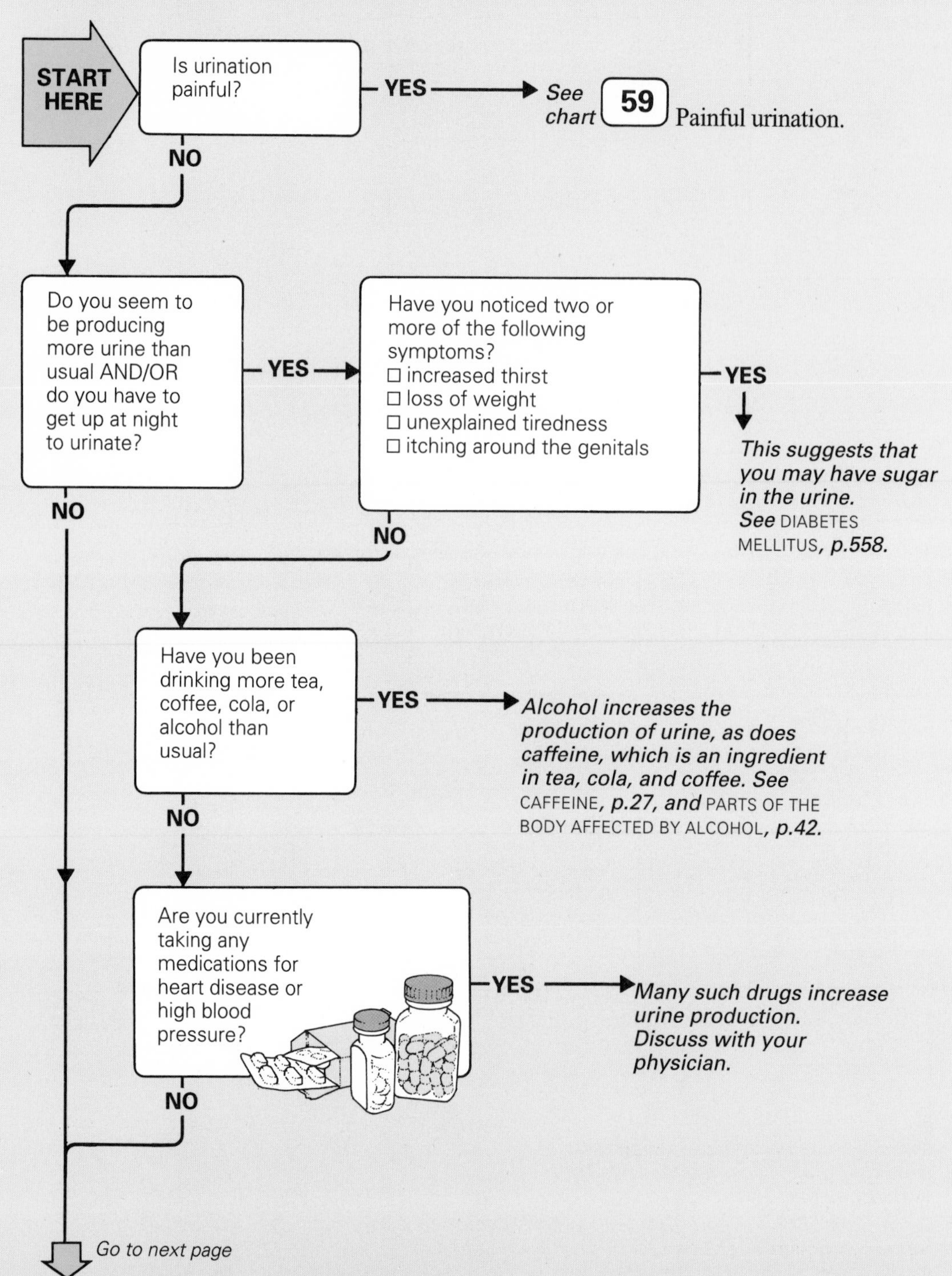

START HERE
Is urination painful?
YES
See chart 59 Painful urination.
NO
Do you seem to be producing more urine than usual AND/OR do you have to get up at night to urinate?
YES
Have you noticed two or more of the following symptoms?
☐ increased thirst
☐ loss of weight
☐ unexplained tiredness
☐ itching around the genitals
YES
This suggests that you may have sugar in the urine. See DIABETES MELLITUS, p.558.
NO
NO
Have you been drinking more tea, coffee, cola, or alcohol than usual?
YES
Alcohol increases the production of urine, as does caffeine, which is an ingredient in tea, cola, and coffee. See CAFFEINE, p.27, and PARTS OF THE BODY AFFECTED BY ALCOHOL, p.42.
NO
Are you currently taking any medications for heart disease or high blood pressure?
YES
Many such drugs increase urine production. Discuss with your physician.
NO
Go to next page

Continued from previous page

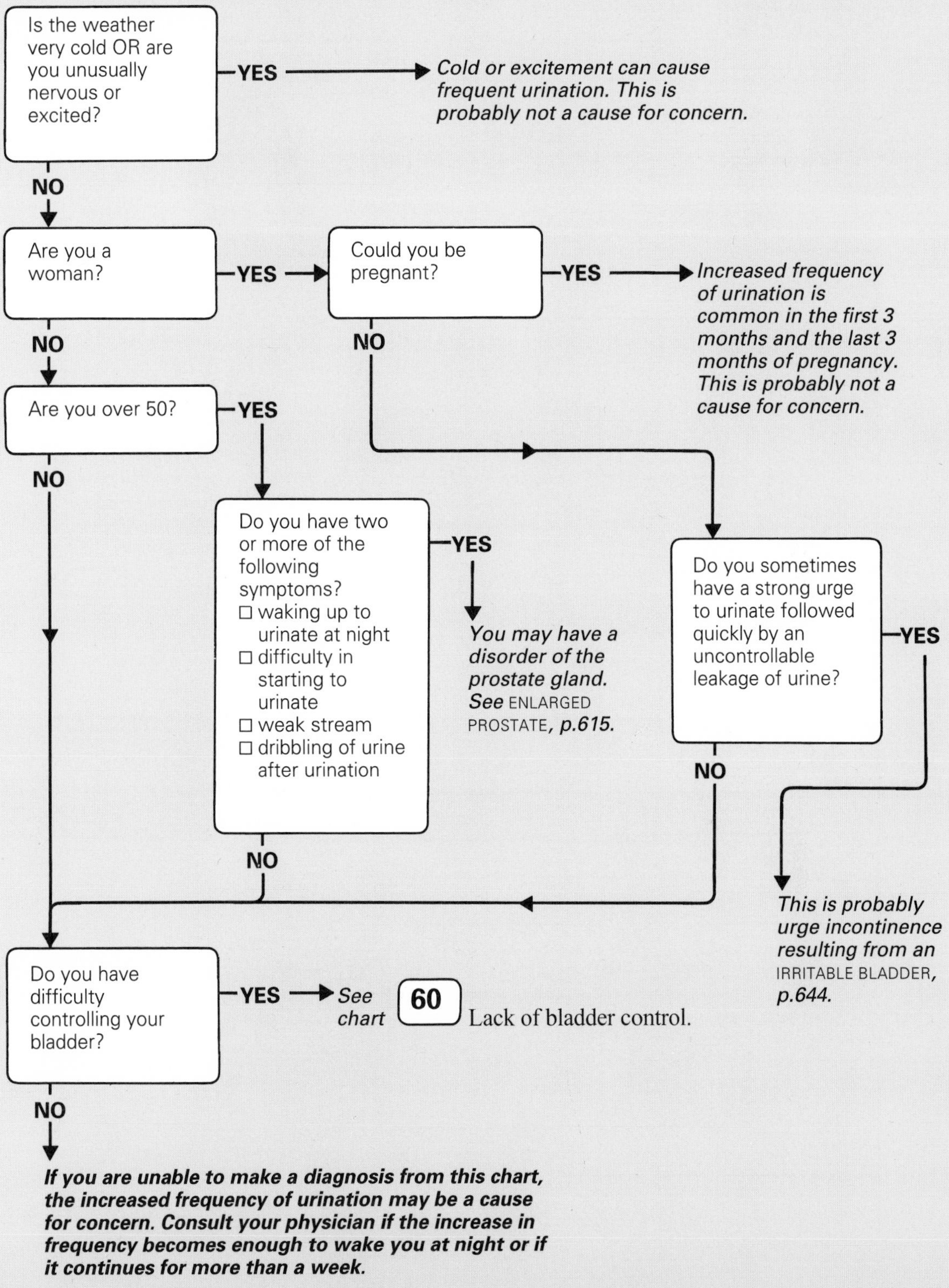

Is the weather very cold OR are you unusually nervous or excited?

YES → *Cold or excitement can cause frequent urination. This is probably not a cause for concern.*

NO ↓

Are you a woman?

YES → Could you be pregnant?

YES → *Increased frequency of urination is common in the first 3 months and the last 3 months of pregnancy. This is probably not a cause for concern.*

NO → (to "Do you sometimes have a strong urge...")

NO ↓

Are you over 50?

YES → Do you have two or more of the following symptoms?
- ☐ waking up to urinate at night
- ☐ difficulty in starting to urinate
- ☐ weak stream
- ☐ dribbling of urine after urination

YES → *You may have a disorder of the prostate gland. See* ENLARGED PROSTATE*, p.615.*

NO → (to "Do you have difficulty controlling your bladder?")

Do you sometimes have a strong urge to urinate followed quickly by an uncontrollable leakage of urine?

YES → *This is probably urge incontinence resulting from an* IRRITABLE BLADDER*, p.644.*

NO → (to "Do you have difficulty controlling your bladder?")

NO ↓

Do you have difficulty controlling your bladder?

YES → *See chart* **60** Lack of bladder control.

NO ↓

If you are unable to make a diagnosis from this chart, the increased frequency of urination may be a cause for concern. Consult your physician if the increase in frequency becomes enough to wake you at night or if it continues for more than a week.

58
GENERAL
all ages

Abnormal-looking urine

Urine that differs from the usual straw color, or that is cloudy or tinged with blood.

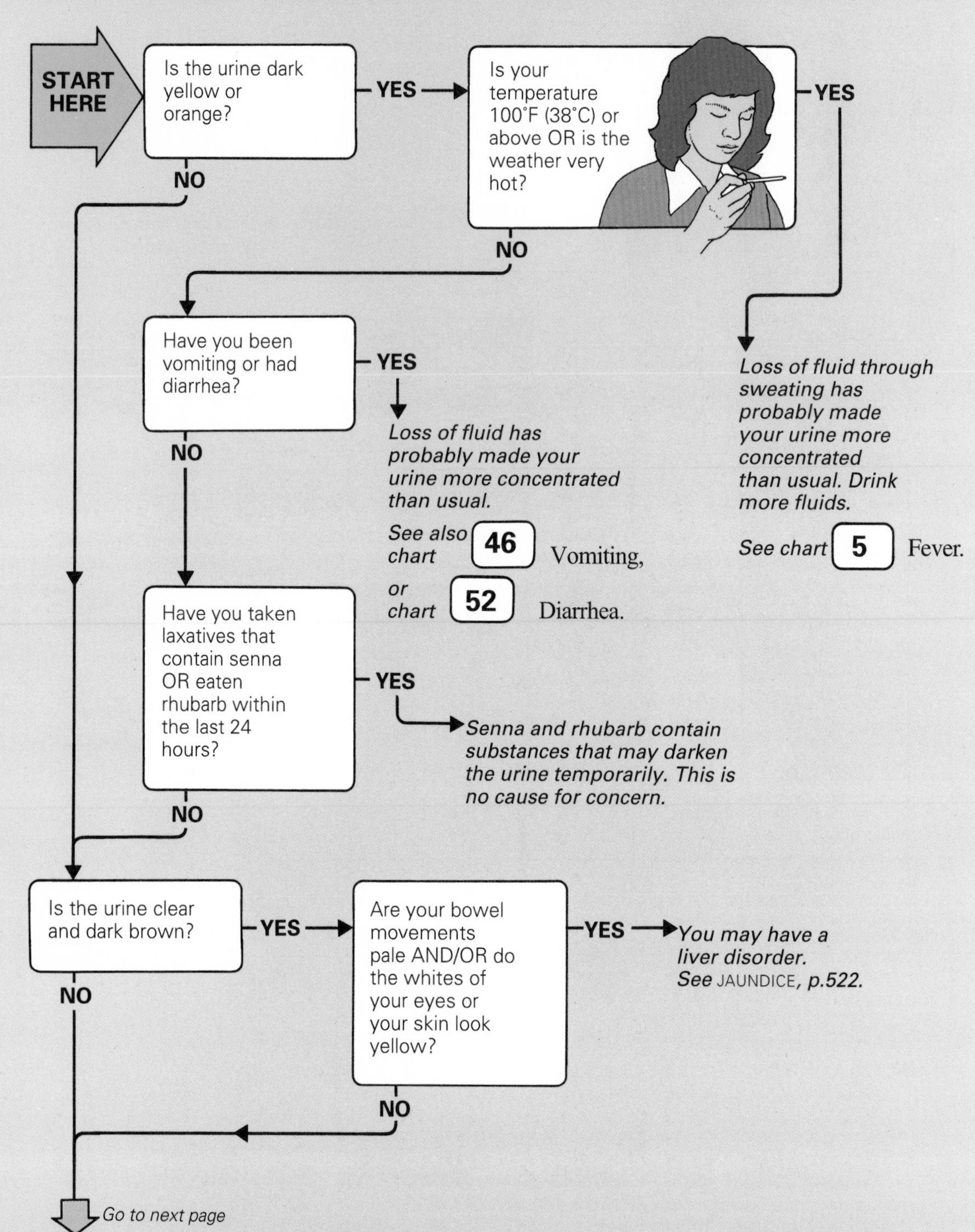

START HERE
Is the urine dark yellow or orange?
YES
Is your temperature 100°F (38°C) or above OR is the weather very hot?
YES
Loss of fluid through sweating has probably made your urine more concentrated than usual. Drink more fluids.
See chart 5 Fever.
NO
Have you been vomiting or had diarrhea?
YES
Loss of fluid has probably made your urine more concentrated than usual.
See also chart 46 Vomiting,
or chart 52 Diarrhea.
NO
Have you taken laxatives that contain senna OR eaten rhubarb within the last 24 hours?
YES
Senna and rhubarb contain substances that may darken the urine temporarily. This is no cause for concern.
NO
NO
Is the urine clear and dark brown?
YES
Are your bowel movements pale AND/OR do the whites of your eyes or your skin look yellow?
YES
You may have a liver disorder.
See JAUNDICE, p.522.
NO
NO
Go to next page

Continued from previous page

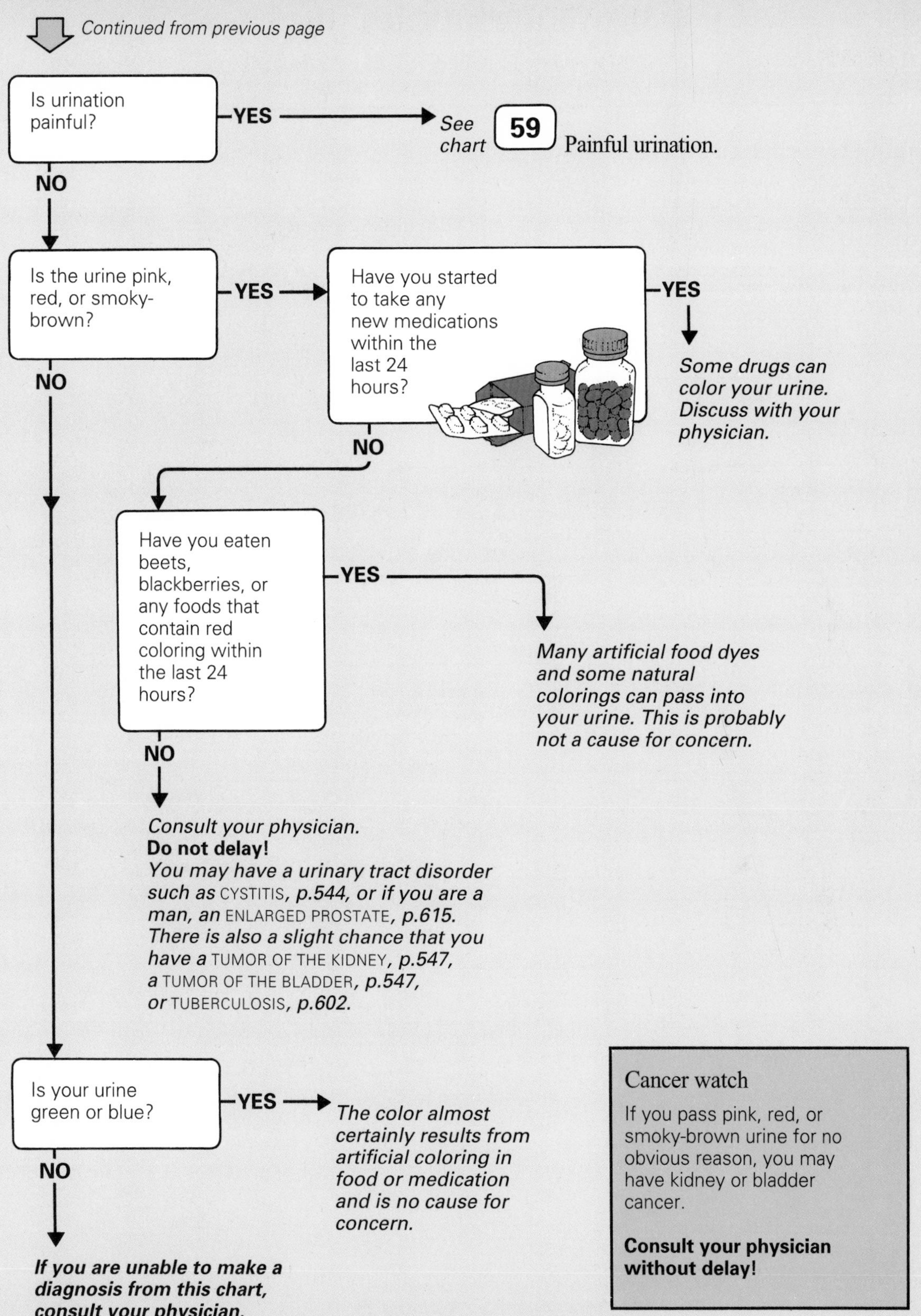

Is urination painful?
YES
See chart 59 Painful urination.
NO
Is the urine pink, red, or smoky-brown?
YES
Have you started to take any new medications within the last 24 hours?
YES
Some drugs can color your urine. Discuss with your physician.
NO
NO
Have you eaten beets, blackberries, or any foods that contain red coloring within the last 24 hours?
YES
Many artificial food dyes and some natural colorings can pass into your urine. This is probably not a cause for concern.
NO
Consult your physician.
Do not delay!
You may have a urinary tract disorder such as CYSTITIS, p.544, or if you are a man, an ENLARGED PROSTATE, p.615. There is also a slight chance that you have a TUMOR OF THE KIDNEY, p.547, a TUMOR OF THE BLADDER, p.547, or TUBERCULOSIS, p.602.
Is your urine green or blue?
YES
The color almost certainly results from artificial coloring in food or medication and is no cause for concern.
NO
If you are unable to make a diagnosis from this chart, consult your physician.

Cancer watch

If you pass pink, red, or smoky-brown urine for no obvious reason, you may have kidney or bladder cancer.

Consult your physician without delay!

Painful urination

Discomfort when urinating, which may be accompanied by pain in the lower abdomen or urinary passage.

START HERE

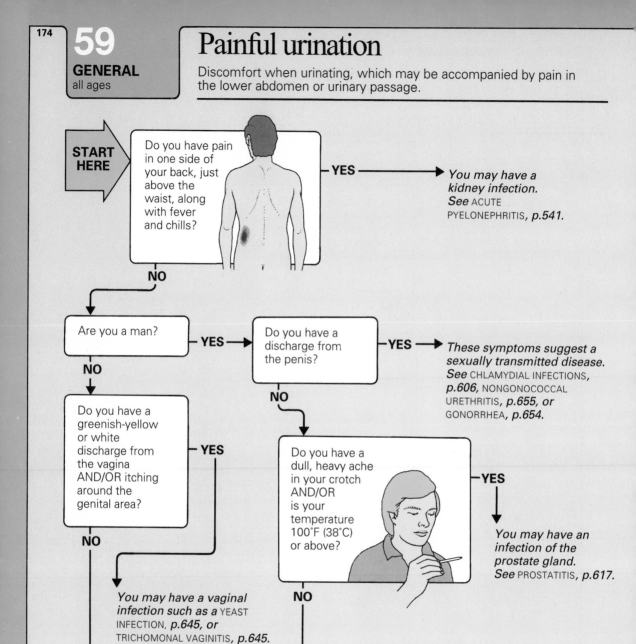

Do you have pain in one side of your back, just above the waist, along with fever and chills?

- **YES** → *You may have a kidney infection. See* ACUTE PYELONEPHRITIS, ***p.541.***
- **NO** ↓

Are you a man?

- **YES** → Do you have a discharge from the penis?
  - **YES** → *These symptoms suggest a sexually transmitted disease. See* CHLAMYDIAL INFECTIONS, ***p.606,*** NONGONOCOCCAL URETHRITIS, ***p.655, or*** GONORRHEA, ***p.654.***
  - **NO** ↓ Do you have a dull, heavy ache in your crotch AND/OR is your temperature 100°F (38°C) or above?
    - **YES** → *You may have an infection of the prostate gland. See* PROSTATITIS, ***p.617.***
    - **NO** ↓ (go to "Are you urinating more frequently than usual?")
- **NO** ↓

Do you have a greenish-yellow or white discharge from the vagina AND/OR itching around the genital area?

- **YES** → *You may have a vaginal infection such as a* YEAST INFECTION, ***p.645, or*** TRICHOMONAL VAGINITIS, ***p.645.***
- **NO** ↓

Are you urinating more frequently than usual?

- **YES** → *Your bladder may be inflamed. See* CYSTITIS, ***p.544.***
- **NO** → ***If you are unable to make a diagnosis from this chart, consult your physician.***

60
GENERAL
0-70 years

Lack of bladder control

Involuntary urination.
For those over 70 see chart 98, **Incontinence in older people.**

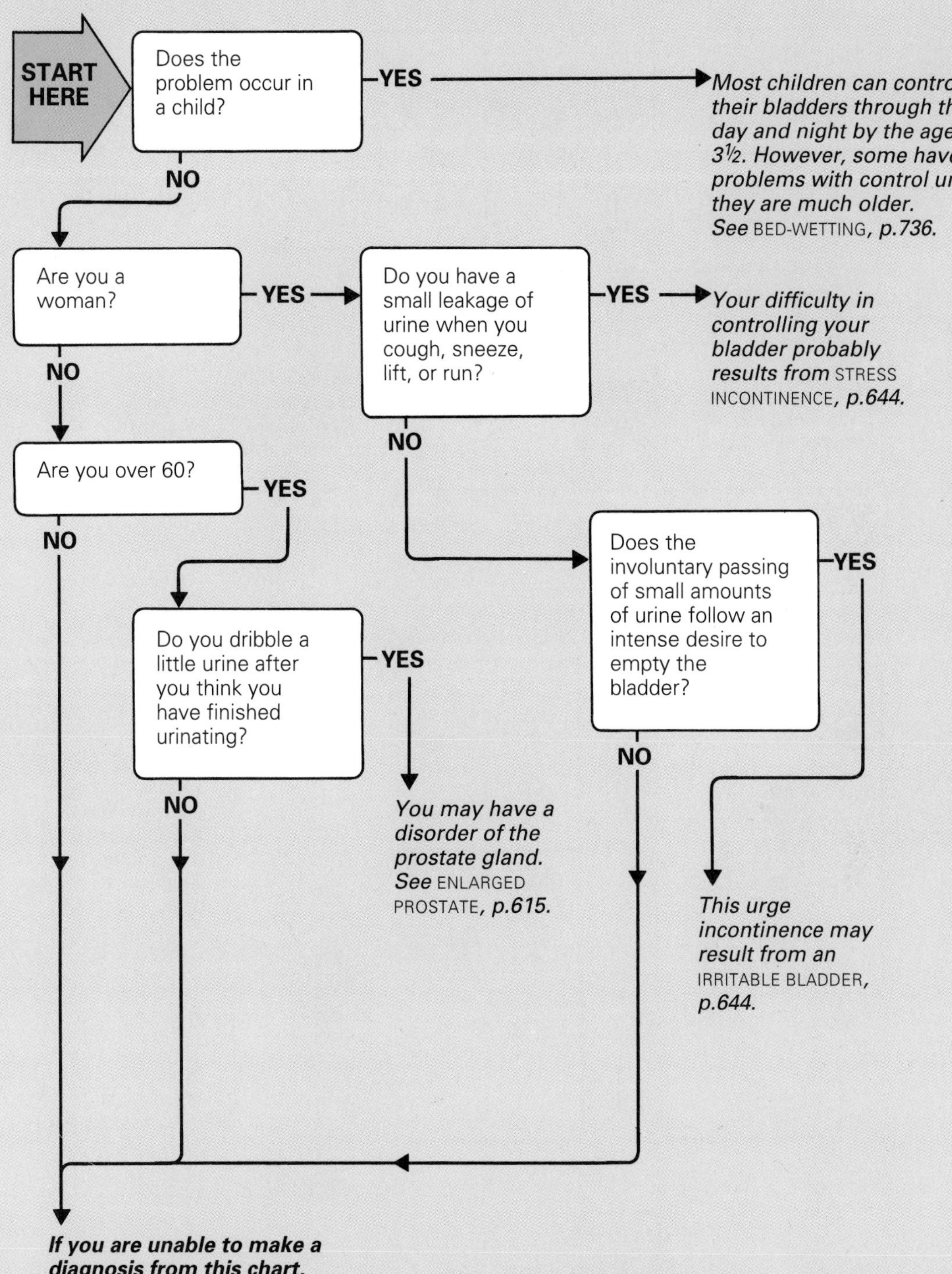

START HERE
Does the problem occur in a child?
YES
Most children can control their bladders through the day and night by the age of 3½. However, some have problems with control until they are much older. See BED-WETTING*, p.736.*
NO
Are you a woman?
YES
Do you have a small leakage of urine when you cough, sneeze, lift, or run?
YES
Your difficulty in controlling your bladder probably results from STRESS INCONTINENCE*, p.644.*
NO
NO
Are you over 60?
YES
NO
Does the involuntary passing of small amounts of urine follow an intense desire to empty the bladder?
YES
Do you dribble a little urine after you think you have finished urinating?
YES
NO
NO
You may have a disorder of the prostate gland. See ENLARGED PROSTATE*, p.615.*
This urge incontinence may result from an IRRITABLE BLADDER*, p.644.*
If you are unable to make a diagnosis from this chart, consult your physician.

61
GENERAL
all ages

Backache

Pain and/or stiffness in the back that may be continuous or intermittent.

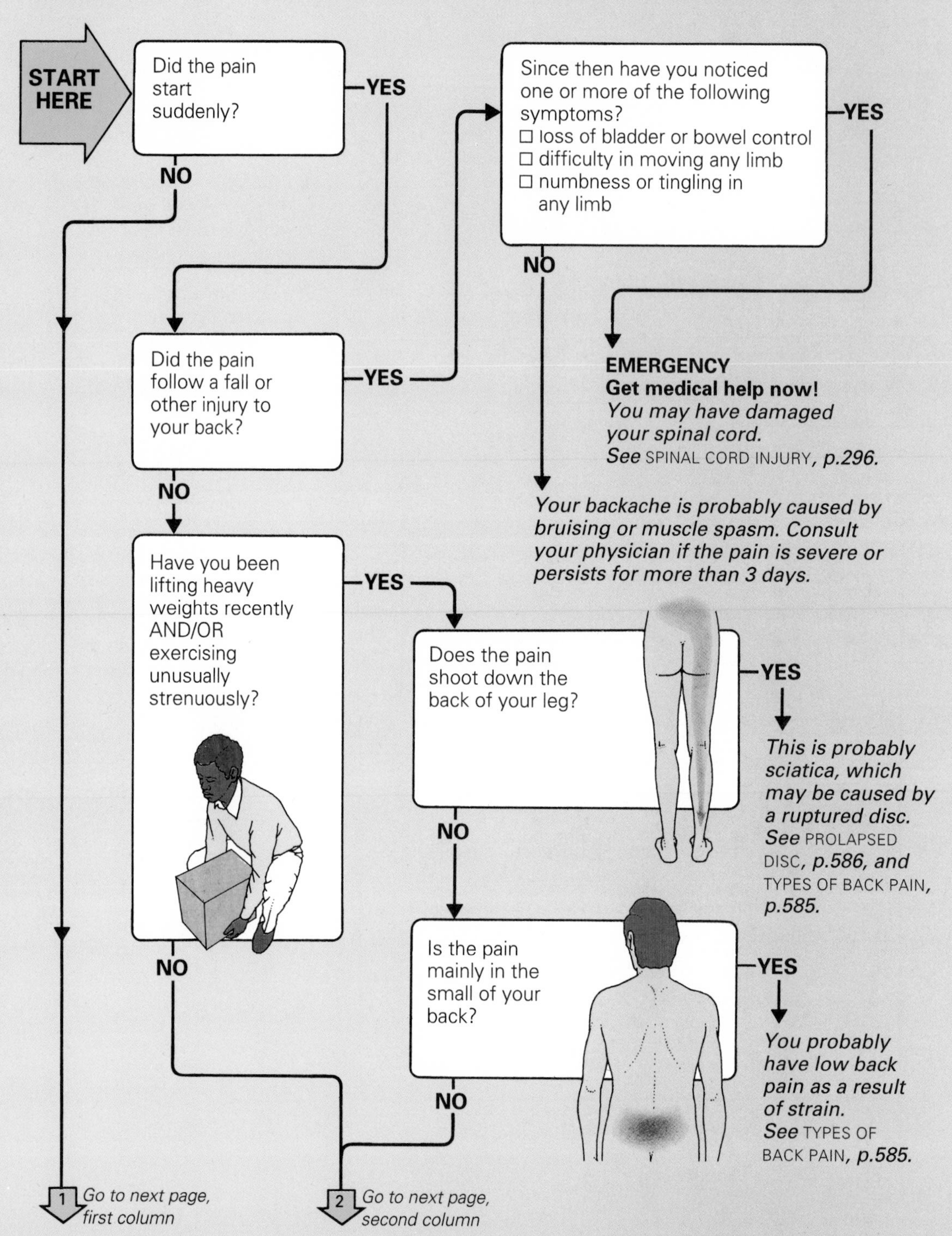

START HERE
Did the pain start suddenly?
YES
NO
Since then have you noticed one or more of the following symptoms?
☐ loss of bladder or bowel control
☐ difficulty in moving any limb
☐ numbness or tingling in any limb
YES
NO
EMERGENCY
Get medical help now!
You may have damaged your spinal cord.
See SPINAL CORD INJURY, p.296.
Did the pain follow a fall or other injury to your back?
YES
NO
Your backache is probably caused by bruising or muscle spasm. Consult your physician if the pain is severe or persists for more than 3 days.
Have you been lifting heavy weights recently AND/OR exercising unusually strenuously?
YES
NO
Does the pain shoot down the back of your leg?
YES
NO
This is probably sciatica, which may be caused by a ruptured disc.
See PROLAPSED DISC, p.586, and TYPES OF BACK PAIN, p.585.
Is the pain mainly in the small of your back?
YES
NO
You probably have low back pain as a result of strain.
See TYPES OF BACK PAIN, p.585.
1 Go to next page, first column
2 Go to next page, second column

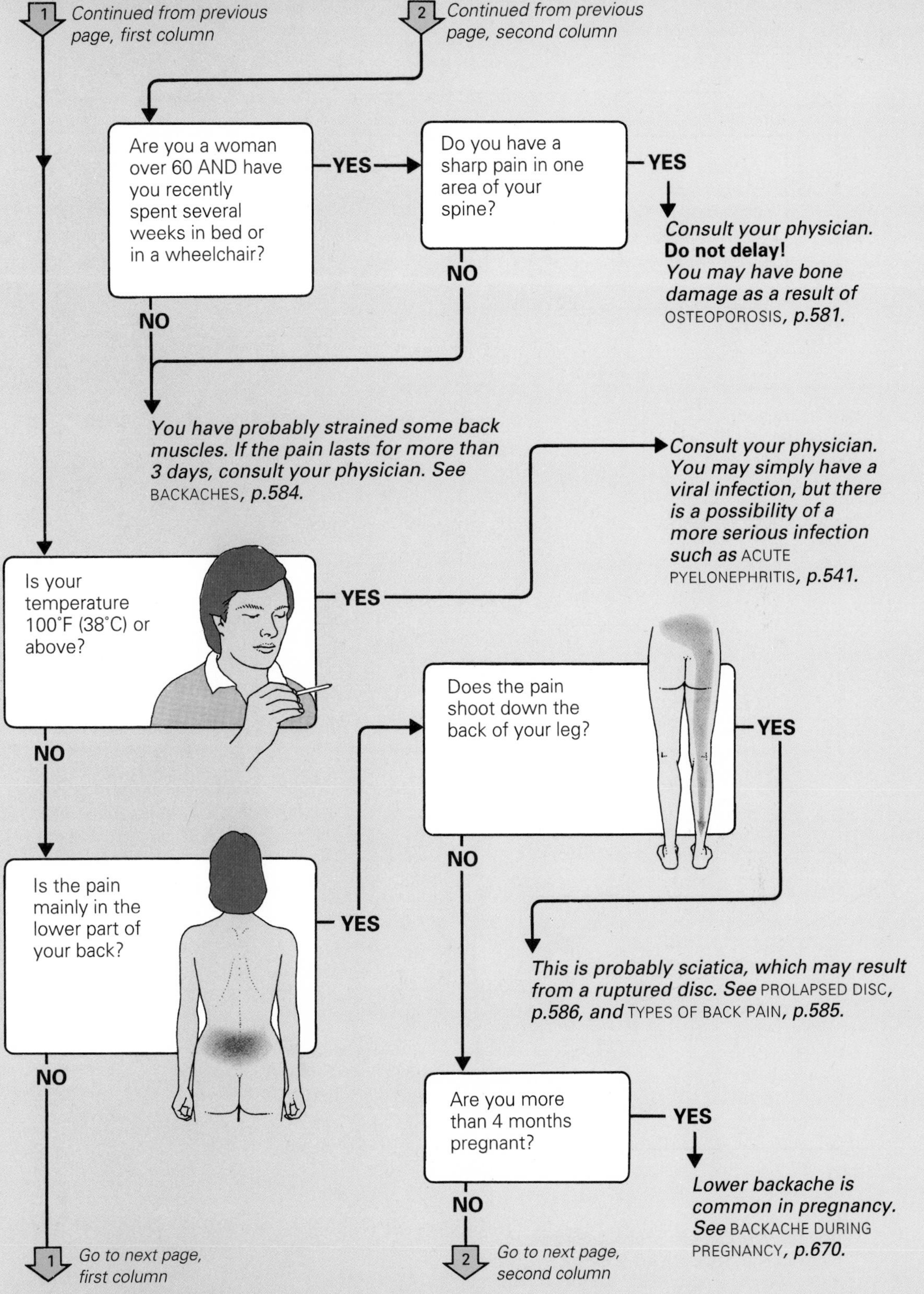

1 Continued from previous page, first column
2 Continued from previous page, second column
Are you a woman over 60 AND have you recently spent several weeks in bed or in a wheelchair?
YES
NO
Do you have a sharp pain in one area of your spine?
YES
NO
Consult your physician. **Do not delay!** You may have bone damage as a result of OSTEOPOROSIS, p.581.
You have probably strained some back muscles. If the pain lasts for more than 3 days, consult your physician. See BACKACHES, p.584.
Is your temperature 100°F (38°C) or above?
YES
NO
Consult your physician. You may simply have a viral infection, but there is a possibility of a more serious infection such as ACUTE PYELONEPHRITIS, p.541.
Is the pain mainly in the lower part of your back?
YES
NO
Does the pain shoot down the back of your leg?
YES
NO
This is probably sciatica, which may result from a ruptured disc. See PROLAPSED DISC, p.586, and TYPES OF BACK PAIN, p.585.
Are you more than 4 months pregnant?
YES
NO
Lower backache is common in pregnancy. See BACKACHE DURING PREGNANCY, p.670.
1 Go to next page, first column
2 Go to next page, second column

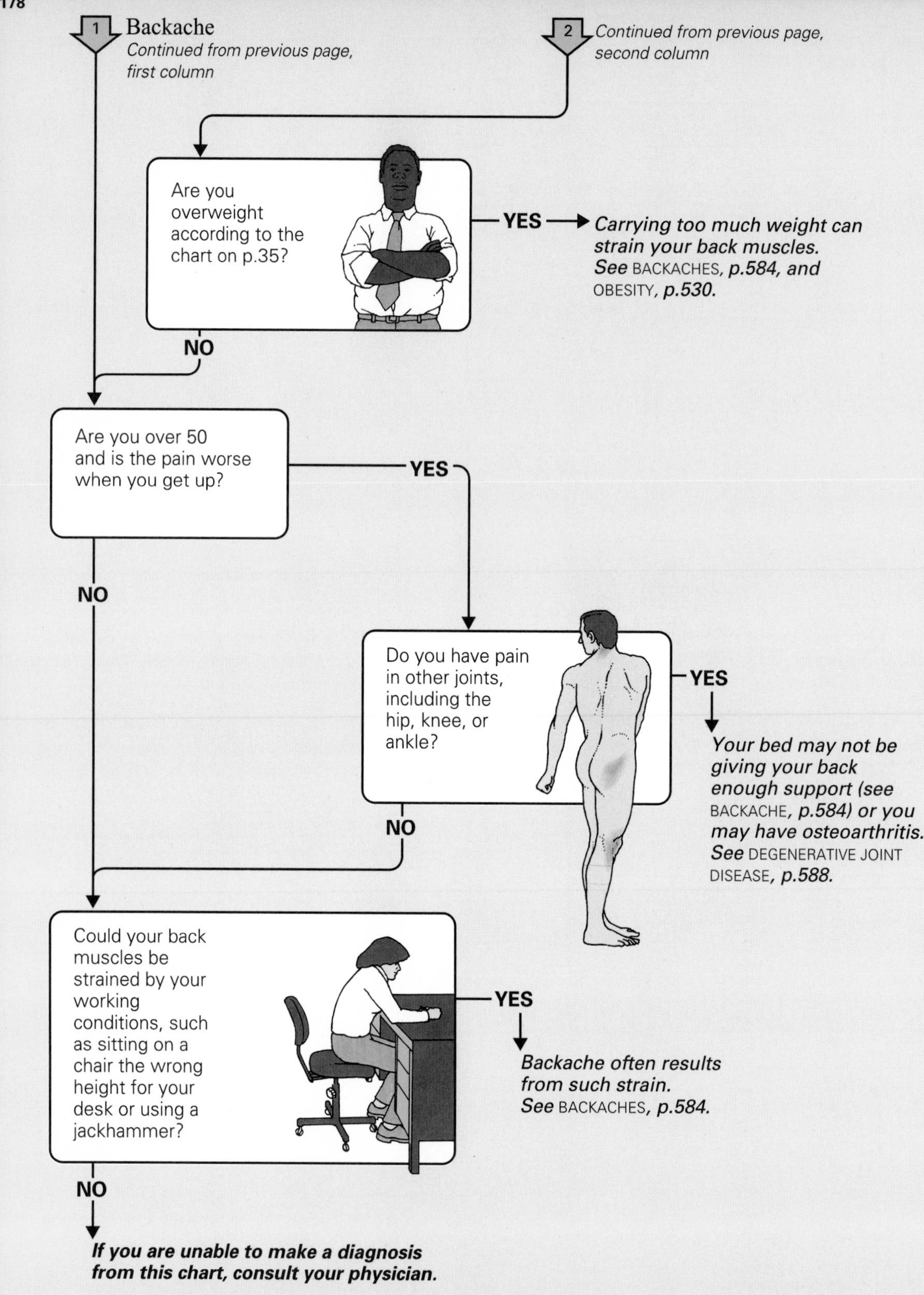

1 Backache
Continued from previous page, first column
2 Continued from previous page, second column
Are you overweight according to the chart on p.35?
YES
Carrying too much weight can strain your back muscles. See BACKACHES, p.584, and OBESITY, p.530.
NO
Are you over 50 and is the pain worse when you get up?
YES
NO
Do you have pain in other joints, including the hip, knee, or ankle?
YES
Your bed may not be giving your back enough support (see BACKACHE, p.584) or you may have osteoarthritis. See DEGENERATIVE JOINT DISEASE, p.588.
NO
Could your back muscles be strained by your working conditions, such as sitting on a chair the wrong height for your desk or using a jackhammer?
YES
Backache often results from such strain. See BACKACHES, p.584.
NO
If you are unable to make a diagnosis from this chart, consult your physician.

62 GENERAL all ages

Cramp

Involuntary, painful tightening of muscles other than abdominal muscles. For abdominal cramps see chart 48, **Abdominal pain**.

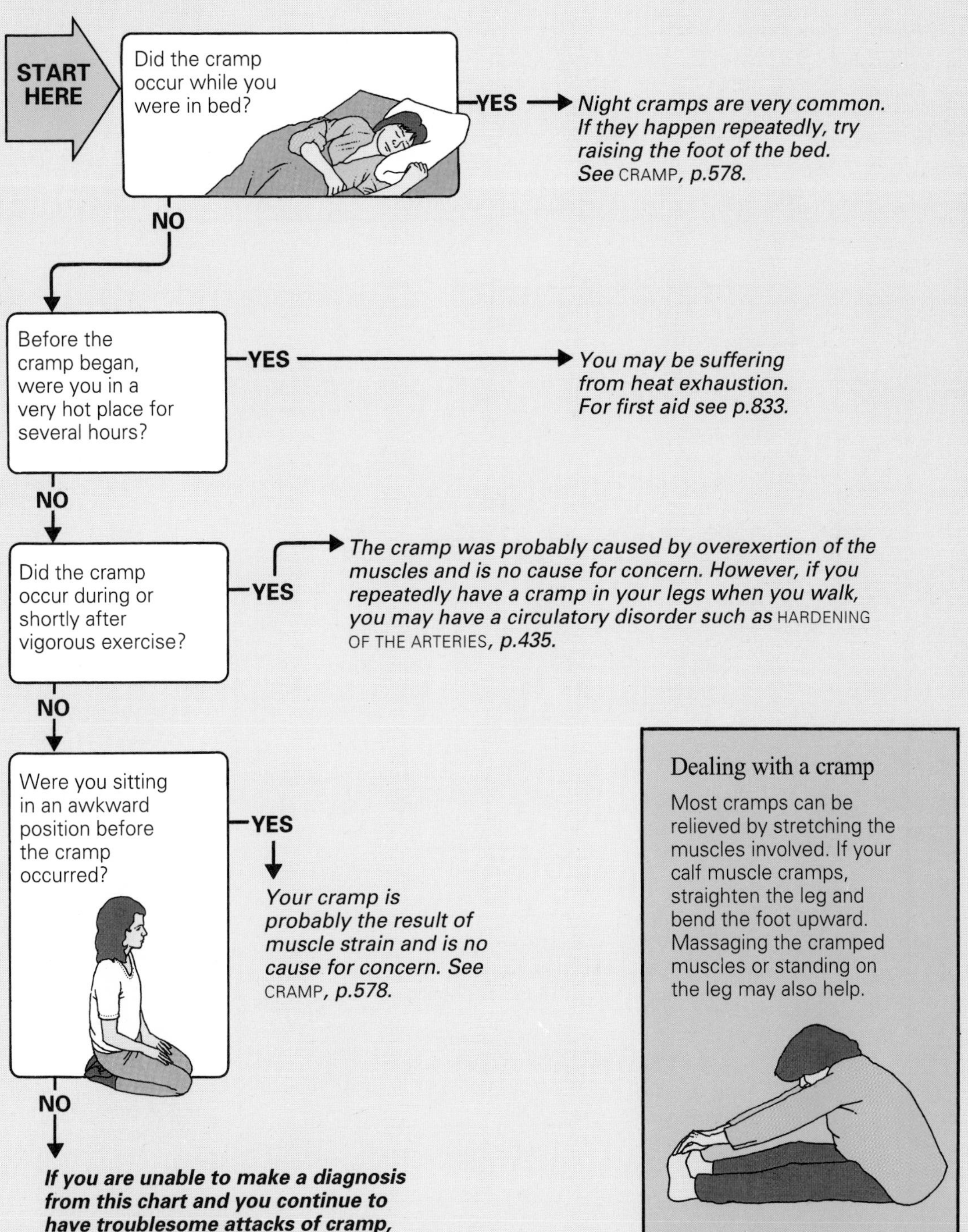

START HERE
Did the cramp occur while you were in bed?
YES → *Night cramps are very common. If they happen repeatedly, try raising the foot of the bed. See* CRAMP*, p.578.*
NO
Before the cramp began, were you in a very hot place for several hours?
YES → *You may be suffering from heat exhaustion. For first aid see p.833.*
NO
Did the cramp occur during or shortly after vigorous exercise?
YES → *The cramp was probably caused by overexertion of the muscles and is no cause for concern. However, if you repeatedly have a cramp in your legs when you walk, you may have a circulatory disorder such as* HARDENING OF THE ARTERIES*, p.435.*
NO
Were you sitting in an awkward position before the cramp occurred?
YES → *Your cramp is probably the result of muscle strain and is no cause for concern. See* CRAMP*, p.578.*
NO
If you are unable to make a diagnosis from this chart and you continue to have troublesome attacks of cramp, consult your physician.

Dealing with a cramp

Most cramps can be relieved by stretching the muscles involved. If your calf muscle cramps, straighten the leg and bend the foot upward. Massaging the cramped muscles or standing on the leg may also help.

63

GENERAL
all ages

Painful and/or stiff neck

Pain or discomfort that may or may not be accompanied by a slight headache.

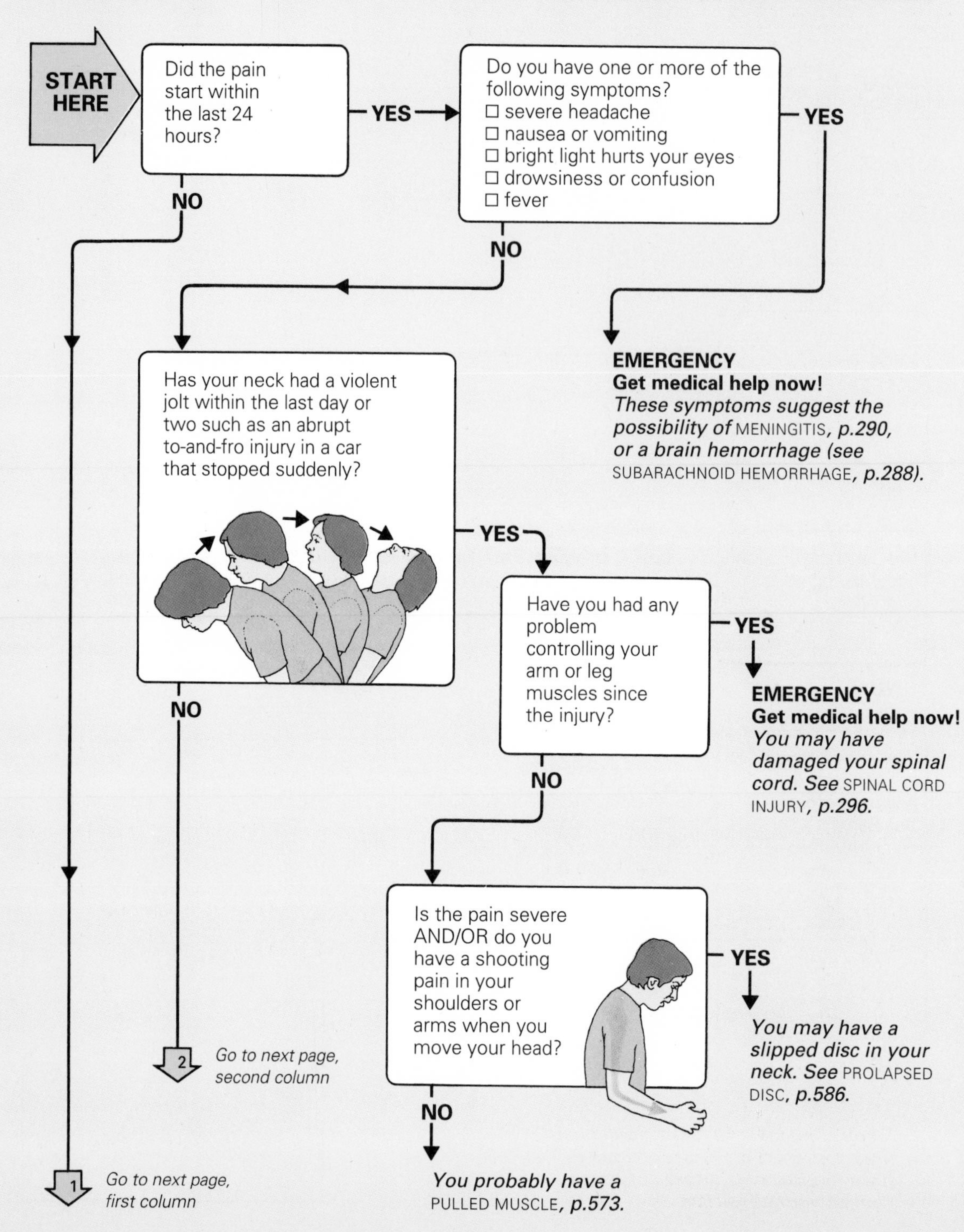

START HERE
Did the pain start within the last 24 hours?
YES
NO
Do you have one or more of the following symptoms?
☐ severe headache
☐ nausea or vomiting
☐ bright light hurts your eyes
☐ drowsiness or confusion
☐ fever
YES
NO
EMERGENCY
Get medical help now!
These symptoms suggest the possibility of MENINGITIS, p.290, or a brain hemorrhage (see SUBARACHNOID HEMORRHAGE, p.288).
Has your neck had a violent jolt within the last day or two such as an abrupt to-and-fro injury in a car that stopped suddenly?
YES
NO
Have you had any problem controlling your arm or leg muscles since the injury?
YES
EMERGENCY
Get medical help now!
You may have damaged your spinal cord. See SPINAL CORD INJURY, p.296.
NO
Is the pain severe AND/OR do you have a shooting pain in your shoulders or arms when you move your head?
YES
You may have a slipped disc in your neck. See PROLAPSED DISC, p.586.
NO
You probably have a PULLED MUSCLE, p.573.
2
Go to next page, second column
1
Go to next page, first column

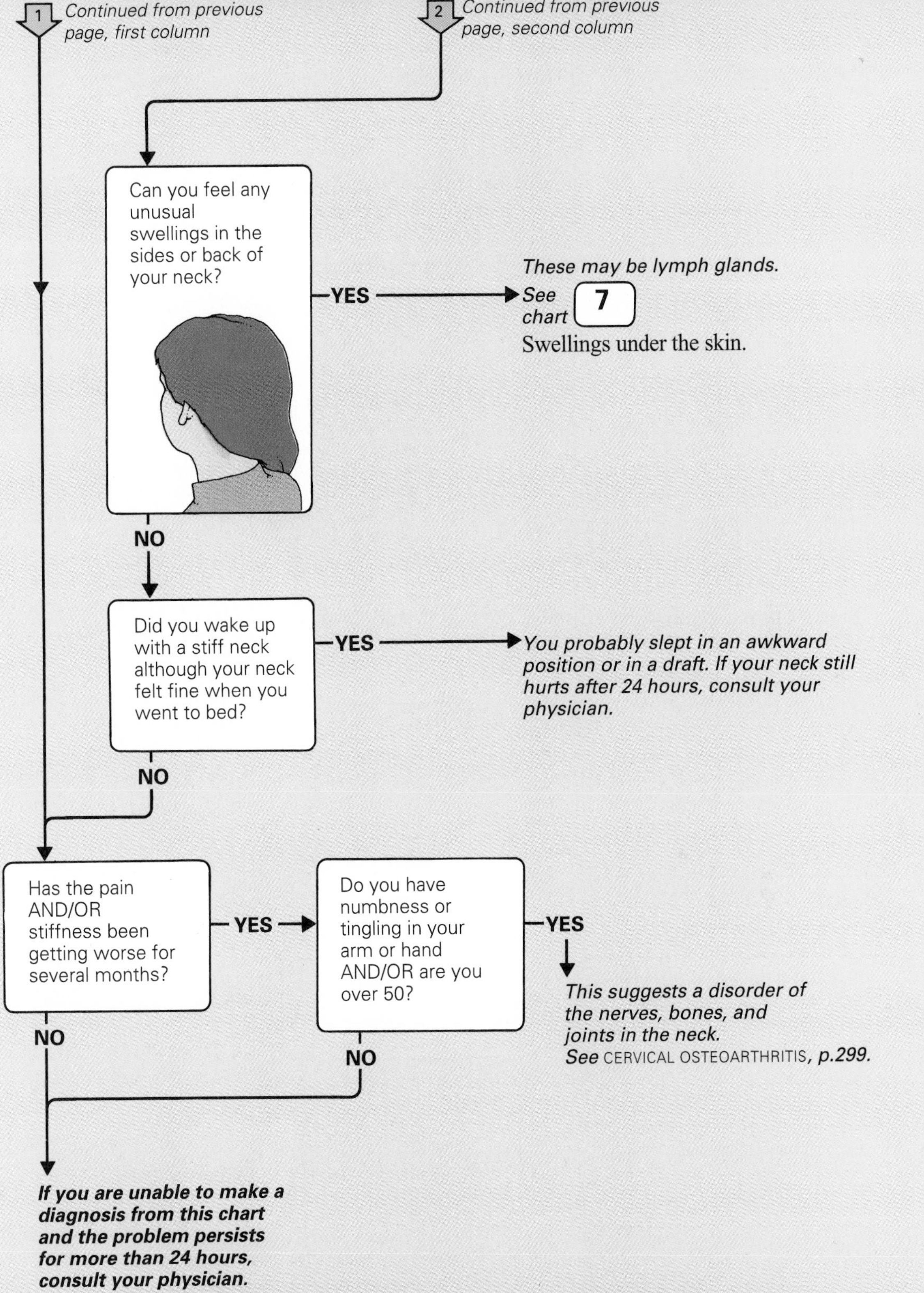

1 Continued from previous page, first column
2 Continued from previous page, second column
Can you feel any unusual swellings in the sides or back of your neck?
YES
These may be lymph glands.
See chart 7
Swellings under the skin.
NO
Did you wake up with a stiff neck although your neck felt fine when you went to bed?
YES
You probably slept in an awkward position or in a draft. If your neck still hurts after 24 hours, consult your physician.
NO
Has the pain AND/OR stiffness been getting worse for several months?
YES
Do you have numbness or tingling in your arm or hand AND/OR are you over 50?
YES
This suggests a disorder of the nerves, bones, and joints in the neck.
See CERVICAL OSTEOARTHRITIS, p.299.
NO
NO
If you are unable to make a diagnosis from this chart and the problem persists for more than 24 hours, consult your physician.

64
GENERAL
all ages

Painful arm or hand

Pain in the arm, elbow, wrist, or hand, but not the shoulder.

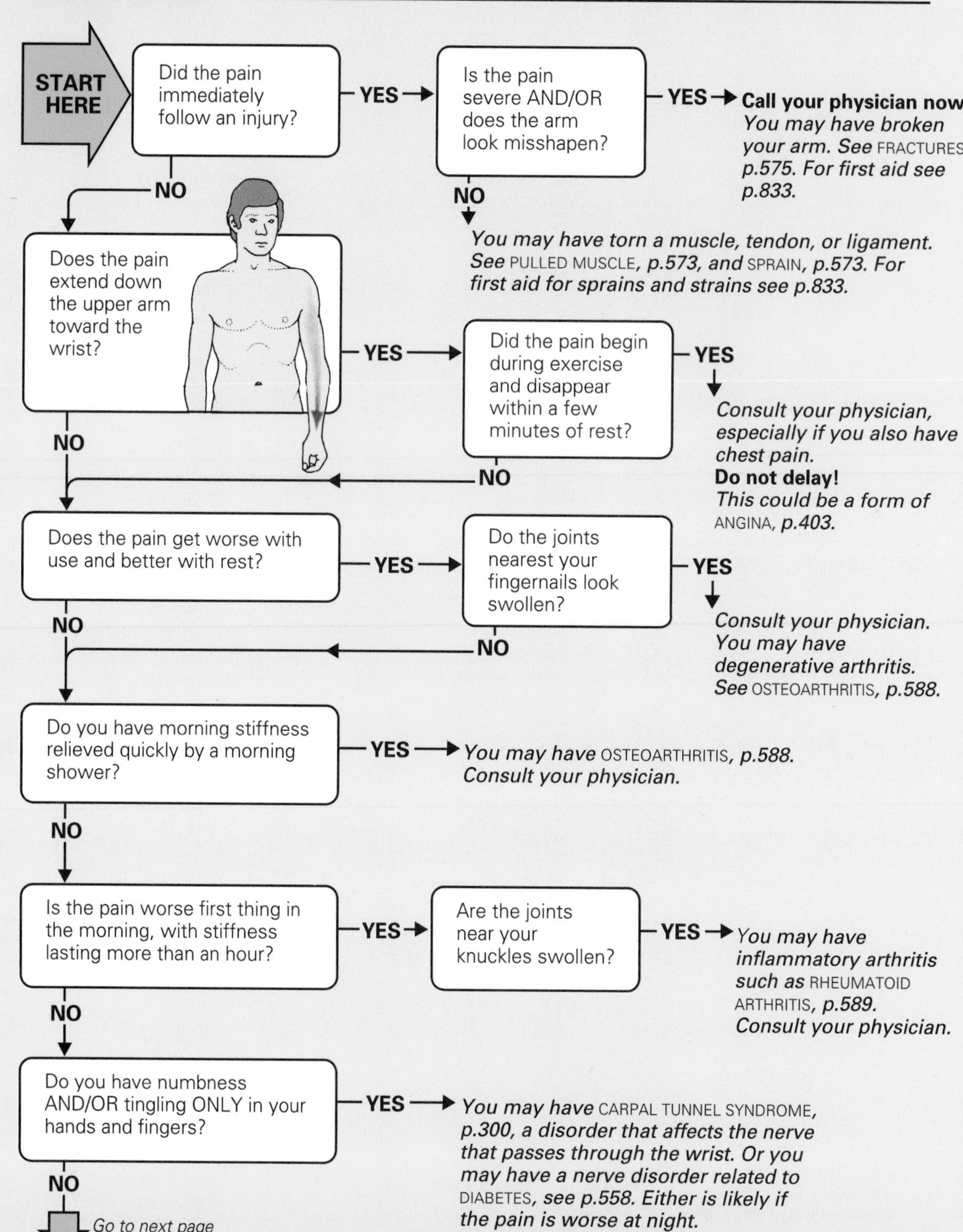

START HERE
Did the pain immediately follow an injury?
YES
Is the pain severe AND/OR does the arm look misshapen?
YES
Call your physician now! *You may have broken your arm. See* FRACTURES, *p.575. For first aid see p.833.*
NO
You may have torn a muscle, tendon, or ligament. See PULLED MUSCLE, *p.573, and* SPRAIN, *p.573. For first aid for sprains and strains see p.833.*
NO
Does the pain extend down the upper arm toward the wrist?
YES
Did the pain begin during exercise and disappear within a few minutes of rest?
YES
Consult your physician, especially if you also have chest pain. **Do not delay!** *This could be a form of* ANGINA, *p.403.*
NO
NO
Does the pain get worse with use and better with rest?
YES
Do the joints nearest your fingernails look swollen?
YES
Consult your physician. You may have degenerative arthritis. See OSTEOARTHRITIS, *p.588.*
NO
NO
Do you have morning stiffness relieved quickly by a morning shower?
YES
You may have OSTEOARTHRITIS, *p.588. Consult your physician.*
NO
Is the pain worse first thing in the morning, with stiffness lasting more than an hour?
YES
Are the joints near your knuckles swollen?
YES
You may have inflammatory arthritis such as RHEUMATOID ARTHRITIS, *p.589. Consult your physician.*
NO
Do you have numbness AND/OR tingling ONLY in your hands and fingers?
YES
You may have CARPAL TUNNEL SYNDROME, *p.300, a disorder that affects the nerve that passes through the wrist. Or you may have a nerve disorder related to* DIABETES, *see p.558. Either is likely if the pain is worse at night.*
NO
Go to next page

Continued from previous page

Do you have numbness AND/OR tingling in your arm or hand, possibly with a stiff neck?

YES → *You may have a disorder that affects the nerves, bones, and joints in the neck. See* CERVICAL OSTEOARTHRITIS, *p.299.*

NO ↓

Is the pain in the elbow, wrist, or finger joints?

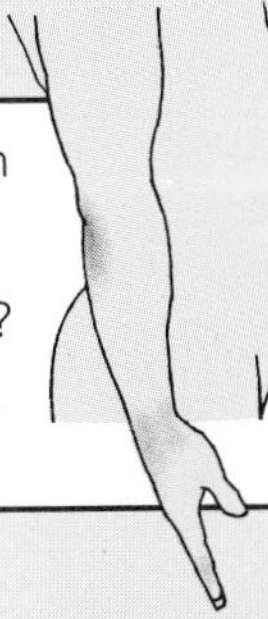

YES → Is the pain accompanied by redness and swelling?

YES → Is only one joint affected?

YES ↓

Is your temperature 100°F (38°C) or above AND/OR have you recently begun to feel sick?

YES ↓

Consult your physician.
Do not delay!
You may have a joint infection. See INFECTIOUS ARTHRITIS, *p.591.*

NO ↓

You may have BURSITIS, *p.592, or* GOUT, *p.537.*

NO (redness and swelling / only one joint) ↓

Do your hand, hands, or fingers turn white, then blue, then red, especially in the cold?

YES ↓

Consult your physician. You may have RAYNAUD'S DISEASE, *p.440.*

NO ↓

Is the pain worse first thing in the morning, with stiffness lasting more than an hour?

YES → Are the joints near your knuckles swollen?

YES ↓

Consult your physician. You may have inflammatory arthritis, such as RHEUMATOID ARTHRITIS, *p.589.*

NO ↓

Does the pain occur only when you bend or use your arm in a certain way, or during certain activities, such as typing?

YES ↓

You may have inflammation of the tendons (see TENDINITIS, *p.578).*

NO ↓

If you are unable to make a diagnosis from this chart, consult your physician.

65 GENERAL all ages

Painful leg

Pain in the thigh and/or calf that may be fleeting or continuous.

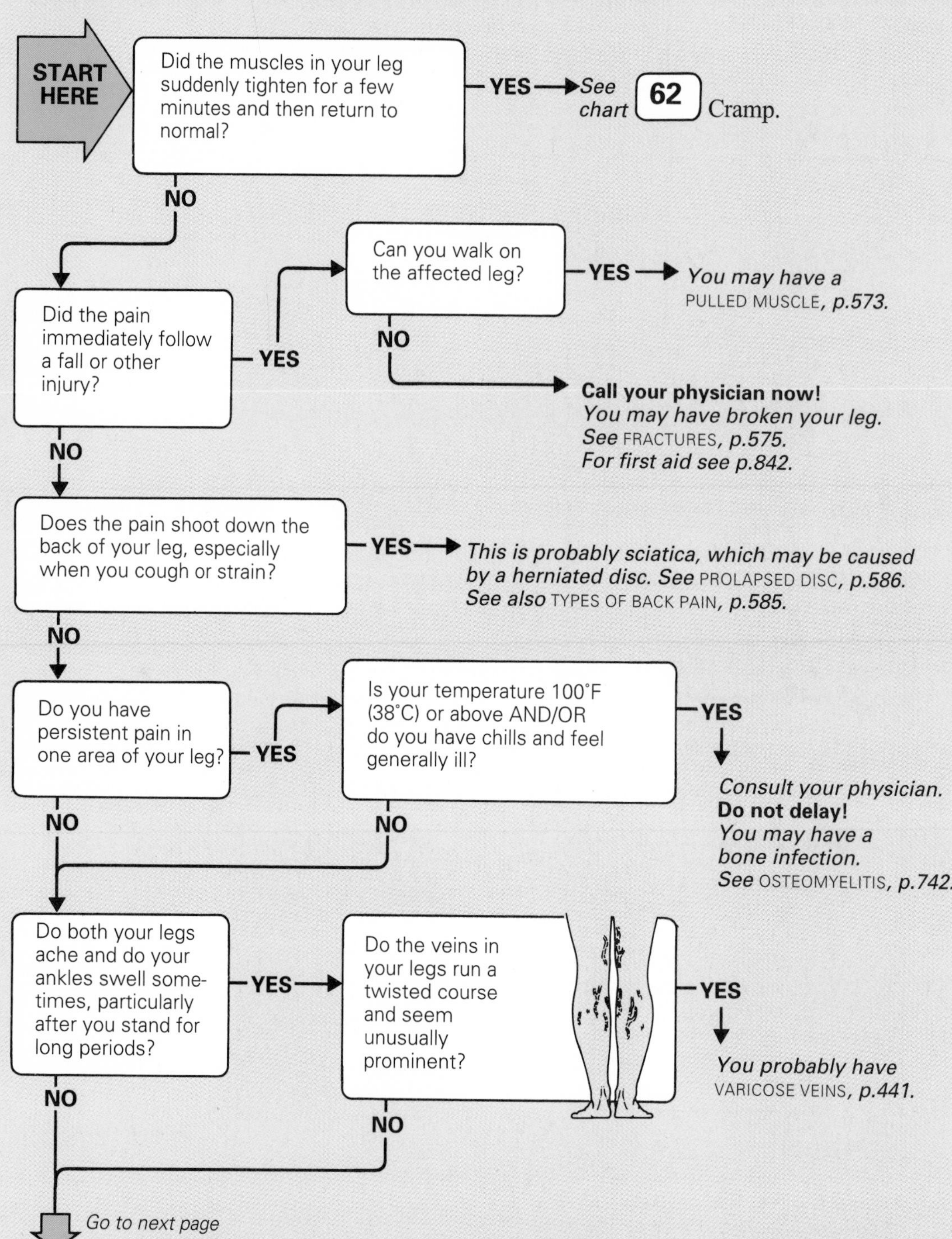

START HERE
Did the muscles in your leg suddenly tighten for a few minutes and then return to normal?
YES
See chart 62 Cramp.
NO
Did the pain immediately follow a fall or other injury?
YES
Can you walk on the affected leg?
YES
You may have a PULLED MUSCLE, p.573.
NO
Call your physician now!
You may have broken your leg.
See FRACTURES, p.575.
For first aid see p.842.
NO
Does the pain shoot down the back of your leg, especially when you cough or strain?
YES
This is probably sciatica, which may be caused by a herniated disc. See PROLAPSED DISC, p.586.
See also TYPES OF BACK PAIN, p.585.
NO
Do you have persistent pain in one area of your leg?
YES
Is your temperature 100°F (38°C) or above AND/OR do you have chills and feel generally ill?
YES
Consult your physician.
Do not delay!
You may have a bone infection.
See OSTEOMYELITIS, p.742.
NO
NO
Do both your legs ache and do your ankles swell sometimes, particularly after you stand for long periods?
YES
Do the veins in your legs run a twisted course and seem unusually prominent?
YES
You probably have VARICOSE VEINS, p.441.
NO
NO
Go to next page

Continued from previous page

Is your hip painful and/or stiff on the same side as the affected leg?

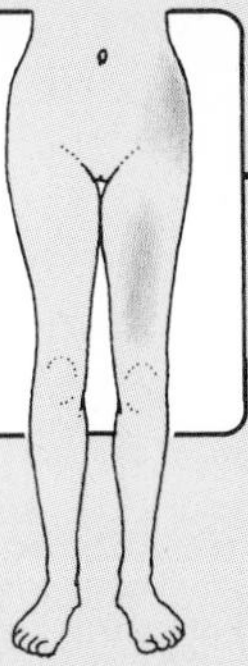

YES → *A disorder of the hip such as* OSTEOARTHRITIS, *p.588, may result in leg pain.*

NO ↓

Is the pain mainly in your calf?

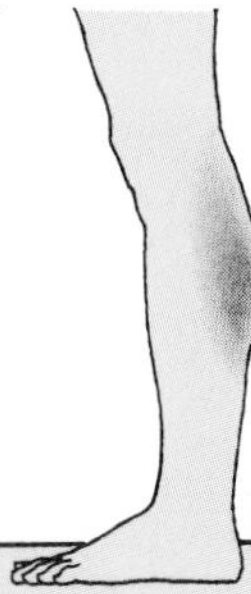

YES → Is your calf swollen, and is it tender when you walk on that foot?

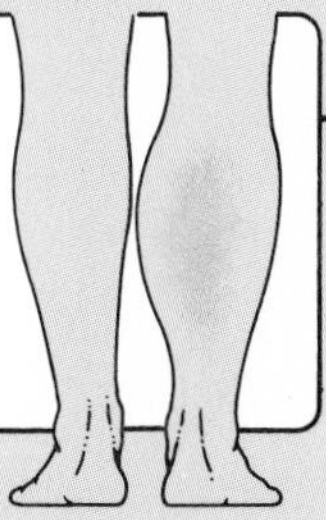

YES → **Call your physician now!** ***You may have a blood clot in your leg. See*** DEEP VEIN THROMBOSIS, ***p.445.***

NO ↓

Is one of your veins red and inflamed?

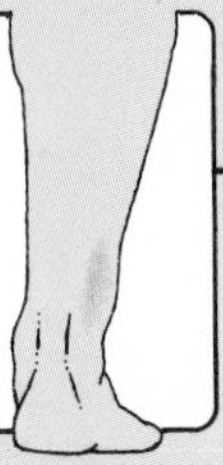

YES → *This may be* THROMBOPHLEBITIS, *p.444.*

NO ↓

Does your leg start to hurt while you walk and does the pain disappear with rest?

YES → *Recurrent pain in the calf during exercise that disappears promptly when you stop may be a sign of a circulatory problem such as* HARDENING OF THE ARTERIES, *p.435, or a sports injury. See* SPORTS INJURIES, *p.577.*

NO → (go to "Did your leg become painful following unusually strenuous exercise?")

NO (from "Is the pain mainly in your calf?") ↓

Did your leg become painful following unusually strenuous exercise?

YES → *You may have a* PULLED MUSCLE, *p.573.*

NO ↓

If you are unable to make a diagnosis from this chart, and the pain persists for more than 48 hours or gets worse, consult your physician.

66

GENERAL
all ages

Painful knee

Pain in or around the knee joint that may be accompanied by swelling.

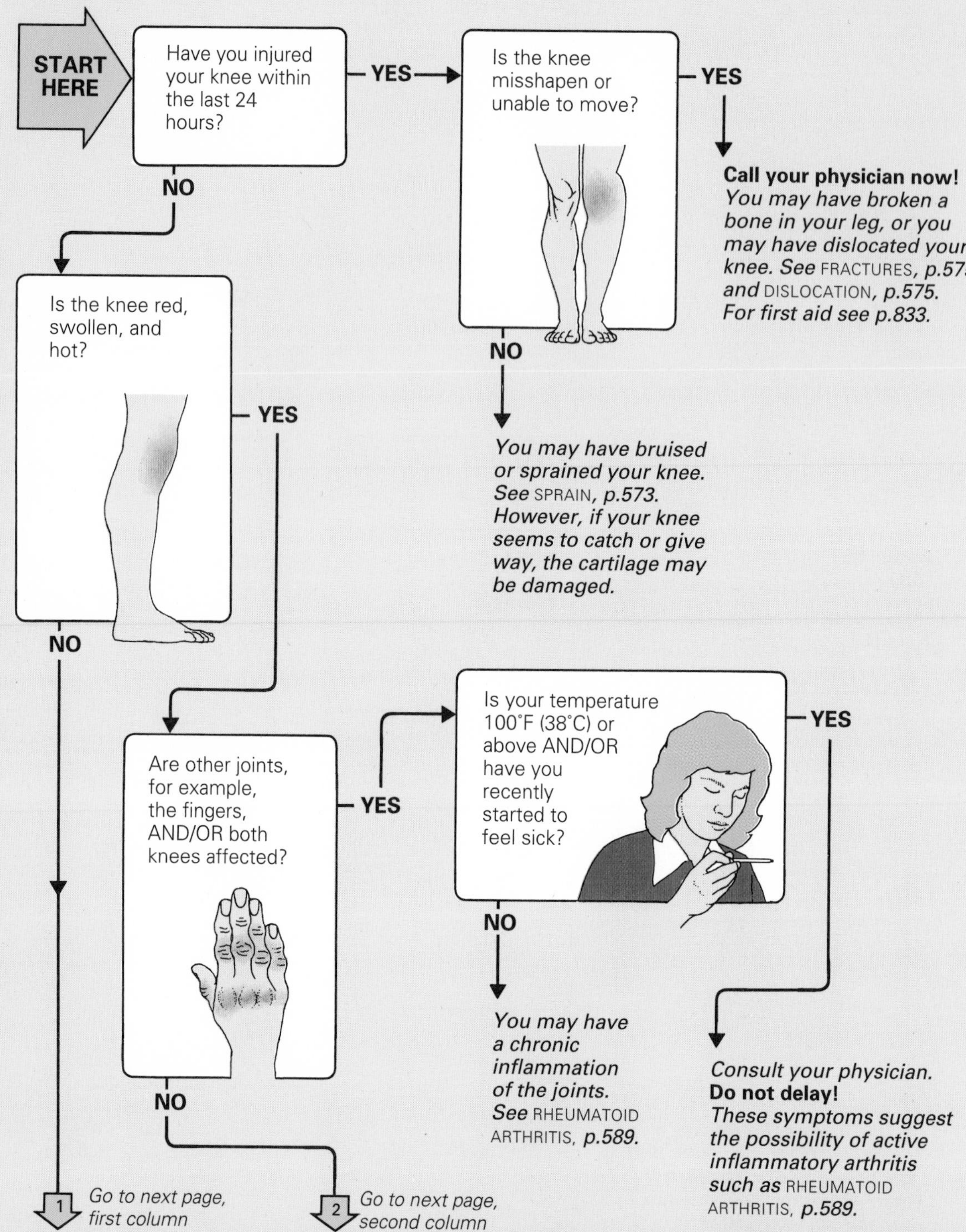

START HERE
Have you injured your knee within the last 24 hours?
YES
Is the knee misshapen or unable to move?
YES
Call your physician now!
You may have broken a bone in your leg, or you may have dislocated your knee. See FRACTURES, *p.575, and* DISLOCATION, *p.575. For first aid see p.833.*
NO
You may have bruised or sprained your knee. See SPRAIN, *p.573. However, if your knee seems to catch or give way, the cartilage may be damaged.*
NO
Is the knee red, swollen, and hot?
YES
Are other joints, for example, the fingers, AND/OR both knees affected?
YES
Is your temperature 100°F (38°C) or above AND/OR have you recently started to feel sick?
YES
Consult your physician.
Do not delay!
These symptoms suggest the possibility of active inflammatory arthritis such as RHEUMATOID ARTHRITIS, *p.589.*
NO
You may have a chronic inflammation of the joints. See RHEUMATOID ARTHRITIS, *p.589.*
NO
NO
1 *Go to next page, first column*
2 *Go to next page, second column*

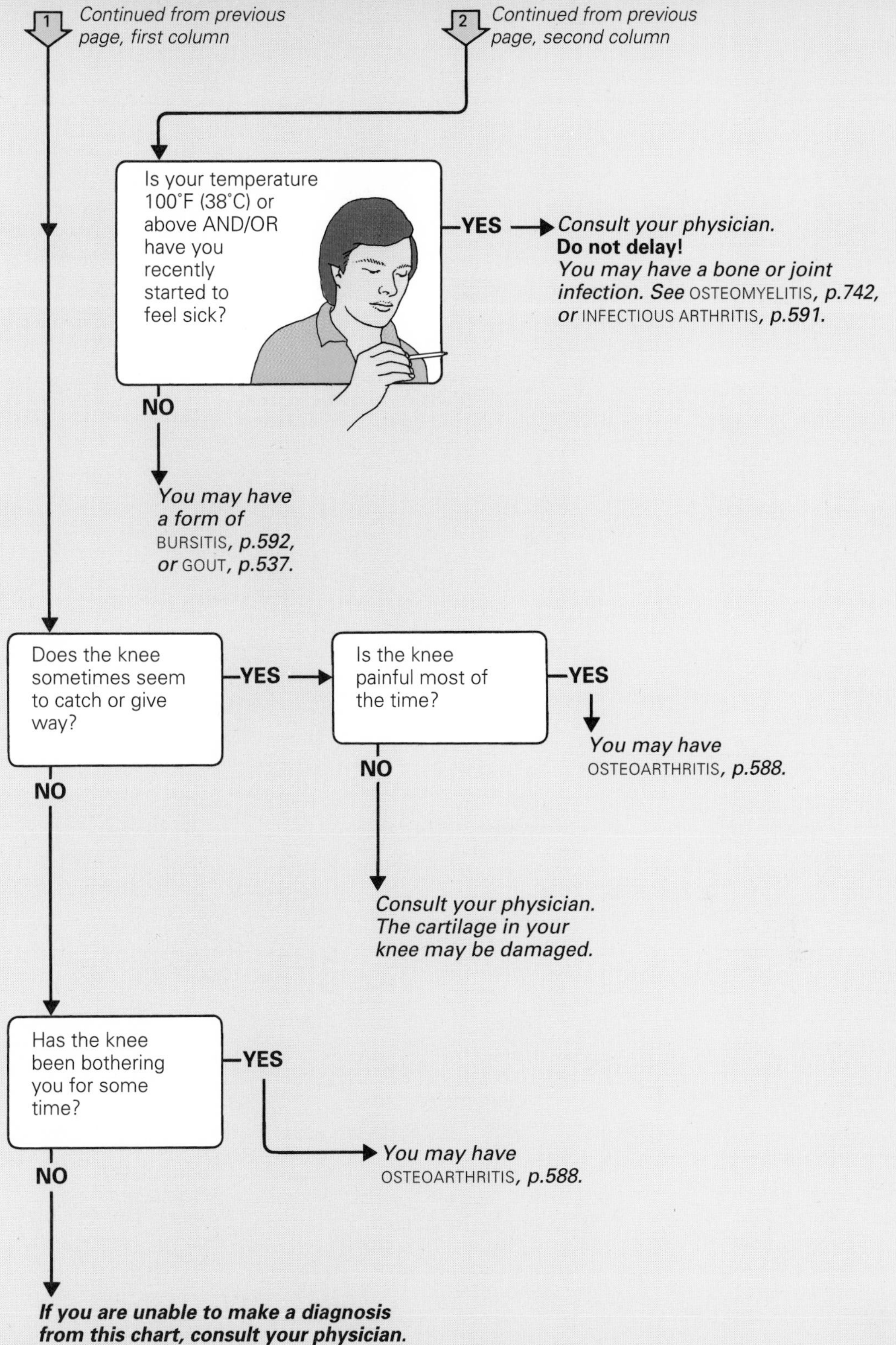

1
Continued from previous page, first column
2
Continued from previous page, second column
Is your temperature 100°F (38°C) or above AND/OR have you recently started to feel sick?
YES
Consult your physician.
Do not delay!
You may have a bone or joint infection. See OSTEOMYELITIS, p.742, or INFECTIOUS ARTHRITIS, p.591.
NO
You may have a form of BURSITIS, p.592, or GOUT, p.537.
Does the knee sometimes seem to catch or give way?
YES
Is the knee painful most of the time?
YES
You may have OSTEOARTHRITIS, p.588.
NO
Consult your physician. The cartilage in your knee may be damaged.
NO
Has the knee been bothering you for some time?
YES
You may have OSTEOARTHRITIS, p.588.
NO
If you are unable to make a diagnosis from this chart, consult your physician.

67
GENERAL
all ages

Painful shoulder

Pain in the shoulder, which may be accompanied by stiffness that limits the movement of your upper arm.

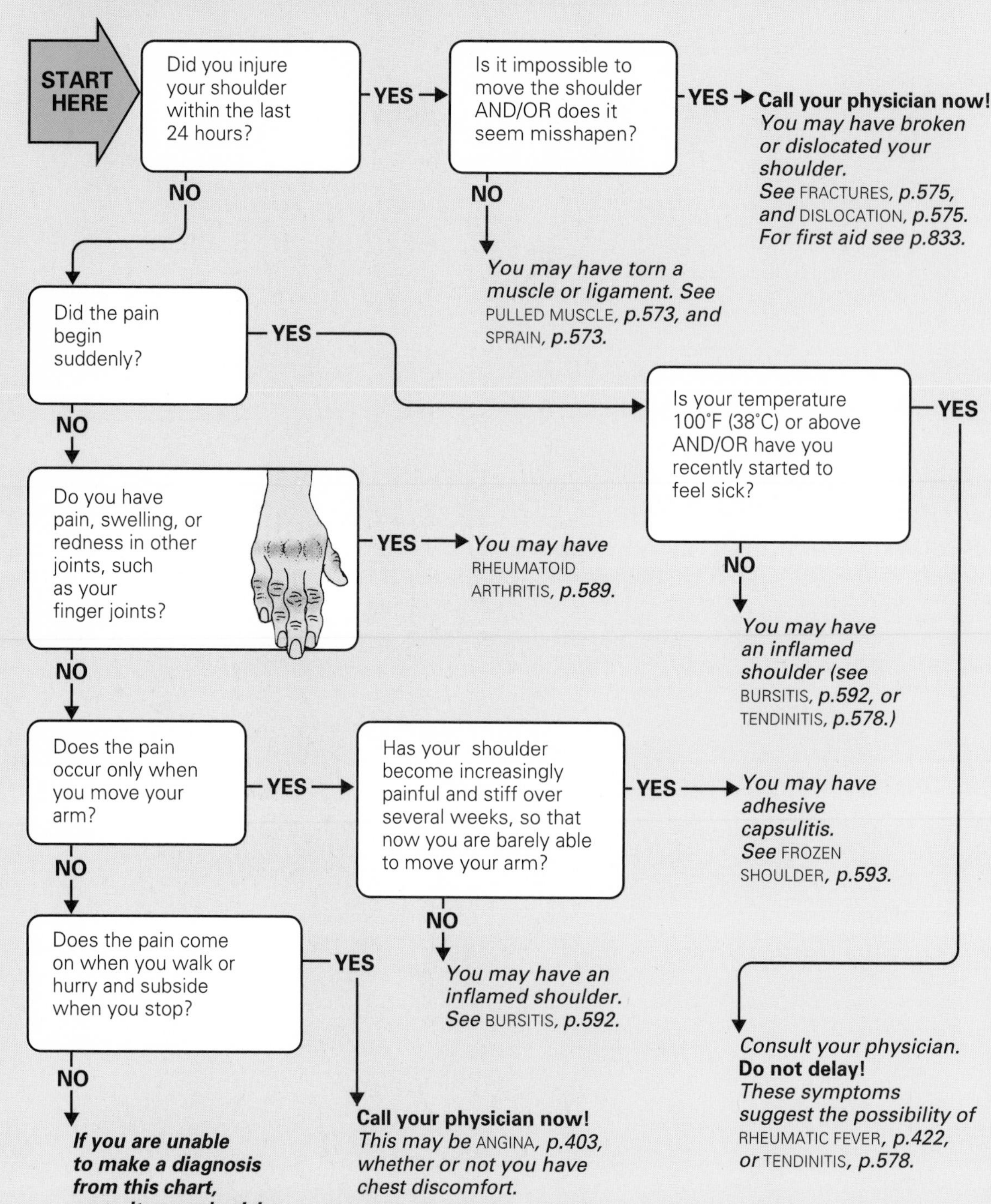

START HERE
Did you injure your shoulder within the last 24 hours?
YES
Is it impossible to move the shoulder AND/OR does it seem misshapen?
YES
Call your physician now!
You may have broken or dislocated your shoulder.
See FRACTURES, *p.575, and* DISLOCATION, *p.575.*
For first aid see p.833.
NO
You may have torn a muscle or ligament. See PULLED MUSCLE, *p.573, and* SPRAIN, *p.573.*
NO
Did the pain begin suddenly?
YES
Is your temperature 100°F (38°C) or above AND/OR have you recently started to feel sick?
YES
Consult your physician.
Do not delay!
These symptoms suggest the possibility of RHEUMATIC FEVER, *p.422, or* TENDINITIS, *p.578.*
NO
You may have an inflamed shoulder (see BURSITIS, *p.592, or* TENDINITIS, *p.578.)*
NO
Do you have pain, swelling, or redness in other joints, such as your finger joints?
YES
You may have RHEUMATOID ARTHRITIS, *p.589.*
NO
Does the pain occur only when you move your arm?
YES
Has your shoulder become increasingly painful and stiff over several weeks, so that now you are barely able to move your arm?
YES
You may have adhesive capsulitis.
See FROZEN SHOULDER, *p.593.*
NO
You may have an inflamed shoulder.
See BURSITIS, *p.592.*
NO
Does the pain come on when you walk or hurry and subside when you stop?
YES
Call your physician now!
This may be ANGINA, *p.403, whether or not you have chest discomfort.*
NO
If you are unable to make a diagnosis from this chart, consult your physician.

68
GENERAL
all ages

Painful ankles

Pain, with or without swelling, in or around one or both ankles.

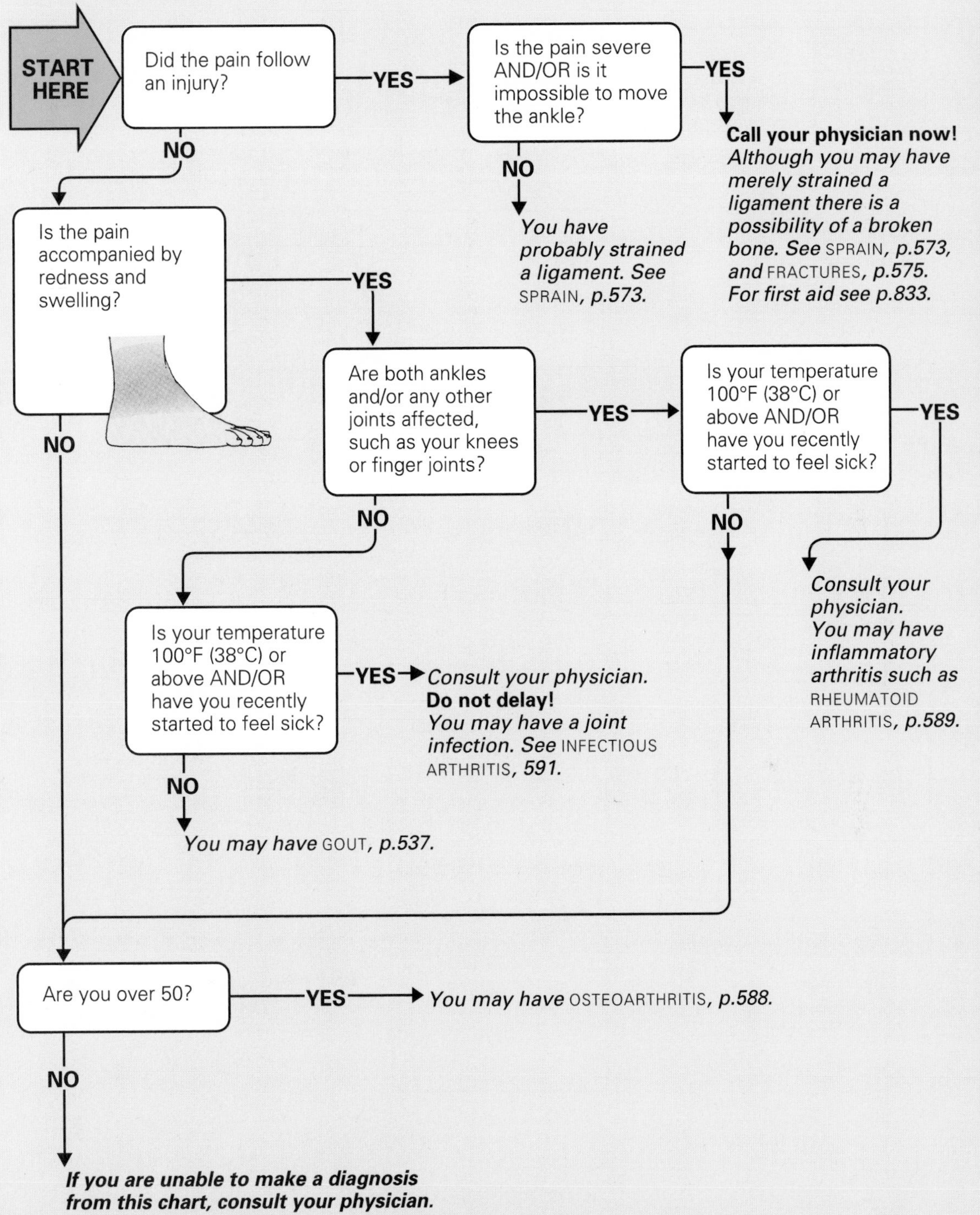

START HERE
Did the pain follow an injury?
YES
Is the pain severe AND/OR is it impossible to move the ankle?
YES
Call your physician now!
Although you may have merely strained a ligament there is a possibility of a broken bone. See SPRAIN, *p.573, and* FRACTURES, *p.575. For first aid see p.833.*
NO
You have probably strained a ligament. See SPRAIN, *p.573.*
NO
Is the pain accompanied by redness and swelling?
YES
Are both ankles and/or any other joints affected, such as your knees or finger joints?
YES
Is your temperature 100°F (38°C) or above AND/OR have you recently started to feel sick?
YES
Consult your physician. You may have inflammatory arthritis such as RHEUMATOID ARTHRITIS, *p.589.*
NO
NO
Is your temperature 100°F (38°C) or above AND/OR have you recently started to feel sick?
YES
Consult your physician. **Do not delay!** *You may have a joint infection. See* INFECTIOUS ARTHRITIS, *591.*
NO
You may have GOUT, *p.537.*
NO
Are you over 50?
YES
You may have OSTEOARTHRITIS, *p.588.*
NO
If you are unable to make a diagnosis from this chart, consult your physician.

69

GENERAL
all ages

Swollen ankles

Swelling or puffiness that may affect one or both ankles.

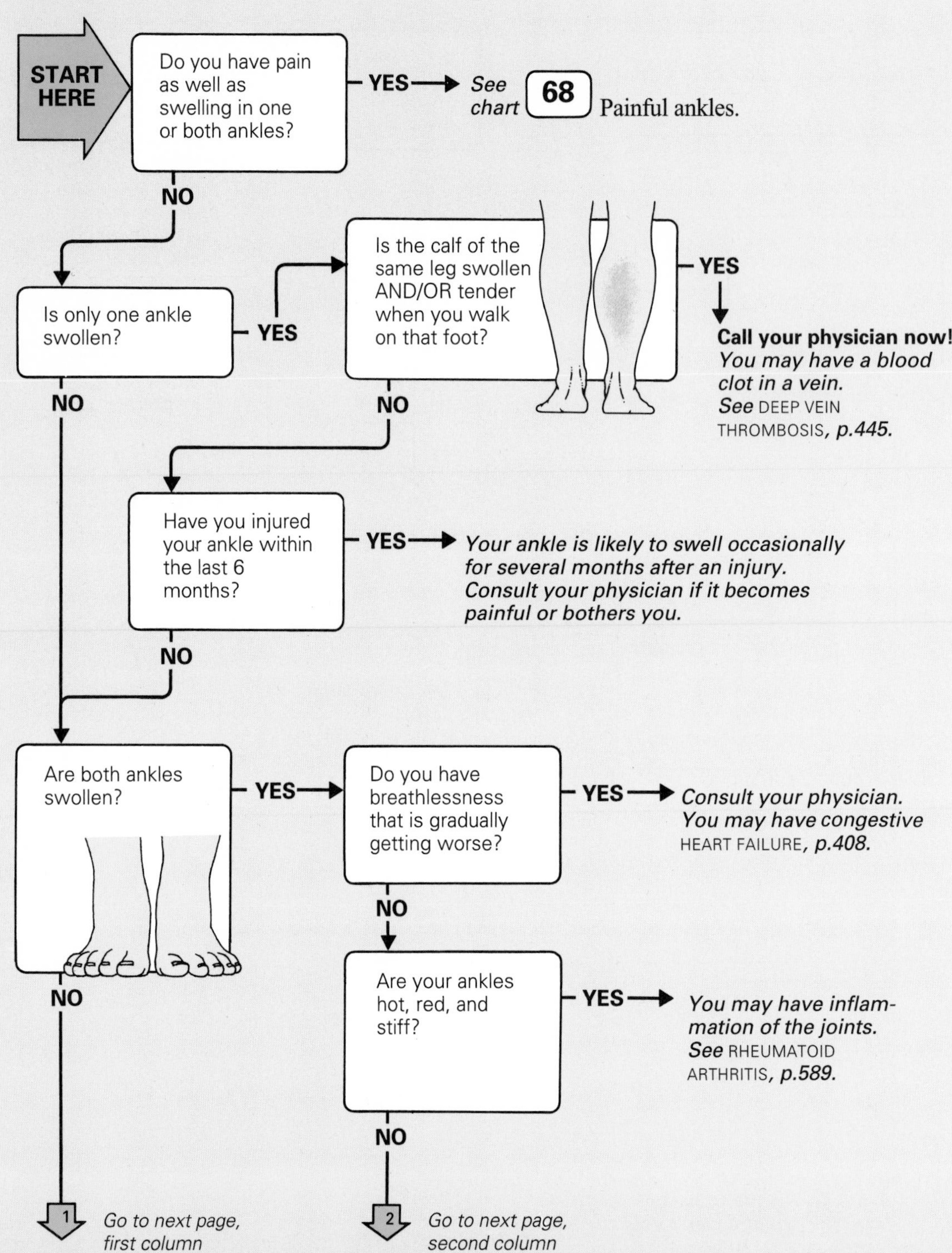

START HERE
Do you have pain as well as swelling in one or both ankles?
YES → See chart 68 Painful ankles.
NO
Is only one ankle swollen?
YES
Is the calf of the same leg swollen AND/OR tender when you walk on that foot?
YES
Call your physician now!
You may have a blood clot in a vein.
See DEEP VEIN THROMBOSIS, *p.445.*
NO
Have you injured your ankle within the last 6 months?
YES → *Your ankle is likely to swell occasionally for several months after an injury. Consult your physician if it becomes painful or bothers you.*
NO
NO
Are both ankles swollen?
YES →
Do you have breathlessness that is gradually getting worse?
YES → *Consult your physician. You may have congestive* HEART FAILURE, *p.408.*
NO
Are your ankles hot, red, and stiff?
YES → *You may have inflammation of the joints. See* RHEUMATOID ARTHRITIS, *p.589.*
NO
NO
1 *Go to next page, first column*
2 *Go to next page, second column*

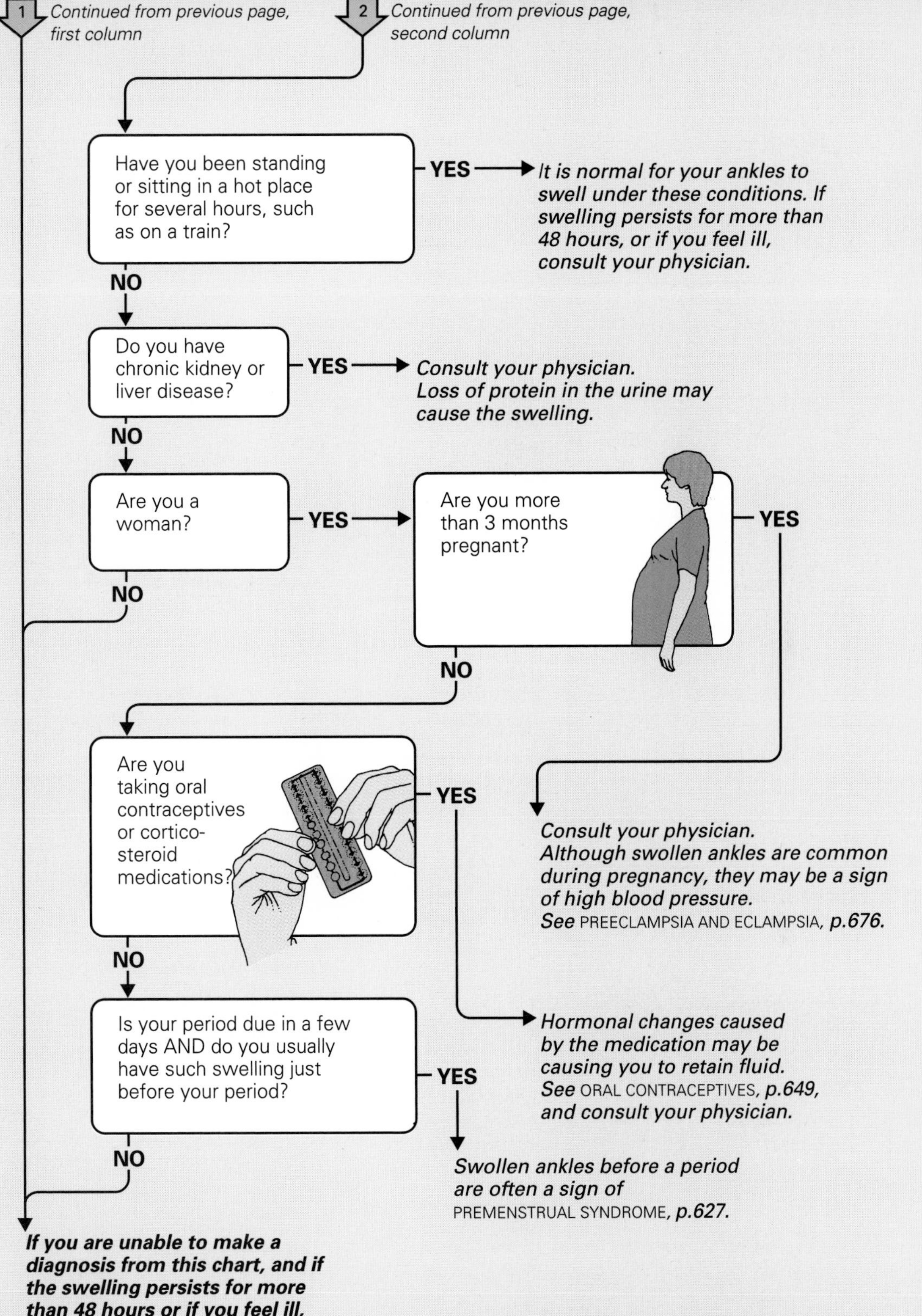
1
Continued from previous page, first column
2
Continued from previous page, second column
Have you been standing or sitting in a hot place for several hours, such as on a train?
YES
It is normal for your ankles to swell under these conditions. If swelling persists for more than 48 hours, or if you feel ill, consult your physician.
NO
Do you have chronic kidney or liver disease?
YES
Consult your physician. Loss of protein in the urine may cause the swelling.
NO
Are you a woman?
YES
Are you more than 3 months pregnant?
YES
Consult your physician. Although swollen ankles are common during pregnancy, they may be a sign of high blood pressure. See PREECLAMPSIA AND ECLAMPSIA, p.676.
NO
NO
Are you taking oral contraceptives or cortico-steroid medications?
YES
Hormonal changes caused by the medication may be causing you to retain fluid. See ORAL CONTRACEPTIVES, p.649, and consult your physician.
NO
Is your period due in a few days AND do you usually have such swelling just before your period?
YES
Swollen ankles before a period are often a sign of PREMENSTRUAL SYNDROME, p.627.
NO
If you are unable to make a diagnosis from this chart, and if the swelling persists for more than 48 hours or if you feel ill, consult your physician.

70
GENERAL
all ages

Foot problems

Pain, irritation, or swelling anywhere in one or both feet, but not in the ankles.

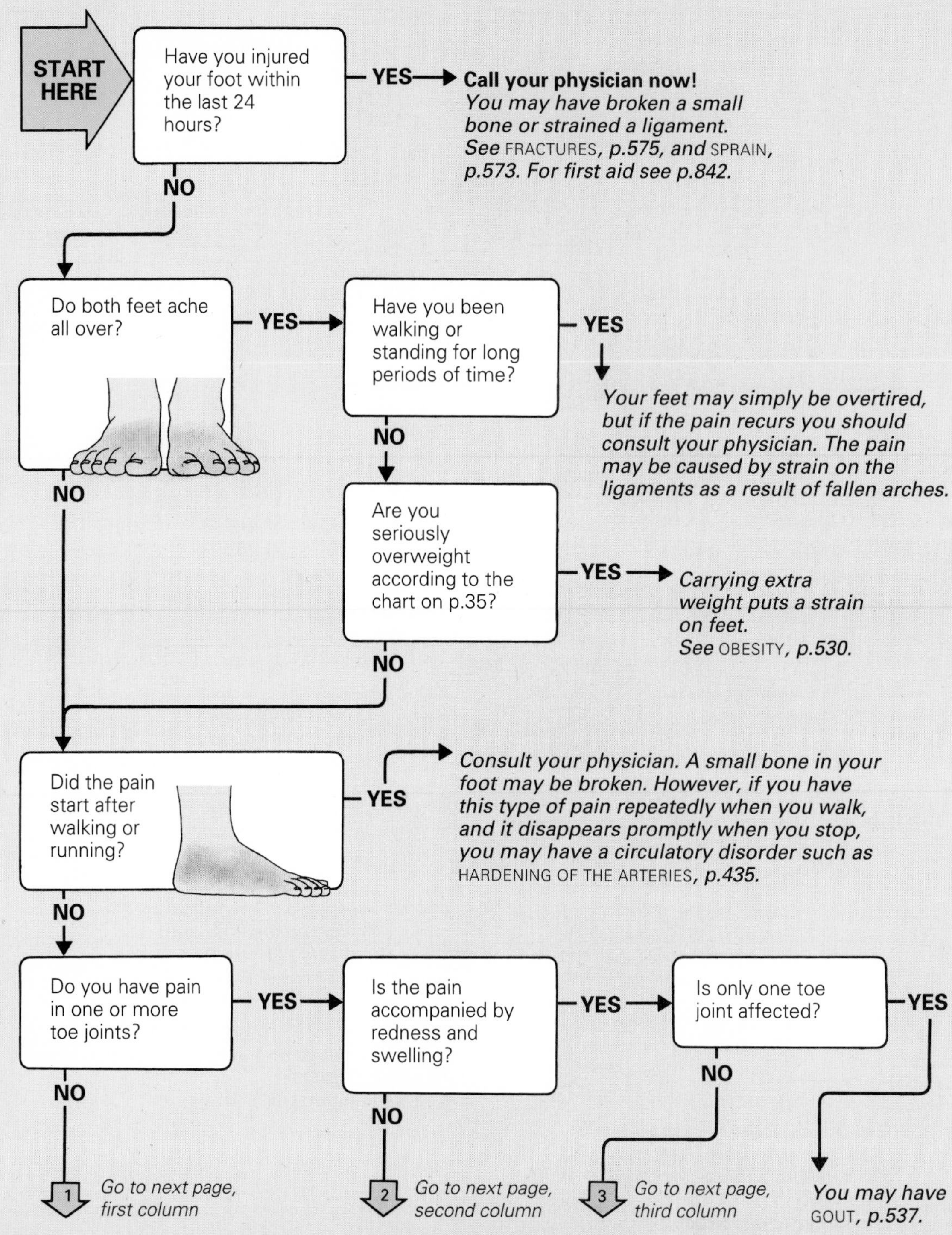

START HERE
Have you injured your foot within the last 24 hours?
YES
Call your physician now!
You may have broken a small bone or strained a ligament. See FRACTURES, p.575, and SPRAIN, p.573. For first aid see p.842.
NO
Do both feet ache all over?
YES
Have you been walking or standing for long periods of time?
YES
Your feet may simply be overtired, but if the pain recurs you should consult your physician. The pain may be caused by strain on the ligaments as a result of fallen arches.
NO
Are you seriously overweight according to the chart on p.35?
YES
Carrying extra weight puts a strain on feet. See OBESITY, p.530.
NO
NO
Did the pain start after walking or running?
YES
Consult your physician. A small bone in your foot may be broken. However, if you have this type of pain repeatedly when you walk, and it disappears promptly when you stop, you may have a circulatory disorder such as HARDENING OF THE ARTERIES, p.435.
NO
Do you have pain in one or more toe joints?
YES
Is the pain accompanied by redness and swelling?
YES
Is only one toe joint affected?
YES
You may have GOUT, p.537.
NO
3
Go to next page, third column
NO
2
Go to next page, second column
NO
1
Go to next page, first column

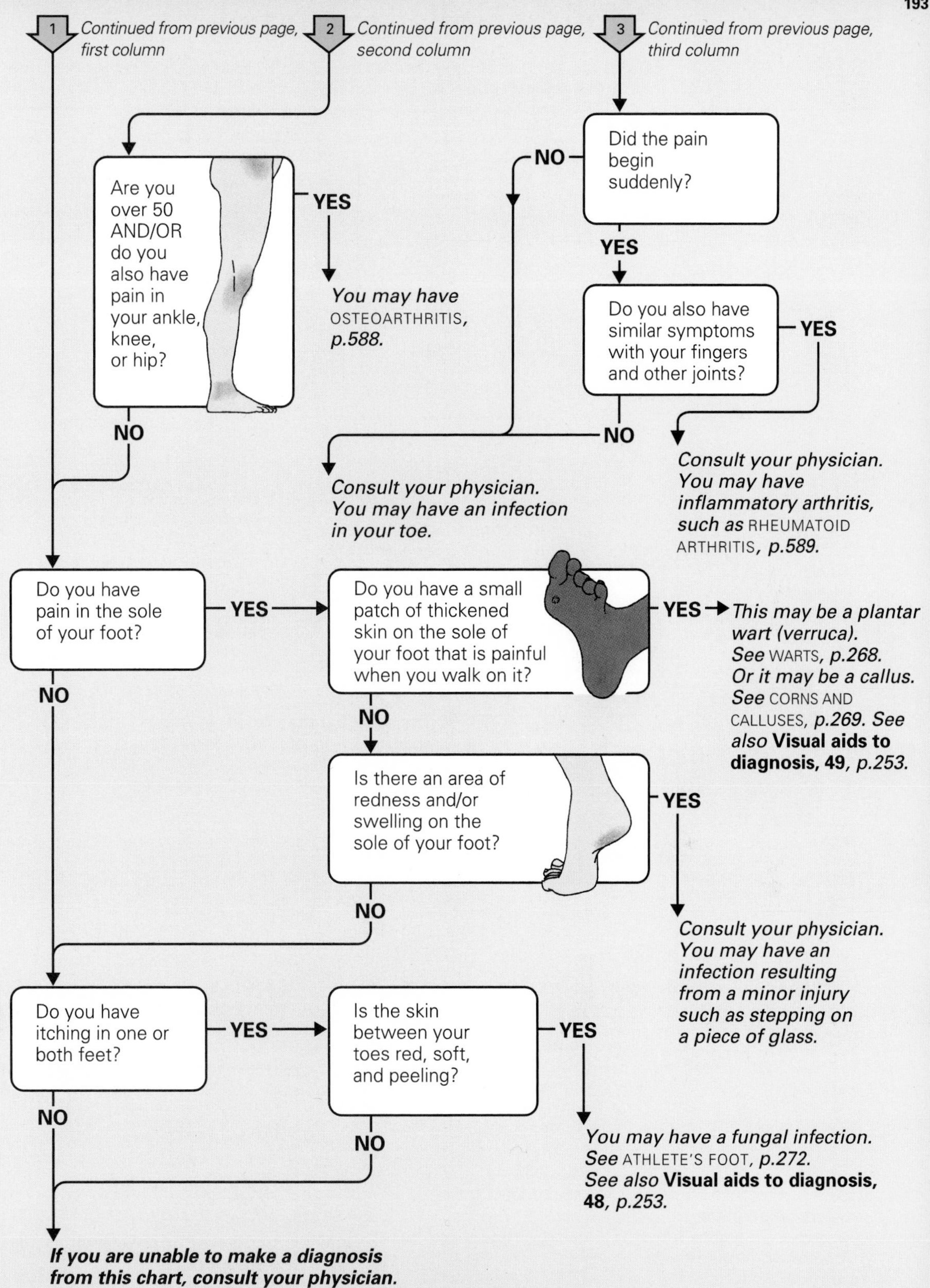
1 Continued from previous page, first column
2 Continued from previous page, second column
3 Continued from previous page, third column
Are you over 50 AND/OR do you also have pain in your ankle, knee, or hip?
YES
You may have OSTEOARTHRITIS, p.588.
NO
Did the pain begin suddenly?
NO
YES
Do you also have similar symptoms with your fingers and other joints?
YES
NO
Consult your physician. You may have an infection in your toe.
Consult your physician. You may have inflammatory arthritis, such as RHEUMATOID ARTHRITIS, p.589.
Do you have pain in the sole of your foot?
YES
Do you have a small patch of thickened skin on the sole of your foot that is painful when you walk on it?
YES
This may be a plantar wart (verruca). See WARTS, p.268. Or it may be a callus. See CORNS AND CALLUSES, p.269. See also Visual aids to diagnosis, 49, p.253.
NO
NO
Is there an area of redness and/or swelling on the sole of your foot?
YES
Consult your physician. You may have an infection resulting from a minor injury such as stepping on a piece of glass.
NO
Do you have itching in one or both feet?
YES
Is the skin between your toes red, soft, and peeling?
YES
You may have a fungal infection. See ATHLETE'S FOOT, p.272. See also Visual aids to diagnosis, 48, p.253.
NO
NO
If you are unable to make a diagnosis from this chart, consult your physician.

71

MEN
all ages

Painful or enlarged testicles

Pain or swelling that may affect one or both testicles, or the whole area inside the scrotum (the supportive bag).

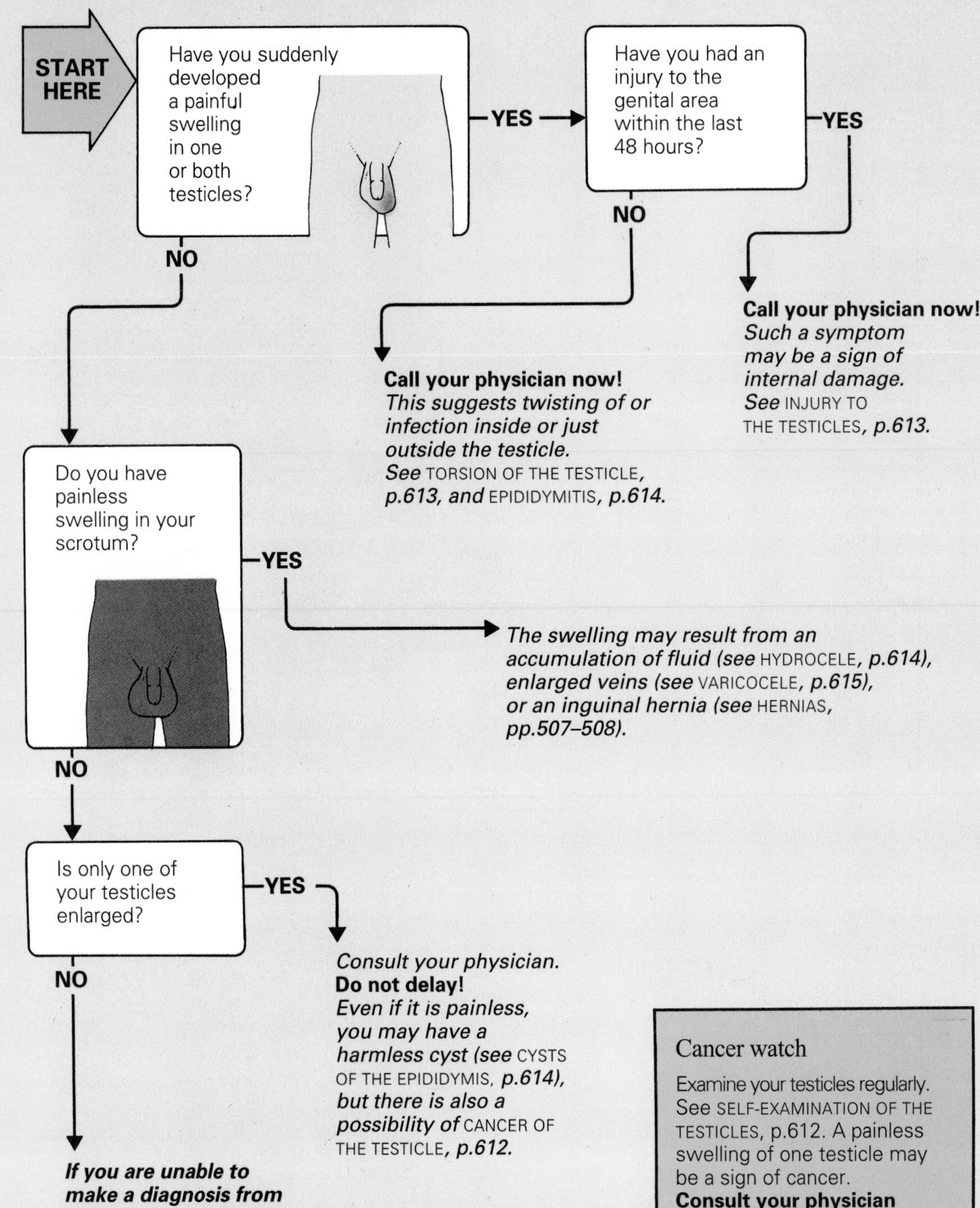

START HERE

Have you suddenly developed a painful swelling in one or both testicles?

YES → Have you had an injury to the genital area within the last 48 hours?

- YES → **Call your physician now!** *Such a symptom may be a sign of internal damage. See* INJURY TO THE TESTICLES, *p.613.*
- NO → **Call your physician now!** *This suggests twisting of or infection inside or just outside the testicle. See* TORSION OF THE TESTICLE, *p.613, and* EPIDIDYMITIS, *p.614.*

NO → Do you have painless swelling in your scrotum?

YES → *The swelling may result from an accumulation of fluid (see* HYDROCELE, *p.614), enlarged veins (see* VARICOCELE, *p.615), or an inguinal hernia (see* HERNIAS, *pp.507–508).*

NO → Is only one of your testicles enlarged?

YES → *Consult your physician.* **Do not delay!** *Even if it is painless, you may have a harmless cyst (see* CYSTS OF THE EPIDIDYMIS, *p.614), but there is also a possibility of* CANCER OF THE TESTICLE, *p.612.*

NO → ***If you are unable to make a diagnosis from this chart, consult your physician.***

Cancer watch

Examine your testicles regularly. See SELF-EXAMINATION OF THE TESTICLES, p.612. A painless swelling of one testicle may be a sign of cancer.
Consult your physician without delay!

Painful intercourse in men

Pain or discomfort during or just after intercourse.

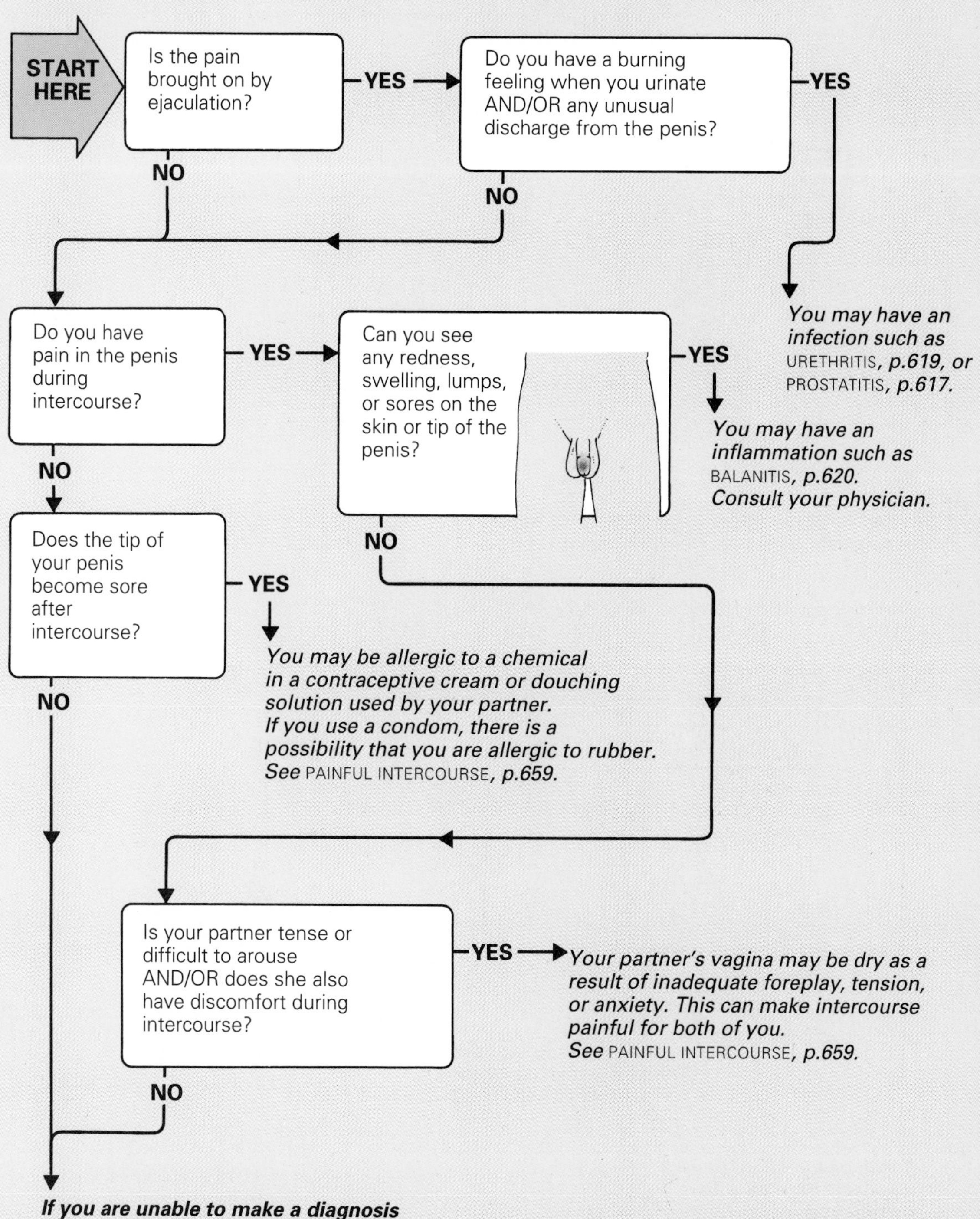

START HERE
Is the pain brought on by ejaculation?
YES
NO
Do you have a burning feeling when you urinate AND/OR any unusual discharge from the penis?
YES
NO
You may have an infection such as URETHRITIS, p.619, or PROSTATITIS, p.617.
Do you have pain in the penis during intercourse?
YES
NO
Can you see any redness, swelling, lumps, or sores on the skin or tip of the penis?
YES
NO
You may have an inflammation such as BALANITIS, p.620. Consult your physician.
Does the tip of your penis become sore after intercourse?
YES
NO
You may be allergic to a chemical in a contraceptive cream or douching solution used by your partner. If you use a condom, there is a possibility that you are allergic to rubber. See PAINFUL INTERCOURSE, p.659.
Is your partner tense or difficult to arouse AND/OR does she also have discomfort during intercourse?
YES
NO
Your partner's vagina may be dry as a result of inadequate foreplay, tension, or anxiety. This can make intercourse painful for both of you. See PAINFUL INTERCOURSE, p.659.
If you are unable to make a diagnosis from this chart, consult your physician.

73
WOMEN

Pain or lumps in the breast

Aches, pain, tenderness, or lumps in one or both breasts that you may notice when you examine yourself as described on p.630.

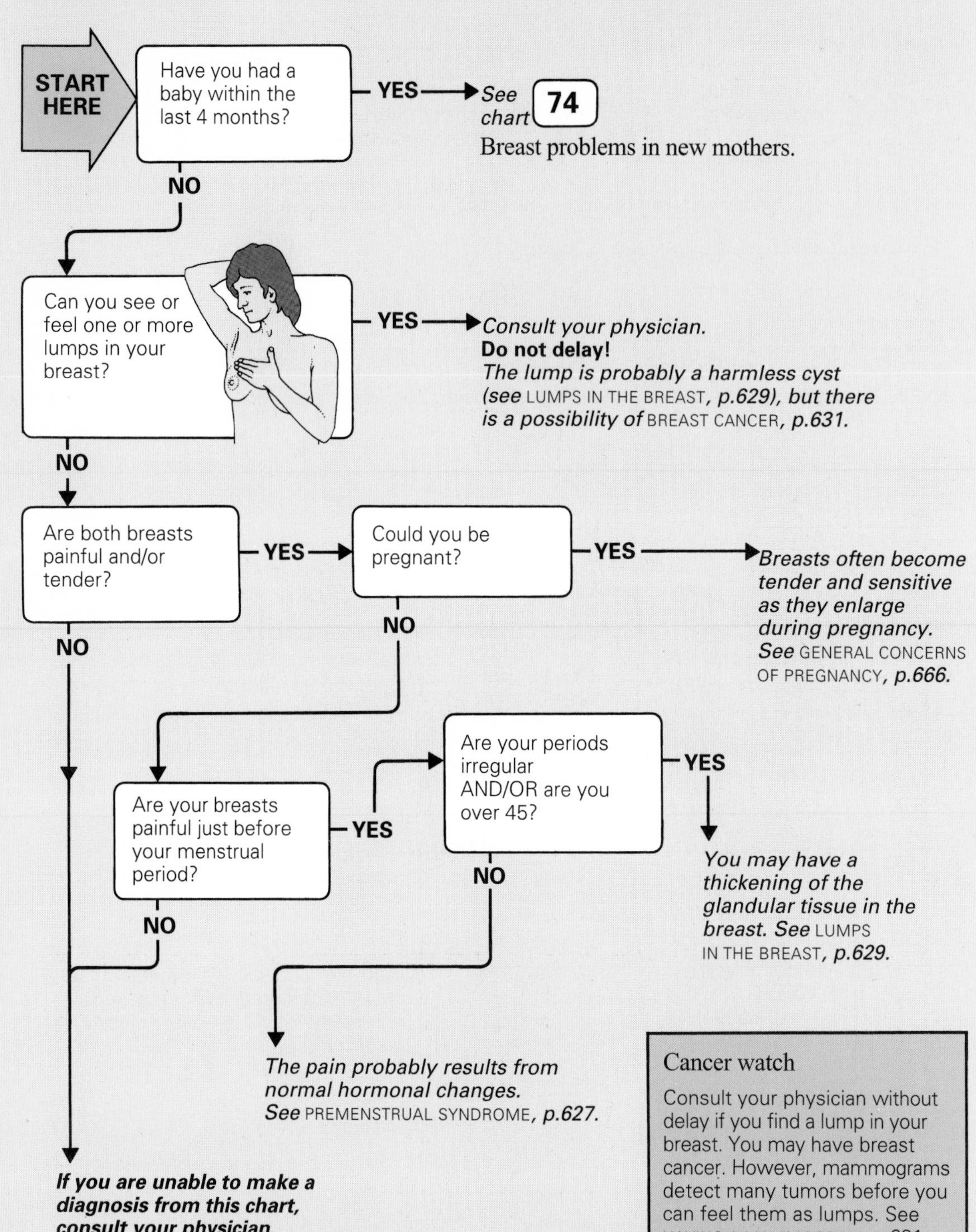

START HERE
Have you had a baby within the last 4 months?
YES
See chart 74
Breast problems in new mothers.
NO
Can you see or feel one or more lumps in your breast?
YES
Consult your physician.
Do not delay!
The lump is probably a harmless cyst (see LUMPS IN THE BREAST*, p.629), but there is a possibility of* BREAST CANCER*, p.631.*
NO
Are both breasts painful and/or tender?
YES
Could you be pregnant?
YES
Breasts often become tender and sensitive as they enlarge during pregnancy.
See GENERAL CONCERNS OF PREGNANCY*, p.666.*
NO
NO
Are your breasts painful just before your menstrual period?
YES
Are your periods irregular AND/OR are you over 45?
YES
You may have a thickening of the glandular tissue in the breast. See LUMPS IN THE BREAST*, p.629.*
NO
The pain probably results from normal hormonal changes.
See PREMENSTRUAL SYNDROME*, p.627.*
NO
If you are unable to make a diagnosis from this chart, consult your physician.

Cancer watch

Consult your physician without delay if you find a lump in your breast. You may have breast cancer. However, mammograms detect many tumors before you can feel them as lumps. See HAVING A MAMMOGRAM, p.631.

74
WOMEN

Breast problems in new mothers

Pain, tenderness, or lumps in the breasts of women who have had a baby within the last 4 months.

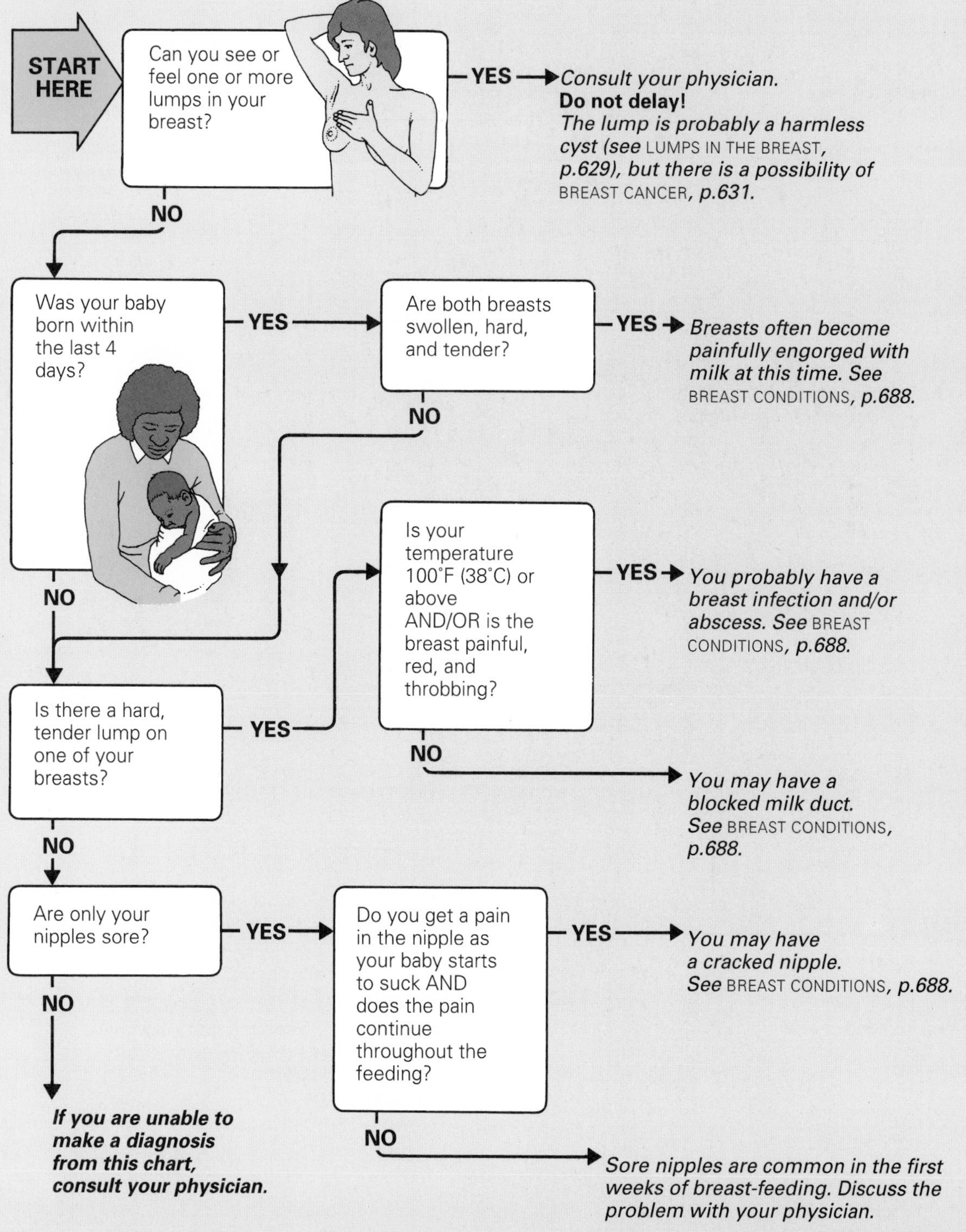

START HERE
Can you see or feel one or more lumps in your breast?
YES
Consult your physician.
Do not delay!
The lump is probably a harmless cyst (see LUMPS IN THE BREAST, p.629), but there is a possibility of BREAST CANCER, p.631.
NO
Was your baby born within the last 4 days?
YES
Are both breasts swollen, hard, and tender?
YES
Breasts often become painfully engorged with milk at this time. See BREAST CONDITIONS, p.688.
NO
NO
Is there a hard, tender lump on one of your breasts?
YES
Is your temperature 100°F (38°C) or above AND/OR is the breast painful, red, and throbbing?
YES
You probably have a breast infection and/or abscess. See BREAST CONDITIONS, p.688.
NO
You may have a blocked milk duct. See BREAST CONDITIONS, p.688.
NO
Are only your nipples sore?
YES
Do you get a pain in the nipple as your baby starts to suck AND does the pain continue throughout the feeding?
YES
You may have a cracked nipple. See BREAST CONDITIONS, p.688.
NO
Sore nipples are common in the first weeks of breast-feeding. Discuss the problem with your physician.
NO
If you are unable to make a diagnosis from this chart, consult your physician.

75
WOMEN

Absent periods

Lack of a period for at least 2 weeks after a period was due.

START HERE

Have you ever had a period?

YES → Could you be pregnant?

YES → *If there is a possibility of pregnancy, perform a home pregnancy test and consult your physician.* ***See*** GENERAL CONCERNS OF PREGNANCY, ***p.666.***

NO → Have you recently had a baby?

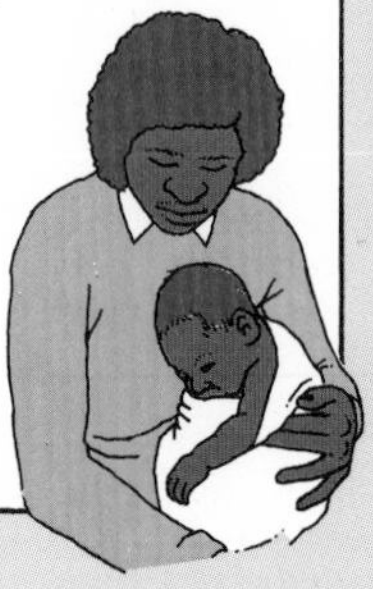

YES → *Periods seldom start until at least 6 weeks after childbirth. Expect an even longer delay if you are breast-feeding.* ***See*** SEX AFTER CHILDBIRTH, ***p.689.***

NO (from "Have you ever had a period?") → *If you have never had a period, but think that your periods should have started by now, consult your physician.*

NO (from "Have you recently had a baby?") → Have you recently been ill or under stress OR have you had a change of environment, such as a new job or a new home?

YES → *Change or stress can affect your periods.* ***See*** ABSENCE OF PERIODS, ***p.624.***

NO → Have you recently stopped taking oral contraceptives?

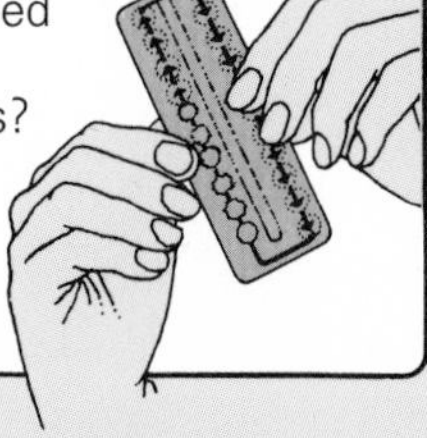

YES → *It often takes several months for periods to begin again after you stop taking oral contraceptives.* ***See*** ABSENCE OF PERIODS, ***p.624.***

NO

Go to next page

Continued from previous page

Have you lost a lot of weight in a short time through a strict diet or vigorous exercise?

YES → *Sudden loss of weight or very strenuous exercise often results in an absence of periods.* *See* ABSENCE OF PERIODS, *p.624.*

NO

Are you over 45?

YES → *It is common for women over 45 to begin skipping periods.* *See* MENOPAUSE, *p.627.*

NO

Do you have two or more of the following symptoms?
- ☐ increased hairiness
- ☐ deepening of the voice
- ☐ unexplained weight gain

YES → *The delay in your periods may be caused by disruption in the production of hormones.* *See* ABNORMALITIES OF THE HYPOTHALAMUS, PITUITARY, AND OVARIES, *p.628.*

NO

Are you currently taking any medications?

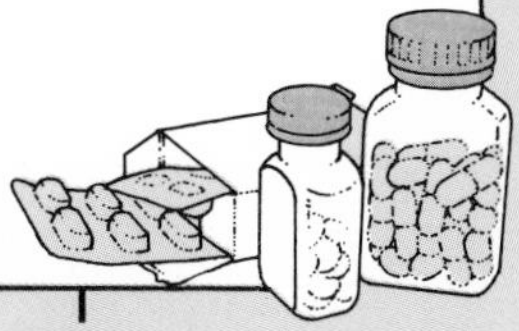

YES → *Some drugs can cause periods to stop. Discuss with your physician.*

NO

If you are unable to make a diagnosis from this chart, consult your physician.

76
WOMEN

Heavy periods

Menstrual periods that last more than 7 days, that have recently become longer, or that now produce more blood than usual.

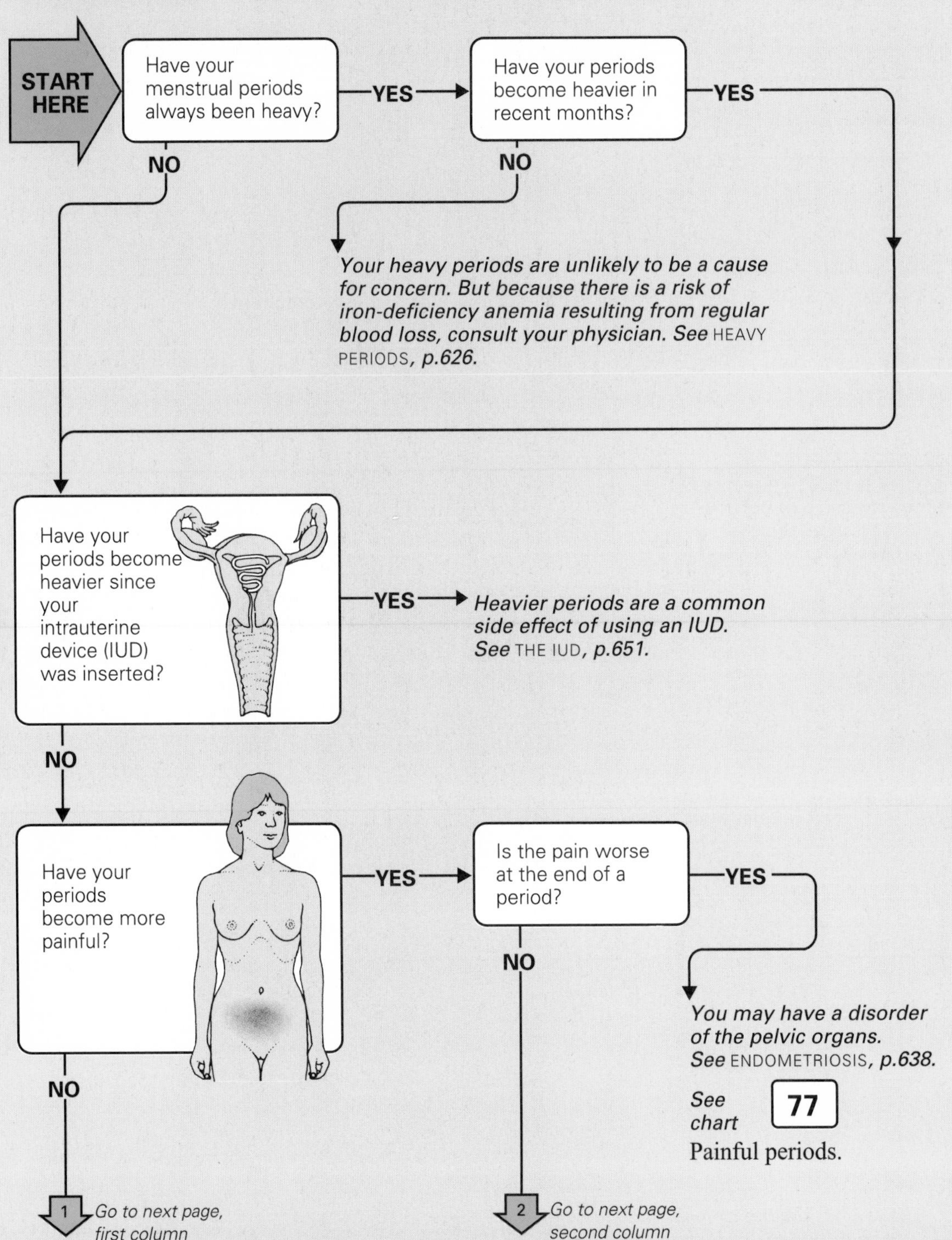

START HERE
Have your menstrual periods always been heavy?
YES
Have your periods become heavier in recent months?
YES
NO
NO
Your heavy periods are unlikely to be a cause for concern. But because there is a risk of iron-deficiency anemia resulting from regular blood loss, consult your physician. See HEAVY PERIODS*, p.626.*
Have your periods become heavier since your intrauterine device (IUD) was inserted?
YES
Heavier periods are a common side effect of using an IUD. See THE IUD*, p.651.*
NO
Have your periods become more painful?
YES
Is the pain worse at the end of a period?
YES
You may have a disorder of the pelvic organs. See ENDOMETRIOSIS*, p.638.*
See chart 77 Painful periods.
NO
NO
1 *Go to next page, first column*
2 *Go to next page, second column*

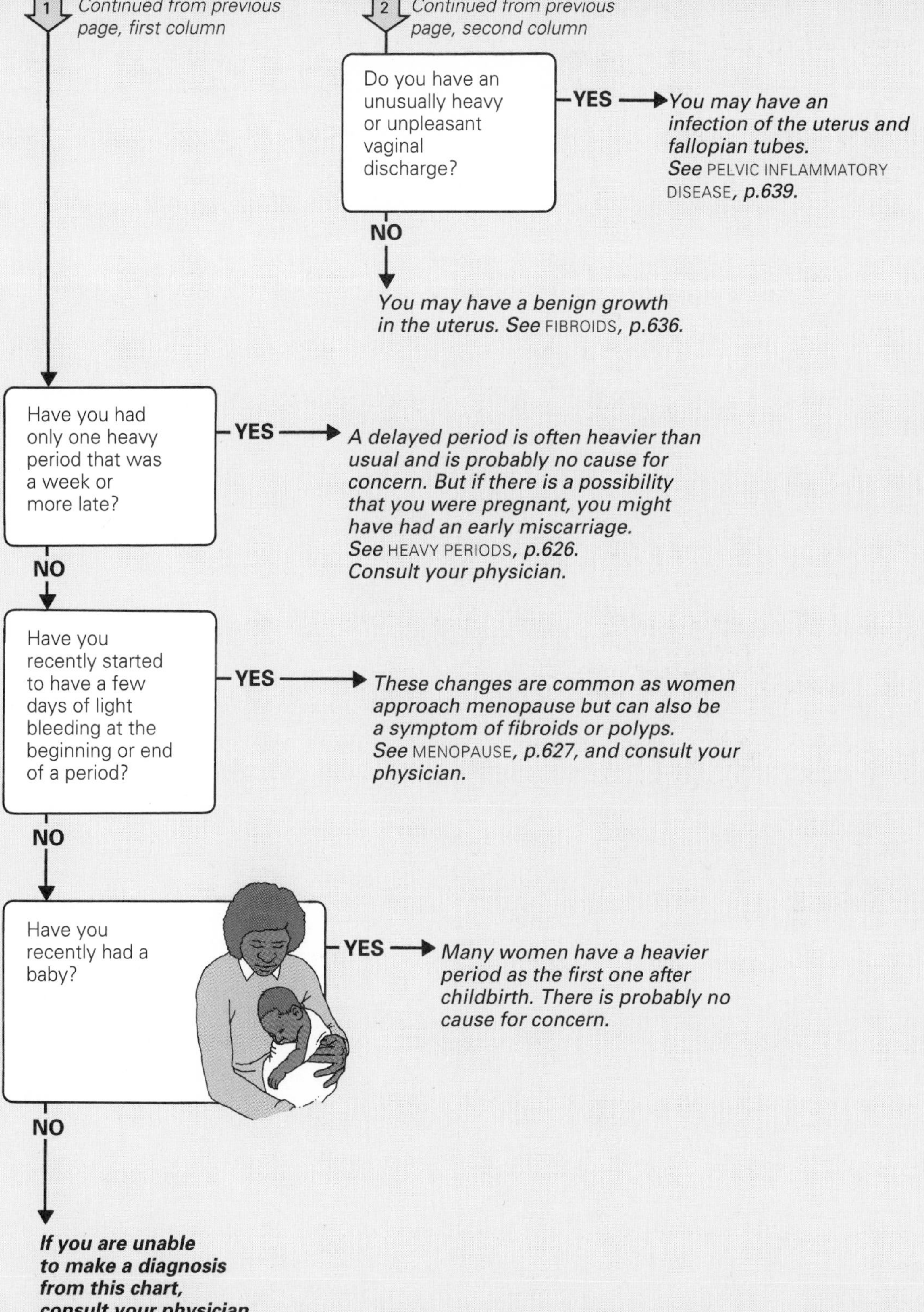

1 *Continued from previous page, first column*

2 *Continued from previous page, second column*

Do you have an unusually heavy or unpleasant vaginal discharge?

YES → *You may have an infection of the uterus and fallopian tubes. See* PELVIC INFLAMMATORY DISEASE, *p.639.*

NO → *You may have a benign growth in the uterus. See* FIBROIDS, *p.636.*

Have you had only one heavy period that was a week or more late?

YES → *A delayed period is often heavier than usual and is probably no cause for concern. But if there is a possibility that you were pregnant, you might have had an early miscarriage. See* HEAVY PERIODS, *p.626. Consult your physician.*

NO

Have you recently started to have a few days of light bleeding at the beginning or end of a period?

YES → *These changes are common as women approach menopause but can also be a symptom of fibroids or polyps. See* MENOPAUSE, *p.627, and consult your physician.*

NO

Have you recently had a baby?

YES → *Many women have a heavier period as the first one after childbirth. There is probably no cause for concern.*

NO

If you are unable to make a diagnosis from this chart, consult your physician.

77

WOMEN

Painful periods

Pain with menstruation, usually a dull ache or cramps in the lower abdomen.

START HERE

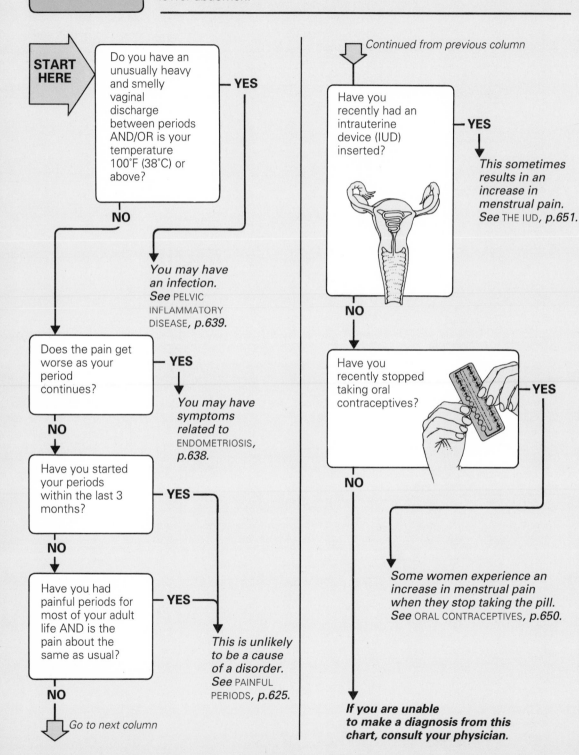

Do you have an unusually heavy and smelly vaginal discharge between periods AND/OR is your temperature 100°F (38°C) or above?

YES — *You may have an infection. See* PELVIC INFLAMMATORY DISEASE, *p.639.*

NO

Does the pain get worse as your period continues?

YES — *You may have symptoms related to* ENDOMETRIOSIS, *p.638.*

NO

Have you started your periods within the last 3 months?

YES — *This is unlikely to be a cause of a disorder. See* PAINFUL PERIODS, *p.625.*

NO

Have you had painful periods for most of your adult life AND is the pain about the same as usual?

YES — *This is unlikely to be a cause of a disorder. See* PAINFUL PERIODS, *p.625.*

NO

Go to next column

Continued from previous column

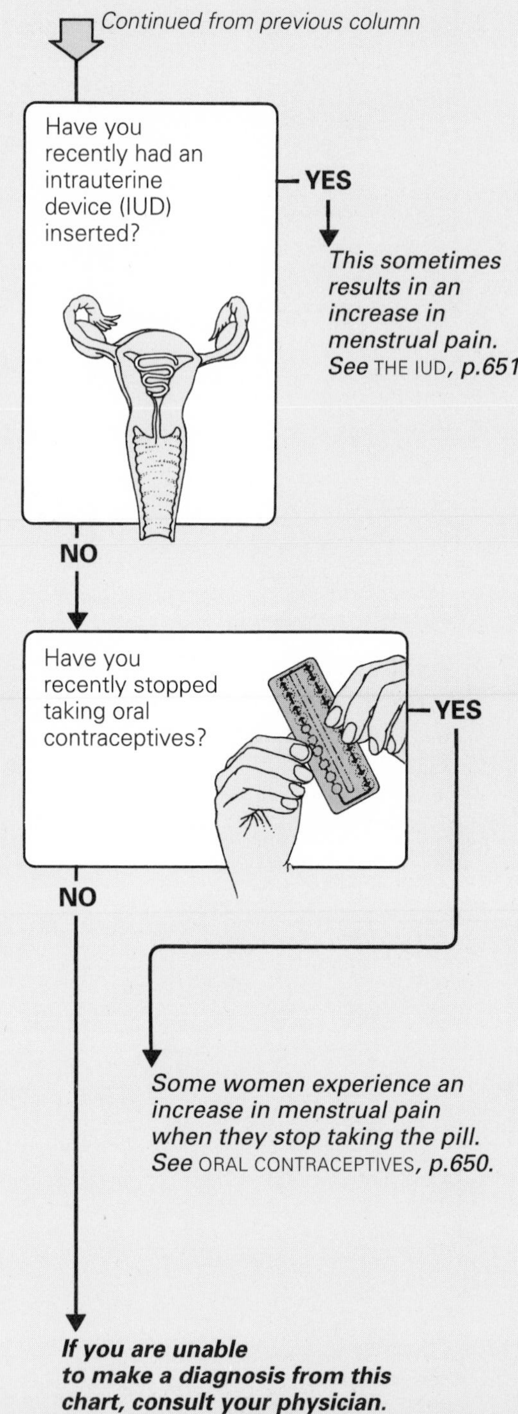

Have you recently had an intrauterine device (IUD) inserted?

YES — ***This sometimes results in an increase in menstrual pain. See*** THE IUD, ***p.651.***

NO

Have you recently stopped taking oral contraceptives?

YES — *Some women experience an increase in menstrual pain when they stop taking the pill. See* ORAL CONTRACEPTIVES, *p.650.*

NO

If you are unable to make a diagnosis from this chart, consult your physician.

Lower abdominal pain in women

Pain below the waist in women of childbearing age.
Use this chart only after consulting chart 48, **Abdominal pain**.

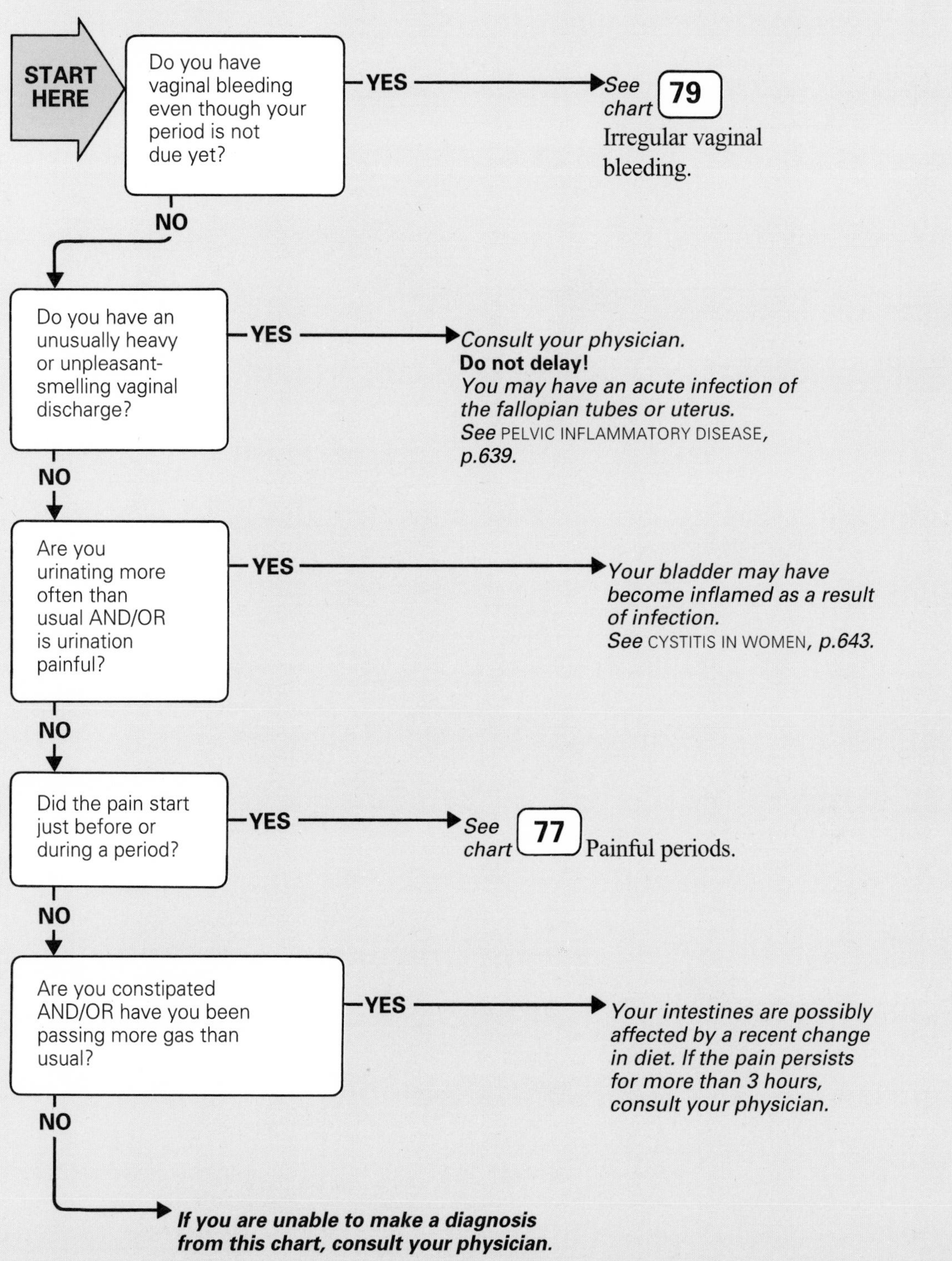

START HERE
Do you have vaginal bleeding even though your period is not due yet?
YES
See chart **79** Irregular vaginal bleeding.
NO
Do you have an unusually heavy or unpleasant-smelling vaginal discharge?
YES
Consult your physician.
Do not delay!
You may have an acute infection of the fallopian tubes or uterus.
See PELVIC INFLAMMATORY DISEASE, *p.639.*
NO
Are you urinating more often than usual AND/OR is urination painful?
YES
Your bladder may have become inflamed as a result of infection.
See CYSTITIS IN WOMEN, *p.643.*
NO
Did the pain start just before or during a period?
YES
See chart **77** Painful periods.
NO
Are you constipated AND/OR have you been passing more gas than usual?
YES
Your intestines are possibly affected by a recent change in diet. If the pain persists for more than 3 hours, consult your physician.
NO
If you are unable to make a diagnosis from this chart, consult your physician.

79
WOMEN

Irregular vaginal bleeding

Any bleeding that occurs between normal menstrual periods, during pregnancy, or after menopause.

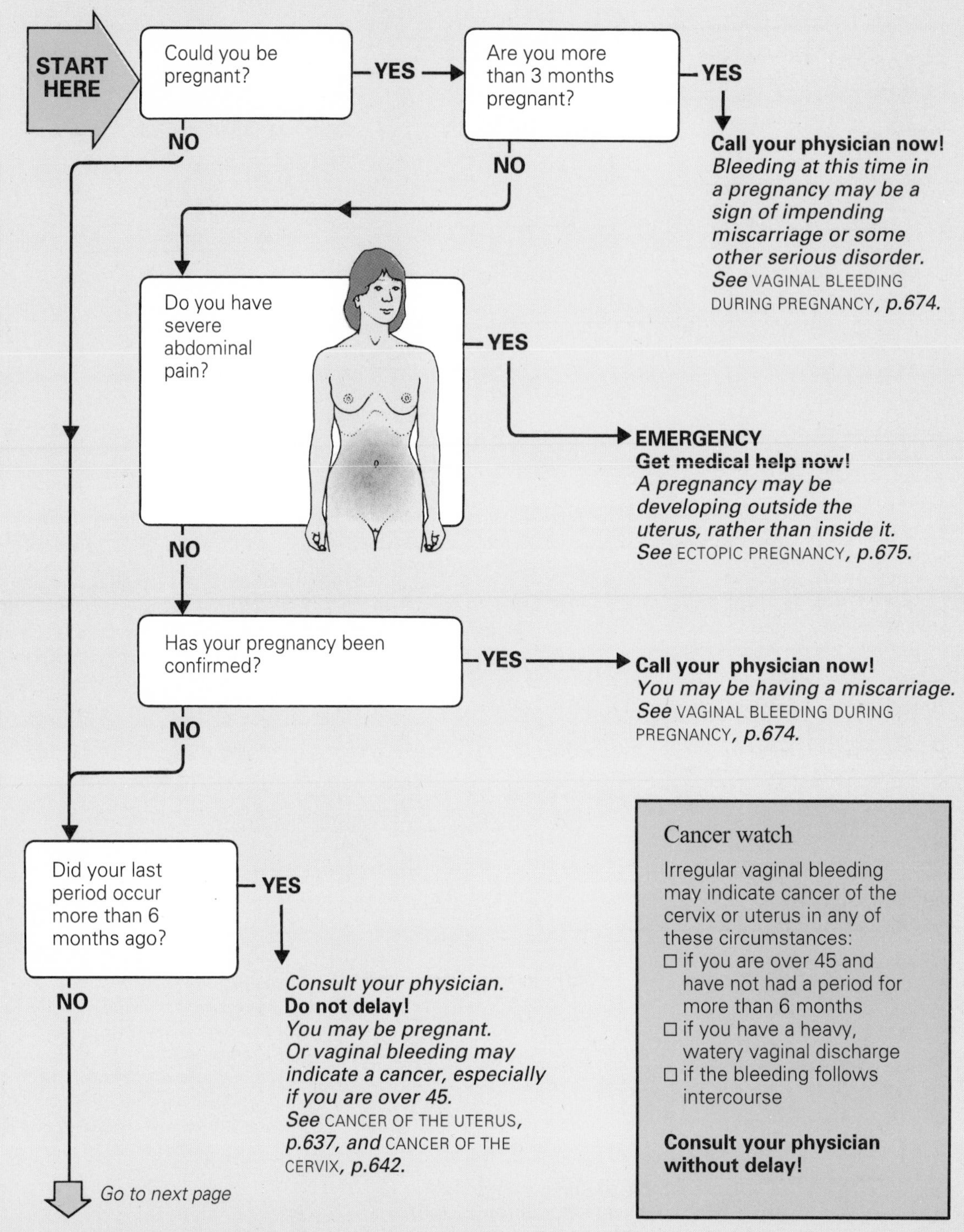

START HERE
Could you be pregnant?
YES
Are you more than 3 months pregnant?
YES
Call your physician now!
Bleeding at this time in a pregnancy may be a sign of impending miscarriage or some other serious disorder.
See VAGINAL BLEEDING DURING PREGNANCY, *p.674.*
NO
NO
Do you have severe abdominal pain?
YES
EMERGENCY
Get medical help now!
A pregnancy may be developing outside the uterus, rather than inside it.
See ECTOPIC PREGNANCY, *p.675.*
NO
Has your pregnancy been confirmed?
YES
Call your physician now!
You may be having a miscarriage.
See VAGINAL BLEEDING DURING PREGNANCY, *p.674.*
NO
Did your last period occur more than 6 months ago?
YES
Consult your physician.
Do not delay!
You may be pregnant.
Or vaginal bleeding may indicate a cancer, especially if you are over 45.
See CANCER OF THE UTERUS, *p.637, and* CANCER OF THE CERVIX, *p.642.*
NO
Go to next page

Cancer watch

Irregular vaginal bleeding may indicate cancer of the cervix or uterus in any of these circumstances:

- ☐ if you are over 45 and have not had a period for more than 6 months
- ☐ if you have a heavy, watery vaginal discharge
- ☐ if the bleeding follows intercourse

Consult your physician without delay!

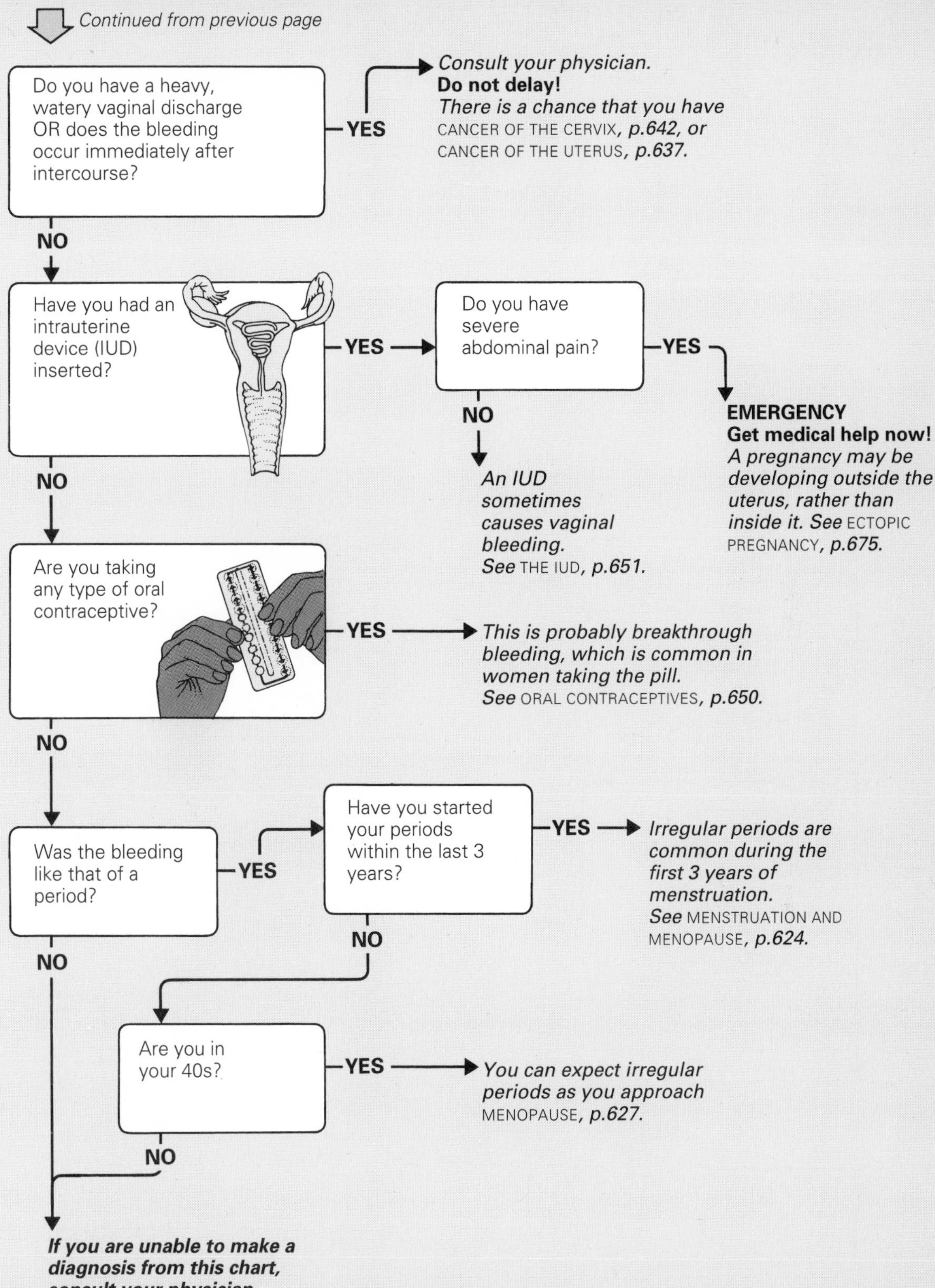
Continued from previous page
Do you have a heavy, watery vaginal discharge OR does the bleeding occur immediately after intercourse?
YES
Consult your physician.
Do not delay!
There is a chance that you have CANCER OF THE CERVIX, p.642, or CANCER OF THE UTERUS, p.637.
NO
Have you had an intrauterine device (IUD) inserted?
YES
Do you have severe abdominal pain?
YES
EMERGENCY
Get medical help now!
A pregnancy may be developing outside the uterus, rather than inside it. See ECTOPIC PREGNANCY, p.675.
NO
An IUD sometimes causes vaginal bleeding.
See THE IUD, p.651.
NO
Are you taking any type of oral contraceptive?
YES
This is probably breakthrough bleeding, which is common in women taking the pill.
See ORAL CONTRACEPTIVES, p.650.
NO
Was the bleeding like that of a period?
YES
Have you started your periods within the last 3 years?
YES
Irregular periods are common during the first 3 years of menstruation.
See MENSTRUATION AND MENOPAUSE, p.624.
NO
Are you in your 40s?
YES
You can expect irregular periods as you approach MENOPAUSE, p.627.
NO
NO
If you are unable to make a diagnosis from this chart, consult your physician.

80
WOMEN

Abnormal vaginal discharge

Fluid from the vagina that differs in color, consistency, and/or quantity from what you would normally have between menstrual periods.

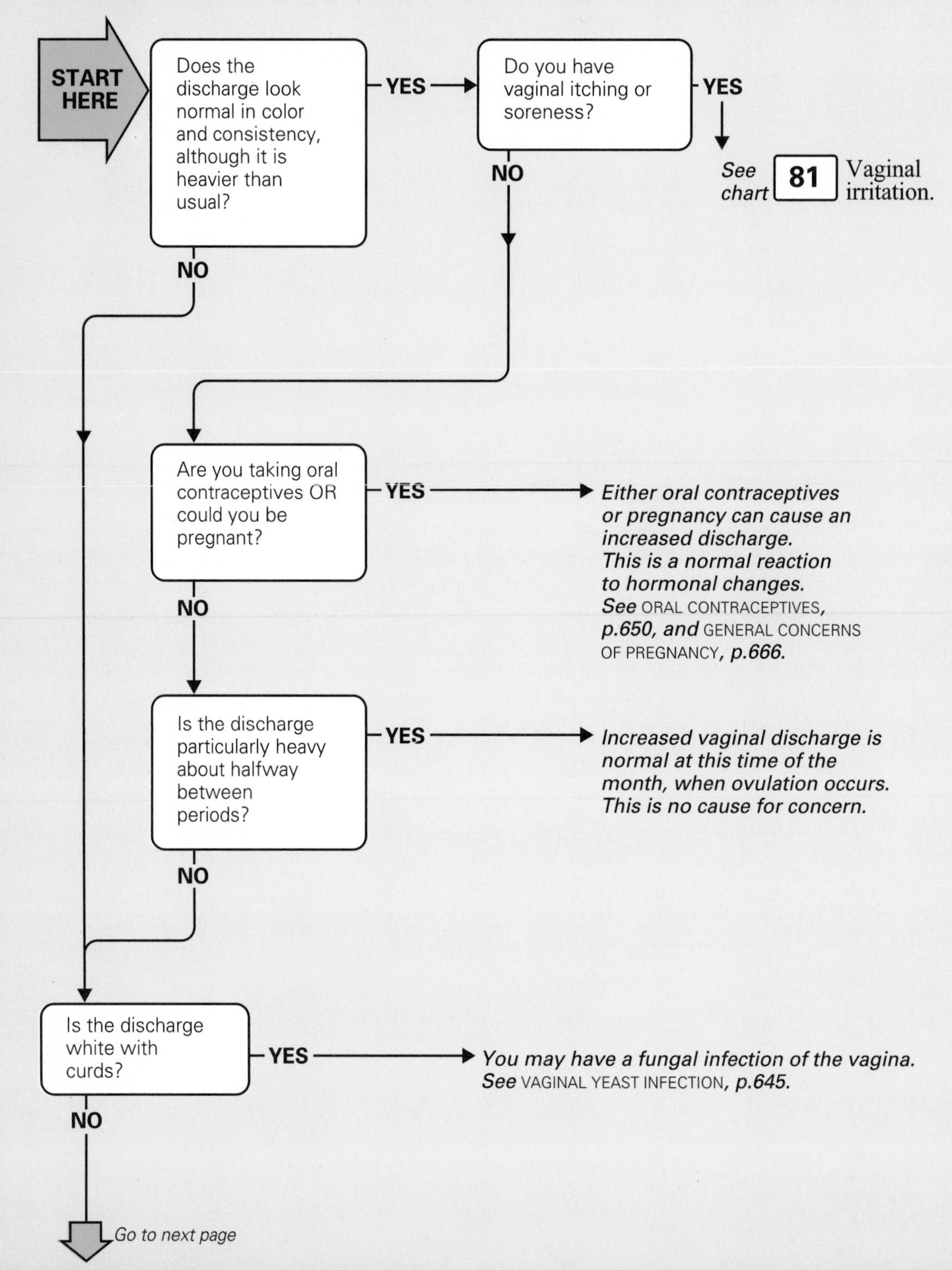
START HERE
Does the discharge look normal in color and consistency, although it is heavier than usual?
YES
Do you have vaginal itching or soreness?
YES
See chart 81 Vaginal irritation.
NO
NO
Are you taking oral contraceptives OR could you be pregnant?
YES
Either oral contraceptives or pregnancy can cause an increased discharge. This is a normal reaction to hormonal changes. See ORAL CONTRACEPTIVES, p.650, and GENERAL CONCERNS OF PREGNANCY, p.666.
NO
Is the discharge particularly heavy about halfway between periods?
YES
Increased vaginal discharge is normal at this time of the month, when ovulation occurs. This is no cause for concern.
NO
Is the discharge white with curds?
YES
You may have a fungal infection of the vagina. See VAGINAL YEAST INFECTION, p.645.
NO
Go to next page

Continued from previous page

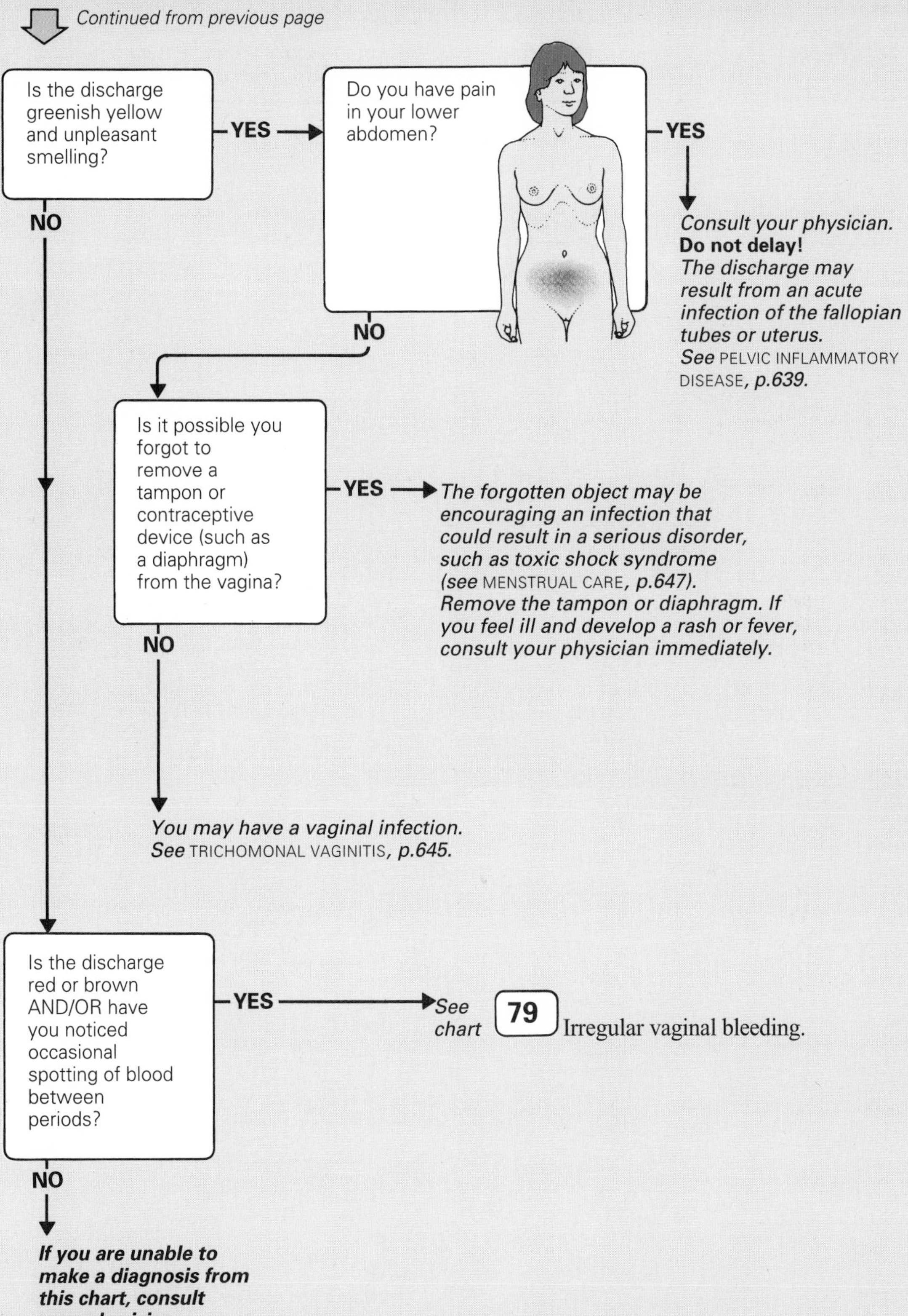

Is the discharge greenish yellow and unpleasant smelling?
YES
NO
Do you have pain in your lower abdomen?
YES
NO
Consult your physician.
Do not delay!
The discharge may result from an acute infection of the fallopian tubes or uterus.
See PELVIC INFLAMMATORY DISEASE, p.639.
Is it possible you forgot to remove a tampon or contraceptive device (such as a diaphragm) from the vagina?
YES
NO
The forgotten object may be encouraging an infection that could result in a serious disorder, such as toxic shock syndrome (see MENSTRUAL CARE, p.647). Remove the tampon or diaphragm. If you feel ill and develop a rash or fever, consult your physician immediately.
You may have a vaginal infection.
See TRICHOMONAL VAGINITIS, p.645.
Is the discharge red or brown AND/OR have you noticed occasional spotting of blood between periods?
YES
See chart 79 Irregular vaginal bleeding.
NO
If you are unable to make a diagnosis from this chart, consult your physician.

81 WOMEN

Vaginal irritation

Itching or soreness in the vagina or around the genital area

START HERE

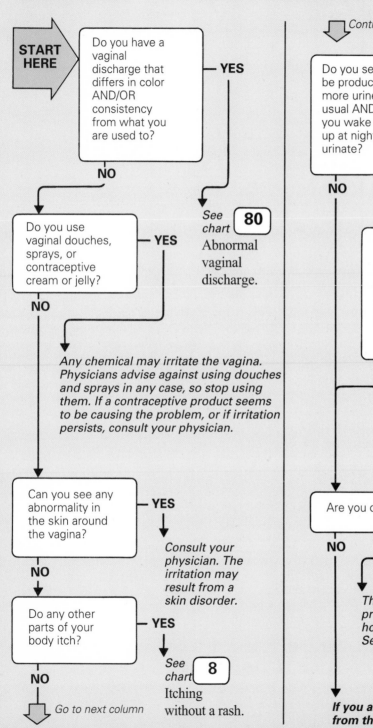

Do you have a vaginal discharge that differs in color AND/OR consistency from what you are used to?

YES — *See chart* **80** Abnormal vaginal discharge.

NO

Do you use vaginal douches, sprays, or contraceptive cream or jelly?

YES — *Any chemical may irritate the vagina. Physicians advise against using douches and sprays in any case, so stop using them. If a contraceptive product seems to be causing the problem, or if irritation persists, consult your physician.*

NO

Can you see any abnormality in the skin around the vagina?

YES — *Consult your physician. The irritation may result from a skin disorder.*

NO

Do any other parts of your body itch?

YES — *See chart* **8** Itching without a rash.

NO

Go to next column

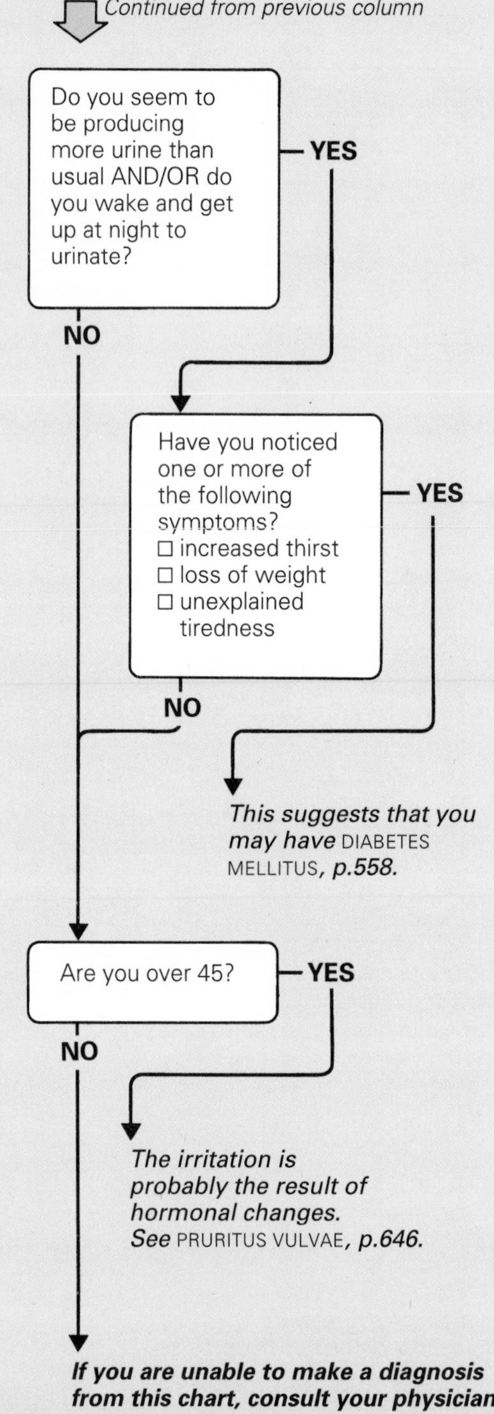

Continued from previous column

Do you seem to be producing more urine than usual AND/OR do you wake and get up at night to urinate?

YES

Have you noticed one or more of the following symptoms?
- ☐ increased thirst
- ☐ loss of weight
- ☐ unexplained tiredness

YES — *This suggests that you may have* DIABETES MELLITUS, ***p.558.***

NO

NO

Are you over 45?

YES — *The irritation is probably the result of hormonal changes. See* PRURITUS VULVAE, ***p.646.***

NO

If you are unable to make a diagnosis from this chart, consult your physician.

82 WOMEN

Abnormal hair growth in women

Any excessive hair on the face, limbs, or torso.

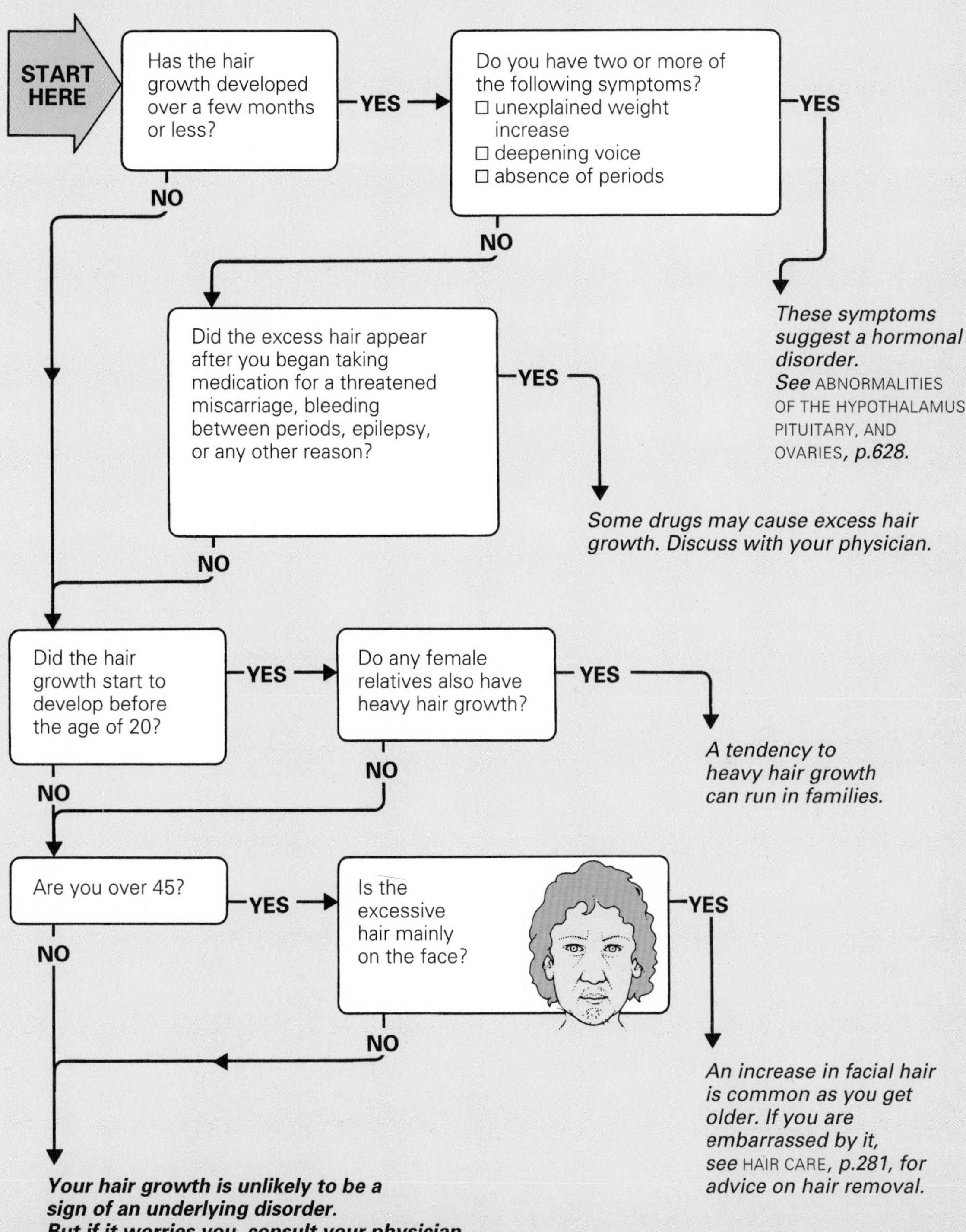

START HERE
Has the hair growth developed over a few months or less?
YES
NO
Do you have two or more of the following symptoms?
☐ unexplained weight increase
☐ deepening voice
☐ absence of periods
YES
NO
These symptoms suggest a hormonal disorder. See ABNORMALITIES OF THE HYPOTHALAMUS, PITUITARY, AND OVARIES, p.628.
Did the excess hair appear after you began taking medication for a threatened miscarriage, bleeding between periods, epilepsy, or any other reason?
YES
NO
Some drugs may cause excess hair growth. Discuss with your physician.
Did the hair growth start to develop before the age of 20?
YES
NO
Do any female relatives also have heavy hair growth?
YES
NO
A tendency to heavy hair growth can run in families.
Are you over 45?
YES
NO
Is the excessive hair mainly on the face?
YES
NO
An increase in facial hair is common as you get older. If you are embarrassed by it, see HAIR CARE, p.281, for advice on hair removal.
Your hair growth is unlikely to be a sign of an underlying disorder. But if it worries you, consult your physician.

83

WOMEN

Painful intercourse in women

Pain or discomfort during or just after sexual intercourse.

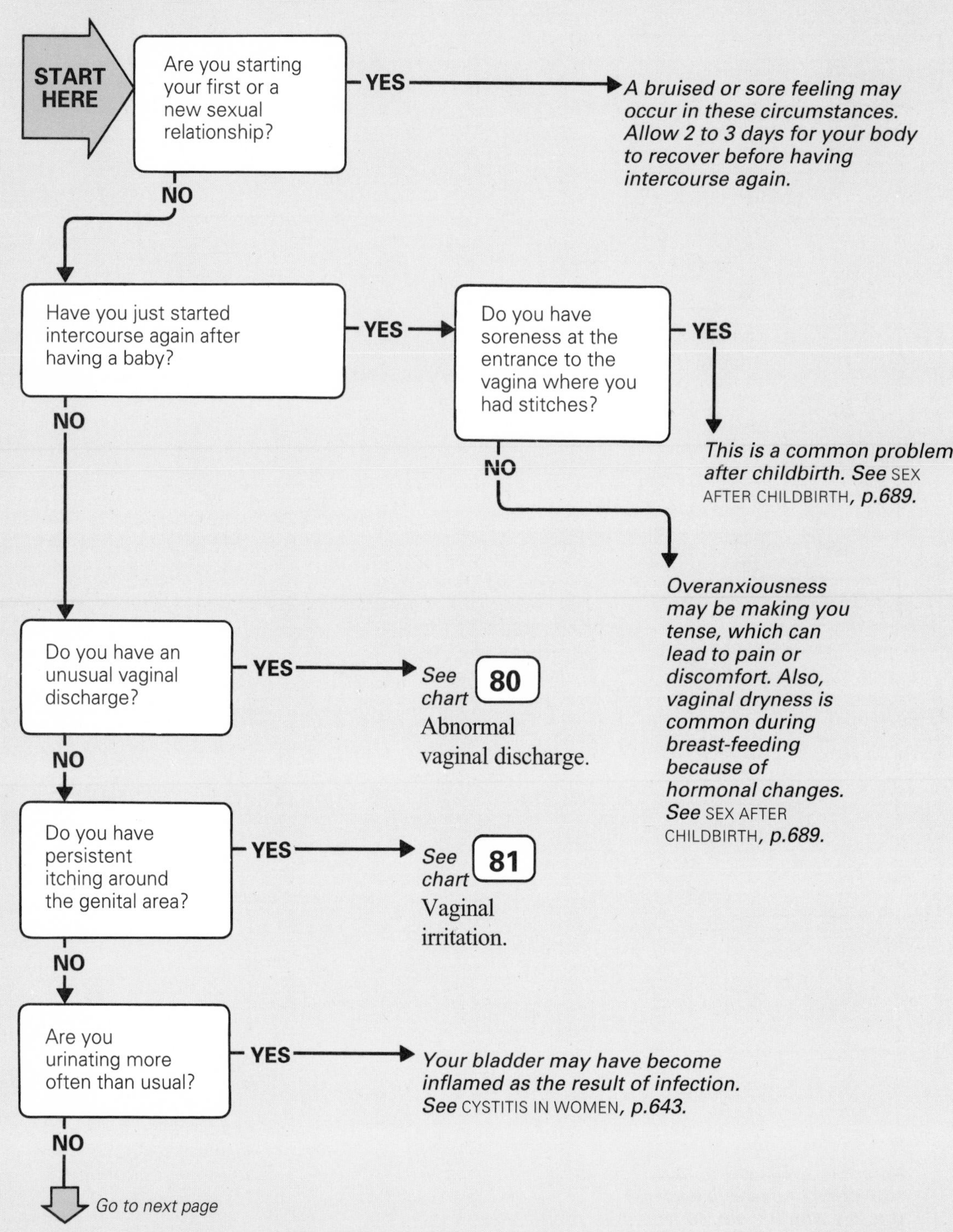

START HERE
Are you starting your first or a new sexual relationship?
YES
A bruised or sore feeling may occur in these circumstances. Allow 2 to 3 days for your body to recover before having intercourse again.
NO
Have you just started intercourse again after having a baby?
YES
Do you have soreness at the entrance to the vagina where you had stitches?
YES
This is a common problem after childbirth. See SEX AFTER CHILDBIRTH, p.689.
NO
Overanxiousness may be making you tense, which can lead to pain or discomfort. Also, vaginal dryness is common during breast-feeding because of hormonal changes. See SEX AFTER CHILDBIRTH, p.689.
NO
Do you have an unusual vaginal discharge?
YES
See chart 80 Abnormal vaginal discharge.
NO
Do you have persistent itching around the genital area?
YES
See chart 81 Vaginal irritation.
NO
Are you urinating more often than usual?
YES
Your bladder may have become inflamed as the result of infection. See CYSTITIS IN WOMEN, p.643.
NO
Go to next page

Continued from previous page

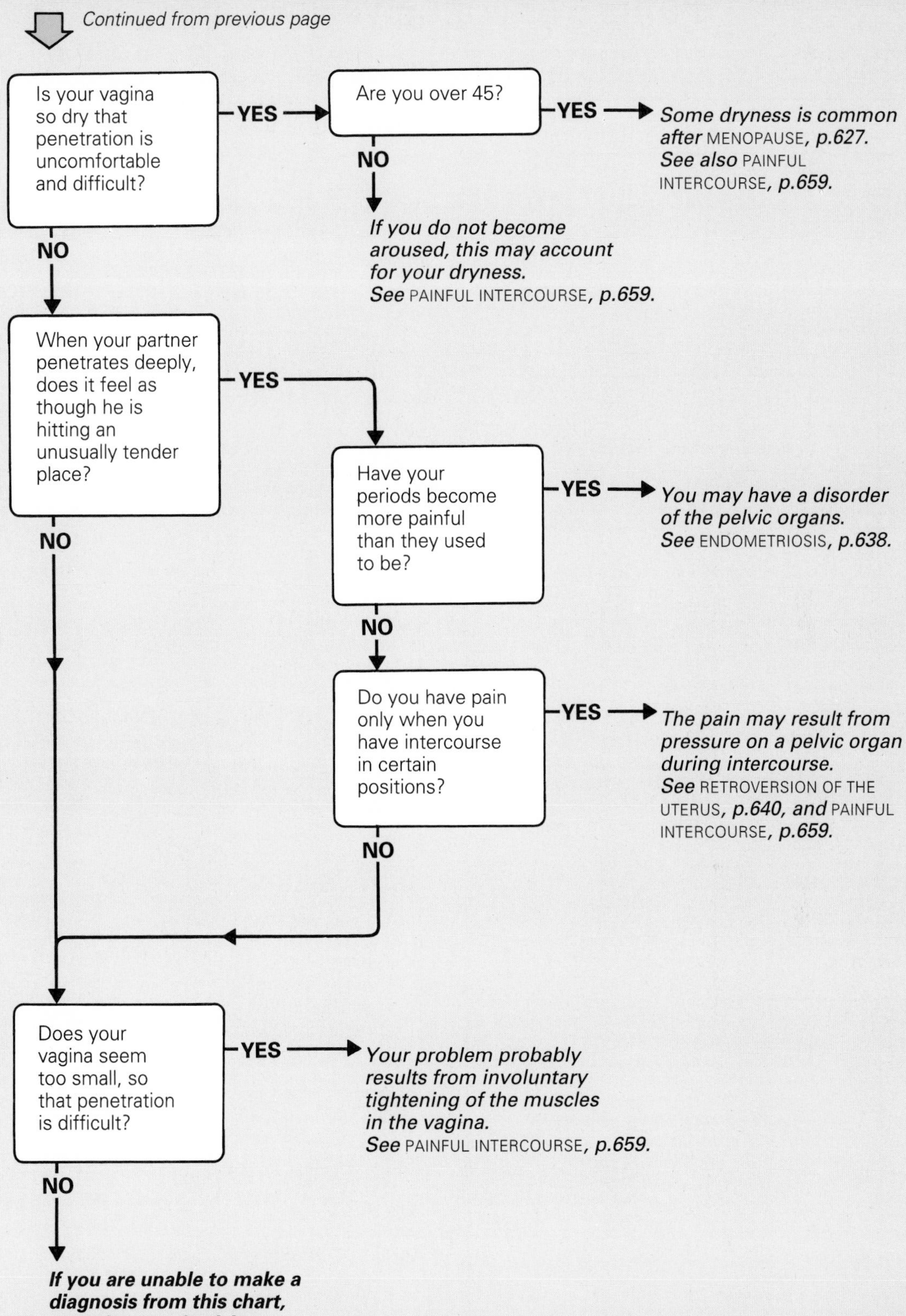

Is your vagina so dry that penetration is uncomfortable and difficult?
YES
Are you over 45?
YES
Some dryness is common after MENOPAUSE, p.627. See also PAINFUL INTERCOURSE, p.659.
NO
If you do not become aroused, this may account for your dryness. See PAINFUL INTERCOURSE, p.659.
NO
When your partner penetrates deeply, does it feel as though he is hitting an unusually tender place?
YES
Have your periods become more painful than they used to be?
YES
You may have a disorder of the pelvic organs. See ENDOMETRIOSIS, p.638.
NO
Do you have pain only when you have intercourse in certain positions?
YES
The pain may result from pressure on a pelvic organ during intercourse. See RETROVERSION OF THE UTERUS, p.640, and PAINFUL INTERCOURSE, p.659.
NO
NO
Does your vagina seem too small, so that penetration is difficult?
YES
Your problem probably results from involuntary tightening of the muscles in the vagina. See PAINFUL INTERCOURSE, p.659.
NO
If you are unable to make a diagnosis from this chart, consult your physician.

84

COUPLES

Failure to conceive

Failure to get pregnant after more than 12 months of trying without contraception. Both partners should read the chart.

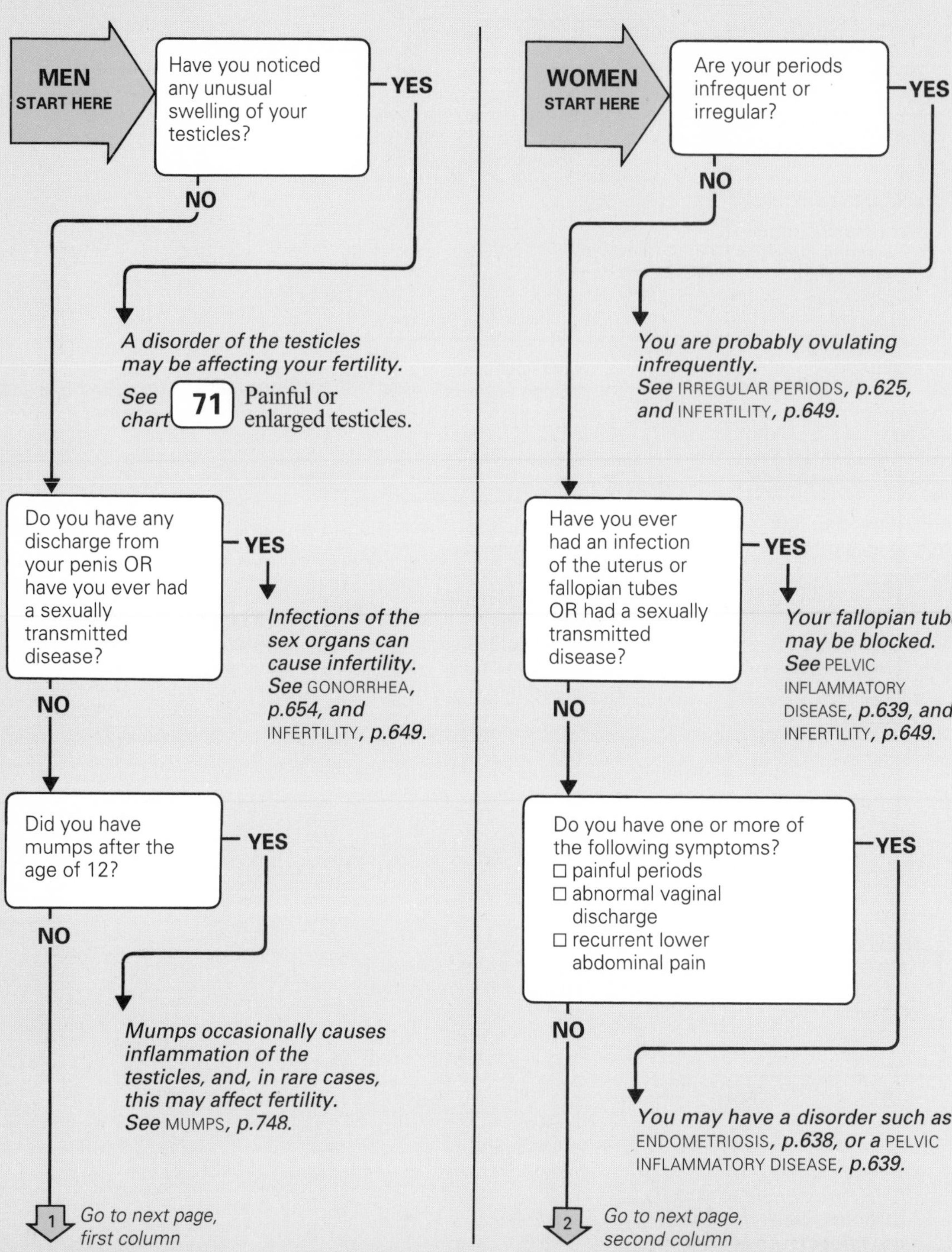

MEN
START HERE
Have you noticed any unusual swelling of your testicles?
YES
NO
A disorder of the testicles may be affecting your fertility.
See chart 71 Painful or enlarged testicles.
Do you have any discharge from your penis OR have you ever had a sexually transmitted disease?
YES
NO
Infections of the sex organs can cause infertility. See GONORRHEA, p.654, and INFERTILITY, p.649.
Did you have mumps after the age of 12?
YES
NO
Mumps occasionally causes inflammation of the testicles, and, in rare cases, this may affect fertility. See MUMPS, p.748.
1 Go to next page, first column
WOMEN
START HERE
Are your periods infrequent or irregular?
YES
NO
You are probably ovulating infrequently. See IRREGULAR PERIODS, p.625, and INFERTILITY, p.649.
Have you ever had an infection of the uterus or fallopian tubes OR had a sexually transmitted disease?
YES
NO
Your fallopian tubes may be blocked. See PELVIC INFLAMMATORY DISEASE, p.639, and INFERTILITY, p.649.
Do you have one or more of the following symptoms?
☐ painful periods
☐ abnormal vaginal discharge
☐ recurrent lower abdominal pain
YES
NO
You may have a disorder such as ENDOMETRIOSIS, p.638, or a PELVIC INFLAMMATORY DISEASE, p.639.
2 Go to next page, second column

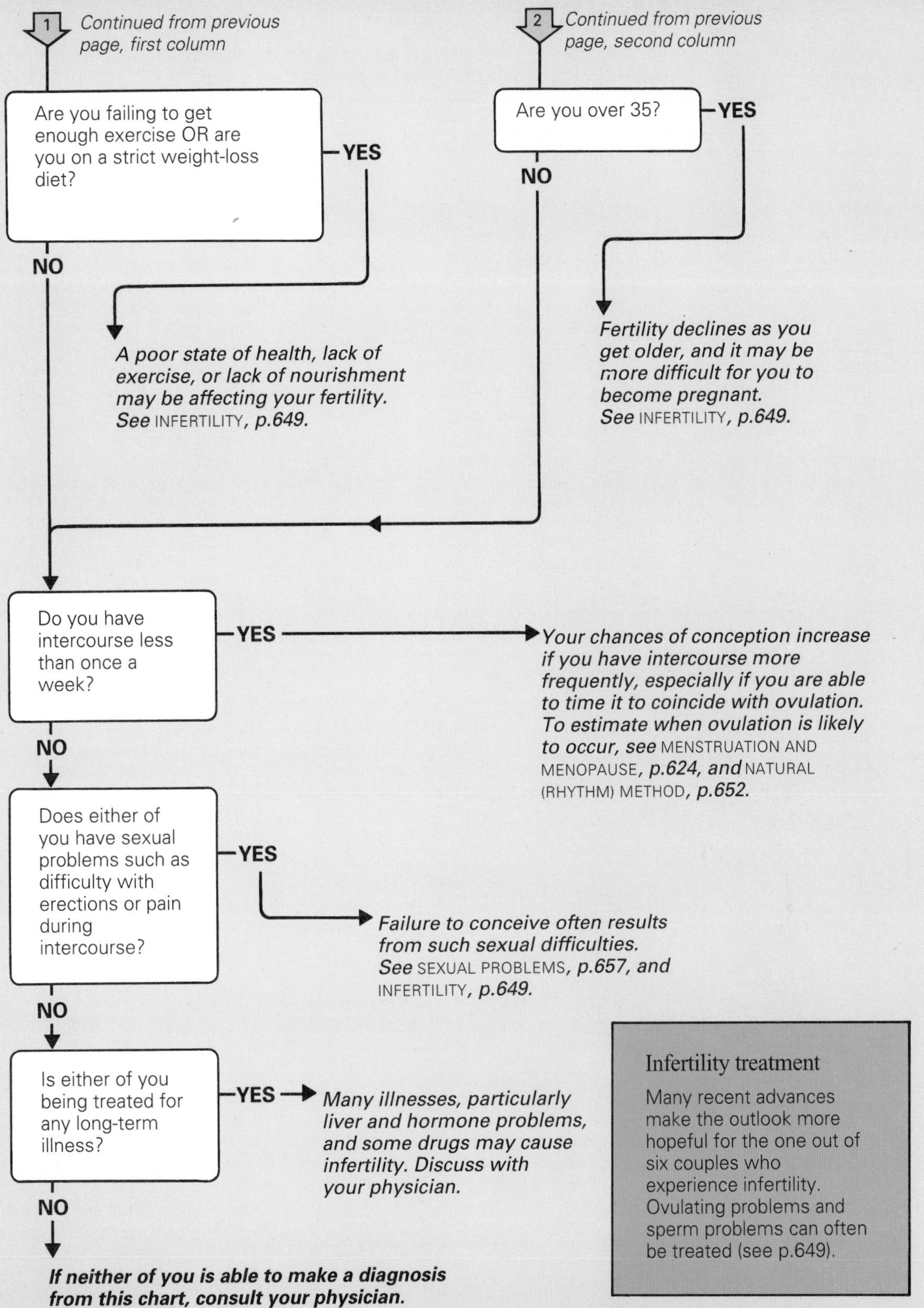

1 Continued from previous page, first column
Are you failing to get enough exercise OR are you on a strict weight-loss diet?
YES
A poor state of health, lack of exercise, or lack of nourishment may be affecting your fertility. See INFERTILITY, p.649.
NO
2 Continued from previous page, second column
Are you over 35?
YES
Fertility declines as you get older, and it may be more difficult for you to become pregnant. See INFERTILITY, p.649.
NO
Do you have intercourse less than once a week?
YES
Your chances of conception increase if you have intercourse more frequently, especially if you are able to time it to coincide with ovulation. To estimate when ovulation is likely to occur, see MENSTRUATION AND MENOPAUSE, p.624, and NATURAL (RHYTHM) METHOD, p.652.
NO
Does either of you have sexual problems such as difficulty with erections or pain during intercourse?
YES
Failure to conceive often results from such sexual difficulties. See SEXUAL PROBLEMS, p.657, and INFERTILITY, p.649.
NO
Is either of you being treated for any long-term illness?
YES
Many illnesses, particularly liver and hormone problems, and some drugs may cause infertility. Discuss with your physician.
NO
If neither of you is able to make a diagnosis from this chart, consult your physician.

Infertility treatment

Many recent advances make the outlook more hopeful for the one out of six couples who experience infertility. Ovulating problems and sperm problems can often be treated (see p.649).

85

CHILDREN
0-5 years

Waking at night

Any waking after your child has gone to sleep for the night that causes the child to cry or call out.

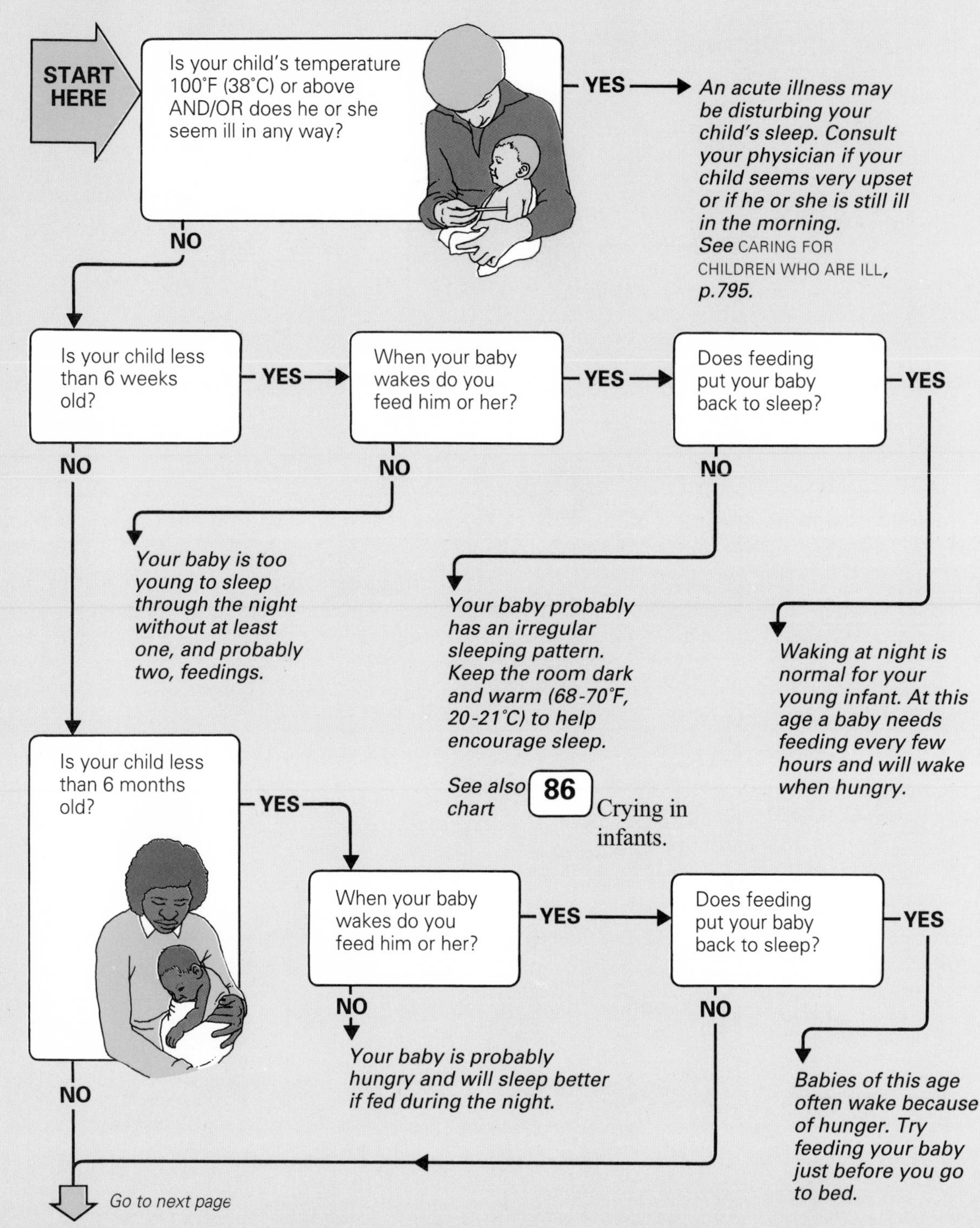

START HERE
Is your child's temperature 100°F (38°C) or above AND/OR does he or she seem ill in any way?
YES
An acute illness may be disturbing your child's sleep. Consult your physician if your child seems very upset or if he or she is still ill in the morning.
See CARING FOR CHILDREN WHO ARE ILL, p.795.
NO
Is your child less than 6 weeks old?
YES
When your baby wakes do you feed him or her?
YES
Does feeding put your baby back to sleep?
YES
Waking at night is normal for your young infant. At this age a baby needs feeding every few hours and will wake when hungry.
NO
Your baby probably has an irregular sleeping pattern. Keep the room dark and warm (68-70°F, 20-21°C) to help encourage sleep.
See also chart 86 Crying in infants.
NO
Your baby is too young to sleep through the night without at least one, and probably two, feedings.
NO
Is your child less than 6 months old?
YES
When your baby wakes do you feed him or her?
YES
Does feeding put your baby back to sleep?
YES
Babies of this age often wake because of hunger. Try feeding your baby just before you go to bed.
NO
NO
Your baby is probably hungry and will sleep better if fed during the night.
NO
Go to next page

Continued from previous page

Is your child less than a year old?

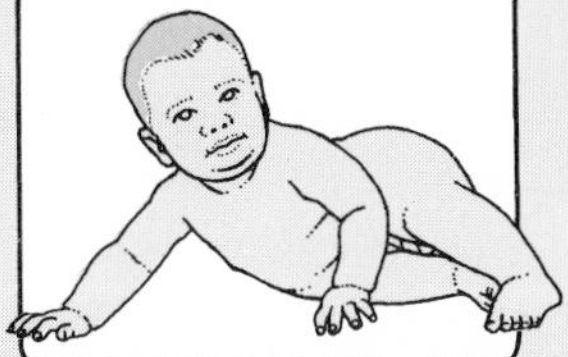

YES →

When you respond to the baby's crying during the night, do you find that the covers have been kicked off?

YES → *Your baby is probably awakened by cold. Warmer pajamas, a sleeping bag, or a warmer room may solve the problem.*

NO ↓

Does your baby's bottom look red or sore or have a rash?

YES → *Your baby probably has* DIAPER RASH, *p.696, which stings when the baby's diaper is wet. This may cause the baby to wake. See also* **Visual aids to diagnosis, 4**, *p.242.*

NO ↓

Does your baby usually sleep through most of the night, but wake early in the morning?

YES → *Your baby probably does not need additional sleep. Change the baby's diaper, give him or her a drink of water, and put a few toys in the crib. This may enable you to get some more sleep.*

NO → *Your baby probably has an irregular sleeping pattern. See* SLEEPING PROBLEMS IN CHILDREN, *p.717.*

(Is your child less than a year old?) **NO** ↓

Does your child seem upset or frightened when he or she wakes up?

YES → *Nightmares may be waking your child. See* SLEEPING PROBLEMS IN CHILDREN, *p.717. A dim light in the room may help if your child seems afraid of the dark.*

NO ↓

Does your child have any source of stress, such as the arrival of a new baby, starting school, or tension in the home?

YES → *Anxiety may be making it difficult for your child to sleep. Extra reassurance and affection during the day may help solve the problem. See* SLEEPING PROBLEMS IN CHILDREN, *p.717.*

NO → ***The child's tendency to wake up probably results from an irregular sleeping pattern and is unlikely to be a sign of any disorder. However, if you are worried by it, consult your physician.***

86

CHILDREN
0-6 months

Crying in infants

Any persistent sobbing, whimpering, or wailing that makes you wonder if your baby is healthy.

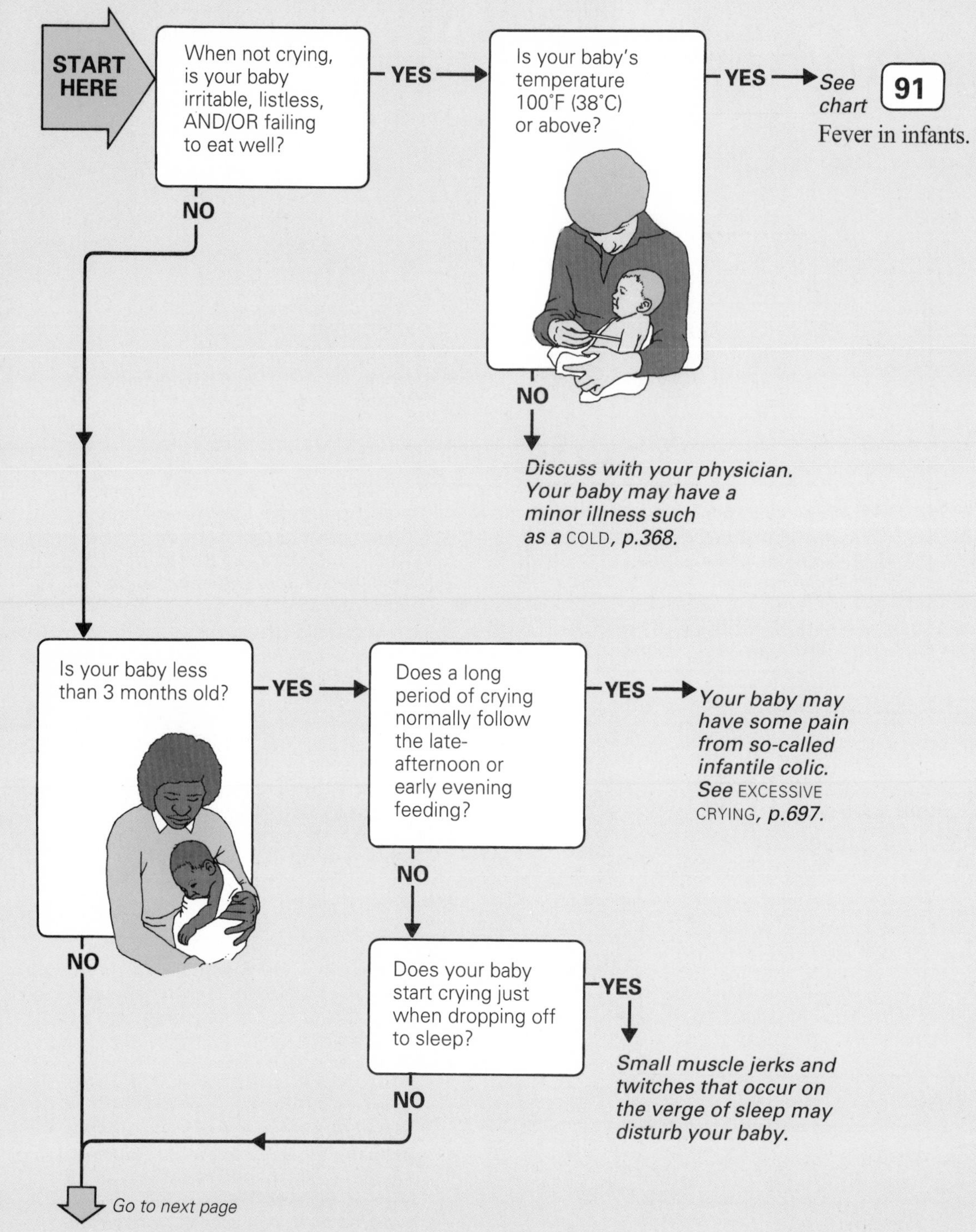

START HERE
When not crying, is your baby irritable, listless, AND/OR failing to eat well?
YES
Is your baby's temperature 100°F (38°C) or above?
YES
See chart 91
Fever in infants.
NO
Discuss with your physician. Your baby may have a minor illness such as a COLD, p.368.
NO
Is your baby less than 3 months old?
YES
Does a long period of crying normally follow the late-afternoon or early evening feeding?
YES
Your baby may have some pain from so-called infantile colic. See EXCESSIVE CRYING, p.697.
NO
Does your baby start crying just when dropping off to sleep?
YES
Small muscle jerks and twitches that occur on the verge of sleep may disturb your baby.
NO
NO
Go to next page

Continued from previous page

Is your baby in a cool room or outside in a buggy on a chilly day?

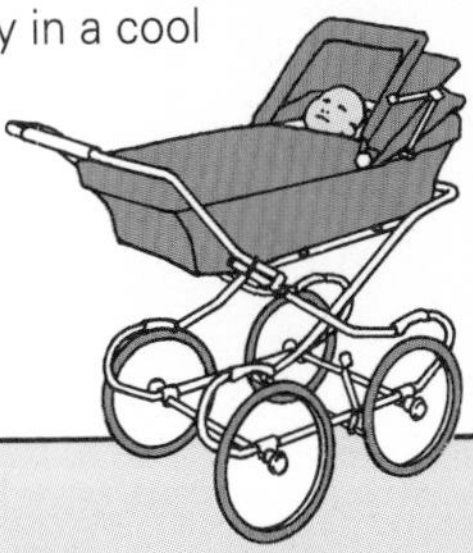

YES → *Your baby may simply be too cold. Moving indoors or warming up the room will probably help.*

NO ↓

Does your baby generally stop crying when you pick up him or her?

YES → *Your baby is probably bored or lonely. Try offering a little more attention or placing the baby where he or she can see you. Some babies settle down better in the presence of a familiar toy or blanket.*

NO ↓

Does your baby's bottom look red or sore or have a rash?

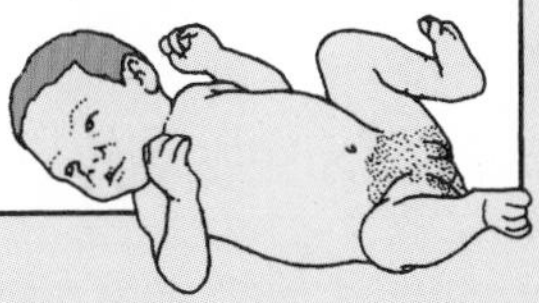

YES → DIAPER RASH, *p.696, may be making your baby uncomfortable. See also* **Visual aids to diagnosis, 4**, *p.242*

NO ↓

Does your baby stop crying after being fed?

YES → Does your baby start crying again less than 2 hours after feeding?

- **YES** → *You may not be providing enough food. If you are breast-feeding, allow your baby to suck more often and longer. If you are bottle-feeding, increase the amount offered. Remember that babies also get thirsty. Offering water between feedings may help to reduce crying. See* FEEDING PROBLEMS, *p.694, and* EXCESSIVE CRYING, *p.697.*
- **NO** → *Your baby probably cries simply because he or she is hungry. Try offering a feeding whenever he or she seems hungry.*

NO ↓

If you are unable to make a diagnosis from this chart and the crying is worrying you, consult your physician.

87
CHILDREN
0-6 months

Vomiting in infants

Regurgitating (burping up) or throwing up stomach contents.

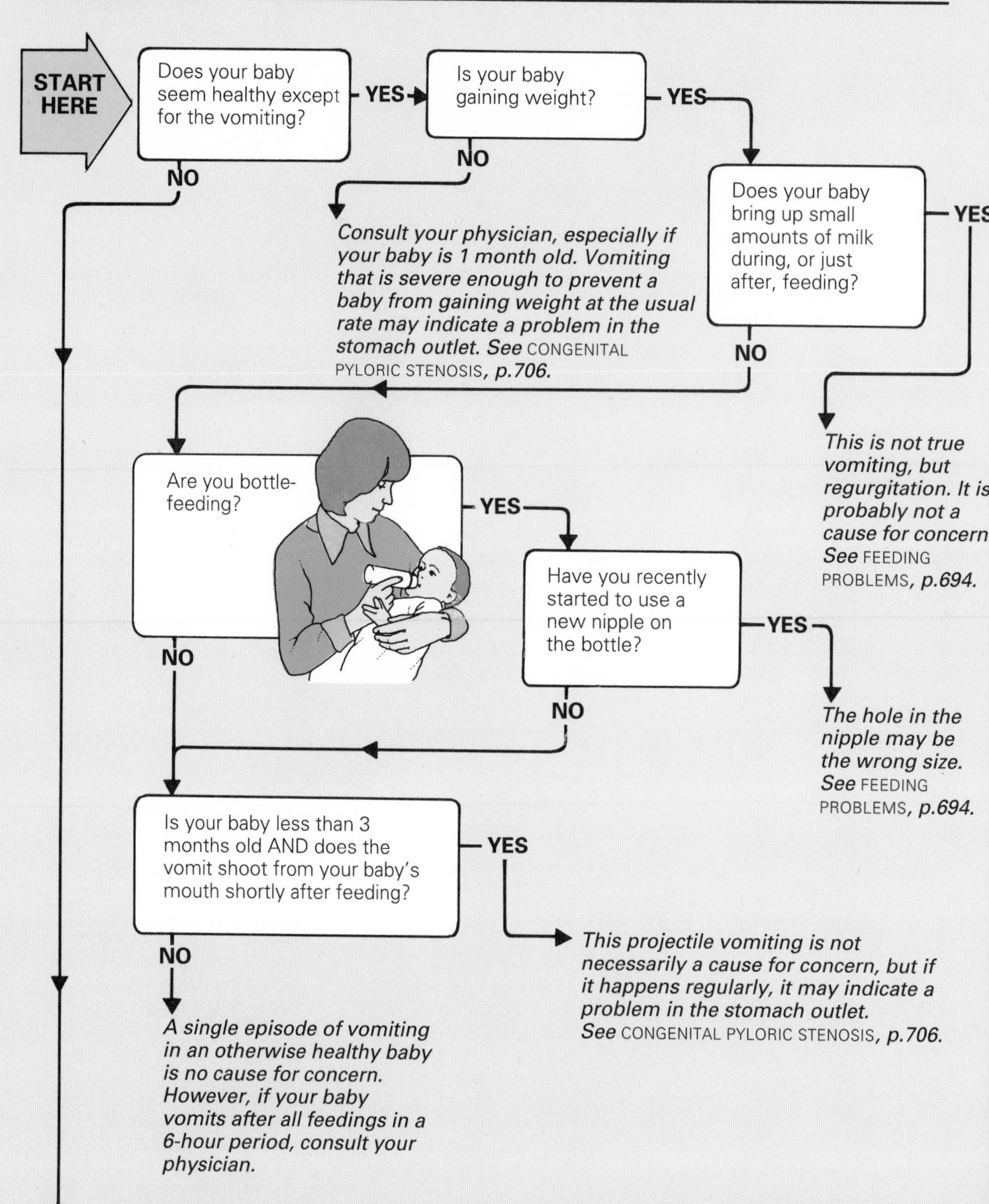

START HERE
Does your baby seem healthy except for the vomiting?
YES
NO
Is your baby gaining weight?
YES
NO
Consult your physician, especially if your baby is 1 month old. Vomiting that is severe enough to prevent a baby from gaining weight at the usual rate may indicate a problem in the stomach outlet. See CONGENITAL PYLORIC STENOSIS, p.706.
Does your baby bring up small amounts of milk during, or just after, feeding?
YES
NO
This is not true vomiting, but regurgitation. It is probably not a cause for concern. See FEEDING PROBLEMS, p.694.
Are you bottle-feeding?
YES
NO
Have you recently started to use a new nipple on the bottle?
YES
NO
The hole in the nipple may be the wrong size. See FEEDING PROBLEMS, p.694.
Is your baby less than 3 months old AND does the vomit shoot from your baby's mouth shortly after feeding?
YES
NO
This projectile vomiting is not necessarily a cause for concern, but if it happens regularly, it may indicate a problem in the stomach outlet. See CONGENITAL PYLORIC STENOSIS, p.706.
A single episode of vomiting in an otherwise healthy baby is no cause for concern. However, if your baby vomits after all feedings in a 6-hour period, consult your physician.

Go to next page

Continued from previous page

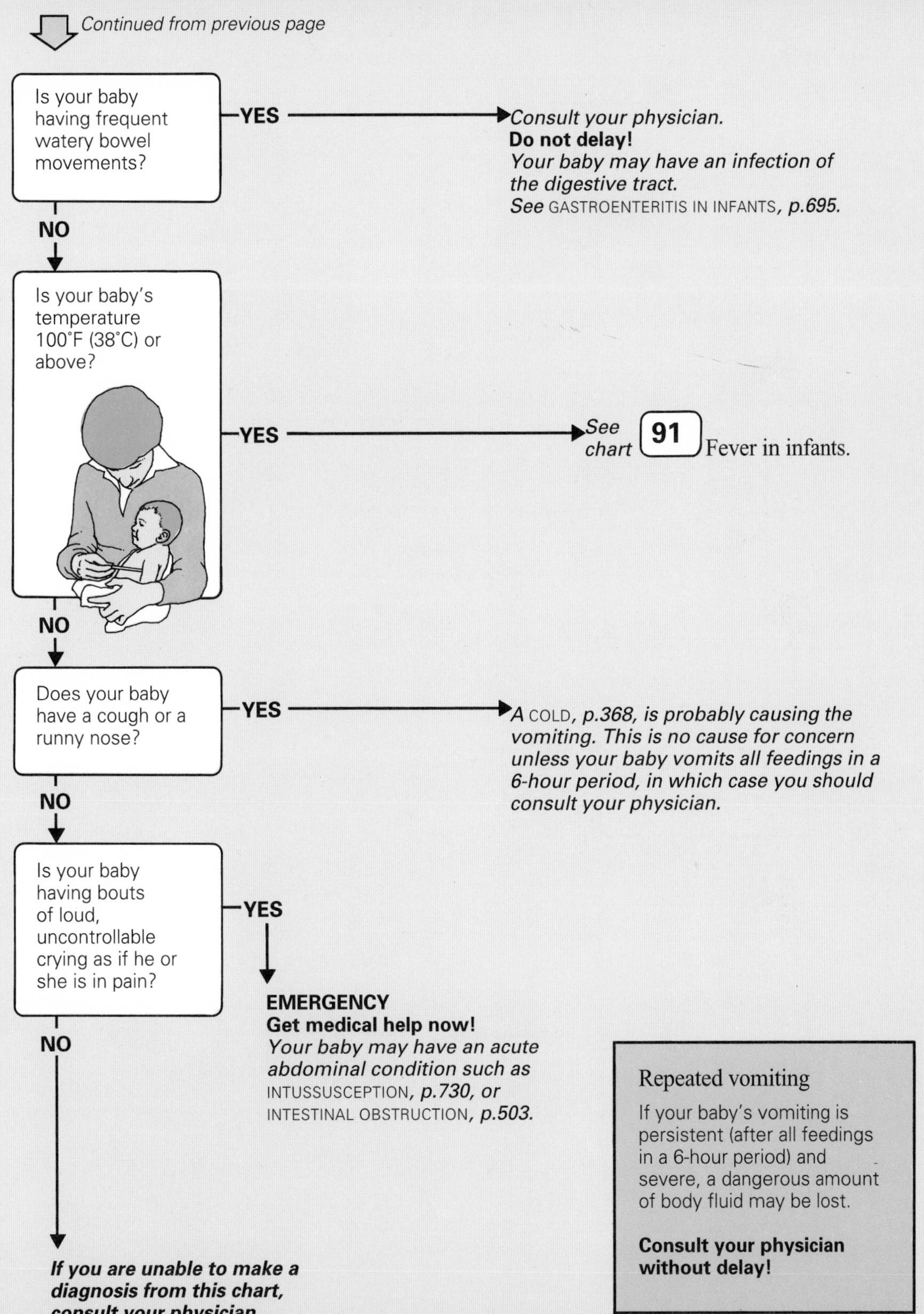

Is your baby having frequent watery bowel movements?

YES → *Consult your physician.*
Do not delay!
Your baby may have an infection of the digestive tract.
See GASTROENTERITIS IN INFANTS*, p.695.*

NO ↓

Is your baby's temperature 100°F (38°C) or above?

YES → *See chart* **91** Fever in infants.

NO ↓

Does your baby have a cough or a runny nose?

YES → *A* COLD*, p.368, is probably causing the vomiting. This is no cause for concern unless your baby vomits all feedings in a 6-hour period, in which case you should consult your physician.*

NO ↓

Is your baby having bouts of loud, uncontrollable crying as if he or she is in pain?

YES ↓

EMERGENCY
Get medical help now!
Your baby may have an acute abdominal condition such as INTUSSUSCEPTION*, p.730, or* INTESTINAL OBSTRUCTION*, p.503.*

NO ↓

If you are unable to make a diagnosis from this chart, consult your physician.

Repeated vomiting

If your baby's vomiting is persistent (after all feedings in a 6-hour period) and severe, a dangerous amount of body fluid may be lost.

Consult your physician without delay!

88

CHILDREN
0-6 months

Diarrhea in infants

Having runny, watery bowel movements that are more frequent than regular bowel movements.

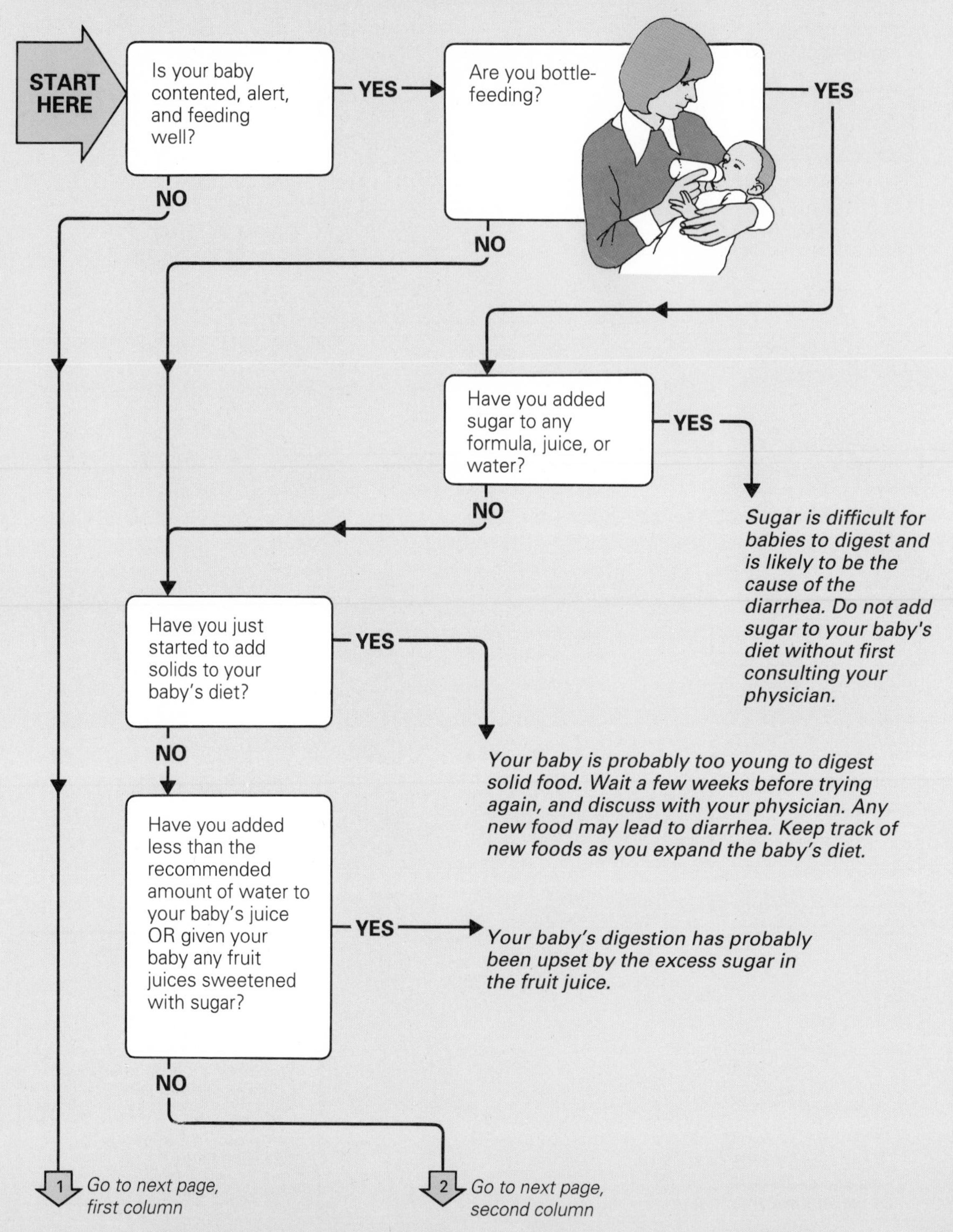

START HERE
Is your baby contented, alert, and feeding well?
YES
NO
Are you bottle-feeding?
YES
NO
Have you added sugar to any formula, juice, or water?
YES
Sugar is difficult for babies to digest and is likely to be the cause of the diarrhea. Do not add sugar to your baby's diet without first consulting your physician.
NO
Have you just started to add solids to your baby's diet?
YES
Your baby is probably too young to digest solid food. Wait a few weeks before trying again, and discuss with your physician. Any new food may lead to diarrhea. Keep track of new foods as you expand the baby's diet.
NO
Have you added less than the recommended amount of water to your baby's juice OR given your baby any fruit juices sweetened with sugar?
YES
Your baby's digestion has probably been upset by the excess sugar in the fruit juice.
NO
1 Go to next page, first column
2 Go to next page, second column

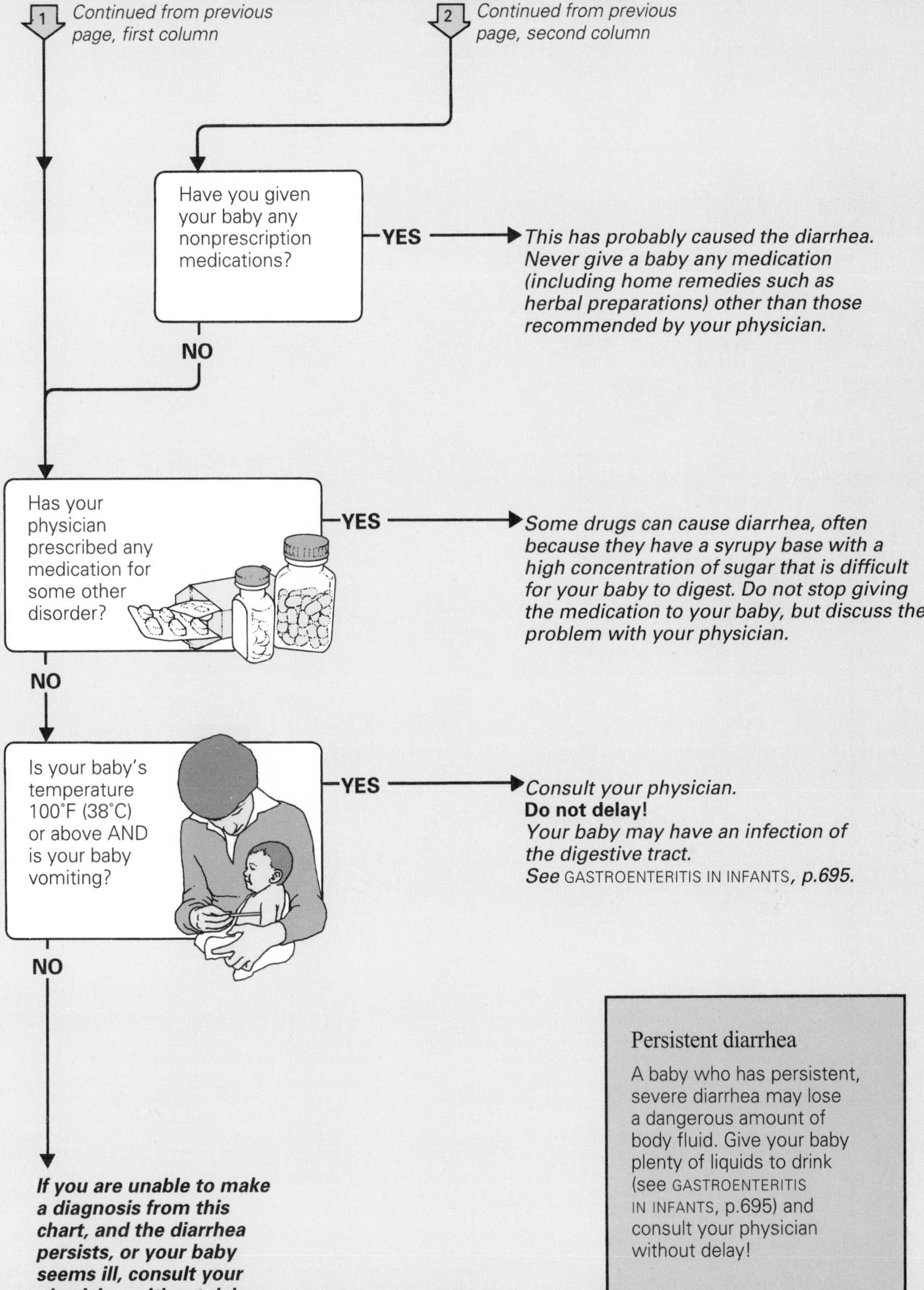

1
Continued from previous page, first column
2
Continued from previous page, second column
Have you given your baby any nonprescription medications?
YES
This has probably caused the diarrhea. Never give a baby any medication (including home remedies such as herbal preparations) other than those recommended by your physician.
NO
Has your physician prescribed any medication for some other disorder?
YES
Some drugs can cause diarrhea, often because they have a syrupy base with a high concentration of sugar that is difficult for your baby to digest. Do not stop giving the medication to your baby, but discuss the problem with your physician.
NO
Is your baby's temperature 100°F (38°C) or above AND is your baby vomiting?
YES
Consult your physician.
Do not delay!
Your baby may have an infection of the digestive tract.
See GASTROENTERITIS IN INFANTS, p.695.
NO
If you are unable to make a diagnosis from this chart, and the diarrhea persists, or your baby seems ill, consult your physician without delay.

Persistent diarrhea

A baby who has persistent, severe diarrhea may lose a dangerous amount of body fluid. Give your baby plenty of liquids to drink (see GASTROENTERITIS IN INFANTS, p.695) and consult your physician without delay!

89

CHILDREN
0-2 years

Skin problems in infants

Any skin spots, discolored areas, or blisters that may be sore or itchy.

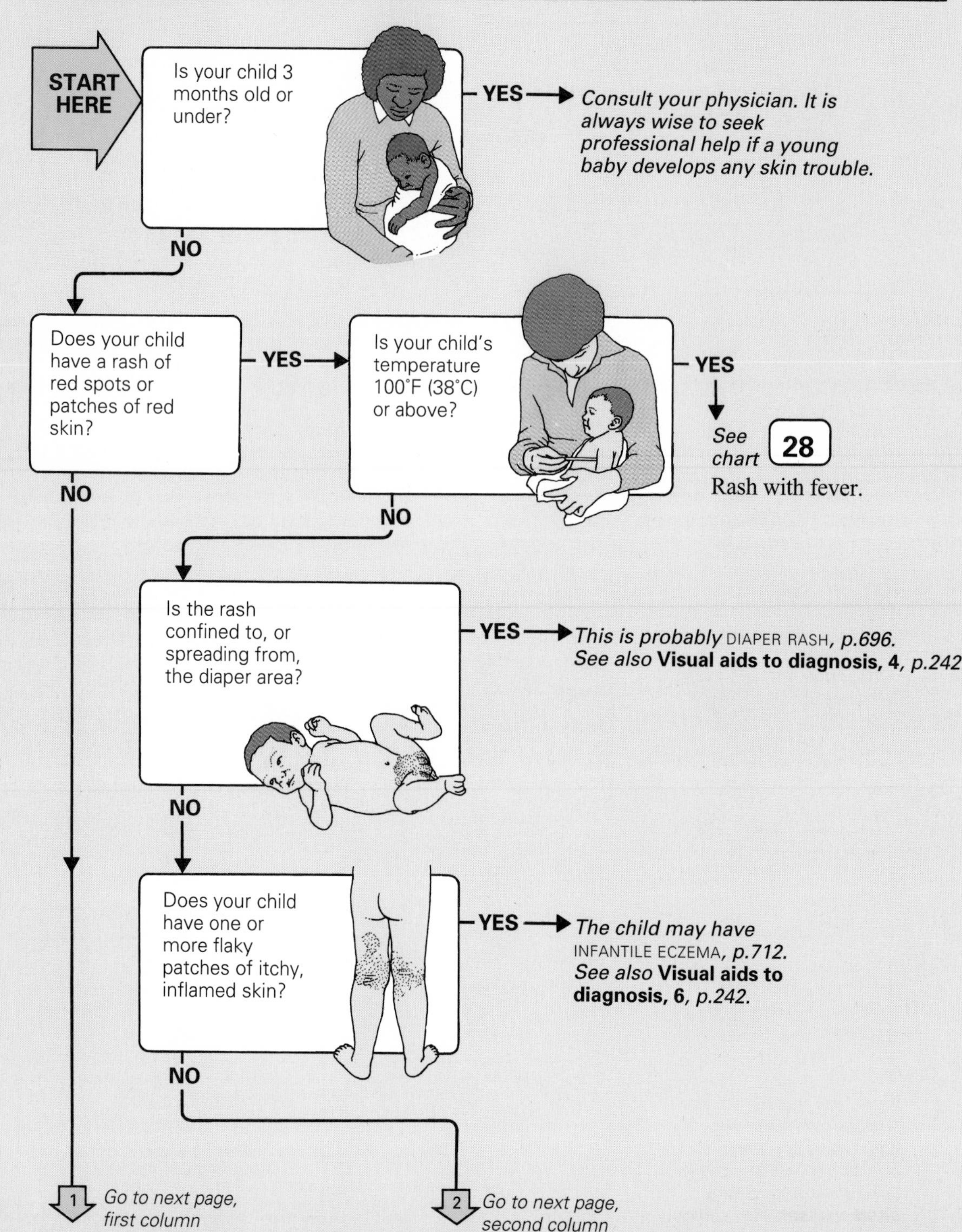

START HERE
Is your child 3 months old or under?
YES → *Consult your physician. It is always wise to seek professional help if a young baby develops any skin trouble.*
NO
Does your child have a rash of red spots or patches of red skin?
YES
Is your child's temperature 100°F (38°C) or above?
YES
See chart 28
Rash with fever.
NO
Is the rash confined to, or spreading from, the diaper area?
YES → *This is probably* DIAPER RASH, *p.696.*
See also **Visual aids to diagnosis, 4**, *p.242.*
NO
Does your child have one or more flaky patches of itchy, inflamed skin?
YES → *The child may have* INFANTILE ECZEMA, *p.712.*
See also **Visual aids to diagnosis, 6**, *p.242.*
NO
NO
1 *Go to next page, first column*
2 *Go to next page, second column*

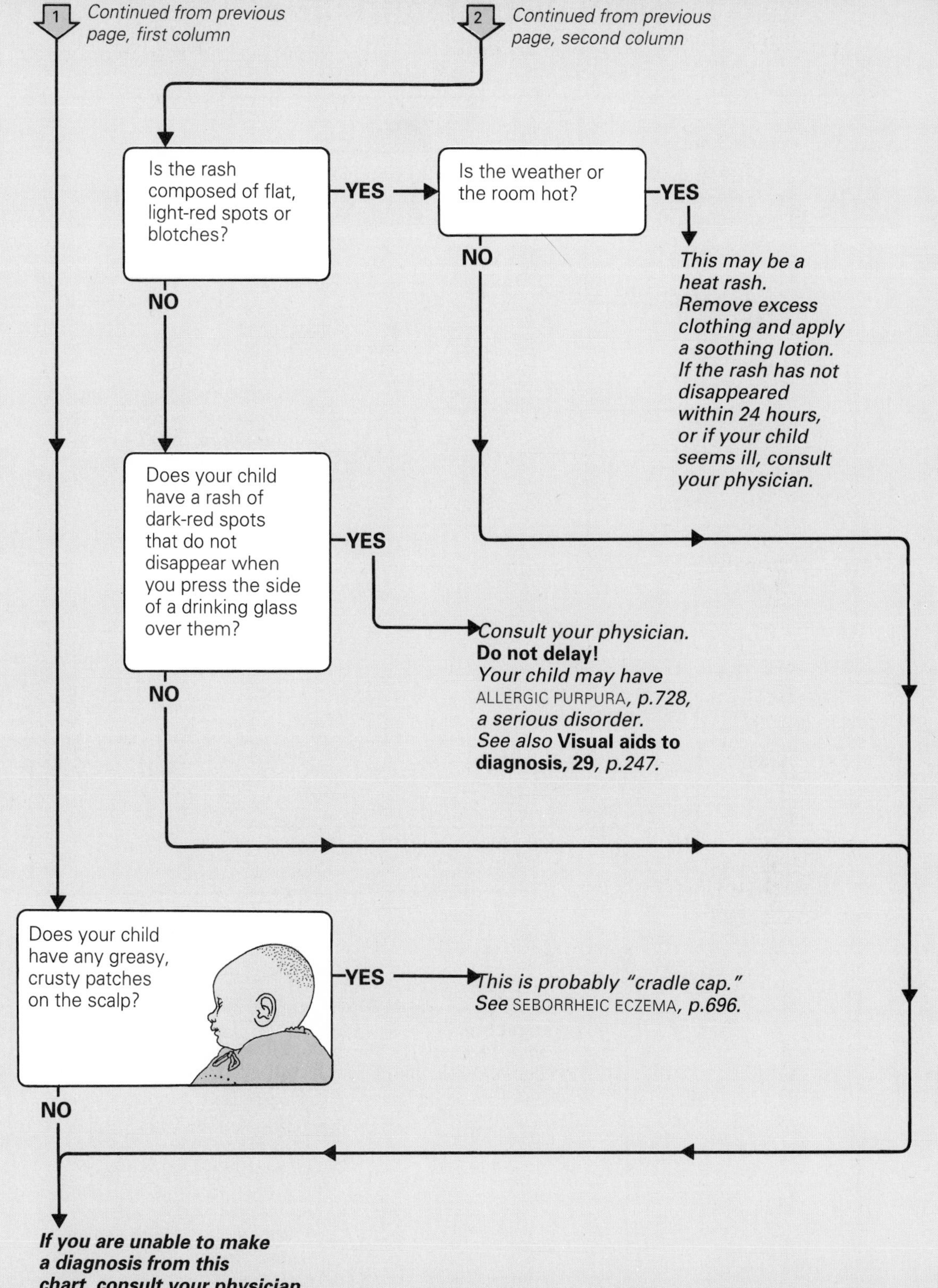

1 Continued from previous page, first column
2 Continued from previous page, second column
Is the rash composed of flat, light-red spots or blotches?
YES
NO
Is the weather or the room hot?
YES
NO
This may be a heat rash. Remove excess clothing and apply a soothing lotion. If the rash has not disappeared within 24 hours, or if your child seems ill, consult your physician.
Does your child have a rash of dark-red spots that do not disappear when you press the side of a drinking glass over them?
YES
NO
Consult your physician. Do not delay! Your child may have ALLERGIC PURPURA, p.728, a serious disorder. See also Visual aids to diagnosis, 29, p.247.
Does your child have any greasy, crusty patches on the scalp?
YES
NO
This is probably "cradle cap." See SEBORRHEIC ECZEMA, p.696.
If you are unable to make a diagnosis from this chart, consult your physician.

90
CHILDREN
0-5 years

Slow weight gain

Failure to gain weight or grow at the expected rate (see the box below right and the growth charts on p.691).

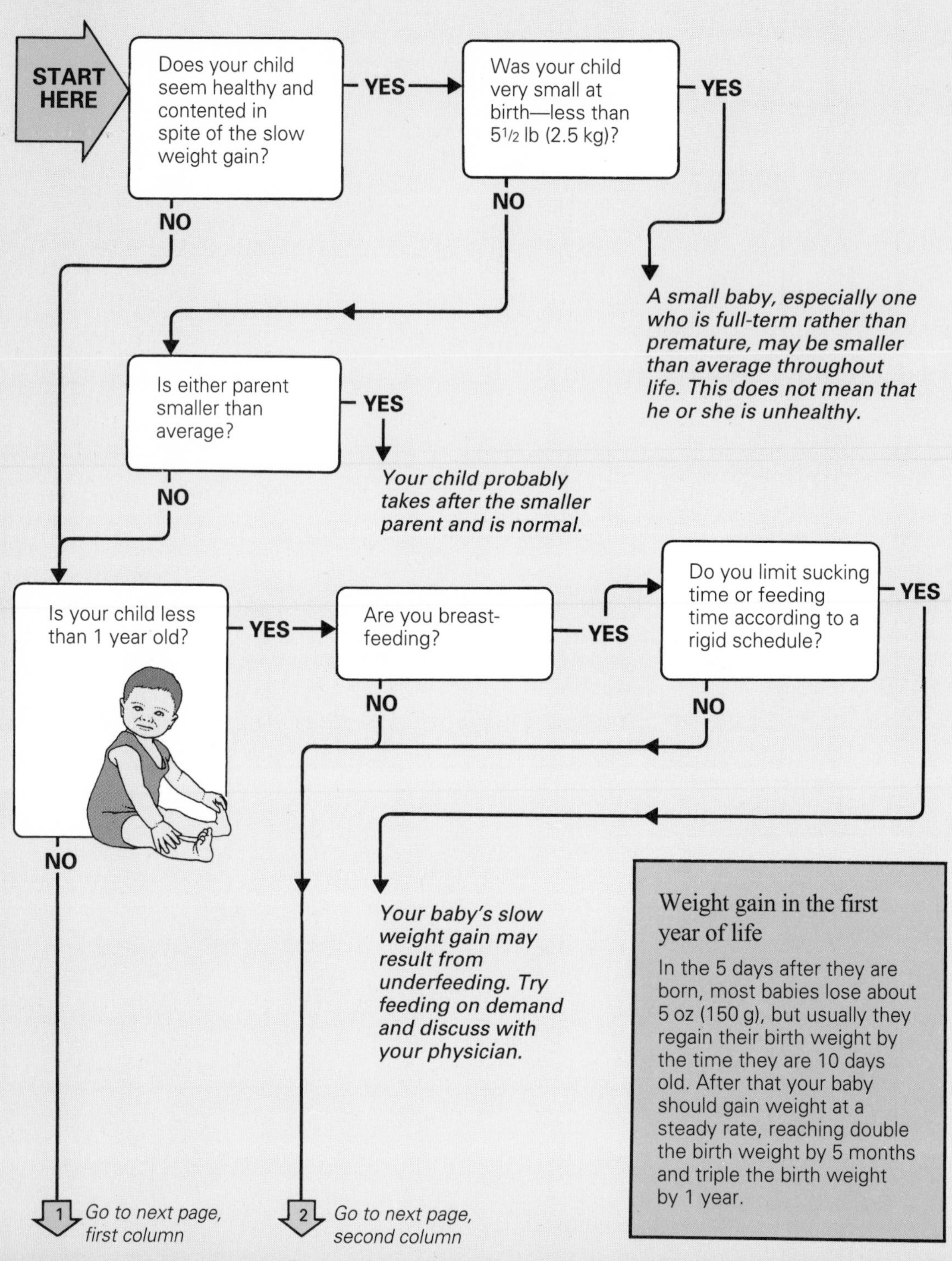

START HERE
Does your child seem healthy and contented in spite of the slow weight gain?
YES
NO
Was your child very small at birth—less than 5½ lb (2.5 kg)?
YES
NO
A small baby, especially one who is full-term rather than premature, may be smaller than average throughout life. This does not mean that he or she is unhealthy.
Is either parent smaller than average?
YES
NO
Your child probably takes after the smaller parent and is normal.
Is your child less than 1 year old?
YES
NO
Are you breast-feeding?
YES
NO
Do you limit sucking time or feeding time according to a rigid schedule?
YES
NO
Your baby's slow weight gain may result from underfeeding. Try feeding on demand and discuss with your physician.
1 Go to next page, first column
2 Go to next page, second column

Weight gain in the first year of life

In the 5 days after they are born, most babies lose about 5 oz (150 g), but usually they regain their birth weight by the time they are 10 days old. After that your baby should gain weight at a steady rate, reaching double the birth weight by 5 months and triple the birth weight by 1 year.

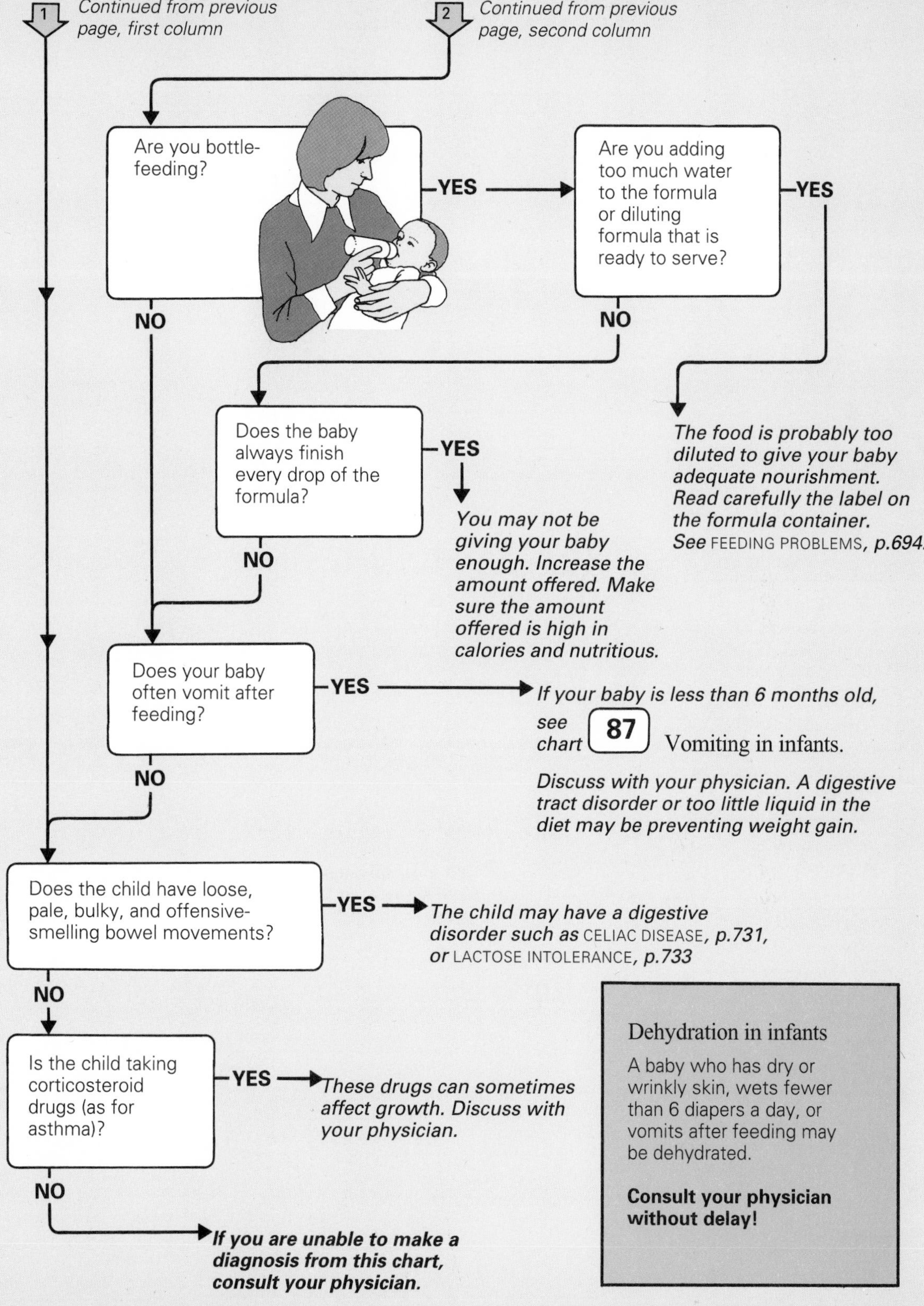

1
Continued from previous page, first column
2
Continued from previous page, second column
Are you bottle-feeding?
YES
Are you adding too much water to the formula or diluting formula that is ready to serve?
YES
The food is probably too diluted to give your baby adequate nourishment. Read carefully the label on the formula container. See FEEDING PROBLEMS, p.694.
NO
NO
Does the baby always finish every drop of the formula?
YES
You may not be giving your baby enough. Increase the amount offered. Make sure the amount offered is high in calories and nutritious.
NO
Does your baby often vomit after feeding?
YES
If your baby is less than 6 months old, see chart 87 Vomiting in infants.
Discuss with your physician. A digestive tract disorder or too little liquid in the diet may be preventing weight gain.
NO
Does the child have loose, pale, bulky, and offensive-smelling bowel movements?
YES
The child may have a digestive disorder such as CELIAC DISEASE, p.731, or LACTOSE INTOLERANCE, p.733
NO
Is the child taking corticosteroid drugs (as for asthma)?
YES
These drugs can sometimes affect growth. Discuss with your physician.
NO
If you are unable to make a diagnosis from this chart, consult your physician.

Dehydration in infants

A baby who has dry or wrinkly skin, wets fewer than 6 diapers a day, or vomits after feeding may be dehydrated.

Consult your physician without delay!

91

CHILDREN
0-2 years

Fever in infants

Temperature of 100°F (38°C) or above, which may make your baby flushed and irritable.

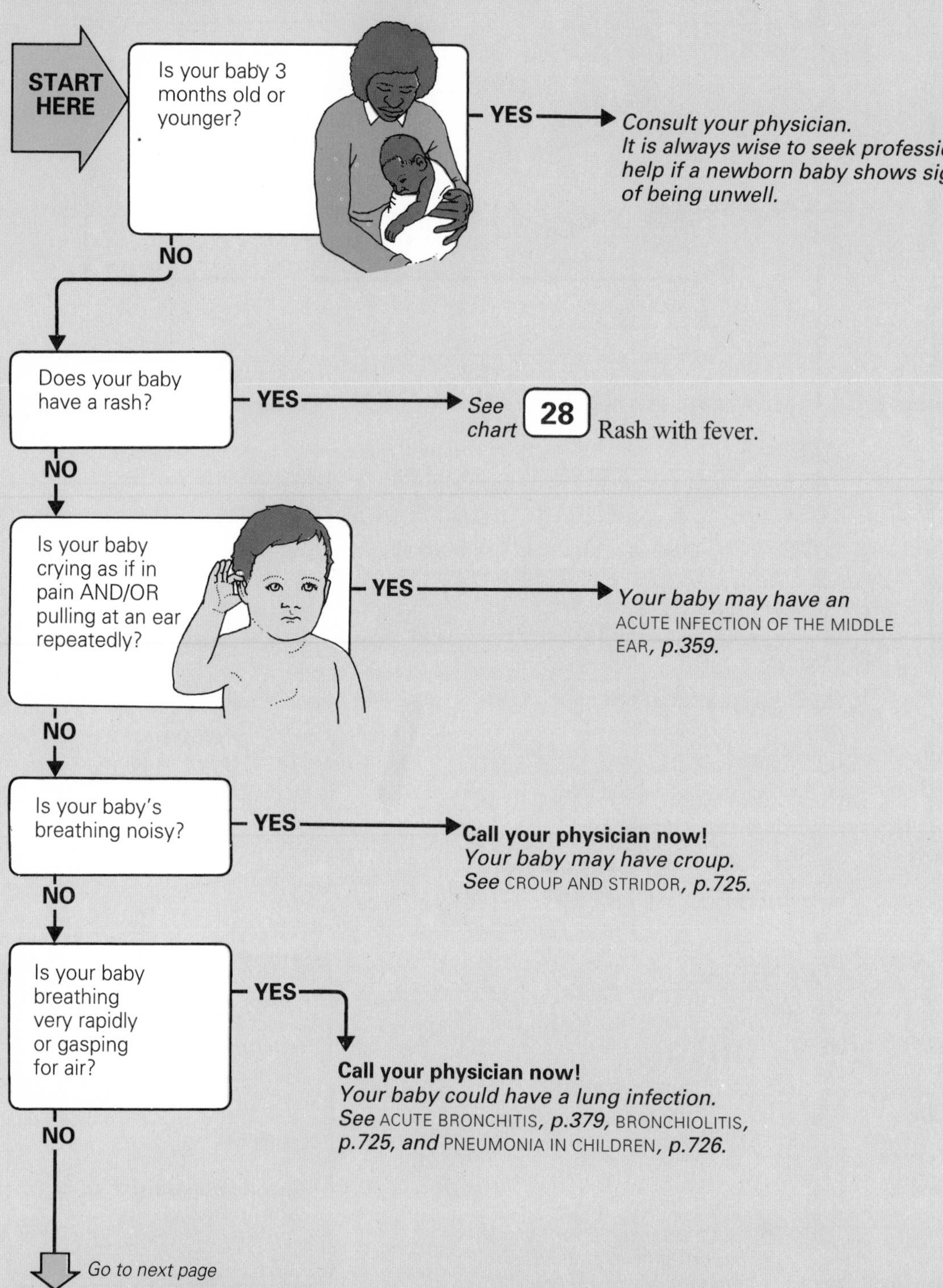
START HERE
Is your baby 3 months old or younger?
YES
Consult your physician.
It is always wise to seek professional help if a newborn baby shows signs of being unwell.
NO
Does your baby have a rash?
YES
See chart **28** Rash with fever.
NO
Is your baby crying as if in pain AND/OR pulling at an ear repeatedly?
YES
Your baby may have an ACUTE INFECTION OF THE MIDDLE EAR, *p.359.*
NO
Is your baby's breathing noisy?
YES
Call your physician now!
Your baby may have croup.
See CROUP AND STRIDOR, *p.725.*
NO
Is your baby breathing very rapidly or gasping for air?
YES
Call your physician now!
Your baby could have a lung infection.
See ACUTE BRONCHITIS, *p.379,* BRONCHIOLITIS, *p.725, and* PNEUMONIA IN CHILDREN, *p.726.*
NO
Go to next page

Continued from previous page

Does your baby have diarrhea?

YES → *Consult your physician.*
Do not delay!
This may be an infection of the digestive tract. See GASTROENTERITIS, *p.491. If your baby is less than 1 year old, see* GASTROENTERITIS IN INFANTS, *p.695.*

NO ↓

Does your baby have a runny nose?

YES → Has your baby been around someone who has an infectious disease in the last 2 weeks?

YES → *Your baby may be developing that infectious disease. See* CHILDHOOD INFECTIOUS DISEASES, *p.744.*

NO ↓ *Your baby probably has a cold with a fever. See* COLDS, *p.368.*

NO ↓

Is the weather or the room hot AND is your baby warmly dressed?

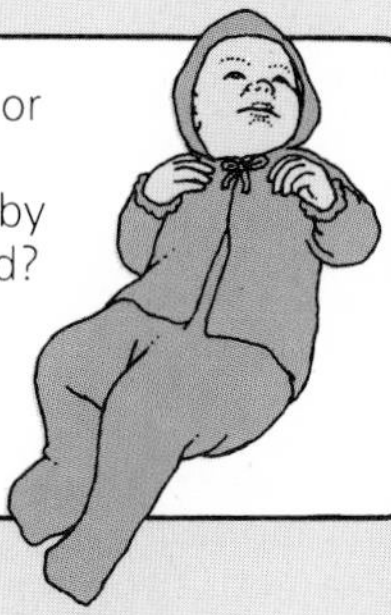

YES → *The fever probably results from overheating. Try removing some of your baby's clothing and offering a drink of water.*

NO ↓

If you are unable to make a diagnosis from this chart, consult your physician. Do not delay if your baby seems very ill or has a temperature of 102°F (39°C) or above.

Seizures

Sometimes a high temperature in an infant can cause seizures (see SEIZURES IN CHILDREN, p.713). If this happens, or if your baby's temperature reaches 102°F (39°C) or above, call your physician immediately. Also see p.796 for advice on dealing with a fever.

EMERGENCY
Get medical help now!

92
CHILDREN
2-14 years

Fever in children

A temperature of 100°F (38°C) or above, which may make your child flushed, irritable, or sleepy.

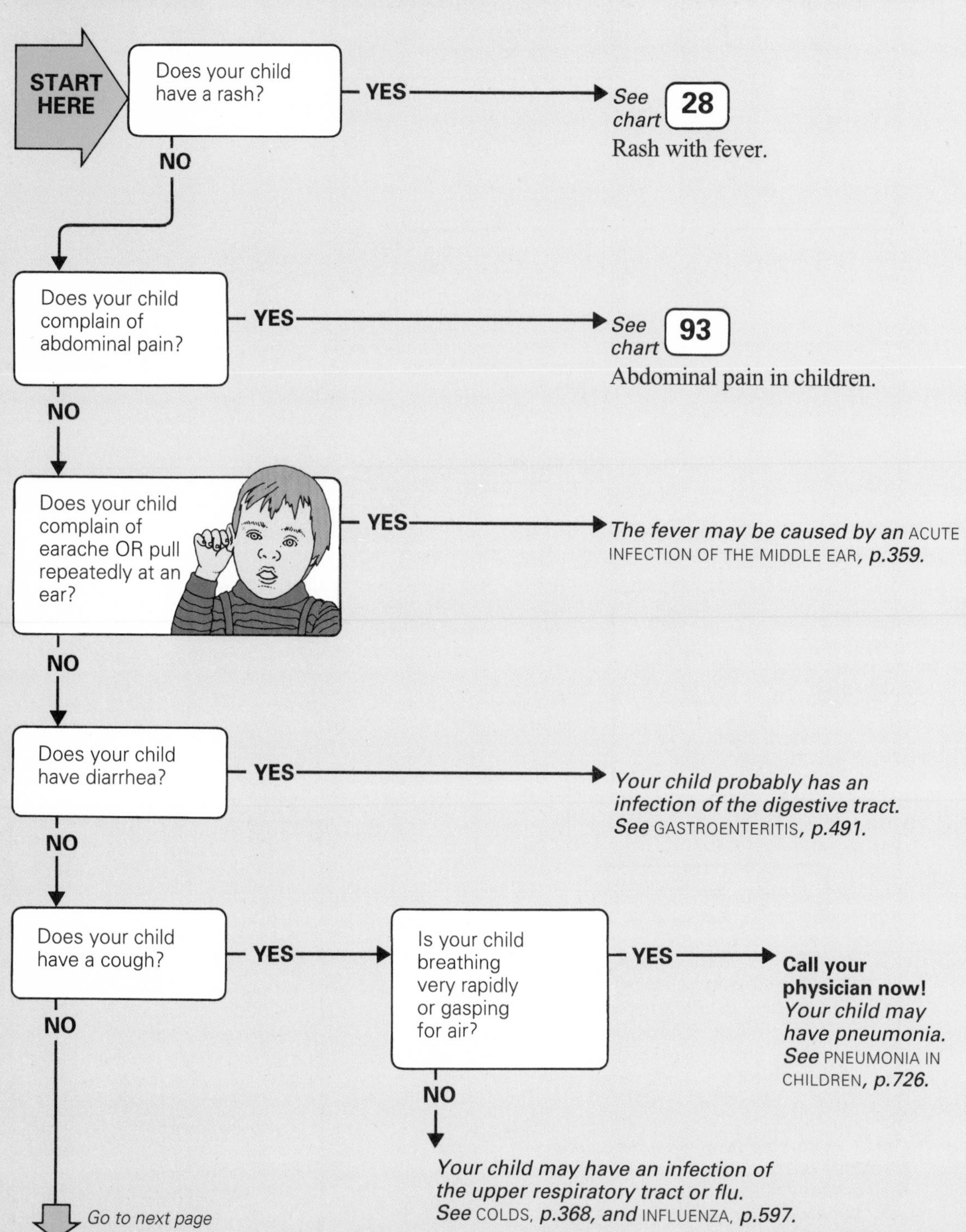

START HERE
Does your child have a rash?
YES
See chart 28
Rash with fever.
NO
Does your child complain of abdominal pain?
YES
See chart 93
Abdominal pain in children.
NO
Does your child complain of earache OR pull repeatedly at an ear?
YES
The fever may be caused by an ACUTE INFECTION OF THE MIDDLE EAR, p.359.
NO
Does your child have diarrhea?
YES
Your child probably has an infection of the digestive tract. See GASTROENTERITIS, p.491.
NO
Does your child have a cough?
YES
Is your child breathing very rapidly or gasping for air?
YES
Call your physician now! Your child may have pneumonia. See PNEUMONIA IN CHILDREN, p.726.
NO
Your child may have an infection of the upper respiratory tract or flu. See COLDS, p.368, and INFLUENZA, p.597.
NO
Go to next page

Continued from previous page

Does your child complain of a sore throat AND/OR is his or her voice faint or hoarse?

YES → *Your child may have an infection of the upper respiratory tract. See* TONSILLITIS IN CHILDREN, *p.723,* PHARYNGITIS, *p.376, and* LARYNGITIS, *p.377.*

NO ↓

Does your child have a runny nose?

YES → Has your child been in contact with anyone who has an infectious disease such as measles?

YES → *Your child may be in the early stages of an infectious disease such as* MEASLES, *p.745.*

NO → *This is probably a fever that accompanies a* COLD, *p.368.*

NO ↓

Is there any swelling between the ear and the angle of the jaw AND/OR is that area painful and tender?

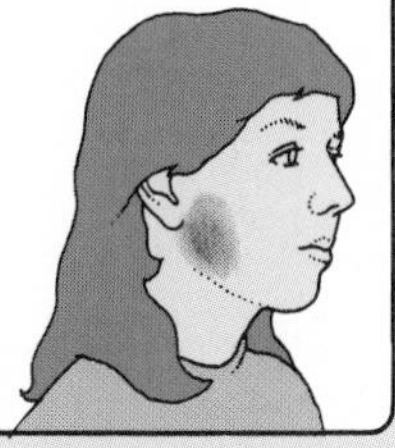

YES → *Your child may have* MUMPS, *p.748.*

NO ↓

Does your child seem very ill and have two or more of the following symptoms?

- ☐ vomiting
- ☐ headache
- ☐ bright light hurts the eyes
- ☐ stiff neck, or pain when trying to bend the head forward

YES ↓

Call your physician now! *These symptoms suggest the possibility of meningitis. See* MENINGITIS IN INFANTS AND CHILDREN, *p.715.*

NO ↓

If you are unable to make a diagnosis from this chart and your child's temperature remains high for more than 6 hours, consult your physician.

Seizures and fever

A high temperature in a child under age 5 may bring on seizures (see SEIZURES IN CHILDREN, p.713). If this happens, call your physician immediately. Also, see p.744 for advice on dealing with a fever.

EMERGENCY
Get medical help now!

Temperature over 102°F

If a child of any age has a temperature of 102°F (39°C) or above, call your physician immediately. Also, see p.744 for advice on dealing with a fever.

Call your physician now!

93

CHILDREN
2-14 years

Abdominal pain in children

Pain in the area between the bottom of the rib cage and the groin, which may vary from a mild stomachache to severe pain.

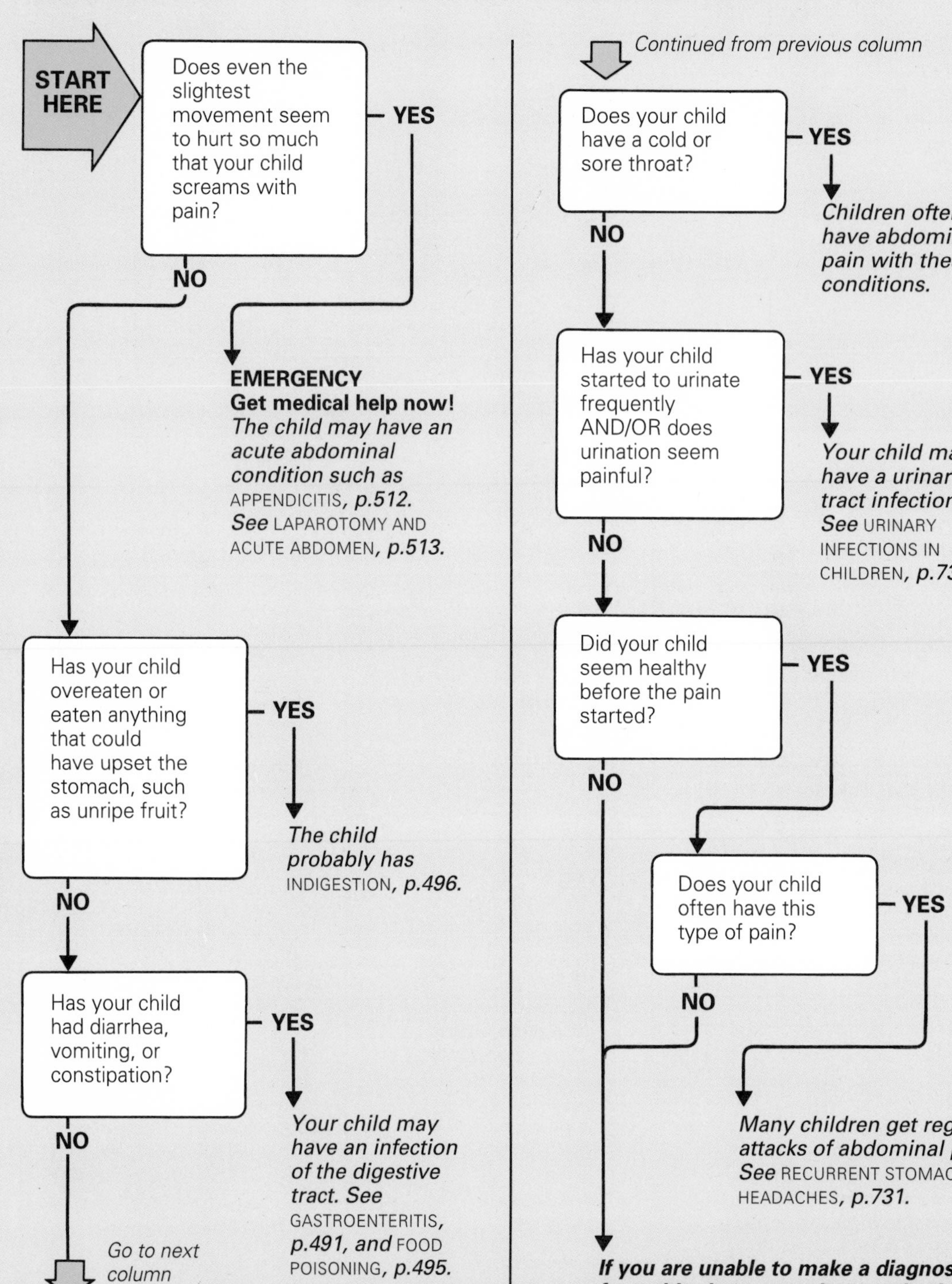

START HERE
Does even the slightest movement seem to hurt so much that your child screams with pain?
YES
EMERGENCY
Get medical help now!
The child may have an acute abdominal condition such as APPENDICITIS, p.512. See LAPAROTOMY AND ACUTE ABDOMEN, p.513.
NO
Has your child overeaten or eaten anything that could have upset the stomach, such as unripe fruit?
YES
The child probably has INDIGESTION, p.496.
NO
Has your child had diarrhea, vomiting, or constipation?
YES
Your child may have an infection of the digestive tract. See GASTROENTERITIS, p.491, and FOOD POISONING, p.495.
NO
Go to next column
Continued from previous column
Does your child have a cold or sore throat?
YES
Children often have abdominal pain with these conditions.
NO
Has your child started to urinate frequently AND/OR does urination seem painful?
YES
Your child may have a urinary tract infection. See URINARY INFECTIONS IN CHILDREN, p.736.
NO
Did your child seem healthy before the pain started?
YES
Does your child often have this type of pain?
YES
Many children get regular attacks of abdominal pain. See RECURRENT STOMACH AND HEADACHES, p.731.
NO
NO
If you are unable to make a diagnosis from this chart, consult your physician.

94
CHILDREN
2-14 years

Itching in children

Irritation of the skin, in one area or all over the body, which makes your child want to scratch.

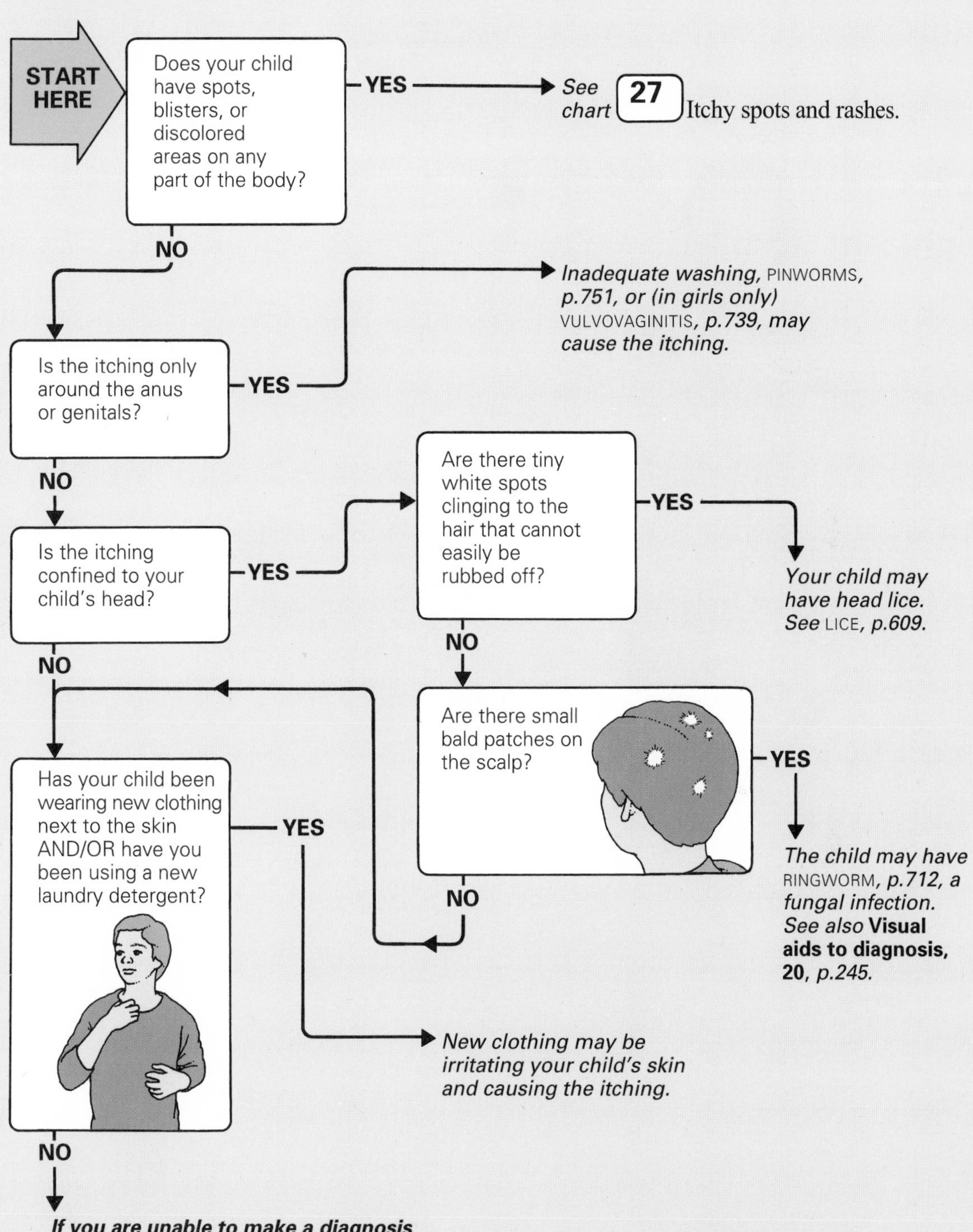

START HERE
Does your child have spots, blisters, or discolored areas on any part of the body?
YES
See chart 27 Itchy spots and rashes.
NO
Is the itching only around the anus or genitals?
YES
Inadequate washing, PINWORMS, p.751, or (in girls only) VULVOVAGINITIS, p.739, may cause the itching.
NO
Is the itching confined to your child's head?
YES
Are there tiny white spots clinging to the hair that cannot easily be rubbed off?
YES
Your child may have head lice. See LICE, p.609.
NO
Are there small bald patches on the scalp?
YES
The child may have RINGWORM, p.712, a fungal infection. See also Visual aids to diagnosis, 20, p.245.
NO
NO
Has your child been wearing new clothing next to the skin AND/OR have you been using a new laundry detergent?
YES
New clothing may be irritating your child's skin and causing the itching.
NO

If you are unable to make a diagnosis from this chart, consult your physician.

95

CHILDREN
2-14 years

Coughing in children

Noisy expulsion of air from the lungs.

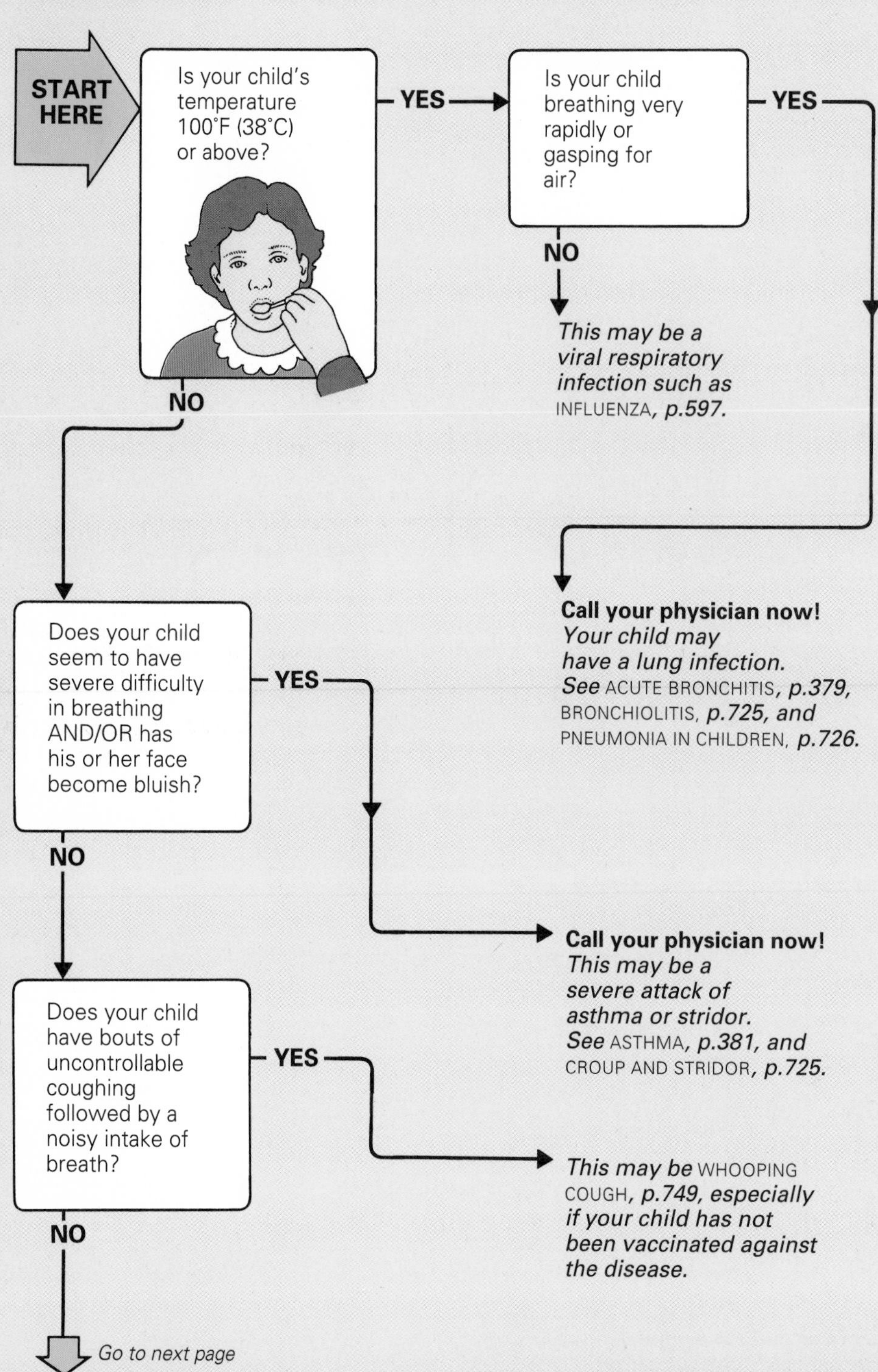

START HERE
Is your child's temperature 100°F (38°C) or above?
YES
Is your child breathing very rapidly or gasping for air?
YES
NO
This may be a viral respiratory infection such as INFLUENZA, p.597.
NO
Call your physician now! Your child may have a lung infection. See ACUTE BRONCHITIS, p.379, BRONCHIOLITIS, p.725, and PNEUMONIA IN CHILDREN, p.726.
Does your child seem to have severe difficulty in breathing AND/OR has his or her face become bluish?
YES
Call your physician now! This may be a severe attack of asthma or stridor. See ASTHMA, p.381, and CROUP AND STRIDOR, p.725.
NO
Does your child have bouts of uncontrollable coughing followed by a noisy intake of breath?
YES
This may be WHOOPING COUGH, p.749, especially if your child has not been vaccinated against the disease.
NO
Go to next page

Continued from previous page

Is your child's breathing harsh or wheezy?

YES → Could your child have choked on or inhaled a small foreign object, such as a peanut, within the last few days?

YES → *This may be causing the coughing. See* INHALED FOREIGN OBJECT, *p.725.*

NO → *Your child may have asthma or croup. See* CROUP AND STRIDOR, *p.725, and* ASTHMA, *p.381.*

NO ↓

Does your child have a runny nose or congestion?

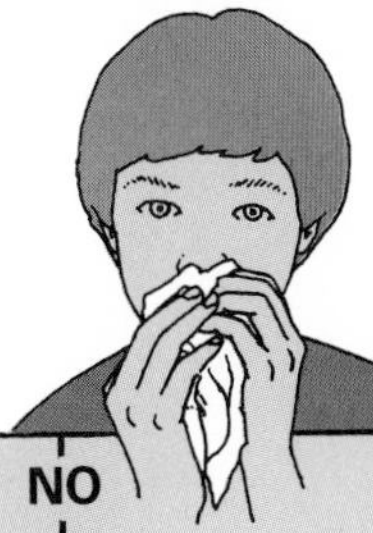

YES → *Discharge from the back of the nose may be irritating the throat, causing your child to cough. See* RECURRENT COLDS IN CHILDREN, *p.727, and* ADENOIDS, *p.724.*

NO ↓

Has your child had whooping cough within the last 3 months?

YES → *Persistent coughing often follows* WHOOPING COUGH, *p.749.*

NO ↓

Does anyone in the house smoke OR could your child be smoking?

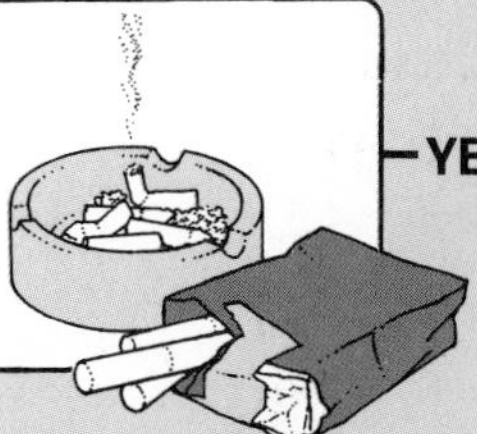

YES → *Smoking, or even living with a smoker, can make your child cough. Quitting smoking will benefit your health and your child's health.*

NO ↓

If you are unable to make a diagnosis from this chart, and the cough persists for more than 2 weeks, consult your physician.

Noisy breathing

Rapid noisy breathing in a child is always a cause for concern, especially if the child is under 3.

Consult your physician without delay!

96

CHILDREN
0-14 years

Swellings in children

Any swellings or lumps in the neck or armpits, which may be tender or painful.

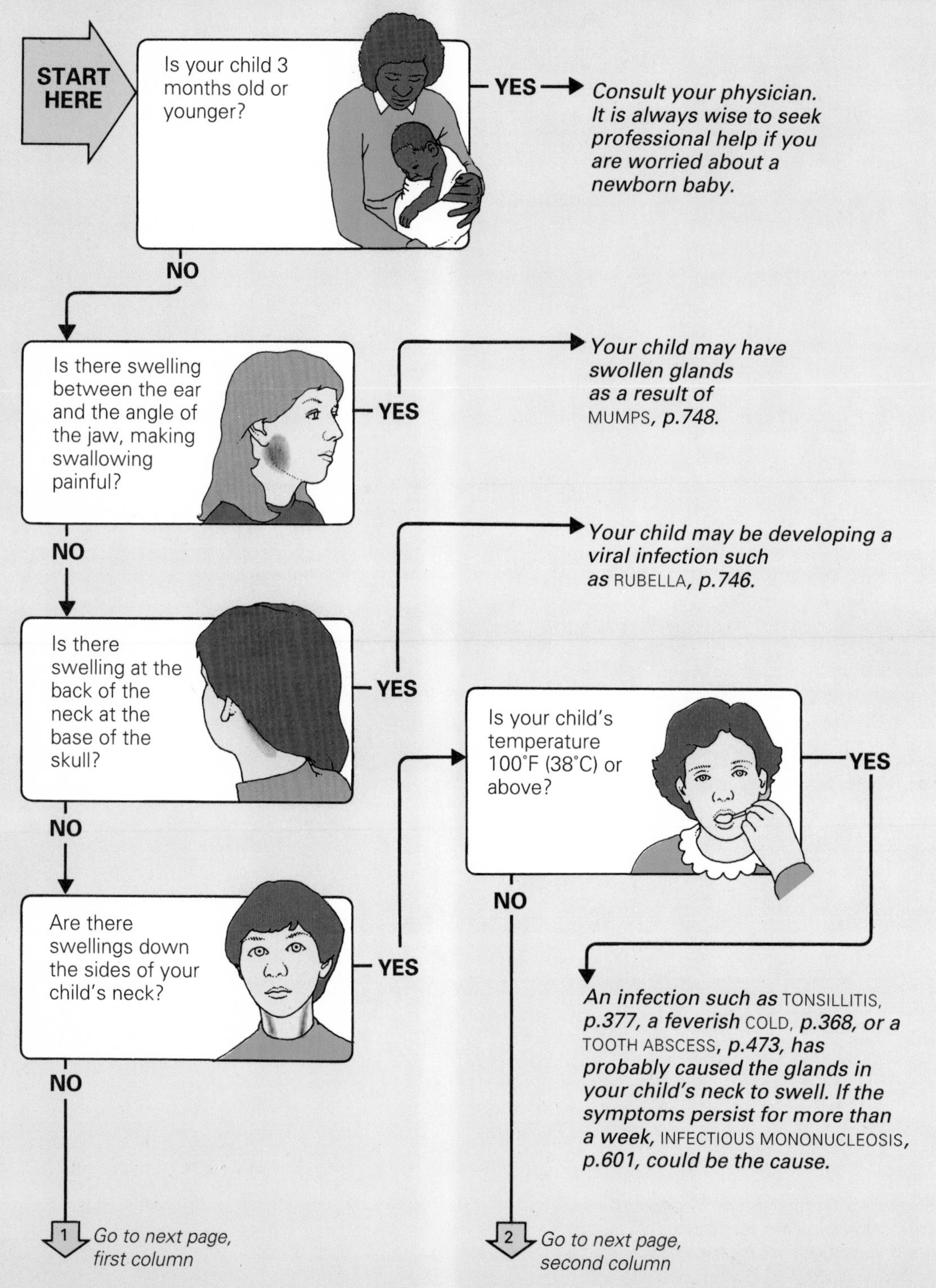

START HERE
Is your child 3 months old or younger?
YES
Consult your physician. It is always wise to seek professional help if you are worried about a newborn baby.
NO
Is there swelling between the ear and the angle of the jaw, making swallowing painful?
YES
Your child may have swollen glands as a result of MUMPS, *p.748.*
NO
Is there swelling at the back of the neck at the base of the skull?
YES
Your child may be developing a viral infection such as RUBELLA, *p.746.*
NO
Are there swellings down the sides of your child's neck?
YES
Is your child's temperature 100°F (38°C) or above?
YES
An infection such as TONSILLITIS, *p.377, a feverish* COLD, *p.368, or a* TOOTH ABSCESS, *p.473, has probably caused the glands in your child's neck to swell. If the symptoms persist for more than a week,* INFECTIOUS MONONUCLEOSIS, *p.601, could be the cause.*
NO
2 *Go to next page, second column*
NO
1 *Go to next page, first column*

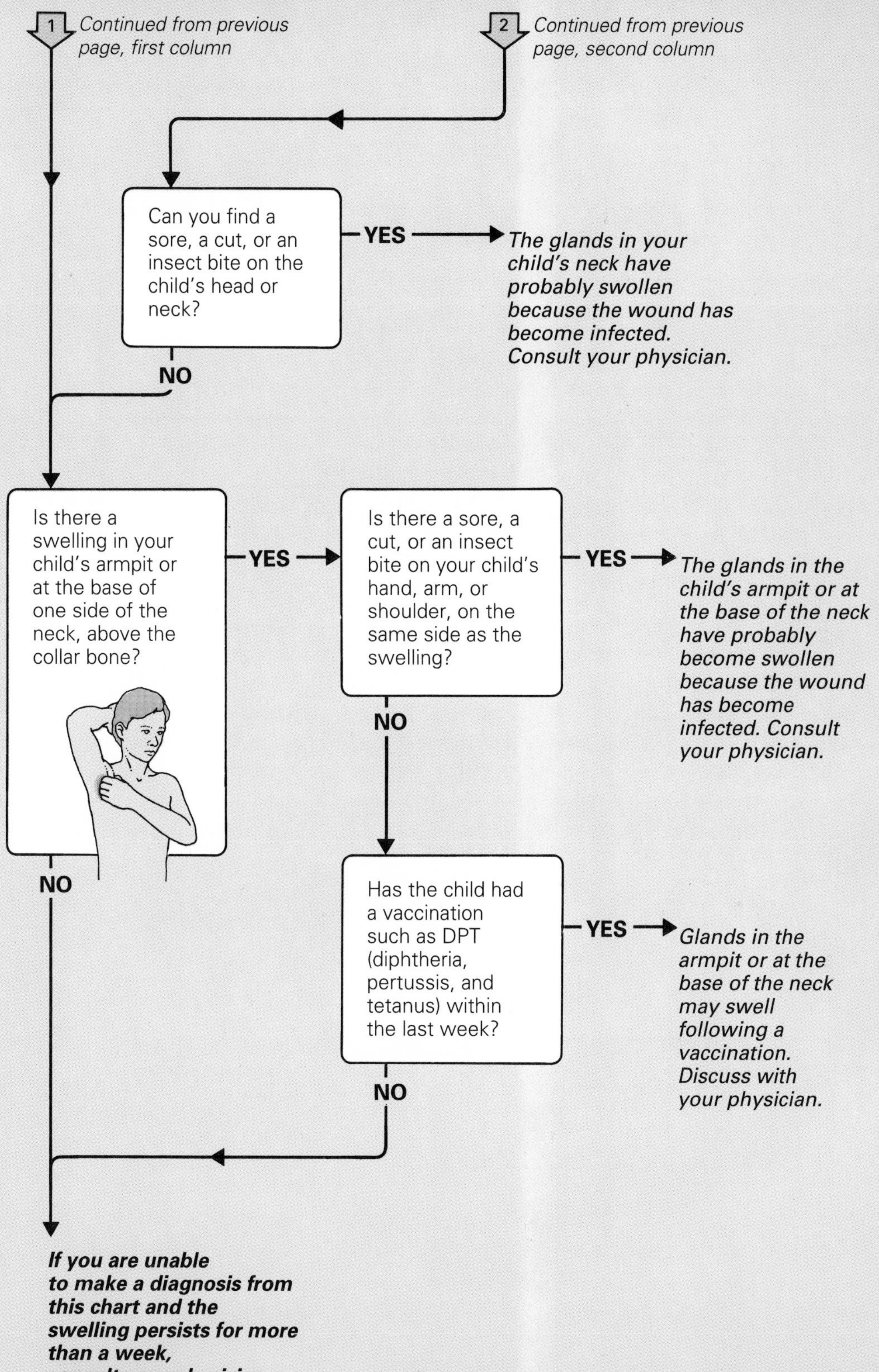

Continued from previous page, first column
Continued from previous page, second column
Can you find a sore, a cut, or an insect bite on the child's head or neck?
YES
The glands in your child's neck have probably swollen because the wound has become infected. Consult your physician.
NO
Is there a swelling in your child's armpit or at the base of one side of the neck, above the collar bone?
YES
Is there a sore, a cut, or an insect bite on your child's hand, arm, or shoulder, on the same side as the swelling?
YES
The glands in the child's armpit or at the base of the neck have probably become swollen because the wound has become infected. Consult your physician.
NO
Has the child had a vaccination such as DPT (diphtheria, pertussis, and tetanus) within the last week?
YES
Glands in the armpit or at the base of the neck may swell following a vaccination. Discuss with your physician.
NO
NO
If you are unable to make a diagnosis from this chart and the swelling persists for more than a week, consult your physician.

97

CHILDREN
0-14 years

Limping in children

Difficulty walking that may be accompanied by pain in the affected hip, leg, or foot, and in a young child may result in a reluctance to walk.

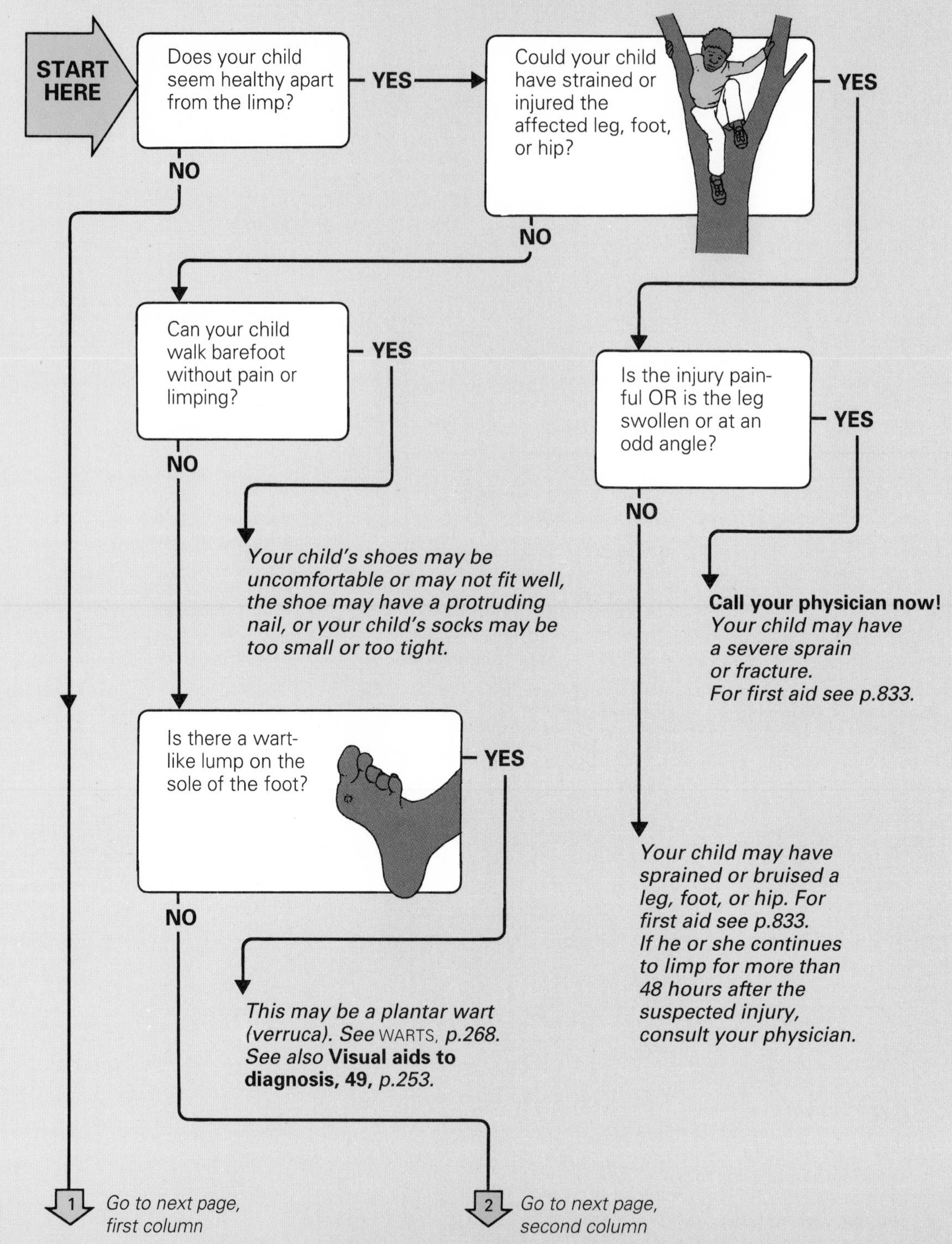

START HERE

Does your child seem healthy apart from the limp?

YES → Could your child have strained or injured the affected leg, foot, or hip?

- YES → Is the injury painful OR is the leg swollen or at an odd angle?
  - YES → **Call your physician now!** *Your child may have a severe sprain or fracture. For first aid see p.833.*
  - NO → *Your child may have sprained or bruised a leg, foot, or hip. For first aid see p.833. If he or she continues to limp for more than 48 hours after the suspected injury, consult your physician.*
- NO → Can your child walk barefoot without pain or limping?
  - YES → *Your child's shoes may be uncomfortable or may not fit well, the shoe may have a protruding nail, or your child's socks may be too small or too tight.*
  - NO → Is there a wart-like lump on the sole of the foot?
    - YES → *This may be a plantar wart (verruca). See* WARTS, *p.268. See also* **Visual aids to diagnosis, 49,** *p.253.*
    - NO → 2 *Go to next page, second column*

NO → 1 *Go to next page, first column*

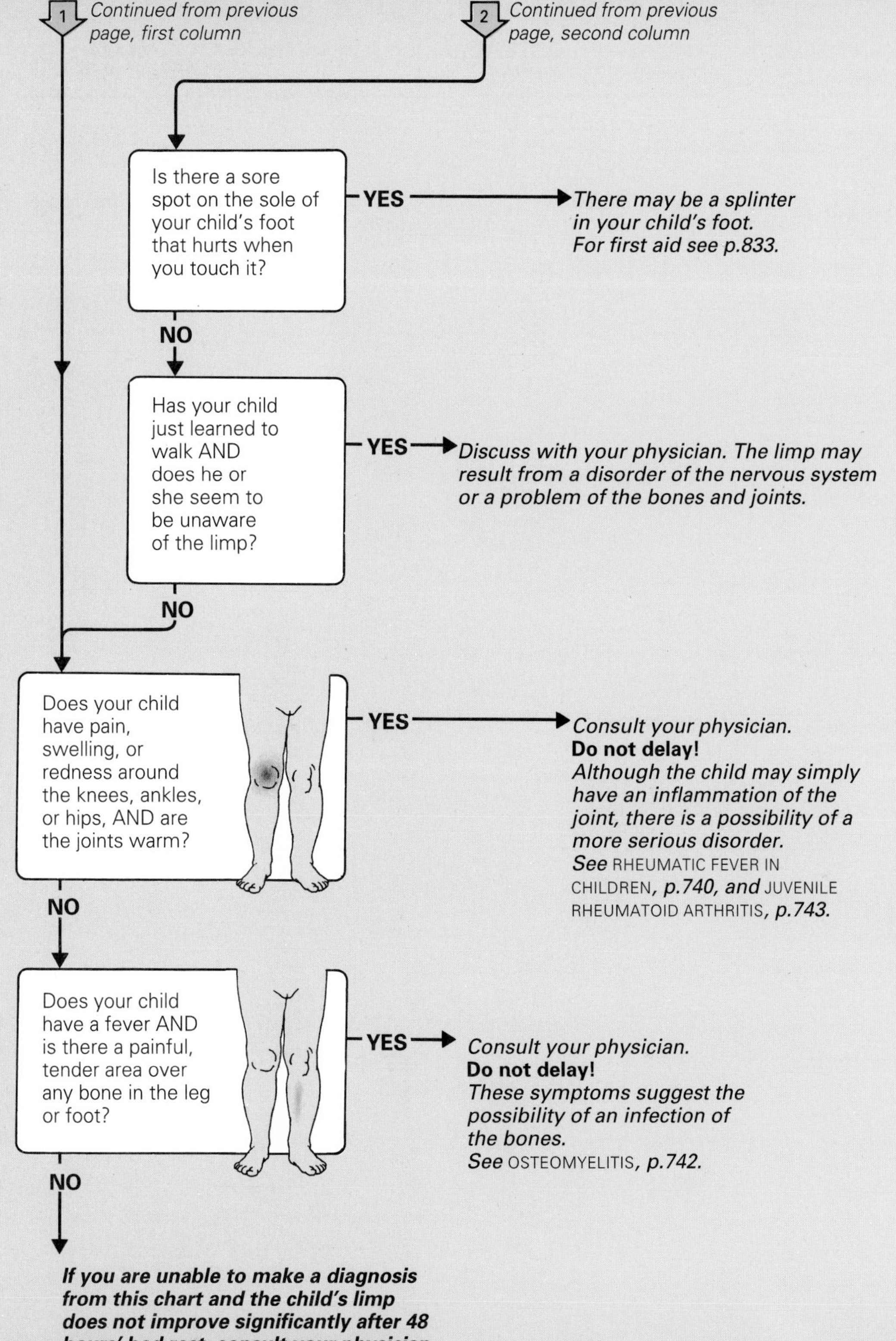
1
Continued from previous page, first column
2
Continued from previous page, second column
Is there a sore spot on the sole of your child's foot that hurts when you touch it?
YES
There may be a splinter in your child's foot. For first aid see p.833.
NO
Has your child just learned to walk AND does he or she seem to be unaware of the limp?
YES
Discuss with your physician. The limp may result from a disorder of the nervous system or a problem of the bones and joints.
NO
Does your child have pain, swelling, or redness around the knees, ankles, or hips, AND are the joints warm?
YES
Consult your physician.
Do not delay!
Although the child may simply have an inflammation of the joint, there is a possibility of a more serious disorder.
See RHEUMATIC FEVER IN CHILDREN, p.740, and JUVENILE RHEUMATOID ARTHRITIS, p.743.
NO
Does your child have a fever AND is there a painful, tender area over any bone in the leg or foot?
YES
Consult your physician.
Do not delay!
These symptoms suggest the possibility of an infection of the bones.
See OSTEOMYELITIS, p.742.
NO
If you are unable to make a diagnosis from this chart and the child's limp does not improve significantly after 48 hours' bed rest, consult your physician.

98

OLDER PEOPLE
over 65 years

Incontinence in older people

Involuntary urination that may vary from a small leak to complete emptying of the bladder.

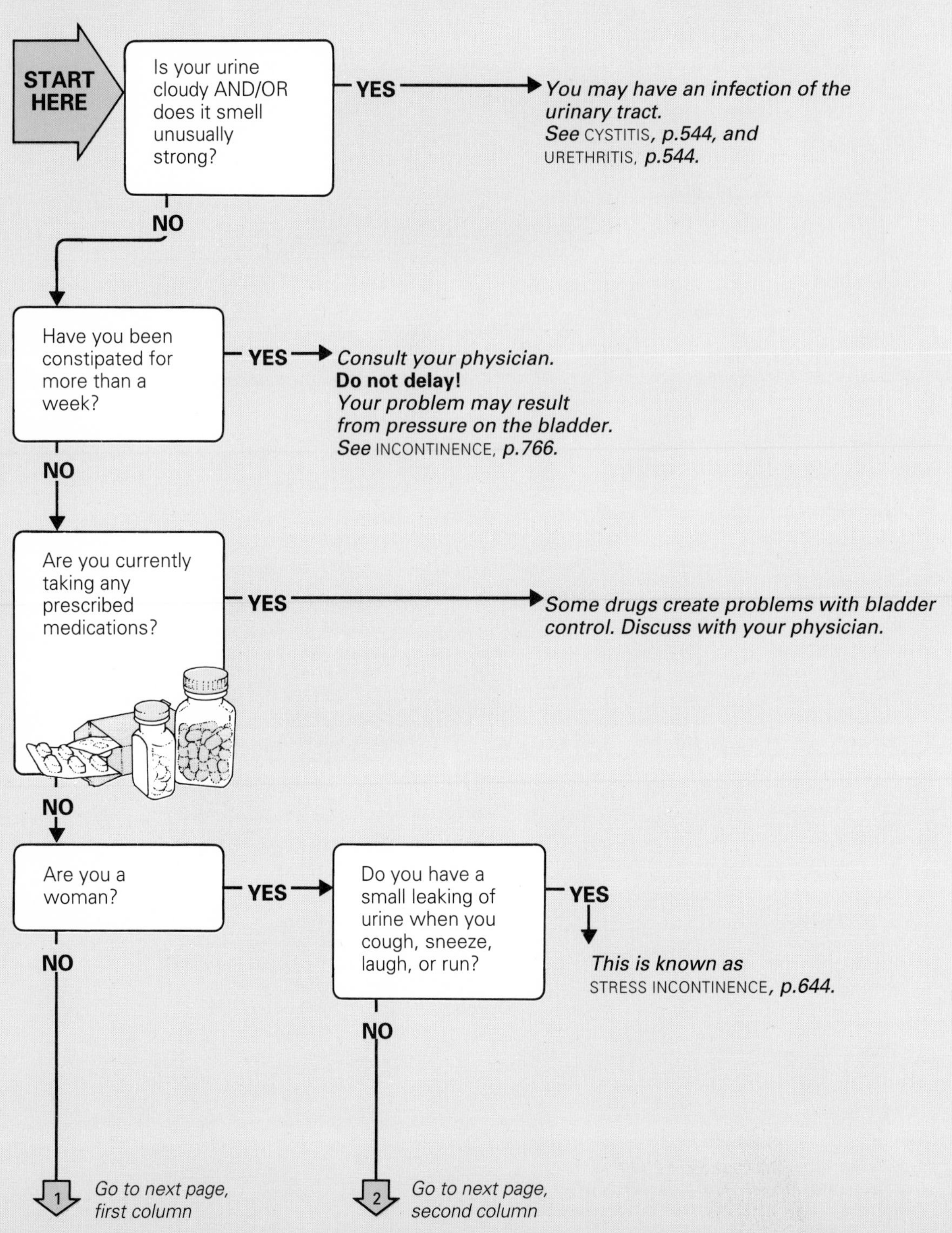

START HERE

Is your urine cloudy AND/OR does it smell unusually strong?

YES → *You may have an infection of the urinary tract.* *See* CYSTITIS, *p.544, and* URETHRITIS, *p.544.*

NO ↓

Have you been constipated for more than a week?

YES → *Consult your physician.* **Do not delay!** *Your problem may result from pressure on the bladder.* *See* INCONTINENCE, *p.766.*

NO ↓

Are you currently taking any prescribed medications?

YES → *Some drugs create problems with bladder control. Discuss with your physician.*

NO ↓

Are you a woman?

YES → Do you have a small leaking of urine when you cough, sneeze, laugh, or run?

- **YES** → *This is known as* STRESS INCONTINENCE, *p.644.*
- **NO** ↓ 2 *Go to next page, second column*

NO ↓ 1 *Go to next page, first column*

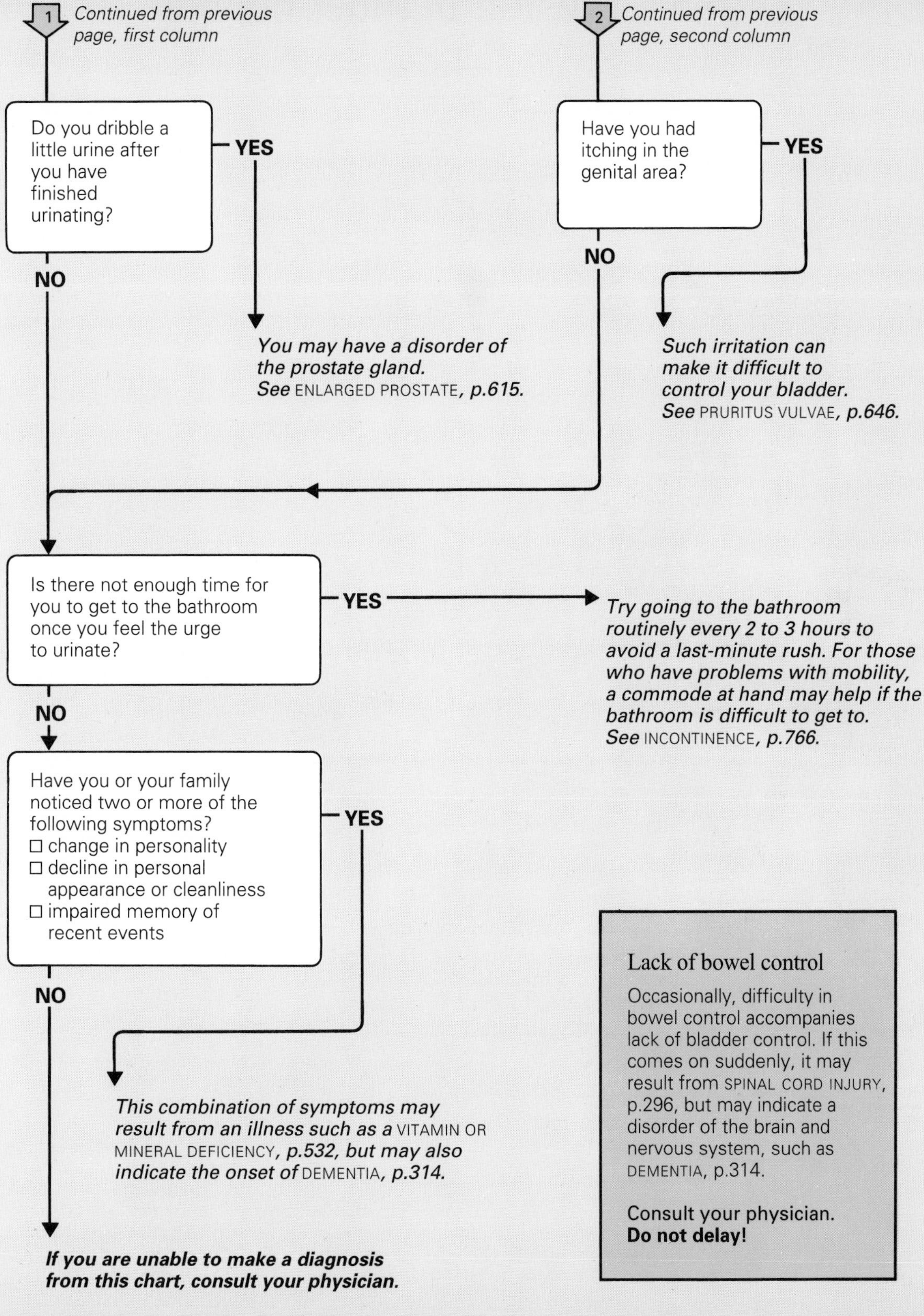

1 Continued from previous page, first column
2 Continued from previous page, second column
Do you dribble a little urine after you have finished urinating?
YES
NO
You may have a disorder of the prostate gland.
See ENLARGED PROSTATE, p.615.
Have you had itching in the genital area?
YES
NO
Such irritation can make it difficult to control your bladder.
See PRURITUS VULVAE, p.646.
Is there not enough time for you to get to the bathroom once you feel the urge to urinate?
YES
Try going to the bathroom routinely every 2 to 3 hours to avoid a last-minute rush. For those who have problems with mobility, a commode at hand may help if the bathroom is difficult to get to.
See INCONTINENCE, p.766.
NO
Have you or your family noticed two or more of the following symptoms?
☐ change in personality
☐ decline in personal appearance or cleanliness
☐ impaired memory of recent events
YES
This combination of symptoms may result from an illness such as a VITAMIN OR MINERAL DEFICIENCY, p.532, but may also indicate the onset of DEMENTIA, p.314.
NO
If you are unable to make a diagnosis from this chart, consult your physician.

Lack of bowel control

Occasionally, difficulty in bowel control accompanies lack of bladder control. If this comes on suddenly, it may result from SPINAL CORD INJURY, p.296, but may indicate a disorder of the brain and nervous system, such as DEMENTIA, p.314.

Consult your physician.
Do not delay!

99

OLDER PEOPLE
over 65 years

Confusion in older people

A loss of clarity about times, places, and events, or a loss of contact with reality. Use this chart only after consulting chart 15, **Confusion**.

START HERE

Has the confusion appeared recently?

- **YES** → Have you recently started a new medication or changed doses of any one you have been taking?
  - **YES** → *Consult your physician, who may change your dose or stop the medication.*
  - **NO** → Did the confusion begin in the weeks following a fall or head injury?
    - **YES** → *Consult your physician.* **Do not delay!** *These symptoms suggest the possibility of bleeding inside the skull. See* SUBDURAL HEMORRHAGE AND HEMATOMA, ***p.289.***
    - **NO** → Have you noticed two or more of the following symptoms?
      - ☐ change in personality
      - ☐ decline in personal appearance or cleanliness
      - ☐ impaired memory of recent events
      - **YES** → ***This combination of symptoms may result from an illness such as a*** VITAMIN OR MINERAL DEFICIENCY, ***p.532, but may also indicate the onset of*** DEMENTIA, *p.314, several minor* STROKES, ***p.772, or a*** BRAIN TUMOR, ***p.301.***
      - **NO** → Is the confusion accompanied by signs of physical illness...
- **NO** → Is the confusion accompanied by signs of physical illness such as a fever, a cough, or lack of bladder control?
  - **YES** → *Consult your physician.* **Do not delay!** *Many types of physical illness may cause confusion in older people.*
  - **NO** → Could you be chilled AND/OR does your abdomen feel unusually cold?
    - **YES** → *This may indicate a dangerous drop in body temperature. See* HYPOTHERMIA, *p.772. For first aid see p.833.*
    - **NO** → Is it possible that you missed a meal?
      - **YES** → *Lack of food can cause confusion. A sweet drink or snack should clear the mind within 10 minutes. If confusion persists, call your physician at once.*
      - **NO** → ***If you are unable to make a diagnosis from this chart, consult your physician.***

Visual aids to diagnosis

The purpose of this section of the book is to help you identify visual signs of illness. The pictures on the following pages show symptoms that appear on the skin in some disorders, the symptoms of skin disorders themselves, and also certain nail and eye problems. The best way to use these pictures is to consider the following suggestions. If you are concerned about any symptom, whether it is visible or not, begin by consulting the appropriate self-diagnosis symptom chart (see p.74). The chart may then refer you not only to an article, but also to one of the visual aid illustrations in this section. Many kinds of skin problems look similar, and you might be misled if you examine a picture *before* you study the chart, so do not use these illustrations as the only step, or even as the first step, in the process of preliminary self-diagnosis. One additional word of warning: if the picture you have referred to does not really look like your own symptoms, it is best to consult your physician. Symptoms vary from case to case, and only a limited number of examples can be given here. Your physician is familiar, in most cases, with the full range of appearances of a disorder's visual signs.

If you are upset by medical illustrations showing sores, rashes, and tumors, you should probably not look at this section. The same is true if you are offended by pictures of any portions of the human body.

Birthmarks

An area of discolored skin present from birth (or soon after) may be called a birthmark. There are two main types of birthmarks: a concentration of tiny blood vessels in the skin (often called red marks), and a patch of discolored skin (a pigmented spot). Birthmarks usually are harmless, but they are often unattractive (see Birthmarks, p.698).

1 Strawberry hemangioma

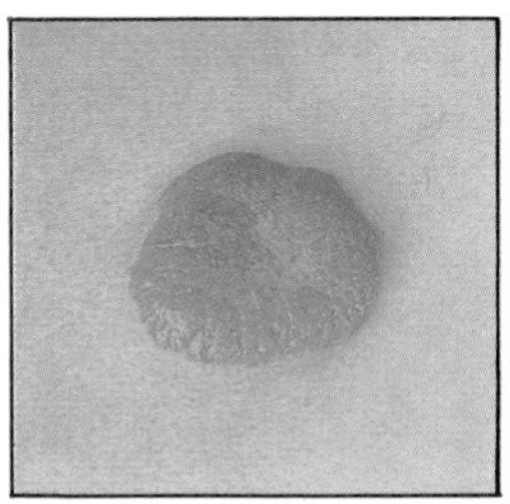

A strawberry hemangioma is a raised, bright-red patch of skin that grows in the first few months of life. After about 6 months the mark begins to shrink and fade. Most of these birthmarks disappear by the time the child reaches 9 years of age.

2 Port wine stain

A port wine stain is another type of birthmark. It usually consists of a flat or pebbled patch of purplish-red skin. Generally this type of birthmark covers a large area and occurs singly, most commonly on the face or limbs. Port wine stains usually remain the same throughout life, though occasionally they may fade a little. If such a stain is considered disfiguring, makeup may be used to cover the stain. A new type of laser works well to eliminate port wine stains.

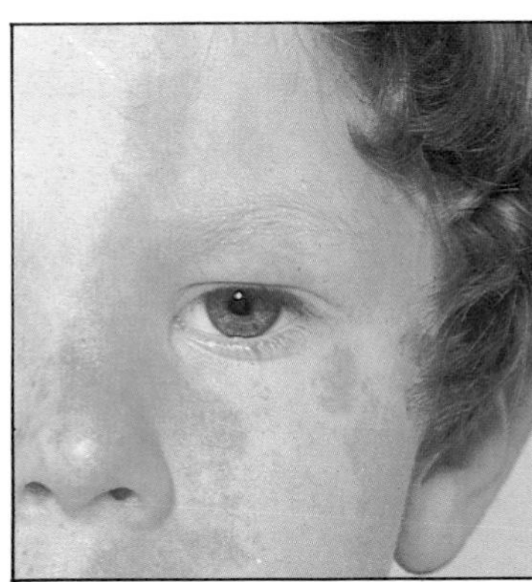

3 Pigmented spot

There are several types of pigmented spots. One, called a "cafe au lait" spot, is a flat patch of regularly darkened skin. It is harmless, but if several are present they should be examined by a physician for a hereditary disorder that may accompany this type of birthmark. Pigmented spots are usually small and occur singly. They tend to remain unchanged throughout life. Makeup can be used to cover them if necessary. In rare cases, especially if a pigmented spot is present at birth and changes later, it may need to be removed surgically.

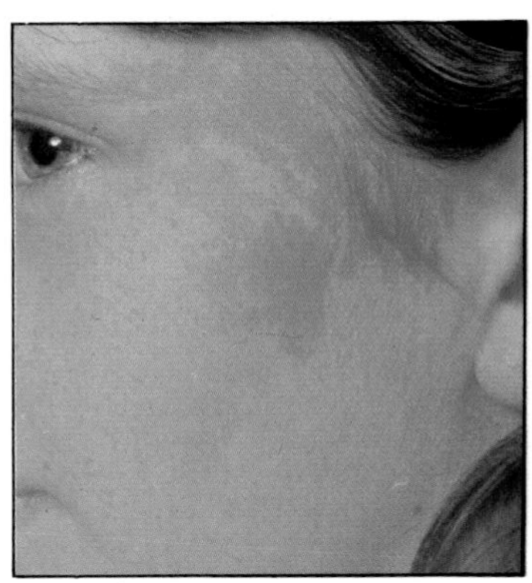

4 Diaper rash

Many babies have this redness around the thighs, buttocks, and genitals at some time. The rash varies in severity from slight redness to severe, bright-red inflammation. Urine, wetness, and stools irritate the skin. The skin also becomes sore and moist. For mild diaper rash, frequent changing of diapers is often sufficient treatment. Wash the baby's buttocks gently without scrubbing. Also, expose the baby's buttocks to warm air for a few hours each day, and apply a zinc oxide cream or over-the-counter diaper cream after every diaper change (see Diaper rash, p.696).

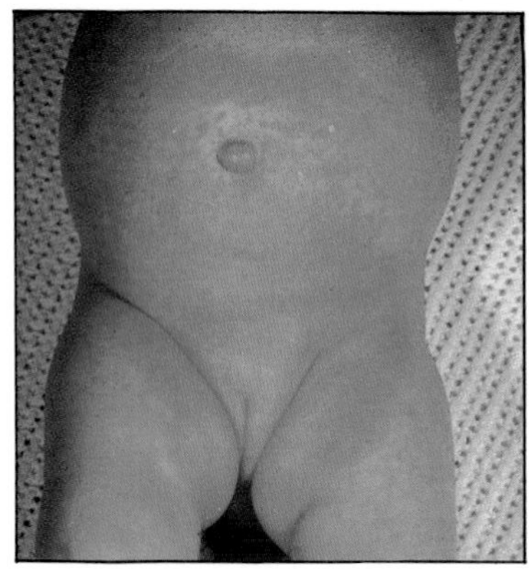

Severe diaper rash (above), if infected, may be treated with an antibiotic or mild corticosteroid ointment. A boy's foreskin may be inflamed, making urination difficult.

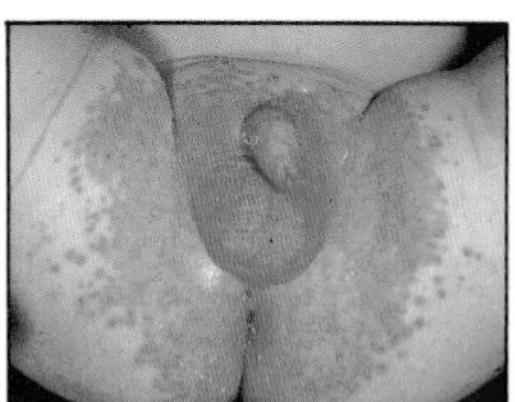

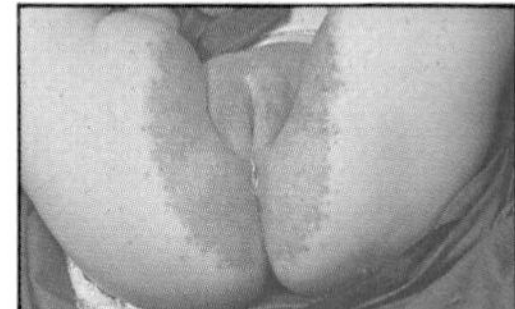

The photographs above show how the inflamed area is limited to the area of skin covered by the diaper.

Eczema in children

There are many types of eczema (also known as dermatitis). All are basically skin inflammations that usually itch. Babies with a tendency to have eczema are very sensitive to irritants. (See the articles on Eczema and dermatitis, p.269, Seborrheic dermatitis, p.269, and Infantile eczema, p.712.)

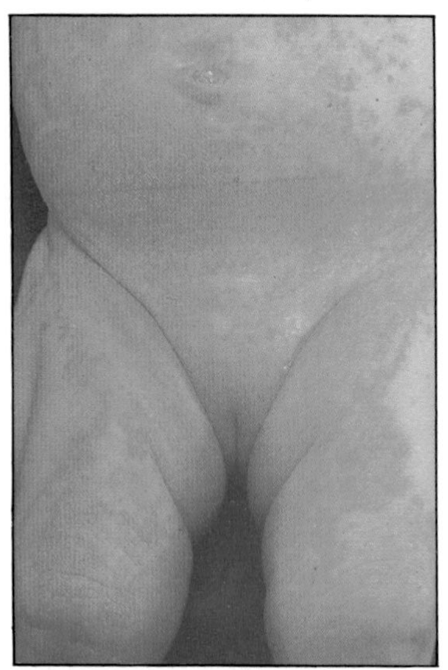

5 Seborrheic eczema in infants

This type of eczema usually takes the form of a red, scaly rash on the face and/or body (as shown above). It may also appear as yellowish, greasy-looking scales on the scalp, where it is known as "cradle cap." Seborrheic eczema appears during the first 3 months of life. Mild cases tend to clear up of their own accord, but occasionally a physician may prescribe a special cream to loosen the scales.

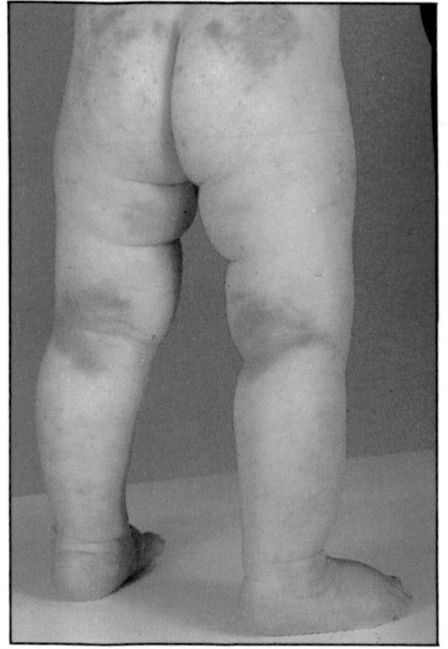

6 Infantile eczema

This red, itchy skin condition (shown in the photograph above) usually appears as a widespread rash in the first year of life, and improves as the child gets older. A mild case requires no specific treatment except regular applications of soothing creams or corticosteroid ointments. Hot water should not be used, but bathing the area with bath oil should do no harm. This type of eczema may persist.

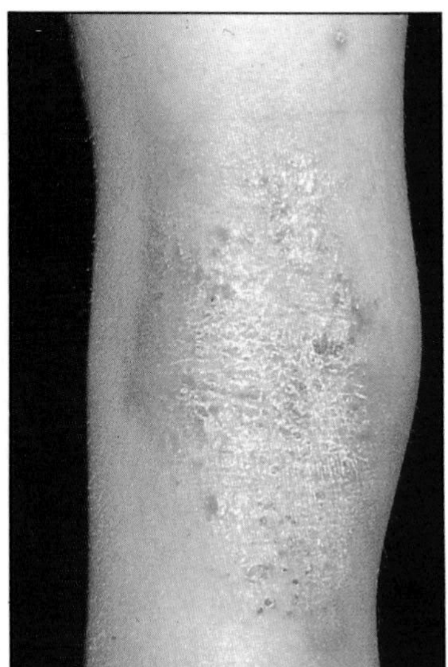

7 Skin changes in recurrent eczema

When eczema becomes a persistent problem, the skin in the affected areas may become dry, leathery, creased-looking, and either darker or lighter than the surrounding skin, as a result of recurrent inflammation and repeated rubbing. Crusting may form if the affected area is scratched. A common site for eczema is on the back of the leg (above). Such long-term skin changes may affect adults and children.

Adult skin problems

There are several types of eczema and dermatitis that occur in adults. Some of them are pictured here.

See the article on Eczema and dermatitis. p.269, for further information and descriptions.

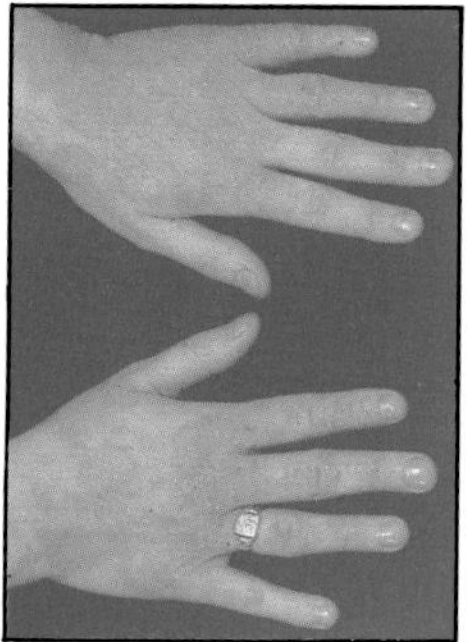

8 Irritant dermatitis

This type of dermatitis is common in adults who have sensitive skin and constantly handle irritant chemicals.

9 Dermatitis in older people

Many older people have dry skin, particularly on the legs, that may crack and itch. Applying moisturizing ointment or cream, avoiding hot water, and bathing with bath oil may help.

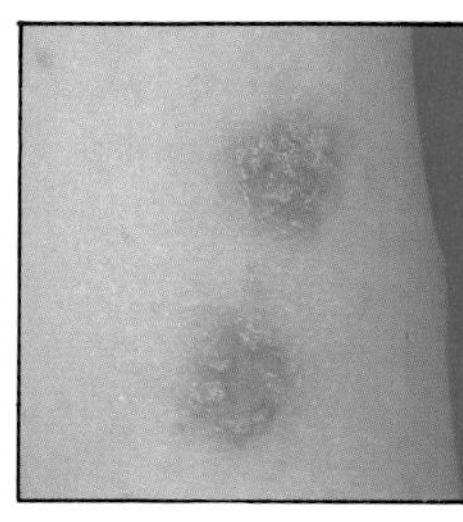

10 Nummular eczema

In nummular eczema, round, red, flaky patches form. The photograph above shows the crusting produced when fluid from the patches oozes and dries. It is relatively rare and may spread.

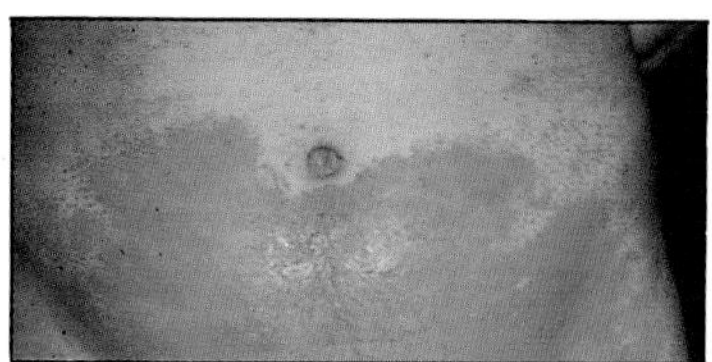

11 Seborrheic dermatitis on the body

Seborrheic dermatitis commonly appears on the scalp, the chest, or lower abdomen (above), as a red, flaky, itchy rash.

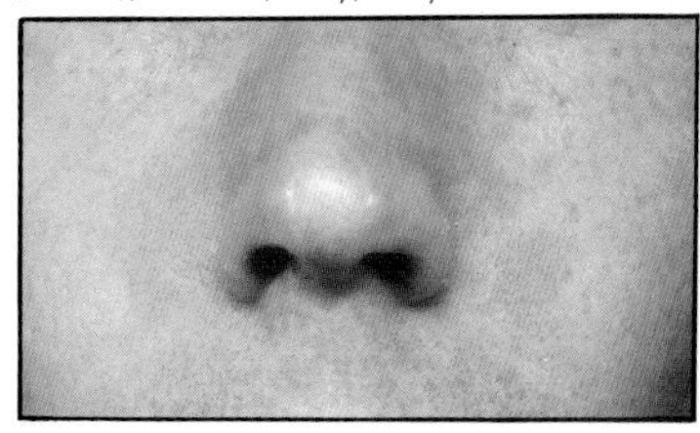

12 Seborrheic dermatitis on the face

Seborrheic dermatitis appears between the nose and cheeks, on the forehead, under the chin, and behind the ears.

Contact (allergic) dermatitis

Some types of eczema or dermatitis are caused by certain substances coming into contact with the skin. Touching the substance produces an itchy, flaky rash that is usually limited to the area of contact. This type of dermatitis may be accompanied by allergies to other substances (see Allergies, p.754). A substance that causes a very strong allergic reaction in one person may not cause any allergic reaction at all in someone else.

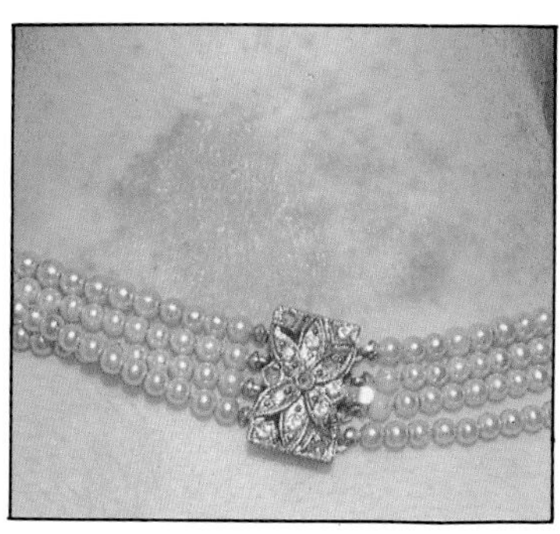

13 Metal contact

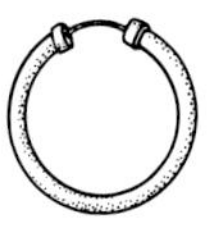

Some metals used to make items such as earrings, necklaces, watchbands, and rings cause contact dermatitis. Pure gold or silver rarely causes a reaction, but other metals may be mixed in. Nickel often causes dermatitis.

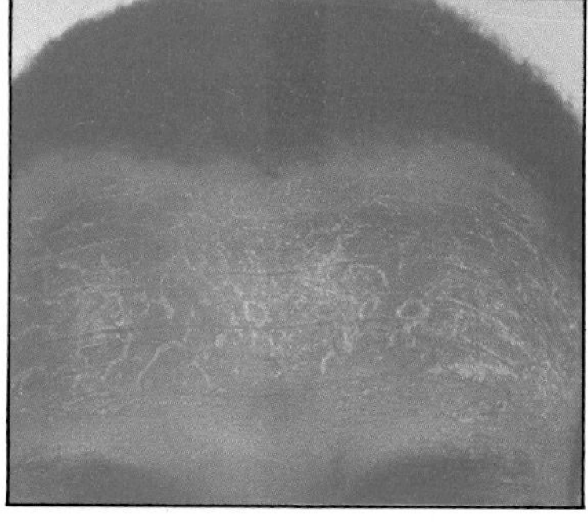

14 Hatband contact

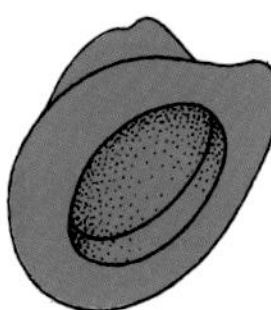

Some substances in fabric can occasionally produce contact eczema. The rash shown above was caused by material in the lining of a hat. The lining in gloves has also been known to cause contact eczema.

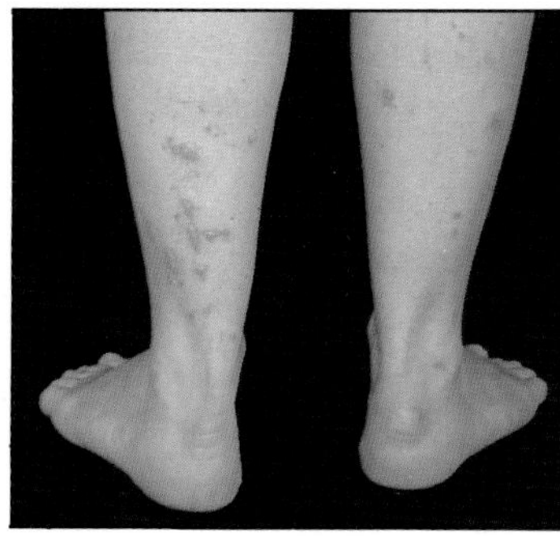

15 Plant contact

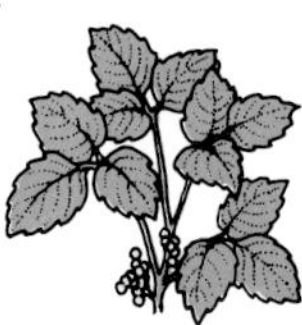

Touching certain plants such as poison ivy, poison oak, and poison sumac may cause severe cases of contact dermatitis. The rash may later spread from the area of contact to other parts of the body (above).

Allergic reactions

Many people have allergic reactions to external factors. Food, drugs, hair dyes, heat, and cold are all known causes. Itchy lumps appear on the skin. They can occur anywhere on the body and sometimes combine to cover large, patchy areas. Allergic reactions can be very uncomfortable but are usually harmless. However, in a severe reaction to hair dye or a sting in the head region, the scalp, face, and throat may swell dramatically, endangering breathing.

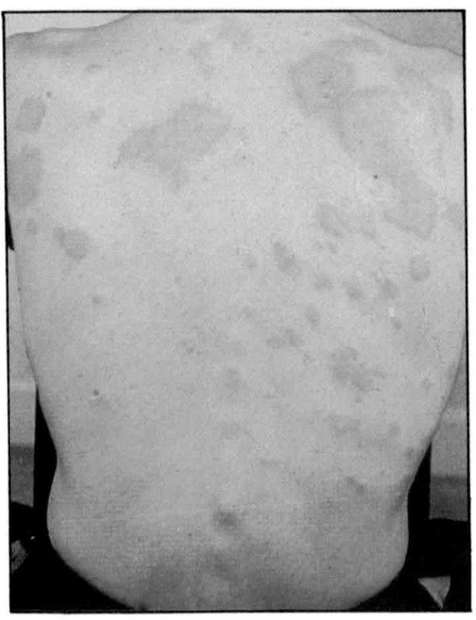

16 Hives

Hives (see p.272) is the most common form of allergic skin reaction. The rash usually takes the form of one or more raised, light-red patches called wheals (above), which have clearly defined edges and are itchy. They can occur anywhere on the body and usually disappear within a few hours, but may recur for longer periods. If the wheals cause persistent discomfort, a physician may prescribe antihistamine drugs.

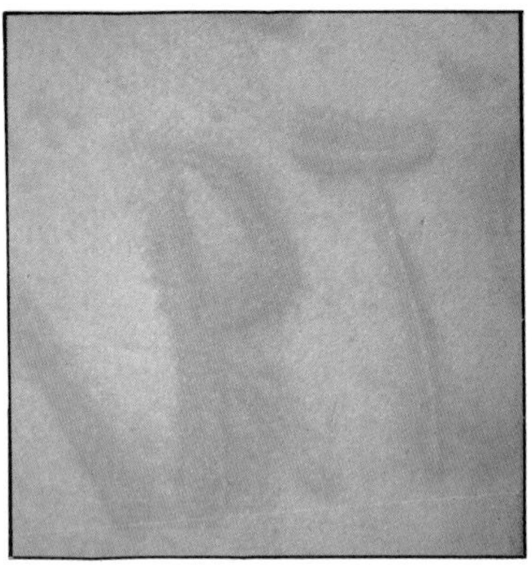

17 Dermographism

Dermographism is a type of hives usually caused by scratching the skin. It consists of long, raised, narrow wheals (above) that exactly follow the lines where scratching or rubbing has occurred. It is relatively easy to confirm the cause of this type of allergic reaction, even though sometimes the wheals do not appear on the skin until several hours after the irritation that caused the marks to form.

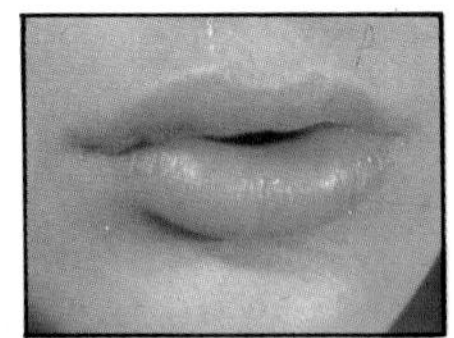

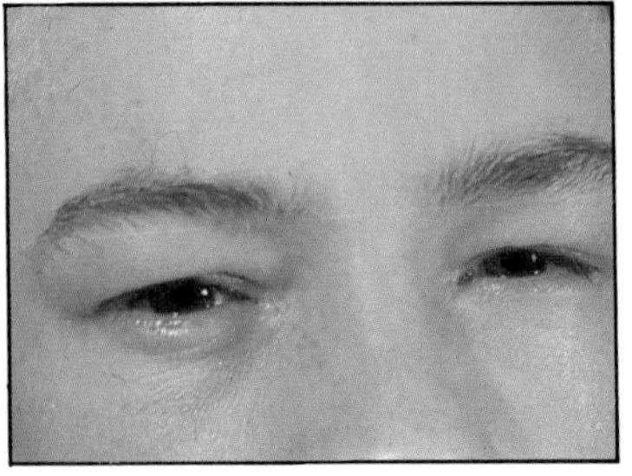

18 Angioneurotic edema

When hives affect the face, considerable swelling may result, especially around the eyes (above) and lips (top). In these circumstances there is a risk that the tissues on the inside of the throat may also swell and cause the person to suffocate. (For further information see the article on Hives, p.272.)

19 Pityriasis rosea

The patches that make up the pityriasis rosea rash have a slightly scaly surface. They look orangy-red in white skin, and dark brown in black skin. The condition is usually itchy and may persist for up to 2 to 3 months. It generally disappears by itself, though cream may be prescribed to relieve itching (see Pityriasis rosea, p.277).

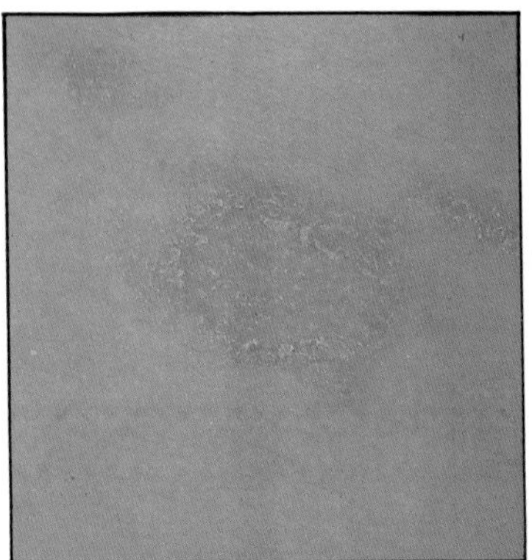

Pityriasis rosea starts as a single, oval patch, known as a herald patch, on the chest or back (above). Over the next few weeks several similar, but usually smaller, patches appear on the trunk (right), the upper arms, and the thighs.

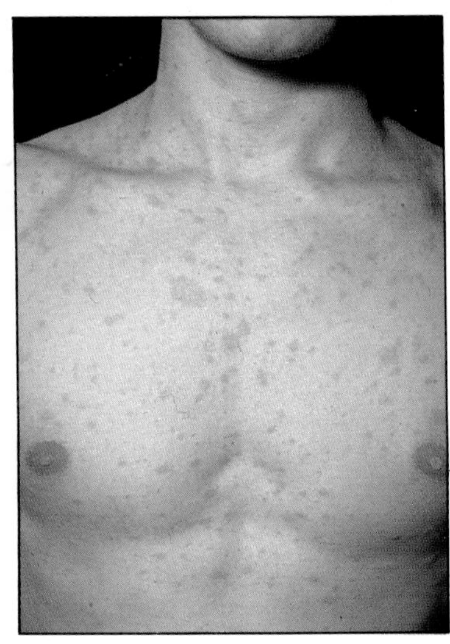

Bacterial and fungal infections

The skin is susceptible to several types of infection. Two of the most common are shown here: ringworm, which is caused by a fungus, not a worm; and impetigo, a fast-spreading bacterial infection. Most similar skin infections do not clear up, or clear up very slowly, unless you use a prescribed medication. It may be difficult for you to positively identify these infections by yourself, so if you seem to have one of them, consult your physician.

20 Ringworm

This fungal infection often appears as a red, itchy rash in the shape of a ring. It usually occurs on warm, moist areas such as the groin or under the breasts or between the buttocks (below). Within 2 weeks of the appearance of the first ring, other rings appear close to the first one. Ringworm is rarely a serious condition, but it heals more rapidly with professional help (see Ringworm, p.712).

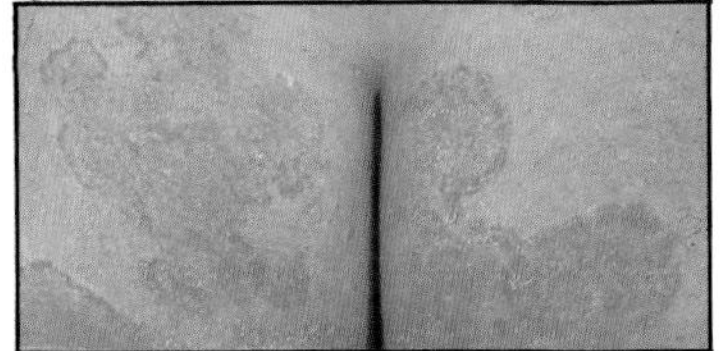

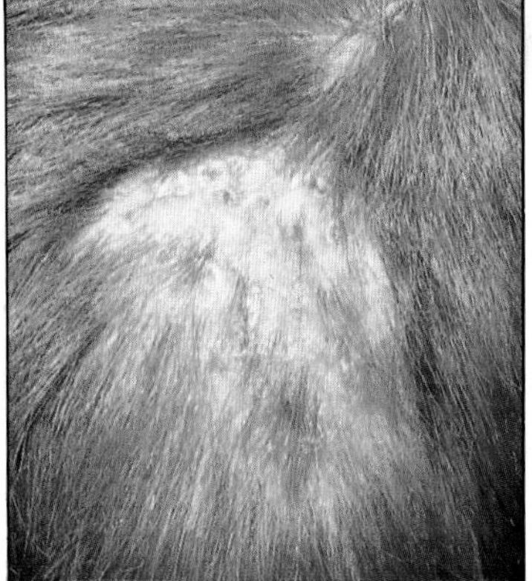

Ringworm on the scalp (above) can lead to temporary bald patches.

21 Animal ringworm

Some types of ringworm fungus that usually live on pets or wild animals can live on human skin. The ring (above) may appear on any part of the body and is likely to be more red or inflamed than the rings caused by human ringworm. It is treated in the same way, however. An infected pet should be treated by a veterinarian.

22 Impetigo

This bacterial infection most commonly affects the area around the nose and mouth. The appearance of groups of small blisters is the first sign of the condition. The blisters then burst to form a yellowish-brown crust. The infected area gradually spreads, and the condition usually has to be treated with antibiotic drugs.

Pictured at right is a case of impetigo at an early stage of the infection. The condition is shown at an advanced stage (far right), after the yellowish-brown crust has formed (see Impetigo, p.273).

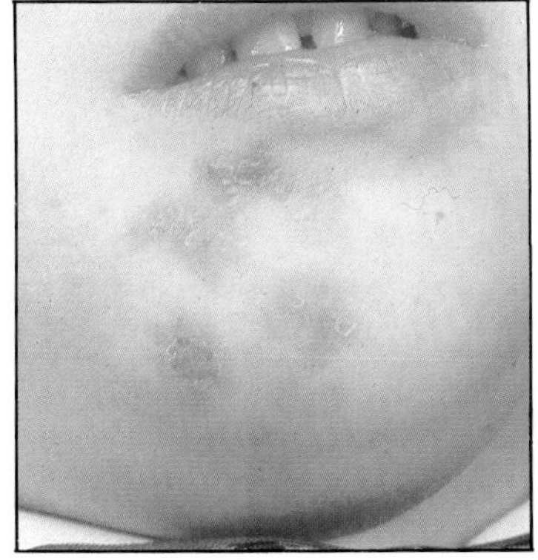

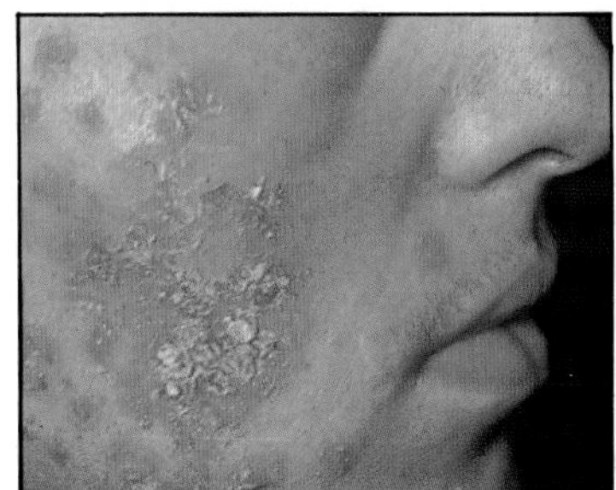

23 Boils

A boil is the result of a hair follicle's becoming infected and inflamed. It starts as a red, usually painful, lump that gradually becomes swollen with pus. A head forms and the pain generally increases, until eventually the boil bursts. Boils may occur anywhere on the body (see Boils and carbuncles, p.267).

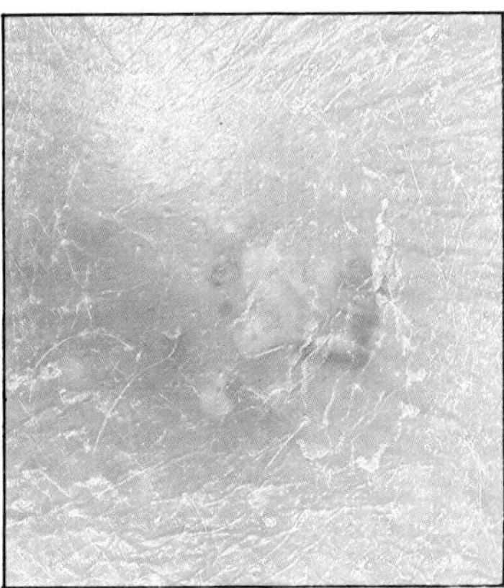

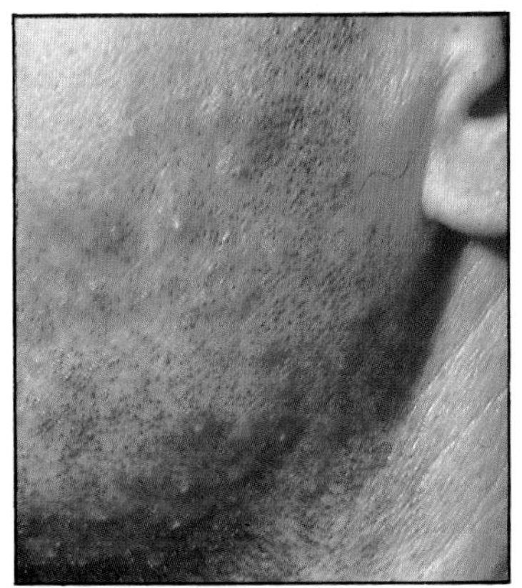

24 Cold sores

Cold sores are small blisters that are often found on the face, around the lips and nose. The blisters contain small areas of infection caused by a virus, herpes simplex. The infection occurs in two stages, as shown in the photographs below. These blisters tend to appear when you are feeling tired and run down, when you have some other infection such as a cold, or when you are exposed to wind or sunshine (see Cold sores, p.484).

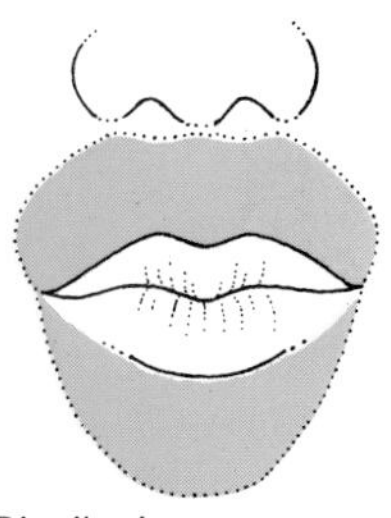

Distribution
Cold sores most commonly develop either around or on the lips.

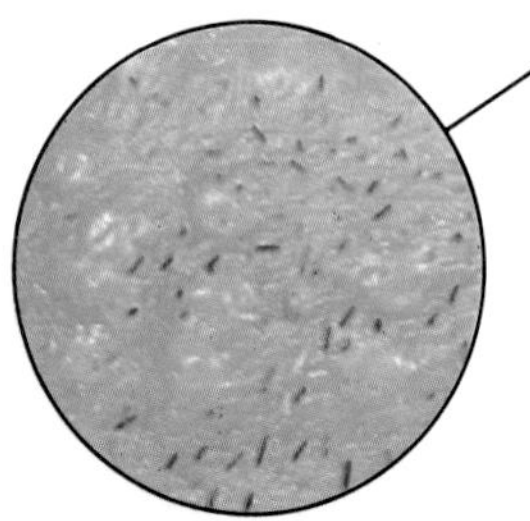

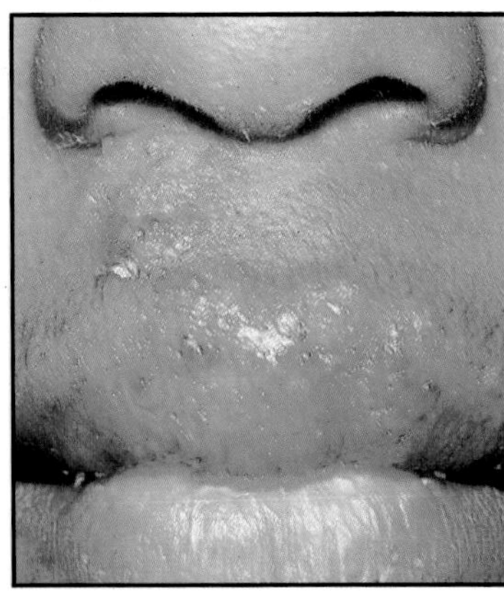

Early stages
In the early stages of cold sores, a group of tiny blisters appears (the inset photograph at left shows the blisters in more detail). Around the blisters is an area of red, inflamed skin. The early stage may produce little or no discomfort in a child; adults tend to have burning, itching, and pain.

Late stage
Within a few days of their appearance the blisters (shown above left) enlarge, burst, and dry out. The yellowish crust that forms (above) is similar in appearance to the crust that forms in impetigo (see p.273). If the cold sore blisters persist or recur, be sure to see your physician.

25 Shingles

Like cold sores (above), shingles is caused by a virus—in this case, a herpes virus, the same one that causes chickenpox (see opposite page). Before the rash appears, there is a burning or stabbing pain in the affected area (see Shingles, p.602).

Distribution
Shingles usually develops along a long, thin area on only one side of the body. The trunk and the face are the most common sites. On the trunk, the shingles rash often affects front and back.

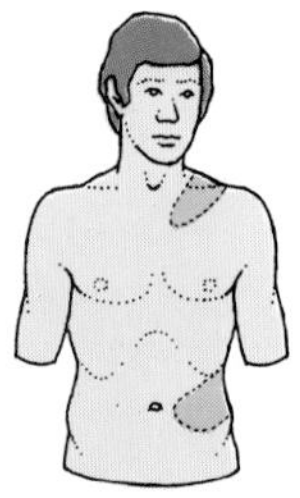

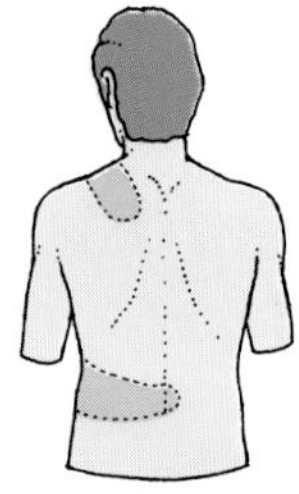

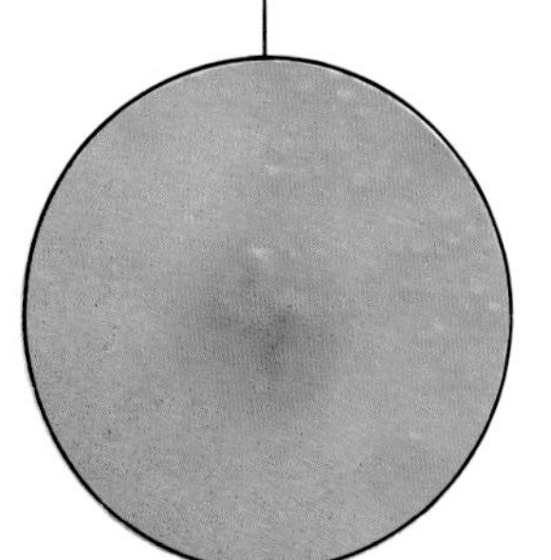

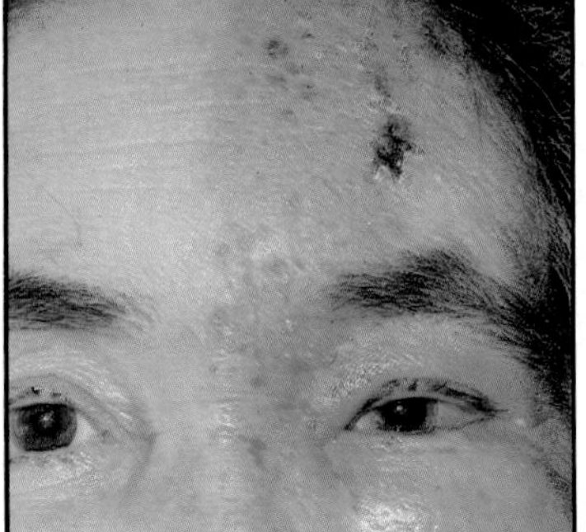

The shingles rash
The rash of shingles consists of numerous small blisters, shown in detail in the photograph at left. Within a week the blisters become dry and scab over. Then they slowly fade away. If the rash occurs near an eye (as shown above), it may cause severe pain, redness, and watering in the eye. If this occurs, see your physician without delay. When the rash affects the trunk (above left), it tends to occur in a long strip. If you have shingles more than once, see your physician.

Common childhood infections

Several infectious diseases are usually caught in childhood. Three common examples—measles, rubella, and chickenpox—are shown below. These three infections each produce a characteristic skin rash that aids identification.

These diseases can have serious complications, including encephalitis and birth defects. Be sure to consult your physician if you or your child appear to have one of them. See also Childhood infectious diseases, p.744.

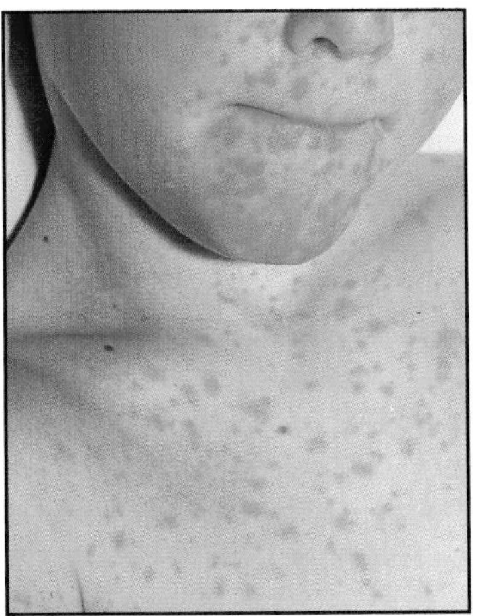

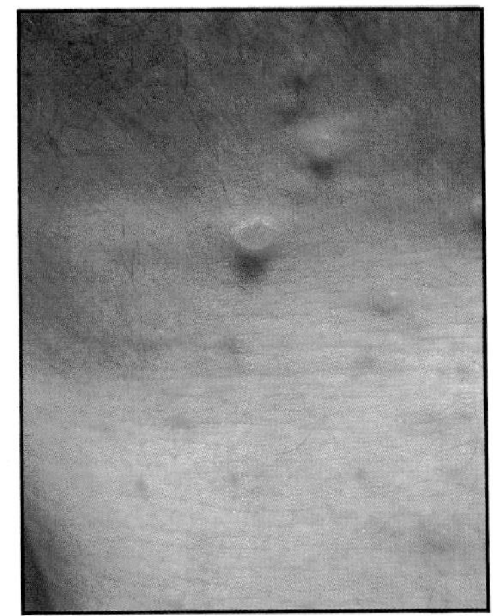

26 Measles

The rash of measles is flat, dark-pink spots that often join to form larger blotches (above). At first, the rash mainly affects the face, usually starting on the forehead and behind the ears. The rash spreads to cover the trunk (left) but it rarely appears on the arms or legs (see Measles, p.745).

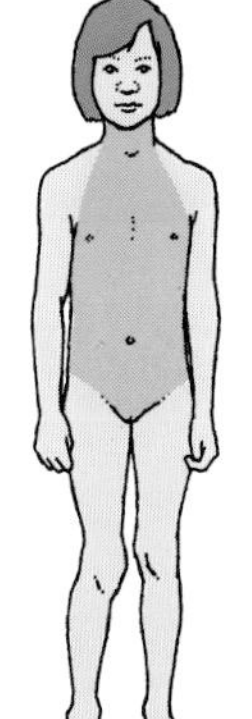

27 Rubella

The rash of rubella, or German measles (above), tends to be less severe than the measles rash (above left). Rubella produces tiny, light-red spots that merge to form an evenly colored patch. The rash usually covers the neck and trunk (left). It usually lasts only a few days (see Rubella, p.746).

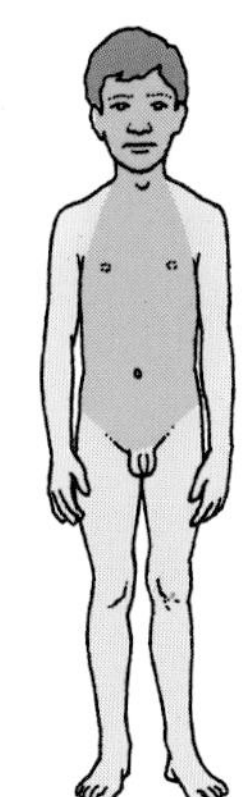

28 Chickenpox

This infection is caused by the same virus that is responsible for shingles (opposite page). The photograph above shows the characteristic small, fluid-filled blisters. The rash covers mainly the face and trunk (left). It can also affect the scalp, the inside of the mouth, the eyes, and the nose (see Chickenpox, p.747).

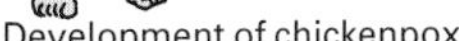

Development of chickenpox
There are three typical stages in the development of the chickenpox rash. In the first, tiny red spots appear. Then the spots enlarge and fill with fluid to form raised blisters. In the third stage the blisters burst, dry out, and crust over. They are very itchy.

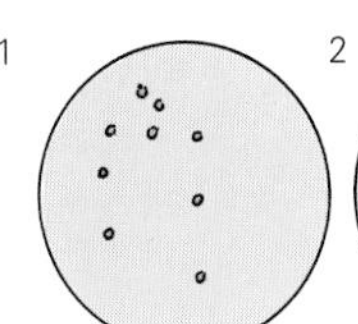

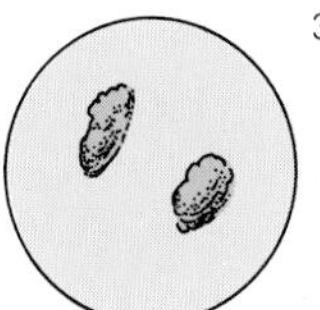

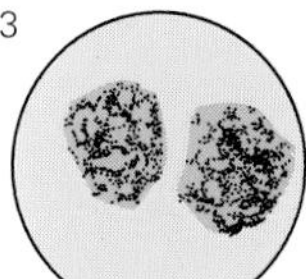

1 Small red spots
2 Fluid-filled blisters
3 Crusted scabs

29 Purpura

A "purpuric" rash may be produced by any of a number of disorders in which blood leaks through the walls of small blood vessels into the skin. The rash consists of many flat, dark-red or purplish spots or blotches. As with other rashes, colors vary by skin tone. See Thrombocytopenia, p.456, Allergic purpura, p.728, and Skin problems of older people, p.770.

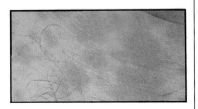

30 Acne

In acne there is persistent, recurrent development of various types of blemishes on the skin. The condition is extremely common during adolescence—slightly more so in young men—and in most cases, but not all, it fades away during the late teens or early twenties. (For further information see Acne, p.271.)

Distribution

Acne pimples commonly appear on the face, mainly around the mouth, and often on the chest, shoulders, neck, and the upper (and occasionally lower) portion of the back.

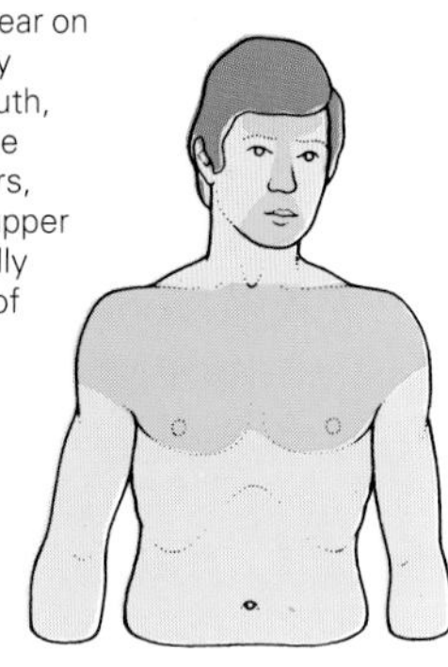

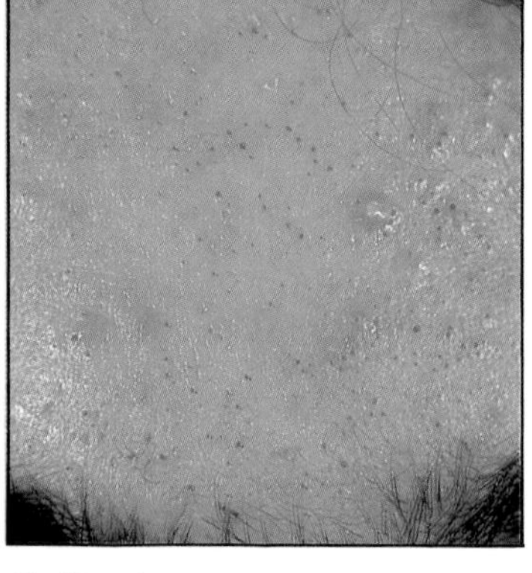

Blackheads

One type of pimple that appears in acne is the blackhead (photograph above). The black area for which it is named is a tiny plug of dark material stuck in a skin pore. Some experts believe the plug is a mixture of keratin and sebum and the color is melanin (the skin pigment). The "black" of the blackhead is not dirt. Blackheads rarely become inflamed unless they are picked at or squeezed.

Pimples

The typical pimples that occur in acne (photograph above) may develop from blackheads (above left). Others develop from whiteheads. If picked or scratched, the pimples may become infected and pus-filled. Some acne pimples are just small red lumps; others have white tops. They tend to develop and then fade over several weeks.

A pimple develops

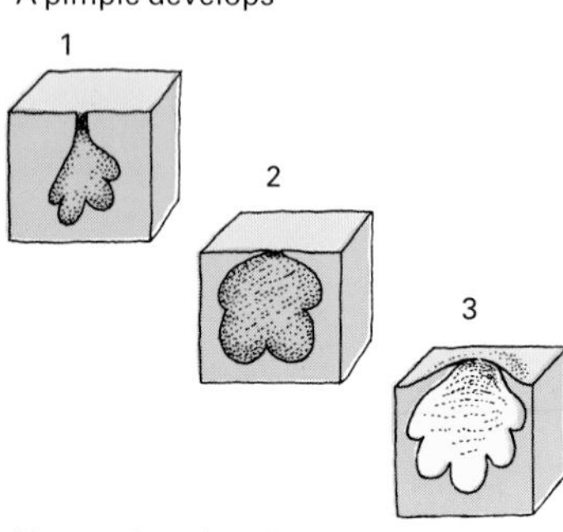

The opening of a sebaceous, or oil-producing, gland near the surface of the skin becomes blocked (1). There is a build-up of oily sebum within the gland (2). This accumulation leads to localized inflammation (redness and swelling) (3).

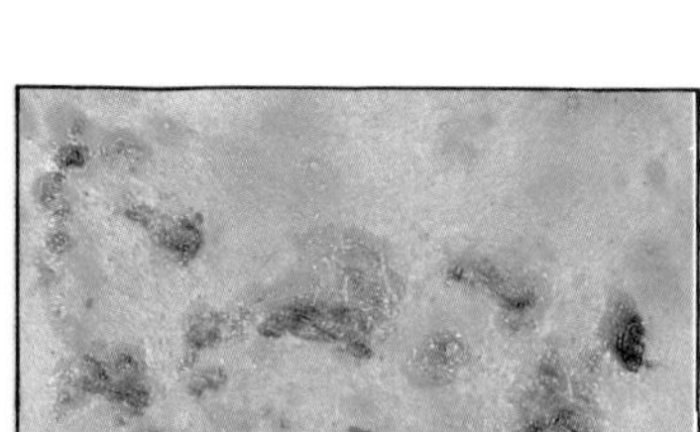

Severe acne

The most severe form of acne produces painful, fluid-filled lumps called cysts under the skin (photograph left). The cysts may be up to ¾ in (about 2 cm) across, often persist for many weeks, and may leave pitted, scarred areas of skin.

31 Rosacea

Rosacea, formerly called acne rosacea, occurs mainly in adults. The skin on the face, principally the cheeks and the nose, becomes abnormally red and flushed. After a time, pus-filled raised spots may also appear in the affected skin. Why this occurs is not known. The rash tends to spread or become more prominent after eating hot or spicy food, or drinking alcohol or beverages containing caffeine. Rosacea is most common in women over 30 years of age (see Acne vulgaris and rosacea, p.271).

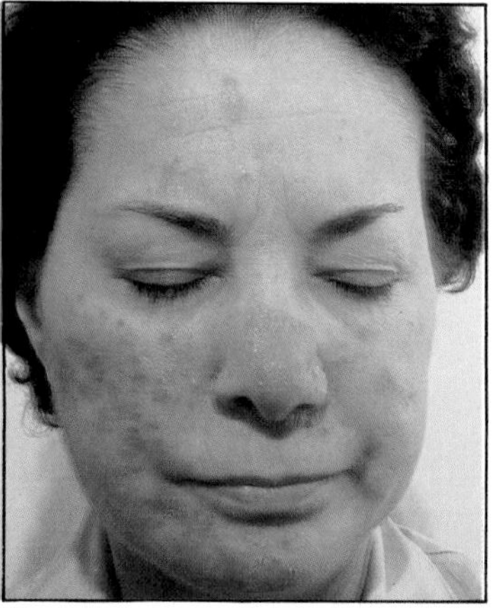

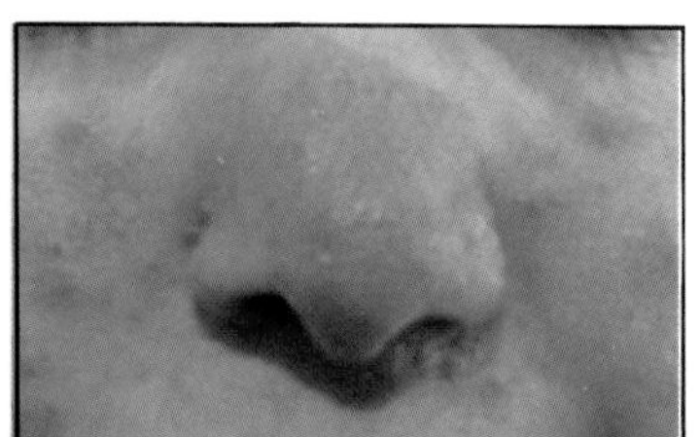

Distribution

Most people who get rosacea have the rash on their cheeks (right). The nose may also be severely affected (shown in more detail above).

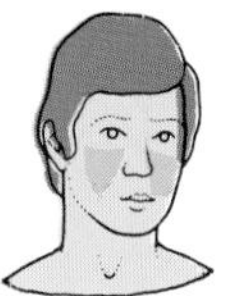

Abnormal skin formation

A number of skin conditions, some of which are shown below, are characterized by a fault in the normal maintenance of skin tissue. Although not always harmful to physical health, these conditions can cause embarrassment because they are unattractive. This often leads to considerable emotional stress.

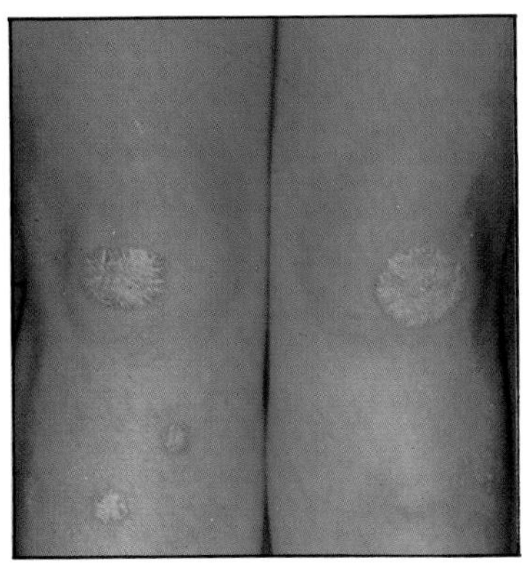

32 Psoriasis

Psoriasis consists of patches of thickened, silvery-white, scaly skin (photograph above). The patches often have a red rim. Skin affected by psoriasis generally causes little itching, but in a few cases it may be sore (see Psoriasis, p.271, for further information).

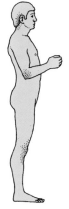

Distribution
Common sites for psoriasis are the knees, elbows, and scalp.

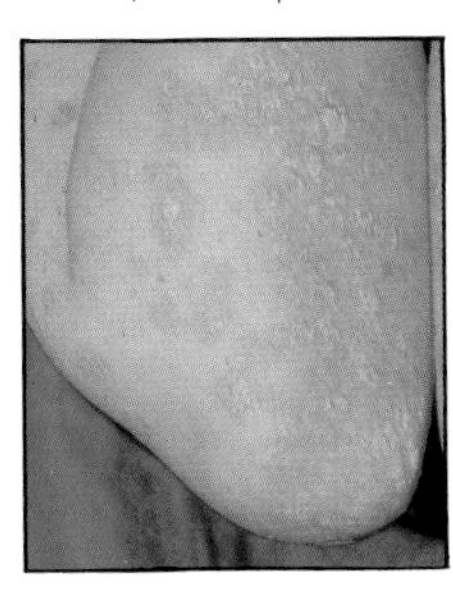

Severe psoriasis
In more severe cases of psoriasis (photograph above) the characteristic small patches join together to produce a more extensive area of affected skin. The fingernails and toenails (see p.282) become stippled, thickened, and roughened.

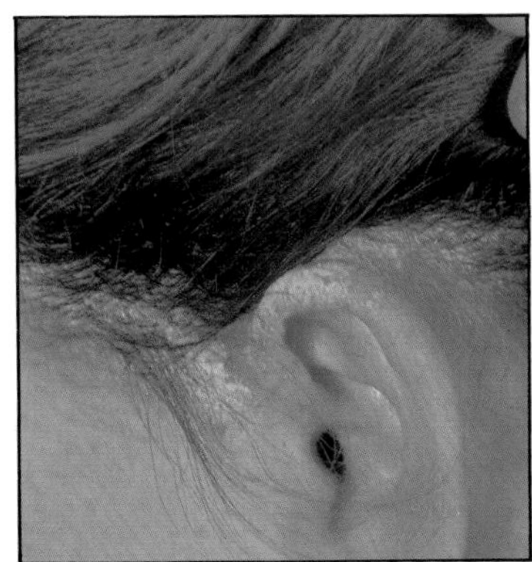

Psoriasis of the scalp
When psoriasis occurs on the scalp, scaly, sometimes lumpy, patches appear. In most cases the hair of the scalp remains unaffected, but sometimes temporary hair loss occurs. It is rare for psoriasis to spread from the scalp to the face.

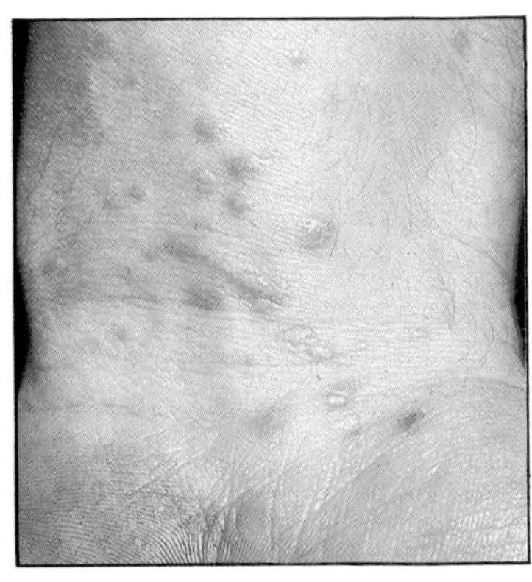

33 Lichen planus

This skin condition is extremely variable in appearance. In one typical example (photograph above), a rash of numerous, tiny, purplish-red lumps appears on the inside of the wrist. The lumps are not scaly, but you may be able to see small white marks on the surface of the skin. The cause of the condition is not known (for further information see Lichen planus, p.278).

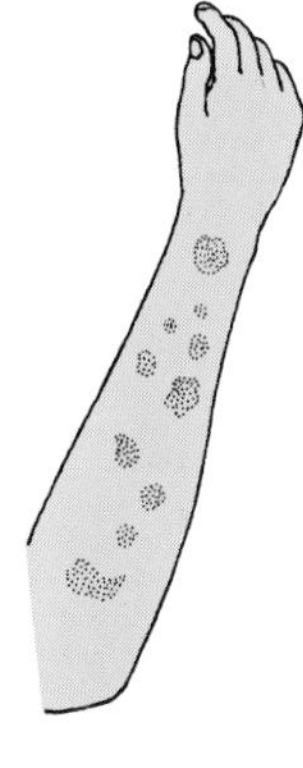

Distribution
Lichen planus may occur anywhere on your body, but the most usual sites are the wrists, arms (above), and legs. It often also appears on the lining of the mouth (see Oral lichen planus, p.485).

Scar tissue

Whenever the skin is damaged, it is repaired by scar tissue. Scar tissue is formed by special cells called fibroblasts that manufacture collagen and other protein substances. The material they produce is stronger and tougher than ordinary skin, but tends to shrink slightly with age.

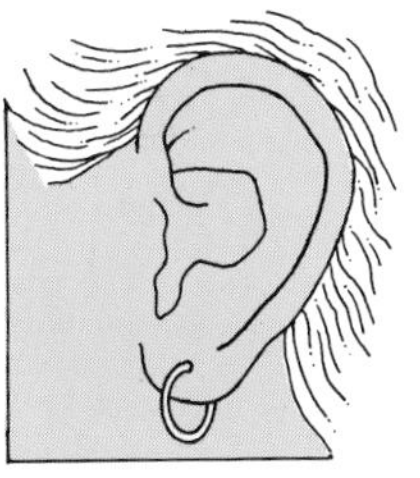

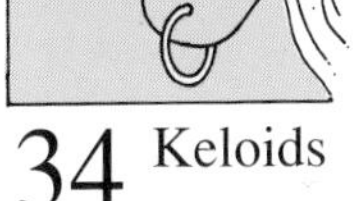

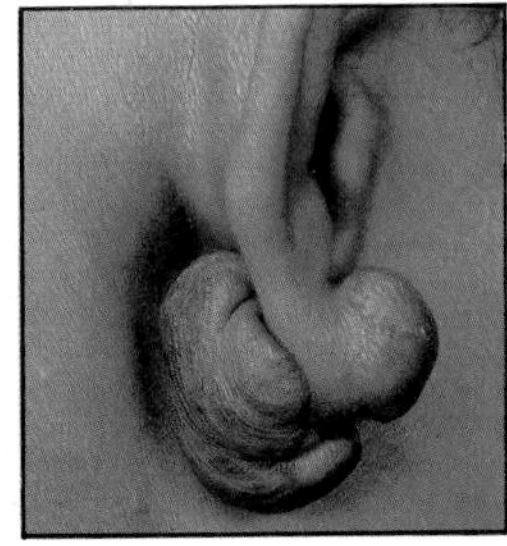

34 Keloids

A keloid is formed because of an abnormality in the mechanism for producing scar tissue. The scar tissue does not stop growing. Keloids can develop after an operation, a vaccination, or an injury. Even an ear lobe pierced for an earring (above left) may form a keloid (above right). The growths are more common in blacks than whites (see Keloid, p.277).

Warts and moles

Warts and moles are not related conditions, but they are sometimes confused because they look alike. Warts are small areas of long-standing viral infection. Moles are areas of skin that are heavily pigmented with melanin, the substance responsible for skin color. Warts vary in appearance. Some common types are shown below. Warts are harmless but may be a nuisance. A mole that is present from birth may develop into a malignant melanoma (opposite page). If this occurs it should be removed by a physician.

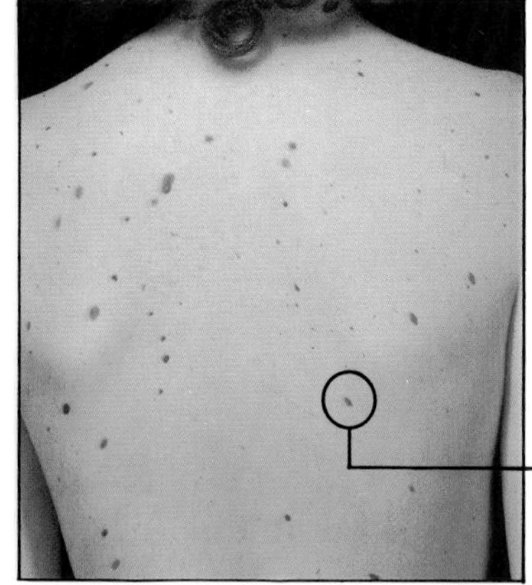

35 Moles

Moles can occur anywhere on the body. They are small, roughly circular areas of skin that are much darker than the surrounding skin. Large moles may have coarse hairs growing out of them. Some moles are present from birth. In some people a few develop during childhood.

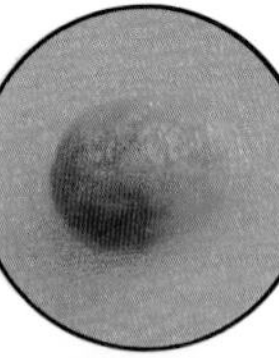

Appearance
The dark patch that constitutes a mole may be flat or raised above the surrounding skin (inset photograph left).

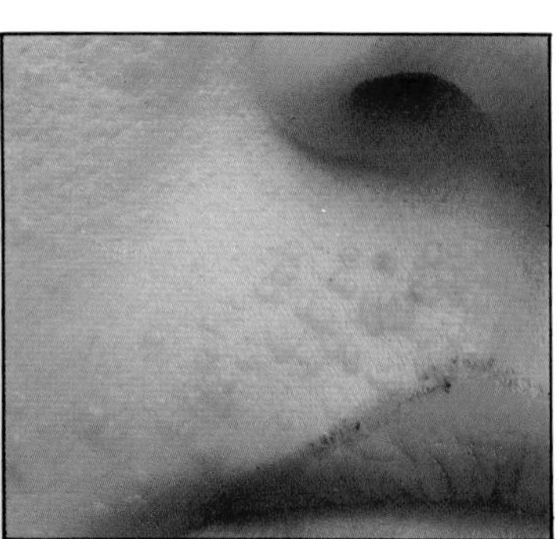

36 Plane warts

Plane warts are flat-topped, brownish spots that usually have a smooth surface. They often appear in groups, and may develop on the face or the back of the hand along the line of a scratch. This type of wart is most commonly seen in children and young adults. Plane warts (photograph above) commonly occur on the skin near the upper lip (see Warts, p.268).

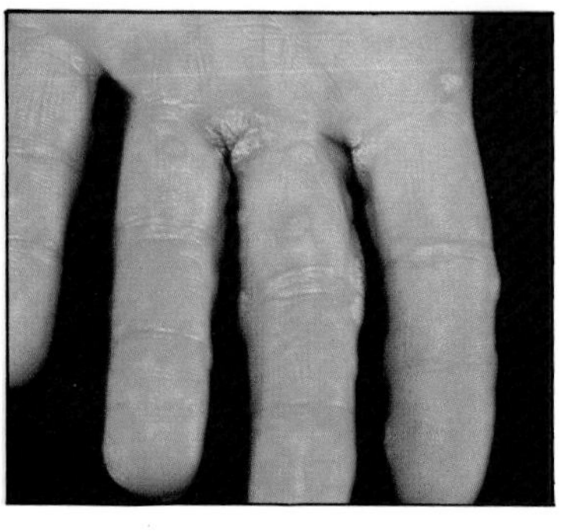

37 Common warts

This type of wart usually grows on the hands (photograph above) or on the feet (where they are known as plantar warts – see p.253). The typical common wart is a hard lump with a roughened, cauliflower-like surface. Tiny black flecks may be visible in the body of the wart.

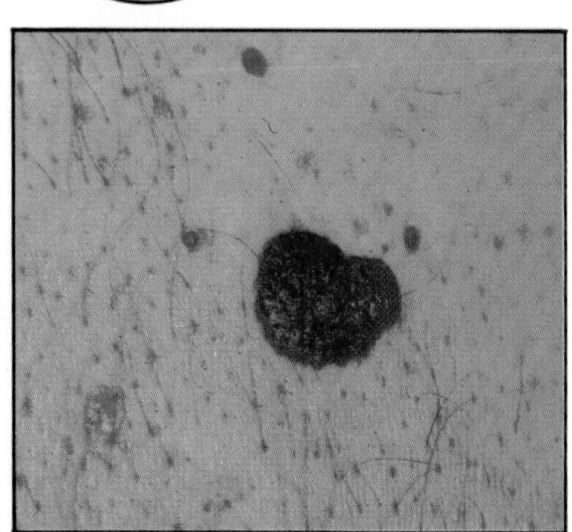

38 Seborrheic keratosis

These growths (above) are dark, sometimes rough-surfaced, lumps that often appear on the skin in large numbers in later life. They are harmless, but because some may look fairly dark and similar to malignant melanoma, you should have your dermatologist check them (see Abnormal skin pigmentation, p.278).

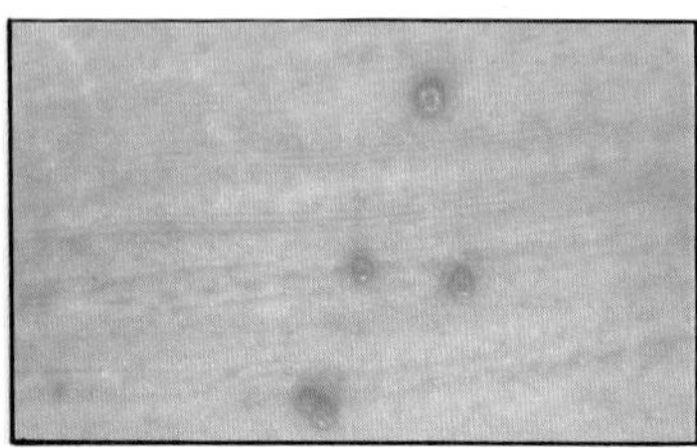

39 Molluscum contagiosum

These tiny, pale lumps are filled with cheesy material. They are not true warts, but like warts, they are caused by a viral infection. They appear in groups, especially in children with eczema, and are passed among adults as a sexually transmitted infection.

40 Sebaceous cysts

These cysts (right) are sometimes mistaken for warts, although they are not related. A sebaceous cyst typically appears as a soft, smooth, yellowish lump just under the surface of the skin. Sometimes a tiny dark dot can be seen in the skin over the center of the cyst. The scalp is a common site for these harmless growths (see Sebaceous cysts, p.276).

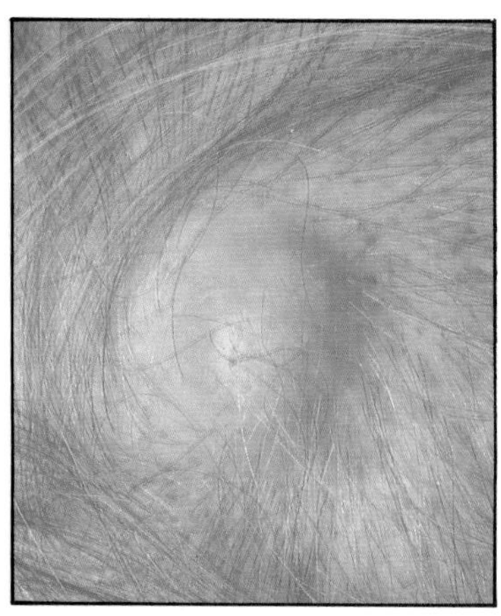

Skin cancers

There are three main types of malignant, or life-threatening, skin growths. These are basal cell carcinoma, squamous cell carcinoma, and malignant melanoma. Skin cancers tend to be somewhat variable in appearance. As with most other malignant growths, early diagnosis and removal offer a good chance of cure. For this reason, always report any suspicious lump, sore, or ulcer on the skin to your physician if it persists for more than a week.

41 Basal cell carcinoma

This type of skin cancer tends to grow very slowly and rarely, if ever, spreads. It is variable in appearance. One common version (right) is the ulcerated (open-sore) form (see Basal cell carcinoma, p.274).

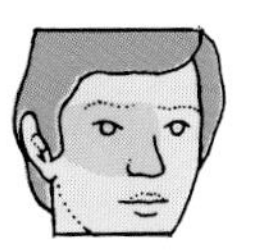

Common sites
Basal cell carcinomas usually appear on the face (left), near an eye, or next to the nose.

Encrusted type
A basal cell ulcer can form a scab (round photograph right). When the scab detaches, the ulcer is revealed again.

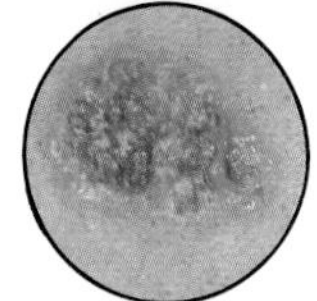

Cystic type
A cystic type of basal cell carcinoma growing on the bridge of the nose appears as a relatively smooth, skin-colored lump (photograph above). The lump gradually enlarges and may have blood vessels visible on the surface.

42 Squamous cell carcinoma

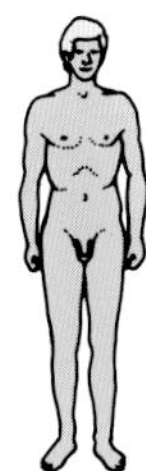

Common sites
Squamous cell growths commonly occur in areas exposed to the sun but may occur anywhere on the body (see Squamous cell carcinoma, p.275).

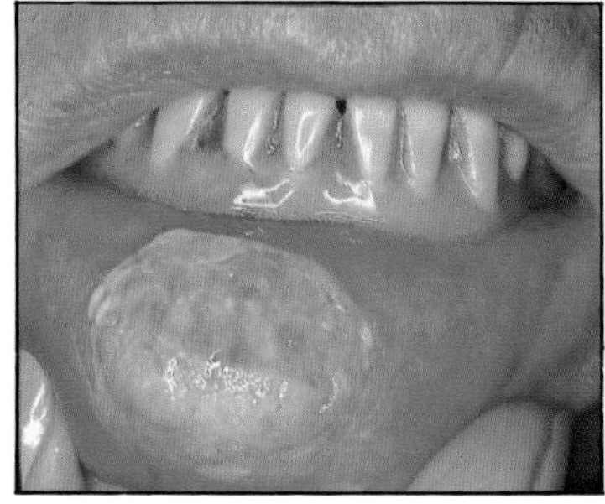

Ulcerated type
A typical ulcerated type of squamous cell carcinoma (above) is a persistent open sore that gradually enlarges.

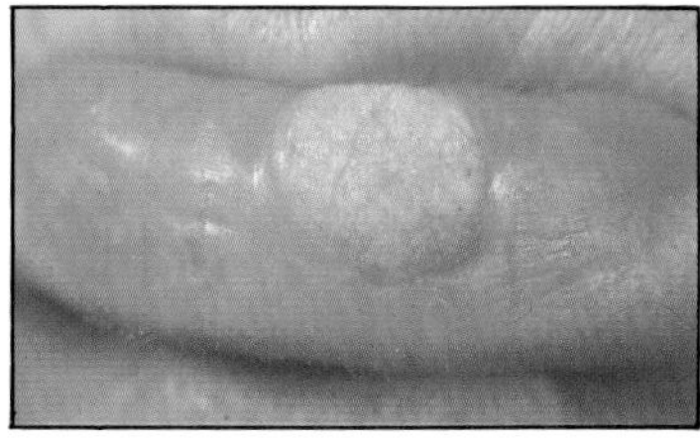

Warty type
Squamous cell carcinoma sometimes appears as a small, hard nodule that gradually enlarges into a wartlike lump (above). Like the ulcerated type (left), the warty type of squamous cell carcinoma is not usually painful.

43 Malignant melanoma

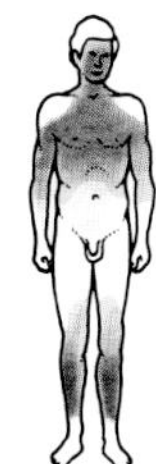

Common sites
Malignant melanomas can occur on any part of the body and are associated with exposure to strong sunlight. The most common sites are the face, upper trunk, and legs. Because they can arise from preexisting moles, see your physician or dermatologist immediately if you notice any of the changes shown (right), or if you discover a new mole.

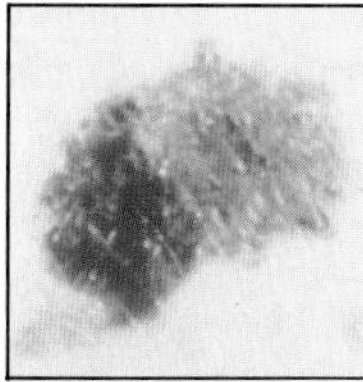

A: Asymmetry
One half of a mole looks different (it may be darker) than the other half.

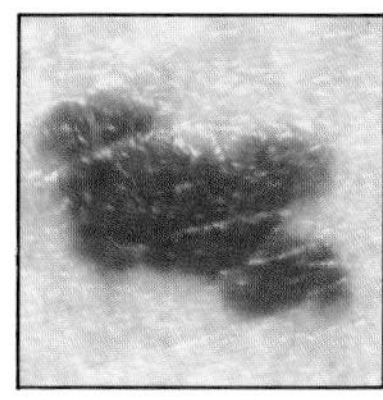

B: Border
The outline of the mole may be irregular or have poorly defined edges. Not all melanomas protrude above the surface of the skin.

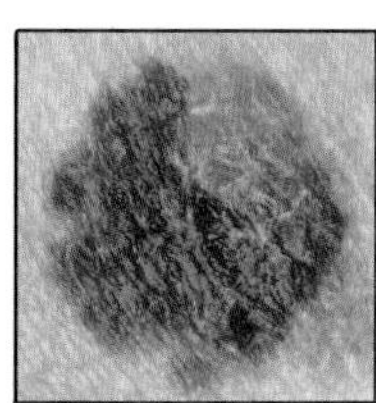

C: Color
Although usually very dark, raised lumps, some melanomas have shades of tan, brown, or even white, red, or blue. Some may bleed.

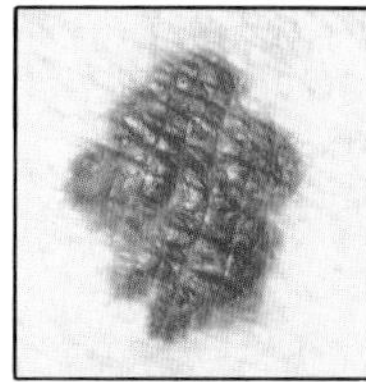

D: Diameter
If the mole grows or is larger than 1/2 in (6 mm) across—about the width of a pencil eraser—consult your physician.

Abnormal skin coloration

In these conditions, there is an abnormality in the natural coloring of the skin. The conditions are not harmful to general health but may, particularly in the case of vitiligo, cause mental or emotional stress because of their appearance (see Abnormal skin pigmentation, p.278).

44 Vitiligo

In vitiligo irregularly shaped patches of skin on certain parts of the body (drawing right) lose their normal color and become much paler than the surrounding skin (photograph right). The nature of the skin surface and its texture do not change. The cause of the condition is not clearly understood, but it may be an autoimmune problem — that is, a disorder of the body's natural defense system. If the appearance of the patches is embarrassing, you can apply a special makeup to hide them.

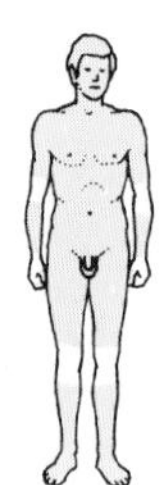

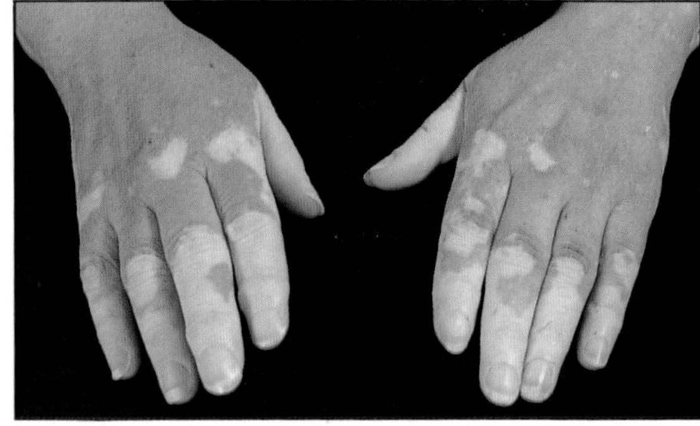

In vitiligo patches of depigmented skin are often symmetrically placed on either side of the body. When vitiligo occurs on the scalp, hairs in the affected area may turn white.

45 Perfume pigmentation

Some perfumes, colognes, and aftershaves contain chemicals that, when exposed to sunlight, temporarily increase pigmentation in the skin where they are applied. The skin returns to normal once you discontinue the use of the chemical. The neck (right) may be particularly susceptible to this effect. Some individuals are more susceptible to this condition than others.

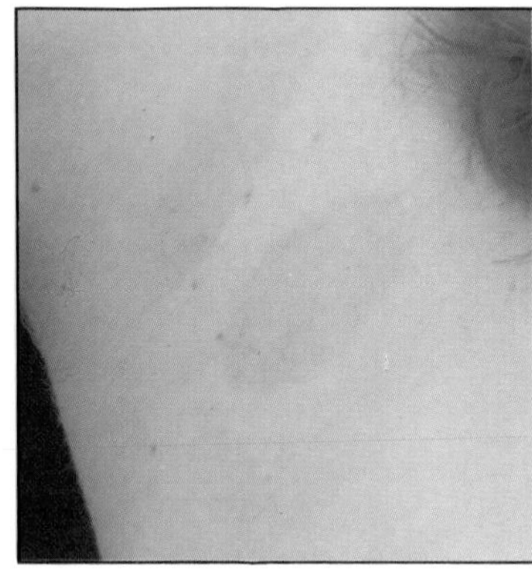

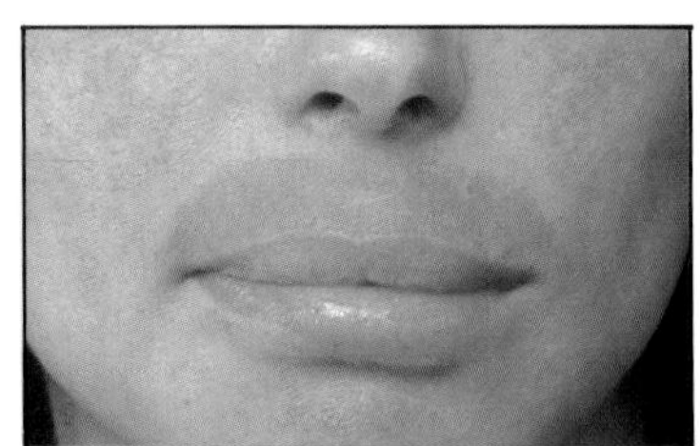

46 Chloasma

This condition may result from hormonal changes such as those caused by oral contraceptives, pregnancy, or cirrhosis of the liver. Patches of skin become darker.

47 Jaundice

Skin color

Jaundice is not a disease, but a sign of one of several underlying diseases (see Jaundice, p.522). It results from a build-up in the blood of bilirubin, a yellowish-brown substance that is normally extracted from the bloodstream by the liver and excreted in bile. In jaundice, the skin takes on a yellowish or greenish tinge (photograph right). The whites of the eyes also turn yellow (far right). The development of jaundice symptoms always requires the attention of a physician.

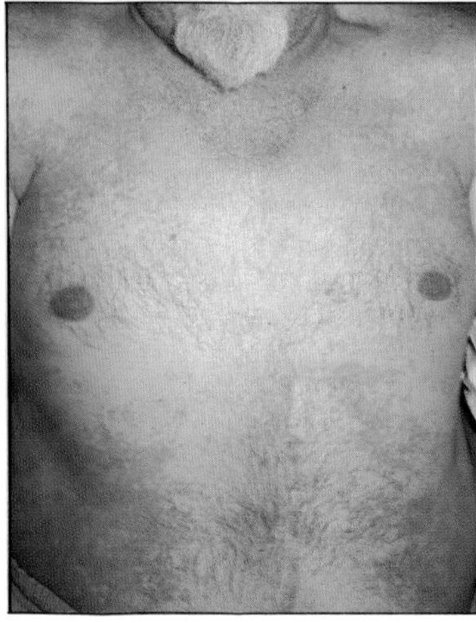

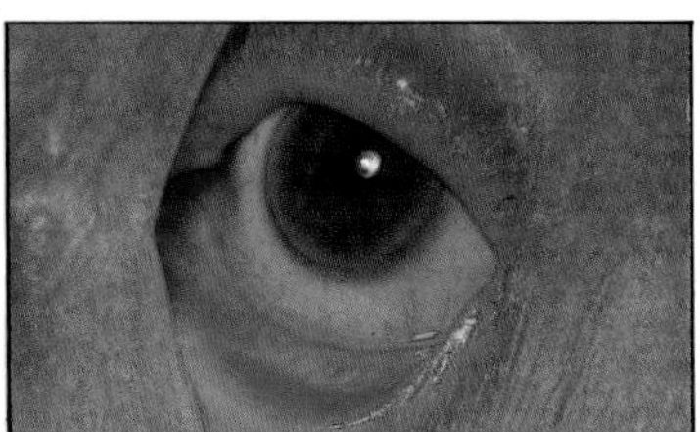

Eye color

Besides yellowing of the skin (left), jaundice also causes the whites of the eyes to take on a yellowish color (above). The change in eye coloration is a more reliable sign of jaundice than yellowing of the skin.

Common foot disorders

Athlete's foot and verrucas (warts) are common and harmless but irritating. Most other foot problems are also minor, but older people and those with diseases that may affect circulation (for example, diabetes) should not neglect sores, cuts, and other foot conditions, because they may become serious without attention.

48 Athlete's foot

Athlete's foot (right) is a fungal infection in which the skin of the foot becomes damp, inflamed, and itchy. The infection particularly affects the skin between and underneath the toes. The skin may peel and crack, sometimes producing sore areas. In severe cases (far right) the nails are also infected and look thickened and discolored (see Athlete's foot, p.272).

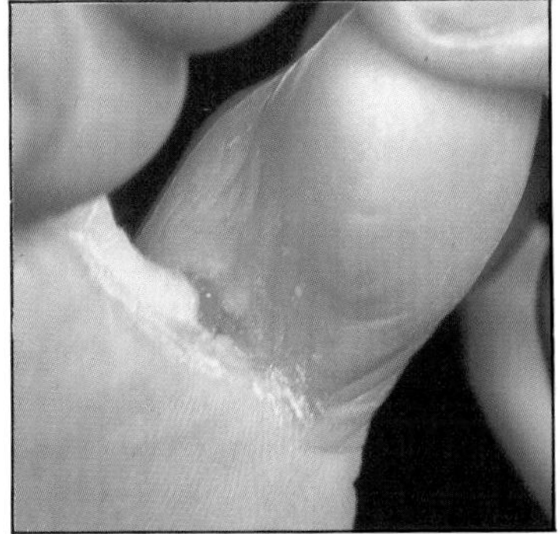

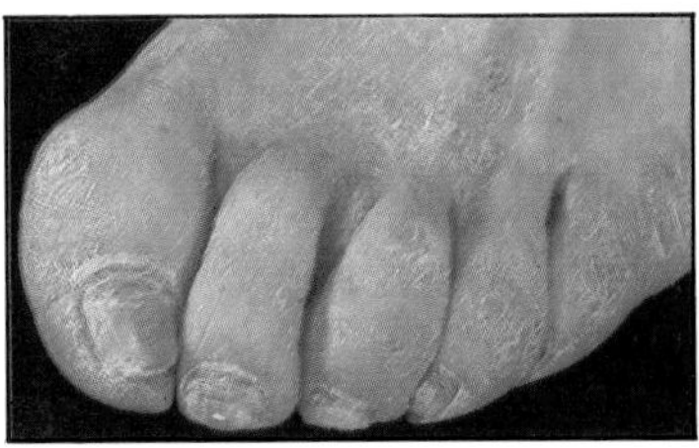

An example of severe athlete's foot that has affected the toenails.

49 Plantar wart

The plantar wart is also called the common wart (or verruca) and appears on the sole of the foot (see Warts, p.268, and Warts and moles, p.250). Unlike other warts, the plantar wart does not usually grow as a raised lump. It is a flat area of hard, tough skin. Despite its flatness, walking on a plantar wart often feels like walking with a stone in your shoe.

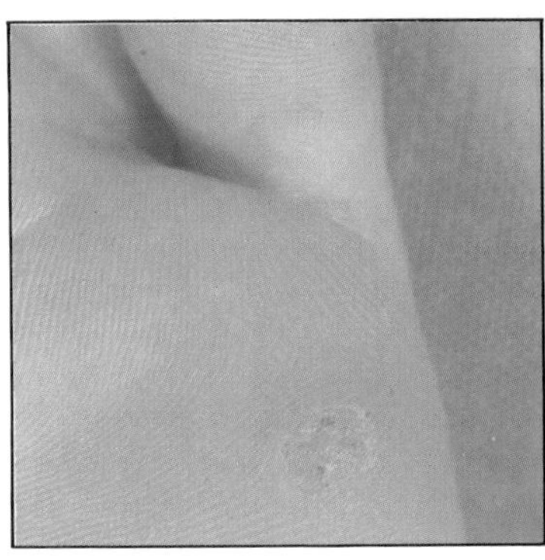

How a plantar wart develops

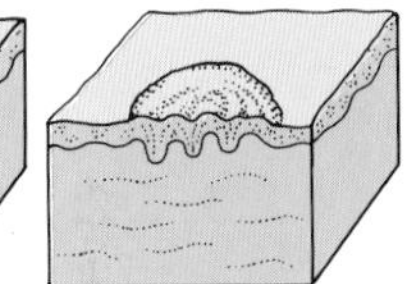

When a plantar wart first grows, it may be a raised lump like a common wart elsewhere on the body (1). It soon becomes pushed into the surface of the skin (2), which makes it more difficult to treat.

Common nail disorders

Some disorders, such as psoriasis, may affect the nails as well as the skin. In other cases, such as paronychia, it is only the nails, and perhaps the cuticles and nail beds, that are involved (see Deformed and discolored nails, p.282).

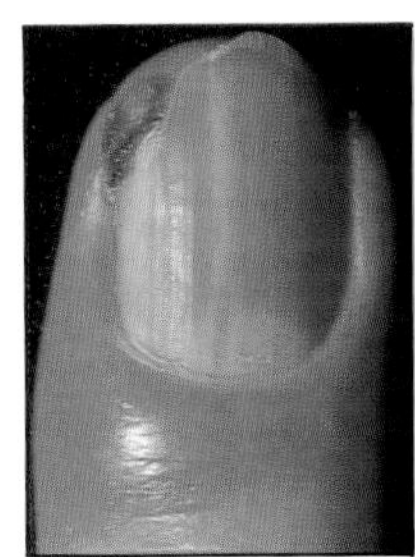

51 Paronychia

In this nail disorder the cuticles and nail fold become swollen and inflamed as a result of infection by bacteria (left) or fungi. If the problem persists, the nail itself may become darkened and deformed (see Paronychia, p.281).

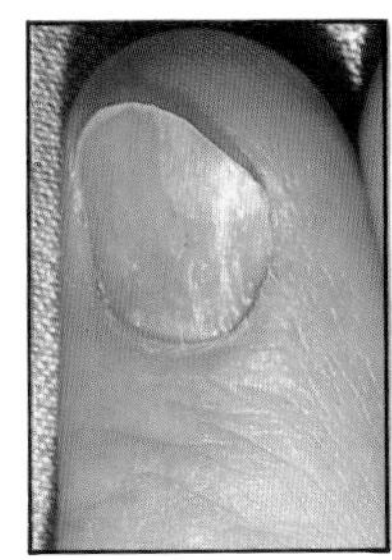

50 Deformed nails

Deformed nails (right) are usually the result of generalized illness, when healthy nail growth is disrupted, or of injury to the nail bed at the base of the nail. Once the cause is removed the nails should grow healthily again, though it may take some months for the deformed portions to grow out completely (see Deformed and discolored nails, p.282).

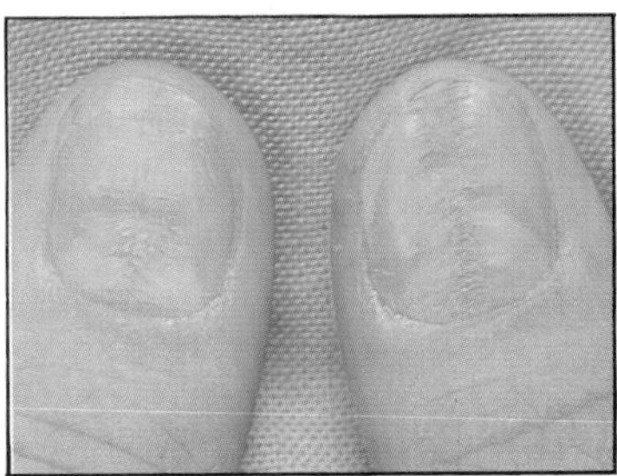

52 Psoriasis of the nails

Psoriasis may cause the nails to become pitted and roughened (above). In other cases, the nails become thickened. Only rarely are the nails alone affected by psoriasis (see p.249 and p.271). Sometimes the nail becomes completely detached.

Common eye disorders

The common eye disorders shown below are all treatable. Styes and conjunctivitis are due to infection of the eye. Corneal ulcers may be caused by either infection or physical injury. Several other eye conditions, among them glaucoma (see p.346), do not produce obvious changes in the appearance of the eye, but do affect vision. Cataracts (see p.345) affect both the appearance and the vision of the eye. Do not ignore unexplained or sudden changes in vision.

53 Stye

A stye (right) is an infected eyelash follicle (see Stye, p.340). A stye resembles a boil (see p.267) in that the follicle (the pit in the skin where the eyelash is formed) becomes inflamed and pus-filled due to a bacterial infection. Styes are uncomfortable and may be painful, but they usually clear up within a week if you apply warm, wet compresses and an antibacterial eye ointment.

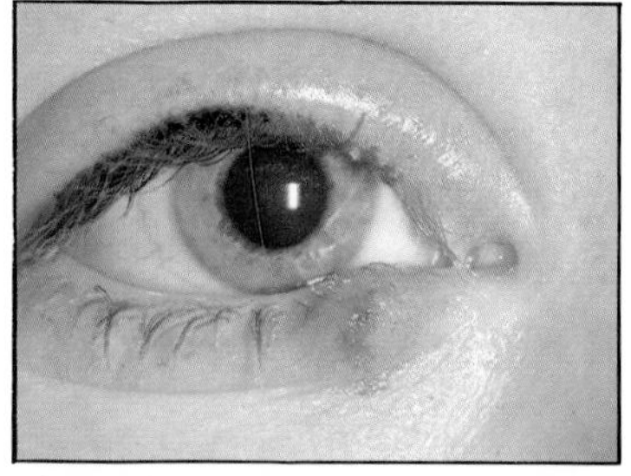

54 Corneal ulcer

An ulcer on the cornea causes pain and discomfort in the eye and may make the white of the eye turn pink or red. In addition, you may be able to see the ulcer as a whitish patch (right), and your vision in that eye may be misted over or otherwise impaired (see Corneal ulcers and infections, p.342). This potentially blinding condition needs immediate medical attention.

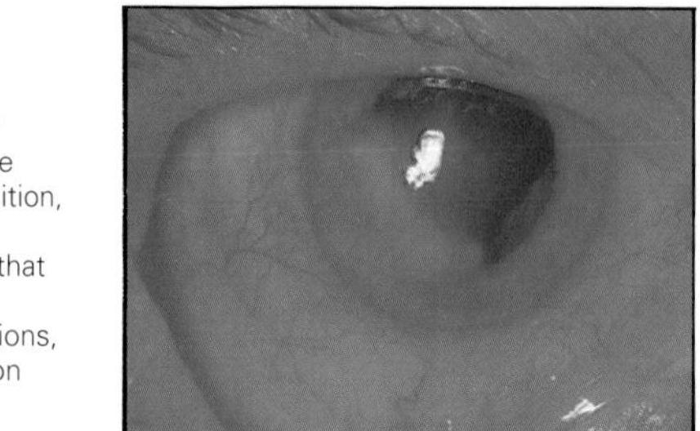

55 Conjunctivitis

In conjunctivitis the surface of the eye and the inside lining of the eyelids, all of which are covered with a membrane called the conjunctiva, become inflamed and sore. The eye looks red and bloodshot, and there may be a discharge that makes it feel sticky and "gummed up." If the lower eyelid is pulled down (below) the redness of the lower eyelid lining is clearly visible (see Conjunctivitis, p.343).

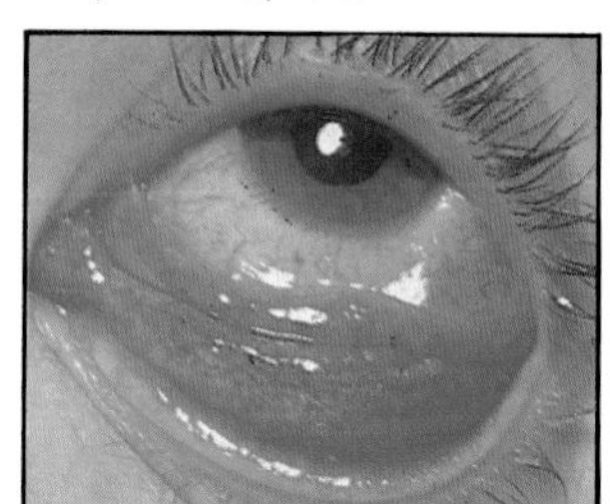

56 Foreign body on the cornea

A speck of grit or other small particle that enters the eye is usually moved to the edge of the eye by blinking, and you can remove it yourself (see Injuries and emergencies, p.848). A corneal foreign body (below) needs expert medical care.

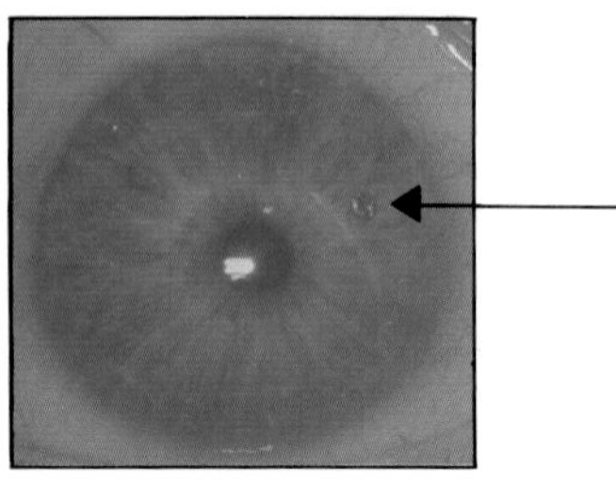

A foreign body stuck in the cornea, the dome-shaped front of the eye (see diagram right and photograph above), is a serious problem if mishandled. DO NOT attempt to move a particle embedded in the cornea. Get a physician to remove it for you.

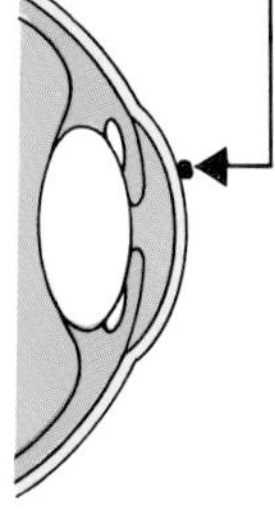

57 Chalazion

A chalazion (also called a meibomian cyst) is a painless swelling on the edge of the eyelid. Chalazions vary in size. Some are so small that they are barely noticeable, but others grow to be as large as a pea. Some become red and swollen (right), probably resulting from infection. Sometimes a chalazion will disappear by itself. In other cases, they have to be removed surgically (see Lumps on the eyelid, p.341).

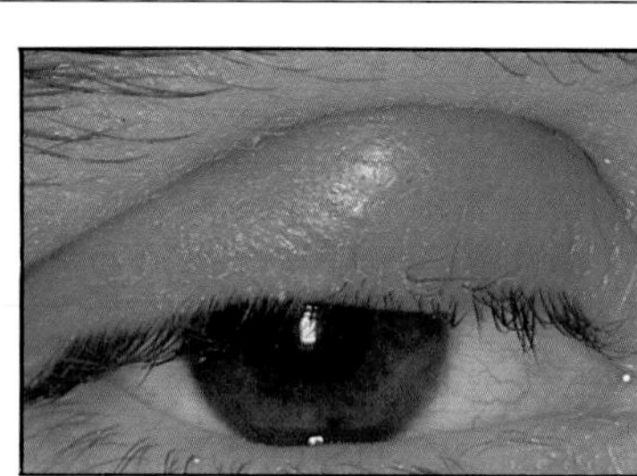

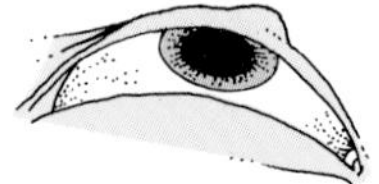

58 Xanthelasma

These are small patches of yellow material that grow in the skin around the eyes, particularly near the nose (right). In most cases they are harmless, but they can signify an underlying disease, so they should always receive medical attention. The patches are painless (see Lumps on the eyelid, p.341).

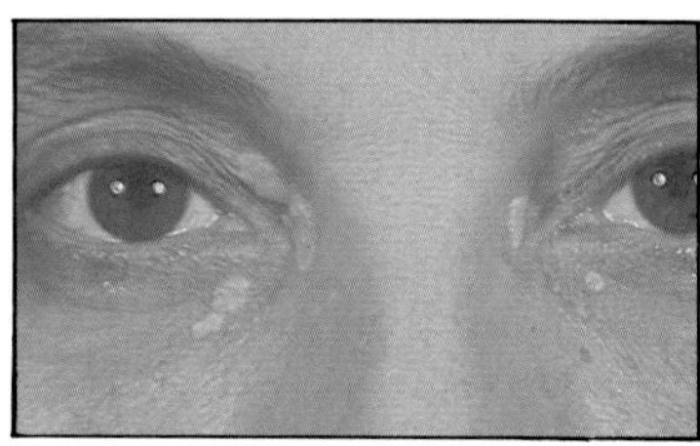

Eye problems in older people

The eye problems covered below occur mainly, but not exclusively, in older people. Entropion and ectropion are unlikely to go unnoticed as they usually cause irritation and discomfort. Cataracts are much more difficult to detect at first.

59 Entropion

In entropion the eyelid turns inward, so that the eyelashes rub on the surface of the eyeball. This irritates and inflames the eye (below) and may cause much pain and discomfort. Entropion can usually be corrected by minor surgery.

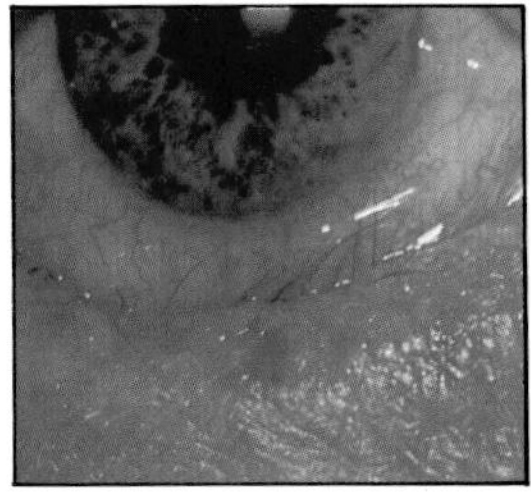

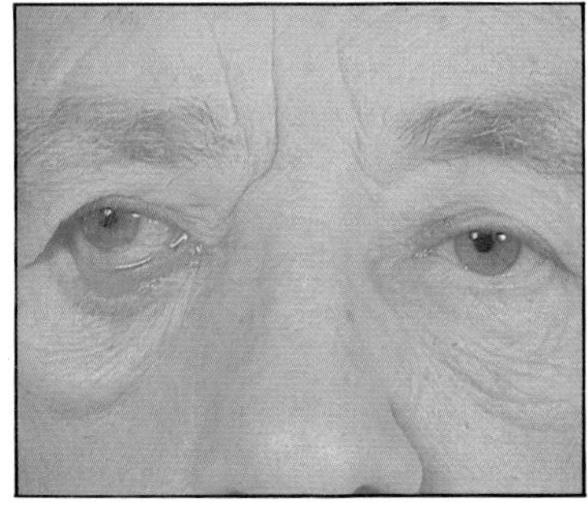

60 Ectropion

In ectropion (see p.341) the lower eyelid becomes slack and hangs away from the eyeball. This gives the appearance that the eyelashes are turned outward (above). The lining of the lid and the eye itself dry out and become sore. Also, tear fluid cannot drain away from the eye properly and runs down the face. Ectropion can usually be corrected by minor surgery.

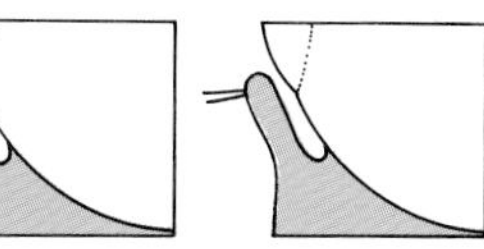

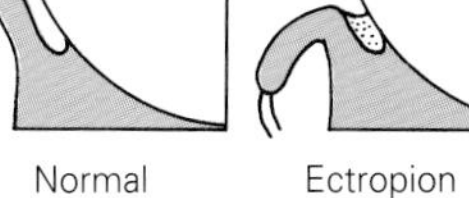

Entropion Normal Ectropion

61 Cataract

A cataract is an opaque area in the normally clear tissue of a healthy lens. In an advanced cataract (below and bottom) a misty circular area within the normally black-looking pupil is large and clearly visible. The upper eyelid has been pulled up slightly to give a clearer view of the cataract (see Cataracts, p.345).

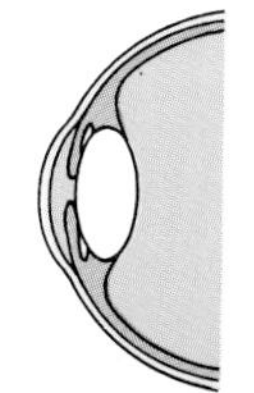

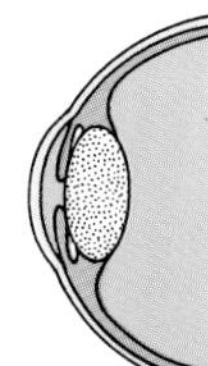

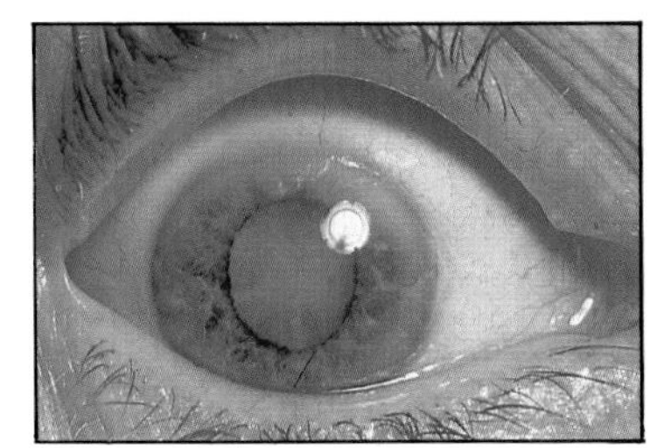

Other eye problems

62 Exophthalmos

Exophthalmos is the technical term for eyeballs that appear to bulge, stare, or protrude (right). Although the eyes appear to be enlarged, the eyeballs themselves are usually unchanged in size. Exophthalmos results from a build-up of tissue behind the eyeball that pushes it forward within its bony socket (far right). An abnormally large amount of the whites of the eyes becomes visible, and it may be difficult to close the eyelids. Exophthalmos is a sign of any one of several underlying disorders (see Exophthalmos, p.352) and needs prompt medical attention.

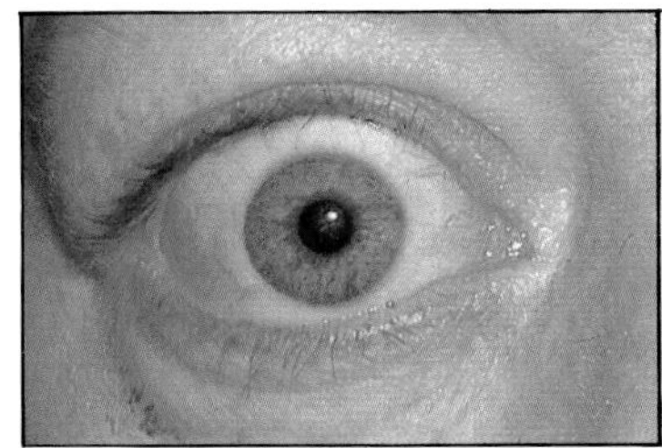

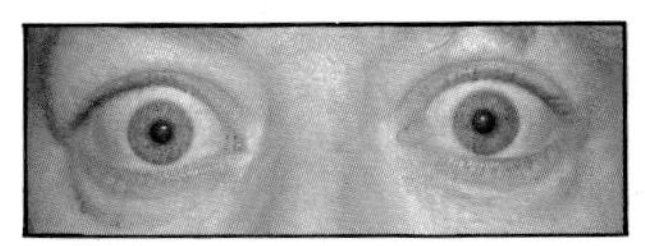

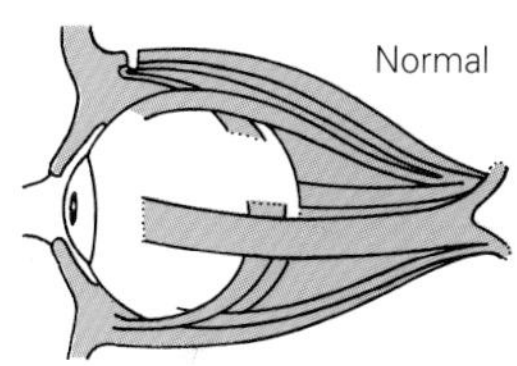

Normal

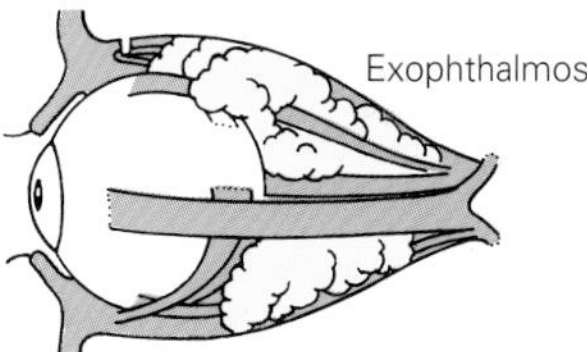

Exophthalmos

63 Ptosis

In ptosis (right) the upper eyelid starts to droop so that the eye will not completely close. Occasionally ptosis affects both eyes. The condition may be present from birth or may develop later. It may signify an underlying disorder (see Ptosis, p.340).

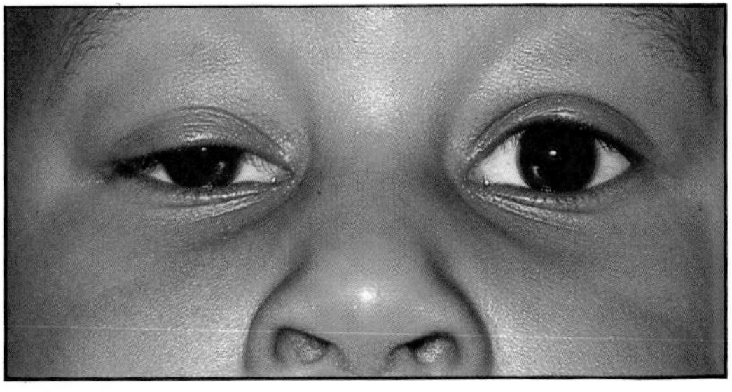

Mouth disorders

One of the disorders that affects the lining of the mouth and the tongue and lips is mouth ulcers (see below). This condition is not usually serious but some ulcerlike growths in the mouth or on the tongue are malignant, or life-threatening. Early detection of any malignant growth is vital, so any lump or raw area that persists for more than about 3 weeks should be closely examined by a physician (see Mouth and tongue, p.483).

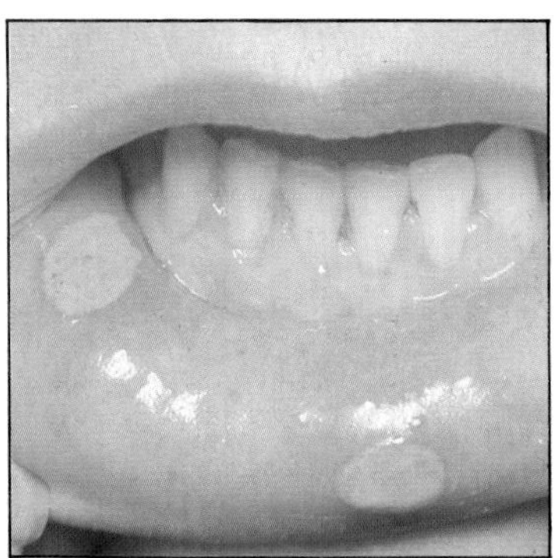

64 Canker sores

These (above) are small, raw, painful areas inside the mouth or on the tongue or lips (see Canker sores, p.483). They may occur as a result of injury (by a toothbrush, for instance) or illness. They usually heal within 7 to 10 days.

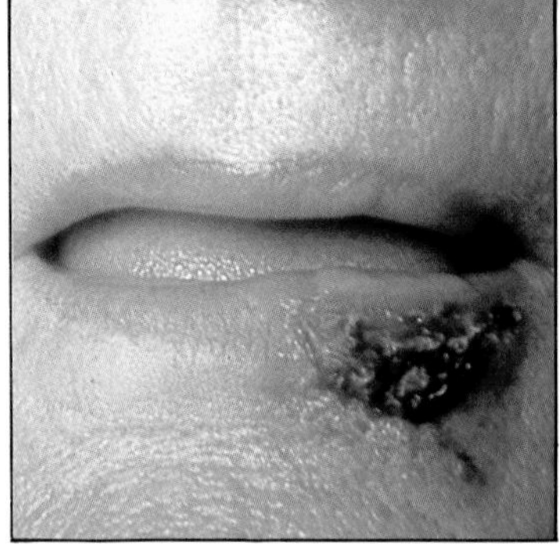

65 Cancer of the lip

The lip is one of the more common sites of cancer on the face. Usually the first sign is a shallow, painless ulcer either on the inside or outside of the lip, or a warty outgrowth (see above). The condition is more common in people who have spent most of their lives outdoors, without covering their faces.

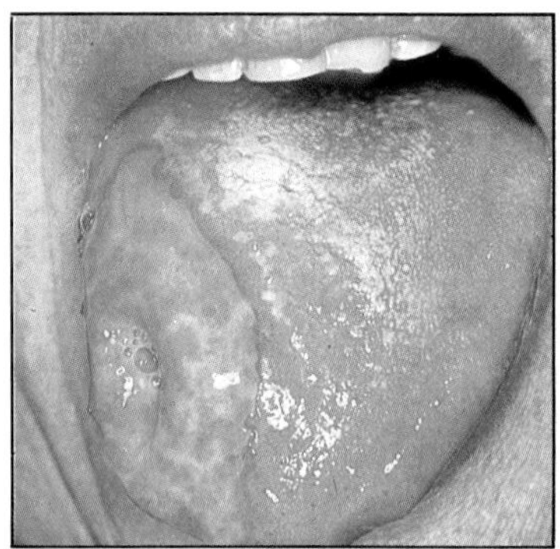

66 Cancer of the tongue

Cancer of the tongue can occur in cigarette and cigar smokers, those who use smokeless tobacco, and in nonsmokers. Any ulcer, crack, or lump on the tongue that persists for more than 3 weeks should be examined by your physician.

Parasites

There are a number of small animals that live on or in human skin and produce characteristic marks there. Some of the more common ones are shown here.

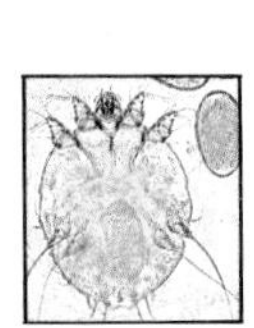
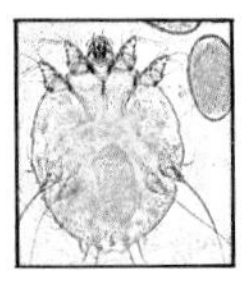

Scabies mite
This tiny, insectlike creature (right) is responsible for the rash of scabies (right center).

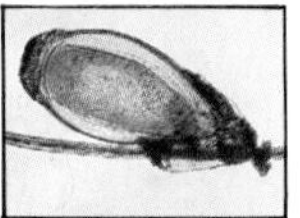

Nits
Nits are the eggs of lice (see p.609). They adhere tenaciously to a strand of human hair (right).

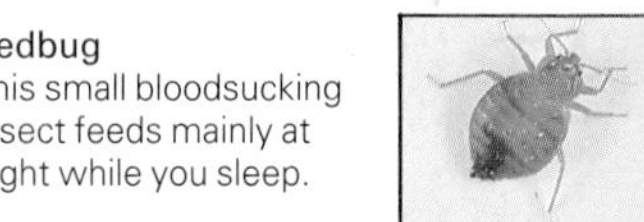

Bedbug
This small bloodsucking insect feeds mainly at night while you sleep.

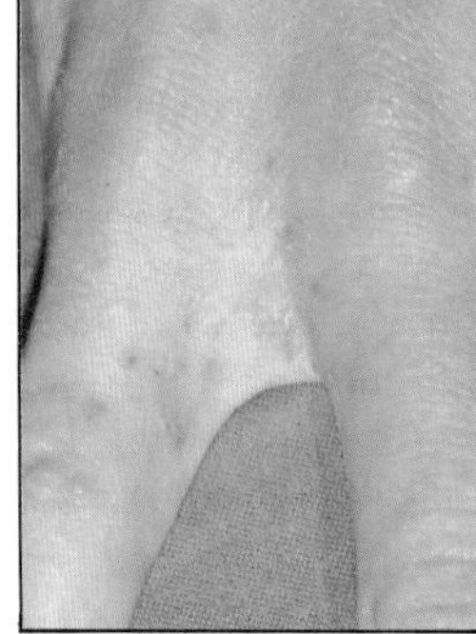
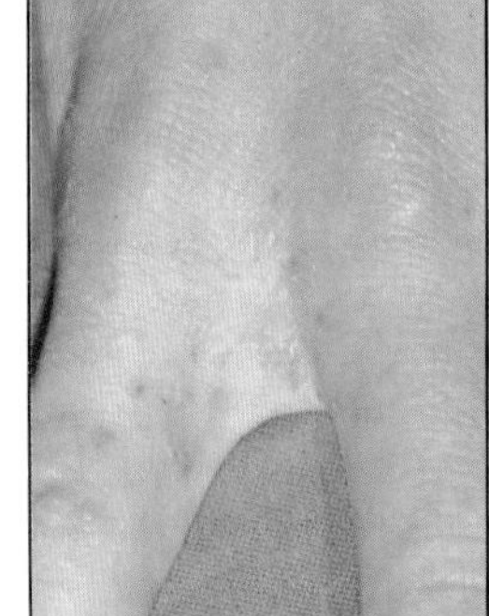

67 Scabies

A typical infestation of scabies shows various marks (above). Sometimes the burrows of the scabies mite can be seen as tiny white lines in the skin, and red lumps may also appear in this area. In most cases there is also a widespread, intensely itchy rash on the trunk. Common sites for this infestation are the hands, wrists, and genitals (see Scabies, p. 609).

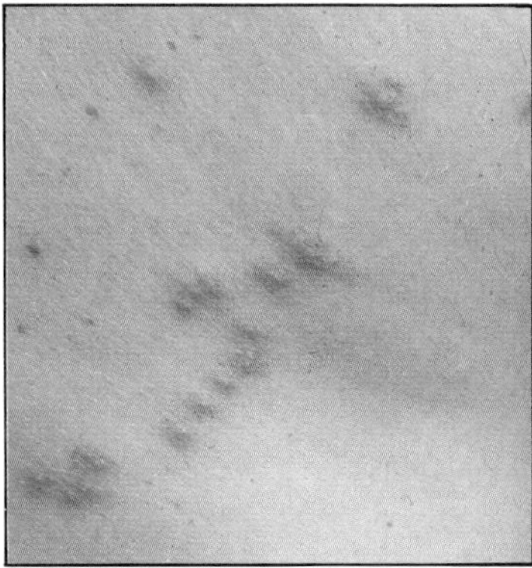

68 Insect bites

Many small insects, including gnats, fleas, mosquitos, bedbugs, and lice, produce small, inflamed, itchy spots where they bite the skin. Sensitivity to such bites varies; some people get large, puffy, red wheals that last for days, while others hardly notice a bite from the same insect. Often several bites (above) appear together (see Lice, p.609, Fleas, p.610, and Chiggers, p.610).

Diagnostic imaging techniques

Introduction

Diagnostic imaging is a branch of medicine that attempts to answer questions about your symptoms that cannot be answered by a physical examination and laboratory tests. For example, after taking a health history and performing a physical examination, a physician may advise a person with a chronic cough to have a chest X ray, or a person who may have had a stroke to have a computed tomography (CT) scan or magnetic resonance imaging (MRI) scan of the head. These tests can often provide the reason for your symptoms or narrow down the possible causes.

Today's advanced imaging techniques began with the discovery of X rays in 1895. X rays are frequently used to examine bones and air-filled organs such as the lungs. In 1952, a new technique called ultrasound used sound waves to examine a fetus in a pregnant woman's uterus. More recently, ultrasound has been used to image almost every organ in the body, including the heart.

Diagnostic imaging advanced in the 1970s with the introduction of CT and MRI scanning, which produce cross-sectional images of any part of your body. By using these techniques, your physician can examine the appearance and function of your internal organs without invasive tests or surgery.

Another advance in diagnostic imaging was the development of endoscopes, which are viewing devices with a lens mounted on a long, flexible tube. Endoscopes allow your physician to look directly inside your body.

Imaging the brain

Your brain is a soft, complex organ enclosed in a bony covering called the skull. A conventional X ray of the head shows only the skull, not the brain inside. For most of the 20th century, physicians imaged the brain first by injecting air into its fluid-filled cavities, or by injecting a dye that would pass through its blood vessels. These techniques often were uncomfortable for the patient, carried a risk of complications, and were limited because they showed abnormalities in the brain only when they were noticeable enough to distort the brain's normal appearance.

Diagnostic imaging improved in the 1970s when computerized scanning was introduced. Since then, there has been progressive development of imaging techniques that produce clear, detailed pictures of the brain.

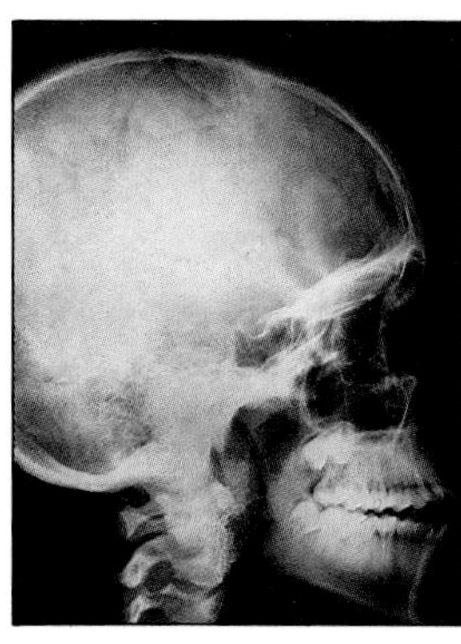

X ray

This X ray of a human skull shows the bone that surrounds and protects the brain but provides very little information about the brain tissue itself. Conventional X rays are often used to detect skull fractures.

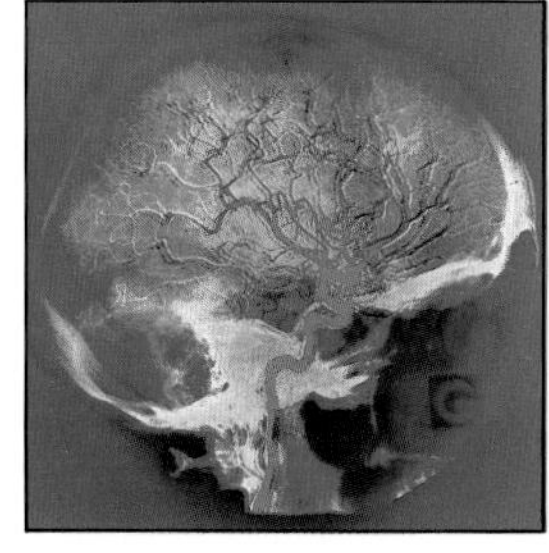

Arteriogram

An arteriogram of the brain is performed by injecting dye into one of the arteries in the neck. The dye reveals the circulation of the blood (shown in red). Physicians can usually diagnose any narrowing or blockage of an artery, or a tumor or cyst that may distort the normal pattern of blood vessels, by using this type of angiography.

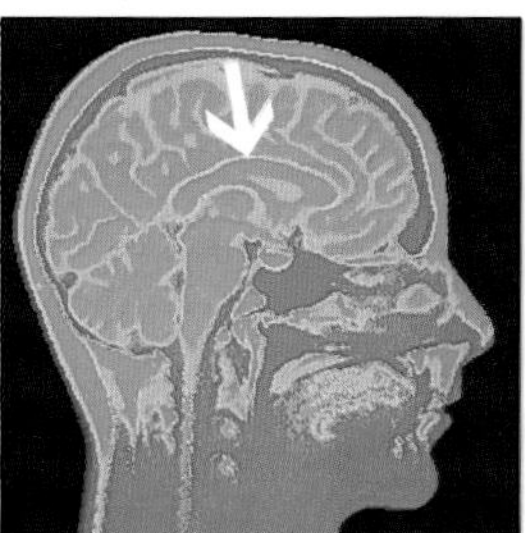

MRI scan

Magnetic resonance imaging (MRI) uses radio waves, a powerful magnet, and a computer to create cross-sectional images. This image shows the cerebral cortex, or outer layer of the brain (top). The curved shadow (arrow) is the corpus callosum, a bridge of nerve fibers that connects the two sides of the brain.

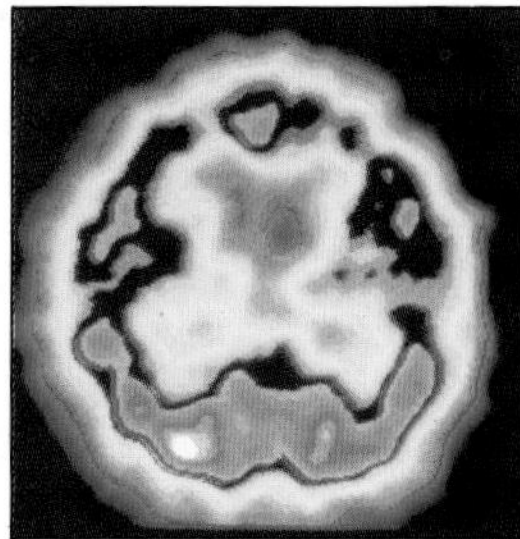

PET scan

Positron emission tomography (PET) scanning shows both the structure of the brain and the amount of chemical activity in different areas of the brain. In this cross-sectional image, low activity is colored blue, medium activity is yellow, and high activity is pink. Too little or too much activity in an area indicates an abnormality.

Conventional X rays

Conventional X rays are high-energy electromagnetic waves that have a shorter wavelength than visible light or radio waves. When a beam of X rays is passed through the body, some parts of the body absorb more radiation than do other parts, which produces a shadow image on the X-ray film. Dense structures, such as bone, allow few X rays to pass through, so the film is only slightly exposed. Such structures appear white on the image. Hollow structures, such as the lungs, allow most of the radiation to pass through, almost fully exposing the film. Such structures appear black on the image.

Hollow and tubular structures—such as the intestines and the blood vessels—can be outlined more clearly on X-ray films if they are filled with a substance that blocks the passage of the rays, such as barium sulfate.

For X-ray examinations of the upper digestive tract, you are asked to fast for a number of hours and then swallow a barium sulfate mixture. The mixture does not allow X rays to pass through, thereby producing clearly outlined images of the esophagus, stomach, and upper intestine. For an X-ray examination of the lower intestine, you are given a barium enema. Other substances that block the passage of X rays (called contrast media) contain iodine and are used to examine blood vessels and the urinary tract.

What happens during an X ray?

First, the X-ray technician will explain the procedure to you, and you may need to remove some of your clothing. He or she will then carefully position the part of your body to be examined between the X-ray machine and the photographic film. The technician may cover other parts of your body with a lead apron to protect them from exposure to the radiation. You will be asked to stay very still so that the photographic image will be as clear as possible. For a chest X ray, you will also be asked to hold your breath.

In some cases, it may be necessary to support or immobilize the part of your body being examined. Also, several images may be taken from various angles; the technician will reposition you and/or the X-ray equipment as necessary. When you are in the correct position in front of the lens, the technician walks behind a protective screen and presses a button that releases the radiation. Your actual exposure to the radiation lasts only a fraction of a second. You cannot feel the X rays pass through your body, and the procedure causes no discomfort.

There is a small risk of tissue damage from exposure to X rays. Because of this, X-ray examinations are performed only when necessary, and pregnant women should not have them, except in emergencies.

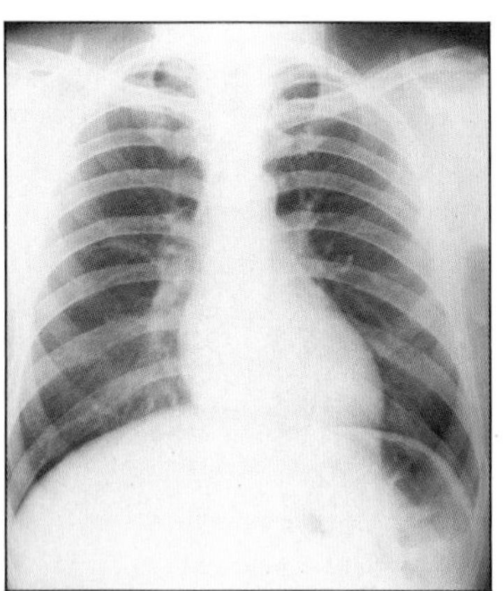

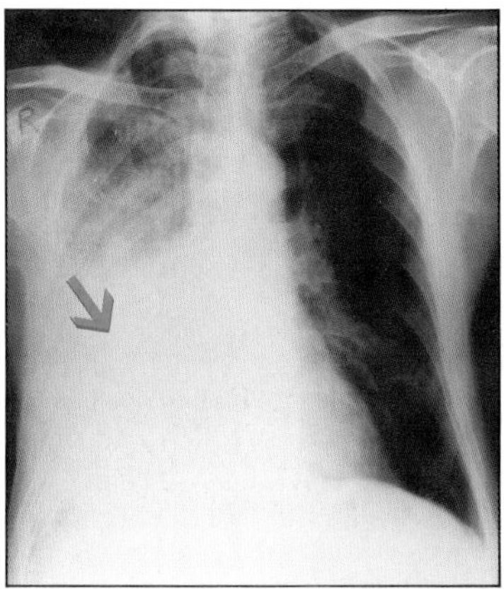

X ray: Chest

The image on the far left shows the rib cage, the lungs and their faintly visible blood vessels, and the pear-shaped shadow of the heart between the two lungs. In lobar pneumonia, one of the lobes (segments) of a lung becomes damaged by a bacterial infection and the lung's normal spongy structure becomes filled with fluid and cells. The image on the near left shows a fluid-filled lobe as a white shadow (arrow).

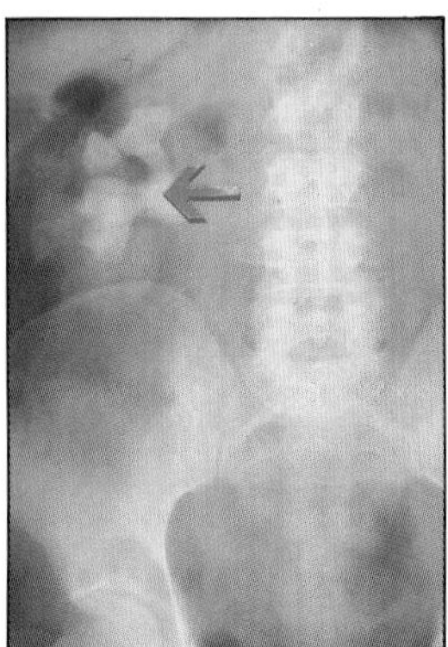

X ray: Kidney

This image of the abdomen shows a large, white "staghorn" (it resembles a stag's antler) calculus, or stone (arrow), in the kidney. The stone gets this irregular shape from the internal structure of the kidney. The dark, circular areas are gas in the intestines.

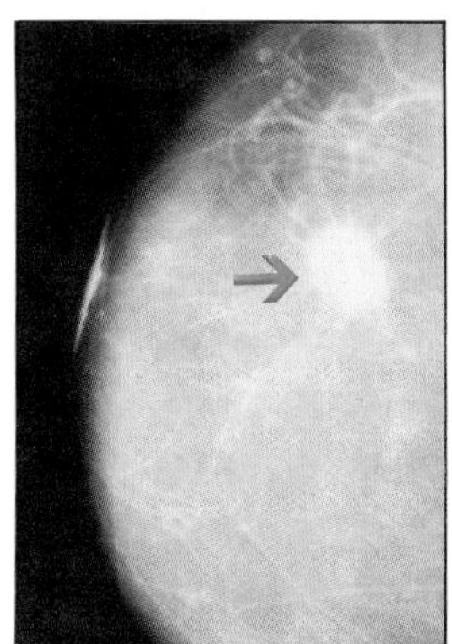

Mammogram: Breast

Mammography uses low doses of X rays to produce an image of the soft tissues of the breast. In this mammogram, the large, circular shadow (arrow) with an irregular outline is a tumor. Many tumors detected by mammography are much smaller than this, and many are benign (not likely to spread).

Angiography

Angiography is a reliable way of imaging arteries. A dye containing iodine, which absorbs X rays, is injected into the artery being examined. The physician injects an anesthetic to numb the skin before he or she makes a small incision (cut) in order to insert a thin catheter into the femoral artery of the upper thigh. (This is called an invasive procedure.) From this point the catheter may then be guided up into the main artery, the aorta, and any of its branches. When the catheter is in position, the dye is injected, and a rapid series of X-ray pictures is taken. These pictures show the dye flowing in the artery and through its branches. Any defects in the wall of the artery (such as an aneurysm) or in the flow of blood will be shown on the pictures.

Angiography is the standard test for diseases of the blood vessels. It is almost always performed before any surgery on a blood vessel.

What happens during an angiogram?

You remove your clothing and wear a hospital gown. During the examination, you will be asked to lie very still on an examination table. As the dye is injected, you will feel a sensation of warmth for a few seconds. The procedure lasts from about 30 to 120 minutes. After the examination, you have to lie flat for a number of hours. There is a very small risk of damage to the artery during the injection and of allergic reaction to the dye.

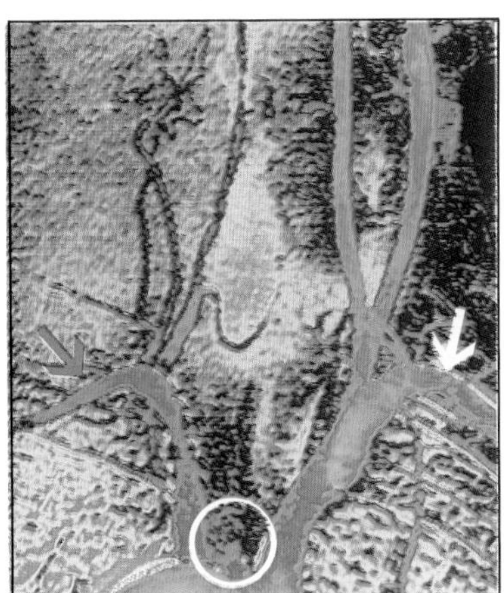

Angiogram: Carotid artery

This angiogram shows the three main arteries that lead from the aorta at the base of the neck. The aorta is the blue curved area at the bottom of the picture. The subclavian artery is visible both on the left (white arrow) and on the right (red arrow) in this image. In between, one of the carotid arteries is blocked completely at its root (circle) and has caused a massive stroke.

Angiogram: Legs

This angiogram of the legs shows the femoral arteries (the thin pink bars, much narrower than the thighbones). In this image, the main artery in the leg has been blocked by a blood clot (circle). New small blood vessels have formed around the blocked section, allowing some blood to get through to the lower part of the artery and to the lower leg.

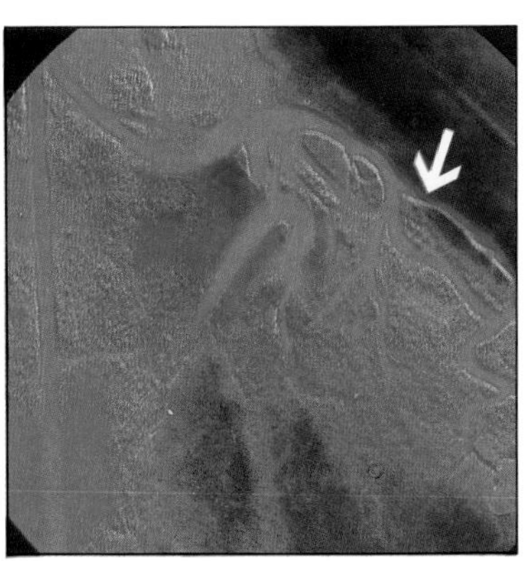

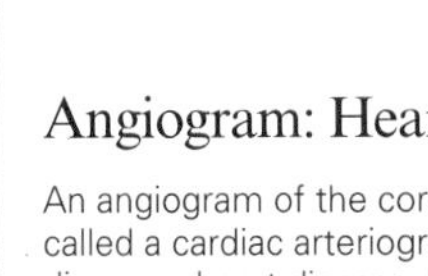

Angiogram: Heart

An angiogram of the coronary arteries, called a cardiac arteriogram, is used to diagnose heart disease. In the image on the left, the dye reveals a narrowed section (called a stenosis) on the circumflex artery (arrow) on the surface of the heart.

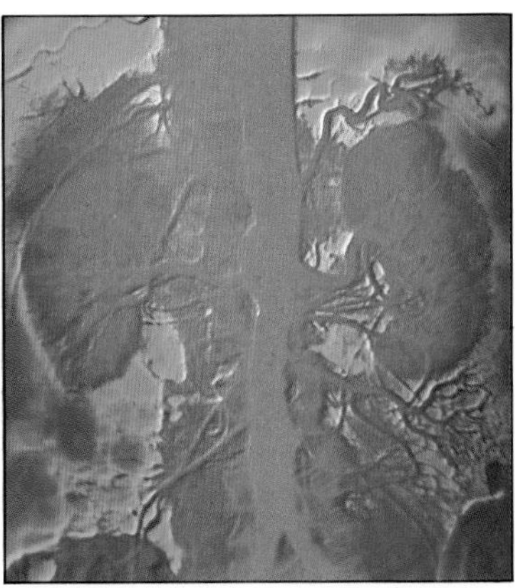

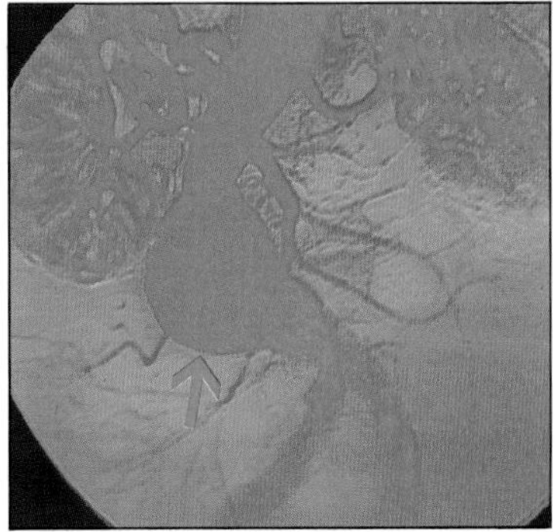

Angiogram: Kidneys

The image at the top is an angiogram of normal kidneys. The bottom image shows a balloonlike swelling called an aneurysm (arrow) in the aorta below the kidneys. An untreated aneurysm may grow until it bursts.

Ultrasound

Ultrasound scanning, originally used to examine the fetus before birth, is now used to diagnose many different conditions, often instead of conventional X rays. In ultrasound, high-frequency sound waves (far above the human range of hearing) are directed (using a device called a transducer) into the body part being examined. Some of these sound waves are absorbed by body tissues and some are reflected back. The image is made by measuring the amount of sound that is reflected by different body tissues. Ultrasound produces clear images of soft and fluid-filled organs, such as the ovaries, but is less useful for examining organs filled with gas or air, such as the lungs. Also, ultrasound waves do not penetrate bone. The images generated by ultrasound scanning can be immediately displayed on a screen; this technique is often used to guide a needle into an organ during a biopsy (removal of a small piece of tissue for microscopic examination). Ultrasound examinations of the heart, which are called echocardiography, may use a single transducer passing a beam of sound through the heart in a straight line, or the transducer may be rotated through an arc of 90 degrees to produce a two-dimensional image.

Doppler ultrasound is a variation on simple ultrasound. It is used to watch the flow of blood through arteries and veins. Doppler ultrasound is based on the principle that flowing blood cells in a blood vessel will reflect sound waves. The speed and direction of blood flow through the vessels can be measured and analyzed. This information is displayed on a screen as a graph. Doppler ultrasound is often used before angiography and in some instances can replace this more invasive procedure.

What happens during an ultrasound scan?

You remove all clothing from the area to be examined. A jelly is spread over your skin so that the transducer makes good contact and can be easily and smoothly passed back and forth over the area. Depending on the type of ultrasound scan being performed, you will either lie on an examination table or sit in a chair near the ultrasound machine. The room is darkened so that images of your body are clearly visible on the screen of a monitor. The sound waves produced by the machine cannot be seen or felt; the only sensation is light pressure from the transducer against your skin. The examination lasts from about 15 to 30 minutes.

Your physician will ask you to fast for at least 12 hours before any scan of the abdominal area. And because a full bladder is needed to examine the pelvic area or a fetus, you are instructed to drink three or four glasses of water about 20 to 30 minutes before this type of examination.

Ultrasound scanning is a very safe procedure that has no apparent side effects and carries no known risks.

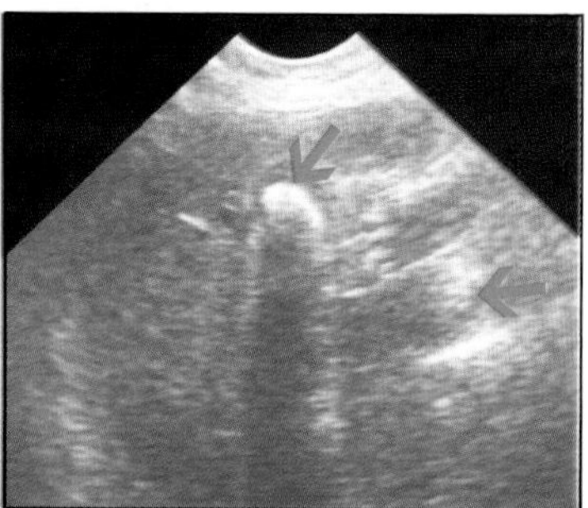

Ultrasound: Gallstones

A close look at this ultrasound scan of the liver and gallbladder (left) shows that there are at least two gallstones (arrows) in the gallbladder.

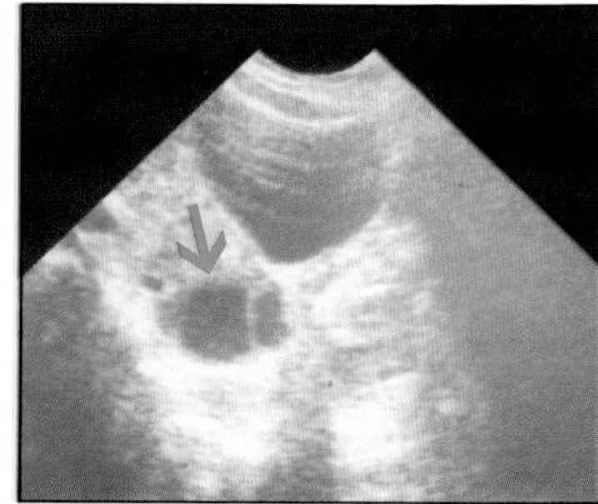

Ultrasound: Female pelvis

This image faintly shows the ovaries and other pelvic organs. The large dark area is the bladder; the smaller dark area (arrow) is an ovarian cyst.

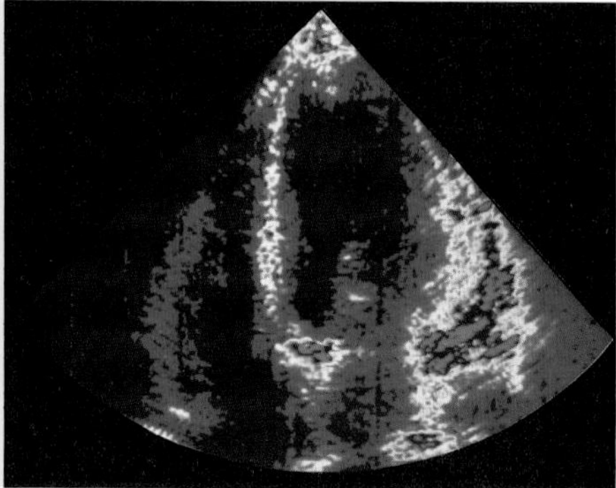

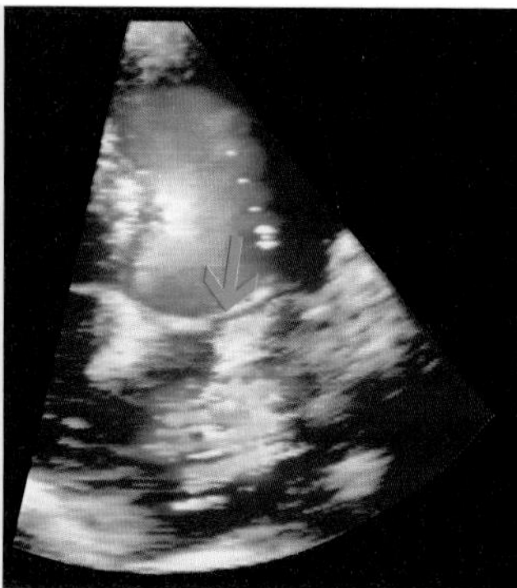

Ultrasound: Doppler blood flow of the heart

The image on the far left shows the heart of a person who has hypertension (high blood pressure), which has caused the muscular wall of the left ventricle (shown in red) to thicken. The black areas are the two main heart chambers. The image on the near left shows blood leaking through a defective mitral valve (located between the ventricle and the atrium). A normal valve is shut tight, but here, a narrow jet of blood, visible as a thin blue line (arrow), is leaking through the valve.

CT scanning

Computed tomography (CT) scanning uses X rays in a different way from a conventional X-ray machine. Instead of taking an X-ray photograph, a scanner sends large numbers of X-ray beams from many directions through the part of the body being examined, records the amount of each beam that has been absorbed, and uses its internal computer to construct an image. The computer produces a series of cross-sectional images of the body (like slices of bread), these images offer clear pictures of all the organs in the part of the body being studied. The computer can form these cross-sectional images horizontally and vertically, and it can also produce three-dimensional views.

Today's CT scanners are able to create much more fully defined pictures of the head and body than conventional X rays, and have reduced the need for uncomfortable, invasive, and potentially hazardous diagnostic procedures such as exploratory surgery.

What happens during a CT scan?

You lie very still on a table inside the circular opening of the scanner. The technician will probably inject a dye containing iodine as a contrast medium (to show blood vessels and any tumors better) into a vein in your arm. If your abdomen and pelvis are being scanned, you will be asked to drink a very weak solution of barium sulfate to expand your intestines. The procedure causes no discomfort, and you will not feel the X rays pass through your body.

The time needed to complete the examination is usually an hour or more, depending on the number of angles and exposures required. If more than one angle is required, you may need to change positions; the technician will reposition you and/or the scanner as necessary.

In some people, there is a small risk of allergic reaction to the contrast medium that is sometimes used. The dye can also damage diseased kidneys.

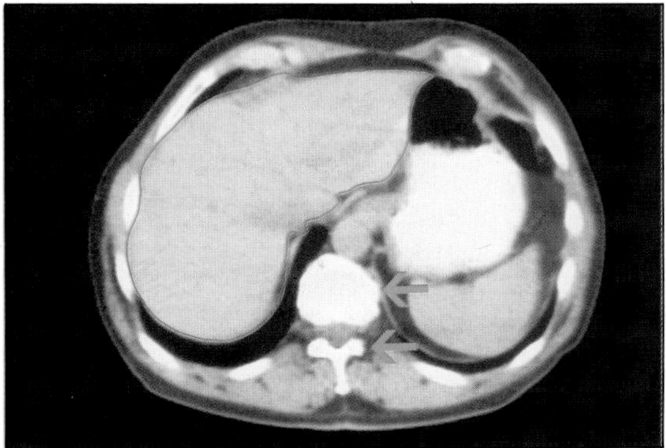

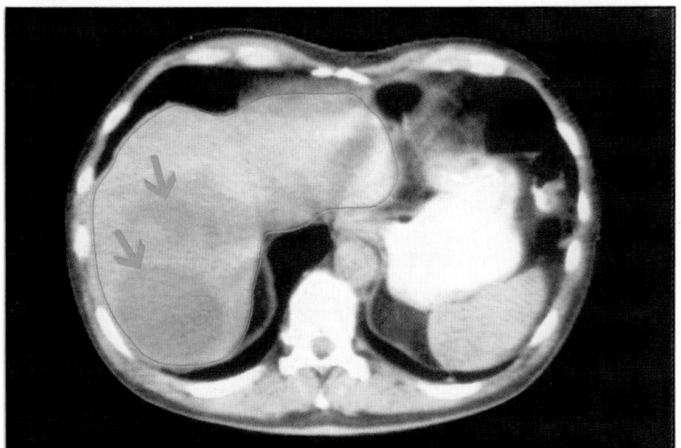

CT scan: Liver

A normal CT scan of the body (top) shows the healthy liver as a large gray shape (outline) occupying more than half the image. The backbone and the spinal cord (red arrows) are in the midline, and the ribs are the pale broken lines surrounding the internal organs. The smaller gray shape is the spleen. The bottom scan shows a liver that has circular patches in one lobe (red arrows). These are abscesses. The image is clear enough to allow a physician to insert a needle into one of the abscesses to perform a biopsy (removal of a sample of tissue for laboratory examination).

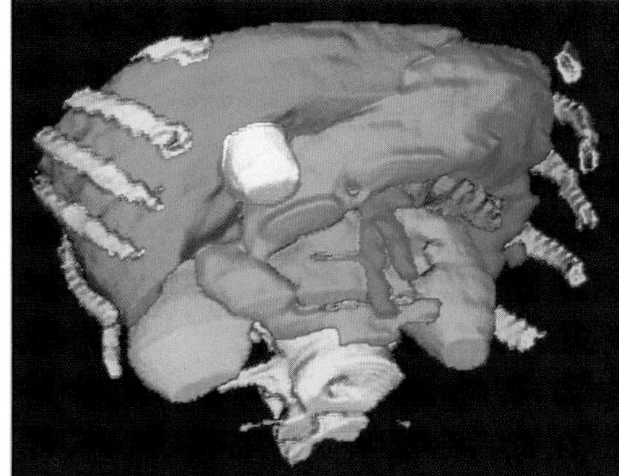

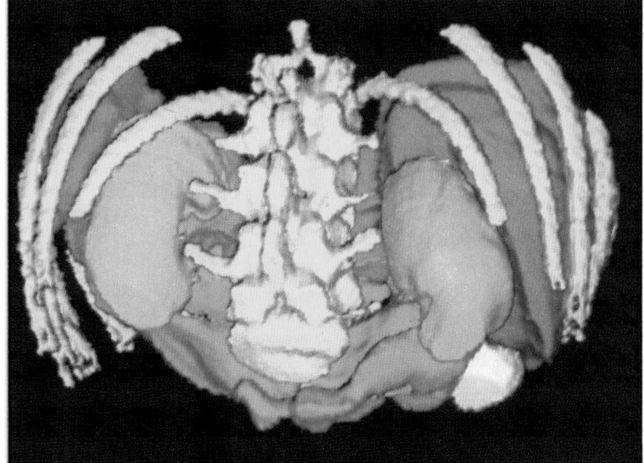

CT scan: Upper abdomen

These three-dimensional CT scans show the organs in the upper abdomen. The images have been colored to help identify the organs shown. The liver is colored reddish-brown; the gallbladder is white; the digestive tract is lavender-pink; the kidneys are blue; and the ribs and spine are yellow.

Magnetic resonance imaging (MRI)

Like CT scanning, magnetic resonance imaging (MRI) uses a computer to construct images from information recorded by the scanner. In MRI, however, the information is not provided by X rays. Instead, the person being examined is placed inside a huge, powerful magnet, which arranges the nuclei of some of the hydrogen atoms in the body in a precise pattern (like iron shavings around a magnet). A pulse of radio waves is then passed through the person's body, moving the nuclei of the aligned hydrogen atoms briefly out of alignment. The nuclei then return to their original pattern, emitting radio signals as they do so. These signals are detected by the machine and analyzed by the computer. The information is then used by the computer to construct an image.

What happens during an MRI scan?

During magnetic resonance imaging, you need to lie very still in a tunnel inside the magnet for up to 1 hour. Some people find this claustrophobic, so ask your physician for tranquilizers beforehand if you feel anxious. The procedure is painless, and you feel no physical discomfort.

During the procedure, the magnet makes loud clanking noises and you may be offered headphones so that you can listen to music that will help block out the noise. A signal button is also provided for you so that if you begin to feel uncomfortable or claustrophobic at any time during the examination you can signal the technician, who will immediately stop the procedure and remove you from the tunnel inside the magnet.

MRI scanning carries no known risks and has no apparent side effects. However, because the scanner creates a very strong magnetic field, you cannot carry or wear any metal objects during the examination. Also, it is important to tell your physician if you have any metal implants such as artificial joints, plates, screws, or clips or electrical devices such as a hearing aid or pacemaker; any of these could be affected by the magnet; a pacemaker might stop completely, causing death.

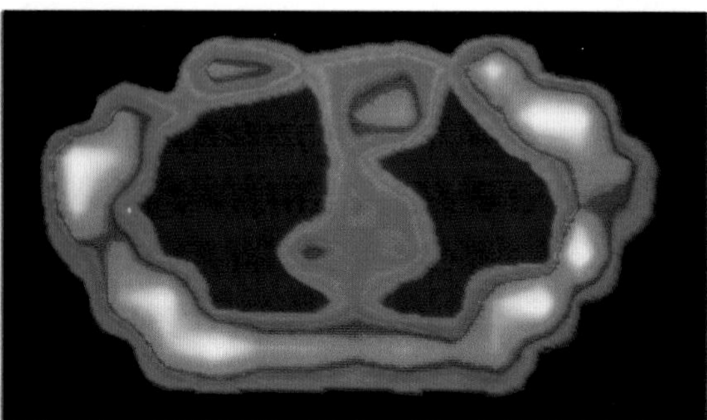

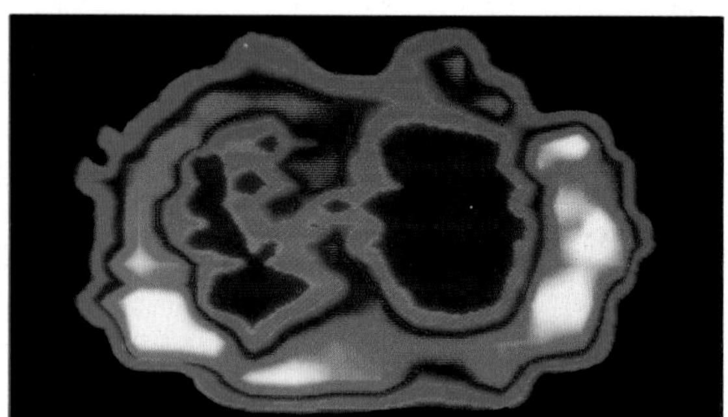

MRI: Chest

These two MRI scans show cross-sectional views of a healthy chest (above) and a chest with a tumor in the left lung (above right). The lungs are the large black areas in the center of each image; the red-yellow areas are the ribs. In the image on the right, the small size of the lung at the left and the large amount of blue in that lung indicate a tumor.

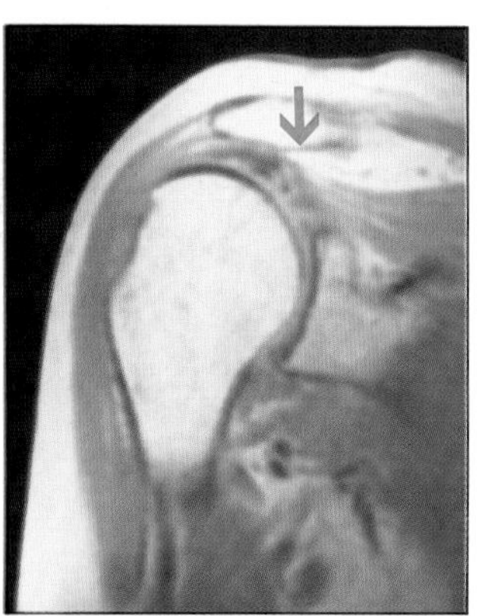

MRI: Shoulder

This MRI scan (left) shows a front view of the shoulder. In the scan, soft tissues such as tendons and muscles are clearly visible. The scan also reveals that there is a tear (arrow) in the supraspinatus tendon, in the upper part of the shoulder.

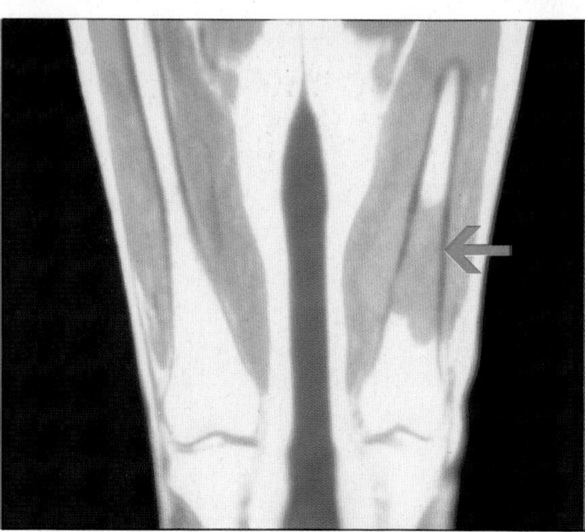

MRI: Legs

The image above shows a normal leg (left) and a femur (thighbone, right) that has a dark area in the lower part of the shaft (arrow) caused by infiltration of the bone by a tumor.

Radionuclide scanning

In radionuclide scanning a radioactive substance called a tracer or isotope is either swallowed or injected into the body. The physician chooses a tracer that confines itself to the organ being examined (for example, iodine concentrates in the thyroid gland). After entering the bloodstream, the tracer travels to the target organ, where it emits very small amounts of gamma rays (similar to X rays), which are detected by an instrument called a gamma camera. The information is then analyzed by computer and constructed into an image of the organ. Radionuclide scanning can also be used with a computer to help form the image in techniques such as single photon emission computed tomography (SPECT), in which cross-sectional images of the body are created by using a gamma camera that rotates around the patient, and PET scans.

What happens during a radionuclide scan?
After the tracer is swallowed or injected, you may need to wait for it to travel through your bloodstream and collect in the target organ—sometimes for several hours—before you are examined by the gamma camera. While you lie or sit on the examination table, the gamma camera is moved close to the area being examined. You must stay very still during the scan, but you may be asked to change positions; the technician will reposition you and/or the gamma camera as necessary. The amount of time the procedure takes varies from about 1 to 5 hours. In some cases, you may need to return for a second or third scan. Radionuclide scanning is a painless procedure, and the tracer quickly breaks down into harmless substances and is eliminated from your body.

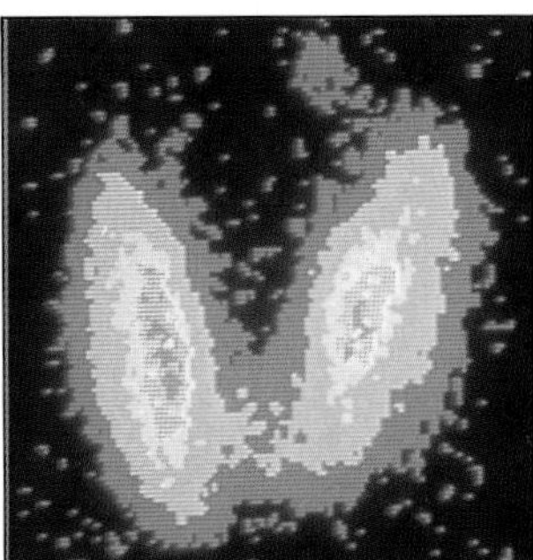

Radionuclide scan: Thyroid scan

Radioactive iodine that you take by mouth or injection travels to the thyroid gland, where the body uses it to make the thyroid hormones. The iodine helps to create a scan that reveals the two equal-sized lobes of the normal thyroid gland as shown in the image on the left.

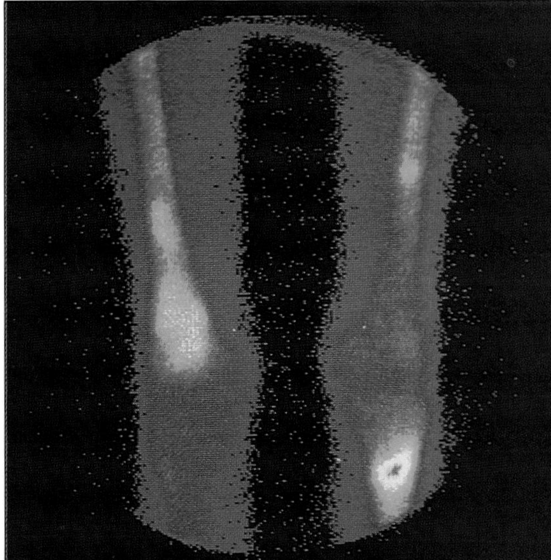

Radionuclide scan: Bone scan of legs

Here, the gamma camera produced an image with bright spots in the lower femur (thighbone, left) and below the knee (right). These bright spots represent cells that have spread through the bloodstream from a cancerous tumor elsewhere in the body.

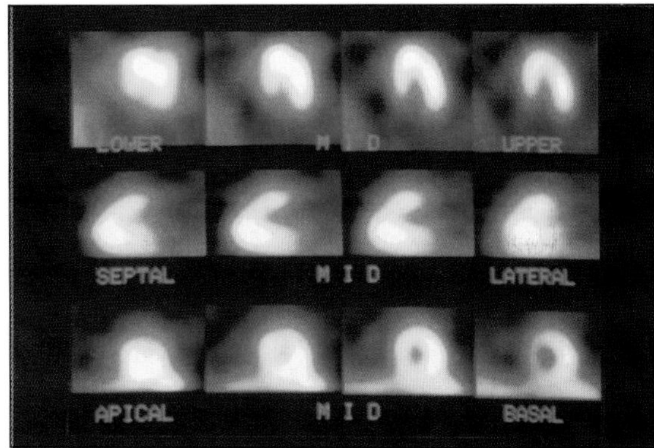

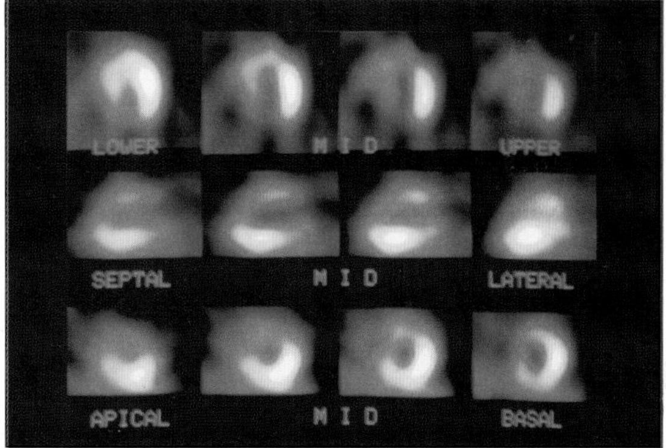

SPECT scan: Heart

The two series of scans shown above, performed during a stress test (see Glossary, p.831), show normal blood circulation (bright yellow areas) in a resting heart (top scan) and large areas of decreased circulation (orange and brown areas) in a heart after exercise (bottom scan). SPECT scans are often performed to determine whether a specific area of the heart has lost its blood circulation or whether the area is not receiving adequate blood flow. During a stress test, factors such as blood flow through the coronary arteries and the heart muscle are monitored while the person performs some type of standardized physical activity, such as walking on a treadmill.

Endoscopy

Endoscopy gives your physician a direct look at the inside of your body. Endoscopes are made of fiber optic (glass-fiber) bundles, are flexible, and have an eyepiece at one end and lenses or a video computer chip at the other so that they can transmit images accurately. An endoscope has a light source, a suction channel, and another channel or tube through which instruments can be passed and manipulated. Endoscopes are used to view the inside of the lungs, the digestive tract, the urinary system, and joints such as the knee. In some cases, the physician inserts the endoscope directly through a natural opening in the body; for example, a bronchoscope is guided into the lungs through the mouth, throat, and trachea. In other cases, such as examination of the arteries, he or she makes a small incision (cut) through which to insert the endoscope and guide it to the area being examined.

What happens during endoscopy?

You remove your clothing and wear a hospital gown. During the examination, you will lie on an examination table. Depending on the type of endoscopic examination, you may be given a mild sedative, either intravenously or by mouth, or a local or general anesthetic. The procedure generally takes from about 30 minutes to 1 hour.

In some cases, you may feel some discomfort; if you receive an anesthetic, you will feel no discomfort.

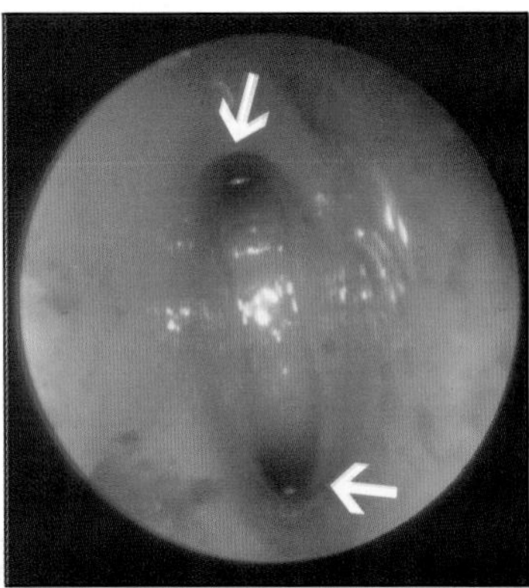

Endoscopy: Uterus

Here is a view inside the uterus through a special endoscope, called a hysteroscope, which is guided into the uterus through the vagina and cervix. The image shows the openings of the two fallopian tubes (arrows) that connect the uterus to the ovaries.

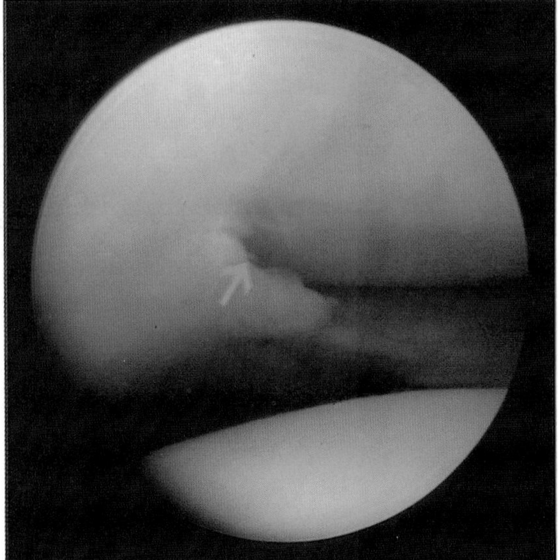

Endoscopy: Knee

The knee joint (above) is seen through a special type of endoscope called an arthroscope. The two large, pale brown areas are the cartilage that covers the ends of the bones in the joint. In this image, one of the cartilages is obviously damaged (arrow).

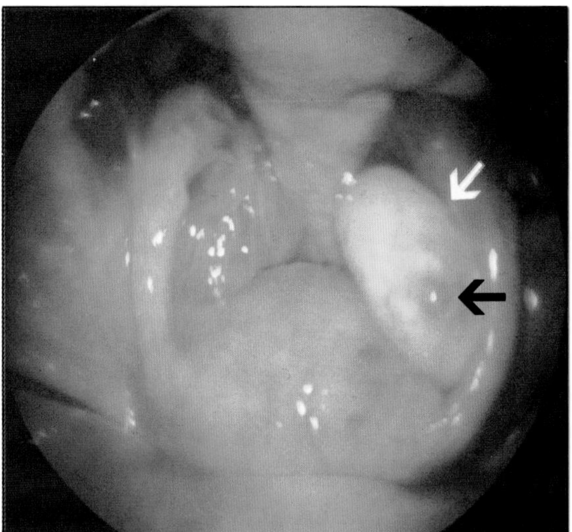

Endoscopy: Ovary

This view through a hysteroscope shows an ovary with a mature ovarian follicle. The ovary is the paler, oval structure toward the right (white arrow). The ovarian follicle is the small, round, darker area within the ovary (black arrow). Inside the follicle is an ovum (egg cell), which will be released during ovulation.

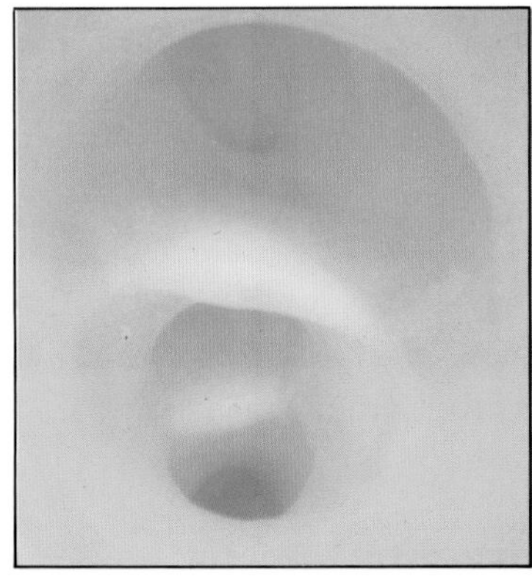

Endoscopy: Arteries

This view through an endoscope shows the inside of a pair of arteries. Two main channels are visible: note how the artery on the bottom divides again into two more branches.

PART THREE

Diseases, disorders, and other problems

Skin, hair, and nail disorders

Introduction

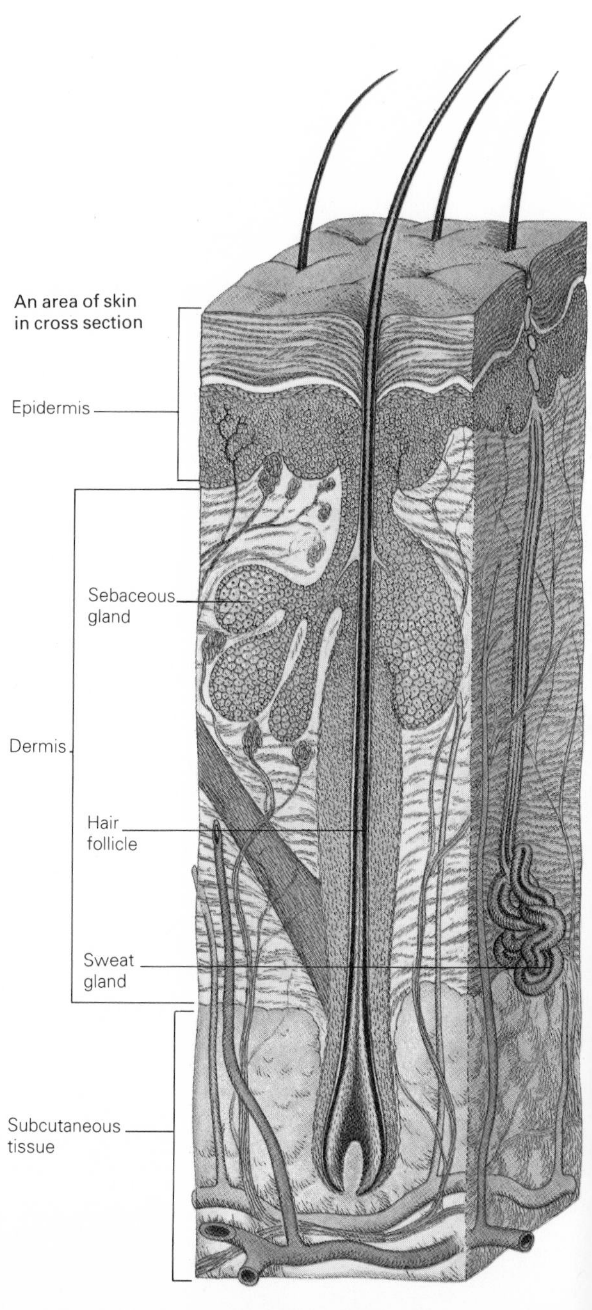

Your skin is one of your largest organs. It is a supple, elastic organ that conserves moisture and heat. In addition, it provides you with information about your surroundings. Buried in your skin are millions of tiny nerve endings called receptors that sense touch, pressure, heat, cold, and pain. Also embedded in your skin are many tiny glands. Sebaceous glands produce an oily substance that helps keep your skin surface supple and helps prevent it from drying and cracking. Sweat glands produce a watery liquid called perspiration to cool you when you are too hot. The process of evaporation (drawing off of moisture into the air) of perspiration from your skin cools you. To help with temperature regulation, the small blood vessels in your skin dilate (widen) to lose heat when you have a fever or in hot weather. This may make you look flushed. The same vessels constrict in cold weather to conserve heat. When the vessels constrict, they move away from the skin, so less blood flows through the vessels. This causes you to look pale.

There are thousands of hair follicles in your skin. These are pits of actively dividing cells that continuously make hairs. There are large, thick, hairs on your scalp and in your pubic region. In addition, there are smaller, fine, hairs all over your body, some that can barely be seen. Your fingernails and toenails are also continuously produced by actively dividing cells. These cells, which are similar to those in hair follicles, are situated under the fold of skin at the cuticle or the base of each of your nails.

Because your skin, hair, and nails are on the outside of your body, you quickly notice any change in their appearance. Most of the problems included here relate mainly to changes in appearance. There may be symptoms such as itching, swelling, or pain. Diseases of the skin, hair, and nails can be irritating and uncomfortable. Their appearance can also be embarrassing. Serious diseases of the skin such as cancer can occur, especially among people exposed to bright sunlight for many years.

See your physician or a dermatologist if you are worried about a skin, hair, or nail problem. Get medical advice before you try any of the many nonprescription preparations that are available at the drugstore.

Skin

Skin is composed of two layers. The surface layer that you see is a thin covering called the epidermis. Below the epidermis is a thicker layer, the dermis. The dermis contains many specialized structures such as hair follicles and sweat glands (see previous page). Below the dermis is a layer of fat that is called subcutaneous tissue.

The surface skin layer, the epidermis, is a very active layer of cells. Cells at its base are continuously dividing to produce new cells, which gradually die as they fill up with a hard substance, keratin. As they die, they are moved up to the skin surface to be shed or worn away by rubbing from your clothes or by washing. In fact, virtually any movement that causes friction also causes some skin cells to be rubbed away. The continuous production of cells at the base of the epidermis keeps up with the continuous loss of cells from its surface. It takes an average of 1 month for any single epidermal cell to complete the journey from base to surface. On parts of the body where pressure and friction are greatest, the epidermis is thicker, and the journey takes longer. A number of skin conditions are caused by problems with the normal turnover of skin cells. In psoriasis, for example, there is an abnormal buildup of surface cells because there are increased numbers of cells being produced and pushed up from the base of the epidermis.

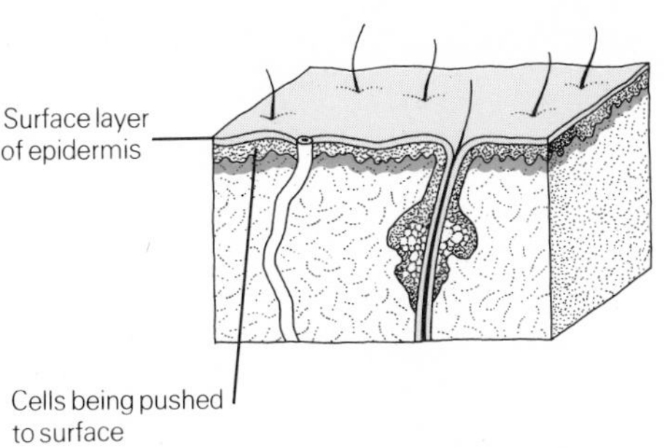

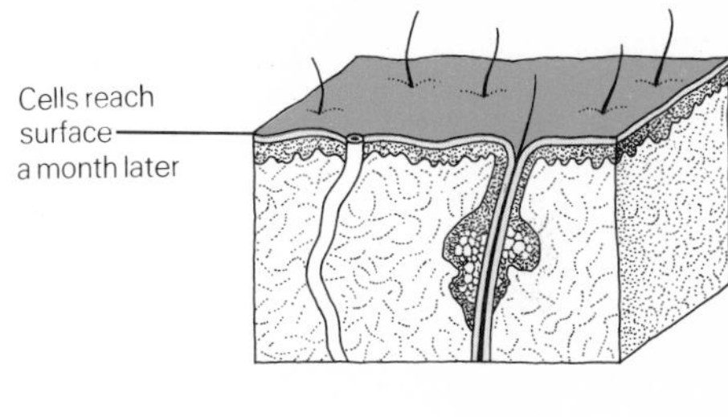

Skin renewal
The skin consists of two layers: the epidermis, a semitransparent layer of cells, and the dermis, a permanent foundation of fat, supportive tissue, and blood vessels. The cells at the surface constantly are being shed and rubbed off. Those at the base of the epidermis are dividing constantly to produce new cells, which, after about a month, reach the surface to replace those being lost.

Boils and carbuncles

See p.245, **Visual aids to diagnosis, 23.**

A boil in the skin is an infection of a hair follicle (a tiny pit in the skin from which a hair grows) by certain bacteria, usually *Staphylococcus*. The follicle becomes inflamed and very painful. White blood cells, which form part of the body's defense system against bacteria, gather at the site to combat the infection. White blood cells, bacteria, and dead skin cells form thick white or yellow pus within the inflamed area.

A carbuncle is either an unusually large, severe boil or a group of boils joined together by small tunnels in the skin.

Boils and carbuncles are both localized infections and usually heal quickly. In a few cases, they are the result of poor resistance to infection or poor hygiene. Boils should not be confused with acne (see p.271).

What are the symptoms?

A boil starts as a red, warm, tender lump, which may throb. Over the next day or two, it becomes larger and more painful. As pus collects, it develops a white or yellow head, or center. The pus is under pressure, which increases the pain and tenderness. Eventually, it either bursts through the skin or, less commonly, disperses inside. The pain is thus relieved and the boil heals with drainage of the pus. When the pus spreads internally, complications may develop.

Boils are extremely common. They affect virtually everybody at some time. Carbuncles are much rarer. Both may recur, because the bacteria that cause the boil or carbuncle may remain on the skin and produce more boils later. There is a risk that if the bacteria find their way from the boil or skin into food, they can multiply and produce toxins that cause food poisoning (see p.495). If you have a boil, wash your hands thoroughly before preparing food and cover the boil with antibiotic ointment and a small bandage.

What should be done?

Most boils burst or dissipate of their own accord within 2 weeks. If you have a boil for longer than this, or if you have recurrent boils, see your physician. The physician may take a sample of your blood and/or urine to rule out the possibility that an underlying disease such as diabetes mellitus (see p.558) is responsible for the boils. Treatment of any underlying disease or condition should stop the boils from recurring.

What is the treatment?

Self-help: To get rid of a boil as quickly as possible, apply a cloth soaked in hot water to the boil every few hours. This will help relieve discomfort and hasten bursting and drainage of the boil.

Professional help: If the boil is about to burst, your physician may make a small cut in the center to allow the pus to drain away. In addition, or perhaps as an alternative, your physician may prescribe an antibiotic to kill the bacteria. The treatment for recurrent boils is usually antibiotics and/or an antiseptic soap. This treatment may need to be carried out for several weeks to eradicate the bacteria that are causing the boils.

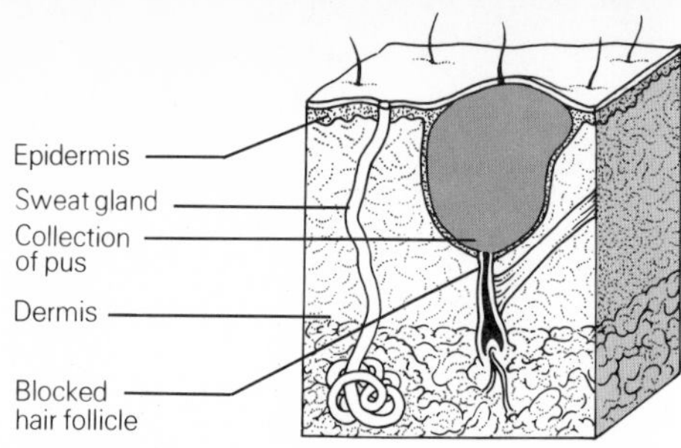

Warts

(including verrucas)

See p.250, **Visual aids to diagnosis, 36–37,** and p.253, **visual aids 49.**

A wart is a lump on the topmost layer of skin produced when a virus invades skin cells and causes them to multiply rapidly. Wart viruses spread by touch or by contact with the skin shed from a wart.

Warts are common in teenagers, less so in children, and even less so in adults. There are no serious health risks associated with warts themselves, but some of the viruses that cause them can also produce cancers.

What are the symptoms?

There are several different types of warts, each produced by a specific virus. The common wart, also called a verruca or a plantar wart when on the bottom of the foot, is a small, hard, horny, white or pink lump with a cauliflowerlike surface. Inside are small, clotted blood vessels that resemble black splinters. The common wart can grow anywhere on your body but is most likely to develop on your hands. On the bottoms of your feet and palms of your hands, a common wart tends to become pushed in so that its surface is level with the rest of the skin. Several warts may appear next to one another on your foot, forming a mosaiclike area 1 in (25 mm) or more across.

Common warts on most parts of the body are usually painless. However, a wart on the bottom of your foot can make you feel as though you are walking on a pebble.

Among the other types of warts are plane warts: small, pale-brown, smooth warts that occur most often on children's faces. Another skin condition caused by a virus is molluscum contagiosum: tiny, white lumps that are often mistaken for warts. The condition, caused by the pox virus, is common among children, and is considered a sexually transmitted condition in adults (see p.654).

What should be done?

Most warts disappear naturally, but this may take years. You may prefer to wait for this to happen. But if you have any warts that you consider unsightly or annoying, try the self-help method described below.

However, there are two cases in which you should consult a physician. One is if you have anal or genital warts. The other is if you develop a wart and you are over age 45; what looks like a wart may be a more serious skin condition, such as skin cancer (see Basal cell carcinoma, p.274, Squamous cell carcinoma, p.275, and Malignant melanoma, p.275).

What is the treatment?

Self-help: There are many folk remedies for removing warts, and some may appear to be effective, but that is only because most warts eventually disappear of their own accord. The best way to treat unsightly warts is to apply a wart remedy in the form of ointment, lotion, or plaster, which are available without a prescription at most drugstores. These strong preparations contain chemicals that destroy the abnormal skin cells. However, the chemicals also affect the surrounding healthy cells, so apply these preparations carefully.

Do not treat warts on your face or genitals with a wart remedy; the skin on these areas is tender and sensitive. And never allow these preparations to get into your eyes.

If you have a wart that does not respond to this treatment, see your physician.

Professional help: Your physician may prescribe a more effective kind of wart preparation, or he or she can remove the wart by freezing it with liquid nitrogen or burning it off with electricity. A few days after this treatment, the wart usually falls off. If it does not, repeated treatment should remove it. As an alternative to freezing or burning, a wart can be scraped off (curettage) after being numbed by a local anesthetic. Warts can also be removed by laser surgery. Anal and genital warts are effectively treated by injecting the drug interferon directly into the warts. Occasionally a wart seems resistant to all forms of treatment and requires several visits to the dermatologist to cure.

Corns and calluses

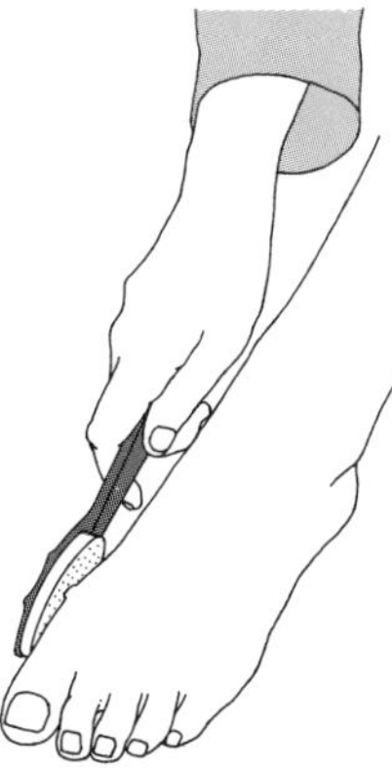

If you are prone to corns or calluses, it may be helpful to use a file or pumice stone to rub away the top layers and ease the discomfort.

Corns and calluses are areas of skin that have thickened because of constant pressure and friction. This causes tenderness in the tissues beneath the thickened skin. Corns are small (less than 5 mm, or ⅕ in) and develop on the toes and feet. Calluses are larger (up to 30 mm, or about 1 in) and commonly form on the ball of the foot or over a bunion (see p.592). Both usually occur after you have been wearing a new or poorly fitting pair of shoes. A callus can also form if you wear high heels, since this type of shoe causes increased pressure on the ball of the foot. Some people apparently have less cushioning tissue than normal between the bones and skin of their feet and thus get calluses and corns very easily. Calluses may develop on your palms, especially if you do heavy manual work.

What are the risks?

Corns and calluses are extremely common. Nearly everyone gets them at some time. But it is unusual for them to become so painful that you have to consult a physician.

If you have lack of feeling in your feet as a result of some disease of the nerves (see Peripheral neuropathy, p.302), this indicates poor circulation, which may be caused by diabetes mellitus (see p.558). In such a case callus formation can be followed by deep ulceration of the area, which may require considerable medical attention.

What is the treatment?

Self-help: Wear shoes that fit comfortably. After several weeks, the corn or callus should disappear. In the meantime, to ease any discomfort, regularly soften your feet with a bland ointment. You may also want to rub away the dead skin with a pumice stone. Calluses on the hands can be softened and trimmed in the same way. To prevent direct pressure, cover the corns with small spongy rings available at your pharmacy. Acid plasters, also available at your drugstore, can be applied to corns to help dissolve them. If these self-help measures do not work, consult your physician, who may decide to trim the corn or callus surgically or chemically.

Eczema and dermatitis

See p.243, **Visual aids to diagnosis, 8–12** and p.243, **visual aids 13–15.**

The word dermatitis means inflammation of the skin. Eczema is a specific form of dermatitis. Some physicians use the word eczema to describe any internally provoked inflammation of the skin, which may affect some people more than others. Dermatitis, on the other hand, also includes conditions that are caused by external factors, such as contact with poison ivy, and affect everybody in the same way.

In addition to inflammation of the skin, eczema is characterized by redness and flaking and/or blistering. Eventually, the skin in the affected area becomes thickened and changes color.

There are many different types of dermatitis and eczema. Several of the more common varieties that adults get follow (see also Infantile eczema, p.712).

Contact dermatitis: This varied condition is caused by a reaction to certain substances that may touch the skin. If you touch poison ivy, for example, a delayed hypersensitivity reaction occurs within 48 hours after contact. The skin becomes red and itchy, even beyond the point of contact, and tiny blisters develop. These may join to form large blisters, which then break and crust over. If minute traces of chemicals from the plant are accidentally transferred from one part of the body to another, contact dermatitis may develop on the second part also.

Some forms of contact dermatitis are much less pronounced. For example, allergy to contact with nickel (on the underside of a wristwatch or earrings, for example) produces a red, flaky, itchy patch of skin, a reaction which may take weeks or even months to develop.

If an irritant remains in constant contact with your skin, the dermatitis will spread.

Seborrheic dermatitis: This type of eczema affects adults and young infants in different ways (for seborrheic eczema in infants, see p.712). In adults, the creases from the sides of the nose to the corners of the mouth may become red, flaky, and itchy. In men, this inflammation may extend to the beard area on the face and the hairy parts of the chest and back. The condition may also affect other skin creases in other parts of the body, such as those found in the groin, armpits, and under the breasts. Seborrheic dermatitis in a mild form also causes dandruff (see p.280).

The cause of seborrheic dermatitis is not known. This condition tends to run in families and usually comes and goes over the course of several years.

Irritant dermatitis: The skin of an older person tends to be dry, particularly on the legs. This can lead to mild redness, flaking, and irritation. If you take hot showers, you may get this type of eczema. People who are constantly using dishwashing liquids, detergents, household cleaners, and shampoos often damage the skin on their hands. The skin becomes dry, rough, and reddened, particularly over the knuckles. It may thicken, crack, flake, and itch. A similar type of eczema occurs among people who expose their hands to other kinds of irritant chemicals, often for a prolonged period.

Dyshidrosis: In this type of eczema, itchy blisters erupt on the palms of the hands and the soles of the feet. Some of the blisters may burst and ooze, and the surrounding areas may become inflamed and tender. Other blisters do not burst but die down to form a flat brown spot under the skin. An attack of this type of eczema usually lasts 2 to 4 weeks and then clears up of its own accord, though attacks tend to recur. At its worst, this type of eczema can be incapacitating.

Nummular eczema: Disks of red, flaking, weeping, itching skin appear on the body, most commonly on the arms and legs. The condition lasts for several months, then usually clears up permanently on its own. Its cause is not known.

What are the risks?

Eczema and dermatitis are not generally dangerous to your health, but they can be a severe nuisance. If blisters burst or if you scratch them, they may become infected.

What should be done?

If you have irritant dermatitis, contact dermatitis of which you know the cause, or a mild form of any eczema, try the self-help measures that follow. If they do not help or if your dermatitis is severe, see your physician.

What is the treatment?

Self-help: Dermatitis on the hand will improve if you wear rubber gloves over white cotton gloves for short periods when in contact with irritants such as dishwater. Dry your hands thoroughly after washing them. Apply an unscented hand cream frequently.

If you avoid whatever is causing contact dermatitis, the condition should disappear within a few weeks. You may speed up the process by using an over-the-counter corticosteroid cream or ointment. However, do not use corticosteroids unless you are certain of the cause of your dermatitis and your skin is no longer exposed to the irritant.

Professional help: Your physician may prescribe a corticosteroid cream to speed up the natural healing process, or he or she may refer you to an allergist or dermatologist to discover the underlying cause. This may involve tests on the blood and skin to determine whether you are allergic to a particular substance.

If your physician suspects you have a contact dermatitis, he or she will discuss the possible causes with you. Then patch tests (applying suspected irritants to the skin) can be used to try to identify the specific cause.

Even when the cause is unknown, corticosteroids are effective. But prolonged use of corticosteroids produces adverse side effects (see Box, this page).

Corticosteroid skin preparations

Inflammation is a major feature of many skin conditions. Corticosteroids are drugs that prevent or reduce inflammation, so they are useful for treating a number of skin conditions. However, there are certain drawbacks to their use:

1 In certain people the corticosteroid clears up the initial problem, but causes a "steroid rash" of flushed, or pink, flaky skin with pus-filled spots. The rash disappears when use of the corticosteroid is stopped.

2 If you use a corticosteroid skin preparation, skin infections such as boils may become worse.

3 If you use too much corticosteroid cream for certain conditions, the original condition will return when you stop the treatment, probably in a more severe form.

4 If you use a corticosteroid cream for too long (several months), it may cause permanent skin changes. The skin thins out, fine blood vessels underlying the skin become conspicuous, and stretchmarks similar to those that occur in pregnancy may appear.

5 The function of your adrenal glands (see p.563) may be diminished by too much corticosteroid medication and this can be life-threatening. If your physician prescribes a corticosteroid-containing skin preparation, or if you purchase one over the counter, make sure you use it *exactly* as directed.

Psoriasis

See p.249, **Visual aids to diagnosis, 32** and p.253, **visual aids 52.**

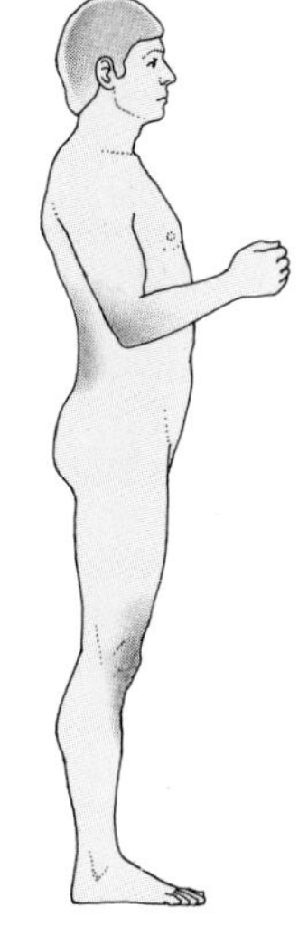

Common sites of psoriasis

As your skin is worn away, it is replaced by new cells produced beneath the surface. In psoriasis the normal rate of cell production is speeded up in some areas, and skin cells pile up faster than they can be shed. The result is an unsightly thickening of the skin. An outbreak of psoriasis is often triggered by emotional stress, damage to the skin, or a period of generally poor health.

What are the symptoms?

Deep pink, raised patches, covered by white scales, appear on your skin. They usually cause no discomfort, but they may be slightly itchy or sore. You may have anything from a single small patch to many large ones. The most common sites are the knees, elbows, and scalp. Less commonly, patches appear under the armpits and breasts, on the genitals, and around the anus. When psoriasis occurs on your hands and feet, it is usually in the form of raised areas with painful cracks or little blisters filled with white fluid. In some cases, your nails become thickened, pitted, and separated from the skin beneath.

Occasionally psoriasis is associated with a form of arthritis that resembles rheumatoid arthritis (see p.589).

What are the risks?

Psoriasis appears most commonly between the ages of 10 and 30, and tends to run in families. In most cases, it does not affect general health. In older people and the very young, however, psoriasis may cause serious distress if the condition is severe and widespread, and if it is not treated.

What should be done?

Many people learn to live with mild forms of psoriasis. In time, you may become familiar with your particular form of the disorder, and you may be able to identify the factors that trigger an outbreak and learn to prevent it. But if you have a severe case, or if it is causing you serious discomfort or distress, consult your physician.

What is the treatment?

Self-help: Sunbathing or using an ultraviolet lamp helps to clear up psoriasis, but a sunburn can make the condition worse. In addition, these treatments definitely increase your risk of skin cancer and should only be used when recommended and monitored by a dermatologist.

Professional help: There are a number of treatments for psoriasis, including tar compounds, anthralin, and corticosteroids, all for application directly to the skin, as well as several medications that are taken orally. The choice of treatment depends on how severe your condition may be and also on how well your psoriasis responds to a test of these various treatments.

You may need treatment with powerful topical drugs. Or you may need intensive treatment with ultraviolet light, sometimes combined with psoralen, a drug to sensitize the skin to light, and possibly with etretinate, a drug related to vitamin A. Another treatment that may work for you is the anticancer drug methotrexate, which slows down cell division. Each of these treatments requires close supervision and monitoring by a dermatologist to minimize the risk of possible side effects.

For most people who have it, psoriasis is a long-term condition, and there is no permanent cure. The condition usually reappears throughout a person's life with varying degrees of severity, although treatment is usually successful in clearing up any individual outbreaks that may occur.

Acne vulgaris and rosacea

See p.248, **Visual aids to diagnosis, 30–31.**

Acne vulgaris, often called simply acne, is a condition in which blemishes of various types appear on the skin. As many adolescents know, it nearly always develops during puberty. For this reason it is discussed under Adolescent health (see p.755).

Rosacea (formerly called acne rosacea) is a condition in which the tiny blood vessels under the skin of the cheeks, nose, and forehead enlarge over a period of weeks or months. The cause is unknown. Some blood vessels are visible as red streaks on the face. In some cases, the skin becomes completely reddened. With rosacea, eating hot spicy food, or drinking alcohol or strong tea or coffee, makes you flush brightly. In some cases, pus-filled spots appear. About half of people with rosacea also get sore eyes from a type of conjunctivitis that develops with the condition (see p.343).

Rosacea is harmless. It affects adults and tends to persist for years, usually coming and going spontaneously.

What should be done?

Your physician may prescribe a topical or oral antibiotic drug. This often improves the condition within a few weeks. However, the condition may recur, and therefore you may require antibiotic treatment again.

Hives

(urticaria)

See p.244, **Visual aids to diagnosis, 16.**

In this very common disorder, red, itchy lumps, known as hives or wheals, develop on the skin. They sometimes have a pale center of variable size, and they often join together to form large, irregular patches. The wheals may occur anywhere on the body.

Hives are sometimes triggered by an allergic reaction to a food such as shellfish, strawberries, nuts, or food additives, or to a drug such as penicillin. Handling certain plants, particularly those with prickly leaves, can also bring on the condition. In other people, wheals form simply when the skin is scratched or exposed to heat, cold, or sunlight. In many cases, it is impossible to pinpoint what triggers the condition. Whatever the cause, tension and stress of any kind usually make hives worse.

Usually, the condition clears up within a few hours and does not cause any other problems, but occasionally it persists or recurs for days or months, even if it is treated.

Some people have a more distressing form of the disorder, called angioneurotic edema. In this condition the tissues underlying the wheals swell, particularly on the face. In severe cases, the lips and skin around the eyes swell enormously. If the swelling spreads to the throat, breathing can become obstructed. Such cases are rare but serious, because it is possible to suffocate under these conditions. Very rarely, hives are a symptom of a more serious disease, such as systemic lupus erythematosus (see p.594). In most cases, however, hives are irritating but harmless.

What should be done?

If your hives result from a food allergy, you may be able to identify the food responsible, because wheals will appear within a few minutes of eating that food. Identification of plants or drugs responsible for the disorder is usually also simple. Wheals will appear when you start to take the drugs and clear up when you finish. But you may not be able to identify the food or substance to which you are allergic if, for example, it is a food dye added to a wide variety of foods. In that case, if the disorder is troublesome, you should consult your physician. He or she may refer you to an allergist for skin tests to identify the causative agent. However, if your lips and the skin around your eyes start to swell, see your physician immediately.

To control hives, your physician may prescribe an antihistamine.

Athlete's foot

See p.253, **Visual aids to diagnosis, 48.**

In this irritating but usually harmless condition, a fungus grows on the skin between and under the toes, especially the fourth and fifth toes. The skin becomes red, flaky, and itchy and smells unpleasant. Sweat or water makes the top layer of skin white and soggy. Other parts of the foot may also be affected by the fungus.

Athlete's foot is slightly contagious. It can be acquired from others through contact with fragments of affected skin that have been shed. It is very common, but it is not usually severe enough to require professional treatment by a physician.

What should be done?

Soggy skin between the toes, without underlying inflammation and itching, does not always harbor athlete's foot but may simply result from sweaty feet. Either condition will benefit from the following self-help treatment.

Self-help: After taking a bath or shower, or swimming, dry between your toes carefully. Do not use the same towel or bathmat as other members of the family or they may become infected. After drying your feet, apply an antifungal cream, spray, or powder, which are available without a prescription. If the

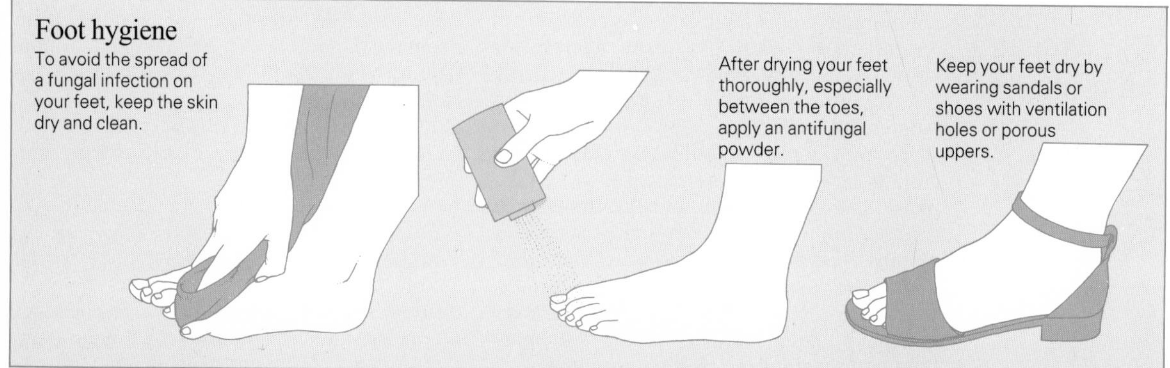

Foot hygiene
To avoid the spread of a fungal infection on your feet, keep the skin dry and clean.
After drying your feet thoroughly, especially between the toes, apply an antifungal powder.
Keep your feet dry by wearing sandals or shoes with ventilation holes or porous uppers.

skin is soggy, use an antifungal powder. Wear absorbent socks made of natural fibers, such as cotton or wool, rather than artificial fibers. Wear open sandals or shoes with porous soles and uppers. Change your socks daily, and air your shoes well when you are not wearing them. Once the skin is dry, an antifungal cream will help. If these measures fail to clear up the problem, consult your physician for further recommendations.

Professional help: Your physician may prescribe a different antifungal preparation from the one that you have been using. Rarely, an oral medication may be prescribed to control infections of the nails, scalp, or other parts of the body.

Impetigo

See p.245, **Visual aids to diagnosis, 22.**

Impetigo is a bacterial skin infection. It can occur almost anywhere but usually appears in the area around the nose and mouth. The infection is contagious (catching), especially among children.

In impetigo, a small patch of tiny blisters appears, but you may not notice them until they break, exposing a patch of red, moist, weeping skin beneath. Gradually, the area becomes covered by a tan crust that looks like brown sugar. The infection then spreads at the edges, and newly infected areas may develop elsewhere.

Impetigo is common and is more prevalent among children than adults. Usually it is not a serious disease, but in a baby it can spread all over the body and make the child very ill. Very rarely, if *Streptococcus* bacteria are the cause of the infection in a baby or child, acute glomerulonephritis (see p.737) can develop.

What should be done?

You should consult your physician. Left untreated, impetigo persists and spreads.

What is the treatment?

Self-help: Until you see your physician, gently wash away the crusts of impetigo with soap and water, so that any ointment your physician may prescribe will be able to contact the affected area and hasten healing. Keep your own soap and towel away from others to avoid spreading the infection. Wash the surrounding skin twice a day to keep it free of bacteria. Children should stay out of school until the condition has healed.

Professional help: Your physician will probably prescribe antibiotics to be taken by mouth or by injection. A new ointment, mupirocin, works very well for impetigo and makes oral antibiotics unnecessary.

Cellulitis

(erysipelas)

Cellulitis is a skin infection caused by *Streptococcus* bacteria that enter the skin through a small cut or sore. The bacteria produce special chemicals called enzymes that break down the skin cells. Any part of the body can be infected. A red, tender swelling develops and spreads gradually for a day or two. Red lines may appear on your skin, running from the infected area along lymph vessels to nearby lymph glands such as those in your groin. Your lymph glands may swell, your temperature rises, and you become feverish and ill.

What are the risks?

If the infection is not treated, the bacteria may get into your bloodstream and cause blood poisoning (see p.452). Consult your physician as soon as you become aware of the infection. Your physician will probably prescribe an antibiotic medication, which should clear up the disorder.

Dermatitis herpetiformis

This rare disorder produces recurrent crops of blisters on the buttocks, back, scalp, and arms or legs, and on the backs of the hands and feet. The blisters usually itch severely and may persist for months or years. If the condition begins in childhood, it tends to recur in adult life, although there may be periods of normal health between episodes. Dermatitis herpetiformis may be related to an allergy to wheat protein (gluten) that may also damage the intestine, resulting in chronic fatty diarrhea. This condition results in considerable weight loss, because you are unable to absorb most essential nutrients. In other cases, the cause is unknown.

What is the treatment?

Dermatitis herpetiformis caused by allergy to gluten can usually be controlled by a gluten-free diet. Ask your physician for advice on diet. If the underlying cause is not known, or even in cases caused by allergy to gluten, treatment with the drug dapsone sometimes improves the rash.

Sunburn

Sunburn is inflammation of the skin and the tissues just beneath it caused by overexposure to the ultraviolet rays of the sun. The affected area becomes red, hot, tender, and swollen, and in severe cases blisters may form. You are much more likely to become sunburned if you have light skin. In addition, a few people are extraordinarily sensitive to the sun because they have a disease or they are taking a drug that makes them particularly sensitive to the sun.

You can become sunburned without sitting under the blazing sun. Ultraviolet rays can and do penetrate a hazy atmosphere in which you may feel comfortable. Also, if you are on the water or on sand, sun rays may reflect off those surfaces and burn parts of your skin that you think are protected.

Sunburn is a special problem throughout the year in the intense sunlight of the southeastern US, southwestern US, and Hawaii. Vacationers are susceptible, because they may unwisely try to get a tan.

Because cold temperatures do not block ultraviolet rays, and snow reflects them the same way that sand and water do, you can also get a severe sunburn while skiing.

What are the risks?

Repeated sunburn, or regular exposure to strong sun over many years, breaks down the elastic tissues in the skin and makes it look prematurely old and wrinkled. In addition, it can produce solar keratoses (roughened red patches) on exposed skin, especially in fair-skinned people. Solar keratoses and/or long-term exposure to strong sun—whether tanning or getting a sunburn—increase the risk of your getting skin cancer (see Squamous cell carcinoma, p.275, and Basal cell carcinoma, below). Sunbathers are at increased risk for melanoma (see p.275).

What should be done?

For those prone to sunburn, a sunblock lotion with an SPF (sun protection factor) of 15 or higher will prevent it. The lotion should be applied to all uncovered areas of the body before prolonged exposure to the sun. It is not advisable to seek a suntan. Try to avoid the sun at its height between 10 AM and 2 PM.

If you do get a sunburn, use the following self-help measures. Protect sunburned skin, even while swimming, by wearing clothing or applying a sunscreen or sunblock lotion, and use a soothing cream. You can take aspirin to relieve discomfort.

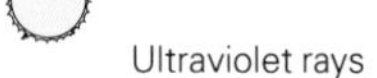

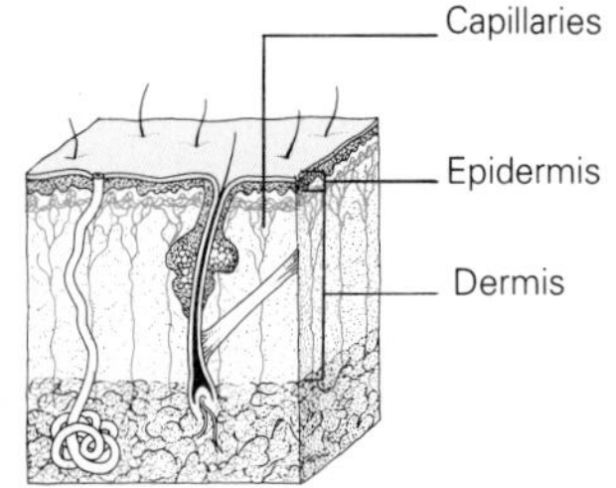

The sun and your skin
The sun's ultraviolet rays can penetrate the semitransparent epidermis and reach the underlying dermis. Blood vessels dilate and let more blood flow near the surface, making the skin look red. Burned skin also looks red.

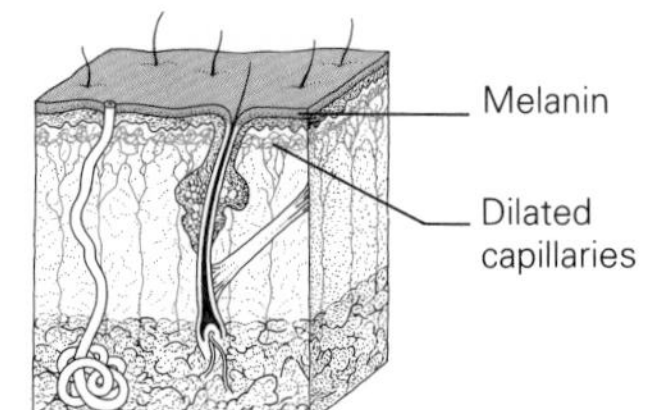

The ultraviolet rays eventually stimulate certain cells to produce more melanin, a skin pigment that protects the underlying tissues. The melanin moves upward toward the epidermis, darkening it.

Basal cell carcinoma

See p.251, **Visual aids to diagnosis, 41.**

Basal cell carcinoma is the most common of the three types of skin cancer. The other two are squamous cell carcinoma (see p.275) and malignant melanoma (see p.275). In basal cell carcinoma, cells just below the surface of the skin become cancerous, and a tumor develops and often becomes an ulcer. The cell damage usually seems to result from long-term exposure to strong sunlight, but it may be many years before skin cancer develops. The ulcer grows slowly as it destroys the tissue at its edges. Unlike many other malignant (life-threatening) growths, it does not spread to other parts of the body until a long time after it forms.

What are the symptoms?

A small, flesh-colored, or sometimes pearly looking lump appears on the skin with enlarged blood vessels (telangiectasias). A common site is the face, especially next to the eye or on the side of the nose. It usually appears as a lump that may grow steadily and within about 6 weeks may become an ulcer with a hard border and a raw, moist center that may bleed. Scabs may keep forming over the ulcer, but they come off and the ulcer does not heal. Sometimes basal cell carcinomas develop as flat sores on the back and chest that grow slowly. This type most commonly affects people with light skin who have spent many years in a sunny climate.

What are the risks?

Because they grow slowly and rarely metastasize, or spread to other parts of the body, basal cell carcinomas cause local destruction of tissue and disfigurement, and this only if they are neglected. A large, untreated basal cell carcinoma will grow relentlessly and can destroy part of a nearby structure such as an eye or ear. However, death from this type of cancer is rare.

What should be done?

To help prevent skin cancer, use a sunblock lotion and protective clothing (see Sunburn, p.274). If you suspect you may have skin cancer, see your physician, who will probably make the diagnosis after a visual examination and a biopsy, in which a small sample of skin is removed for examination. A basal cell carcinoma can be removed in a number of ways. It may be cut out by conventional surgery or by a laser, frozen by cryosurgery, destroyed with a cautery device (high-frequency electric current), or destroyed by radiation therapy. All these methods have a high success rate. Another method of removing these skin cancers is called Moh's surgery. Progressive layers of skin and surrounding tissue are cut out and examined microscopically for the presence of cancer.

After treatment, your physician will probably want to see you regularly, because a small percentage of these cancers recur, usually within 2 years. If this happens, the cancer will have to be treated again. People with skin cancer are at higher risk for more skin cancers in the future.

Squamous cell carcinoma

See p.251, **Visual aids to diagnosis, 42.**

This is one of three types of skin cancer. The other two are basal cell carcinoma (see previous article) and malignant melanoma (see next article). In squamous cell carcinoma, underlying skin cells are damaged, and this leads to the development of a life-threatening tumor, or lump. This tumor has the ability to spread throughout the entire body. As with the other types of skin cancer, many years of exposure to strong sunlight seems to be the main cause.

What are the symptoms?

A firm, fleshy, hard-surfaced, sometimes scaly lump develops and grows steadily. In some cases, it looks like a wart. In others it looks like an ulcer, but the ulceration never heals completely. A squamous cell tumor usually appears on a place constantly exposed to sunlight, including the ears and the hands.

What are the risks?

You are most at risk of having skin cancer if you have lived in a sunny area or worked outdoors for many years, have light skin, and are middle-aged or older.

If the cancer is allowed to reach an advanced stage, it may metastasize, or spread to other parts of the body. If this happens, the outlook is poor. Usually, the treatment is effective if the problem is detected early.

What should be done?

To help prevent skin cancer, use a sunblock lotion and protective clothing (see Sunburn, p.274). Go to your physician without delay if you develop a lump that does not heal in 2 weeks. Your physician may want you to have a biopsy, in which a small sample of the suspected tumor is removed for analysis.

Most squamous cell tumors are removed by cutting them away. A skin graft (see next page) may be needed to cover the scar. Other treatments include cryosurgery (freezing), Moh's surgery (see previous article), and radiation therapy. Most patients are completely cured if treated early, and regular checkups are recommended for 5 years.

Malignant melanoma

See p.251, **Visual aids to diagnosis, 43.**

Malignant melanoma is the most serious of the three types of skin cancer (see also Basal cell carcinoma, p.274, and Squamous cell carcinoma, previous article). This is because malignant melanoma often metastasizes, or spreads, throughout the body. Changes in the underlying skin cells that produce melanin, or skin-coloring pigment, cause a malignant, or life-threatening, tumor to develop. This cancer develops sometimes from pigment cells in a mole present since birth, sometimes in a mole that developed later, and often from pigment cells in what for years simply looks like ordinary skin to you.

What are the symptoms?

A melanoma may develop on any skin surface, even under a nail. It may begin as a flat spot or a bump, usually with some black or brown pigment visible. Often, you can see other colors such as gray, red, blue, and white within a melanoma as well. Occasionally, however, there is no dark pigment at all. Often melanomas appear asymmetric (one half does not look the same as the other, in either shape or color). The edges of a melanoma may be jagged, notched, or blurred, as opposed to a normal mole, which usually has a smooth, distinct edge. Melanomas are usually greater than ¼ in (6 mm) in diameter, but may be smaller. A melanoma may also develop within an existing mole. See a dermatologist about any flat or raised mole that is growing, bleeding, or itching.

What are the risks?

Malignant melanoma is becoming more common in the US and Europe, although it is still rarer than other forms of skin cancer. The increase in occurrence is probably the result of the longtime popularity of sunbathing, because the condition is generally most prevalent among middle-aged or older people with light skin who live in sunny areas such as the southwestern US, southeastern US, and Hawaii and who sunbathe.

Melanoma rarely occurs before adolescence. When it does, it may occur in a mole that has been present from birth. Because the cancer may spread quickly, early recognition, diagnosis, and treatment are essential. Otherwise the outlook is poor.

What should be done?

To help prevent skin cancer, use a sunblock lotion and protective clothing (see Sunburn, p.274). A change in a mole may not signal cancer, but may result from some minor injury. In the same way, a change in the pigment of an area may be caused by a harmless skin condition. However, if you develop any of the symptoms described, you should take no chances and should see your physician immediately. Even if the physician thinks the mole or paler skin is harmless, he or she may still recommend that you have it removed and tested. If the diagnosis of malignant melanoma is confirmed, a surgeon will remove the cancer along with surrounding normal skin. In addition, any nearby lymph glands may be removed, because the cancer can spread through them. A skin graft (see Box, p.279) to cover the area is often done at the same time, especially if the melanoma was large. In some cases, anticancer drugs are also used.

Varicose ulcers

(venous ulcers)

If you have poor circulation in your legs, which becomes more likely as you grow older, the blood flow through the lower parts of your body, especially your calves, ankles, and feet, becomes sluggish. You may already have varicose veins (see p.441). In this situation, any small injury or crack in the skin is unlikely to heal because the tissues are filled with stagnant fluid and are not getting enough blood. The injury or crack enlarges and gradually becomes a varicose ulcer. The condition is more common in older people and in pregnant women. Obesity and lack of movement may aggravate the condition.

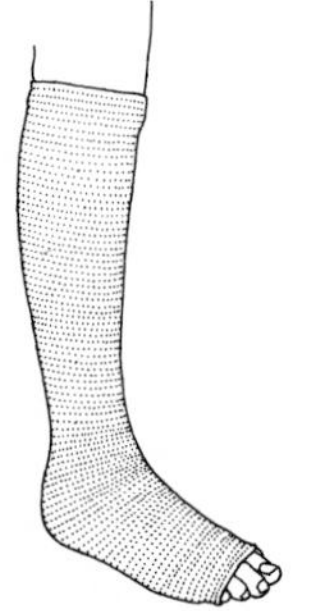

An elastic bandage can speed up sluggish blood flow.

What are the symptoms?

The ulcer is shallow, may weep, and may be infected. Once it has formed, it may remain unchanged or constantly keep healing and recurring. The most common site for a varicose ulcer is the skin on the inside of the leg, just above the ankle. The skin around the ulcer becomes red, then brownish purple, flaky, and itchy, and the ankles often swell. Varicose ulcers may persist for months or even years and may, in uncommonly severe cases, require amputation.

If you think you have a varicose ulcer, see your physician and use the self-help measures described below.

What is the treatment?

Self-help: Whenever you sit and relax at home, raise the affected ankle. Sleep with your feet higher than your chest. This can be done by raising the foot of your bed about 8 in (20 cm). Avoid standing for long periods of time, and exercise by walking regularly.

Professional help: Your physician may suggest that you wear an elastic bandage or thick elastic stocking during the day. If the ulcer is severe, the physician or nurse may teach you to clean it frequently with a mild antiseptic and cover it with a dressing.

If the ulcer does not heal, your physician may coat it with a white paste and then bandage it. In some cases this treatment does not clear up the problem, and you may be advised to rest in bed for a few weeks. Your physician will advise you on how to rest in the proper position and how to keep your ulcer clean. More serious complications require hospitalization. To hasten healing, a skin graft (see Box, p.279) may be needed.

Sebaceous cysts

A sebaceous gland is a very small gland that lies just beneath the skin and produces an oily, waxy substance to keep the skin supple. A sebaceous cyst develops when the gland's outflow is obstructed and it fills with a thick "cheesy" fluid that slowly accumulates. The cyst then grows slowly over many years. It can be seen as a pale lump beneath the skin.

See p.250, **Visual aids to diagnosis, 40.**

Sebaceous gland

In some cysts there is a narrow pore connecting the cyst and the skin surface.

Sebaceous cysts usually occur singly. They are often painless and harmless, are common, and are often first noticed in young adults. The cause of these cysts is not known, but some are produced by acne (see p.271).

What are the risks?

If bacteria enter the pore, the cyst becomes infected. It then becomes enlarged, red, inflamed, and tender. It may eventually burst and release foul-smelling pus. After this, the inflammation recedes but the cyst still remains and may enlarge and become reinfected later. The cyst may also break beneath the skin. This causes a great deal of redness and pain. As the cyst heals, scar tissue may develop, and this may make it difficult to remove the cyst through surgery.

What should be done?

Most people with small sebaceous cysts simply accept them. If a sebaceous cyst becomes infected, or if you want a cyst removed because it is unsightly, see your physician. Antibiotics and warm, moist compresses are usually prescribed for an infected cyst. An obtrusive sebaceous cyst can be removed by surgery in a simple outpatient operation, for which you may be given a local anesthetic. However, if even a small part of the cyst is left behind, which is sometimes unavoidable, it can recur.

Ichthyosis

Ichthyosis is an inherited skin condition. In infancy or early childhood the skin is extremely dry, especially on the hands, and is broken up into diamond-shaped plates that resemble fish scales. Often the skin is darker than normal. Some types of ichthyosis improve considerably during adolescence.

What should be done?

There are various ointments, creams, and special soaps your physician can recommend to make the skin less dry. Cold weather makes this skin condition worse, probably because a decrease in relative humidity makes the air drier.

Pityriasis rosea

See p.244, **Visual aids to diagnosis, 19.**

The cause of this skin rash is unknown, although some physicians think that a virus is responsible. It starts as one or more large, red, scaly spots, generally on the trunk. Over the next few days the spots grow and new ones appear on the trunk and upper part of the arms (the same area that a T-shirt would cover) and sometimes the upper part of the legs. The spots become oval patches of copper-colored skin with scaly surfaces, which often itch. This condition may persist for 4 to 8 weeks. A slight sore throat may occur as the rash develops. Pityriasis rosea affects mainly children and young adults.

What should be done?

Pityriasis rosea is not dangerous, but you should see your physician to be sure that you do not have some other similar, but more serious, skin disorder such as secondary syphilis. Your physician may advise you to wait for the rash to disappear naturally. You can relieve any minor itching by applying cold cream to the rash. If the rash is very bad, your physician may prescribe a corticosteroid cream, and severe itching can be treated with antihistamine tablets. During the worst weeks of the condition, you should avoid taking any hot baths or hot showers.

Keloid

See p.249, **Visual aids to diagnosis, 34.**

A keloid is scar tissue that grows excessively. The keloid can occur after an operation, a burn, a vaccination, severe acne (see p.271), or even the piercing of an ear lobe. At first the scar seems normal, but after several months it grows and becomes noticeably larger and thicker. Occasionally, for unknown reasons, a keloid develops after a very minor scratch.

Keloids are harmless growths, but they can itch and cause discomfort. They sometimes cause deformity. They are fairly common in people with black skin, but less so in those with light skin.

What should be done?

Some keloids stop growing, or even disappear, for no apparent reason. If you want one treated for cosmetic reasons, an injection of corticosteroid medication or a corticosteroid ointment or cream may make the keloid smaller. A keloid cannot simply be cut out. This would leave a scar that could turn into another keloid. Removing the keloid and treating the new scar with corticosteroid injections sometimes results in only a small scar. Radiation therapy is occasionally used to treat keloids.

Lichen planus

See p.249, **Visual aids to diagnosis, 33.**

Lichen planus is an itchy skin rash of unknown origin. It is either small, shiny, reddish spots that appear suddenly, often on the wrists, or patches of thickened, discolored skin that gradually fade and leave a brown mark. Another type of lichen planus is a light, lacy pattern of slightly raised tissue in moist areas such as the vulva and also the inside of the mouth (see Oral lichen planus, p.485). Lichen planus can also make fingernails and toenails ridged.

Lichen planus is most common in middle-aged people. If you suspect you have it you should consult your physician, because there are many other skin conditions, some of them serious, that resemble lichen planus.

What is the treatment?

Most of the time, a dermatologist can diagnose lichen planus on sight. If the diagnosis is in doubt, you may need to have a biopsy, in which a sample of skin is removed and examined. Corticosteroid ointment usually relieves the irritation and reduces the rash. If the ointment does not clear up the rash, consult your physician again.

Discoid lupus erythematosus

(DLE)

Discoid lupus erythematosus (sometimes called DLE) is a chronic skin disorder of unknown cause. It usually takes the form of a red, itchy, scaling rash on the bridge of the nose and cheeks—often called a "butterfly" rash. Other areas (particularly those exposed to sunlight) may also be affected, either with or without facial involvement. On the body, the rash usually occurs as circular patches. The condition may last for several years, with intermittent improvement and worsening. When patches of the rash heal, the skin is often left thin, pale, and scarred.

DLE may occur on its own or it may be a sign of systemic lupus erythematosus, or SLE (see p.594), a more serious, generalized disorder. People with DLE alone have the rash but remain well otherwise; those with generalized SLE have numerous additional symptoms. DLE is more common in women than men and usually develops between the ages of 30 and 40.

What should be done?

You should consult your physician to determine whether your rash is caused by DLE or SLE. If you have only DLE, he or she may recommend that you protect the affected areas from sunlight by using a barrier cream (a sunscreen, sunblock, or zinc oxide) or with clothing. In many cases this is the only treatment needed. If this does not work, a corticosteroid cream usually produces a dramatic improvement. However, long-term use of corticosteroids may cause adverse side effects (see Box, p.270), and the rash may reappear when the corticosteroids are stopped. For these reasons your physician may prescribe other drugs instead, such as chloroquine or dapsone.

Abnormal skin pigmentation

See p.252, **Visual aids to diagnosis, 44–46** and p.251, **visual aid 43.**

Normal skin contains cells called melanocytes that produce the brown skin-coloring pigment melanin. There are several conditions in which melanocytes are either abnormal or abnormally distributed. Sometimes they are fewer or less active than usual; this results in a pale area that does not tan. Alternatively, they may be more numerous or more active than usual. This results in a darker area of skin that tans easily.

Albinism: This is a rare inherited condition. The melanocytes are unable to make melanin, so an albino is very pale skinned and has white hair and pink or very pale blue eyes. Albinos are advised to wear dark glasses and to avoid sunlight, because sun hurts their eyes and burns their skin easily.

Abnormal suntan: Certain diseases (see Addison's disease, p.564), and some drugs can provoke a "suntan" without exposure to sun. See your physician if this happens.

Vitiligo: In vitiligo, pale irregular patches of skin with no pigment (color) appear, often symmetrically placed on either side of the body. The patches may grow, shrink, or stay the same size.

Tinea versicolor: This uncommon fungal infection causes patches of paler or darker skin to develop on the trunk. In addition, the affected skin may flake.

Chloasma: Hormonal changes during pregnancy or while taking oral contraceptives cause some women to develop patches of darker skin on the face, particularly over the cheeks. The condition disappears after childbirth or when the pill is stopped.

Moles: These are small dark areas of skin composed of dense collections of melanocytes. Some moles have hairs growing from them. Very occasionally, one may become malignant (see Malignant melanoma, p.275). If you have a mole that changes in size, shape or color, or begins to itch or bleed, you should see your physician.

Seborrheic keratoses: These are round or oval patches of dark skin up to about 1 in (1 to 3 cm) across. They are common and often develop after middle age. They have a crusty, greasy surface.

What should be done?

Most of these conditions are harmless, but if you are concerned, consult your physician.

Self-help: You can find a number of non-prescription depigmenting creams available for lightening skin, but follow the instructions carefully and do not use such a preparation for more than a few weeks at a time. The darker your skin is, the more care you should take in using these preparations. Covering the discolored area with cosmetics may take care of the problem.

Professional help: There are specific treatments available for some of these conditions. Vitiligo may be improved by ultraviolet lamp treatment combined with drug therapy. Tinea versicolor may be treated by an antifungal lotion. Moles may be surgically removed. Special cosmetics can be used to cover various skin blemishes.

Plastic surgery

Plastic surgery is done to repair or reconstruct a part of the body that has been injured (by, for example, a burn) or that is malformed (for instance, a cleft lip and palate). It may involve transferring skin or deeper tissue such as muscle or bone to replace whatever is lacking in the wound or deformity. Aesthetic, or cosmetic, plastic surgery may be performed to enhance a person's appearance.

Skin grafts

An accident or an extensive operation, such as removal of a larger skin tumor, may result in a wound that cannot be stitched together. In such a case, a skin graft might be used. This skin is taken from elsewhere on the person's body and thus is not subject to rejection, as occurs in other forms of transplantation (see p.432). Usually a split-thickness graft is used, shaving off part of the skin from a location such as the thigh. The shaved graft (about 15 thousandth of an inch thick) attaches to the wound bed; the remainder of the thigh skin at the site of removal heals by regrowing the surface layer in 2 weeks.

A full-thickness graft is occasionally used on the face or hand because it has a better texture than a shaved graft, resulting in a better appearance and durability. The supply of skin is limited since the donor area would also need a skin graft if it could not be stitched together.

The grafts are completely removed from the donor site and reattached. The transplanted graft must live without a blood supply until new blood vessels grow into the tissue. In some cases it is important that the new tissue still possess a blood supply, such as when the wound bed cannot supply enough nutrition for a graft to "take." Skin transferred with a preserved blood supply is called a skin flap. Flaps may also include deeper tissue, such as muscle and bone. Blood vessels to a flap may be severed and then reconnected to vessels near the wound by using microsurgical techniques.

Cosmetic (aesthetic) surgery

Facelifts (operations to improve sagging skin of the face and neck), remodeling of the nose (rhinoplasty), eyelid surgery, and other operations to enhance a person's appearance have gained increased popularity in recent years. Plastic surgery is also used to recreate a new breast after an operation for cancer (see p.633). Often, the patient's muscle and fat are used (as a flap). Silicone implants are also commonly used in breast replacement; however, leakage of silicone has been associated with many side effects.

Many operations have lasting results. They do not, however, alter the aging process, which continues. Some patients, especially after a facelift, may decide to have another such operation several years later.

Although these operations are not considered dangerous, they do carry some risk. Occasionally, a patient feels worse than before surgery. There can be rare and life-threatening complications. Liposuction, a means of sucking excess fat from under the skin, may produce considerable blood loss or other complications.

Ask your physician to recommend a plastic surgeon who is skilled at the procedure you are considering. A plastic surgeon should review your expectations to check if they are realistic and should explain the risks of disappointment. The surgeon can help you decide whether you are a good candidate physically and psychologically for the surgery you are considering.

Hair and nails

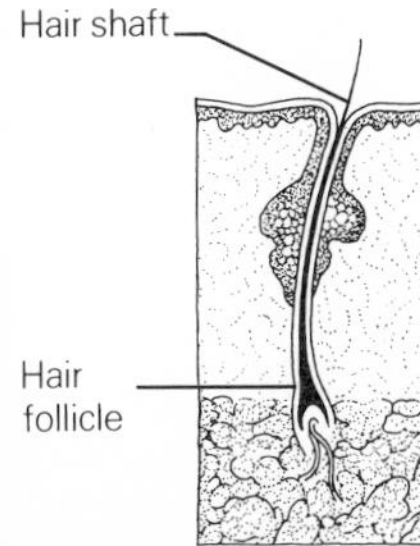

Hair and nails are dead, hardened structures that are very similar chemically to the surface layer of your skin. Hairs grow from follicles, which are pits of actively dividing cells that occur in varying numbers in your skin. Nails grow from special folds in your skin. The substance that gives both hair and nails their hardness is a protein called keratin, which is found in smaller amounts in the top epidermal layers of the skin.

Because hair has little real function in human beings, disorders that affect it generally cause cosmetic and psychological problems rather than medical problems. Similarly, nail conditions can be unsightly and irritating but are not harmful to your physical health. Nevertheless, appearance is usually of some importance to a feeling of well-being, so you should talk to your physician about hair and nail problems.

Dandruff

Dandruff comes from small flakes of dead skin on the scalp, which appear whenever the skin cells of the scalp grow unusually fast. The two main causes of this are a mild form of seborrheic dermatitis (see p.269), or, less commonly, psoriasis (see p.271) of the scalp. The hairs are not affected. Dandruff does not endanger health. It is simply unattractive.

What is the treatment?

Self-help: Use an antidandruff shampoo daily that contains one or more of the following ingredients: tar, selenium, sulfur, salicylic acid, zinc, and ketoconazole. Follow the instructions on the container. Massage the shampoo well into the scalp, and rinse. This should clear up the dandruff within 2 weeks, but the condition often recurs.

Professional help: If the shampoo does not work, your physician may prescribe a lotion containing a corticosteroid. Use the lotion only as directed, and you should have less of a problem with dandruff.

If the scaling is thick and sticks to your scalp, your physician may prescribe a lotion containing one or more of the ingredients mentioned above. The lotion loosens the dead skin and allows an antidandruff shampoo to work more effectively on removing the dead skin cells from the area.

Ingrown hairs

Ingrown hairs are a feature of two different conditions: pilonidal sinus and pseudofolliculitis barbae. A pilonidal sinus becomes inflamed when one or more hairs become trapped beneath the skin just above the cleft of the buttocks, possibly causing an ulcer from which fluid or pus may leak. The condition is most common in young men, particularly those who have a lot of body hair.

Pseudofolliculitis barbae is the condition in which facial hairs become trapped, which may lead to the development of small swellings or pustules. The problem occurs almost exclusively in black males.

What should be done?

If you have a painful swelling between your buttocks, you should consult your physician. Sometimes a pilonidal sinus in its early stages of development can be successfully treated simply by removing the fluid and trapped hairs. Usually, however, the sinus needs to be cut out surgically.

The skin of the buttocks should be kept clean and dry to help prevent the condition from recurring.

If you are a black male with pseudofolliculitis barbae, probably the most effective remedy is to grow a beard.

Baldness

(including alopecia areata)

Baldness that occurs naturally in men generally runs in families. The front hairline may recede first and often meets a balding patch at the crown.

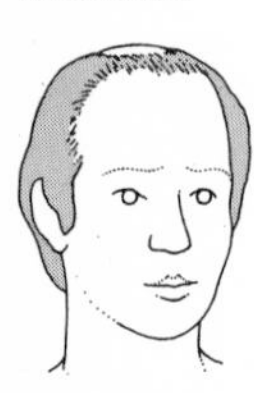

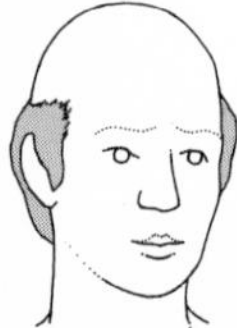

In the vast majority of cases, baldness is a natural process. Baldness tends to run in families, on either the mother's or father's side. The usual pattern is for the front hairline to recede while hair thins at the top of the head. In some men these balding areas eventually meet, and continued thinning may eventually occur over the whole scalp.

In most women, there is a gradual but slight loss of hair throughout life. Again, this is a normal process, although it may be distressing. For men or women, hair loss may follow any major stress, surgery, illness, or accident, but generally the hair grows back over the following weeks or months.

Rarely, baldness is caused by some underlying disorder. In certain severe or prolonged illnesses, such as thyroid diseases (see p.565) and iron-deficiency anemia (see p.450), not only is some hair lost but also the remaining hair becomes fine and lusterless, giving the appearance of extensive loss. Usually, effective treatment of the underlying disease restores hair to normal. Certain diseases that affect the skin, such as lupus erythematosus or lichen planus, may destroy the hair follicles. Patches of permanent baldness may persist. Some forms of treatment, particularly radiation therapy and chemotherapy used for cancer, can cause thinning or loss of hair. The hair usually grows back after the treatment.

Finally, alopecia areata is a specific disease that can cause complete hair loss, although it usually causes only patchy loss. Round, bald patches appear suddenly where the hair follicles are temporarily damaged. The exposed scalp, which has normal skin, may contain a few fine, white hairs and/or "exclamation mark" hairs, which are narrower at the base than at the tip. In addition, the fingernails may become pitted. A more severe, but rarer form of alopecia causes permanent hair loss all over the body, including the armpits, pubic area, eyebrows, and eyelashes.

What should be done?

Some people think of their balding as an acceptable part of the aging process. If you do not, there are three main options: buying a hairpiece, trying drug treatment, or having surgery. Treatment with a lotion containing the drug minoxidil (developed as a treatment for high blood pressure) produces a fine growth of downy hair in some men and women, but the hair disappears if the treatment is stopped. The growth occurs on the crown of the scalp, and it takes 6 to 12 months of treatment to produce noticeable hair. Surgery involves either shifting sections of scalp or transplanting plugs of hair. Experienced surgeons obtain good results, but infection may result.

Baldness caused by alopecia areata often stops within a few months. Your physician may advise you to wait for this natural recovery or may attempt to hasten it by injecting corticosteroids into the scalp. The effectiveness of this treatment is variable.

Hair care

To keep your hair in good condition, handle it gently and carefully. You should not brush, comb, or dry your hair roughly or excessively. Excessive brushing (100 strokes each night, for example) simply pulls hair out at the roots. Long hair may look unhealthy and have "split ends" simply because the free ends of long hair are older than the free ends of short hair. Also, hair that grows while you are ill is likely to be of poor quality. When you recover, the condition of the new hair should improve.

Moderate use of cosmetic hair styling will usually not damage your hair seriously. However, tight ponytails, frequent brushing, corn-rowing, permanent curling or straightening procedures, dyeing, and bleaching all damage the hair to some extent.

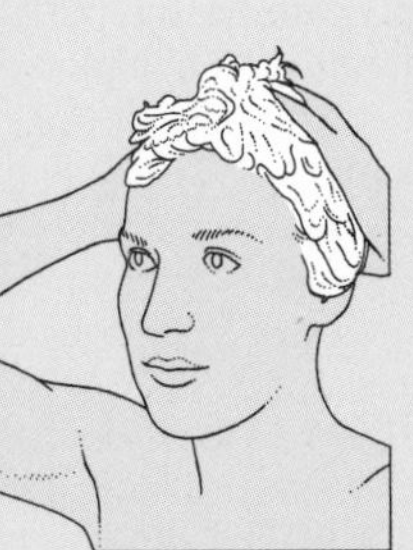

Washing your hair
One application of shampoo should be enough. You can use a mild shampoo designed for your type of hair (oily, dry, etc) and can usually dilute the shampoo by half. Use warm rather than hot water, wet your hair completely, apply the shampoo, and massage gently but thoroughly. Rinse with clean water. If you wish, use a special rinse or conditioner at this stage.

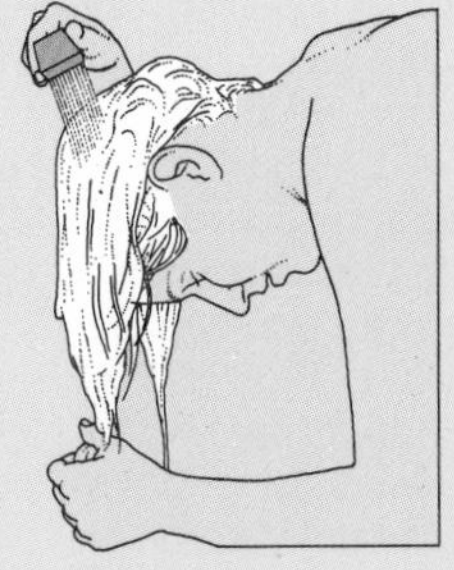

Wrap your dripping hair in a towel to dry it; then remove the towel and comb your hair out gently with a wide-toothed comb.

Drying your hair
Hand-held or hood dryers are unlikely to damage hair if they are used properly, but heated rollers or curling irons should not be too hot or used too frequently. The best way to dry your hair is to let it dry on its own.

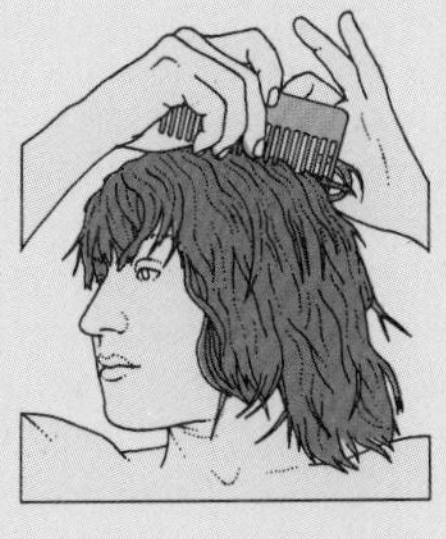

Removing unwanted hair
Many women regularly remove hair from certain areas, and most men shave their faces daily. Hair is usually removed if it is considered unsightly. Whether hair is unsightly or not is a matter of personal preference. Removal of unwanted hair is unlikely to improve hygiene or health.

Most methods of removing unwanted hair do not remove it permanently. Those methods that are most commonly used are described here.

Shaving: suitable for most parts of the body, may irritate and coarsen the skin if used on a woman's face. Contrary to popular belief, the hair does not grow thicker as a result of shaving.

Depilatory creams and sprays: suitable for all parts of the body, but may irritate skin.

Plucking: normally used for small areas such as eyebrows, often individual hairs. Has long-lasting results (usually a month or more).

Waxing: suitable for most areas; like plucking, has long-lasting results. Often done for customers by beauty salons.

Electrolysis: Usually permanent. Should only be done by an expert, generally on small areas (especially of the face).

Paronychia

(including whitlow)

See p.253, **Visual aids to diagnosis, 51.**

A paronychia is an infection of the skin adjacent to a nail; either the cuticle at the base of the nail, or the fold at the side of the nail. It occurs particularly in people who spend a lot of time with their hands in water. The infection may be caused by bacteria or fungi. Bacteria usually cause acute (sudden) infections. Fungi, particularly *Candida*, which also causes oral thrush (see p.484), are usually responsible for chronic infections that develop slowly and are less painful, but may be very persistent.

What are the symptoms?

In acute paronychia, your cuticle or nail fold becomes swollen, red, and painful. The cuticle may lift away from the base of your nail, and if you press on it pus may come out from beneath it. When the nail fold is affected, a blister of pus (often called a whitlow) develops alongside the nail. Chronic infections produce similar, but less severe, symptoms. Often the skin around several nails is affected. The nail roots are no longer protected by the cuticles, and they are damaged. This causes deformed or discolored nails (see next article). Occasionally, the nails themselves are attacked by the fungi and become thick, whitish, and powdery.

What should be done?

You can prevent paronychia by protecting your hands when they are immersed in water. Wear rubber or synthetic gloves over white cotton gloves or rubber gloves with a dusting of talcum power inside if you need to immerse your hands in water. Your physician may treat an acute bacterial infection in the early stages with antibiotics. If pus has collected, your physician may pierce the blister, which will allow pus to drain, relieve the pain, and facilitate healing.

Paronychia is usually caused by bacteria (*Staphylococcus* or *Pseudomonas*), sometimes the result of a yeast (*Candida*), and only rarely caused by a true fungus. If the infection is chronic, your physician will determine the cause of the infection and treat you with an antifungal cream if the cause is a fungus or with an antibiotic if the cause is bacterial. Stop pushing back, manipulating, or otherwise damaging your cuticle. The cuticle serves as a seal to prevent an infection from getting under your nail. Results of treatment for paronychia vary.

Deformed and discolored nails

(including ingrown toenails)

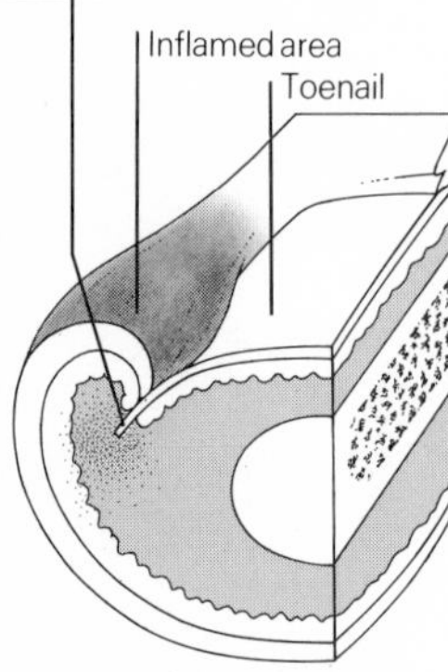

An ingrown toenail curves into the sides of the toe and can be very painful.

See p.253, **Visual aids to diagnosis, 50–52.**

Nails usually become deformed and/or discolored by injury or illness. Injury to the nail-forming area beneath the cuticle, which in the foot is sometimes caused by continuous pressure from poorly fitted shoes or by a decrease in the circulation from arteriosclerosis (see p.435), can lead to thickening of the whole nail. Many disorders can produce nail deformities. Psoriasis (see p.271), lichen planus (see p.278), and chronic paronychia (see previous article) can cause the trimmed end of the nail to separate from the underlying skin. Bacteria entering this space may make the nail turn blackish green. Iron-deficiency anemia (see p.450) can make nails spoon-shaped. Lung cancer (see p.392), chronic lung infection, and congenital heart disease (see p.702) can cause clubbing, or knobby enlarged ends of the fingers and toes, and the nails may grow around these ends. After any illness, temporary poor nail growth may cause a crosswise groove to appear in your nails, which gradually disappears.

Discoloration of a nail is caused by various illnesses. The nail bed appears pale in anemia (see p.450) and bluish gray in certain heart and lung diseases. Small, black, splinterlike areas appear under the nails with infections of the heart valves (see p.421).

An injury to the nail, or very rarely a vitamin or mineral deficiency, can cause one or more small white patches to appear in the nail and move out with the nail as it grows. Finally, the nail of the big toe sometimes curves under at the sides, catches in the flesh and digs in, causing pain as the nail grows. This is an ingrown toenail. It is believed that the nail causes an injury to the skin that does not heal. Infection can result.

What should be done?

Deformities and discoloration caused by an underlying illness grow out after the illness is over. Nails badly damaged by injury usually grow again naturally in about 9 months. A nail that persistently grows in a deformed way should be examined by your physician, who may be able to correct the problem.

If you have an ingrown toenail, try the following self-help measures. Wear loose-fitting socks and shoes, keep the area clean and dry, and cut the nail straight across the top. If the pain increases or persists see your physician, especially if you have diabetes mellitus or other circulatory problems.

Occasionally, your physician may recommend a minor operation to remove the ingrowing edge of the nail and the toe's nail fold next to it. After the operation, your discomfort will be relieved, but follow your physician's recommendations for preventive care, so that the condition does not recur.

Nail care

For healthy nails, follow these guidelines:

1 Protect your hands from prolonged immersion in water, especially soapy water.

2 Keep nails short to prevent them from getting split, which tends to trap dirt.

3 Trim your nails regularly with scissors, taking care to cut the toenails straight across rather than in a curve (which may damage the skin at the corners of the nail).

4 Leave cuticles alone. Pushing cuticles back damages them and exposes the nail fold to infection.

5 Nail polish remover makes nails weak and brittle. Do not use it more than once a week.

6 Tell your physician about any pain, redness, or swelling around a nail. This is especially important for older people and those with diabetes, in whom nail infections, especially of the feet, need early treatment to avoid complications.

7 If you have difficulty trimming your toenails, perhaps because of poor vision or arthritis, you should have them trimmed regularly by a podiatrist, physician, nurse, or family member.

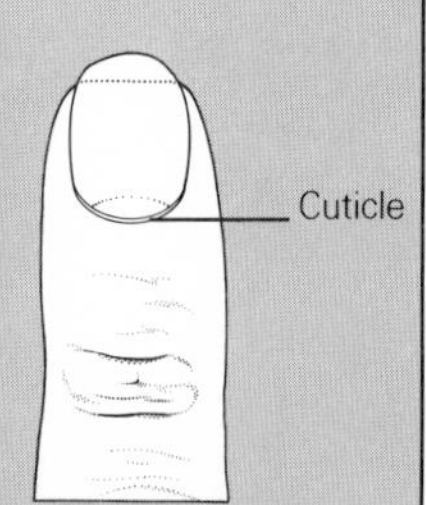

Trimming the nails
Trim your nails straight across to avoid damaging the skin at the corners.

Disorders of the brain and nervous system

Introduction

Imagine the most complex and sophisticated electronic computer ever built. Your brain is far more complex and sophisticated. Your entire nervous system is even more complex. It has two parts: a central system and a peripheral system. The central system is your brain and your spinal cord, both containing nerve fibers. The vast network of nerves throughout the rest of your body is your peripheral system. The peripheral nerves connect with the spinal cord at different levels, and it is through the spinal cord that information flows from these nerves to the brain and back again. This system controls all your conscious activities, and it also automatically maintains posture and muscle tone by a system of reflexes. Some peripheral nerves, known as cranial nerves, connect directly to the brain through openings in the skull. These nerves serve functions such as vision, eye movement, hearing, and facial movement and feeling.

Control of the diameter of blood vessels, intestinal movements, and the actions of the other internal organs are regulated by another system of nerves, called the autonomic nervous system. This system also controls the heartbeat, blood pressure, and body temperature. Virtually all the activities of the autonomic nervous system are unconscious, meaning that they occur without voluntary control.

Like the rest of the body, the nervous system is vulnerable to various problems. Defects in the part of the circulatory system that supplies the brain with blood (vascular disorders) can damage brain cells. The brain can also be damaged by injuries, toxic substances, infections, degeneration, structural defects, and tumors. Because of their complexity, damage to the brain, spine, or peripheral nervous system can cause extremely varied symptoms. The symptoms may include headache, dizziness, loss of balance or coordination, weakness, numbness, tremors, memory loss, difficulty thinking or understanding words, seizures, and loss of consciousness.

When you have symptoms suggesting a nervous system disorder, your physician or a neurologist, a physician who specializes in the nervous system, will try to uncover the cause and choose a treatment.

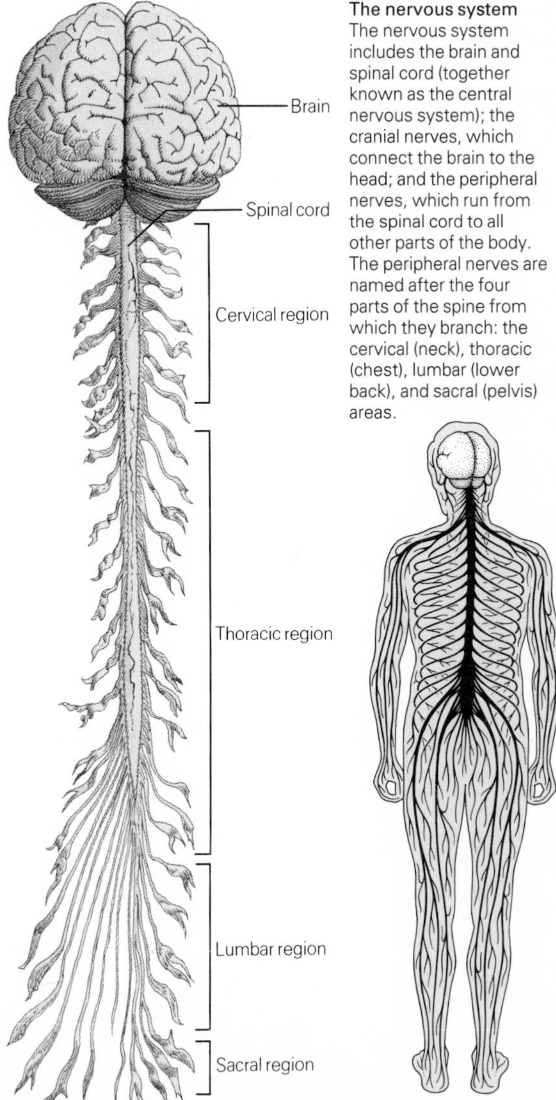

The nervous system
The nervous system includes the brain and spinal cord (together known as the central nervous system); the cranial nerves, which connect the brain to the head; and the peripheral nerves, which run from the spinal cord to all other parts of the body. The peripheral nerves are named after the four parts of the spine from which they branch: the cervical (neck), thoracic (chest), lumbar (lower back), and sacral (pelvis) areas.

The brain

The brain lies well protected within the rigid, bony case of the skull. It has three main parts: the paired cerebral hemispheres, the cerebellum, and the brain stem. The cerebral hemispheres are responsible for controlling such "higher functions" as speech, memory, and intelligence. Some of these functions are controlled by specific areas; for example, the speech center controls speech. If the speech center is damaged by a stroke, the ability to translate thoughts into words is affected. Other functions such as memory cannot be localized and seem to be controlled by centers in the cerebral hemispheres generally.

The cerebellum is located under the cerebral hemispheres. It controls certain subconscious activities, especially coordinating movement and keeping your balance. The brain stem merges into the top of the spinal cord and maintains the vital functions of the body, such as breathing and circulation. Nerve signals travel up and down the spinal cord, which links the brain to the rest of the body.

The diagram (right) shows some of the better-defined areas of the brain and their functions.

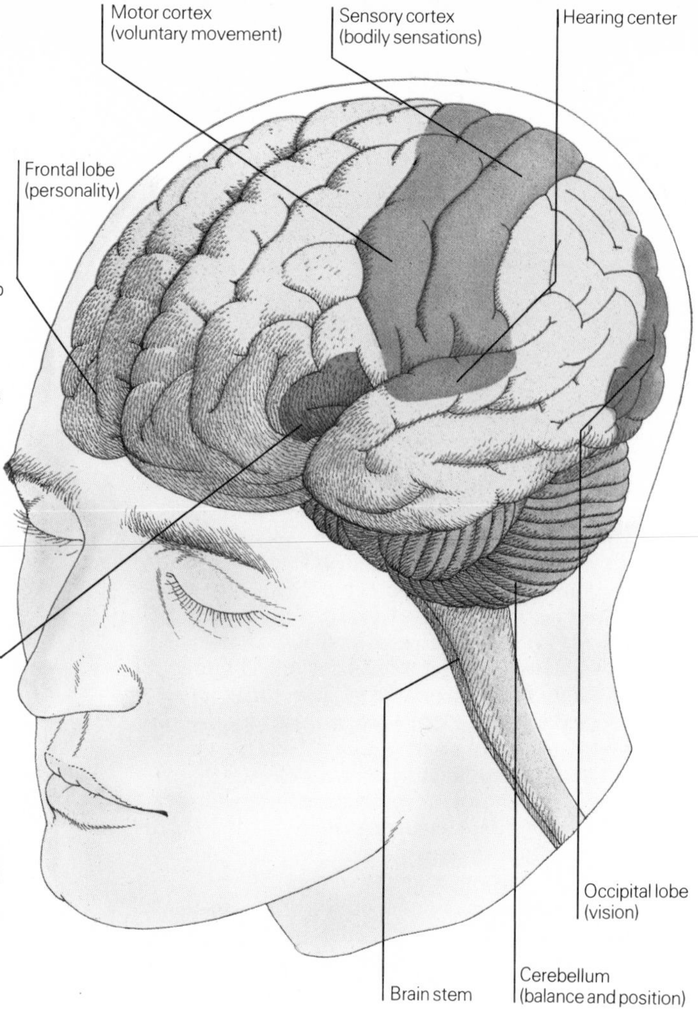

Motor cortex (voluntary movement)
Sensory cortex (bodily sensations)
Hearing center
Frontal lobe (personality)
Speech center
Occipital lobe (vision)
Brain stem
Cerebellum (balance and position)

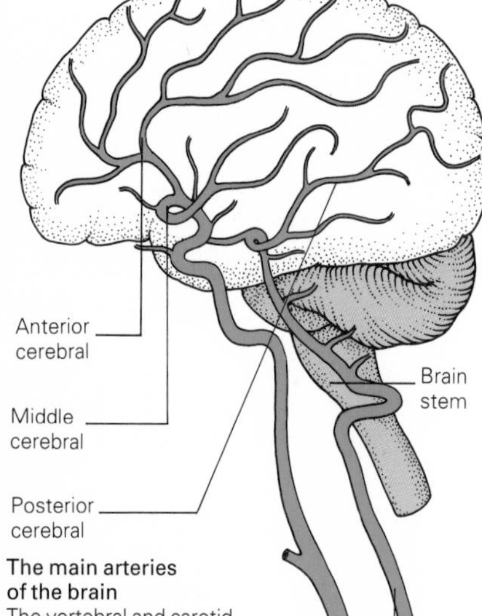

The main arteries of the brain
The vertebral and carotid arteries run up the neck on each side to supply the brain with blood. At the bottom of the brain, they form a circle from which other arteries—the anterior cerebral, the middle cerebral, and the posterior cerebral—run to all parts of the brain.

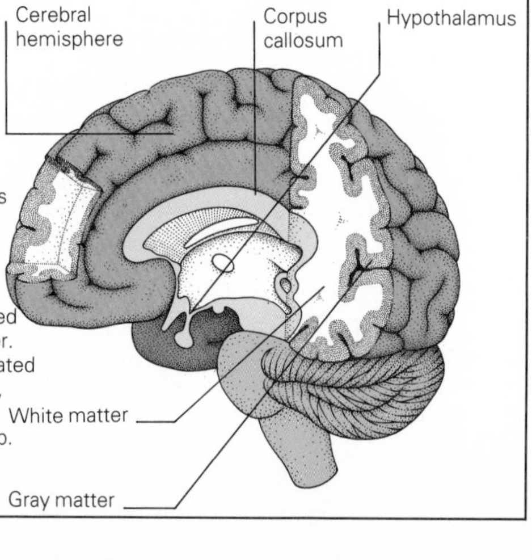

Cerebral hemisphere
Corpus callosum
Hypothalamus
White matter
Gray matter

Inside the brain
A cross section of the brain reveals the corpus callosum, which links the cerebral hemispheres. Each hemisphere has a core of white matter surrounded by a layer of gray matter. The hypothalamus, located at the base of the brain, is related to appetite, sexual desire, and sleep.

Vascular disorders

Four major blood vessels supply your brain with blood to provide it with essential nutrients and oxygen. There are the two carotid arteries in the front of your neck and the two vertebral arteries running up the back in the bony canals in the neck section of your spine. These major arteries join to form the brain's vascular system, a roughly circular arrangement of blood vessels at the base of your brain. Arterial branches from the circle supply blood to all areas of the brain. Areas that depend on only a single branch artery are especially vulnerable to any disturbance in the flow of blood.

The following articles deal with the principal ways in which the brain can be affected by defects in this system. These disorders, such as stroke, which are caused by inadequate blood supply or by bleeding into the brain tissue from diseased arteries, are marked by highly dramatic life-threatening episodes. Professional medical attention is urgently needed for anyone who may have just had a stroke.

Stroke

A stroke occurs when part of the brain is damaged because its blood supply is disturbed. As a result, the physical or mental functions controlled by the injured area are permanently damaged or sometimes may be partially restored via alternate pathways. The disturbance may be from one of three types of vascular disorders: cerebral thrombosis, cerebral embolism, or cerebral hemorrhage.

The first of these, cerebral thrombosis, can happen when an artery that supplies blood to the brain is narrowed, most usually from atherosclerosis (see p.398). A plaque, or large deposit of cholesterol, at the narrowed and roughened portion of the artery may break open and make a place where the blood can coagulate and form a thrombus, or clot. This thrombus may grow until it partially or completely blocks the artery.

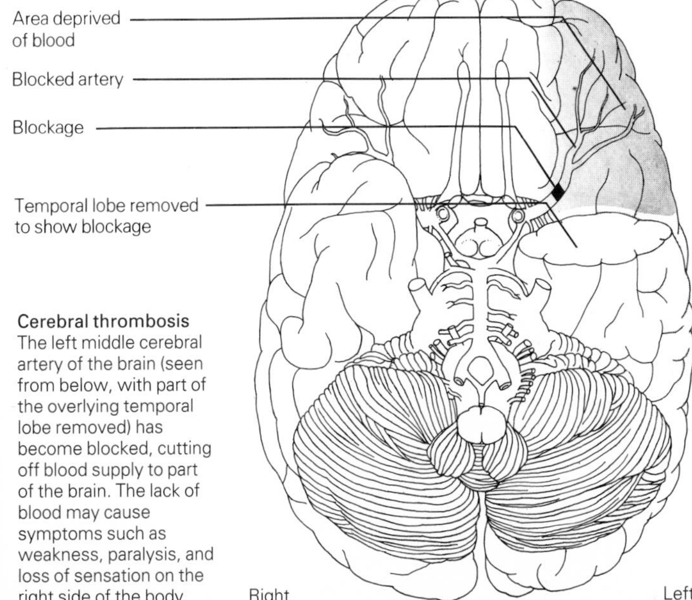

Cerebral thrombosis
The left middle cerebral artery of the brain (seen from below, with part of the overlying temporal lobe removed) has become blocked, cutting off blood supply to part of the brain. The lack of blood may cause symptoms such as weakness, paralysis, and loss of sensation on the right side of the body.

A cerebral embolism is also a blockage, but it is caused by an embolus, which is a clump of material in the bloodstream. The embolus may be a bit of debris from a section of an artery where atherosclerosis has occurred, or a small clot from a diseased heart. It is carried in the bloodstream until it becomes wedged in a place where it obstructs the crucial flow of blood that goes to an area of the brain. In some cases where injury has occurred, fat or air may enter damaged arteries and pass through the bloodstream to cerebral vessels, causing a stroke.

In a cerebral hemorrhage the artery is not blocked; it bursts or leaks. Blood spreads from the rupture into the surrounding brain tissue until the bleeding stops because blood pressure falls or because blood clots seal the leak. The initial effects of a hemorrhage may be more severe than those of a thrombosis or embolism, but the long-term effects of all three types of stroke depend on which part and how much of the brain is affected.

What are the symptoms?

Many of the symptoms of stroke are extremely frightening. You may wake up and find you cannot speak or move part of your body. Or you may, while conscious, feel an arm or leg become heavy, numb, or uncontrollable.

Sometimes a stroke begins with sudden loss of consciousness. Among the many other possible symptoms of a stroke are headache, numbness, blurred or double vision, confusion, and dizziness. Often the functions of only one side of the body are affected. This

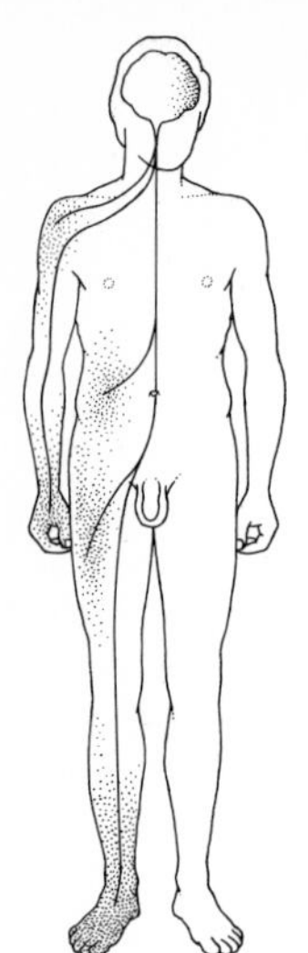

Each side of the body is controlled by the opposite side of the brain. This means that damage to the left side of the brain may result in paralysis and loss of sensation in the right side of the body.

is because damage is usually limited to one side of the brain, and each side of the brain controls only one side of the body.

There are specific areas of the brain that control movement and sensation in definite parts of the body or functions such as vision, memory, and speech. Thus there is a characteristic pattern of symptoms that indicate which cerebral artery is malfunctioning. For example, you may have weakness or numbness in your arm or hand, or on one side of your face. If the stroke affects the brain stem (which connects the brain and spinal cord), then actions such as swallowing may be affected. A stroke often causes loss of some or all sensation in the parts of the body affected. In any event, the symptoms of a stroke, unlike those of a transient ischemic attack (see next article), persist for at least 24 hours, and usually longer.

What are the risks?

Strokes and coronary artery disease (see p.400) are two of the most common causes of death in the US. Both problems are often the result of atherosclerosis (see p.398) and high blood pressure (see p.411).

Most people who have strokes are over 65 (more often men than women), have blood vessels that are narrowed by atherosclerosis, and have high blood pressure. Abnormally high blood pressure can cause a stroke at any age by weakening arterial walls.

Whether or not your blood pressure is high, you are more likely than others to suffer a stroke if you smoke heavily. Strokes also seem to be more prevalent among people with diabetes and people with a high level of cholesterol in their blood.

About one in three strokes is fatal, one in three causes permanent damage or disability, and one in three has no lasting ill effects. If you survive a stroke, you may be partially paralyzed for a number of weeks before improvement becomes apparent. Even a mild stroke is a danger signal; it may be the first of a series of strokes.

What should be done?

If you develop symptoms that suggest you may have had a stroke, get medical help immediately. Rapid evaluation and treatment are essential if an attempt is to be made to limit the extent of damage to the affected area of the brain. You will probably need to be admitted briefly to a hospital. To assess your condition fully, your physician will probably require a CT (computed tomography) scan of the brain and continuous monitoring of your heart rhythm by electrocardiogram (ECG). Along with these tests, your physician may want you to have special X rays of the cerebral arteries called arteriograms. These X rays outline the anatomy of the cerebral blood vessels and can help your physician determine the cause and location of the abnormalities producing your symptoms, aiding in decision making on how best to treat you. Surgery to prevent further strokes is sometimes possible if the source of the embolus is traced to a carotid artery in the neck. Ultrasound scans of your heart and the carotid arteries in your neck may also help your physician decide on the source of an embolus. For a more complete discussion of diagnostic tests for embolism, read the article on transient ischemic attack (see next article).

If someone loses consciousness, it may be because of a stroke. Whatever the cause, call immediately for emergency medical assistance and carry out first-aid measures (see Injuries and emergencies, p.837) while you wait for help to arrive.

Remember that in cases of stroke an apparently unconscious person often senses what is going on around him or her. So do not panic, but try to speak words of comfort; they may be helpful.

What is the treatment?

Self-help: You can do nothing in the first week after you have had a stroke, but you can do much to guard against strokes or prevent them from recurring. Have your blood pressure checked regularly. If it is high, be sure to take the medication your physician prescribes. Do not smoke or eat too much fat, and exercise regularly.

Professional help: Your physician's first priority is to discover the exact cause of the stroke so as to be able to give treatment that will minimize brain damage. He or she will usually arrange to admit you to the hospital for a series of diagnostic tests and initiate therapy, which may include both medication and physical therapy.

Several techniques are now available for imaging the brain without discomfort or risk to the patient. Examination using a CT scanner or magnetic resonance imaging (MRI) can often show the exact regions of the brain affected and whether the stroke was from an infarction (blockage) or hemorrhage.

If within a few hours of the onset of symptoms your physician learns that the stroke resulted from a thrombosis or an embolism, investigational treatment may be given with thrombolytic drugs. These drugs dissolve the blood clot and thereby restore blood flow to the part of the brain affected by the stroke. However, the treatment carries certain risks. Bleeding may occur in the damaged part of the brain or elsewhere in the body. Research studies are under way to evaluate this type of treatment and so help physicians identify the patients most likely to benefit from it.

If the cause of the stroke proves to be an embolism from a blood clot in the heart, without any accompanying bleeding into the brain tissue, treatment may consist of anticoagulant drugs to reduce the risk of further emboli as far as possible.

If the cause of the stroke is a narrowed carotid artery, treatment to prevent further strokes may be possible by surgery on the diseased section of the artery. This treatment is also considered when transient ischemic attacks (TIAs, see next article) occur despite therapy with aspirin.

Severely damaged nerve tracts can never be regenerated, but sometimes professionals can help you teach unaffected parts of your brain to assume control of a function lost because of a stroke. Impaired movements or speech may be improved greatly by therapy, especially if you can approach the process with a positive attitude. However, if a stroke victim is older, is in failing health, and has dementia, treatment may be confined simply to rehabilitation.

Prevention of further strokes is of prime importance. You will probably be warned not to smoke and may need to have regular doses of drugs to keep your blood pressure down. Your physician may prescribe aspirin or other drugs that prevent clotting or reduce platelet stickiness in areas of atherosclerotic damage. Surgery may be advisable if one of the main arteries is severely narrowed; such surgery will improve the blood supply to the brain and reduce the likelihood of further strokes. If the affected artery is in the neck, the blocked or narrowed section may be cleared by surgery called carotid endarterectomy (removal of the obstructing clot and the thickened lining).

In some cases, particularly those in which clots originating in the heart are the cause of a stroke, your physician may prescribe anticoagulant drugs for the rest of your life. These so-called "blood thinners" help prevent clots from forming around irregularities in your arterial walls or inside your heart.

Transient ischemic attack

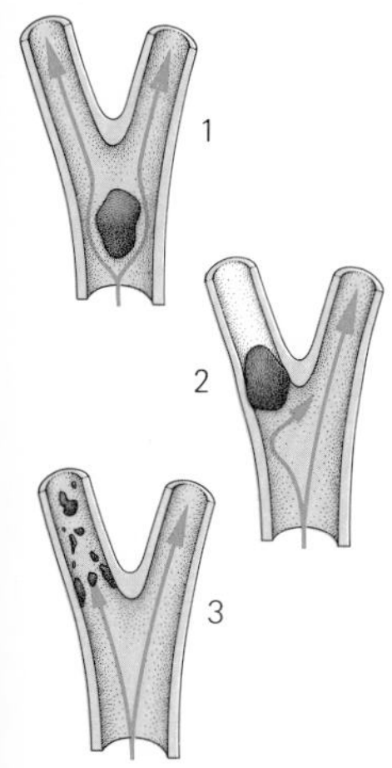

A transient ischemic attack often is caused by a clump of blood cells (1) blocking off a small artery in the brain (2). The attack is only temporary; the clump is soon broken up and swept away (3), restoring blood flow.

During ischemia tissues do not get enough oxygen because blood flow through vessels that supply those tissues is impeded. An ischemic attack in the brain resembles a stroke resulting from a cerebral embolism (see previous article), but a transient ischemic attack differs in that the symptoms last for less than 24 hours. A sudden onset of weakness and numbness down one side of the body, for example, may last a few minutes or hours and then disappear, but the symptoms of a stroke last for more than 24 hours. It is important to understand this difference. But transient ischemic attacks are often signals of an impending stroke. Therefore, they should be quickly evaluated by a physician to attempt to avoid a stroke that may occur later and cause more serious and lasting damage.

The narrowing or obstruction of arteries to the brain can be caused by several factors. Most often, however, an ischemic attack occurs because a small clot or a piece of plaque (see Atherosclerosis, p.398) breaks away from the wall of an artery or heart valve and is carried into the brain. As the fragment of clot or plaque (called an embolus) passes through blood vessels in the brain, it temporarily impedes the flow to an area of brain tissue and causes strokelike symptoms. The exact symptoms will vary, depending primarily on the portion of the brain affected. Circulation may soon be restored, however, and the temporarily deprived tissues recover. The block is therefore transient, or short-lived. But the problem is likely to recur.

What are the symptoms?

The symptoms are like those of a stroke, but they do not last long. They may include headaches, dizziness, tingling, numbness, blurred or double vision, confusion, or loss of the use of part of one side of the body. If the embolus makes its way into an artery that supplies an eye, there may be temporary blindness in that eye.

What are the risks?

Recurring transient ischemic attacks often warn of an impending stroke. Nearly half of those who have transient ischemic attacks are apt to have a stroke within 5 years after they have their first attack.

What should be done?

If you have had strokelike symptoms or sudden loss of vision in one eye, do not delay in consulting your physician, who will examine you and who may then refer you to a neurologist. The first diagnostic step will be to try to identify the source of a possible embolus. A likely source of emboli is one of the two carotid arteries in your neck. To search for signs of narrowing of the carotid arteries, your physician may listen with a stethoscope to various places in your neck. Your physician may also listen with a stethoscope placed on your chest to pick up any sounds of an abnormal heart valve or irregularity in heartbeat rhythm. You may then need to have a portable electrocardiogram (Holter monitor) and also tests of the neck arteries and heart (when rhythm changes exist) using ultrasound techniques. If these tests suggest that one of your carotid arteries is narrowed or blocked, and surgery is recommended, more tests may be done using X rays and a dye injected into the circulatory system. These arteriograms give accurate pictures of the blood vessels that may be the source of the problem.

What is the treatment?

The purpose of treatment is to try to prevent a future stroke. The preventive measures used depend mainly on your age and general state of health. Medical treatment may consist simply of an aspirin tablet once a day for the rest of your life. Aspirin is a good weapon against recurrent attacks, since it acts as an anticoagulant, reducing the likelihood of blood clot formation. More powerful anticoagulant drugs have reduced the number of strokes in people with abnormal heart rhythms. In some cases surgery may be recommended to remove the fatty material that is the cause of the narrowing.

Subarachnoid hemorrhage

As with cerebral hemorrhages (see Stroke, p.285), the cause of a subarachnoid hemorrhage is a ruptured blood vessel. The disorder differs from a cerebral hemorrhage because the blood spreads over the surface of the brain rather than seeping down into the brain tissue.

The surface of the brain is covered by three thin, membranous layers called the meninges. The outside membrane, the dura mater, adheres to the skull; the innermost one, the pia mater, adheres to the brain; and the middle one, the arachnoid, is much closer to the dura mater than to the pia mater. The space between the arachnoid and the pia mater is called the subarachnoid space and is normally filled only with a liquid called cerebrospinal fluid. A subarachnoid hemorrhage occurs when blood leaks into the subarachnoid space. This is usually caused by a burst aneurysm (see p.436) in a cerebral artery wall. The blood either remains in the fluid or pushes its way through the pia mater and into the brain tissue.

Site of lumbar puncture

Needle

Bottom of spinal cord

Cerebrospinal fluid

Backbone

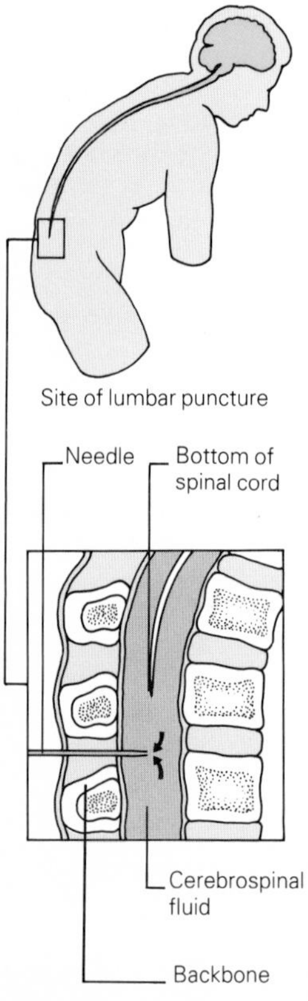

Close-up of lumbar puncture

What are the symptoms?

The main symptom is a sudden headache, which is likely to be far more painful than an ordinary headache (see p.303) or even a migraine (see p.304). A stiff neck and virtual inability to endure bright light (photophobia) often follow, and there may also be faintness, dizziness, confusion, drowsiness, nausea, and vomiting. A major hemorrhage can cause sudden loss of consciousness.

What are the risks?

Subarachnoid hemorrhage most often occurs in people aged 40 to 60 and is slightly more common in women. Anyone with high blood pressure (see p.411) or diabetes mellitus (see p.558) may be more susceptible.

Up to 45 percent of major episodes (those that cause unconsciousness) are fatal, and 1 in 3 people who survive have additional episodes. There is a risk of permanent brain damage resulting from the pressure of blood on the brain surface. In many cases, either blood spreads into the brain tissue, causing strokelike symptoms, or the blood vessels constrict, causing similar problems.

What should be done?

If you develop a sudden severe headache accompanied by a stiff neck and extreme sensitivity to light, go to a hospital emergency department immediately. If someone complains of a sudden headache and then lapses into unconsciousness, call 911 (or your local emergency medical services system) or get that person to a hospital emergency department immediately. While waiting for help, follow the first-aid instructions given in Injuries and emergencies (see p.837).

With an unconscious person, the physician's first step is to restore circulation and breathing. The next step is to do a CT scan to distinguish between the two possible causes. If the scan is normal your physician may want to do a lumbar puncture, a test that involves taking a specimen of cerebrospinal fluid. The easiest place to take the specimen and check it for blood is in the lumbar region, at the base of the spine.

What is the treatment?

If blood is found in your cerebrospinal fluid, your physician's main concern will be to

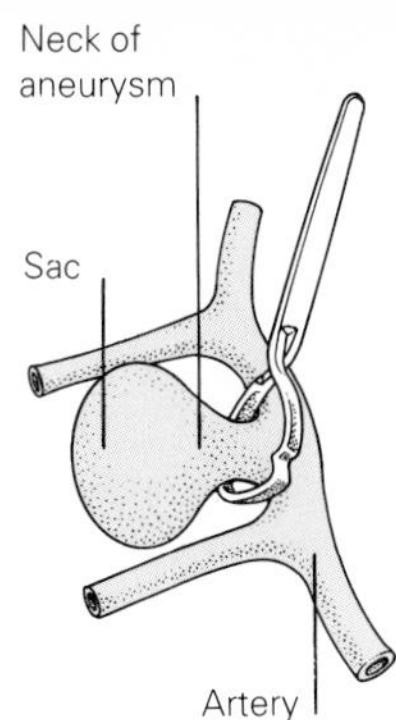

During surgery a small clip is placed around the narrow neck of the aneurysm. Other treatments include using a catheter to carry drugs to the area.

prevent further bleeding. No drug treatment can heal a burst artery, but if you survive the first few days after a subarachnoid hemorrhage, the rupture that caused the problem has probably been sealed (at least temporarily) by natural clotting of blood, and healing is under way. The initial treatment includes complete bed rest. Medication may be prescribed to facilitate relaxation, prevent seizures, and control narrowing of blood vessels (called vasospasm). In some cases if your blood pressure is very high, medication may be administered to lower it. Special X rays of the arteries that supply the brain, called arteriograms, are done to locate the source of the bleeding and to identify any additional aneurysms that may be present. If an aneurysm proves to be the cause of the bleeding, you will need surgery to prevent a future, possibly fatal, recurrence. Depending on your condition, this surgery may be done in the first few days or may be delayed for about 2 weeks. The surgeon will place a tiny clip across the neck of the aneurysm, closing it to further blood flow.

What are the long-term prospects?

If you regain consciousness after a major episode and survive for 6 months without further problems, you are probably out of danger. Chances of full recovery from surgery, if it is advised, are also good. Residual damage from an episode varies according to which areas of the brain are affected. Partial paralysis, weakness, or numbness may linger or be permanent, as may vision and speech problems (for further information, see Stroke, p.285). You should have your blood pressure checked regularly and have high blood pressure controlled.

Subdural hemorrhage and hematoma

In subdural hemorrhage blood leaks from vessels in the dura mater, the outermost of the three meninges, or membranes that cover the brain. It differs from extradural hemorrhage (see next article) in that the ruptured blood vessels are usually small veins that break on the underside of the dura mater. Because the blood pressure in veins is less than in arteries, less blood is likely to leak out. The blood tends to seep quite slowly into the space between the dura mater and the arachnoid (the middle of the three meninges) and causes a hematoma, or collection of clotted blood.

Among eventual symptoms of subdural hemorrhage are drowsiness, confusion, weakness or numbness down one side of the body, imbalance, and persistent or recurrent headaches and nausea. During a period of days or weeks such symptoms may start gradually, come and go, but eventually become worse.

Subdural hemorrhage usually occurs as a result of a head injury (see Brain injury, p.294). It occurs most often in older people who have fallen. The older person may have forgotten about the accident by the time symptoms develop, complicating the process of diagnosis.

Subdural hematoma
A subdural hemorrhage is bleeding between the dura mater and arachnoid, two of three layers covering the brain. It results in a subdural hematoma, which may cause symptoms similar to those of stroke or dementia.

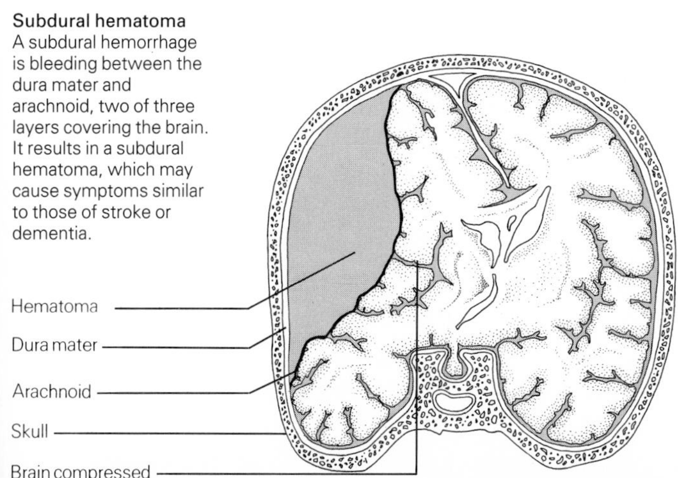

What should be done?

Consult your physician without delay if you develop the symptoms described above. Because they are similar to those of a minor stroke (see p.285), if you remember any such incident be sure to tell your physician that you have recently injured your head, even if only slightly.

If any member of your family shows signs of mental deterioration and abnormal drowsiness, be sure that he or she consults a physician. The affected person will be given diagnostic tests such as a CT scan or MRI (magnetic resonance imaging, see p.295) scan, to find the cause of the symptoms. If the problem is diagnosed as subdural hematoma, treatment depends on the size of the hematoma and may include surgery to remove the clot. In some instances where the hematoma is small, your physician may not recommend surgery because the blood is gradually absorbed. Your physician will follow your progress closely. Rehabilitation therapy is usually helpful after subdural hemorrhage or subdural hematoma.

Extradural hemorrhage

Extradural hemorrhage occurs when blood vessels rupture in the dura mater, the outermost of the three meninges, or membranes that cover the brain. Blood then flows outward between the dura mater and the skull. The problem usually results from a head injury that causes some of the blood vessels in the outer surface of the dura mater to burst (see Brain injury, p.294). Because these vessels are usually arteries, a substantial amount of blood leaks into the space between the dura mater and the skull. The symptoms of an extradural hemorrhage are likely to appear within 24 hours of the injury (see also Subdural hemorrhage and hematoma, previous article). Even if the original injury seemed trivial when it happened, the effects of the injury are not. Symptoms of an extradural hemorrhage may include a sudden severe headache; nausea, which often leads to vomiting; increasing drowsiness, all of which ultimately may lead to unconsciousness, coma, and death. Prompt treatment is essential.

What are the risks?

Head injuries are very common, but only about 10 percent of them require hospital admission, and only 1 to 2 percent cause extradural hemorrhage as a complication. Pressure on the brain mounts as blood fills the space between brain and skull.

What should be done?

If you or anyone in your presence shows symptoms of an extradural hemorrhage, get emergency medical help fast, especially if there has been a blow to the head within the past several hours or the last day. Unless the person is treated promptly, there is a danger of permanent brain damage or death. The person will be admitted to the hospital immediately for diagnostic tests and general treatment for head injury (see Brain injury, p.294). If tests indicate the presence of extradural hemorrhage, surgery will be necessary to stop the bleeding. When the operation is done promptly, it usually results in complete recovery.

Infections

Infections of the nervous system are less common than infections of other systems, such as the respiratory system, because the brain and spinal cord have no contact with the outside. Those infections that do occur gain entry through the bloodstream, the air spaces in the ears or sinuses (the cavities in the bones of the skull), or through fractures caused by head injuries. Many nervous system infections cause obvious, serious illness. Early diagnosis is important, since prompt treatment can save a life and prevent long-term damage to the nervous system. Become familiar with the symptoms of this type of infection in the pages that follow, so that you can act quickly and decisively if necessary.

Meningitis

Meningitis is an inflammation of the meninges, the membranes that cover the brain and spinal cord. There are three meninges. First is the outside membrane, the dura mater, which adheres to your skull. Next is the middle layer, the arachnoid. Finally, there is the innermost membrane, the pia mater, which adheres to the brain. The cause of infection of these membranes is usually an invasion by either bacteria or viruses. There are a number of ways that infection can reach the meninges. For example, infectious agents may spread through the bloodstream from some other part of the body, such as the lungs, where there is an infection. They can also spread to the brain from an infected middle ear or infected sinuses. If you have a head injury involving a fractured skull, this provides an easy entry for infection. There are many forms and degrees of meningitis. Much depends on the microorganism (bacteria or fungus) or virus that has caused the disease.

What are the symptoms?

When the infection is caused by bacteria, fever, headache, nausea and vomiting, a stiff neck, and photophobia (being bothered by bright light) usually develop over the course of a few hours. An occasional additional symptom is a deep red or purplish skin rash. If the infection continues unchecked, you become drowsy and may eventually lose consciousness and go into shock.

The symptoms of meningitis may be less obvious in infants and young children. For a

The brain and spinal cord are surrounded by cerebrospinal fluid, contained between two of three sheets of tissue called the meninges.

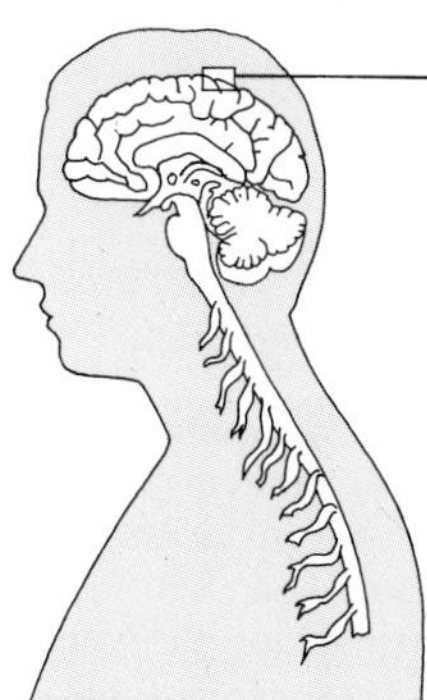

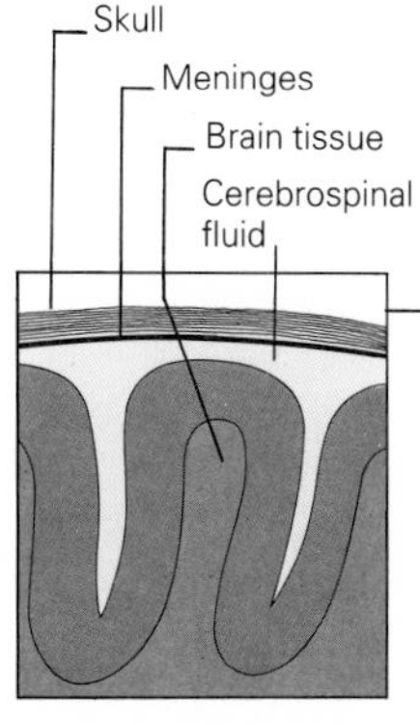

Meningitis occurs when the cerebrospinal fluid becomes infected, causing inflammation of the meninges.

full discussion of the differences, read the article on meningitis in infants and children (see p.715). Older people and those with illnesses that compromise the immune system may also fail to show all of the typical symptoms of meningitis.

When meningitis is caused by a virus, symptoms are milder than with bacterial meningitis. You may have a fever, headache, or a sore neck.

What are the risks?

Meningitis is uncommon in the US. The most common form of meningitis, a viral infection, spreads from person to person through the air. It therefore tends to occur in epidemics, as do many viral illnesses, often in winter when people are in close contact indoors. Viral meningitis is uncomfortable but usually does not result in permanent damage to the nervous system. Most of the time, improvement in the person's condition occurs over a period of days to weeks.

Bacterial meningitis may also occur in epidemics, but sporadic cases of this form are more commonly seen. The sooner treatment of bacterial meningitis is started, the better the results. Untreated bacterial meningitis can be fatal; several deaths have occurred recently in US college students. With rapid appropriate treatment, most people recover completely, but a few are left with permanent damage including deafness, blindness, and/or mental deterioration.

Infants and older people are most in danger of either failing to recover or of being left with lasting damage. The reason for this may be that infants and older people have weakened immune systems.

What should be done?

If you or anyone in your family develops symptoms of meningitis, particularly a combination of fever, severe headache, stiff neck, and photophobia (being bothered by bright light), consult your physician without delay. A tentative diagnosis of meningitis can be confirmed by an examination of a sample of cerebrospinal fluid, the liquid that surrounds your central nervous system. This sample will be taken in a hospital. If the sample, which is obtained by a lumbar puncture (see illustration on p.288), looks cloudy and contains pus cells, the meninges are probably infected.

If a bacterium is causing the infection, tests on the liquid sample should make it possible to identify the agent, and this will help your physician plan treatment aimed at eliminating the organism involved.

What is the treatment?

If the infection is bacterial, you will be given large doses of antibiotics that will be infused directly into a vein. You will have to be hospitalized until the meningeal infection has cleared up. While you are in the hospital, you will be kept in bed and given fluids and medicine for fever and pain in addition to the antibiotics. You can expect to be hospitalized for at least a week or two.

When meningitis is caused by a virus, antibiotics are usually not effective. The body's immune system will mount a response to the virus that usually leads to complete recovery within a few weeks. Supportive treatment during the course of the infection includes bed rest, fluids, and medication for fever and pain.

Encephalitis

Encephalitis is inflammation of brain cells. It is usually caused by a viral infection. In some cases, the virus is one that has caused a generalized infectious disease such as mumps (see p.748), measles (see p.745), or infectious mononucleosis (see p.601). The herpes simplex virus (see Cold sores, p.484) or retroviruses like HIV may cause encephalitis without causing symptoms in other parts of the body. In some instances encephalitis actually results from the body's own immune response to the virus rather than as a result of the viral invasion itself. Other infectious agents may also cause encephalitis, such as the bacteria that cause Lyme disease, or parasites such as the agent that is transmitted in Africa by the tsetse fly and is known to cause sleeping sickness.

What are the symptoms?

The severity of encephalitis varies enormously. In mild cases the symptoms are those of any viral infection: fever, headache, and loss of energy and appetite. In more severe cases brain function is more obviously affected, causing irritability, restlessness, and drowsiness. In the most severe cases there may be loss of muscular power in the arms or legs, double vision, and impairment of speech and hearing or balance. The drowsiness may deepen into a coma.

What are the risks?

Mild encephalitis is common and may not even be noticed. About 1 in 1,000 cases of measles causes mild encephalitis. Severe episodes are rare. The risks vary with age and the kind of infectious agent that causes the disease. Encephalitis in infants and older people can be fatal, but those in other age groups are more likely to recover completely, although sometimes only after a serious and prolonged illness.

Although there is a risk of permanent brain damage, only a small percentage of cases of encephalitis have serious consequences. In some of these cases, particularly with the herpes simplex virus, problems with memory may persist for a time.

What should be done?

If you develop these symptoms, consult your physician, who will probably order various diagnostic tests, including blood tests, a CT or MRI scan of the brain (see p.295), and an electroencephalogram (EEG). An essential test for diagnosis of infection of the nervous system is an examination of cerebrospinal fluid (see illustration on p.288). With the advent of specific antiviral therapy for certain viruses (such as the herpes virus), a brain biopsy may be recommended to help make a diagnosis.

What is the treatment?

Some of the most dangerous types of encephalitis (the type that results from the herpes simplex virus, for example) may now be treated with drugs such as acyclovir or adenine arabinoside. These infections were otherwise always fatal.

Because most of the other viruses that cause encephalitis do not usually respond to antibiotic drugs, the basic treatment consists of measures to ease the symptoms and allow the body's natural defenses to overcome the infection. In most cases, you are simply kept comfortable and well nourished. Sometimes corticosteroid drugs can help suppress brain swelling. If you are unconscious, you will be fed through a nasogastric tube, and your breathing may be assisted by a ventilator.

Recovery from a severe episode may be slow, and you may need special therapy to relearn basic skills such as clear speech.

Polio

(poliomyelitis)

Polio, or poliomyelitis, is a viral infection that affects muscle-controlling nerves. It used to be universally feared, with parents dreading the "polio season," which occurred in summer. This is because in a small proportion of cases the disease caused permanent paralysis or death. But with modern preventive vaccination the disease has been almost eliminated in developed countries. There is only an occasional case in the US, because children are routinely given doses of antipolio vaccine from early infancy onward (see Immunization, p.748). If you or members of your family are about to travel abroad, ask your physician about extra preventive doses of the vaccine.

Where polio exists, it is spread by personal contact and also by eating or drinking contaminated foods or liquids. Its early symptoms are headache, sore throat, and fever. These are followed by pain in the neck and back muscles. In severe cases, muscular weakness may then lead to paralysis.

With antipolio vaccine readily available, everyone should be protected against polio. Children are routinely immunized in stages. If you or a member of your family has not been immunized, consult your physician. Travel to developing countries poses special risks as do rare epidemics of the disease.

Years after extensive paralysis with some recovery the person may have "postpolio" deterioration with new weakness and pain in some of the partially recovered muscles. There is no treatment for postpolio symptoms other than trying to keep active.

Epidural abscess

An epidural abscess is a collection of pus in the space between the skull or spinal bones and the dura mater, which is the outermost of the three meninges, or membranes that cover the brain and spinal cord. The pus usually results from a bacterial infection or accumulates because of an injury. As the pus collects it exerts pressure on the nerve tissue. In rare cases, toxins, or harmful chemicals that are produced by bacteria, may cause damage to the dura mater. Multiple abscesses occur in some cases.

What are the symptoms?

An abscess over the spinal cord can cause loss of muscular power in the legs and numbness of the entire lower part of the body.

An abscess in the brain may have the same symptoms as a stroke (see p.285), causing weakness on one side of the body or difficulty with speech. Headaches, confusion, and seizures may also occur.

The development over a period of a few hours of muscular weakness or a loss of sensation in the legs is a medical emergency,

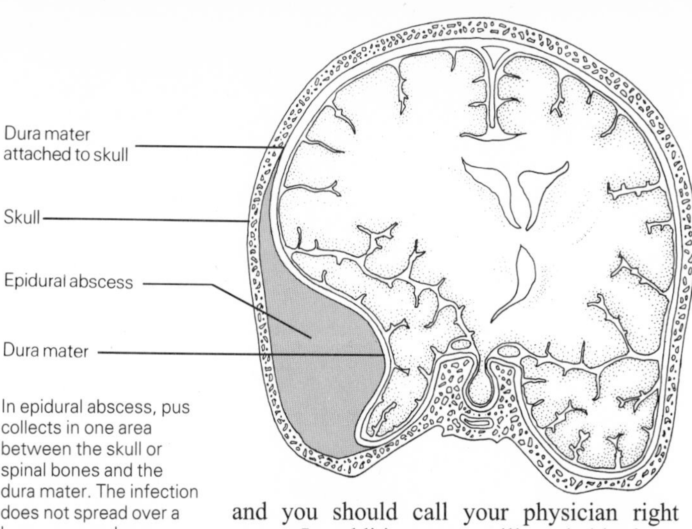

In epidural abscess, pus collects in one area between the skull or spinal bones and the dura mater. The infection does not spread over a larger area or damage more nerve tissue, because the dura mater is closely attached to these bones.

and you should call your physician right away. In addition, you will probably have general symptoms caused by the infection, such as fever and chills.

What are the risks?
Epidural abscesses are rare, because the infections that cause them can now be treated with antibiotics. Such infections include acute infection of the middle ear (see p.359) and sinusitis (see p.373).

What should be done?
If you suspect that you have an abscess, consult your physician, who will ask you about any history of infection, and may order diagnostic tests. Among them may be blood tests to identify the invading bacteria and a CT scan or MRI (magnetic resonance imaging, see p.295). An X-ray examination of the spinal cord (myelography) may also be needed in some cases.

What is the treatment?
Your physician will probably prescribe an antibiotic. In some cases, however, an antibiotic does not solve the problem and surgery is necessary to drain the abscess. For example, if the abscess is putting pressure on the brain or spinal cord, a surgeon will relieve the pressure to prevent permanent damage. The surgeon makes an opening in the skull or in the vertebral bone through which pus can be removed. After the operation, antibiotic treatment is continued. If the original cause of infection is treated, you have a good chance of full recovery.

Structural disorders

A structural disorder of the nervous system is one in which a portion of the system is in some way physically distorted, malformed, or damaged. The cause may be an injury, a tumor, or a disorder of the nerves themselves or the bones and coverings that surround the system. While the skull protects the brain from external damage, the brain may also be damaged because of the inflexibility of the protective bones that make up the skull. For example, a small tumor on the brain cannot expand outward because of the skull, and so the growing tumor may compress the brain and cause severe problems.

Like many other conditions of the nervous system, structural disorders often cause symptoms in areas far from the actual problem. This is because the nervous system is a far-reaching interlinked network that connects various parts of the body. Spinal cord injury may paralyze your arms, cause loss of bowel control, or lead to a number of other problems depending on what part of the cord is injured.

Arteriovenous malformations

Arteriovenous malformations are congenital (from birth) abnormalities of blood vessels that can occur in any part of the brain or spinal cord. Many are small but others can be large and form a convoluted (twisted) pattern in the brain tissue.

What are the symptoms?
Most arteriovenous malformations cause no symptoms for years. When symptoms do occur, they usually consist of bleeding, seizures, or headaches. Bleeding may occur into the subarachnoid space (see Subarachnoid hemorrhage, p.288) or into the brain tissue itself. Seizures are often localized, involving only one part of the body (see Epilepsy, p.306), and the particular part of the body involved and the symptoms associated with it depend on the location of the arteriovenous malformation in the brain.

What are the risks?
The most important risk of arteriovenous malformation is bleeding into the brain, spinal cord, or subarachnoid space. The result of this bleeding can be permanent damage to the brain tissue or death.

What should be done?
Imaging tests of the brain or spinal cord such as CT scans or MRI (see p.295) usually reveal an arteriovenous malformation. It is likely that you will need a special X-ray test called an arteriogram, in which dye injected into blood vessels shows on X-ray films the pattern and origin of the blood vessels that make up the arteriovenous malformation.

Some arteriovenous malformations can be removed by a neurosurgeon. In some cases, it is possible to tie off or inject material into the blood vessels that supply the malformation, cutting off its blood flow. In many cases these treatments are not completely successful and symptoms recur. You may not have surgery if your arteriovenous malformations are located in parts of the nervous system that are inaccessible without risk of serious neurological injury. Small malformations may be treated with radiation therapy.

Brain injury

A substantial blow to the head can sometimes damage the brain, jolting and bruising it even though the skull is not fractured. As a result, the brain tissues may swell, which can produce symptoms as pressure on the brain increases since outward expansion is obstructed by the rigid confines of the skull. If the skull is fractured, brain damage is even more likely. In either case, the extent of the damage and whether any loss of function will be temporary or permanent depend on the type and force of the injury.

What are the symptoms?
The symptoms depend on the force of the blow and exactly what part of the head is damaged. Generally, however, a minor injury is followed almost immediately by a headache. A simple headache that clears up within a day or two usually signals minimal, if any, damage, rapid repair of brain tissues, and, in all but rare cases, complete recovery. A more severe injury usually causes immediate unconsciousness, which may last only a few seconds or persist for weeks. Prolonged unconsciousness is called a coma.

A person who has been temporarily knocked out is dazed and confused upon regaining consciousness. There may also be amnesia, or loss of memory. He or she may also experience headaches or mental lapses, as well as muscular weakness or paralysis (including difficulty with speech). Such symptoms tend to disappear gradually as healing progresses, but in extreme cases there may be residual damage that leads to lasting physical or emotional problems such as paralysis, abnormal irritability, depression, or decreased mental alertness.

What are the risks?
In a small percentage of head injuries, the damage is severe enough to cause permanent mental and physical disability. These severe head injuries are most often caused by traffic accidents (especially those involving injury to people riding on motorcycles), industrial accidents, falls, fights, explosions, or gunshot wounds.

Because of the alarming number of head injuries that occur in motorcycle accidents, many states have enacted mandatory helmet laws for motorcyclists. Those who drive or ride as passengers on motorcycles, even in states that do not require helmets, should always wear a helmet to help avoid possible head and brain injury.

A severe head injury may rupture one or more of the blood vessels to produce a subarachnoid, subdural, or extradural hemorrhage (see pp.288, 289, and 290). The symptoms of cerebral hemorrhage resulting from an injury may not appear until hours, days, or even weeks after the injury occurs. If the skull is fractured, there is a serious additional danger. Infectious agents may enter through the fracture and infect brain tissues, causing meningitis (see p.290).

Finally, there is at least a possibility that lasting brain damage from a serious injury in the form of scarring may cause occasional seizures (see Epilepsy, p.306). This happens in about 5 percent of head injuries, excluding those caused by gunshot wounds. About 33 percent of those who survive gunshot head injuries subsequently experience seizures.

What should be done?
If you are present when someone loses consciousness because of an injury, follow the first-aid instructions in the Injuries and emergencies section (see p.837) and call for medical help immediately. An injured person who does not lose consciousness but has other symptoms of brain injury should see a physician as soon as possible.

If you were in an accident and you do not remember precisely what happened, it will help if someone who saw the accident can describe it to your physician.

If you develop a headache for no apparent reason and begin to feel weak or mentally confused, think back over the past few days. Have you recently hit your head or had a

Brain death

Today's intensive care technology allows physicans to maintain heartbeat, breathing, blood pressure, and other vital functions in patients with severe brain damage. Such treatment is used in the hope that with the passage of time, the brain will recover from injury, infection, or chemical damage from drugs or other substances such as poisons.

In some circumstances, damage to the brain is such that functional recovery is impossible; that is, some patients remain in a permanent state of coma. They need to be fed, helped with elimination, and protected from bedsores (see p.792), but they are still capable of breathing. This condition is called a "persistent vegetative state," and current medical and nursing ethics require that supportive care be given to these patients.

In other cases the damage to the patient's brain may have destroyed the vital centers that control breathing and blood pressure. Such patients can be maintained indefinitely by life support machines that perform vital functions. If tests show that all the brain stem centers are not functioning and if the cause of the brain damage is known to be irreversible, then, even if the patient's heart is still beating, a diagnosis of brain death may be made. Brain death is the medical, legal, and ethical equivalent of loss of heartbeat and breathing. The life support machines may be withdrawn if the person has left clear and convincing instructions in writing that he or she would want them withdrawn. The rigorous tests that must be applied in these difficult situations vary from state to state (see also Dying and death, p.800).

Brain-imaging techniques

As a result of modern technology, various techniques are now utilized for producing detailed two-dimensional images of the brain; both its structure and functioning. The chief imaging techniques are computed tomography (CT) scanning, digital subtraction angiography, positron emission tomography (PET) scanning, and magnetic resonance imaging (MRI).

As aids to diagnosis, these techniques provide more accurate and specific information than any methods previously available. Conventional X rays, for example, reveal little of the brain's internal structure. But today's brain-imaging techniques not only can detect structural abnormalities such as tumors, but also can suggest whether or not the brain is functioning normally.

A CT scan of the head

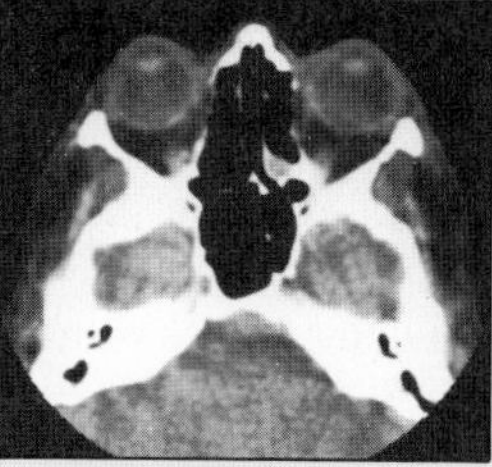

Computed tomography (CT) scanning

CT scanning (computed tomography) involves passing numerous X-ray beams through the brain from various angles and at different levels, measuring their absorption and penetration, and then integrating the data (by use of a computer) to produce a composite picture. From this composite picture, individual "slices" of the brain can be selected and displayed on a screen for examination. These slices, which can be from any level of the brain, seen from any direction, reveal internal structures much more clearly than do normal X-ray pictures. White matter (nerve fibers) and gray matter (nerve cells) show up fairly well, but CT scans provide an especially good image of the fluid-filled spaces (ventricles) within the brain. Tumors, too, are often clearly outlined.

Digital subtraction angiography

Digital subtraction angiography is a refinement of regular angiography. In digital subtraction angiography a radiologist inserts a catheter in an artery in the groin (or occasionally in the arm) and then passes the catheter into the arteries that supply blood to the brain. A radiograph of the brain is then made. After this a small amount of radio-opaque contrast material (which is impervious to X rays) is injected through the catheter and a series of radiographs taken. This makes the blood vessels of the cerebral circulation visible on the radiograph. The radiograph taken without contrast is then "subtracted" from the X rays taken with contrast so that only the blood vessels are shown, producing a very clear picture.

Positron emission tomography (PET) scanning

PET scanning is a way of evaluating the functioning of the brain, which varies under different conditions. Unlike CT scanning and MRI, which give only structural pictures of the brain, PET provides information about how the brain is working. It produces a two-dimensional "map" that differentiates those areas where a lot of chemical activity is taking place from those of lesser activity. PET shows the chemical activity that takes place in tumors but not in scar tissue. So PET can differentiate between a recurring tumor and scar tissue from surgery or radiation therapy.
Along with mapping tumors, PET scanning can be used to locate the origin of epileptic activity inside the brain, and is used in research to examine brain function in various mental illnesses.

Magnetic resonance imaging (MRI)

The principle behind magnetic resonance imaging (MRI) is that some of the water molecules of the body, when placed in a very strong magnetic field, will become aligned with the magnetic field. Radiofrequency waves are then passed through the body and cause some of these molecules to become unaligned with the magnetic field. The picture generated by MRI clearly delineates the gray and white matter of the brain, so the MRI is now the premier type of imaging in the US for most central nervous system disorders including multiple sclerosis, seizures, tumors, infarctions, aneurysms, and degenerative brain diseases. MRI scans can often reveal abnormalities that simply are not depicted on CT scans.

slight accident? In any case, you should consult your physician. Depending on the severity of the symptoms and the results of your physician's observations, you may need some diagnostic tests to discover the extent of the damage. The first of these may be a brain scan (a CT scan or MRI scan, p.295).

What is the treatment?

Self-help: Medications should never be taken by someone who has been knocked unconscious unless a physician has been consulted and has recommended them. If you have had a fairly severe blow, your physician may want you to spend a night in the hospital for observation, to check for complications. Two or 3 days of rest after a slight accident should be sufficient treatment. Most minor damage is self-healing.

Professional help: An unconscious person should be in the hospital, because intensive professional care is of vital importance. In cases of severe swelling, medications such as mannitol or corticosteroids may be given, or a surgeon may operate to place a device in the brain that measures increased pressure caused by the accumulated fluid and may relieve some of that pressure. In some cases of skull fracture, surgery is performed to relocate bone fragments displaced by the injury.

What are the long-term prospects?

Recovery from severe brain injury usually takes many weeks, but chances for complete recovery of lost functions can only be described as fair. People with closed head injuries (those involving no fracture) may be left with memory and thinking disorders, personality changes, slurred speech, or muscular weakness in an arm or leg. Encouragement and support from family and friends are a vitally important part of the recovery process for people with brain injuries, many of whom will also need a great deal of occupational, psychological, and physical therapy to help them overcome paralysis, muscle weakness, poor coordination, and other problems.

Spinal cord injury

The vertebrae, the bones that protect your spinal cord, are separated from each other by disks of flexible cartilage. The disks permit a certain amount of bending and twisting of your back. Injuries that primarily affect the bones or cartilage of the back are discussed in another section of this book (see Backaches, p.584). This article is concerned only with injuries that affect your spinal cord.

The nerve pathways that in part make up the spinal cord transmit nerve impulses between your brain and body. This allows you to control your movements and detect sensations such as touch or heat. If the spinal cord is damaged by an accident, part or parts of the body below the point of injury may be affected. The damage to the spine may be only temporary, but the injury usually leads to some degree of permanent disability since these nerve pathways help control many body actions and functions. Prompt medical care by experts is a key factor in reducing the likelihood of permanent damage and disability resulting from spinal cord injuries.

What are the symptoms?

The area of the body affected depends on the location of the damage to the spinal cord. There may be numbness and weakness, or paralysis of all muscles below the level of the injury, including those that control your bowels and bladder. Sometimes muscles on only one side of the body are affected by the injury. Pain is not always a symptom of injury to the spinal cord, but accompanying injury to nearby bone and nerves sometimes causes severe pain.

Unlike the symptoms of certain types of brain injury (see previous article), which may become apparent only after some time has passed, symptoms of spinal cord damage almost always appear immediately after the injury that causes them.

What are the risks?

Spinal cord injuries are all too common today. Most spinal cord injuries result from automobile and motorcycle accidents, diving accidents, other sports injuries, explosions, knife wounds, and gunshot wounds.

Injury to the spinal cord in the neck can be fatal if it damages the nerves there that control breathing, or it can result in total paralysis of both arms and legs, as well as general numbness from the neck down. Injuries to other parts of the spinal cord are not usually fatal but may be permanent and cause severe disability. Numb parts of the body become especially susceptible to various kinds of injury. The reason is that if you are paralyzed, you cannot feel a warning pain if you hurt yourself.

What should be done?

Serious injury to the spinal cord requires immediate hospitalization. If a person who

The spine and its nerves

Nerve signals from the brain go to the spinal cord and pass to the peripheral nerves. These nerves emerge from the spinal cord as two roots (the posterior and the anterior roots) in the gap between each vertebra; then they join together to relay nerve signals to and from specific parts of the body. The peripheral nerves that emerge in the cervical region of the spine serve the neck and the arms; those that emerge in the thoracic region serve the rib cage and the abdominal wall; and those from the lumbar region serve the legs. The nerves that emerge from the sacral region control the bowels and the bladder.

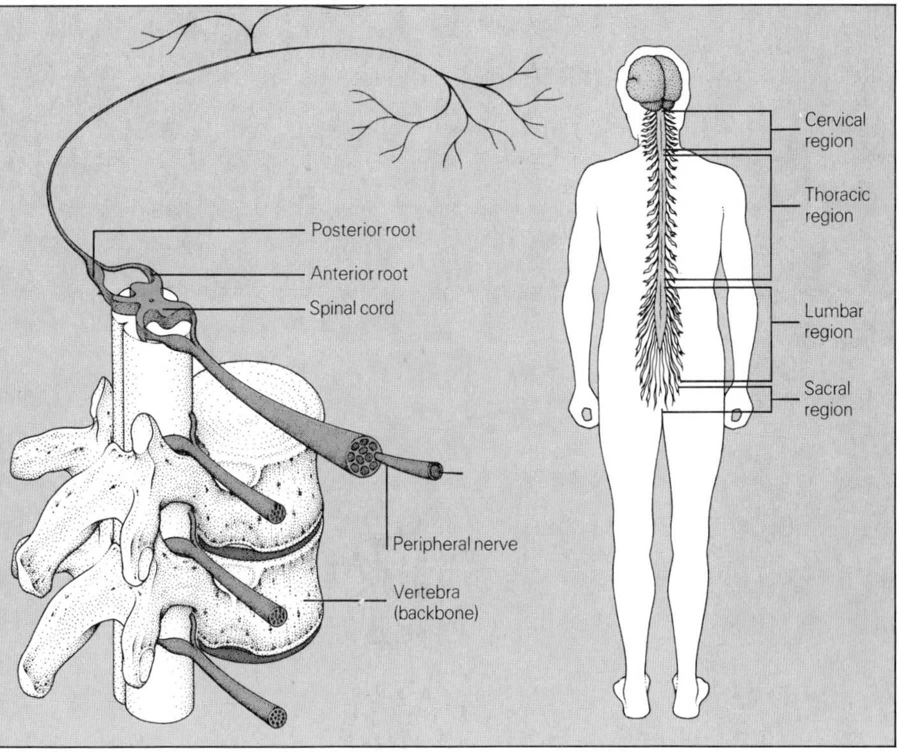

has had an accident is unable to move the legs or experiences numbness, get professional help immediately. Do not try to move the injured person. A wrong kind of movement can cause more damage to nerve pathways. Ambulances are equipped with special stretchers for carrying the injured, and the most helpful thing you can do is have someone get assistance while you stay with the injured person, and let him or her know that help is on the way (see Injuries and emergencies, p.842, for first aid).

Remember that many of the symptoms of a back or neck injury are extremely frightening. You can help the injured person by staying calm and reassuring him or her.

As soon as possible, the spine will be X rayed to determine the site and extent of damage. The physician will test the lower parts of the body for numbness and check if the injured person can move them.

In some cases a CT or MRI scan (see p.295) of the spine or a test called a myelogram is performed to find out if pressure on the spinal cord can be relieved by surgery. In a myelogram a dye that can be seen on an X ray is injected into the fluid that surrounds the spinal cord before the spine is X rayed. Visible on the X ray, the dye usually shows any defects and obstructions.

What is the treatment?

Self-help: The best treatment for injury is prevention. Never dive into water head first until you are sure it is deep enough. Let yourself down into the water feet first. If you must jump in, do so feet first. It is still possible to break your back, but you should not damage your neck in this manner. Always wear a seat belt in an automobile, drive within the speed limit, and do not drink and drive. Wear a safety helmet while riding a motorcycle or a bicycle.

Spinal cord injury with lasting effects will inevitably cause a drastic change in your life. If you have had such an injury, you will have to stay in the hospital or a rehabilitation facility for a long time; several months is not uncommon. With the aid of various medical professionals, you will learn new ways to move around and to cope with daily life.

Some modifications may be necessary in your home. For instance, you may not be able to walk up and down stairs. You should do everything possible to resume your former working routine, but if this is not possible, ask your physician or a social worker for information about programs for vocational rehabilitation.

Professional help: The treatment of suspected spinal damage starts from the time of the injury. If there is severe damage to vertebrae, surgery is sometimes performed, but bed rest is also recommended to promote healing. Treatment within a few hours of the injury with corticosteroid drugs may improve the chances of partial or complete recovery. At first you will be kept fairly immobile and under constant observation to see if your symptoms improve. You may require a surgical procedure to stabilize or realign the damaged vertebrae. While under observation, you will need intensive nursing care. You will have to be fed, turned regularly to prevent bedsores, and helped with emptying your bladder and bowels. See Caregiving at home, p.786.

This stage may last several weeks, after which, if you remain disabled, a team of physicians, nurses, physical therapists, and occupational therapists will start the process of rehabilitation. Their goal is to teach you to make good use of the strength left in your muscles. Various mechanical and electrical aids are available to help develop physical skills and increase independence. The goals and manner of any such treatment depend in a large part on your motivation and on the precise location and the degree of injury. Counseling and guidance are usually available to help you cope with a variety of problems, including sexual problems. You will probably need considerable help in learning to deal with your disability. To live as normal a life as possible, you need to be highly motivated. Therefore, it is important that you try to be very patient with yourself. Try to maintain a positive attitude and be willing to work at rehabilitation over a long period of time.

It may be 3 or 4 months before the degree of disability and possibilities for future recovery can be fully assessed. You and your family may find support and practical help from a self-help organization for people with spinal injuries.

In recent years, increasing attention has been given in the US to the rights of the disabled. Curbs are being lowered, bathrooms and building entrances made more accessible, and job barriers removed.

Bell's palsy

Bell's palsy is a disorder of the facial nerve, usually only temporary, in which the muscles it controls on one side of the face become paralyzed. There are two facial nerves, one on each side, that run out of the brain through a small hole in the skull, just behind the ear. Bell's palsy occurs when one of those nerves becomes swollen and is pinched near the point where it leaves the skull. It is not known what causes the swelling or why only one of the two facial nerves is usually affected.

What are the symptoms?

The characteristic symptom of the disorder is weakness of one side of the face. The corner of the mouth droops, it may become impossible to close one eye, and facial expressions such as smiles or frowns are distorted since there is decreased movement of the muscle from forehead to mouth on the paralyzed side of the face. In some cases, the taste buds may be impaired.

The attack usually comes on suddenly, often overnight, and it is sometimes accompanied by pain either in the ear or on the affected side of the face.

What are the risks?

Bell's palsy occurs at any age, and it is fairly common. A middle ear infection (see Acute infection of the middle ear, p.359) or a sore throat sometimes seems to occur with it.

Though it is disfiguring, Bell's palsy is not a dangerous condition. The main physical risk is irritation of or injury to the eye. The eye does not close properly, so it is exposed to dust, and it may become abnormally dry. The eye may also develop ulcers if it is left unprotected (see Corneal ulcers, p.342).

Embarrassment over the strange appearance of his or her face can cause the person troubling emotional effects. The family and friends of a person with Bell's palsy should understand if he or she is reluctant to go out in public or has even stronger adverse reactions to the problem.

What should be done?

If you have symptoms of Bell's palsy, consult your physician, who will probably be able to recognize this disorder by simply looking at you. Treatment with adrenal corticosteroids or corticotropin (a hormone produced by the pituitary gland) may be recommended by some physicians in the hope of speeding recovery. However, though this treatment is often used, no conclusive evidence confirming the effectiveness of this treatment has been reported. Rarely, an operation to relieve pressure on the nerve may be suggested. However, no treatment has been proved to be entirely effective, and in most instances your physician will tell you that you simply must wait to see what happens.

You may begin to recover within 2 to 3 weeks, and if this occurs your recovery will probably be complete. However, the first signs of returning muscle function may not appear for 2 months or longer. In such cases, recovery will not be complete, but may be satisfactory for most people. Until you have sufficiently recovered from this disorder, you may need to wear a protective eye patch and apply artificial tears to the affected eye at regular intervals.

In the rare cases in which facial disfigurement persists, an operation may help improve facial appearance and relieve the physical disability. An operation may be helpful in cases involving emotional distress.

Cervical osteoarthritis

Cervical osteoarthritis is a disorder that affects some of the 7 cervical vertebrae, which are in the neck. It also affects the flexible discs of cartilage that are sandwiched between these vertebrae. Bony outgrowths develop on the vertebrae, and are frequently accompanied by a hardening of the ligaments and platelike discs. As a result, the neck becomes stiff and the nerve pathway fibers emerging from the upper part of the spinal cord, especially those that run between the cord and the arms and hands, are subjected to an abnormal amount of pressure (see Neuralgia, p.310).

The cause of cervical osteoarthritis is unknown. It is particularly prevalent among middle-aged and older people. Men and women seem to be equally susceptible to cervical osteoarthritis.

What are the symptoms?

The main symptom of cervical osteoarthritis is a stiff, sore neck. Pressure on the nerves that lead from the affected area to your hands and arms may cause such symptoms as muscle weakness, tingling, a pins and needles sensation, numbness, and, occasionally, pains in the shoulders or arms.

Pressure put on the spinal cord from increasingly severe osteoarthritis within the neck or displacement of the discs may damage tracts going to distant parts of the body. As a result, there may be a gradual weakening of the legs and sometimes problems with bladder control.

Sometimes, too, blood vessels that run through the neck vertebrae to the brain can become constricted because of cervical osteoarthritis. This condition can cause symptoms such as headache, dizziness, or unsteadiness, especially if you try to bend your neck backward.

What are the risks?

Cervical osteoarthritis is a common disorder. Minor symptoms of the disease cause discomfort but present no serious problems. Many people who have it do not need to see a physician. In most cases the symptoms do not get worse. If they do, and if lower parts of the spinal cord become affected, there is a risk of serious and irreversible damage. Rarely, in very severe cases, the lower half of the body may become paralyzed.

What should be done?

If minor symptoms persist and seem to be getting worse, consult your physician, who, after examining you, may arrange for an X ray of your neck. He or she may also refer you for a test called electromyography (EMG), which can indicate impairment of nerves and muscles. If your legs appear to be weakening, you may also have an MRI scan of your neck or back, or an X-ray test called myelography to determine the extent of pressure on the spinal cord.

What is the treatment?

Most people with cervical osteoarthritis discover that their symptoms vary in severity from day to day, and they learn to avoid moving their head sharply, tipping their head back, or making any other movement that creates pain or discomfort. If the symptoms are troublesome and persistent, the first treatment that your physician may recommend is the use of a supportive collar and physical therapy with cervical (neck) traction, diathermy (heat treatment), and massage. During the day you may need to wear a rigid plastic collar. You may substitute a more comfortable, soft collar at night. The collar prevents extreme movements of the head and supports it in a position that minimizes pressure on the cervical nerves and blood vessels. The collar is usually worn for about 6 to 12 weeks, and in some cases there is prolonged improvement. While you are wearing the collar, you may be advised to take nonsteroidal anti-inflammatory drugs (NSAIDs) including aspirin. Your physician may also prescribe a very mild tranquilizer in order to relax you and keep your neck muscles from tightening up and causing still more discomfort.

If the symptoms persist, or if new ones develop, you may require traction or an operation if progressive muscle weakness is detected. Surgery involves an enlargement of the constricted bony spinal canal, a fusing together of some of the cervical vertebrae, or both. Either or both of these procedures usually give some relief from the symptoms, but you will be left with a reduced ability to move your neck.

Carpal tunnel syndrome

(including other nerve entrapment syndromes)

At certain points in the body, nerves run through confined spaces where they can become severely pinched if surrounding tissues become swollen. A major nerve particularly subject to this kind of damage is one that carries signals between the brain and the hand. As it travels through the wrist, this nerve passes through a tunnel formed by the wrist bones (known as the carpals) and a tough membrane on the underside of the wrist that binds the bones together. The tunnel is rigid, so that if tissues within it swell for some reason, they press on and pinch the nerve. This leads to the condition called carpal tunnel syndrome.

The condition is fairly common, occurring frequently in pregnant or menopausal women. There is evidence that a change in the balance of hormones during these periods leads to an accumulation of fluid and consequent swelling of the wrists. Carpal tunnel syndrome may also be sports-related, brought on by activities that involve strenuous or repeated use of the wrists, such as racquetball, handball, or weight training. Similar problems may occur with occupations that require repeated actions that include bending of the wrist.

Similar, but much rarer, nerve entrapment disorders may occur at the ankle—called tarsal tunnel syndrome—or at the elbow (where the ulnar nerve may be trapped and compressed).

Cross section through the wrist
Pressure of swollen tissue on the median nerve where it passes through the carpal tunnel can result in loss of sensation in part of the hand, mainly in the thumb and the next three fingers.

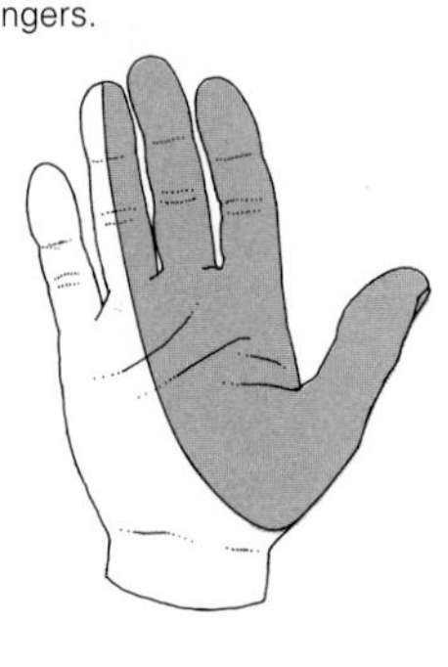

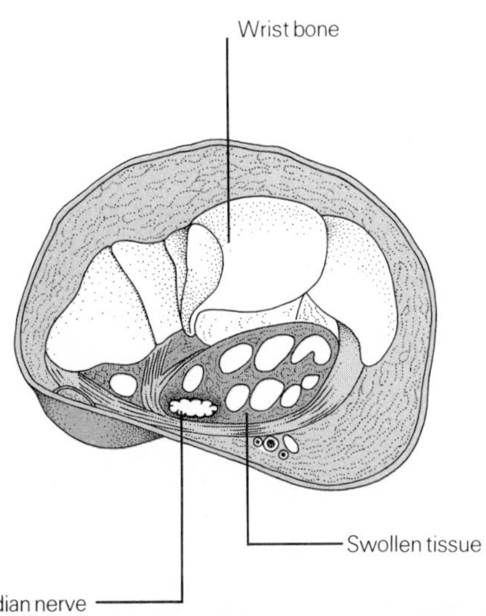

What are the symptoms?

The symptoms of carpal tunnel syndrome are tingling and intermittent numbness of part of the hand, often accompanied by pains that shoot up the forearm from the wrist. The symptoms are generally worse at night and may be severe enough to wake you from a deep sleep. If you hang your hand over the side of the bed and rub or shake it, the pain may lessen. If the condition is very severe it can result in permanent numbness and weakness of the thumb and one or more fingers. One or both hands may be affected.

The principal symptom of tarsal tunnel syndrome is an intermittent burning pain or numbness in the sole or toes of the affected foot that may spread upward to the calf. The problem is often aggravated by standing or walking and usually also becomes worse as the day progresses.

If the ulnar nerve becomes trapped and compressed at the elbow, you may experience tingling or numbness in your little (and sometimes also your ring) finger.

What is the treatment?

In some cases the condition clears up of its own accord. In others a splint worn on the affected wrist at night seems to help. To help combat inflammation, your physician may inject a corticosteroid drug into the fibrous tissue covering the tendons and some nerves at the wrist. But if there is weakness or you are in pain and the condition persists, the best treatment is an operation. The surgeon frees the pinched nerve by cutting through the tough membrane, creating more space. This can be done by open surgery or by arthroscopy (using a small viewing tube). This procedure usually is successful in giving immediate relief, is performed on an outpatient basis, and leaves a barely noticeable scar on the inside of the wrist.

Whether you have tarsal tunnel syndrome or its equivalent in the elbow, the treatment is the same as that for carpal tunnel syndrome. Some people with tarsal tunnel syndrome find that walking barefoot helps to relieve the painful symptoms.

Brain tumor

An abnormal growth, or tumor, in the brain is a serious matter, whether the growth is benign (unlikely to spread) or malignant (likely to spread and threaten life). This is because the protective bones of the skull make it impossible for any type of tumor to expand outward so that the soft brain tissue becomes dangerously compressed as the growth progresses. Since both are very dangerous, the distinction between benign and malignant brain tumors is sometimes less important than it is in other parts of the body.

What are the symptoms?

As a tumor enlarges, it causes increased pressure inside the skull. The result is progressively severe headaches, which are often most painful when you are lying down. The headaches are later accompanied by nausea and vomiting. Sometimes vomiting caused by a brain tumor seems to occur suddenly, without even a warning spell of nausea. Because the buildup of pressure can affect the nerves inside the skull, including those affecting eye movement, you may have double vision. Weakness or loss of sensation of the face can occur, as can other symptoms, depending on the location of the growth in the brain. They include weakness down one side of the body, general unsteadiness, loss of the sense of smell, loss of memory, or even a major personality change. The presence of a brain tumor may also cause epileptic seizures (see Epilepsy, p.306).

What are the risks?

Tumors that originate in the brain are much less common than those that originate in the breast, lungs, or intestinal tract. However, spread of other cancers to the brain, creating secondary tumors, is relatively common. Such secondary tumors (those that have metastasized, or spread, from elsewhere in the body) are more common in later life, when most cancers are most likely to occur. If untreated, tumors of the brain will lead to permanent damage of the brain. Many types of brain tumors are fatal, despite optimal treatment. If a benign growth is discovered and treated early, however, there is often an excellent chance for full recovery. In some cases benign tumors may not require any treatment unless they cause symptoms.

What should be done?

If you have any of the characteristic symptoms, especially a headache that is persistent and progressively severe and is also accompanied by vomiting, seizures, impaired mental functioning, or progressive loss of vision, hearing, speech, or use of your extremities, consult your physician. He or she may refer you to a neurologist for diagnostic tests. This array of tests may include X rays (including X rays of the chest, since secondary brain tumors frequently arise from cells that have migrated from malignant tumors of the lung), CT scans, magnetic resonance imaging (MRI), possibly angiography, or an electroencephalogram (EEG).

What is the treatment?

Surgery to remove a benign tumor is often possible and may be completely successful. Even when the tumor involves a crucial part of the brain and is incurable, it is sometimes possible to remove a portion of the growth to reduce pressure and relieve symptoms. Surgery, whether for full or partial removal of the tumor, is sometimes followed by a course of radiation therapy to kill any remaining tumor cells.

Surgery may not be as successful in the case of malignant brain tumors. However, in selected instances surgery can effectively remove a single metastatic tumor in the brain. When this is not feasible, there are ways of relieving your symptoms and making you more comfortable. Corticosteroid drugs may help diminish the swelling of brain tissue, and thus the pressure, around the growth. Anticonvulsant drugs can be prescribed to control seizures related to the growth. There are also various analgesics available that reduce the pain of severe headaches. Physicians are currently trying to prolong the survival of patients who have some types of malignant brain tumors by using chemotherapy or radioactive disks implanted surgically into the tumor.

Spinal cord tumor

Tumors of the spinal cord are similar to brain tumors (see previous article), but they produce different symptoms. Persistent back pain is the most characteristic symptom. Sometimes sensations of numbness or coldness and muscle weakness in one or both arms or legs may develop, and you may have difficulty in urinating or moving your bowels. The precise symptoms depend on what part of the spinal cord and which nerves are damaged by the tumor.

Spinal cord tumors are even more rare than brain tumors. If you have symptoms suggesting the possibility of a growth on your spinal cord, your physician will probably refer you to a neurologist for an examination, and for a CT scan, magnetic resonance imaging (MRI) scan of the spine, and possibly a myelogram. If a tumor is found that cannot safely be removed, surgical removal of parts of the surrounding vertebrae will relieve pressure on the spinal nerves and pathways, alleviating pain and other symptoms. Following surgery, radiation therapy may be prescribed to retard further growth of the tumor. As with brain tumors, further treatment depends on factors such as the type, size, and site of the growth.

Peripheral neuropathy

Damage to peripheral nerves, which are nerves throughout the body leading from the brain and spinal cord, is called peripheral neuropathy. The damage sometimes occurs as a complication of a generalized illness such as diabetes mellitus (see p.558), alcoholism (see p.329), certain vitamin deficiencies (see p.532), or tumors in distant parts of the body. There are many other possible causes of peripheral nerve damage, including some hereditary conditions, toxic effects of some drugs, and overexposure to certain toxic chemicals (especially arsenic, mercury, lead, and the organic phosphates found in many insecticides). Avoiding toxic chemicals, injuries, and excessive intake of alcohol, along with observing good nutritional and exercise habits, can help you prevent neuropathy.

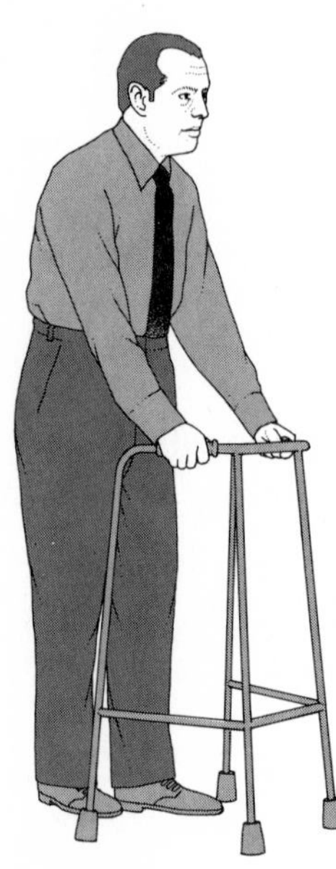

Using a walker

What are the symptoms?

In most forms of peripheral neuropathy, symptoms begin gradually, over many months. A dramatic exception is Guillain-Barré syndrome (see next article). The typical pattern is a tingling sensation that begins in the feet and later occurs in the hands, spreading slowly along the arms and legs to the trunk. In the same way, numbness may develop. Often the skin becomes very sensitive, and you may have pain (see p.310). In some cases there is a gradual weakening of muscle power throughout the body, usually in the muscles of the feet, legs, and hands.

What are the risks?

Peripheral neuropathy is relatively common among alcoholics and people with diabetes. Cases caused by a buildup of toxic chemicals are rare in the general population, but occur more often among farm workers and others who work where there is considerable exposure to chemicals.

One of the risks associated with peripheral neuropathy is that if a numbed part of your body is injured, you may be unaware of the injury until infection or ulceration occurs. Numbness in the fingers can reduce dexterity and make you more susceptible to accidents and injuries. A gradual wasting away of the muscles can eventually progress to the point where it impairs function severely.

What should be done?

Because slow damage to the nerves improves very gradually and may become irreversible, early diagnosis is important. If your hands and feet are tingling, and especially if any of the factors that can cause this condition are applicable to you, see your physician, who will probably refer you to a neurologist for tests. The neurologist will take your medical and personal history and will examine you for signs of numbness, muscle weakness, and changes in your reflexes. The neurologist will test for any correctible vitamin or metabolic deficiencies that can affect nerve function. He or she may send you for electromyography (EMG), a procedure that tests nerve and muscle function, and a nerve conduction velocity measurement. If any members of your family have had similar symptoms, the neurologist may want to review their medical records or examine them to look for possible hereditary conditions that might be involved. Sometimes, a biopsy of a small sensory nerve in the ankle called the sural nerve may be recommended.

What is the treatment?

If the cause of nerve damage is a vitamin deficiency or another treatable disorder, control of the underlying problem can halt or reverse the progress of the neuropathy. If toxic chemicals or drugs are the cause, you will be advised to stop your exposure to those substances. This may require a change of occupation or a change in medications.

In severe cases where muscles have been badly weakened, aids to mobility and independence, such as physical therapy, walking with a cane or other support, and bath rails may be prescribed. You will also be warned to be alert to any wounds on your numb arms or legs and to consult your physician immediately whenever you have a severe bruise or an open sore. Be sure to take good care of your feet and toenails and wear shoes that fit well to prevent pressure sores and infections.

Guillain-Barré syndrome

This is an uncommon and acute form of peripheral polyneuropathy (affecting multiple nerves), which can follow virtually any type of viral infection or even an immunization. Why it occurs is not clear. Some physicians think it may be caused by an unpredictable allergic reaction to the virus that caused the illness or to the vaccine used in the immunization. The symptoms appear within about 3 weeks after the causative illness or the immunization, and they are often severe. Within hours, a sensation of tingling, then numbness, then weakness, or even paralysis may spread from your hands and feet to the rest of your body. Often, the paralysis affects your breathing, and intensive hospital care becomes necessary.

Unlike chronic forms of peripheral neuropathy (see previous page), the nerve damage of Guillain-Barré syndrome is usually only temporary. Treatments such as plasmapheresis (which removes damaging antibodies from the blood) may improve the outlook for a full recovery from severe episodes of the syndrome, but you may need physical therapy for many months to return to normal health completely. Even with optimal treatment, about 10 percent of individuals will develop a chronic neuropathy resulting in varying degrees of impairment.

Neurophysiologic disorders

Many diseases have an apparent cause, such as a tumor, a blood clot blocking a blood vessel, or an infection causing inflammation. However, neurophysiologic disorders of the central nervous system do not appear to have any such structural cause; instead, these disorders seem to result from some fault in the way the brain and its blood vessels work. Symptoms of these so-called functional disorders include headaches, dizziness, blackouts, and seizures.

The reasons for such disorders as migraine and epilepsy, and even the common headache, remain largely unknown despite intensive research. This is why the conditions themselves are usually identified by their characteristic symptoms rather than by the processes that produce them. One achievement of modern medical research, however, has been the discovery of effective ways to relieve the symptoms of many of these disorders, even though actual cure is not yet possible.

There is reason to hope for even greater advances in the future. Scientists have focused much research on the chemistry and electrical nature of the nervous system. The result has been a gradually growing understanding of how the nervous system works. From this understanding will spring new drugs and methods of treating these disorders of the nervous system.

Headache

Headaches are sometimes a symptom of a disease or disorder such as influenza or subarachnoid hemorrhage; in fact, about one fourth of the disorders discussed in this book include headache as a possible symptom. Most headaches, however, occur independently of any other disorder, develop gradually (often without apparent cause), clear up in a few hours, and leave no aftereffects. In other words, the majority of headaches, however painful, are likely to be only temporary, brought on by strain on muscular tissues, or by changes in blood vessels in the head and neck, or both.

There are many other factors that, either alone or combined, can give you headaches. These include stress, too little or too much sleep, overeating or drinking, and a noisy or stuffy environment.

Brain tissues themselves never ache. They are insensitive to pain, since the brain does not contain pain receptors. Sensitivity in this area exists only in the meninges (the membranes that cover the surface of the brain), the skin, muscles, and blood vessels that cover the skull, and the many nerves that run from the brain to the head and face.

You may not be able to figure out what has caused a particular headache. From a physiological standpoint, however, there are two common causes of headache pain. The first is strain on facial, neck, and scalp muscles, often caused by tension. The second is swelling of blood vessels in the head area that results in stretching of their walls. These two types are called tension headaches and vascular headaches, respectively. If you have been under emotional stress, for example, you may think that worry or grief caused your headache. This is true, but only indirectly. The stress may result in contraction of muscles around the head and neck, causing pain. Similarly, if you have spent several hours concentrating on paperwork, your headache may come from a hunched-over position, not from the mental effort.

The typical hangover headache that follows an episode of drinking too much alcohol may result from a widening of the blood vessels around the brain. Alcohol is a vasodilator, which means that it acts to dilate (widen) the blood vessels in your body. In addition, a tension-type pain may also develop because vascular pain can result in tightening of the head and neck muscles, producing a mixed type of headache.

What should be done?

If you have had headaches from time to time for several years, you probably know already what brings them on. You probably also know the most effective way of relieving them. However, if you do not usually have headaches but have recently developed severe head pains, your first priority is to find out what might be causing them.

As a starting point, consult the self-diagnosis symptom chart on Headache (see p.98). This is especially important if you have other symptoms in addition to headache. Take your temperature. If it is higher than normal, your headache may be caused by a virus infection such as influenza (the most common cause of headache). If you have recently had a head injury and you feel drowsy or nauseated, you could have a subdural hemorrhage (see Subdural hemorrhage and hematoma, p.289). If it is painful to bend your head forward and you have been nauseated or have been vomiting, you could have a subarachnoid hemorrhage (see p.288). If you have a fever, light hurts your eyes (photophobia), and it is painful to bend your head forward, you may have meningitis (see p.290). If your symptoms match any of these cases, you should go to an emergency department immediately.

A headache that occurs alone and disappears overnight is probably no cause for concern. But if you have headaches that sometimes last for more than 24 hours or that recur as often as 2 or 3 times each week, consult your physician. After examining you, the physician may refer you to a neurologist for diagnostic tests to make sure you do not have an underlying disorder of the central nervous system.

What is the treatment?

Self-help: Recurrent tension headaches usually indicate stress in your life, and you should discuss with your physician the circumstances that seem to provoke your headaches to see whether they can be reduced or eliminated altogether. Alcohol and tobacco are also potential causes of headaches, as are some types of physical activity that strain neck muscles.

Simple tension headaches can usually be relieved by taking a painkiller such as aspirin, acetaminophen, or ibuprofen. The following measures may also help. First, try to relax. Stretch and massage the muscles of your shoulders, neck, jaws, and scalp. Take a hot bath, lie down, and place a warm, dry cloth or, if it feels better, a cold, wet one, over the aching area. Drink plenty of fruit juices or other nonalcoholic liquids. A good night's sleep is often the best treatment.

Professional help: If you need to take a painkiller several times a week for recurrent headaches, you should consult your physician for help in trying to find the underlying cause. In some cases, recurrent headaches are a feature of depression. Your physician will also want to make sure that the painkillers you are taking will not harm your general health and are not addicting.

Migraine

If you have migraine, you have periodic headaches usually starting on one side, generally with other symptoms such as nausea, vomiting, and disturbed vision, that almost completely incapacitate you for as long as they last. In spite of intensive medical research, it is not known why some people are subject to migraine headaches or what triggers them.

Certain factors do appear to be involved in many cases. For instance, susceptibility to migraine headaches tends to run in families, leading to the strong suspicion that there is an inherited, or genetic, aspect of the disorder. In some cases, certain foods, including cheese, chocolate, caffeine, and red wine, provoke attacks. Often there is a relationship between the recurrent headaches and menstruation or stress. Sometimes even the anticipation of relaxation *after* stress seems to be a cause of migraine headaches. They can also be related to psychological illness. But your own migraines may seem to be unrelated to any of these factors.

The biological cause of migraine is unknown. For some reason the arteries leading to the brain first become narrowed, then become dilated (widened); the change in the diameter of the arteries seems to produce the pain. Narrowing of the arteries also reduces the blood supply to parts of the brain, and this probably explains the other symptoms of migraine such as disturbed vision, strange sensations or lack of any sensation, and weakness or even brief paralysis.

What are the symptoms?
In migraine, severe headaches are both preceded by and accompanied by other symptoms. The nature of each episode varies from person to person, but there is usually a warning period during which you feel abnormally tired and out of sorts. This period is followed by nausea, vomiting, and sometimes diarrhea. You may find bright lights almost unbearable (a condition called photophobia). You may also have some sort of visual disturbance, usually worse in one eye, such as a misting over or a zig-zag distortion. Early warning symptoms can last for varying amounts of time, from several minutes to several hours.

When the headache comes, the warning symptoms tend to fade away. You are likely to have intense, gripping pain, which starts at one side of your forehead but gradually spreads back. The pain usually then begins to throb, and your entire head begins to ache. While you have the migraine headache, your eyes may be bloodshot and you look pale and sick. In some cases the pain is centered between the nose and eye, and both the nose and eye tend to run.

The length of each migraine and the timing of headaches and headache-free periods are unpredictable, but you can learn to predict the nature and duration of each of your own headaches, based on previous experience with the disorder.

Other less common symptoms experienced by some people are numbness or tingling in one arm or down one side of the body, dizziness, ringing in the ears, and temporary mental confusion.

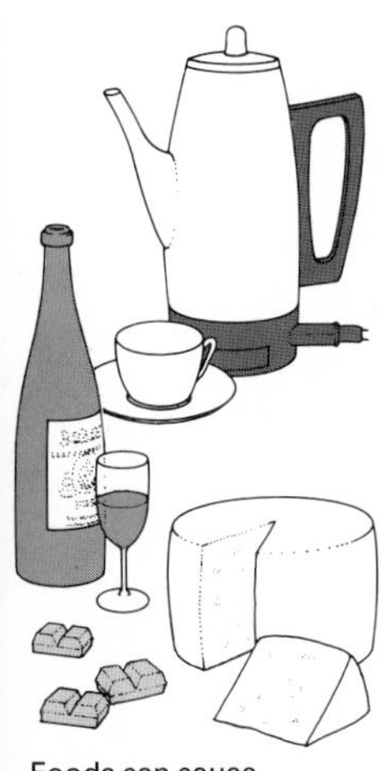

Foods can cause migraine
Many foods, notably cheese, chocolate, red wine, and/or coffee, trigger migraines in some people.

What are the risks?
Migraine is a common complaint. Migraine headaches rarely start before puberty and rarely does a first attack occur after about age 40. In fact, some people stop having migraines after reaching middle age. You are most likely to have migraine if it runs in your family; migraine headaches are more common in women.

Although migraine headaches cause considerable pain and suffering, they are not dangerous. It is unsafe, however, to attempt to drive or operate machinery while in enough pain to be distracted. In a few people some numbness, weakness, or visual disturbance has been known to become permanent. However, this is an extremely rare occurrence.

What should be done?
If you have recurrent severe headaches that you cannot control with simple painkilling drugs such as aspirin, consult your physician. He or she will probably be able to make a diagnosis based on your description of your symptoms. In some cases diagnostic tests designed to exclude other causes of headache may be performed.

What is the treatment?
Self-help: You may be your own best physician since you have the time and incentive to study your case in great detail. Keep a diary in which you record not only the time of onset and length of each migraine episode, but also any other relevant aspect of your life. Try to be objective. Record your meals, snacks, and consumption of alcohol, caffeine, and soft drinks. Write down the time you go to bed and the time you get up (some people get a migraine in the morning after an unusually long time in bed). Once you have a careful record of this kind, some cause for your headaches may become apparent and you can take preventive action. For example, you may find that you tend to have headaches just after periods of extra hard work or stress. In that case try to pace yourself differently. Avoid a crowded schedule, and leave yourself time for relaxation.

For some women, oral contraceptives appear to be the trigger factor. If you have migraine headaches and you are on the pill, talk to your physician. Changing or stopping the type of medication, or changing your contraceptive method (see Contraception, p.649) may eliminate the headaches.

As you come to recognize the early warning signs of a migraine, you may be able to prevent it. The moment you suspect that a migraine is coming, take whatever drug you and your physician have found most effective. It is far easier to abort a migraine in its early stages than it is to control the pain once the headache has reached its peak.

Professional help: Migraine cannot be cured but its symptoms can be relieved, often dramatically. Treatment taken in the early stages of a migraine is most effective.

Treatment may be with painkillers such as acetaminophen; with drugs that narrow the blood vessels (vasoconstrictors), such as ergot preparations; or with medications that control nausea and vomiting, including antihistamines and phenothiazines. In unusually severe and long-lasting episodes, intravenous or intramuscular injections may be required to terminate the headache. Different drugs are effective in different people, and so it may take several months of trying different medications before you and your physician find the one that suits you best. You must take the medication only when necessary, and exactly as prescribed, because an overdose of this kind of medication can have unpleasant side effects, including headaches as bad as or worse than the ones you are trying to avoid.

Severe recurrent migraine may require preventive treatment on a regular basis. Several drugs have proved effective for this purpose, including ergot preparations, beta blockers, and calcium channel blockers. These medications may, however, have adverse side effects and must be taken only under close medical supervision.

Alternative approaches to migraine prevention include relaxation therapy, yoga, and biofeedback.

Cluster headache

This is a variant of migraine that is characterized by sporadic episodes of extreme pain on one side of the head. Typically, an episode begins during the night, waking its victim with an intense, nonthrobbing pain that is usually centered in and around one eye. The affected eye is red and waters profusely, and the nostril on that side produces a flow of clear fluid or is stuffed. The pain often lasts several hours then disappears, only to return within a few more hours or at the same time the next day. After several days of these repeated episodes (the cluster) the headaches disappear and they may not recur for several years.

The condition is more common in men than in women.

What should be done?

The sudden onset of a severe headache with pain centered primarily around one eye may have several causes, including acute glaucoma (see p.346). If this is your first episode, contact your physician immediately.

If you have recurrent episodes of cluster headache, your physician may give you ergot medications to take by inhaling a spray or by placing a pill under your tongue, where it will rapidly dissolve. Other treatments include the use of antihistamine or corticosteroid drugs or inhalation of oxygen. For some patients whose cluster headaches occur with greater frequency, preventive treatment with lithium, calcium channel blockers, or ergot derivatives may be recommended.

Epilepsy

There are many forms of epilepsy, each with its own characteristic symptoms. Whatever its form, the disorder is caused by a problem in communication among the brain's nerve cells. Normally, such cells communicate with one another by sending tiny electrical signals back and forth. In a person who has epilepsy, the signals from one group of nerve cells occasionally become too strong—so strong that they temporarily overwhelm neighboring parts of the brain. It is this sudden, excessive electrical discharge that causes the basic symptom of epilepsy, which is called an epileptic seizure.

It is not known what causes the brain's communication system to misfire in this fashion, or why seizures recur in some people. Exhaustive research, including the testing of great numbers of people with epilepsy, has shown that roughly two out of three people with epilepsy have no identifiable structural abnormality in the brain, that is, there is nothing visibly wrong. The epilepsy of the remaining one third can generally be traced to an underlying problem such as brain damage at birth, a severe head injury, a stroke, or a brain infection. Occasionally the condition may be caused by a brain tumor (see p.301). This is especially likely when the epilepsy appears for the first time in adulthood.

What are the symptoms?

The basic symptom of epilepsy is a brief, abnormal phase of behavior called a seizure. It is important to realize that a single such episode does not indicate that you have epilepsy. By definition, epileptic seizures recur. There are many forms of the disease, but two major (and most familiar) types of generalized (widespread) epilepsy are petit mal and grand mal seizures.

Petit mal epilepsy is most commonly a disease of childhood that does not usually persist past late adolescence. A child may have this form of epilepsy if he or she suddenly stops whatever activity is going on and stares blankly around for a few seconds (sometimes up to half a minute). During the blank interval, known as a petit mal seizure, the child is unaware of what is happening. There may be a slight jerking movement of the head or an arm, but a person having a petit mal seizure does not generally fall to the ground. When the seizure ends, the child often does not realize that the brief blank interval has occurred. In typical cases the child has many episodes each day. Such children are sometimes thought simply to be "day dreamers."

The characteristic symptom of grand mal epilepsy is a seizure affecting the entire body. The person may cry out, then fall to the ground. Then the body stiffens. Next it twitches or jerks uncontrollably. This may last for 1 or 2 minutes and is usually followed by a period of deep sleep or mental confusion. During a seizure some people lose bladder and bowel control. In some cases, the seizure does not stop after 1 or 2 minutes but continues. This is an emergency because the continuing seizures may interfere with breathing, and, if untreated, result in permanent brain damage. It is important to obtain medical help immediately.

In many cases the person gets a warning of an impending seizure known as an aura. The aura can occur just before the seizure or as much as several hours before it strikes. It may be a sense of tension or some other vague feeling, but some people with epilepsy have auras with specific sensory features such as an impression of a distinctive odor, distorted vision, or a bodily sensation, particularly in the stomach.

Other types of epilepsy may begin in one section of the brain. The electrical nerve discharge may spread to produce a grand mal seizure or be restricted to the region in which it starts. These types of seizures are called focal, or partial, seizures, and the symptoms that result depend on the part of the brain where the discharge begins. A person with focal motor epilepsy does not necessarily lose consciousness; the seizure begins with uncontrollable twitching of a part of the body, and the twitch gradually spreads. The thumb of one hand, for instance, may start to jerk, followed by a jerking of the entire arm and then of the rest of that side of the body, after which there may be a more generalized seizure of the entire body.

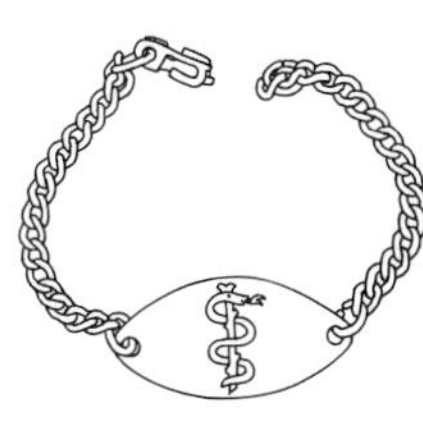

If you have epilepsy, you may wish to wear a bracelet engraved with information about it. If you have a seizure, those around you will know what is wrong and be able to get appropriate help.

A person with temporal lobe or partial complex epilepsy is likely to have an aura lasting only a few seconds. Then, without being aware of it, the person with temporal lobe epilepsy does something entirely out of character, such as becoming suddenly angry, or laughing for no apparent reason, or interrupting normal activity with unusual behavior. Strange chewing movements of the mouth are apt to occur throughout any such episode. Those with partial complex epilepsy have a feeling of being detached or begin daydreaming, often repeatedly during the course of a day.

What are the risks?

Between 1 percent and 2 percent of the population of the US has some form of epilepsy. The disease may occur at a higher rate than this in some families. Both sexes are equally susceptible. Petit mal epilepsy occurs mainly in children, and epilepsy generally is more common in children than in adults.

Isolated, nonrecurring seizures are quite common in children, as a result of the high fevers caused by infectious diseases (see Seizures in children, p.713). A child who gets such seizures and no others does not have epilepsy. If you have any doubts about the nature of the seizures of your child, speak with your physician.

Drug treatment can control most forms of epilepsy, and people with epilepsy can generally lead virtually normal lives. If you have epilepsy that is not well controlled, a seizure could be dangerous to you and others under certain circumstances such as climbing a ladder, working with machinery, or driving a car. You should not drive at all unless your seizures are well controlled. Consult your physician about when it is safe for you to drive, and find out about possible legal restrictions on driving from the agency in your state that issues drivers' licenses.

If you have seizures and go swimming, you should never swim alone. Always swim with someone who has lifesaving skills and can help you if a seizure occurs. If you take baths instead of showers, it is best not to lock the bathroom door when you are bathing. If you have a seizure, somebody would then be able to come to your aid quickly.

Even in a relatively safe situation, you can be injured during a seizure. When your jaw clenches, for instance, you may accidentally bite your tongue badly. Also, sharp objects are a danger if you fall during your seizure. Bumping your head or another part of your body is also possible.

What should be done?

If you think someone in your family may have epilepsy, consult your physician, who

Dealing with an epileptic seizure

An epileptic seizure may cause loss of consciousness and violent, convulsive movements of the arms and legs. The most important thing you can do if someone has a seizure is to make sure that the person is not in physical danger.

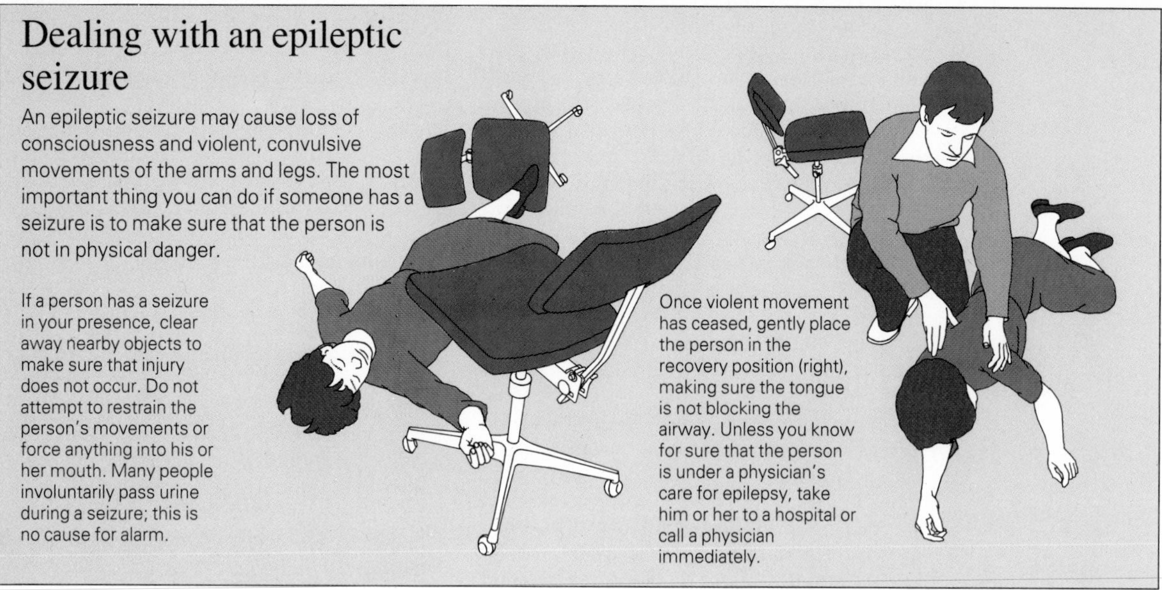

If a person has a seizure in your presence, clear away nearby objects to make sure that injury does not occur. Do not attempt to restrain the person's movements or force anything into his or her mouth. Many people involuntarily pass urine during a seizure; this is no cause for alarm.

Once violent movement has ceased, gently place the person in the recovery position (right), making sure the tongue is not blocking the airway. Unless you know for sure that the person is under a physician's care for epilepsy, take him or her to a hospital or call a physician immediately.

will want a full description of the seizures from both the observer and the affected person, who may be a young child. The physician will also want to know how often the seizures occur. If there has been no recent illness or injury that might cause seizures, your physician can probably diagnose the condition as epilepsy based on the given facts. An electroencephalogram (EEG) test will probably be performed to determine the type of epilepsy and help guide the proper choice of medication. If there is a possibility that some identifiable brain damage or infection is causing the seizures, there may also be a skull X ray, blood tests, a CT or MRI scan of the brain, and, in cases where infection is suspected, a lumbar puncture.

What is the treatment?

Self-help: If you have epilepsy and are taking medicine for it, be sure that you take the drugs exactly as prescribed. If you vomit up pills for any reason, take another dose. However, if you miss a dose, do not compensate for it by taking more the next time. In such instances, you should contact your physician. He or she will recommend the best course of action.

Once the diagnosis of epilepsy is confirmed, ask your physician about how to obtain a bracelet, card, or tag that will tell strangers that you have epilepsy. Some forms of identification include a telephone number or advice on what action any observer should take to help you during a seizure. Wear your bracelet or tag or carry your card at all times.

Professional help: Epilepsy cannot be cured. (Rare cases of seizures caused by curable brain damage, metabolic imbalances, tumors, or infection are not epilepsy.) Anticonvulsant drugs taken as directed, however, effectively prevent most epileptics from having seizures. There are many such drugs, and your physician will prescribe one or more for you. You will need to take medication at regular intervals, and perhaps for the rest of your life if you have persistent episodes. A child with petit mal epilepsy may grow out of it in time, and if this occurs your physician will let you know when the drugs are no longer necessary. Consult your physician if you have any questions.

Anticonvulsant drugs occasionally have unpleasant side effects, especially if they are taken in large amounts. So you should see your physician from time to time for checkups and possibly blood tests to see if the dosage of the prescribed drug needs to be adjusted. If the drug is not completely effective, your physician may increase the dose or may prescribe a different type of anticonvulsant. If your condition is from an underlying disorder, that disorder will also require treatment. As the disorder improves, you should have fewer seizures.

How to help someone who has a seizure

Some epileptic seizures are momentary blackouts, and the posture of the body remains virtually unaffected. Just guide the person gently toward a safe place if any such minor seizure occurs in a potentially dangerous situation—while crossing the street, for example. Just remember that no matter how active he or she may seem to be, the person with epilepsy is actually unaware of what he or she is doing and should be gently guided away from danger, not forcibly restrained or scolded.

Someone who has a grand mal seizure will start to twitch or jerk and may fall to the ground. If this happens, do the following:

1. Guide or push the person to a safe place only if he or she is in immediate danger—on a ladder, for example. Otherwise, do not attempt to move the person.

2. Move nearby objects so that they cannot cause injury. Do not hold down or restrain the person. Do not put anything into the person's mouth. The force of the jaws clamping down on an object can break the jaw or the teeth. In either case serious injury may result.

3. Loosen the person's collar and try to pull the jaw forward and extend the neck so he or she can breathe easily. During the active phase of a seizure, breathing may be much reduced, but artificial respiration is virtually impossible, and the person with epilepsy will breathe normally as soon as the muscles relax again at the end of the seizure.

4. Most seizures last only a minute or two. If a seizure continues for more than about 3 minutes, or if another seizure starts a few minutes after the first, summon medical help immediately. The person may be carrying a card or tag that gives emergency information.

5. Many people with epilepsy fall asleep after a seizure. If this happens, place him or her in a recovery position (see illustration, previous page) and allow the person to wake naturally. If possible, move him or her to a quiet place to allow undisturbed sleep, and check from time to time to be sure that everything is all right.

6. If the person does not have a card or tag, or if he or she is not known to have epilepsy, take the person to a physician or emergency room when the seizure has passed.

Aphasia

Aphasia is a speech disorder that is almost always a consequence of damage to the language centers of the brain. The disorder is characterized by partial or total loss of the understanding of words and, depending on the extent of brain damage, the impairment of certain language functions and not others. For example, spoken but not written word skills may be affected, or particular categories of words (such as names) may present the greatest difficulty. Sometimes, even though the person's own speech is impaired, his or her comprehension of the speech of others remains unaffected; aphasic patients are often able to repeat words that they cannot otherwise "find" for themselves.

Superficially, aphasia may resemble another major type of speech disorder known as dysarthria, which is caused by lack of control over the muscles of the lips, tongue, and face. Something as simple as temporary loss of sensation in the mouth following injection of an anesthetic by a dentist may produce dysarthria, but the disorder can also result from injury to the nerves or to the area in the brain responsible for controlling the muscles used in speech. People who have dysarthria are able to understand what they hear and can read and write without difficulty even though they may be unable to pronounce a single intelligible word.

Because aphasia usually results from a localized brain disorder (though occasionally it is a symptom of psychiatric disturbance), management of the disorder begins with the physician's identification of the underlying cause. When aphasia is a feature of brain damage from a stroke, the outcome depends on the amount of damage done to the speech center of the brain. However, some degree of spontaneous improvement in the weeks and months following a stroke is likely to occur, and speech therapy may help the person recover his or her communication skills.

Dizziness

(vertigo)

Dizziness, or vertigo, may result from a number of causes, some of which are the result of nervous system disorders. Dizziness is a sensation of either spinning around yourself or of being stationary while everything around you spins. Dizziness is not a disease. It is a symptom of a disturbance in the brain and/or the organs of balance in your inner ears (see How you keep your balance, p.355).

Dizziness may be infrequent and mild, or you may have it very often and be so severely affected that you feel nauseated, vomit, lose your balance and fall down, or even faint.

The term vertigo is often incorrectly used to mean fear of heights. The correct term for fear of heights is acrophobia.

Dizziness is sometimes caused by a specific disease such as labyrinthitis (see p.364) or Meniere's disease (see p.363). More often, however, the disorder that causes it is minor and temporary, as is the dizziness. In many cases it is impossible to determine the cause of the problem. Dizziness is especially likely to occur in older people (see Aging and the senses, p.771) and may result from medications taken for other conditions.

What should be done?

If you have severe, prolonged, or repeated episodes of dizziness, consult your physician, who may arrange for special diagnostic tests to determine whether anything is seriously wrong. The best way to deal with dizziness is to lie down until it (and your nausea, if any) goes away. If there is no identifiable underlying cause of persistent episodes of dizziness, your physician may prescribe a drug that helps to stabilize the balancing mechanism in your inner ears. He or she can also recommend special exercises that can reduce the likelihood of your becoming dizzy when you shift your head position.

Neuralgia

Neuralgia is pain from a damaged nerve. Several possible kinds of damage can lead to this disorder. The trouble may be temporary and mild, or it can be chronic and severe, as in sciatica (see p.585), peripheral neuropathy (see p.302), low back pain (see p.585), and trigeminal neuralgia (see p.770), a facial pain that mainly affects older people. The pain of neuralgia, shooting along the affected nerve, tends to be sharp and hard to bear. It usually lasts only a few seconds, but several episodes may occur in quick succession.

Treatment of neuralgia depends on the location of the damaged nerve or nerves and on the cause of the damage. If you have occasional episodes that are only mildly painful, you can usually relieve the pain with analgesics such as aspirin. If the pain becomes intolerable, consult your physician, who may prescribe a stronger painkiller. Your physician may refer you to a neurologist, a physician who specializes in problems of the brain and nervous system, for diagnostic tests and further treatment. In certain severe cases of neuralgia in the face, an operation to destroy the damaged nerve may be advisable. Also, drugs that change nerve conduction may be prescribed.

Dystonia

Dystonia is a condition that was until recently poorly recognized by physicians, many of whom thought that the symptoms had a psychiatric origin. The condition may take many forms, all of which are characterized by the occurrence of unwanted sustained muscle contractions. Any part of the body may be affected. The muscles around the eyes may squeeze shut (blepharospasm), or speech, chewing, or swallowing may be affected. The neck may turn or jerk involuntarily to one side (torticollis), or the hand may spontaneously produce unwanted postures or movements. Usually the condition starts in adults and affects only 1 or 2 body parts (focal dystonia), but sometimes it begins in childhood and spreads to other parts of the body until adulthood (generalized dystonia). In all its forms the condition probably affects about 1 person in 4,000. In most cases, the cause is unknown, but is believed to be a chemical disturbance in a part of the brain that controls automatic movement.

What is the treatment?

For many people with dystonia, correct diagnosis helps them come to terms with what is usually a permanent affliction. Drug treatment may help about a third of people with dystonia. The eyes can be reopened by weakening the surrounding muscles by injections of tiny amounts of a nerve toxin, or by cutting the nerves; in a small number of cases surgery to the neck may help.

Tics

A tic is a repetitive habitual movement such as blinking or hair tossing that can develop at any time during childhood, but most commonly does so around age 7. As many as one fourth of normal children develop a trivial tic of this kind. These tics are harmless and will eventually disappear. Tics tend to be more pronounced if the child is tired or tense. It is best to ignore the tic; focusing attention on it is only likely to make it worse. However, you should consult your physician if a tic persists for a long time or becomes unusually pronounced or severe.

A very few children develop more severe and persistent multiple tics, which may sometimes be accompanied by vocal tics such as coughing, barking, or grunting or even the involuntary utterance of swear words. When this behavior occurs (usually in boys), the condition is known as Tourette syndrome. Such behavior can disrupt a child's education and family relationships, all the more so if the child's classmates, teachers, and parents believe that it is deliberate. Correct diagnosis, with repeated explanations to teachers that the tics are caused by disease rather than mischievousness, can reduce the social impact of what is otherwise a benign condition. In some cases, tranquilizers can dramatically reduce the tics, but a balance must be struck between benefits and possible side effects.

Sleep apnea syndrome

Sleep apnea syndrome is a disorder characterized by interruption of breathing for a limited time during sleep. This may result from dysfunction of central respiratory control in the brain or from obstruction of the airway. The obstructive form of sleep apnea is more common in overweight people.

What are the symptoms?

Symptoms of sleep apnea include excessive sleepiness during the day; heavy snoring; brief lapses of breathing during sleep that end spontaneously, often with a snort; restlessness; fatigue; headaches; and difficulty with concentration and memory.

In some people, sufficient loss of oxygen in the blood occurs at night to lead to hypertension, lung disease, disturbed rhythm and pumping function of the heart, seizures, or personality changes.

What is the treatment?

Self-help: Keeping your body weight within recommended ranges is important. People who have sleep apnea usually improve after losing weight. Avoiding alcohol and excessive use of sleep-inducing medications is also important. Driving may be dangerous.

Professional help: Your physician will first ask you how and when you sleep. He or she may want to speak to another member of your household who has seen you asleep. Your physician will review any medications you are taking and may refer you to a neurologist or a sleep disorders specialist. You are likely to undergo testing of your blood to exclude conditions such as thyroid disease and to be referred for a night-long recording of your brain waves and other tests.

Medication such as protriptyline or medroxyprogesterone may be prescribed. Medications that you take for other conditions may need to be modified. If these measures are insufficient and your apnea is caused by mechanical obstruction, a machine that provides pressure to open the airway may be recommended or surgery to relieve or bypass the obstruction may be necessary.

Myasthenia gravis

This is a rare disease that mainly affects women in their 20s. It occurs because of faulty transmission of nerve impulses to the muscles they control. Symptoms of muscular weakness usually appear first and most noticeably in the face. Your eyelids droop, you may see double, and you may have difficulty talking, chewing, and swallowing because of an inability to control the movements of your lips and other parts of your mouth. If your arms or legs are affected, you may at times be almost unable to stand up or to perform such simple tasks as combing your hair. The degree of weakness varies considerably from hour to hour, day to day, and even year to year. The cause of the fault in transmission of nerve impulses is complex, but it is thought to be caused by an autoimmune problem. In such problems, your immune system, which usually protects you, turns against some of your tissues. In about one fifth of cases, the trouble appears to be related to the development of a growth in the thymus, a gland in your chest that plays a key role in immunity.

What should be done?

If you think you may have myasthenia gravis, consult your physician, who, after examining you, may want you to have blood tests and chest X rays in order to make a diagnosis. If you have the disease, treatment with special drugs that restore transmission of nerve impulses to the affected muscles should greatly improve your condition. Surgery may be required to remove any thymus growth. Sometimes a treatment called plasmapheresis (which washes antibodies from the blood) facilitates recovery from acute attacks.

Although myasthenia gravis cannot usually be cured, treatment can minimize the symptoms of the disease so that you can lead a more normal life.

Degenerative disorders

Grouped under this heading are a number of diseases in which nerve cells degenerate and die, usually very slowly, taking months or years. The symptoms of the various diseases differ widely, depending on the area of the brain or spinal cord in which the degeneration of the nerve cells occurs. The results are distressing and sometimes even tragic. But there is hope because scientific research into causes and possible treatments is gradually increasing our understanding of these disorders. With this new understanding it is reasonable to hope for more and increasingly effective treatments.

Parkinson's disease

(paralysis agitans, shaking palsy)

Parkinson's disease is caused by gradual deterioration in certain nerve centers inside the brain. The centers affected are the ones that coordinate movement, particularly semiautomatic movements such as swinging your arms while walking. Deterioration of these nerve centers upsets the delicate balance between two body chemicals, dopamine and acetylcholine, which are essential for controlling the transmission of nerve impulses within this part of the nervous system. The lack of control that results from this imbalance produces the symptoms of Parkinson's disease. Much of today's research is directed toward finding ways to slow the degenerative process that underlies the disease and ways to restore the brain's capacity for making dopamine.

Nobody knows what causes the more common forms of the illness. In rare cases the nerve degeneration results from such factors as carbon monoxide poisoning or high levels of certain metals in body tissues. Sometimes Parkinson's disease is the result of an earlier infection of the brain, such as encephalitis (see p.291). High doses of certain drugs used in treating psychiatric conditions such as schizophrenia (see p.319) sometimes produce the symptoms of Parkinson's disease.

What are the symptoms?

One characteristic symptom is a type of tremor (sometimes incorrectly called "palsy," which actually means paralysis). There is an involuntary, rhythmic shaking of the hands, the head, or both, which is often accompanied by a continuous rubbing together of thumb and forefinger. Such tremors are most severe when the affected part of the body is not consciously in use. Once you begin consciously to move the involved body part the tremor disappears or diminishes. If the disorder becomes worse, there is a gradual loss of most semiautomatic physical movements such as the natural swinging of the arms that makes walking smooth, or the ability to write legibly or move your mouth and tongue so as to speak clearly. Your arms and legs may feel heavy and stiff. It becomes increasingly difficult to initiate new movements or to change from one position to another. You feel no pain, numbness, or tingling, but simply a decreasing ability to move. You may fall frequently because it is difficult to keep your balance while walking. Simple activities such as rising from a chair can become difficult. Other symptoms include excessive salivation, abdominal cramps, and sometimes in the later stages of the disease, deterioration of memory and thought processes.

What are the risks?

Most people who have Parkinson's disease are older or in late middle age. Men are slightly more susceptible than women, and there is some evidence that Parkinson's disease runs in families. Because the disease does not affect nerves that supply the heart or other vital organs, it is not directly life-threatening. The slowly progressing disability that results from the disease, however, can lead to depression.

What should be done?

There is no immediate cause for concern if, after age 50, you develop a mild tremor. There are many causes of tremors and many people develop a tremor as they grow older. Consult your physician if a tremor interferes with your daily activities, if you have other symptoms of Parkinson's disease, or if the tremor becomes worse. Special diagnostic tests are not always necessary. Your physician may be able to make a diagnosis based on a general physical examination.

What is the treatment?

Self-help: Encouragement and support from family and friends can be very helpful.

Practical changes in the house, such as bathrail supports, special banisters along regular routes, and chairs with high arms, will help you get around more easily and be more comfortable. Try to exercise on a regular basis and keep your spirits up by remaining or becoming engaged in activities. For further ideas on modifying your home to care for an older family member, see Caregiving at home, p.786.

Professional help: Drug treatment can do much to relieve the symptoms of Parkinson's disease, particularly stiffness and immobility. In mild cases drugs are not usually prescribed because they may have some troublesome side effects.

Your physician may want to see you periodically to observe the progress of your condition. If treatment with drugs becomes necessary, medications that reestablish the balance of dopamine and acetylcholine within the affected area of the brain are usually prescribed. Some of these drugs tend to make the mouth unpleasantly dry, but that may seem more like a benefit than a side effect if excessive salivation is a symptom of the disease in your case. New drugs are constantly being developed, but none has yet proved to be completely effective against the tremor that occurs in the disease. If tremors become a serious problem, it is sometimes possible to operate on the portion of the brain that is responsible for the problem, especially in younger people.

Another surgical treatment currently being evaluated is the transplantation into the brain of tissue capable of synthesizing dopamine, the lack of which accounts for most of the symptoms of the disease. Transplantation of a small part of one of the patient's own adrenal glands has offered variable results, with some patients reporting prolonged and substantial improvement and others being disappointed. Transplantation of brain tissue taken from aborted fetuses has also been attempted in people with Parkinson's disease, but the results in these cases have been inconsistent and the treatment has been criticized on ethical grounds. Long-term evaluation of transplant surgery is required before it can be considered part of the standard range of treatments for Parkinson's disease.

What are the long-term prospects?

As yet no treatment has been found that slows down the progression of Parkinson's disease, but the relief from symptoms offered by the various treatments that are now available has enabled many people with this disease to continue normal activity for many years.

Amyotrophic lateral sclerosis

(ALS, motor neuron disease, Lou Gehrig's disease)

This condition, also called Lou Gehrig's disease, occurs when certain nerve cells die. These are the motor neurons that run from the brain stem and spinal cord to the muscles and control the muscles' movements. The affected muscles cannot be stimulated and used, and they gradually waste away. The affected part of the body becomes increasingly weak. The disease can cause difficulty in swallowing, breathing, walking, or any other activity powered by the muscles. Thus it can interfere with virtually any of the body's physical functions.

Amyotrophic lateral sclerosis occurs most often in people over 40. Little is known about its cause, and it cannot be cured. Treatment is directed at easing symptoms and helping you to remain relatively mobile and independent. There are specialized treatment centers in many states that offer comprehensive support services, research studies, and symptomatic therapy.

Huntington's chorea

Huntington's chorea is a very rare degenerative nerve disease that starts in early middle age. Uncontrollable body movements called chorea gradually develop over time and are followed by mental deterioration. Sometimes the symptoms of mental deterioration occur first. No treatment has yet been discovered to halt the progress of the disease or control its symptoms. The word "chorea" literally means "dance." The term therefore serves as a rough description of the swift, jerky movements that occur in people who have this disease.

Huntington's chorea is an inherited disorder that seldom produces symptoms before age 30. Advances in genetics have revealed much about the disease, and most people who know that the disease has affected members of their family can now be tested to find out whether they are carrying the defective gene. For some prospective parents potentially at risk, this may mean a reassurance that they do not carry the gene so they will not pass it on to their children. However, these tests are not 100 percent reliable, and physicians and patients are still debating the most appropriate age and circumstances to undertake testing. Individual counseling is imperative (see Genetic counseling, p.664), so that if the test proves to be positive, support for the inevitable depression that results is available. Individuals at risk should carefully weigh the decision to have genetic testing and discuss the issues thoroughly with their spouse, family, and physician or genetic counselor.

Friedreich's ataxia

This is an exceedingly rare inherited disease in which certain groups of nerve fibers gradually deteriorate. The main symptom is ataxia, or loss of coordination of movement and balance, especially when walking. Gradually it also becomes difficult for the affected person to stand still, to speak, and to use his or her arms. The arms may begin to shake just when he or she intends to move them. This is called an intention tremor. Symptoms usually appear between ages 5 and 15. There is no treatment. Friedreich's ataxia runs in families, so if you have relatives with the disease, seek advice from your physician before starting your own family (see Genetic counseling, p.664).

Dementia

(including Alzheimer's disease, presenile dementia, and senile dementia)

Dementia is a disorder of the brain in which there is a progressive loss of memory and other intellectual functions so that the mind gradually ceases to function normally and the affected person slowly becomes increasingly confused, incapable of sensible conversation, unaware of his or her surroundings, and generally incapacitated.

Dementia may occur at any age. It is often called "presenile" when it occurs before age 65 and "senile" in those over 65. But the vast majority of people over 80 retain normal brain function.

What are the causes?

Dementia may result from any of several underlying causes. In some cases, it is from brain damage caused by narrowing and blockage of the arteries that supply blood to the brain. Deprived of an adequate blood supply, the cells in many small regions of the brain degenerate and die. At one time, this degeneration of the arteries and the natural consequences of aging were thought to be the principal causes of senile dementia, whereas presenile dementia was thought to be caused mainly by Alzheimer's disease. However, research has now shown that Alzheimer's disease is responsible for nearly 80 percent of dementia cases at all ages.

The underlying cause of Alzheimer's disease is not known, but in families in which several individuals have developed the disease before age 65, there is a genetic factor. Wide publicity has been given to research reports suggesting a link between Alzheimer's disease and water supplies that contain high levels of aluminum, but most physicians remain unconvinced that any form of toxicity from metals is relevant. Current studies have established the precise physical effects of the disease on brain tissue. The brain becomes shrunken from the loss of nerve cells, and the nerve tracts become distorted as the protein called amyloid is deposited in the person's brain.

Dementia also sometimes occurs—usually in young or middle-aged people—as a result of rare neurological disorders such as Creutzfeldt-Jakob disease (which is caused by a virus), a brain tumor, or infections associated with acquired immune deficiency syndrome (AIDS).

Dementia is by definition progressive and incapacitating, but when it begins in the presenile years, the mental deterioration tends to advance more rapidly and to be more widespread and severe than when the onset occurs later in life.

In people over 65, the early symptoms of senile dementia may resemble the forgetfulness typical of aging, and many older people may worry that they are becoming demented. However, do not assume that signs of confusion or impaired intellectual capacity in someone over 65 are always from senile dementia. There may be an underlying, and treatable, cause. It has been estimated that 10 percent to 20 percent of people over 65 who have an intellectual impairment have reversible conditions. Important causes of confusion in older individuals are side effects from medication and another illness, which may place added stress on the brain's already depleted reserves. For example, depression (p.321), chest infections (see Lungs and chest, p.379) or urinary tract infections (see p.541), stroke (see p.285), heart attack (see p.406), and hypothermia (see p.772) can result in mental confusion, and so can a low blood sugar level (see Hypoglycemia, p.562). Symptoms that resemble senile dementia are sometimes caused by long-term abuse of alcohol or other drugs or by vitamin deficiency (see p.532), hypothyroidism (see p.567), syphilis (see p.655), or brain disorders such as tumors (see p.301) or subdural hemorrhage and hematoma (see p.289). Very often many of these symptoms will decrease in intensity when the condition is properly treated.

What are the symptoms?

The earliest signs of dementia may be so subtle that even the most perceptive physician fails to notice them. More often it is an observant relative, friend, or employer who first becomes aware of a certain lack of initiative, forgetfulness, and irritability on the part of the affected person. Most characteristic of dementia at the onset is the gradual loss of memory, especially for recent events. You may notice that the person cannot remember what has happened a few hours (or even moments) earlier, although he or she can recall what happened many years ago. As weeks and months pass, the person's powers of reasoning and understanding dwindle, and he or she may lose interest in all familiar pursuits, even in such simple activities as watching television or seeking news of relatives and friends. Eventually this disorder may cause a complete disintegration of the personality.

Dementia often leads to emotional and physical instability. Many people swing between apathy and aggression, and tears and laughter, at the slightest provocation (or even no perceptible provocation). Odd, unpredictable behavior may appear, along with uninhibited and antisocial actions. A person's table manners may deteriorate, personal cleanliness is sometimes neglected, and usual politeness abandoned. Some people may even become violent if their impulsive behavior is frustrated.

A few affected individuals lose their sexual inhibitions, as well, which can lead to their making inappropriate, embarrassing physical advances to persons of either sex.

More unusual disturbances of thought and intellect, including apraxic disorders (in which there is an inability to coordinate muscles and movements), and problems with space perception may also occur in severe cases of presenile dementia and in dementia caused by Alzheimer's disease.

In the advanced stages of dementia, there is generalized stiffness of the muscles, with slowness and awkwardness in all movements. Eventually the person may lose all ability to perceive, think, speak, eat, control the bladder or bowels, or move. This gradual collapse of the individual's intellectual and physical capabilities may progress slowly, lingering over 10 years or more.

What are the risks?

The older a person is, the greater is his or her likelihood of having symptoms of dementia. About 10 percent of people over 65 have some intellectual impairment, and it is estimated that there are about 650,000 people in the US who have senile dementia. In the general population, about one family in every 10 includes at least one older member who has this condition.

There are risks whenever mentally impaired people live alone, especially after they have progressed beyond an early stage of dementia. Because of forgetfulness and a decreased ability to concentrate, there is danger of fires, falls, and other accidents. Combined with possible physical disabilities such as impaired hearing or vision, mental confusion makes it difficult for some older people to take medications as prescribed, to cross streets safely, or even to use the bathroom. Without some supervision a person with dementia may eat poorly and neglect personal hygiene. It also can be distressing if, as often happens, the person becomes incontinent (see p.766).

If a relative of yours is in the early stages of senile dementia and insists on traveling alone, even locally, you can help minimize the danger involved. Be sure that he or she always carries some identification such as a bracelet inscribed with his or her name and address. At the very least, give your relative a piece of paper or card with your address and telephone number on it, and make sure that he or she always carries it.

What should be done?

If you suspect that a relative or close friend is showing signs of dementia, gently persuade (or take) him or her to see a physician. After taking a personal history, making a physical examination, and testing memory and reasoning power, the physician will probably look for symptoms of an underlying disease, such as vitamin B_{12} deficiency, that might be causing the mental deterioration. Further series of laboratory tests and a CT (computed tomography) scan (see p.295) or magnetic resonance imaging (MRI) test may be done to look for the unmistakable signs of brain shrinkage associated with Alzheimer's disease. In addition, the physician may check for the presence of looped or tangled nerve fibers that are also characteristic of

Alzheimer's disease, and to exclude other causes of dementia.

All cases of dementia should be investigated thoroughly, since some can be cured and others helped to a certain extent. Drug treatments for Alzheimer's disease are currently being evaluated in the US and in Europe, but despite some optimistic reports published in newspapers, none has been shown to have any substantial effect on the course of the disease.

Whatever the age of the individual with dementia, a consistent approach to treatment is necessary. Even in the earliest stages of the condition, when many people affected by dementia are still able to live alone, some form of daily attendance is important to guard against potential disasters, such as turning on the kitchen stove and wandering away. Friends and relatives can help by organizing memory aids, lists, and routines, and by making sure that the person has adequate food and warmth. It is essential to maintain a regular mealtime schedule because dementia patients often forget to eat. They eat so little that they may become undernourished (even to the point where they develop a deficiency disease) and emaciated.

If you assume responsibility for the care of a relative suffering from dementia, do not hesitate to seek assistance from community services. In many places, there are day-care centers where people with dementia are supervised for several hours and provided with lunch and some kind of occupational and activity therapy.

Your physician may also be able to arrange for your relative to be admitted to a nursing facility for brief periods so that you can have occasional relief from your responsibilities. Rehabilitation hospitals also may be helpful in improving the affected person's physical and mental abilities. Your physician can give you advice about how to cope with such specific problems as incontinence (see p.766).

Eventually, however, your relative may require the skilled and constant care that is available only in high-quality nursing facilities. If your physician strongly recommends this form of care, you may be doing the person the best possible service by following your physician's recommendation.

Other neurological disorders

Multiple sclerosis

Nerve tracts, or pathways, in the brain and spinal cord are sheathed in a covering called myelin. The myelin sheath acts as an insulating material and enables speedy passage of electrical impulses along the nerves. If a sheath becomes inflamed and swollen, and if this affects a number of nerve tracts in different parts of your central nervous system, you may have the disease known as multiple sclerosis. Any part of the brain or spinal cord can be affected. The underlying cause of multiple sclerosis is not known, but there is evidence that a reaction of the body's own immune system occurs that causes destruction of some myelin segments. Current research is evaluating whether this immune destruction occurs as a result of a viral infection or a disorder of the body's immune system.

What are the symptoms?

Myelin is so widespread in the nervous system and the nervous system so widespread in the body, that multiple sclerosis can show up in many different ways. Most commonly, it begins with a vague, brief symptom that clears up completely within a few days or weeks. For example, you may get a feeling of tingling and numbness or weakness that may affect only one spot, one arm or leg, or one side of the body. Temporary weakness of an arm or leg may cause you to drop things or drag your foot. This type of symptom may be very apparent after a hot bath or exercise.

Other possible indications of multiple sclerosis include ataxia (unsteadiness of movement), temporary blurring of vision, slurred speech, and either difficulty or lack of control in urinating. All symptoms disappear after the first episode in most cases, and often there are no further problems.

But for some people there are repeated episodes. In these instances recovery may be less complete after later episodes, and permanent disability with progressive weakness of arms and legs or loss of vision may develop. Other problems may also occur, including muscle spasms, skin ulcerations, urinary tract infections, constipation, and mood changes. The periods between episodes are called remissions, and during remissions some people who have the disease continue to function in their usual activities for as long as 20 to 30 years.

What are the risks?

Most cases of multiple sclerosis are sporadic, although some studies have shown small increases in risk when a brother or sister (particularly an identical twin) or a parent has the illness. In the majority of cases, the first episode of the disorder occurs between ages 20 and 40. It is rare for the disease to begin before age 10 or after age 60. Multiple sclerosis occurs slightly more often in women than it does in men.

Some studies have shown an increase in relapse rate in women during the 6 months immediately following a pregnancy. Other studies have not found this to be true, and in all cases the majority of women studied had no change in their neurological condition because of a pregnancy. Most women with multiple sclerosis who want and are physically able to care for a baby can have children if they want to.

Repeated episodes of multiple sclerosis can lead to neurological impairment that significantly limits activity, but most people with this illness continue to lead active, productive lives.

What should be done?

If you have symptoms of multiple sclerosis, your physician may refer you to a neurologist, whose diagnosis in most cases will be based on your medical history and the findings of a neurological examination. Also, magnetic resonance imaging (MRI, see p.295) may reveal signs of damage to the nerve pathways, and special tests on the condition of nerve impulses may be needed. The most common of these is the visual evoked response test, in which the patient watches a changing black-and-white checker-board pattern projected onto a screen. While this is happening, electrodes placed at the back of the head detect the electrical activity of the brain's vision center; this electrical activity is the visual evoked response. People with multiple sclerosis often exhibit an abnormal visual evoked response even when they have no other symptoms.

Other diagnostic tests include examination of the cerebrospinal fluid removed from the spine by a lumbar puncture. Analysis of the fluid may reveal characteristic patterns of proteins indicating the presence of an inflammatory reaction in the central nervous system. Blood tests may be performed to exclude other conditions that may cause symptoms very similar to those of multiple sclerosis, including vitamin deficiencies, infections, and vascular inflammations such as lupus cerebritis.

What is the treatment?

Self-help: Limiting excess weight gain may help maintain function and reduce some of the fatigue that affects most people with multiple sclerosis. Support groups such as those sponsored by local chapters of the National Multiple Sclerosis Society can be important sources of information, referrals, and comfort.

Professional help: No therapy has been conclusively shown to prevent acute episodes of multiple sclerosis. When a relapse of this disease occurs, and the person has difficulty walking or talking, many physicians treat the patient with corticotropin or corticosteroid drugs. These medications are less likely to help older patients or those with the progressive form of multiple sclerosis. The drug beta-interferon is used to slow the course of the disease. A number of other medications that affect the immune system have been tried as treatments in clinical studies, including cyclophosphamide, azathioprine, copolymer-1, and cyclosporine, with varying success. Plasmapheresis, a treatment that filters proteins from the blood, is also being evaluated in clinical studies.

Although there is no cure for multiple sclerosis, a number of therapies can help affected people maintain their daily activities. Medications are available that can greatly reduce the stiffness or spasticity of arms and legs, help to restore lost bladder control, and in some cases alleviate pain, tremor, fatigue, and depression.

Occupational and physical therapy with home exercise programs can strengthen and maintain motion in joints of weakened arms and legs. Braces can maintain mobility in some people with multiple sclerosis who have limited weakness; supporting devices and motorized wheelchairs allow more severely affected people to continue working and pursuing active lives.

Any new treatment that you may hear about will not and should not be used until it has been evaluated in strictly controlled research trials. The natural tendency for episodes of multiple sclerosis to clear up by themselves makes evaluation of any new treatment very difficult.

Only a limited number of people are crippled by multiple sclerosis. Many people have transient symptoms that pass without leaving ill effects and may not return for many years. Many others are left with minor disabilities but lead almost normal lives. About 70 percent of multiple sclerosis patients are actively engaged in normal activities 5 years after the diagnosis.

Behavioral and emotional problems

Introduction

There are many good reasons for hope for people who suffer from emotional disorders and mental illness. For example, there are new, clearer ways of diagnosing them. Even for severe mental illness there are new treatments and combinations of treatments that bring better results.

The stigma against emotional disorders and mental illness is lessening. Studies show that an estimated 15 percent of Americans suffer from emotional disorder or mental illness. A recent public opinion survey of Americans showed that 14 percent of us recognize either that we or someone we know has a mental illness. Celebrities talk openly about their experience of mental illness, including alcoholism.

Another factor that helps diminish stigma against persons with mental illness is the growing evidence of an organic, or physical, basis for these disorders. They are not just "all in your mind." Schizophrenia, the depressive disorders, and the anxiety disorders run in families, like hypertension and diabetes, and treatment requires both medication and life-style changes.

In general, if you are able to cope with your life during periods of emotional stress, you can call yourself mentally healthy. If you lose that ability you are ill, at least to some extent. The articles in this section are intended to help you recognize some warning signs of the common mental disorders, not only in yourself but also in others. Current ideas about the causes of emotional problems include environmental factors, chemical imbalances in the brain, or both.

Some people are overwhelmed by minor crises such as marital arguments. Others retain their balance in much more difficult circumstances. Such mental health is not necessarily inborn. You can cultivate it in yourself and thus stand a better chance of coping well.

Mental disorders

The chemistry of the brain plays an important part in mental disorders. The changes in behavior that you see in people with mental disorders may be the result of long-standing emotional problems. Medications may be used along with psychotherapy in treating the disorders discussed below. But most cases of mental disorders such as manic-depression, anxiety, or schizophrenia are thought to be a mixture of biological and emotional factors. Some people irritate easily, are oversensitive, and may lack energy. When under stress, such people may become unduly depressed or anxious. Most of us have swings in mood from elation and energy to lethargy and withdrawal to some extent. Under stress, some people may become manic-depressive. Most people, however, overcome these effects and cope with emotional problems by themselves or with the help of psychotherapy. If you have the characteristics cited above, you are not necessarily on the verge of a mental illness.

It is estimated that 30 to 60 percent of most physicians' patients consult their physicians mainly because of an emotional problem. The physical disorders of many others are related to psychological stress. Many people who consult a physician are either anxious and temporarily in need of help or have what can be physical symptoms of emotional problems, including palpitations or indigestion.

When your physician feels that your problems are mainly of emotional origin, you

Psychiatric terms

A special vocabulary relates to emotional disorders and mental illness and their treatment. Many terms used in these pages have clearly defined meanings for medical professionals, but others sometimes find it difficult to distinguish among them. Here are definitions of nine special psychiatric terms:

Psychiatrist: A psychiatrist is a physician who has been trained to diagnose and prescribe for any illness and who has special training in the diagnosis and treatment of emotional problems.

Psychologist: A psychologist has been trained in human psychology, but not in medicine. There are many kinds of psychologists and generally they are involved in psychological testing and statistical analysis. There are also clinical psychologists who practice psychotherapy.

Psychoanalyst: A psychoanalyst probes into and analyzes the unconscious mind. The approach of the psychoanalyst is that people's problems are caused by their life experiences.

Psychotherapy: Psychotherapy is the term for several types of treatment of mental disorders by verbal means, including suggestion, analysis, and persuasion (see also the box, Psychotherapy, p.323).

Neurosis: This is a nonmedical term for emotional disorders that are not as severe as psychoses. The role of physical factors is not strong for these disorders. People with neuroses have symptoms such as anxieties or fears that they recognize as irrational but cannot overcome.

Personality disorder: When a person's emotional problems have affected and distorted the shape of the whole personality, that individual has a personality disorder. Examples include paranoid personality disorder, in which the person is very suspicious in all personal relationships; schizoid personality disorder, in which the person leads a very isolated life; or obsessive-compulsive personality disorder, in which a person is very meticulous, rigid, and controlling, and obsesses over some idea.

Psychosis: A person who is psychotic has difficulty distinguishing reality from fantasy and is either occasionally or constantly incapable of rational behavior. Psychoses usually have a biological basis.

Psychosomatic: A psychosomatic disorder, sometimes called a psychogenic disorder, is a set of symptoms caused by a mental or emotional problem. The symptoms can often be cured by treatment of an underlying psychological problem or conflict.

Antisocial personality disorder (psychopathic): Individuals with antisocial personalities have no sense of conscience and generally manipulate people and rules according to their own self-centered priorities.

may be referred to a psychiatrist. But it is sometimes difficult to determine whether symptoms are the result of physical or mental illness, or both. If you or a family member have symptoms that you suspect might be totally or even partly caused by emotional difficulties, be sure to tell your physician.

It is only when people lose touch with reality and behave in bizarre and perhaps life-threatening ways that they can be considered psychotic rather than neurotic. People with psychoses may require initial treatment in the hospital, where they are less likely to harm themselves or others.

Schizophrenia

Schizophrenia is a general name for a group of emotional disorders that are all forms of psychosis, in which the person has problems telling fact from fantasy and therefore behaves irrationally. Schizophrenia alters a person's thought patterns, reactions to others, and behavior so severely that he or she undergoes a change in personality.

For a diagnosis of schizophrenia to be confirmed, the person must show signs of fragmentation (disorganization) of the personality for at least 6 months. Also, the 6-month period must include at least one episode of delusions (false ideas), hallucinations (sensory experiences that originate in the mind), or significant thought disorders. Schizophrenia should not be confused with multiple personality disorder.

Some physicians think that schizophrenia is an inherited disorder; others believe that it is the result of a profound disturbance in early mother-child relationships. Symptoms usually appear in late adolescence or early adulthood. The disorder may be lifelong, but acute episodes tend to occur at times of emotional stress or personal loss.

What are the symptoms?

For most people with schizophrenia, an episode begins with a gradual, or occasionally sudden, withdrawal from day-to-day activities. The content of the person's speech may become increasingly vague, and he or she may seem unable to follow a simple conversation. An acute bout can happen unexpectedly. Often the onset is so gradual that it is difficult to know when psychotic symptoms appear. Among such symptoms are seemingly disconnected remarks, along with blank looks.

Schizophrenics often believe that others hear and "steal" their thoughts. Those with schizophrenia may have delusions, ranging from a single idea such as the conviction they are Theodore Roosevelt to complex systems of related beliefs. Sometimes they fear they have lost control of bodily movement as well as thought, as if they were puppets. They frequently believe they hear voices, often hostile ones. Less commonly, they have hallucinations of odd physical sensations, fearing that they have been poisoned or otherwise attacked by others. In time many people with schizophrenia build up a set of beliefs in a fantasy world. In this way they flee from reality and withdraw from what they perceive to be an overwhelmingly threatening world. They may express exaggerated feelings of happiness, bewilderment, or despair. They may laugh at a sad moment or cry without cause.

In an early phase of schizophrenia the person may have symptoms similar to those of manic-depressive illness (see p.323). As schizophrenia deepens, however, the person may become very detached toward other people. The detached person is then more likely to behave strangely and to neglect his or her appearance. There are several types of schizophrenia with similar symptoms, but the only practical distinction that most physicians now make is between paranoid schizophrenia and other types. The main symptoms of a person with paranoid schizophrenia are constant suspicion and resentment, accompanied by an irrational fear that people are hostile or even plotting to destroy him or her.

What are the risks?

Schizophrenia, the most common type of psychosis, usually begins between ages 15 to 30. Males and females are about equally affected by the disorder.

For unknown reasons schizophrenia is more common in certain geographic areas such as inner cities of the US. Throughout the world schizophrenia has an average lifetime prevalence of almost 1 percent. It tends to run in families, and, as mentioned earlier in this article, chemical changes in the brain may also play a role.

People who have bouts of schizophrenia in its most severe forms may physically harm themselves or others, or may try to commit suicide (see p.322).

What should be done?

If you suspect that someone in your family is schizophrenic, try to get the person to see a physician. It probably will not be easy. People who are becoming mentally ill often refuse to admit it. But medical care is vital. Do not leave alone a person who at that time seems extremely disturbed. The presence of a relative or friend will reassure that person. Keeping him or her from self-destructive behavior until help arrives may be essential. However, if you feel threatened, leave the person and wait for help. People with symptoms similar to those of schizophrenia may be admitted to a hospital for a preliminary period of observation.

What is the treatment?

Severe cases are treated in a hospital. Treatment usually involves the use of drugs, psychotherapy, and rehabilitation.

The most effective drugs are regular doses of antipsychotic drugs designed to reduce symptoms so that the person can benefit from psychotherapy. As symptoms gradually disappear, doses are reduced. Some people, however, need long-term medication. They may either take oral medication regularly or be given an injection every 2 to 4 weeks to ensure compliance.

As soon as the person's symptoms are controlled by medication, he or she is ready to be helped by psychotherapy. Techniques of psychotherapy vary, but the goal is the same: to help the person understand the emotional factors underlying the disorder and

What is a nervous breakdown?

The term "nervous breakdown" is often used by the public as a general term to say that a person has had a serious emotional problem that interferes with functioning. In other words, a person who has a nervous breakdown becomes unable to deal with ordinary life because of overwhelming emotional problems.

"Nervous breakdown" is not a medical term and is not used by a physician to describe the diagnosis of a patient who has a mental disorder. Terms such as depression or anxiety are more useful.

Sadly, people who are known to have some severe emotional problem are often feared and avoided by others in the community and sometimes by friends and family. But just as with any other illness, help, concern, and support will greatly benefit the person with a mental disorder, society, and yourself. Ignorance and prejudice can only be harmful to everyone concerned.

how they contributed to the current episode. Medication and psychotherapy play major roles in helping the person get back in touch with reality. For treatment to be effective, the family needs to be closely involved.

The final stage of treatment is rehabilitation, which helps people who are recovering from a bout of schizophrenia to regain normal skills and behavior patterns. In the early stages of hospital treatment, people with schizophrenia are generally given increasingly complex tasks and pressures, which eventually approximate the tasks and pressures of the world outside. Those with schizophrenia need assistance from day centers or other community care once they are released from the hospital, but these resources are not always available.

What are the long-term prospects?

Many people recover from an episode of schizophrenia well enough to return to varying degrees of independence. But they may have further episodes, especially if they do not take their medication as prescribed. In some people the condition becomes chronic. About 10 percent remain impaired for life. The outlook improves if you follow your physician's advice about medication, and if the family is involved in your treatment.

Depression

Most people feel low or sad occasionally, but people are not considered mentally ill if they are able to continue with a daily routine. However, when depression seriously affects a person's job or interpersonal relationships, psychiatrists consider these individuals to have a depression. Such depression may persist, deepen, and eventually interfere with the ability to lead a normal life. If you or someone in your family has occasional periods of blues that last a few days or weeks, you probably don't have a depression.

Serious depression can occur after a specific emotional blow such as the death of someone you love, the end of a marriage or love affair, or a financial loss. Depression is an excessive emotional reaction to loss. Sometimes the losses are internal, such as loss of self-esteem or loss of hope.

People at particular stages in life seem especially susceptible to depression. Late adolescence, middle age, and the years after retirement are critical periods. Many people find the transition from adolescence to adulthood difficult, especially when there are intense family conflicts or educational or work pressures. Loss of fertility or virility in middle age may seem like loss of sexuality, a loss that can trigger depression; conversely, depression can cause a loss of interest in sex. A person in late middle age may brood over the realization that he or she can advance no further in a career.

Depressive illness among older people is extremely common. This may be related to many factors, including the death of friends, a recognition of the physical limitations of aging, and the realization that death is in the foreseeable future.

Severe depression may be accompanied by a chemical change that affects the way the brain functions. Physicians disagree, however, as to whether these chemical changes cause the depression in question or are the result of a deep, prolonged depression.

What are the symptoms?

Symptoms of depressive illness include overriding melancholy and other changes. It is common for the depressed person to become apathetic about the outside world or withdrawn. It is also common for the person to have difficulty concentrating. He or she may also lose interest in or have trouble with eating, sleeping, and sex. Sometimes indigestion, constipation, and headaches appear. A depressed person may be preoccupied with his or her body and have imaginary physical illness. All depressed people have severe psychological symptoms. They may lose touch with reality, may feel guilty and worthless without cause, may believe that they are being persecuted, and may have hallucinations. When acute anxiety (see p.324) accompanies the depression, the resultant restlessness and agitation may mask the more common symptoms.

Intensity of symptoms often varies with the time of day. Typically, a depressed person wakes up early with almost no mental energy but improves as the day progresses. But some people have the worst symptoms at night. As the disorder progresses, depression may deepen until it never lifts. The person then becomes totally withdrawn and may spend most of the the time in bed.

What are the risks?

About 15 percent of the population is likely to experience at least one period of depression severe enough to require medical help. Often, however, symptoms may not be specifically identified as a depressive illness. Some types of depression tend to run in

Suicide

About 30,000 people killed themselves in a recent year; many times that number try but fail to commit suicide. Those who fail often want to fail; an unsuccessful attempt at suicide may be a lonely, frustrated, or ill person's way to attract attention. Keep in mind that someone who tries to commit suicide and fails may try again and succeed. So if anyone you know seems emotionally disturbed and threatens to commit suicide, try to get him or her to see a physician immediately. Call your physician or a hospital for help. While waiting for help, encourage the suicidal person to talk, and listen patiently without passing judgment. Do not leave such a person alone; wait with them at least until professional help arrives.

If you find someone who is unconscious or semiconscious, whatever the cause, call 911 or an ambulance, or take the person to a hospital emergency department. Disturbed individuals often seek death by taking an overdose of sleeping pills. If you find medication or a container anywhere near the person, be sure to give these items to the hospital staff or the ambulance crew. Meanwhile apply first aid (see Injuries and emergencies, p.837).

If someone feels suicidal

- He or she may appear lonely and withdrawn.
- He or she may talk about suicidal intentions.
- He or she may have hoarded pills, or become obsessed making a will or paying insurance policies.
- He or she may have lost a loved one or a job and feel that life is not worth living.
- Try to get the person to talk to someone. Never ignore a verbal threat of suicide.

If you feel suicidal

- Try to be honest about your problems if they are caused by alcohol or drugs.
- Think instead of ways you could seek treatment or change your circumstances.
- Talk to a close friend or a counselor about your feelings and intentions.
- If you still feel suicidal, go to a hospital emergency department. Tell the staff about your problem.

families. Families and physicians often do not recognize depression until the condition is greatly advanced.

The most serious risk of depression is suicide (see Box, above). Although they are too common in all age groups, depression and suicide are particular problems of older people. Sometimes depression can resemble and be confused with dementia (see p.314). This confusion is common but particularly counterproductive since depression is often reversible with effective treatment. The family of a depressed older person may think that he or she has senile dementia and seek no treatment for depression. Young people may express their depression in rebellion or in antisocial behavior.

What should be done?

If you recognize the symptoms in other people, try to persuade them to accept medical help. If you are feeling low and unable to cope, see your physician.

What is the treatment?

Self-help: Productive activity—including a vacation, a hobby, or sports—may help you pull out of a mild depression, as may spending time with others. Regular exercise has been shown to be effective for mild to moderate depression. Continue these measures and consult your physician if your feeling of depression persists or gets worse. If a member of your family seems to be severely depressed, try gentle but firm persuasion to get him or her to a physician. Threats of suicide should always be taken seriously and considered an emergency.

Professional help: Treatment depends on the type and severity of symptoms. If you go to your family physician with symptoms of depression, he or she may refer you to a psychiatrist for treatment. Treatment may consist of medication, psychotherapy, or a combination of both. Antidepressants, which are often used in treatment of depression, can usually begin to provide relief within 2 to 3 weeks. In severe cases a psychiatrist should always be involved, especially when there is a risk of suicide. The physician may advise hospitalization, because in a hospital you can be monitored more easily, you can be prevented from harming yourself, and drug treatment and psychotherapy can be supervised. In rare cases of persistent illness, electroshock therapy may be recommended.

What are the long-term prospects?

People with depression almost always recover. Prompt treatment speeds recovery and lessens suffering. Unfortunately, some types of depression tend to recur. Yet many people who have repeated episodes of severe depression manage to function by getting treatment in the early stages of each episode. Some people with recurring episodes of depression need long-term medication or psychotherapy; others need both.

Manic-depression

(bipolar disorder)

A healthy person has mood swings that shift from moderate liveliness to moderate lethargy, depending largely on circumstances. A person who has the disorder called manic-depression has extreme mood swings, and the relationship between the moods and what is actually happening is not direct.

Manic-depressive illness tends to be cyclical, with periods of unexplainable elation and overactivity (mania) irregularly alternating with deep depression (see previous article). Periods of normality, sandwiched between the extremes, may last for a short time or for years.

Extreme stress or a death may trigger a sudden episode of mania or depression. Often, however, there is no single direct cause, but a gradual accumulation of setbacks. Very rarely manic-depression is caused by a severe infection, a stroke (see p.285), or a brain injury (see p.294).

What are the symptoms?

Close associates of a person with this disorder are likely to be first to recognize the beginning of the manic phase, which starts gradually with hypomania, an output of accelerated energy. People in this phase begin to wake up earlier and earlier in the morning, until they find themselves getting out of bed before sunrise. At the same time, their work output often falls because they are easily distracted and restless. They may be promiscuous sexually, go on spending sprees, and enthusiastically start (but rarely finish) new projects. They are often irritable and may have sudden attacks of rage.

The object of a spending spree is usually to try to feel better by spending money on oneself. Psychotherapists think that this type of short-term lift just masks the underlying depression. In other words, the manic phase is probably a defense against the real problem of depression. Often people with manic depression demonstrate grandiosity (exaggerated thinking) and have a very high opinion of their abilities.

If mania develops, total elation may result in wilder speech, full of rhyming, punning, and illogical word associations. Some people sing and dance or laugh uproariously for no reason. At times anger or underlying sadness may break through in fleeting moments of withdrawal or a total break with reality.

Psychoanalysis

Psychoanalysis is the original technique on which most psychotherapy is based. It was developed by a physician, Sigmund Freud, in Europe in the late 19th century. The technique is based on Freud's theory that adult behavior is largely determined by early childhood conflicts. There are many variations on Freud's basic theory and technique, but all have the same goal: to help the person recall memories buried deep in the subconscious mind. The idea is that once the causes of a problem are remembered and understood, the person may then be able to change long-standing but unhealthy patterns of thought and behavior.

Treatment of this kind requires many meetings with the analyst, during which such matters as present and past dreams, recollections, thoughts, and feelings are discussed, analyzed, and interpreted. Full treatment involves a few hour-long sessions per week for at least 2 or 3 years, although some courses of psychoanalysis may take double this amount of time or more. (In psychoanalysis and other forms of psychotherapy, an "hour" session is usually 50 minutes.)

Psychotherapy

Psychotherapy is treatment by verbal means. The basis of psychotherapy is the relationship between therapist and patient and an attempt on the part of the therapist to remain objective during treatment. It is important for the therapist to have undergone psychotherapy personally, so as not to confuse the patient's problems with his or her own. The psychotherapist adopts a friendly yet professional manner toward the person, offering understanding and support.

Psychotherapy may consist of crisis intervention, short-term treatment, or longer-term treatment. Crisis intervention is psychotherapy aimed at helping you get through a sudden tragedy. Short-term psychotherapy may be effective for emotional disorders, and the exploration of childhood experience is usually not attempted. Longer-term psychotherapy may be necessary to resolve long-standing emotional conflicts and self-destructive behavior. Behavior therapy rejects the idea of delving into the causes of a problem in favor of specific goals for changing behavior. A newer kind of psychotherapy is cognitive therapy, which may help people change the ways they think about problems.

Because they lack concentration, manic people often forget to eat, so they tend to lose weight and become exhausted. Eventually, they may have delusions of grandeur or intense anger at their inability to carry out wild schemes.

The depressive phase is like depression (see previous article), but the symptoms are more severe. The onset may be gradual or very sudden, with the person becoming increasingly withdrawn. Sleep is frequently disturbed. Although there may be early morning wakefulness, late rising becomes habitual. Sex drive decreases, speech and movement slow down, and imagined problems multiply. Some people with manic-depression become unable to face the world, and simply stay in their rooms. This may in turn lead to a break with reality, delusions, and psychosis (see the Box on Psychiatric terms, p.319).

What are the risks?

Manic-depressive illness is rarer than depression. It is thought to occur in about 3 percent of the population. More than one family member may be afflicted, and men and women are equally susceptible to it.

Although someone with this disorder may threaten suicide during depressions, he or she may lack the energy to carry it out. The danger increases with emergence from deep depression, when renewed energy may accompany a continuing death wish. In the manic phase, outrageous behavior may ruin social and professional relationships, and lack of judgment can become serious enough to lead to financial disaster.

What should be done?

If you suspect someone you are close to has manic-depression, persuade him or her to see a psychiatrist. You will need patience and persistence in most cases. If necessary, ask your physician for advice as a first step. If you think that you may be becoming manic-depressive, see your physician without delay. Manic-depression disorder can be treated with psychotherapy and medications.

What is the treatment?

Mild cases often can be treated by medication. The person should also be treated by a psychiatrist (see Box on Psychotherapy, p.323). In severe cases, especially when there is a risk of suicide or if irrational behavior gets out of hand, treatment in a hospital is necessary.

As the treatment in the hospital begins to show results, occupational therapy is added to the treatment to prepare the person for a return to everyday life. If somebody in your family has been in the hospital for this disorder, you will probably be told both how to recognize signs of an impending episode and how to reduce the strain on the patient and lessen the risk of further episodes. After release from the hospital, many people with manic-depression must continue to take medications to prevent recurrent episodes of illness. Many people with severe manic-depression have been restored to near-normal health by long-term treatment with the medication lithium carbonate. This reduces the frequency and severity of episodes. The dosage must be carefully controlled, and regular laboratory tests and checkups to help prevent potentially harmful side effects are an essential part of treatment with lithium.

What are the long-term prospects?

Not long ago most people who had one episode of manic-depressive illness could expect to have more episodes, which might become increasingly severe. However, this gloomy outlook can now often be brightened by long-term treatment combining both psychotherapy and medication.

Anxiety

For most people, anxiety is a temporary reaction to stress. It becomes a disorder only when it persists and prevents you from leading a normal life. Some anxiety states are caused by severe stress, but in some people only slight stress may be involved. The stress may be cumulative. People who have "free-floating" anxiety live in a constant state of apparently causeless anxiety. In reality they are not aware of the actual cause, which may be unconscious.

Psychiatrists have found that there are several different anxiety disorders. These include phobias (see next article) and obsessive-compulsive disorders (p.326). If you have an episode of anxiety, you will probably feel apprehensive and tense, and be unable to concentrate, to think clearly, or to sleep well. You may have frightening dreams and occasional symptoms of fear such as a pounding heart, sweating palms, trembling, or diarrhea. Some people in a state of anxiety find it hard to breathe, as if their lungs are under constant pressure. And they may become convinced that they have heart or stomach trouble when in fact they are physically healthy (see Hypochondriasis, p.327). A man may have trouble maintaining an erection or may have premature ejaculation (see p.657). In "panic attacks," which can occur at any time, the symptoms occur suddenly and intensify alarmingly, in a vicious circle of escalating symptoms.

What are the risks?

Anxiety disorders are very common. They are slightly more common in women than men, and adolescents and older people are especially susceptible. If severe anxiety is not treated, depression may result (see p.321).

What should be done?

If your anxiety is caused by a specific stress, try to understand what's causing it. If you cannot find a way to deal with the stress, or if your severe anxiety persists, consult your physician, who will examine you to see whether he or she can help you with standard medical treatment. If not, you may be referred to a psychiatrist. The first time you have an anxiety attack, you may think you are having a heart attack. To be on the safe side, call your physician. If he or she is not available, call for help to get you to a hospital emergency department.

What is the treatment?

Self-help: Various methods of relaxation can lessen the severity of anxiety symptoms. When you feel tense and troubled, try doing relaxation exercises or some physical activity such as swimming, jogging, or brisk walking.

Professional help: Your physician may suggest that you talk to a psychiatrist to look into the causes of your anxiety. The psychiatrist will determine which of the anxiety disorders you have and recommend treatment. Various forms of psychotherapy are often helpful, as are medications such as antianxiety drugs (minor tranquilizers) or antidepressants. Usually a combination of therapy and drug treatments is helpful to people with anxiety disorders.

What are the long-term prospects?

You need to understand the causes of anxiety to treat it, so it may be necessary to see a psychiatrist to help you understand the psychological conflicts involved. You may be able to avoid symptoms, or at least minimize them, by continuing to do relaxation exercises even when you are not actively anxious. Maintain contact with your physician so he or she can respond to your needs if your attacks are recurring.

Phobias

(phobic disorders)

A phobia is an irrational fear of a specific object or situation. For instance, you may dread the sight or touch of a spider, or you may have a morbid fear of heights (acrophobia). Such fears do not usually prevent you from leading a normal life. Fear of confined spaces (claustrophobia) is more of a problem, because you may try to avoid cars, trains, and elevators. Some phobias, however, may make normal life virtually impossible. A common example is agoraphobia, which is generally defined as fear of open spaces. For those with agoraphobia an open space may be not just a park or field but anywhere outside their own home. The phobia may also involve extreme shyness—a fear of society that is closely associated with the withdrawal symptoms of depression (see p.321). If you suffer from agoraphobia or any other phobia, the need to face the situation that you fear can bring on the symptoms of anxiety, including a racing heart, sweating hands, rapid breathing, and a feeling of nausea.

What is the treatment?

Self-help: Try to face your fear to help overcome it. See a psychiatrist if you are unsuccessful after trying persistently, or if your fear interferes with everyday living or one of your goals.

Professional help: If your symptoms are those of a general anxiety state, treatment is similar to treatment for anxiety. For agoraphobia associated with depression, many physicians prescribe antidepressant drugs and psychotherapy.

Two types of therapy may be used—behavior therapy or psychodynamically oriented psychotherapy. In the behavior therapy approach, the therapist uses desensitization, in which the therapist helps the person with a phobia gradually to increase his or her exposure to the source of fear while simultaneously teaching the individual to become deeply relaxed. As an example of desensitization, someone who is afraid of flying may be taught the process of deep muscle relaxation and then progressively shown pictures of airplanes, asked to imagine flying in an airplane, taken to an airport, and finally taken up in an airplane.

Psychodynamically oriented psychotherapy not only treats the symptom (the phobia) but also helps the person understand and resolve the emotional conflicts underlying the phobia. Phobias reflect unconscious fears, and the object of the phobia is only a symbol of the unconscious fear. Thus, agoraphobia is often linked to underlying dependency fears. Individuals with agoraphobia are afraid to leave home because of irrational fears that they will be unable to cope with life. Claustrophobia may represent a fear of being emotionally trapped. Thus, the real fear may not be what you think it is.

Psychosomatic illness

Almost every physical disorder has some connection with emotional factors. Even accidental injuries such as broken bones seem to happen more often to children from unhappy families than to others. A psychosomatic disease, sometimes called a psychogenic disease, is one in which emotional factors are not merely involved, but are dominant. This appears to be the case, for example, in many skin disorders, migraine, some types of asthma, and some gastrointestinal disorders.

The term "psychosomatic" should not be used to suggest that these illnesses are imaginary. The symptoms are actually being experienced by the person. They are real. Disorders with symptoms that are caused entirely by a mental disorder are called hysteria (see p.327).

You know from experience that your state of mind affects your body. For instance, your heart beats faster when you are excited or frightened, a stomach ache often follows an emotional scene, and fear can make you sweat. These are simple examples of the interaction of the body with the mind under conditions of stress. There are far more complex links known, such as one between chronic anxiety and some disorders of the skin, though the mechanism of the linkage is not clearly understood.

There is much to be learned about the ways in which our emotions cause physical illness. It may be that emotional stress is a final factor or "last straw" in precipitating health problems in people who may already have some genetic susceptibility to a certain disease. Significantly, a tendency to develop disorders such as asthma, dermatitis, irritable colon, or migraine under stress seems to run in families.

What is the treatment?

If you develop an illness that is known to be associated with or aggravated by stress and emotional problems, your physician will ask many questions regarding your personal life. Straightforward medical treatment and reassurance that you do not have a serious disease may relieve your symptoms. If it does not, your physician may begin to concentrate on helping you to handle the stresses of your day-to-day life. The knowledge that you can probably avoid or lessen certain symptoms by avoiding certain emotional strains may be helpful. For example, relaxation exercises, together with a change in your daily routine, can be particularly helpful in treating circulatory disorders such as some types of high blood pressure. If the problem persists, you may want to seek an evaluation by a psychiatrist.

Obsessive-compulsive disorder

A compulsion is an unreasonable need to behave in a certain way. An obsession is an unpleasant or irrational idea or thought that lodges in the mind. Obsessional mental activity often leads to compulsive behavior.

At one time or another most people have minor obsessions and compulsions. One day, you may not be able to get a popular tune out of your head. You are obsessed with it. Or you may irrationally feel compelled to walk to work every day on the same side of the street. You may check several times to make sure you turned off the oven. However, when these thoughts and acts become so intense and persistent that they interfere with normal life, you probably need to get psychiatric help. In such cases the person has an obsessive-compulsive disorder.

What are the symptoms?

Obsessions take hold gradually. Being intensely interested in a topic such as politics, religion, or hygiene does not qualify. True obsessions are unwelcome, intrusive, irrational thoughts that are upsetting. The thoughts are often sexual or religious. If, for instance, you have become obsessed with the idea that burglary is rampant, you may feel a compulsion to test your front door again after you have already locked it securely. This is a relatively harmless compulsion. Some people, however, might carry this too far by getting out of bed repeatedly during the night to test the door over and over again.

Compulsive disorders center on irrational fears. Some people become obsessed with fear of "germs" and wash their hands endlessly. Such a person may realize his or her behavior is irrational, but attempts to resist an overwhelming compulsion cause intense anxiety, which can be relieved only by giving in to the compulsion.

What should be done?

If you feel that any of your ideas or actions are slipping out of control, consult your physician, who will probably refer you to a psychiatrist for therapy. Treatment for mild cases of this disorder is usually based on an effort to reassure you while trying gradually to discover what lies behind your compulsive behavior. Compulsions can sometimes be treated by a type of therapy that is known as desensitization (see Phobias p.325). Psychotherapy may also be used. A medication called clomipramine has been approved specifically to treat obsessive-compulsive disorder. Many psychiatrists believe that the anxiety that underlies such symptoms should be treated with psychotherapy, and in some cases also treated with medication.

For many people, antidepressant and tranquilizer medications also help reduce depression and anxiety, which are symptoms that commonly accompany an obsessive-compulsive disorder.

Hypochondriasis

Most healthy people are barely conscious of the internal workings of their bodies. However, you may be excessively aware of them, concentrating on them so much that they seem to be a constant cause for worry. This is called somatization if you focus on specific body functions or symptoms such as pain. It is called hypochondriasis if you have fears of being ill. Mild cases of somatization are common. Concern about your health becomes an emotional problem, however, if it causes you to lose interest in virtually everything but your presumed ailments.

This disorder usually occurs as a complication of an underlying condition such as anxiety or depression (see p.321).

The severe hypochondriac usually buys and uses great quantities of nonprescription medications, repeatedly visits physicians, and may decide to try various types of unproven medication. The person tends to interpret the symptoms of anxiety as signs of severe illness. If the depression is severe, the person may be convinced that his or her body is degenerating—that, for instance, the person has a relentless fear that he or she has cancer.

What should be done?

If you are constantly worried that you have a serious illness, and you are not convinced by your physician's repeated reassurances, try to accept that you may have an emotional problem. Try to admit the possibility and discuss it with your physician. If your physical concern is caused by underlying anxiety or depression, successful treatment of that disorder will usually clear up the hypochondriasis. Get regular checkups from your physician. Also, try to live as full a life as possible despite your symptoms.

Organic psychosis

Schizophrenia (see p.319) is a psychosis with a mixture of organic (physical) and psychological factors. When a psychosis has a clear physical origin, it is called an organic psychosis. These are very common. For example, acute alcohol intoxication—when a person cannot tell what is real and what is not—is an organic psychosis. A psychosis may be caused by some physical factor such as a brain illness, an infection such as syphilis (see p.655), or a reaction to a drug. In such cases the psychosis is said to be "organic."

Organic psychoses cause obvious signs of illness such as a dazed expression and confused speech. Visual hallucinations (seeing imaginary objects or events) are common. The only satisfactory treatment is to address the underlying physical problem. Antipsychotic drugs such as major tranquilizers may give some temporary relief.

Conversion disorder

(hysterical neurosis)

Conversion disorder, also called hysterical neurosis, is an overreaction to an experience or situation. However, the illness known as conversion disorder occurs when someone (who may or may not be normally "high-strung") reacts to severe stress by developing physical symptoms without any organic disease. Such people do not realize that their symptoms are caused by hysterical neurosis. They, and usually their family and friends, simply assume they have been afflicted by a genuine physical disorder. The problem is often a kind that helps the person to escape from a stressful situation. For example, if you see a terrible accident where you work, you may develop a weakness of the legs that prevents you from leaving home the next day or even for much longer. Or a total loss of memory (amnesia) may follow an accident that you want to forget.

Hypochondriasis (see p.327) also is associated with physical symptoms, but usually vague ones. Conversion disorder involves very specific symptoms, such as blindness in one eye, that have a hidden symbolic meaning (you become blind to avoid seeing a problem in your life).

What are the symptoms?
Conversion disorder is characterized by bodily symptoms resembling those of a physical disease such as paralysis, loss of sensation (numbness), blindness, convulsions, or fainting. Amnesia in various forms may also occur.

What should be done?
If you suspect that the disability of someone in your family is caused by a reaction to some experience or situation, consult your physician. Never directly accuse anyone of faking symptoms. Because conversion disorder is extremely difficult to diagnose, your physician will probably order tests to rule out the possibility of physical causes for the symptoms. If the cause of the symptoms appears to be conversion disorder, the person will probably be referred to a psychiatrist or other specialist.

What is the treatment?
The goal of treatment is to discover the underlying problem and help the person solve it. No standard treatment will work when the symptoms are caused by conversion disorder. Everything depends on sympathetic, patient psychotherapy. Drugs probably are of secondary importance in the treatment of conversion disorder.

Antisocial personality disorder

A person with an antisocial personality disorder is incapable of accepting the rules and restraints that are normally imposed by the outside world. People with such a disorder may be superficially charming but their underlying motivation is selfish, ruthless, and often cruel. They may lie, steal, or threaten to gain their own way. Often they seem unable to learn from experience and continue to generate hostility in those around them. Many such people are obviously irresponsible, unable to hold down jobs, and incapable of having satisfactory relationships. Some individuals affected achieve material or creative success in spite of their disorder. Most, however, are almost constantly unhappy. A fair number become violent when they are frustrated, or they habitually break the rules that create and maintain social order. Such people may spend much of their lives in prison or under supervised psychiatric care.

It is possible to treat the associated disorders to which affected individuals are susceptible, such as severe depression, alcoholism, and drug addiction. But the basic personality remains the same. These conditions are treatable, but only if the person is so unhappy that he or she is motivated to want to change. Many of them are not sufficiently motivated.

If you think the behavior of someone in your family may reflect an antisocial personality disorder, consult your physician, who can help in encouraging the person to seek further guidance.

Addictions and abuses

Drug dependence, including alcohol dependence, is the compulsive, long-term use of a substance taken for pleasure, or to prevent painful effects of not taking it. Emotional disorders may result in addictions in which the person's craving for a drug is uncontrollable. The necessity to have whatever it is that the addict craves prevents him or her from living a normal life. Some addictions can lead to serious illness or death. Three of the many possible types of addiction are singled out for discussion in the following pages: alcohol, drugs, and gambling.

Alcohol is a drug too, but it is discussed separately because, although addiction to alcohol has some characteristics in common with addiction to other drugs, alcoholism is a particularly common disorder.

Abuse of and addiction to drugs is a growing problem. There are many dangerous drugs available both legally and illegally in the US. It is virtually impossible to generalize about what causes addiction and how it develops. A genetic component may exist in certain instances of alcoholism. However, psychotherapy may help some people to stop drinking or abusing other drugs.

Nicotine and caffeine (see p.27), the most widespread of all addictions, are not included in this group of articles. For a general discussion of smoking, along with some ideas on how to quit, see p.51. For more information on the effects of tobacco use, read also the section on disorders of the respiratory system (see p.366) and disorders of the heart and circulation (see p.396).

Alcohol abuse and dependence

People who abuse or become dependent on alcohol often begin to drink heavily to relieve personal, business, and/or social stress. They generally find the relief they are looking for, at least in the short term and at the cost of occasional hangovers. They gradually begin to drink whenever they feel tense. The more they drink, the less tension they can tolerate without alcohol.

You should consider yourself an alcoholic, or in danger of becoming one, if you have reached a point where you need to drink not only to relieve tension but also to make yourself feel "normal." The illness and resulting disability are severe and require immediate treatment if drinking has begun to affect your health and interfere with your personal or work life, or both.

Some people can drink more, and more often, than others before reaching this stage. This difference depends in part on your tolerance for alcohol. The shift from social drinking to alcoholism can happen almost imperceptibly over many years, or it can occur with dramatic speed. Drinking habits also vary widely. Some alcoholics are binge drinkers, who go on sprees with nondrinking periods in between. Others drink constantly and are never completely sober. Some drink only wine, or gin, or beer, while others will drink anything alcoholic.

What are the symptoms?

Family and close friends of people who are becoming alcoholics may not notice the early symptoms. At first the person just seems to have a tendency to drink too much, and this appears to be confined to social occasions. Later, however, drinkers may admit that they have blackouts, which can mean they wake up in the morning with no memory of what happened the night before or have no recollection of what occurred during previous drinking episodes. If this happens to you or to someone in your family, recognize a blackout as a sign of addiction.

In later stages an alcoholic may become secretive about drinking. Glasses of fruit juice may be secretly spiked with alcohol. Bottles may be hidden around the house. Alcoholics often feel guilty about their addiction and may become irritable and aggressive. Another symptom is repeated assertions that they are giving up drinking altogether, alternating with denials that they have a drinking problem. Denial is the major defense employed by alcoholics. They may become depressed, jealous, resentful, or even paranoid, which means the person has unreasonable fears that others are hostile or plotting against him or her. Eventually there is likely to be a loss of memory and concentration, along with an inability to meet the demands of a job. Physically, chronic alcohol abuse may cause a flushed and veiny face, bruises on the body, arms, and legs, a husky voice, trembling hands, and chronic gastritis (see p.497).

What are the risks?

Alcoholism is more common in men than in women, although much of the difference in the past has resulted from a lack of diagnosis and reporting of women alcoholics. In the US an estimated 9 percent of adult males and about 4 percent of adult females are alcoholics. People with alcoholic parents seem to be particularly susceptible, probably because of environmental rather than genetic factors. Some people have symptoms of alcoholism in adolescence or even earlier, but most active alcoholics are between 35 and 55.

Alcoholism can affect every system of the body. Although the exact figures are not known, it is thought that at least 1 in 5 long-term heavy drinkers eventually develops cirrhosis of the liver (see p.524). Heavy drinking makes the liver susceptible to inflammation and may cause serious diseases of the stomach, heart, and brain. Because alcoholics seldom eat adequately, they are likely to develop vitamin deficiencies, particularly of vitamin B (see p.532).

A pregnant woman who is an alcoholic or a heavy drinker subjects her fetus to the risk of being physically and mentally retarded if she continues to drink alcohol throughout pregnancy. The association between maternal intake of alcohol and a variety of developmental abnormalities in the newborn has been firmly established and is called fetal alcohol syndrome. According to some estimates, a woman with alcoholism has at least 4 chances in 10 of having a baby with fetal alcohol syndrome. But even sporadic or binge drinking at critical stages of pregnancy may also affect your child. Women who drink may have a higher risk of spontaneous abortion, premature births and stillbirths, and low birthweight babies.

While no safe level of alcohol intake during pregnancy has been established, the US Food and Drug Administration has concluded that 2 drinks daily increases the risk of abnormalities in fetal growth and development. In fact, many physicians now advise all women planning pregnancy to abstain totally from alcohol while trying to conceive and during pregnancy.

Another danger associated with alcoholism and heavy drinking is traffic accidents. An estimated 50 percent of automobile accident fatalities in the US are alcohol-related.

People with alcoholism also are difficult to live with because they are often irritable and sometimes violent. As a result, the alcoholic risks breaking up his or her family. The same problems of irritability and impaired judgment that affect the alcoholic's home life can also result in loss of a job.

What should be done?

If you detect signs of an early stage of alcoholism in yourself, cut down on the amount and frequency of your drinking for your family's sake as well as your own. If you find that this is impossible to do, seek help immediately. Get in touch with a physician or a recognized addiction treatment program. If someone close to you shows symptoms of alcoholism but denies that he or she is drinking too much (as often occurs), consult a physician about the problem. You cannot force someone to seek help, but persuasion by a physician, social worker, or other professional is sometimes effective. You should attend Alanon meetings to learn how you can help yourself and your family member. Psychotherapy can help people deal with the underlying cause of drinking, but the person must be sober and want to quit before psychotherapy can help.

What is the treatment?

Treatment is a planned, organized intervention to help the person in trouble achieve good physical and mental health and function well without resorting to alcohol or other drug use. Comprehensive treatment, administered by physicians and other health professionals, usually consists of a complete physical, mental, and psychosocial examination of your emotional health, family situation, and occupational stresses. The treatment team monitors and assists in the detoxification (withdrawal) of the drug or drugs of dependence. Next is dealing with the medical and psychological consequences of past drug use, as well as any related disorders, such as depression. Counseling of patient and family about the nature of addiction and the need to find positive alternatives to using drugs is a high priority.

You may be treated as an outpatient or in a hospital, or a combination of both. Treatment depends on the severity of the addiction, the condition of your general health, and the nature of your social support system (whether you can get any practical help you need from people who care about you). The length of treatment also varies from person to person. Usually the sooner the addiction is diagnosed and intervention takes place, the earlier treatment can be completed, and the greater the chances for recovery.

Battered women

Physical abuse of a female partner by a male partner (whether married or not) occurs in all social classes, as does child abuse (see p.718). Beating or other violence is often associated with alcohol abuse, and the man is almost always the aggressor.

Men who abuse women tend to be passive, dependent people who find it difficult to talk about their feelings or to express their anger in less violent ways. Very often they are men who did not have a close relationship with their mothers and so did not learn to form a warm, intimate relationship with a woman. These men have severe emotional disorders but rarely have the strength to confront their problems or deal with them in a constructive fashion.

No matter what causes the violence, the woman should take steps to end it. The best solution is to leave and to seek legal protection. However, this is seldom easy, especially if you have children and few financial resources. Even for women with more money, obstacles may be in the form of social pressure and emotional insecurity.

It is vital for a woman who is being abused to realize that she is not alone and many others have the same urgent problem. Call the police and insist on prompt, respectful treatment of your complaint. Press charges against the abuser. Go to a hospital emergency department for treatment of any serious injuries; the hospital will not only treat you but also provide evidence for any necessary legal proceedings. If you are ready to leave your abusive partner and cannot stay with family or friends, try to locate a women's shelter where you can stay with your children in a protected setting. A hospital social worker, social service agencies, and religious groups may provide assistance.

Drugs of abuse and their effects

A drug can be defined as a nonnutritional chemical substance that can be absorbed into the body. The word "drug" is commonly used to mean either a medication or something taken (usually voluntarily) to produce a temporary (usually pleasurable) effect. Sometimes, the two categories overlap. Morphine may be prescribed as a medical treatment for relief of pain. Obtained and used by an otherwise healthy person, morphine gives a temporary sense of well-being. Some drugs, including morphine and nicotine, are strongly addictive and harmful. Such apparently innocent substances as tea and coffee may be addictive (more accurately, the caffeine that they contain may be addictive) and are capable of harming some people.

All nonmedical use of drugs carries an even greater risk in pregnant women and should be avoided to safeguard the health of the woman and the fetus.

Type of drug	What it does	Visible signs of use	Some long-term effects
Amphetamines, often called speed or uppers.	Speeds up physical and mental processes.	Weight loss, dilated pupils, insomnia, trembling.	Paranoia and violent behavior.
Barbiturates, often called downers.	Produces extreme lethargy and drowsiness.	Blurred and confused speech, lack of coordination and balance.	Disruption of sleeping pattern; double vision; risk of death from overdose, especially when used in conjunction with alcohol.
Cannabis, including marijuana and hashish, often called pot, grass, or hash.	Relaxes the mind and body, heightens perception, and causes mood swings.	Red eyes, dilated pupils, lack of physical coordination, lethargy.	Possible brain, heart, lung, and reproductive system damage.
Cocaine, often called coke, blow, or crack.	Stimulates nervous system and produces heightened sensations and sometimes hallucinations.	Dilated pupils, trembling, apparent intoxication, agitation, rapid breathing, elevated blood pressure.	Ulceration of nasal passages and perforated septum (area separating the nostrils) if drug is snorted; generalized itching, which can produce open sores.
Opiates, including opium, morphine, heroin, and methadone as well as synthetic painkillers.	Relieves physical and mental pain, and produces temporary euphoria.	Weight loss, lethargy, mood swings, sweating, slurred speech, sore eyes, drowsiness.	Constipation; extreme risk of infection (including hepatitis and HIV, if drug is injected); absence of periods in women; possible death from overdose.
Psychedelic drugs, including lysergic acid (LSD) and mescaline, as well as "designer drugs," such as MDMA.	Unpredictable. Usually produces hallucinations, which may be pleasant or frightening.	Dilated pupils, sweating, trembling, sometimes fever and chills.	Possible irresponsible behavior; a single drug-taking episode may cause chronic psychological problems.
Volatile substances such as inhaled fumes of glue or cleaning fluids.	Produces hallucinations, giddiness, euphoria, and unconsciousness.	Obvious confusion, dilated pupils, flushed face.	Risk of brain, liver, or kidney damage; possible suffocation from inhalation.

Both during treatment and in the recovery stage of the addiction, including any period of relapse, self-help groups such as Alcoholics Anonymous, which is listed in the phone book, can be essential for the patient's progress and well-being. The entire family may need self-help.

What are the long-term prospects?

The general outlook for a person with alcoholism is highly variable. If you are an alcoholic and you are determined to give up alcohol, you can do so, with appropriate help. Admitting that you need help is always the crucial first step.

Drug abuse

People start taking drugs (including alcohol) for one of two reasons. Either the drugs are prescribed by a physician to treat some physical or mental disorder, or they are purchased illicitly to provide a pleasurable effect, or to avoid or diminish unpleasant feelings or experiences, such as pain.

Whether or not a drug is addictive varies considerably, not only from drug to drug, but from person to person. Drugs can cause physical dependence, which means that your body gets so used to the drug that your body chemistry is actually changed. When the drug is withdrawn there may be severe physical symptoms, which persist until the body adjusts to doing without the drug. Almost all sleeping pills, for example, alter the sleep rhythm so that unless the drug is taken, sleep is disturbed and restless. A drug is usually regarded as causing true physical dependence when its withdrawal causes a significant degree of discomfort.

Many drugs cause psychological dependence too, in that they produce such pleasurable and satisfying sensations the user feels unable to manage without them and is driven to take the drug again and again. Drugs that are most disruptive to our social structure are alcohol, heroin and other opioids, and cocaine. These cause severe physical and psychological dependence so that the user feels compelled to take them not only to recapture the pleasant feelings but also to avoid physical discomfort.

Many myths surround the use of certain drugs, particularly marijuana and cocaine. These include the incorrect belief that the drugs are not addictive or that they somehow can enhance performance. Recent research proves that such beliefs are false.

The body eventually builds up tolerance to many drugs that cause dependence, so that gradually increasing doses must be taken either to maintain the pleasurable effects of the drug or to prevent any unpleasant ones. If the addict's need for the drug is not satisfied, withdrawal symptoms will result. In some cases the withdrawal symptoms can be harmful, or even fatal, and withdrawal from the drug should be medically supervised.

Who is at risk?

Not everyone who takes an addictive drug, whether for social or medical reasons, becomes dependent on it. Formerly there was a theory that genetic differences between people made them more or less likely to become addicted to drugs. Most physicians now believe that drug addiction is much more the result of an interaction between an individual's personality and his or her life circumstances. The escape route may be alcohol or tranquilizers, or in a different age group or culture, cocaine or heroin. Whatever the drug, it provides only a temporary solution to problems, and dependence on the drug increases until it becomes a central part of the individual's life.

What are the symptoms?

Every type of drug produces its own kind of mental and physical symptoms (see Table, previous page). In general, any addiction is likely to cause a gradual deterioration of the person's standards of work, personal relationships, or both. The behavior of those dependent on drugs is often erratic and their moods may be changeable, with periods of restlessness and irritability alternating with extreme drowsiness. There is often a loss of appetite, unreasonable fatigue, and surliness. If someone close to you has some of these symptoms, it does not necessarily indicate drug dependence. But if he or she also spends increasing amounts of time away from home and seems to be always out of money for no apparent reason, you may have cause for suspecting drug abuse.

What are the risks?

There are no reliable statistics available on the total number of people dependent on drugs in the US. This is due in part to the fact that many addicts never receive treatment and continue to obtain their drugs illegally. It has been estimated that 2 million Americans have tried heroin at one time. A considerably greater number have tried cocaine; more than 4 million people use cocaine regularly and are all addicts or potential addicts. With some drugs, an addict can build up a tolerance for the drug that eventually becomes dangerously close to a fatal dosage.

Apart from the obvious risks to mental health from the effects of the drugs themselves, abuse carries other serious risks. Users of injected drugs often share needles or fail to sterilize them before use and, as a result, hepatitis, HIV infection (which causes AIDS), and other blood-borne disorders are common among addicts. The high cost of illegal drugs may lead addicts into crime including prostitution, with a high risk of sexually transmitted diseases.

Also, with illegal drugs, there are no controls over the purity or strength of the drug. Drugs may be too pure and thus too strong or may be combined with poisonous substances.

What should be done?

Anyone who is addicted to a drug needs help, but addicts are unlikely to seek help themselves unless they are desperate. If you are concerned about drug abuse in yourself or anyone else, consult your physician or a drug counseling center.

What is the treatment?

Treatment is essentially the same as for alcoholism, especially since many people are addicted to other drugs in addition to alcohol. See "*What is the treatment?*" on p.330. Self-help groups such as Cocaine Anonymous (which is similar to Alcoholics Anonymous) are also available for those trying to recover from drug dependency.

Addictive gambling

Obsessive gambling is an addiction, not a compulsion. Gambling gives pleasure to the gambler, and many people enjoy an occasional fling at betting. Obsessive gamblers are people who cannot resist the pleasurable excitement of a card game, the craps table, betting on horse races or other kinds of sports events, and similar games of chance. Unlike the casual gambler, those who are addicted to gambling no longer play primarily in order to win. Their gambling is an addiction because they cannot resist the constant repetition of periods of exciting tension that gambling provides, whether or not they are likely to gain anything from taking the risk. As a result, many obsessive gamblers gamble so recklessly that they gamble away all their own resources as well as those of their families.

This addiction is more common than is generally recognized. It may affect more than 1 million people in the US, and some estimates are as high as 3 million. Addictive gambling seems to affect about five times as many men as women.

What should be done?

If you have an obsessive gambler in your family, try to get him or her to see a psychiatrist and undergo psychotherapy. Groups such as Gamblers Anonymous may also be helpful. If your family member has a problem but refuses to get help, consult your physician for advice.

Addiction to tranquilizers

Despite increasing awareness of the dangers of drug abuse, many people still expect that their problems can be solved by taking drugs. So it is not surprising that many people prefer to ease their anxieties by taking tranquilizers rather than by dealing with the cause of their stress. It is true that in the past many physicians prescribed these drugs too readily, without understanding how rapidly patients can become dependent on them.

People who take minor tranquilizers (benzodiazepines) daily for 3 to 6 weeks physically become dependent on (addicted to) them. Ask your physician if he or she can substitute a drug with a lower potential for withdrawal symptoms. Drugs such as diazepam (Valium) should be taken only for as brief a period, and in as low a dosage, as possible. They should be used with caution by people undergoing the stress of a bereavement or divorce, for instance. The longer you have been taking the drug and the higher the dose, the more difficult withdrawal may be. You and your physician need to decide together when and how to decrease and stop taking the drug. Withdrawal should be slow, with the dose being gradually reduced over a period of at least 8 to 12 weeks, and often much longer, depending upon the amount previously used. Withdrawal symptoms may develop, including tachycardia (rapid heart beat), tremor, abdominal cramps, and sweating; these symptoms may last for at least 3 months, and sometimes for a year or longer. If a person suddenly stops taking a benzodiazepine, then several withdrawal symptoms, seizures, and death may occur. People with severe withdrawal symptoms may need hospitalization, especially if they have any history of seizures. Family support is vital for anyone struggling to withdraw from tranquilizers. Psychotherapy should be employed to treat the emotional problems underlying the person's addiction.

Eye disorders

Introduction

Many people consider sight to be the most important of the five main senses. Your eyes tell you more than your other senses do, and the part of the brain that deals with sight is larger than the parts that deal with other senses.

The eye is a complex and delicate structure (see the illustration opposite). Each eyeball is a sphere about 1 in (25 mm) in diameter. Three concentric layers of tissue cover the eyeball. The tough outermost layer is the sclera, which is visible as the white of the eye. Its exposed surface at the front of the eye has a transparent covering, the conjunctiva, which also lines the inner surface of the eyelids. At the front of the eye, the sclera and conjunctiva join the cornea, a dome-shaped transparent structure sometimes called the "window" of the eye.

Beneath the sclera is the choroid, a layer rich in blood vessels that supply the eye tissues with oxygen and nutrients. Toward the front of the eye, this layer forms the ciliary body. From the front of the ciliary body extends a circular curtain containing muscle fibers, the iris, which varies in color from person to person. In the center of the iris is an opening, the pupil, which looks like a black disk. Through this opening, light enters the eye. The amount of light is controlled by the contraction or dilation (widening) of the pupil, a movement that is regulated by the muscles of the iris.

Immediately behind the iris and pupil is a transparent body, the crystalline lens, which is attached by fibers to the ciliary body. Muscles thicken or narrow the lens, enabling the eye to focus on objects at varying distances. The space between the cornea and the lens is filled with a watery substance called aqueous humor. Behind the lens is a jellylike substance called the vitreous humor, which makes up the bulk of the eyeball.

The innermost layer, the retina, lines the rear three fourths of the eyeball. The retina includes a layer of light-sensitive nerve cells that are called the rods and cones because of their shapes. Light passes through the pupil and lens to the retina in such a way that it forms an upside-down image of whatever you are looking at. The rods are very sensitive to light intensity and enable you to see in dim light. The cones detect color and detail. There are 125 million rods and 7 million cones in each eye. Between them, the rods and cones transform the sensations of color, form, and light intensity that they receive into nerve impulses. These impulses are then transmitted along retinal nerve fibers to the optic nerve, a stalklike collection of nerves that connects the rear of the retina to the brain. The brain interprets the impulses received from each eye, reverses the images, and integrates them into one three-dimensional image.

The eye disorders covered in this section are arranged in four groups. The first consists of errors of refraction such as nearsightedness and farsightedness. The second group is concerned with disorders of those parts of the eye that you can observe, mainly the eyelids, eyelashes, sclera, iris, and lens. The third group deals with two forms of glaucoma, a disease that arises from a problem with drainage of aqueous humor. The final group is concerned with disorders that affect the structures in the inner layer of the eye, including the retina and its blood supply. The muscles and other tissues that surround the eyeball in its bony socket, which is known as the orbit, are also covered in this section. For first-aid treatment of eye injuries, see Injuries and emergencies, p.848.

Drugs and the eye

Drugs used to treat eye conditions can have side effects that also affect the eye. Although most side effects are inconvenient rather than dangerous, some can be serious and may occasionally cause cataracts (see p.345), glaucoma (see p.346), or blindness. Thus, drugs used to treat eye conditions should be administered only by a physician.

The eyes can also be affected by some drugs used to treat general disorders. For example, corticosteroids can cause cataracts, while phenothiazines (major tranquilizers) and chloroquine (an antimalarial, antirheumatic drug) can cause retinal changes. Such side effects do not occur in all cases, but consult your physician if you are taking drugs for a disorder and are having eye problems.

The eye

The main parts of your eye are many and complex. The bony socket, which provides support and protection, is not shown.

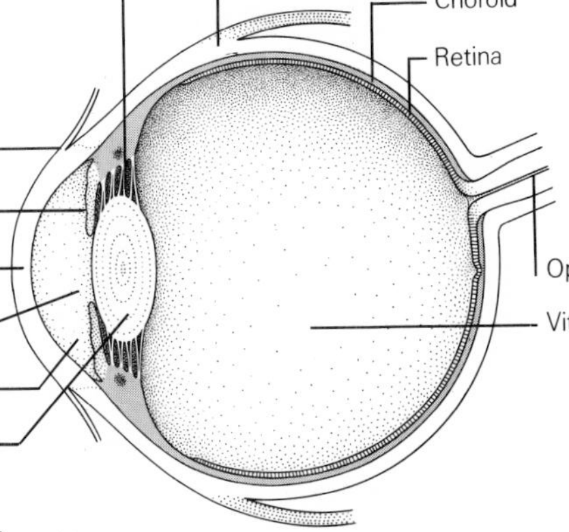

Seeing
When your eye focuses on an object, an image of the object is projected through the pupil and onto the retina. The image is upside-down but is interpreted correctly by your brain, which receives it via the optic nerve.

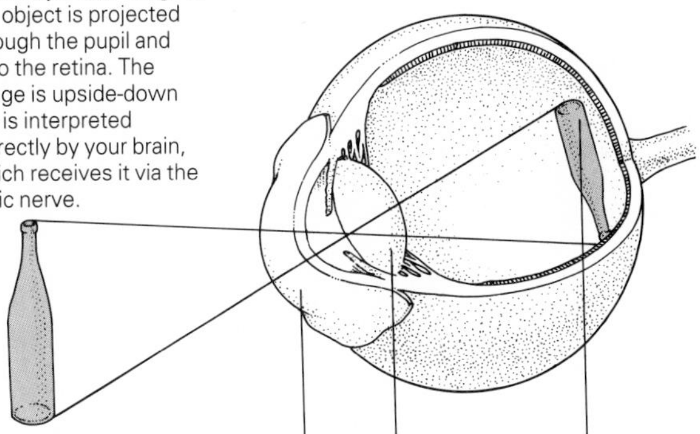

Sight in 3-D
Each of your eyes sees a slightly different view of the same object. Your brain coordinates the two views to form a three-dimensional image.

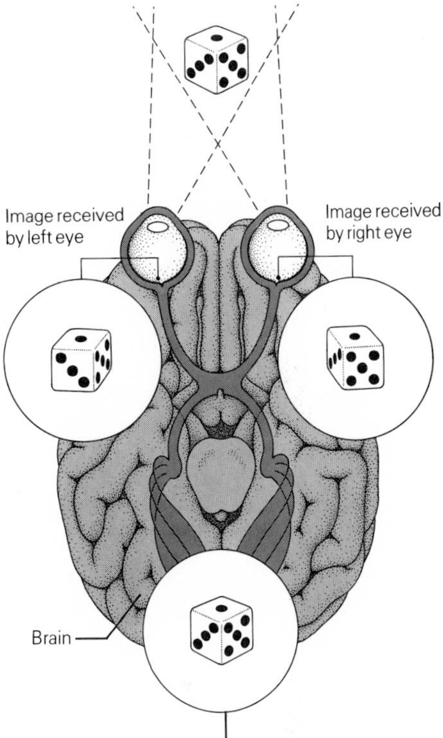

Color blindness

Color blindness is the very common condition of being unable to distinguish between certain colors. Literal color blindness, or seeing everything in shades of gray, is extremely rare.

All the colors are made up of combinations of the three colors red, green, and blue in the light rays that enter the eyes. Certain cells in the retina, which are called cones, contain a light-sensitive substance that responds best to either red, green, or blue light. But if you have an inherited defect of color vision, you may have either a partial or complete lack of one or more of the light-sensitive chemicals in the cones of the retina.

The forms of color blindness that apparently occur most often involve an inability to distinguish between similar shades of reds or greens.

Defects of color vision affect men far more often than women. The defects are usually hereditary and present from birth. They are inherited through the mother's side of the family. They can be caused by an eye disease later in life, but this is much less common.

There is no cure for color blindness, but it is usually mild and does not seriously interfere with day-to-day life. For example, with traffic signals, you memorize the fact that the red light is on the top; green, on the bottom.

Errors of refraction

Refraction and sight
The cornea and the lens act as convex lenses to refract, or bend, light rays from an object and focus them on the retina. These focused rays form the image you see.

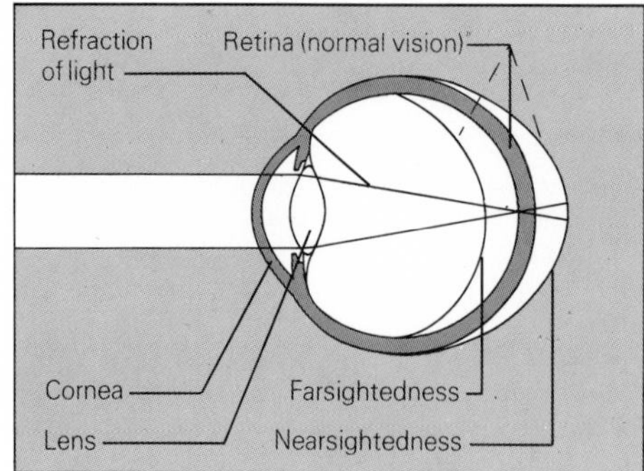

Refraction is the way that light from objects is focused through the eye into an image on the retina. In a normal eye, the point where the light focuses is exactly at the retina, and it is this precise focusing that produces a clear image. In some people, however, the eye focuses the light either behind or in front of the retina, so that the image is blurred.

The four most common disorders of refraction are nearsightedness (myopia), farsightedness (hypermetropia), astigmatism, and presbyopia. Any of these disorders can be present in one or both eyes.

Near-sightedness

(myopia)

In nearsightedness the eye is too long from front to back, or the focusing power of the cornea and lens is too great. As a result, images of distant objects are focused in front of the retina and are blurred. Nearby objects, however, are seen clearly. The eye cannot counteract blurring of distant objects as it sometimes can in farsightedness (see next article).

Correcting nearsightedness
In nearsightedness the cornea and lens focus the light rays from a viewed object short of the retina, producing a blurred image. A concave lens in front of the eye corrects the problem.

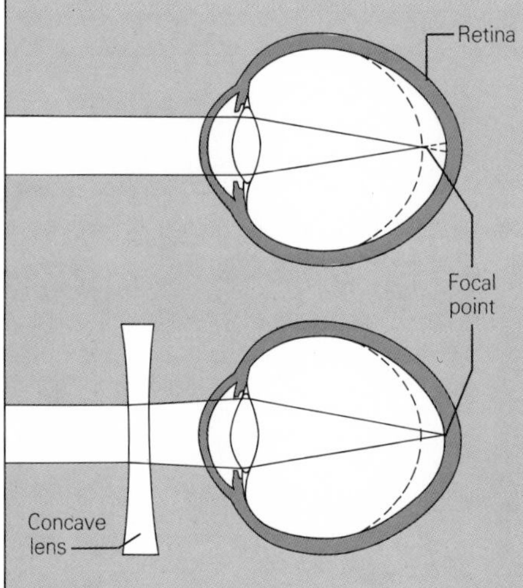

Nearsightedness is very common; about one person in five needs glasses for this problem. It usually develops at about the age of 12 and may worsen until about age 20. It tends to run in families.

What should be done?

If you think you are nearsighted, consult an ophthalmologist (see p.338). If vision tests confirm your suspicion, glasses or contact lenses with concave (inwardly curved) lenses will be prescribed. These will move images of distant objects backward onto the retina and bring them into clear focus. Once you have reached the age of about 30, your nearsightedness is not likely to get any worse, but you should still visit your ophthalmologist every few years to make sure.

Surgical procedures are being developed to try to correct nearsightedness. In radial keratotomy, small radial cuts (like the spokes in a wagon wheel) are made into the cornea to modify its shape. The risk of early and late complications of radial keratotomy seems to be low, but the complications are potentially very serious, and years of follow-up will be needed to determine results and safety. Surgery may be appropriate for people who cannot tolerate, or whose vision cannot be corrected by, glasses or contact lenses.

Far-sightedness

(hypermetropia)

In farsightedness the eye is too short from front to back or there is a weakness in the focusing ability of the cornea and lens. In either case, the eye focuses images of objects at a distance behind the retina, and they appear to be blurred. If the defect is not too severe, the young eye can overcome it naturally by what is called accommodation. The ciliary muscles contract to increase the convexity of the lens, which brings the point of focus forward onto the retina and produces a clear image. Farsightedness is generally present at birth and is usually diagnosed during childhood. It tends to run in families.

What are the symptoms?
Many people with mild farsightedness have few or no symptoms. Rarely, with severe farsightedness, people have eyestrain (aching in the eye), because they constantly must use the ciliary muscles to see clearly. Older people, who cannot accommodate well in general, have continuously blurred vision with moderate to severe farsightedness and may also have eyestrain. Neither symptom permanently damages vision.

What should be done?
If you have symptoms, see an ophthalmologist (see next page). If an examination shows that you are farsighted, he or she will prescribe glasses or contact lenses with convex (outwardly curved) lenses to reinforce the focusing power of the cornea and lens of your eye so that you can see more clearly.

As you get older, usually after age 40, the ciliary muscle may gradually weaken. Because of this you may need to get stronger glasses every few years.

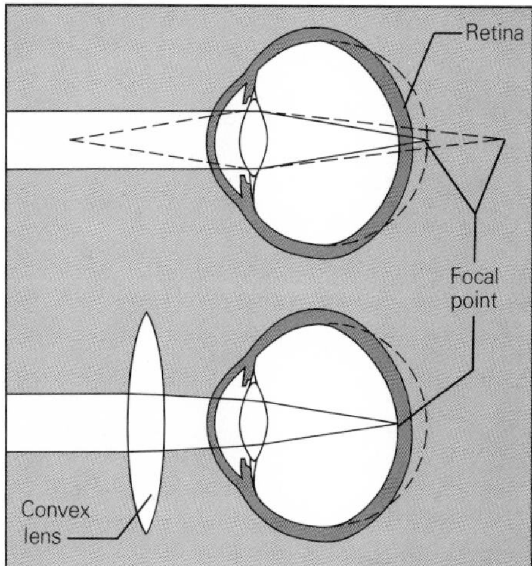

Correcting farsightedness
In farsightedness, the cornea and lens focus the light rays from a viewed object beyond the retina, producing a blurred image. A convex lens in front of the eye corrects the problem.

Presbyopia

At rest, your eye is focused for distance vision. To focus on closer objects, the ciliary muscles of the eye thicken the lens and make it more convex (outwardly curved), a process that is known as accommodation. With age, the lens of the eye hardens; its ability to focus on close objects is reduced. This deterioration is called presbyopia.

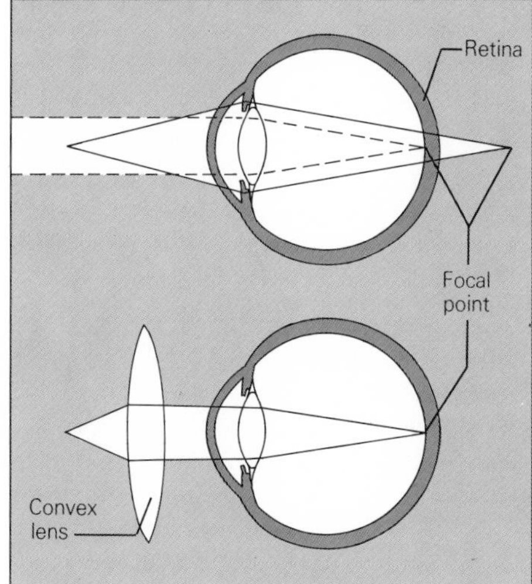

Correcting presbyopia
Presbyopia in people whose eyesight was once normal is corrected the same way as is farsightedness. A convex lens adjusts the focal point.

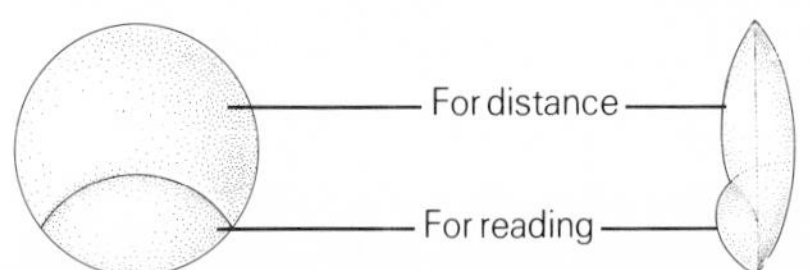

Bifocals
A bifocal lens is a combination of two lenses. The lower one is for reading and other close work. The upper lens helps you see distant objects.

Most people first notice the condition when they are in their mid-40s. It gradually becomes increasingly pronounced. If it is not corrected, you can read printed matter only by holding it farther and farther away from your eyes, until eventually you cannot see well enough to read even at arm's length. If you are nearsighted (see previous page), you may need to take off your glasses to read print at a normal distance.

What should be done?
If you find that close objects are slightly blurred unless you hold them away from you, consult an ophthalmologist (see next page). If you have presbyopia, you will need glasses. These will reinforce the lens and enable you to see close objects clearly.

You will need slightly stronger glasses every few years to compensate for the decreasing power of your own lenses. This continues until you are about 65, when accommodation by the eyes virtually ceases.

If you are also nearsighted (see previous page), farsighted (see previous article), or astigmatic (see p.339), and are already wearing glasses for distance vision, you can avoid the need for two pairs of glasses by getting bifocals. In bifocals, the upper part of each lens is for distance viewing and the lower part for close vision. Some newer types of bifocals gradually increase strength from the middle of the lens to the bottom, without a visible line between the lenses.

Going to the ophthalmologist

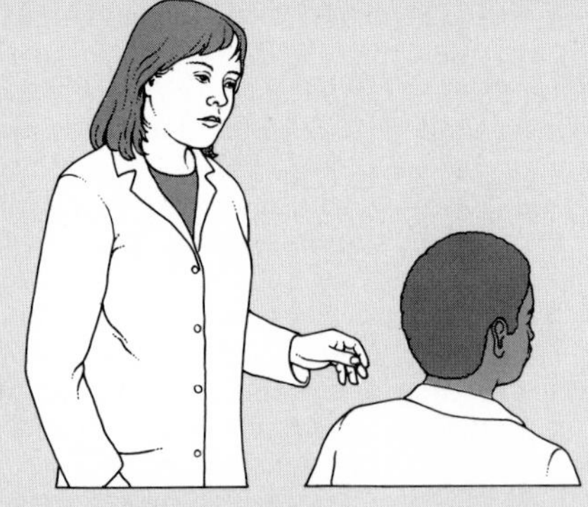

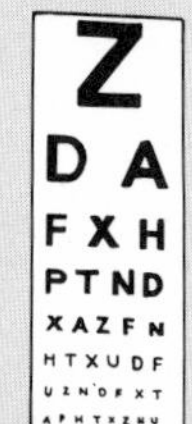

Eye chart
The letters on an eye chart are a standard size and should be read from a distance of 20 ft (6 meters).

When should you go?

Even if there is nothing apparently wrong with your eyes, you should have regular vision tests. Ideally, you should do this once every few years. If you are over 40, your eyes should be tested more often, preferably every 2 years. This is because some serious eye diseases, such as certain types of glaucoma (which can cause blindness), have no symptoms in the early stages and can be detected only by an eye examination. If they are detected early, these diseases usually can be treated.

You should report any sudden changes in your eyesight immediately to your physician.

Three kinds of professionals with different training and skills can be involved in testing the eyes and correcting vision. Ophthalmologists are physicians (medical doctors, or MDs) who specialize in the diagnosis and treatment of eye disorders and in eye surgery. They can prescribe glasses, contact lenses, and drugs and perform surgery. Optometrists are trained and licensed to test vision and can prescribe glasses or contacts. However, an optometrist is not an MD and in some states cannot prescribe drugs. Opticians are trained only to fit glasses and sometimes contact lenses after they have been prescribed by either an ophthalmologist or an optometrist.

What happens?

An ophthalmologist can test your eyes in various ways. He or she will test the acuity, or sharpness, of your vision by asking you to read the rows of letters on an eye chart. The letters vary in size from row to row. The top row has one large letter; the next row, smaller letters; the next, still smaller, and so on.

The result is given as two figures (for example, 20/40). The first refers to the distance at which you read the letters—usually 20 feet. The second is related to the distance at which a person with normal vision can read the smallest letters that you were able to read correctly at 20 feet. The result 20/40 means that you were able to read letters at 20 feet that a person with normal vision would be able to read at 40 feet. The results may be different for each eye. Poor reading of the chart may indicate a disorder of refraction, usually nearsightedness (see p.336) or farsightedness (see p.336). It could also mean a serious eye disease such as macular degeneration (see p.349).

The ophthalmologist checks your lids and may use a slit-lamp (a machine with a bright light and magnifier) to check the surface of your eyes. The intraocular pressure (the pressure inside your eyes) is checked for glaucoma.

The physician also looks at each eye through an instrument called an ophthalmoscope. He or she examines the backs of the eyes to see if you have an internal eye disorder such as retinal detachment (see p.350), or whether there are signs of general disorder, such as high blood pressure. The muscles that control the movements of the eyes will probably also be tested, to detect crossed eyes.

If a disorder of refraction is discovered, glasses or contact lenses may be prescribed. Eye diseases may be treated with medications and/or surgery.

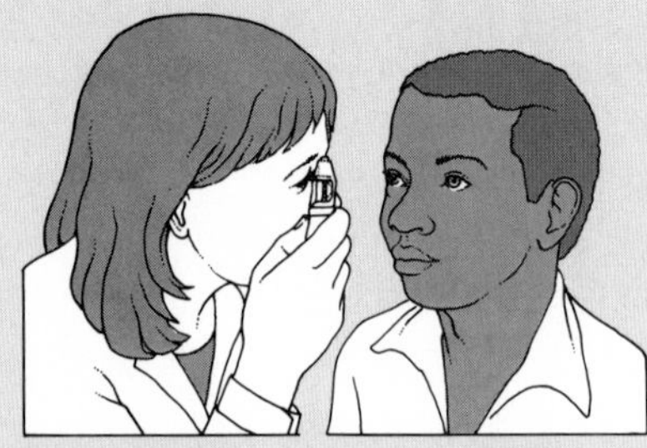

Examining your eye
The physician examines the back of your eye by shining the light from an ophthalmoscope through your pupil and lens.

How do you get glasses?

If your test shows that you need glasses, the physician will give you a prescription, which can be used to make glasses. You choose the type of lenses (glass or plastic, tinted or clear) and the frame you want. The necessary head measurements for the frames are then made by an optician or optometrist. Plastic lenses are lighter than glass. However, they also scratch more easily and must be more carefully cleaned and cared for.

Any necessary adjustments to the frame can usually be made when you pick them up. Wear the glasses for a trial period; if you find the lenses are not satisfactory, return to your fitter for checking and adjustment and contact your ophthalmologist, if necessary.

Astigmatism

Astigmatism is distorted vision caused by an uneven curvature of the cornea, the outside front portion of your eye. One person may see vertical lines out of focus; another, horizontal lines. Diagonal lines may also be out of focus. Astigmatism sometimes occurs in conjunction with farsightedness (see p.336) or nearsightedness (see p.336).

What should be done?

If you suspect that your vision is distorted in the way that is described here, see an ophthalmologist (see previous page). If tests establish that you have astigmatism, your physician will prescribe glasses or contact lenses shaped to the curvature required to correct the unevenness of the cornea. The lenses will help correct the problem and enable you to see clearly.

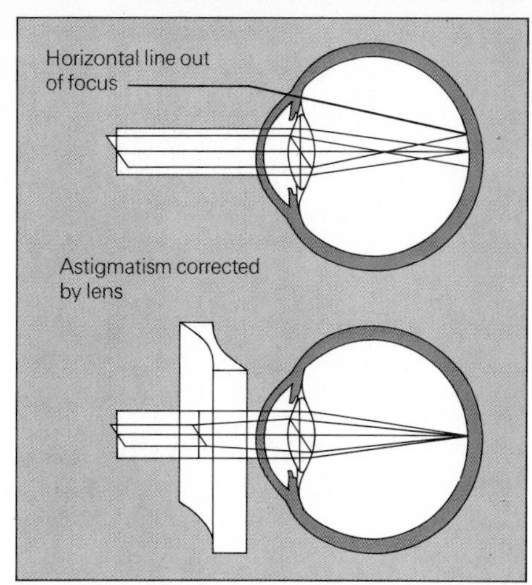

Contact lenses

Contact lenses are a popular alternative to glasses. Each contact lens is a circular plastic lens that fits closely over the front of the eye to help correct errors of refraction.

The three main types of contact lenses are hard lenses, gas permeable hard lenses, and soft lenses. Hard lenses are made of tough plastic and are inexpensive and durable but many people find them difficult to wear. Gas permeable hard lenses are more comfortable than hard lenses but are less durable and more expensive. Soft lenses are the most comfortable and are easy to wear from the beginning; but they are expensive and easily damaged and you have to replace them every 12 to 18 months. So-called "extended-wear soft lenses," including some disposable types, may be kept in the eye for several days, or sometimes even longer, but using contact lenses in this way increases the risk of eye infection and irritation.

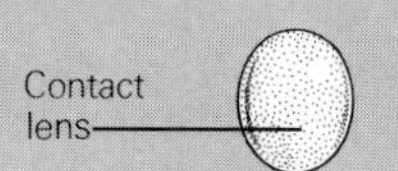

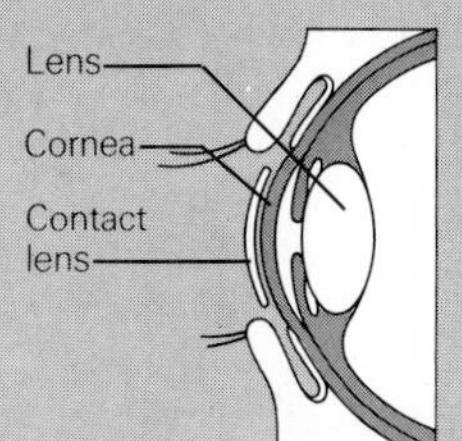

Contact lenses go directly over the cornea and work the same way glasses do.

How do you get contact lenses?

First, go to an ophthalmologist for a thorough eye examination. The ophthalmologist will look for two things: whether contact lenses are appropriate for your eyes (if you have dry eyes, for example, you may not be able to wear them); and which type of lens you should wear. Once you are wearing contact lenses you will probably be advised to have your eyes checked at least once a year, or more often if you note any problem.

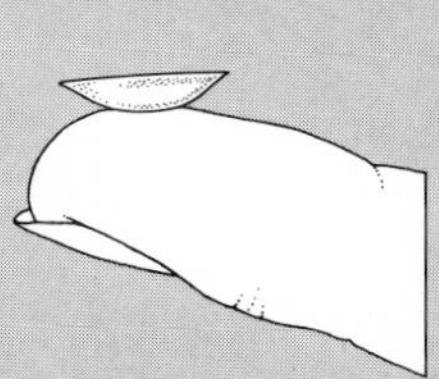

Inserting contact lenses
With clean hands, rinse your contact lenses thoroughly with the proper antiseptic solution after taking them out of their storage solution. Place a lens you have lubricated cup side up on the tip of your forefinger.

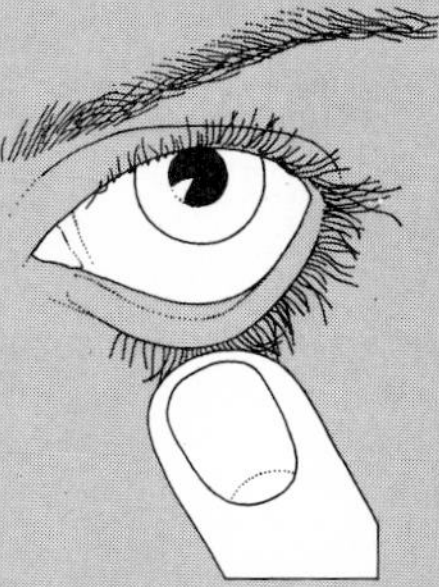

Hold your lids apart with your other hand.

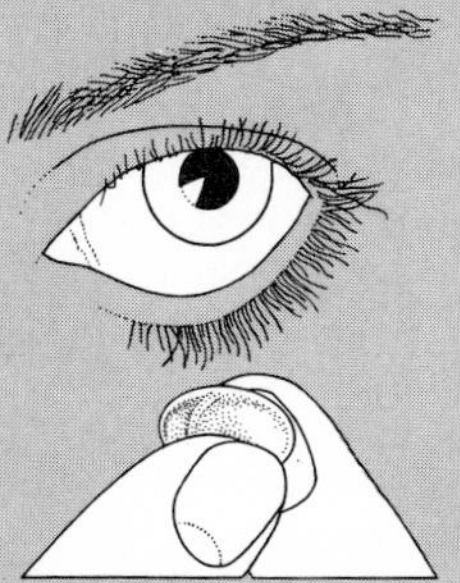

Look straight ahead or at the contact lens as you bring it up to your eye.

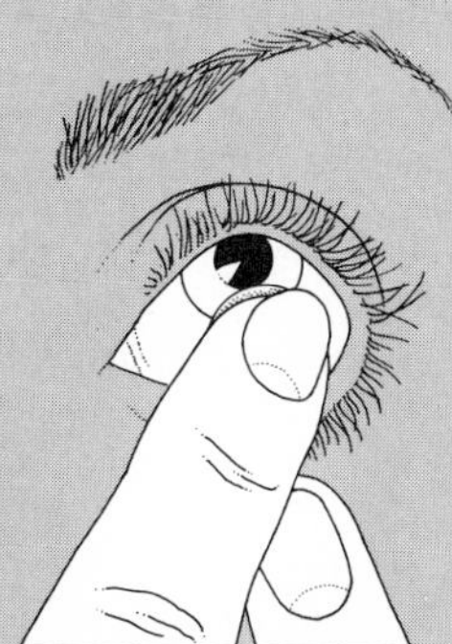

Place the lens gently over the center of your eye. Look downward and release your lids.

Eyelids and the front of the eye

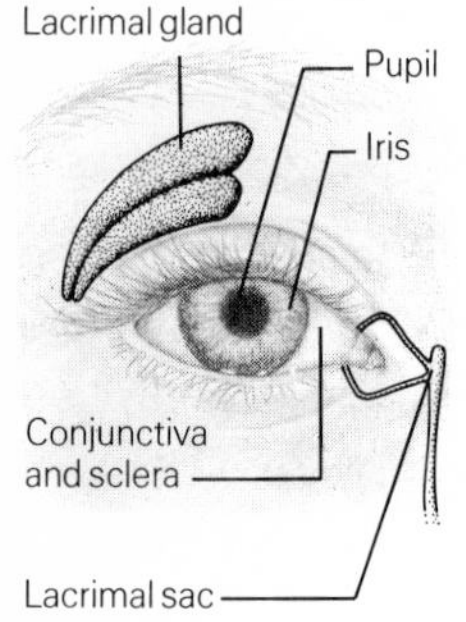

The visible eye represents only about one tenth of the surface area of the entire eyeball. The eyelids act as protective covers for this segment of the eye. Muscles in the eyelids open and close them and act with fibrous and elastic tissue in the eyelids to keep them snug against the eyeball. The edges of the eyelids are lubricated by a row of small glands, called the meibomian glands.

The exposed surface of the eye (except for the cornea, which covers the iris and pupil) and the inner surface of each eyelid are lined with a sensitive transparent mucous membrane called the conjunctiva. They are also covered with a thin film of watery fluid called tears, which is produced in part by the lacrimal glands above each eyeball. Apart from their use in expressing emotion, tears have two main functions: to lubricate the eye so that the lid can move over it smoothly as you blink and to wash away foreign bodies. Tears drain away from each eye along two channels called the canaliculi. A tiny hole at the inner edge of each lid marks the opening of the channels. The channels lead to the lacrimal sac at the side of the nose, and from there the tear fluid passes down into the nose, where it helps keep nasal tissues moist.

Ptosis

See p.255, **Visual aids to diagnosis, 63.**

Ptosis is drooping of the upper eyelid so that it partially or completely covers the eye. The condition is caused by weakness of the muscle that raises the lid. Ptosis may be present from birth, in which case it usually does not grow worse with age. It may run in families. It can also occur at any age, if the nerve that controls the lid muscle or the muscle itself has been damaged. The nerve can be affected by injury; by one of several diseases, including diabetes mellitus (see p.558); or by a brain tumor (see p.301), in which case the ptosis may be accompanied by double vision. Muscle weakness can be caused by muscular dystrophy (see p.741) or myasthenia gravis (see p.311).

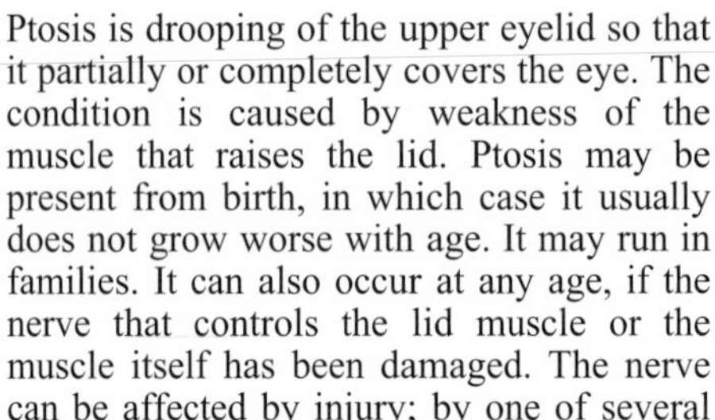

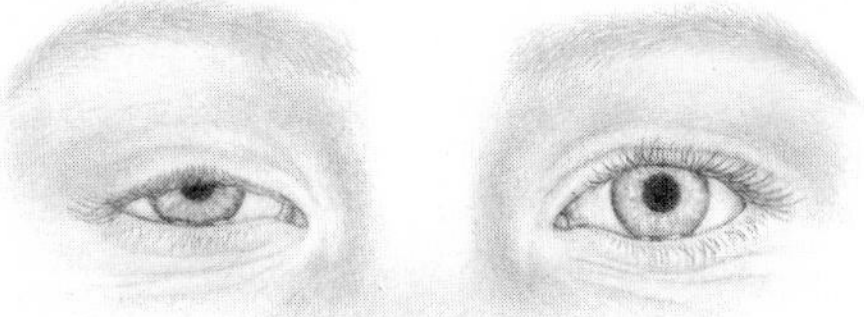

Consult your physician if a previously normal upper eyelid starts to droop and partially cover the eye. This may be a symptom of a muscular disorder such as myasthenia gravis.

Ptosis may affect one or both eyes and may vary in severity during the course of the day. The condition may also occur as age weakens the fibrous tendons of the muscles of the upper eyelids.

Ptosis can be unattractive, and if it is severe it will block the vision of the affected eye or eyes. If ptosis occurs, consult your physician. Successful treatment of any underlying disease will help to improve the ptosis. In cases where vision is impaired, an operation to raise the lid can be performed.

Stye

See p.254, **Visual aids to diagnosis, 53.**

Like all hairs, eyelashes grow from follicles, which are pits in the skin. It is common for one of these follicles to become infected. When that happens, a red, painful swelling like a boil (see p.267) develops on the edge of the eyelid around the base of the eyelash. A white head of pus appears on the swelling, which is known as a stye.

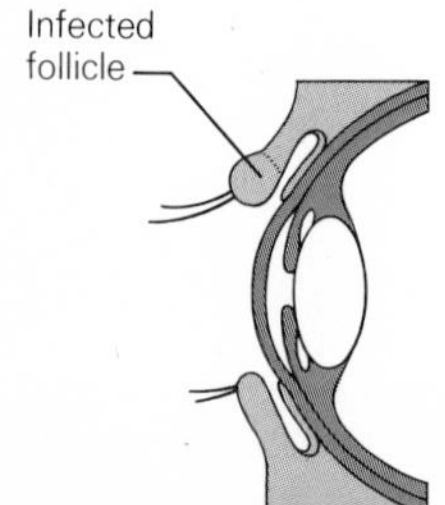

A stye can be very painful, particularly if it is touched. Within a few days after a stye forms, it usually bursts and drains, which relieves the pain.

The stye subsides about 7 days after it first appears, and the eyelid returns to normal. However, styes often recur within a short period, and sometimes several develop on the lids at the same time. In either case, this may occur because the bacteria that caused the initial stye have spread and infected other eyelash follicles.

What should be done?

You can hasten the relief of pain by helping the stye drain earlier. As soon as the inflammation appears, apply warm, moist compresses to it frequently. When these applications draw the pus to a head, do not squeeze the stye, but simply allow the stye to open and release the pus on its own. Wash the eyelid carefully to remove all pus.

If styes continue to recur, talk to or see your physician, who will examine you and perform tests to pinpoint the cause of the infection and prescribe an antibiotic.

Lumps on the eyelid

See p.254, **Visual aids to diagnosis, 57–58.**

The most common kinds of lump that can develop on the eyelid are styes (see previous article), chalazions, papillomas, and xanthelasma.

A chalazion is a painless swelling on the edge of the lid. It is caused by the inflammation (swelling) of one of the meibomian glands, which lubricate the lid edge. Small chalazions usually disappear naturally within a month or two. You can speed up the process and get rid of them sooner by applying mild pressure with warm, moist compresses (warm water on a clean washcloth or gauze). Larger chalazions, which may grow to the size of a small pea, may not disappear on their own and are treated surgically. An incision is made in the eyelid and the contents of the chalazion are removed. This operation is not usually complicated, requires only a local anesthetic, and can be done in a physician's office or a hospital outpatient department. A chalazion can become infected, in which case it becomes more swollen, red, and painful. If an infection occurs, you will want to get professional help as quickly as possible. Treatment may consist of an incision (cut) in the eyelid to allow the pus to drain.

A papilloma is a harmless outgrowth of skin, ranging in color from pink to skin color, anywhere on the eyelid or the edge of the lid. It may increase in size very slowly. If it is large and seems unattractive, it can be removed surgically with local anesthesia. If it is small and inconspicuous and you do not want to have it removed, there is no medical reason to do so.

In xanthelasma, yellow patches of fatty material accumulate beneath the outer skin of the lids, especially near the nose, for no definite reason (but xanthelasma is associated with elevated levels of cholesterol). If the patches are unattractive they can be removed, but they may recur.

Other less common lumps that may occur on the lid include a form of birthmark called a hemangioma (see p.698) and a tumor known as a basal cell carcinoma (see p.274).

Entropion

(inturned eyelashes)

See p.255, **Visual aids to diagnosis, 59.**

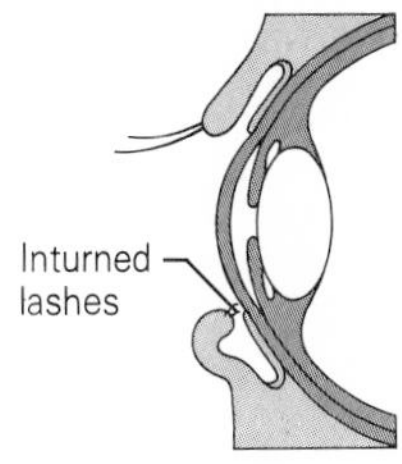

In entropion the lid edge of either eyelid, most often the lower lid, turns inward so that the lashes rub on the surface of the eyeball—the conjunctiva and the cornea. This continuous rubbing causes irritation and may cause conjunctivitis (see p.343) and/or corneal ulcers (see next page). Persistent entropion can also damage the cornea and cause problems with vision.

The condition usually affects older people. As you grow older the fibrous tissue on the lower lids may become lax, which allows the muscle in the lid margin to contract abnormally. It is this laxity and contraction that can pull the edge of the lid toward the eye. Less commonly, scarring (such as that from an injury) on the inner surface of the eyelid can pull the lid edge inward.

What should be done?

If your eye is already irritated when the condition occurs, see your physician to have it treated. Otherwise, turn the lid outward and keep it in this position by attaching one end of a piece of adhesive tape to the skin beneath your lower lashes and the other end to your cheek. After a few days, remove the tape and see if the condition clears up of its own accord. If it does not, consult your ophthalmologist, who may arrange for you to have an operation on the eyelid (usually under a local anesthetic).

Ectropion

(outturned eyelashes)

See p.255, **Visual aids to diagnosis, 60.**

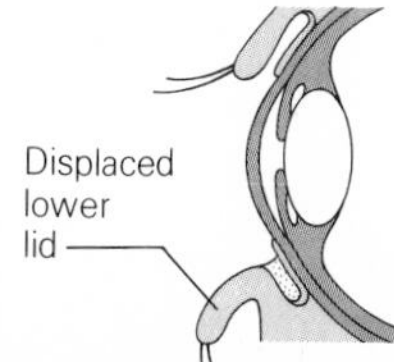

In ectropion the edge of the lid is turned outward away from the eyeball, so that the exposed surface of the eyeball and the lining of the lid become dry and sore. Also, the tears that normally lubricate the lining of your eyelids and the front of the eye may be prevented from entering the tear canals in the lower lid. If this happens, the tears will run down your cheek.

What are the risks?

Ectropion usually occurs in older people because the tendons of the muscle in the lower lid that keep the lid snug against the eyeball become stretched. The condition can also be caused at any age by a scar on the lower lid or cheek that has contracted and pulls down the lid. If ectropion is not treated, corneal ulcers (see next page) may develop on the exposed cornea and damage it.

What should be done?

Ectropion rarely disappears without any treatment, so you should consult your ophthalmologist, who will arrange for you to have an operation on the tissues beneath the eye. This is a minor surgical procedure that requires only a local anesthetic.

Blepharitis

Blepharitis is an inflammation of the lid edges that causes a persistent and unattractive redness and scaliness of the skin on and around the edges of the lids. The disorder has a seborrheic form, which is sometimes but not always accompanied by dandruff (see p.280). In some cases bacteria infect the area and make the condition worse.

In severe cases, small ulcers may develop on the lid edges, and eyelashes may fall out. Often flakes from the lid enter the eye and cause an inflammation called conjunctivitis (see next page).

What should be done?

Try to treat the condition by washing away the scales, morning and night, with warm water or a mild baby shampoo. If this treatment does not improve the condition within 2 weeks, consult your physician, who may prescribe an antibiotic ointment for you to rub into the edges of your lid after washing. This should clear up the condition. If not, an operation may be necessary.

Blepharitis is a disorder that often recurs and needs repeated treatment. It is not, however, a threat to general health.

Dry eye

Dry eye results from a deficiency of tear production. The white of the eye may become red and swollen, and the eye feels hot and gritty. Usually both eyes are affected. Dry eye often occurs in people who have rheumatoid arthritis (see p.589) or Sjögren's syndrome. In many instances it occurs for no obvious reason; that is, it may not be a symptom of disease.

The condition most often begins in middle age and affects women more than men. It usually does not threaten sight, but you may also have a dry mouth, joint pains, and not enough digestive juice in your stomach.

To relieve the discomfort, your physician will probably prescribe artificial tear drops that you can apply to your eye. You may have to use the drops for the rest of your life.

Watering eye

Continuous watering (tearing) of the eye may be caused by an irritation that results in increased tear production or by a blockage in the lacrimal or nasolacrimal tear ducts that drain tears from the eye into the nose. Sometimes blockage follows an injury to the bone at the side of the nose. Sometimes it occurs in long-standing sinusitis (see p.373). Occasionally it results from a foreign object in the eye. But often the cause is unknown. Usually only one eye waters.

Blockage of the tear duct can lead to infection of the lacrimal sac, as bacteria build up inside the duct. This causes a red and painful swelling in the skin on the side of the nose. In some babies the tear duct fails to open after birth, which causes tearing and a discharge from the eye.

Watering of the eye resulting from blockage is an unusual problem. It usually occurs in middle age or later.

What should be done?

If your eye keeps watering, see your ophthalmologist, who will examine your eyes to try to determine the cause.

In an infant, if the nasolacrimal duct is blocked and the condition is in an early stage, the blockage may open and the tearing resolve. In some cases, if the infant's excess tearing does not disappear, the blockage may be cleared by inserting a probe or by irrigating the eye while the child is either sedated or under a general anesthetic.

If blockage of the duct or sac is at a stage that is too advanced for these procedures, as is usually the case in adults, you may need an operation. The operation that is performed creates an artificial duct that bypasses the blockage. If the lacrimal sac is infected, you may have to take antibiotics (as an oral medication or as eyedrops) to clear up the infection before surgery is performed.

Corneal ulcers and infections

The cornea is a transparent section of the eye's outer covering at the very front of the eye. Because of its position, it is very susceptible to injury and infection.

When an ulcer (an open sore) occurs on the cornea, infection can follow, and the reverse is also true. When an ulcer forms first, it is usually the result of a foreign body striking or scratching the cornea. The ulcer then becomes infected by bacteria, viruses, or fungi. If there is no ulcer or injury, an infection of the cornea may be caused by a virus, herpes simplex, the virus that also produces cold sores (see p.484) around the mouth. If you have a cold sore, never put your fingers on your eyes after touching your mouth.

See p.254, **Visual aids to diagnosis, 54.**

What are the symptoms?

You will feel discomfort or pain in the eye, and the sharpness of your vision will be impaired to some degree. The effect on your vision is determined by the size of the ulcer. The white part of the eye will be reddened. In cases of infections other than those caused by herpes simplex, the ulcer is sometimes visible, if you look closely, as a whitish patch. Herpes simplex infections produce what is called a dendritic ulcer, which has a branching pattern and is invisible to the naked eye. The symptoms are much more pronounced in bacterial infections than in viral or fungal infections.

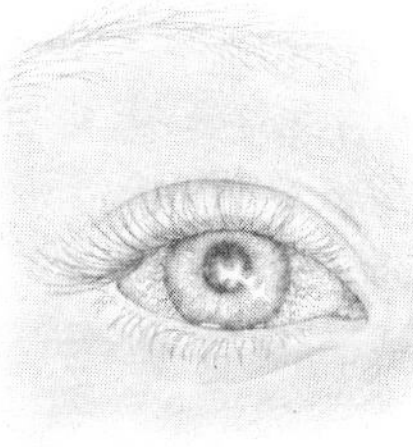

A corneal ulcer caused by bacteria may be visible as a white patch on the cornea.

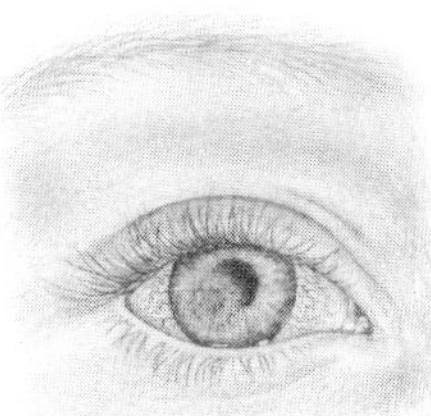

A dendritic ulcer of the cornea from herpes simplex is usually not visible to the naked eye. But it can be made visible with a special stain.

What are the risks?

Many of those affected by corneal ulcers are people whose eyes are exposed to a spray of particles, such as wood shavings or grit from car engines. If an ulcer is not treated promptly, a scar can form on the cornea and sometimes reduce vision. An infected ulcer may perforate the cornea, cause pain and loss of vision, and allow infection to enter the eyeball, causing blindness.

What should be done?

Because of the serious risks involved, as soon as you suspect you have a corneal ulcer or infection, see an ophthalmologist. If the physician suspects a herpes simplex infection, he or she may apply drops to the eye that stain and reveal any dendritic ulcer present, which can confirm the diagnosis.

Ulcers caused by injury to the cornea with a bacterial infection from the injury are treated with antibiotics, given as drops, ointment, tablets, or injections. For herpes simplex viral infections and the ulcers they produce, other specific antiviral drops and ointments are prescribed. Fungal ulcers are more difficult to treat. Dendritic ulcers tend to recur from time to time.

If scars from ulceration drastically reduce vision, you may need a corneal transplant —an operation to graft a new cornea onto the eye (see Transplants, p.432). If an ulcer has perforated the cornea, immediate surgery is required to seal the hole.

Conjunctivitis

See p.254, **Visual aids to diagnosis, 55.**

Conjunctivitis (commonly called pink-eye) is inflammation of the conjunctiva, a transparent membane that lines the eyelids and covers the outer eye up to the edge of the cornea. The disorder can result from an infection, an allergy, or an irritant.

An infection may be introduced by contaminated fingers, towels, handkerchiefs, or washcloths touching the eye. In babies up to about 3 days old it is sometimes acquired from contact with the lining of the mother's birth canal. This condition, known as ophthalmia neonatorum, may be very serious and result in blindness.

In all cases of infectious conjunctivitis, the white part of the eye turns red and feels gritty. There is then a discharge of yellow pus from the eye. Overnight the pus forms a crust. Bacterial infection usually produces a discharge of pus; viral infection usually causes a more watery discharge.

Allergic conjunctivitis is caused by an allergy to pollen, cosmetics, or other substances. There is usually a long-standing redness and itchiness of the white of the eye, without any discharge of pus. A form that occurs more often in children and young adults, especially severely in the pollen season, is a form of hay fever (see Allergic rhinitis, p.370). Less commonly, there is a sudden white puffiness and itchiness of the conjunctiva, usually during the pollen season, that disappears after a few hours.

Conjunctivitis is very common. It is an annoying disorder but, except in rare instances of ophthalmia neonatorum, it is not usually serious.

What should be done?

If you think that you or your child may have conjunctivitis, see your physician immediately. If the symptoms are those of infectious conjunctivitis, avoid spreading the disease. Wash your hands after you touch your eyes, and use your own separate washcloth and towel.

In cases of infectious conjunctivitis caused by bacteria, your physician may prescribe antibiotic drops or ointment to apply to your eyes after you have bathed away any discharge from the lids with warm water. One or 2 weeks of this treatment should clear up the condition. Viral infections usually disappear on their own. Certain types of ophthalmia neonatorum may need treatment in the hospital.

If you can identify the cause of allergic conjunctivitis, it may be possible to avoid the disorder. Consult your physician about using antihistamine medications or other non-prescription drugs that may relieve this form of the disorder.

Subconjunctival hemorrhage

A subconjunctival hemorrhage is a red patch on the white of the eye caused by leakage of blood from a small blood vessel. The condition is harmless, common, and may occur suddenly without an obvious cause.

One or sometimes several subconjunctival hemorrhages may develop as a result of a minor injury to the eye, or of an infection, or after a bout of coughing, sneezing, or straining, or any other activity that raises the pressure in the veins of the head and neck. The hemorrhages usually disappear without treatment within 2 to 3 days. However, if they are associated with injury, you should see an ophthalmologist promptly to ensure that no serious eye injuries occurred, including any underlying injury.

Small subconjunctival hemorrhages are painless and are no cause for concern. However, if you are uncertain about the cause of a red patch on the white of the eye, or if such a patch is painful, you should consult your physician for a definite diagnosis. If you are taking anticoagulant drugs (blood thinners) and experience a subconjunctival hemorrhage, you should immediately contact your physician to see if you need to change the dosage of your medication.

Scleritis

Scleritis is inflammation of the sclera, the outermost layer of tissue that covers the eyeball and that you can see as the white of the eye. The inflammation sometimes accompanies rheumatoid arthritis (see p.589) or certain disorders of the digestive system, including Crohn's disease (see p.508). It can affect one or both eyes.

The symptoms are a dull, severe pain in the eye and one or more areas of intense redness on the white of the eye. The inflammation can occur at the back of the eye, in which case there may be some loss of vision.

Scleritis is a rare disorder that occurs mainly in people between about 30 and 60. If the condition is not treated, there is a risk that the inflamed tissue of the sclera will become perforated, or opened. It is essential that you see your physician right away if you suspect you have scleritis.

What is the treatment?

In mild or moderate cases of scleritis, the inflammation can usually be cleared up with anti-inflammatory medications such as corticosteroids, usually in tablet form. In severe cases, your physician may prescribe immunosuppressive drugs. If the sclera has become perforated, an operation will be needed to repair the damage.

Iritis

Iritis is inflammation of the iris (the part of the eye that determines eye color) and sometimes also of the ciliary body, which is behind the iris. In this disorder microscopic white blood cells from the inflamed area and excess protein that leaks from the small blood vessels inside the eye float in the aqueous humor, the fluid between the iris and the cornea. If there are many floating cells, they may become attached to the back of the cornea or they may settle to the bottom of the aqueous humor. One or both eyes may be affected by this inflammation. Iritis is sometimes called uveitis.

What are the symptoms?

There is a feeling of discomfort or pain in the eye, which becomes reddened. The discomfort may be worse in bright light. The symptoms, which may be mild or severe, are accompanied by a slight reduction in vision.

What are the risks?

Iritis is a fairly rare disorder. It can occur at any age, but is most common in young adults.

If it is treated early, iritis is generally not a serious problem. However, if you do not consult a physician because your symptoms are mild, complications will develop. So many white cells may accumulate in the aqueous humor that they block or scar the opening through which the liquid drains from the eye. This can cause glaucoma (see p.346). This complication may also develop if the back of the inflamed iris sticks to the front of the lens and aqueous humor is trapped behind the iris. Long-standing iritis can also cause cataracts (see next article).

What should be done?

At any sign of unexplainable redness or discomfort or any loss of vision in an eye, however slight, see your ophthalmologist. If you have iritis, the earlier you begin treatment the easier it is to clear it up and the less likely it is that complications will occur.

What is the treatment?

Eye drops or ointment is given to reduce the inflammation. In severe cases, a drug may be injected into the outer layer of the eye after the use of a local anesthetic or you may be given anti-inflammatory medications such as corticosteroids. You may also be given eye drops that dilate the pupil to prevent the back of the inflamed iris from sticking to the front of the lens. The swollen iris can block the flow of fluid, producing a rise in pressure in the eye that endangers sight but that is controlled by medication.

Even when it is treated early, iritis often recurs. In most cases, however, it eventually disappears completely and with it goes any slight impairment of vision.

Cataracts

See p.255, **Visual aids to diagnosis, 61.**

A cataract is an opaque, cloudy area that occurs in the normally clear lens of the eye. Over a period of time, the cataract blocks or distorts light that is entering the eye and progressively reduces vision. In some cases the loss of vision is only slight and never becomes severe enough to warrant treatment. Cataracts usually occur in both eyes, but in most cases one eye is more severely affected than the other.

The most common cause of a cataract is deterioration of the lens in aging. Other causes include iritis (see previous article), injury to the eyeball (in which case only the injured eye is affected), and diabetes mellitus (see p.558). Less commonly, cataracts run in families, and in some cases they are present at birth or shortly after birth.

What are the symptoms?

The main symptom is a blurring of vision in the affected eye. In some cases, it is worse in bright sunlight. In advanced cases, the lens may become white, opaque, and readily visible through the pupil. If you can observe a cataract in the eye of a family member, it is already at an advanced stage. A very advanced cataract may produce painful inflammation and pressure inside the eye.

What are the risks?

Cataracts are fairly common, and you are more likely to develop them as you get older. The disorder may lead in time to severe deterioration of vision, but this can be corrected by surgery.

What should be done?

If your vision deteriorates or becomes distorted, see an ophthalmologist. Your physician may recommend removal of the cataract if glasses fail to improve your vision.

What is the treatment?

The only treatment possible for a cataract is an operation to remove the affected lens. This is the most common of all operations on the eye. If your vision is not too badly affected, your ophthalmologist will probably not operate but will make sure that you get glasses that help you see as well as possible.

With a cataract that appears to be causing inflammation and pressure in the eye, removal of the affected lens is essential. This is also necessary for an infant or young child with a cataract that is reducing vision. An ophthalmologist usually also recommends an operation for an adult if vision gets worse because of the cataract to the point that everyday activities become difficult or if you need good vision in both eyes for your job and new glasses cannot adequately improve your vision.

A local anesthetic is required for a cataract removal operation. The entire lens may be taken out, but usually only the substance within the lens is removed, by use of a hollow needlelike ultrasonic device, and the transparent posterior (rear) capsule of the lens is left in the eye.

Unless you were originally severely nearsighted, surgery that only removes the cataractous lens from the eye makes the eye significantly farsighted (see p.336), so vision is poor. In the past, this farsighted condition after cataract removal surgery was corrected with heavy eyeglasses with thick lenses that could be difficult to tolerate and looked rather ugly. A contact lens can be used but frequently is hard for older people to care for, wear comfortably, insert, and remove. Today, correction is usually by implantation of a replacement lens into the eye and the (depending on the implant type) prescribing of a regular pair of bifocal glasses. After the defective natural lens has been removed during the cataract operation, a plastic one is inserted in its place. This procedure is now well established, and the risk of complications is low. An implant may not be recommended for patients with other eye disorders that could increase the risks. Ophthalmologists are still cautious about recommending implants for very young people and infants. Sometimes after cataract and implant surgery the posterior capsule behind the implant gradually becomes cloudy and the vision in the eye may slowly decrease. If this happens the ophthalmologist may need to use a special type of laser to open the cloudy capsule.

Sometimes after cataract surgery vision is not as good as was anticipated. This may often result from a defect in the retina at the back of the eye, which was obscured before the operation by the opacity of the lens. The most common retinal defect is macular degeneration (see p.349).

Glaucoma

Medical myths

Glaucoma inevitably leads to blindness

Wrong. Prompt treatment of the disease is extremely effective in halting any deterioration of sight.

Glaucoma is one of the most common and severe eye disorders in people over 60. Early treatment is vital, or the condition can ultimately lead to blindness.

The ciliary body in the eye constantly produces a fluid called aqueous humor, which circulates from behind the iris, through the pupil, and into the chamber between the iris and the cornea. In a healthy eye the fluid drains out of the eye through a network of tissue between the iris and the cornea, which is called the drainage angle. From there it flows into a channel that leads to a network of small veins on the outside of the eye. In some eyes the drainage angle does not work properly. As a result, the aqueous humor either flows away more slowly than it is produced or fails to flow away at all, and pressure builds up in the eye. Part of the extra pressure is exerted, via the lens, onto the vitreous humor, the jellylike fluid that fills the eyeball behind the lens.

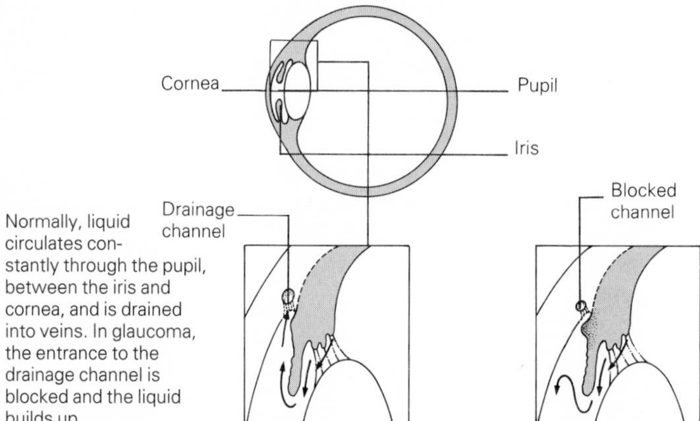

Normally, liquid circulates constantly through the pupil, between the iris and cornea, and is drained into veins. In glaucoma, the entrance to the drainage channel is blocked and the liquid builds up.

The increased pressure in the eye causes pressure on retinal nerve fibers and sometimes also causes the collapse of tiny blood vessels that nourish the light-sensitive cells of the retina and the fibers of the optic nerve, both of which play a vital part in vision. The cells and nerve fibers begin to die from the pressure, and vision begins to fade in certain areas.

The cause, extent, and type of glaucoma can vary considerably. Certain drugs such as antidepressants and anticholinergics (which you may be taking for asthma or irritable bowel syndrome) may provoke the onset of the condition; if you are taking one of these medications, it is vital to check with your physician. The two most common types of the disease, both of which are described here, are acute glaucoma (also known as angle closure glaucoma) and chronic glaucoma (also known as open angle glaucoma).

Acute glaucoma

(angle closure glaucoma)

Glaucoma is a disorder in which the circulation of aqueous humor, a fluid in the eye that is produced by the ciliary body, is blocked. The blockage occurs in a network of tissue between the iris and the cornea that is called the drainage angle. Pressure builds in the eye because the aqueous humor cannot flow away, and this affects the functioning of both the retina and the optic nerve, which are essential to vision. For more about glaucoma in general, read the previous article. In acute glaucoma, the drainage angle becomes blocked suddenly. This type of glaucoma occurs mainly in farsighted older people. In farsightedness the distance between the cornea and the iris is shorter than normal, so the drainage angle is narrower. With age, the lens of the eye gradually enlarges and pushes the iris forward, and this narrows the angle further. In some cases where the drainage angle is extremely narrow, blockage can occur at any time. The outer edge of the iris blocks the drainage angle when the iris contracts to enlarge the pupil. This occurs naturally when you need to see in dim light or as part of your body's reaction to emotion. Aqueous humor, which is produced in the chamber behind the iris, cannot then drain away, and pressure builds up in the eyeball. The iris may recede from the drainage angle after the light has increased or the emotion has passed. If the liquid fails to drain, the pressure in the eyeball continues to build, which causes acute glaucoma.

Usually, only one eye is affected at first, but once you have glaucoma the other eye is highly susceptible.

What are the symptoms?

In some cases there are short preliminary episodes months or weeks before a fully developed episode of acute glaucoma occurs. The episodes usually occur in the evening, when the light is dim, and last for as long as the iris blocks the drainage angle. Your vision becomes blurred, you may see halos around lights, the cornea begins to look hazy (as pressure in the eyeball forces aqueous humor into it), and often there is some pain and redness in the eye.

In a fully developed episode, the same symptoms occur but they persist and become worse. Pain, often severe, may be felt in the head as well as in the eye. The pain is often accompanied by vomiting and extreme weakness. The cornea appears increasingly hazy and sometimes it even looks gray and granular. In addition, the eyeball may be painful and hard to the touch.

What are the risks?

Acute glaucoma is not a common condition. In the 40 to 65 age group, 1 person in 1,000 has it. In the over-65 age group, 1 person in 500 may have the condition. Men and women are equally susceptible. About half of those who have the disease seek medical attention because of the warning symptoms that occur before a fully developed episode.

Acute glaucoma tends to run in families, partly because its predisposing factors, such as farsightedness, also run in families. If you are over 40, farsighted, and have two or more blood relatives who have (or have had) the disease, you should be especially aware of the possible symptoms.

If a fully developed episode of acute glaucoma is treated early, vision in the eye usually returns almost to normal. But once an episode is well under way, the fibers of the optic nerve at the back of the eye are damaged, which causes some permanent loss of vision. If glaucoma is neglected, you are likely to become blind in the affected eye.

What should be done?

Because of the risks to sight, early treatment is essential. Most people seek treatment anyway, because of the extreme discomfort of the symptoms. At the first signs of an episode consult your physician or an ophthalmologist immediately. If the episode occurs outside of office hours, contact a physician on call or go to the emergency room. The physician will probably arrange for you to see an ophthalmologist.

What is the treatment?

The physician may prescribe eye drops to encourage the iris to separate further from the drainage angle and to decrease production of watery fluid (aqueous humor). You may also need a pill or injection of a medication (such as acetazolamide) to decrease aqueous humor production. Also you may receive a dehydrating (drying) agent, in the form of a liquid (glyterine) or an intravenous drip (mannitol).

Usually, this treatment brings down the pressure in the eye within hours. Then, an operation called an iridotomy may be performed to prevent any further attack. The operation can be done with a laser beam. A tiny artificial channel for the drainage of aqueous humor is made through the iris. The channel goes through the outer edge of the iris. Since your other eye may be affected by glaucoma later, you will probably be advised to have an iridotomy performed later on that eye. Iridotomy usually prevents further attacks of glaucoma. Sometimes, however, an iridectomy (cutting-type surgical operation) is needed to make the opening in the iris.

If you do not get immediate treatment, the iris may become stuck to the drainage angle and cause a permanent obstruction. If this occurs, you will need a more complex operation, possibly a trabeculectomy. In this procedure, aqueous humor is allowed to drain more freely. Either a general or a local anesthetic is used. When it is only partially successful, it is sometimes possible to perform a second operation. If not, lifelong drug treatment, along with the partial drainage achieved by the operation, often keeps the pressure under control.

Chronic glaucoma

(open angle glaucoma)

In chronic glaucoma, the outflow from the eye of a fluid called aqueous humor, which is produced constantly by the ciliary body in the eye, is blocked gradually over a period of years. Aqueous humor builds up in the eye, and eventually creates an internal pressure that affects the nerve fibers and blood supply to the retina and the optic nerve, both of which are essential to vision. The aqueous humor normally drains out of the eye through a network of tissue between the iris and the cornea. This network is called the drainage angle, and it is there that the blockage occurs.

As the disorder progresses, it becomes increasingly more difficult for the aqueous humor (which normally flows from behind the iris, through the pupil, and into the chamber between the iris and the cornea) to drain out of the eye through the drainage angle. The blockage causes a slow and steady buildup of internal pressure on the rest of the eyeball. For a more detailed description of how glaucoma occurs, read the introduction to this section (see p.346).

Unlike acute glaucoma (see previous article), chronic glaucoma often is not detected without an eye examination. This is because the blockage occurs and the pressure builds up so slowly. In most cases of chronic glaucoma, both eyes are affected by the disorder, one soon after the other.

Medical myths

Watching too much television or working for a long time with inadequate light can harm the eyes.

Wrong. Extensive use of your eyes does not damage them any more than extensive walking damages your legs. However, your eyes can get tired, and you should read in adequate light.

What are the symptoms?

The development of the disorder is so gradual that the only symptom that occurs in the early stages is too slight to be noticeable. This is the loss of small areas of peripheral vision in one eye, on the side near the nose, caused by pressure in the eyeball that damages the fibers of the optic nerve. The loss passes unnoticed because the peripheral vision of the other eye compensates for it. Gradually, other areas of peripheral vision are lost, the lost areas increase in size, and the disorder affects the other eye. At some point in this process, you will become aware of the loss of part of your vision, but this occurs late, and the lost vision cannot be restored.

What are the risks?

Chronic glaucoma is more common than acute glaucoma (see previous article). It may affect 1 to 2 percent of the population over age 40. The risk increases from middle age onward. The disease tends to run in families, so you are more likely to get it if you have relatives who have it. If the disease is allowed to continue unchecked, all your peripheral vision in both eyes is lost. The ability to see straight ahead gradually diminishes until it disappears altogether and you become totally blind in both eyes.

What should be done?

Since any vision that is lost through the disease cannot be regained, the sooner you receive treatment for chronic glaucoma the better. In the early stages of this type of glaucoma, it is impossible to tell that you have the disease unless you are tested for it. For this and other reasons, you should have regular eye examinations by a qualified physician. Be sure to go to an ophthalmologist for a checkup every 2 years after you reach age 40. Such examinations will include tonometry testing, a procedure that measures the pressure within the eyeball, a check of the optic nerve, and, if necessary, a peripheral vision test and check of the drainage angle.

What is the treatment?

The treatment for chronic glaucoma is to try to bring down the pressure in the eyeball. Your physician will prescribe eye drops that allow better aqueous outflow from the eyes and/or drops or tablets to reduce the production of aqueous humor. These drops and tablets generally have to be taken for life, and you will also need to have regular checkups by your ophthalmologist to be certain that the drugs are working. Taking the drugs soon becomes part of your daily routine, and if you continue to take them and have regular examinations usually you will not have any further loss of vision.

If drugs fail to reduce the pressure in the eye sufficiently or fail to prevent progressive visual loss, the ophthalmologist will probably recommend a laser procedure to the drainage angle (laser trabeculoplasty) to try to increase aqueous flow through the angle. Some drugs have to be continued after the surgery. If drugs and laser surgery do not control the chronic glaucoma or if the damage is extensive, the ophthalmologist will probably recommend an operation to make a hole to drain the aqueous humor from the eye.

Back of the eye and orbit

The function of the back of the eye is to receive the light that is focused by the front of the eye and transform it into nerve impulses. These impulses then pass along the optic nerve, which leads from the back of the retina to the areas of the brain that control vision. The impulses are in a "code" that is determined by the details of what the eye sees. The brain "decodes" this message and you see what the eye saw an instant before.

The eye structure that receives the light is the retina, a layer of light-sensitive nerve cells that lines the back three fourths of the eyeball. The nerve cells consist of rods and cones. They are particularly well adapted for detecting light.

The cones detect fine detail and color. They are most highly concentrated in the macula, which is an area in the center of the retina at the very back of the eye. This is why you have to look straight at an object to see it clearly. Most of the rods are located around the edges of the macula. They detect much less detail and no color, but are sensitive to the intensity of the light entering the eye.

The bony socket in which each eyeball lies is called the orbit. The eyeball swivels in the orbit by means of muscles attached to the outside of the eyeball and the inside of the orbit. Either an imbalance in the pull between these muscles or a defect in the nerves that control them causes the disorder known as crossed eyes. Only the adult form of the disorder is covered in this section; crossed eyes in a child have a different cause (see Crossed eyes, p.353).

Macular degeneration

The macula, the area of the retina near the optic nerve at the back of the eye, is the part of the eye that distinguishes fine detail at the center of the field of vision. In some older people the macula and its functioning begin to deteriorate and the sharp central vision is lost. The exact cause of this degeneration is not known, but some have suggested a dietary or vitamin deficiency or long-term exposure to certain types of light. In most cases, both eyes are affected, either simultaneously or one after the other. Macular degeneration is a leading cause of blindness in older people.

Macular degeneration usually develops very gradually and imperceptibly and is painless. For these reasons, you may not notice it coming on, particularly in its early stages. Eventually, you will notice difficulty with reading and other activities requiring sharp vision. Once you have macular degeneration, any sudden deterioration in your vision may be caused by a leak of fluid or blood at the back of the eye, and in some of these cases laser surgery (see Box, next page) performed early may help restore some vision or help prevent further deterioration. In most cases, however, the loss of central vision is irreversible, but the peripheral vision remains.

An extensive range of low-vision aids is now available for people to use when glasses alone are no longer helpful. Use of large-type books, audiocassettes, and magnifying lamps may help improve the quality of life for the person with macular degeneration.

Diabetic retinopathy

In some people who have diabetes mellitus (see p.558), many of the small blood vessels of the retina, the layer of light-sensitive cells in the back of the eyeball, become constricted and plugged. The disorder usually occurs in both eyes. The remaining vessels may then leak blood into the retina and cause a permanent reduction in sharpness of vision. In addition, fragile new blood vessels grow on the retina and in many cases they leak blood into the vitreous humor, the jellylike bulk of the eyeball. This dims or obliterates vision. In both kinds of blood leakage, blood is usually reabsorbed by the retina, but scar tissue forms on the retina, and this may cause permanent, partial loss of vision. All people with diabetes should have their eyes checked regularly by an ophthalmologist.

Treatment frequently is effective in controlling retinopathy. The vessels that leak blood can often be plugged or shrunk by laser surgery (see Box, next page), and any bleeding into the vitreous humor that has not cleared up can be treated by using special instruments to drain the eye of vitreous humor and replace it with a substitute.

The disorder can recur, but with repeated treatment vision can usually be maintained.

Retinal detachment

The retina is a delicate layer of light-sensitive cells that lines the rear three fourths of the eyeball. Beneath the retina is a layer of blood vessels called the choroid, which provides the outer retina with nutrients and oxygen.

Retinal detachment occurs when the retina lifts away from the choroid. A hole in the retina causes the detachment in most cases. The hole forms either because of degeneration of the retina or because the vitreous humor (the jellylike bulk of the eyeball) has shrunk away from the retina and torn it. The hole usually forms near the front edge of the retina. Fluid seeps through the hole and starts to detach the retina from the choroid. If the condition is not treated, this process continues, and more and more retina is lifted away. Eventually the retina is attached only at the front of the eye, to the ciliary body (an extension of the choroid), and at the rear of the eye, to the end of the optic nerve. Both eyes may be affected, but rarely at the same time.

What are the symptoms?

The only symptoms are abnormalities of vision in the affected eye. Since the other eye is almost always normal, it may compensate for the affected eye, so that early symptoms may not be noticed. The first signs of a detached retina may be flashes of light, which may occur shortly before a hole is formed in the retina. Floating, black, often cobweblike shapes may be seen when the hole is actually formed. Once detachment starts you may notice the loss of part of your peripheral vision in the affected eye. This often appears as a narrow black "curtain" coming from the top, the bottom, or one side of the eye. If detachment continues unchecked, the loss of vision spreads. The vision that remains becomes progressively blurred.

What are the risks?

Retinal detachment is rare. It occurs mainly from middle age onward, and men and women are equally susceptible. You are particularly at risk if you are nearsighted (see p.336), because your retina is likely to be stretched by the shape of your eyeball. If your eye is injured, or if you have the lens of your eye removed because of a cataract (see p.345), you are also at risk. If the disorder is neglected, there is a risk of permanent blindness in the affected eye.

What should be done?

If you experience any of the symptoms described, see your ophthalmologist without delay. The ophthalmologist will be able to detect retinal detachment by looking into your eye through an instrument called an ophthalmoscope.

What is the treatment?

If a hole in the retina is discovered before detachment has started, you may need to have an operation to seal the hole permanently. This is done by freezing (cryotherapy) or by a laser beam after a sedative or local anesthetic has been given. If retinal detachment has already begun, a different kind of operation done under a local or general anesthetic may be necessary. In this procedure, the fluid between the retina and the choroid may be drained away, which allows the retina to sink back against the choroid and regain its blood supply. The hole in the retina is sealed, and the wall of the eye may be buckled inward to bring the retina into contact with the underlying tissues.

If the operation is performed before detachment has started or when it has occurred only around the front edge of the retina, your vision will probably return to

Laser photocoagulation surgery on the eye

The development of the laser has enabled ophthalmic surgeons to treat successfully many eye disorders that once led inevitably to blindness. One type of laser surgery known as photocoagulation can be used to treat retinal holes and tears (see the article on this page), diabetic retinopathy (see previous page), and macular degeneration (see previous page).

The technique of laser photocoagulation depends on the ability of the laser to produce a very narrow beam of extremely intense light. When this beam is focused onto the retina, it produces a tiny circular burn. Any blood vessel that crosses this target area is blocked.

When an ophthalmologist uses laser photocoagulation, he or she may need to make several thousand tiny burns on the retina to make abnormal vessels caused by diabetes shrink and disappear. The burns may be repeated in several treatment sessions. The procedure usually produces minimal or no discomfort and you may be given only a sedative or a local anesthetic. In either case you will remain conscious throughout the operation and will see a bright flash of light every time the surgeon makes a burn with the laser.

normal. If the detachment is more extensive and your central vision has been impaired, the full field of vision may be restored, although central vision will be permanently blurred to some extent.

Following retinal detachment in one eye, there is a considerable risk that the condition will develop in the other eye. After the operation, you should see your ophthalmologist regularly to have the other eye examined. This will enable any weak areas in the retina that are likely to develop into a hole to be detected at an early stage and possibly treated by means of surgery.

Retinal artery occlusion

The blood required by the retina (in the back of the eyeball) is supplied by the central retinal artery, a tiny vessel that enters the back of the eye near the optic nerve. Sometimes, usually in middle-aged or older people, the artery or one of its branches becomes blocked. This is caused by a blood clot resulting from thrombosis or by an embolus, a tiny piece of a blood clot or of a fatty deposit that has traveled from the heart or from a diseased blood vessel elsewhere in the body (see Arterial embolism, p.438). The clot or embolus cuts off all or part of the retina's blood supply. If the artery is blocked, there is immediate blindness in the involved eye. If a branch of the artery is blocked, only part of the vision of that eye, usually the upper or lower half, blacks out.

If you suddenly lose all or part of the vision in one eye, you should see your ophthalmologist or go to a hospital emergency department immediately. If the blockage can be treated within a few hours, it may be possible to restore some of the sight in the eye. This is done by certain techniques to try to cause the clot or embolus to move farther along the blood vessel to a position where less of the retina is affected.

Retinal vein occlusion

The central retinal vein carries blood away from the retina and, therefore, plays a key role in circulation within the eye. In rare cases, mainly from middle age onward, the vein or one of its branches can become blocked by a blood clot. When this happens, blood leaks out of the blocked vessel and causes blurred vision. The blurring may occur gradually, but in most cases it happens quite suddenly without warning.

Retinal vein occlusion may occur in the early stages of chronic glaucoma (see p.348) or it may occur with high blood pressure (see p.411). The disorder can also be caused by a blood disease in which the blood is thicker and tends to clot more readily than normal, such as polycythemia (see p.460), but this is rare.

Sometimes the retinal artery occlusion (see above) and the loss of vision tend to be worse and more permanent. In retinal vein occlusion alone, the vision may improve as the clot is reabsorbed. If reabsorption does not occur, the blurring is permanent. In some cases your ophthalmologist may suggest laser surgery.

The early signs of retinal vein occlusion can sometimes be detected by examining the eye with an ophthalmoscope. This examination is performed during a routine eye examination, which is one good reason for having such a test regularly (see Going to the ophthalmologist, p.338). Effective control of any underlying problem such as high blood pressure may then control the disorder.

Choroiditis

Choroiditis is inflammation of the choroid, a layer of blood vessels beneath the retina, in the back of the eyeball. The retina and the vitreous humor, the jellylike filling of the eyeball, may also become inflamed. When the inflammation subsides, the choroid is left scarred. Often the exact cause of the disorder cannot be determined. In some cases, infectious agents, such as tuberculosis, may be the cause. In other cases, abnormal changes in the immune system produce proteins that attack the choroid (and sometimes other parts of the eye). The inflammation causes blurred vision and sometimes also causes reddening of the eye and discomfort.

If you or your child have these symptoms, see your ophthalmologist without delay. The ophthalmologist will probably arrange blood tests and imaging procedures, which may include ultrasound and CT examinations. Corticosteroid drugs may be prescribed in an attempt to clear up the inflammation and the blurred vision, or if infection is causing the condition, your physician may prescribe an antibiotic drug to treat the infection.

Tumors of the eye

Tumors are abnormal growths of tissue. They may be malignant (likely to spread and threaten life) or benign (unlikely to spread).

Malignant melanoma

This is a type of eye tumor similar to a form of skin cancer (see Malignant melanoma, p.275). It occurs mainly in the choroid (the layer of blood vessels beneath the retina) or the ciliary body (an extension of the choroid in the front of the eye). Such tumors occasionally grow in the iris. Only one eye is affected, and the problem rarely occurs in young people. More than half of these tumors are discovered during a routine examination by an ophthalmologist. The rest are discovered because of a gradual loss of some vision in the affected eye. The ophthalmologist may arrange for you to have fluorescein angiography (a type of imaging that involves an injection of fluorescent dye into the eye), echography (ultrasound), and other tests to show the nature and extent of the tumor. Studies are being done to compare various types of treatment of malignant melanoma, including removal of the affected eye and different types of radiation or vaccination to stimulate immune responses.

Secondary tumors

In some cancers, tumors metastasize, or spread, through the bloodstream from the primary growth and grow in other parts of the body. Such secondary tumors in the eye develop during the late stages of the primary cancer. If these tumors grow behind the eyeball, they may cause bulging of the eye (see Exophthalmos, below). If they grow inside the eye, they may cause blurred vision. Their effect on vision varies according to exactly where they are located in the eye, their rate of growth, and whether one or both eyes are involved. A secondary tumor in the eye can be destroyed, or at least sometimes controlled through the use of radiation therapy, but it may already have caused some permanent loss of vision. The primary tumor must be treated separately.

Retinoblastoma

A retinoblastoma is a malignant tumor of the retina that occurs in one or both eyes, usually in a child under age 5. The child may not have any symptoms. If the central vision of only one eye is affected, the child may have crossed eyes, which is one reason why crossed eyes should be examined by a physician (see p.338). If the tumor is not discovered and treated early, it may become visible through the pupil as a white area in the interior of the eye. The disease is often inherited. If you know that it runs in your family, seek genetic counseling (see p.664) before having children. If you already have a child, tell your physician about the family history of retinoblastoma so that your child can have regular eye examinations by an ophthalmologist. If this type of tumor is detected early, treatment with radiation therapy, a laser, or freezing can be effective. If the tumor is advanced, the eye will have to be removed to try to prevent secondary tumors from spreading to other parts of the body and endangering the child's life. Even after the eye is removed, the child may need radiation treatments and chemotherapy.

Optic neuritis

In some people, generally between ages 20 and 40, the optic nerve in one eye becomes inflamed. The inflammation causes a gradual or sudden blurring of vision in the eye. In severe cases, the blurring progresses within a few days to temporary blindness. Other symptoms may include seeing the color red as though it were faded and pain when the eye is moved. If your physician thinks you may have optic neuritis, he or she will refer you to an ophthalmologist to confirm the diagnosis and to rule out other possible causes of recent loss of vision. Multiple sclerosis sometimes is a cause of optic neuritis.

In most cases optic neuritis without complications clears up without treatment, although sometimes a course of treatment with corticosteroids is used. Some impairment of vision may persist, and the optic neuritis may recur in the same or the other eye.

Exophthalmos

Exophthalmos is a bulging forward of one or both eyeballs. In most cases, both eyes are affected. The condition may be caused by a swelling or growth of tissue in the bony orbit in which the eyeball lies. The eyeball is pressed forward, which exposes an abnormally large amount of the front of the eye. The eye then tends to become dry and feel gritty. Eye movement may be restricted, which can cause double vision. In severe cases, the eye is pressed forward so much that its blood supply and nerve functioning are

See p.255, **Visual aids to diagnosis, 62.**

restricted and vision becomes seriously blurred. The bulge may also prevent the lid from closing completely. You may feel uncomfortable about the changed appearance of your eye.

The most common cause of the swelling is related to an overactive thyroid gland (see Hyperthyroidism, p.565). Other cases are caused by a tumor behind the eyeball (see Tumors of the eye, previous page) or inflammation of the tissue behind the eyeball (see Orbital cellulitis, next article).

Blood tests, X rays, echography, CT scans, and an examination of the eye and particularly the orbit are performed to find out what is causing the disorder.

What is the treatment?

If a thyroid gland disorder is related to the exophthalmos, that disorder will be treated. This may not control the exophthalmos, however, and corticosteroid drugs may be prescribed. Surgery may be necessary to stitch together portions of the lid to prevent corneal ulcers (see p.342). In severe cases, an operation may be needed to relieve the pressure behind the eyeball. If a tumor is present, surgical removal may be necessary.

Orbital cellulitis

The bony orbit in which the eyeball lies is filled with soft tissue. Bacteria may enter the tissue, usually from infected sinuses around the nose (see Sinusitis, p.373), or from a boil near the eye, and cause infection. This is called orbital cellulitis.

The pressure of the swollen tissue pushes the eyeball forward, giving your eye a staring appearance (see Exophthalmos, previous article). Other symptoms are severe pain and redness in the eye, swollen eyelids, and usually a fever. In rare cases the eye exudes pus. Outwardly, the redness of the eye and surrounding tissue may resemble conjunctivitis (see p.343). If there is pressure and inflammation of the blood vessels and nerves that supply the eye, you may lose some vision. There is also a risk that the infection may spread to the brain and cause meningitis (see p.290).

Treatment consists of high doses of antibiotics taken intravenously. If infected sinuses are the source of the problem, you may need an operation to have them drained to relieve the infection and obtain a sample of the drained substance for testing. If pus pockets form in the orbit they may be surgically drained for the same reasons.

Crossed eyes in adults

Normal eyes move together, so that both look at an object at the same time. This is essential for good, clear vision. Crossed eyes (a very general term) occur when this coordination is absent. One eye looks at the object, and the other looks elsewhere.

Crossed eyes usually develop in infancy or early childhood (see p.721), usually as the result of a disorder that causes uncoordinated contraction of the eye muscles. After childhood, crossed eyes almost always occur for a different reason. In most cases, crossed eyes that develop after childhood are caused by a disorder that affects either the nerves between the brain and the eye muscles or, less commonly, the muscles themselves.

Each eye is controlled by 6 muscles. An underlying illness affecting the control of these muscles can cause crossed eyes.

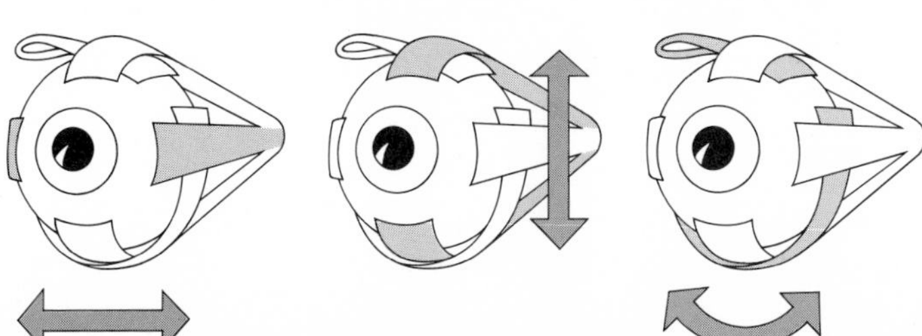

Disorders that can cause crossed eyes include diabetes mellitus (see p.558), high blood pressure (see p.411), temporal arteritis (see p.439), brain injury (see p.294), and muscular dystrophy (see p.741).

In almost all cases, double vision occurs; you may also have the symptoms of the underlying disorder.

What should be done?

If you start to see double and have never had crossed eyes, see your physician. As a temporary measure to prevent double vision, cover one eye with a patch, which you can buy at a drugstore. To discover the underlying cause of the problem, the physician will probably take your blood pressure, ask you to provide urine and blood samples for testing, and possibly arrange for you to have various X rays.

Depending on the underlying causes of the condition, the double vision may gradually disappear within a few months. If the problem remains to some extent, it may be corrected by special glasses. Otherwise, an operation may be necessary.

Disorders of the ear

Introduction

The ear is the organ of hearing and it also plays a role in maintaining balance. It has three parts—the outer, middle, and inner ear. The outer ear includes the ear that we see—folds of skin and cartilage known as the pinna—and the ear canal, a passage about ¾ in (20 mm) long that leads from the pinna to the eardrum. The opening of the canal is surrounded by cartilage, which is covered with skin that contains wax-producing glands and hairs. The deeper part of the canal is lined by a thin membrane and surrounded by bone. The eardrum is the thin membrane that is stretched across the end of the outer ear canal. It separates the outer ear from the middle ear.

The middle ear is a small cavity between the eardrum and the inner ear. It is bridged by three small, connected bones. These bones are named the hammer, anvil, and stirrup because of their shapes. The hammer is attached to the inner lining of the eardrum. The stirrup is attached by a ligament to the oval window, an opening that leads to the inner ear. The anvil lies between the hammer and the stirrup, and is attached to both of them.

One of the openings in the middle ear leads into the mastoid portion of the temporal bone (the bone that contains all of the internal organs of the ear). Two openings lead into the inner ear. One opening, the eustachian tube, leads to the back of the nose. The eustachian tube permits equalization of air pressure on the inside of the eardrum with air pressure on the outside. Sometimes the tube becomes blocked during a cold. When it becomes clear again, the sudden equalization of air pressure makes you feel as if the ear has "popped."

The inner ear consists of two structures that contain membrane-lined, fluid-filled chambers: the labyrinth and the cochlea. The labyrinth is involved in balance. It consists of the semicircular canals, three connected tubes bent into half circles and connected to the vestibular nerve (which is essential to balance). The cochlea, which plays a role in hearing, starts on the inner side of the oval window and curls around like a snail's shell. The auditory nerve attaches to the labyrinth and the cochlea, meeting up with the vestibular nerve to connect the hearing and balance functions of the inner ear to the brain.

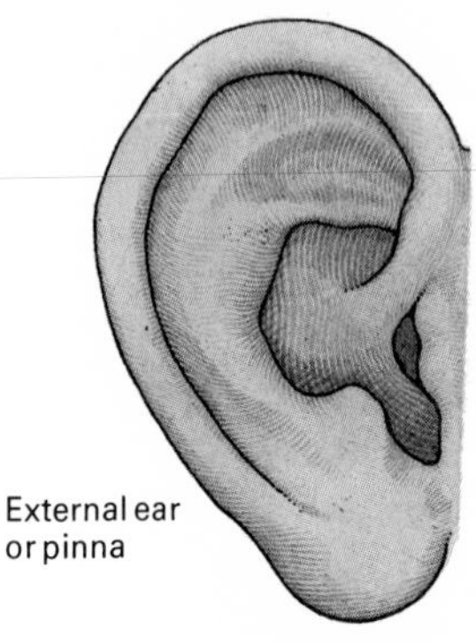

The structure of the ear
The outer ear collects sound waves and funnels them into the middle ear, which passes them on to the inner ear. The inner ear converts the waves into nerve impulses and transmits them to the brain. The inner ear also contains the mechanism for keeping your balance.

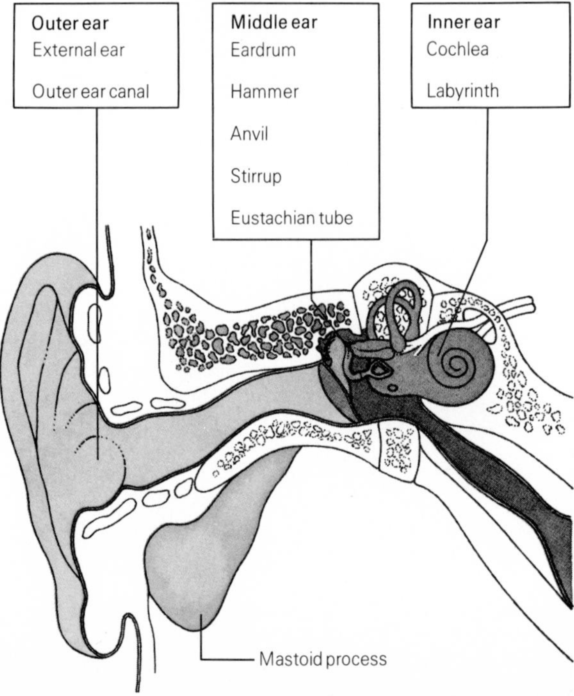

How the ear works

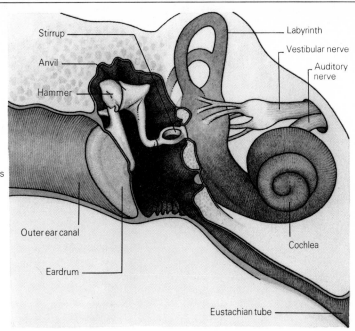

How you hear

A sound starts as a disturbance of the air, which produces sound waves. The visible ear helps to channel these waves down the outer ear canal, so that they hit the eardrum and make it vibrate. The vibrations pass through the hammer, anvil, stirrup, and oval window into the fluid in the cochlea. Tiny hairs that line the cochlea change the vibrations in the fluid into electrical nerve impulses, which are transmitted to the brain along the auditory nerve.

Most sounds reach you through this route, but this type of hearing is supplemented by vibrations conducted through the bones of the skull to the inner ear. You hear your own voice mainly through this vibration type of hearing.

How you keep your balance

Your brain constantly monitors the position and movement of your head and body so that you can keep your balance. In the inner ear is a structure called the labyrinth, which monitors the position and movement of the head by means of three semicircular canals. Each canal is at right angles to the other two, so no matter which way you move your head—nod it (A), shake it (B), or tilt it (C)—one or more of the semicircular canals (below right) detects the movement and relays the information to the brain. The utricle and saccule portions of the semicircular canal tell you the direction of the pull of gravity. The brain coordinates these facts with more information from your eyes, and from the muscles in your body and your arms and legs, to assess your exact position and the movements you need to make to keep your balance.

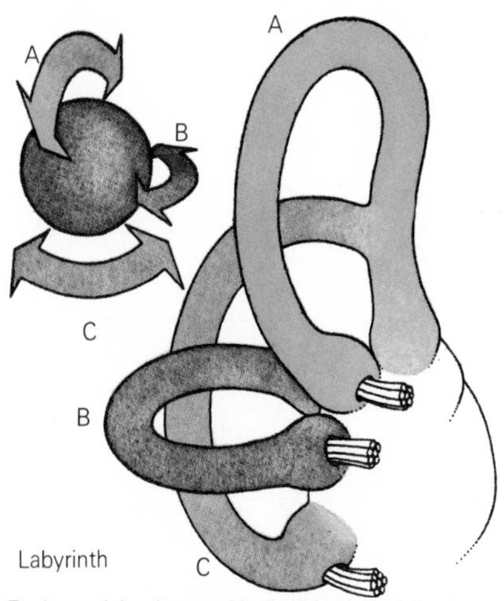

Each semicircular canal in the labyrinth detects movement in one of the three directions shown above left.

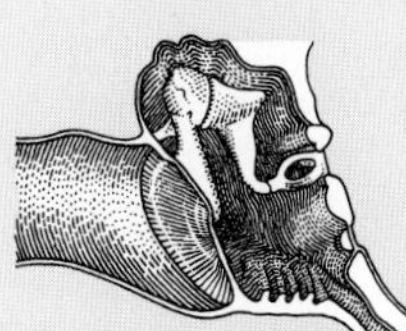

Conductive hearing loss
In conductive hearing loss, sounds do not reach the inner ear because of a mechanical defect in the middle ear.

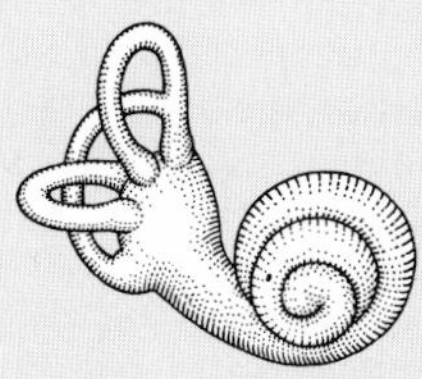

Sensorineural hearing loss
In sensorineural hearing loss, sounds reach the inner ear but are not passed on to the brain.

Hearing loss and vertigo

There are two kinds of hearing loss, conductive and sensorineural. Conductive hearing loss is caused by a mechanical failure that keeps sounds from reaching the inner ear. For example, this mechanical failure may occur because of wax blockage in the outer ear (see next page). Sensorineural hearing loss is caused by nerve failure. Although sounds reach the inner ear, they are not perceived because the appropriate nerve impulses do not reach the brain. Sensorineural hearing loss is usually caused by damage to the cochlea or the auditory nerve. This sometimes happens in old age (see Aging and the senses, p.771). However, loud music, machinery noise, viral infections, heredity (family tendency), or side effects from medications can cause this type of damage to hearing at any age.

Vertigo is a false sense that you or your surroundings are spinning around. Vertigo often causes loss of balance. It is usually a symptom of disorders of the inner ear, the part of the ear that senses movement and maintains balance.

The outer ear

The lining of the outer ear canal is an extension of the skin of the visible ear, so most disorders of the outer ear are skin disorders. While the symptoms that you experience may be very annoying or distressing, these disorders are generally not as serious as middle and inner ear diseases, since they do not affect the delicate mechanisms of hearing and balance.

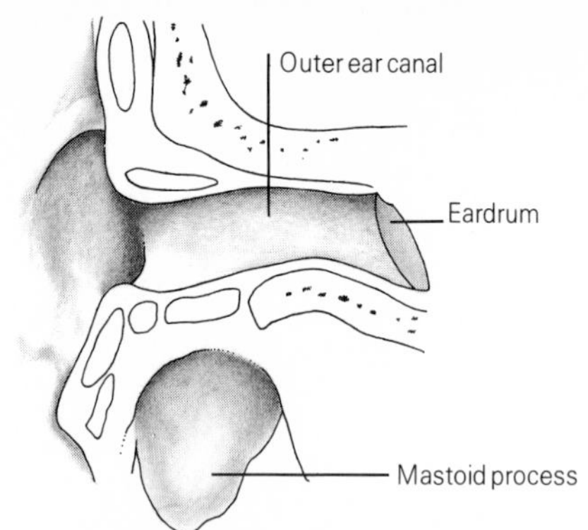

Wax blockage

Glands in the outer ear canal produce wax to protect the canal. The amount of wax produced varies from person to person. Some people produce so little wax that it falls out and never accumulates in the canal. Others produce enough wax to block the canal in one or both ears every few months.

The symptoms of wax blockage are a feeling that the ear is plugged, partial hearing loss, ringing in the ear, and sometimes earache. No serious risks are involved.

Removing ear wax
A physician uses a syringe to put warm water in the ear. The water flows along the ear canal, bounces off the eardrum, and flows back along the bottom of the canal, helping clean out any blocking wax.

What is the treatment?
Self-help: The best self-help for wax blockage is prevention. If you work in very dusty conditions, which can trigger wax blockage, consider wearing ear plugs.

Do not try to remove the wax with a stick or swab. It is easy to pack ear wax against the eardrum and cause damage. Over-the-counter liquids are available to loosen wax. Follow the instructions on the label and check with your physician.
Professional help: After examining your ear, your physician may soften the wax with eardrops before removing it. When wax is very difficult to remove, the physician may decide to dislodge it with a probe or electric suction apparatus.

Protruding ears

Most people's ears lie almost flat against the sides of their heads, but in some people they protrude to some degree. In extreme cases, the ears may stick straight out from the sides of the head. Protruding ears are not a risk to your physical health, but occasionally they can be a source of psychological distress. For some people these feelings of distress may become quite intense.

If you have protruding ears and are bothered by their appearance, discuss this with your physician. The belief that the protrusion can be countered by strapping or taping your ears to the sides of your head at night is not true. Mild protrusion may be concealed easily either by letting your hair grow longer or by changing your hair style so that your hair covers your ears. In extreme cases, your physician may recommend an operation. The surgical procedure for correcting protruding ears is relatively simple. An incision is made near the crease of skin behind your ear, the ear is pulled back flat against your head, and the incision is sewn up. Scars from the operation are behind the ear, and in most cases are not visible.

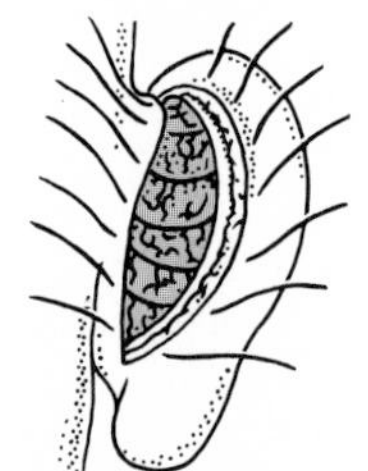

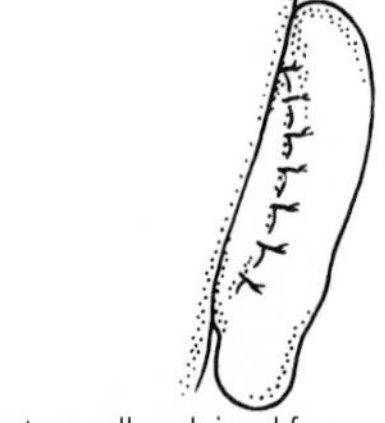

The simple surgery
The ear is pulled back after a strip of skin has been removed from behind it. This surgery is not usually advised for children under 5, since their ears are not yet fully developed.

Infections of the ear canal

(otitis externa)

Infections of the ear canal may take one of two forms: a localized infection such as a boil or abscess, or a generalized infection that affects the whole lining of the ear canal. Ear infections can occur after swimming. Persistent, excessive moisture in the ear canal can make the canal more susceptible to infection. Polluted water from lakes and rivers can cause infection by direct contact with the ear canal. Another cause of both localized and generalized infections is scratching inside the ear to relieve itching or while attempting to remove ear wax.

The first symptom of infection may be itching in your ear, usually followed by pain. Sometimes yellowish-green pus seeps from the ear. If the pus blocks your ear canal, you may lose some hearing. When you have this kind of ear infection, it will hurt to touch the ear, but not to move your head.

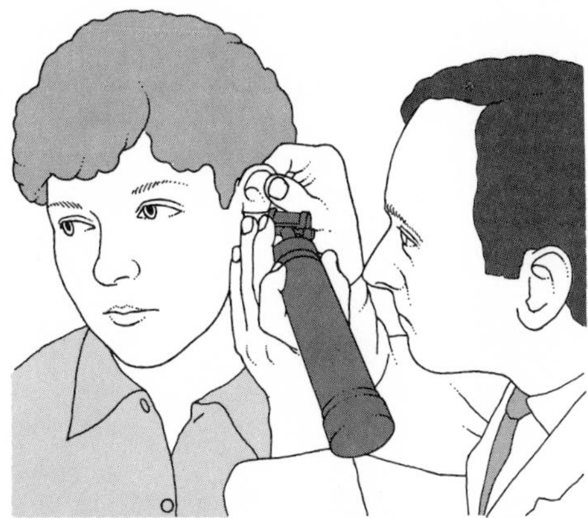

Examining the ear canal
A physician examines the ear through an otoscope. Pulling the top of the ear up and back straightens the canal and gives a clearer view of the entire canal.

Infections of the ear canal appear most often in young adults. If you do not seek treatment for such an infection, it may spread and affect underlying cartilage and bone.

What is the treatment?

Self-help: Take aspirin and place a warm, clean cotton pad or a heating pad over your ear to help relieve pain until you see your physician.

Professional help: Your physician will probably look into your ear with an otoscope and may prescribe an antibiotic-corticosteroid ear drop. Your physician may also put in a wick to make sure that the medicine is reaching the ear canal if the canal is very swollen. If the infection has not cleared up in a week, he or she will take a sample of any pus. The sample will be sent to a laboratory to see what has caused the infection. Your physician will then prescribe an appropriate oral antibiotic. Then he or she will probably clean your ear with a suction device or a cotton-tipped probe. This usually relieves irritation and pain. Gentle daily cleaning of the ear and taking prescribed drugs should clear up the condition.

You must keep the infected ear dry. This means no swimming, and wearing either cotton covered with petroleum jelly as an earplug or a shower cap in the tub or shower.

The infection may recur and require treatment for many weeks if it has been caused by fungi, or if you develop an allergy to your medication. If this happens, your physician may prescribe a corticosteroid cream or ear drops.

Tumors of the outer ear

Ear tumors
Tumors on the visible part of the ear can be removed by surgery.

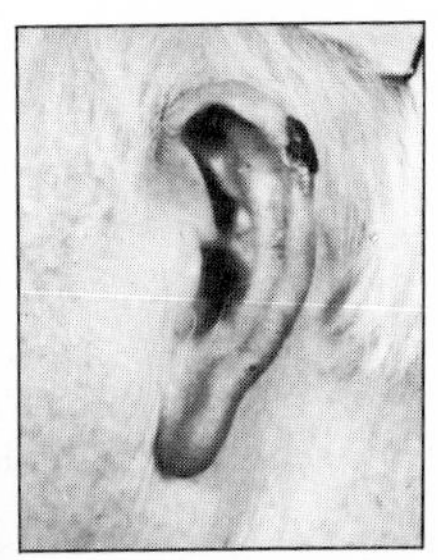

Like all tumors, those of the outer ear may be either benign (unlikely to spread) or malignant (likely to spread and threaten life).

On the visible portion of the ear, a benign tumor occurs as a painless lump. In the canal, it occurs as a hard growth of bone tissue called an osteoma. With an osteoma, there may be no symptoms, or an accumulation of wax, discomfort, and hearing loss.

Malignant tumors on the visible ear occur as wartlike growths, like benign tumors, or as ulcers or bleeding sores that fail to heal. Malignant tumors of the outer ear are almost always skin cancers. The cells multiply uncontrollably. The ulcers or sores may bleed and eventually become painful. Malignant tumors in the ear canal cause intense earache and bloody drainage when they are in an advanced stage. The dangers of a malignant tumor are the same as those of any malignant growth. If you notice any of the symptoms described here, you should see your physician immediately.

What is the treatment?

Benign tumors can be removed by a minor surgical procedure. Malignant tumors located on the visible part of the ear require surgery, radiation therapy, or both. During surgery, the tumor and all or some of the visible portion of the ear are removed. The operation is sometimes followed by radiation therapy. Tumors in the canal may require an operation known as a mastoidectomy or temporal bone resection. This operation is usually followed by radiation therapy.

The middle ear

The most common disorders of the middle ear are infections and damage to the eardrum. Infections of the middle ear are commonly caused by bacteria or viruses, which enter the middle ear through a perforated eardrum or along the eustachian tube from the back of the nasal cavity. The delicate bones within the middle ear that conduct sound to the inner ear are very vulnerable to damage, so some degree of conductive hearing loss (see p.355) is a common symptom in many types of middle ear disorders.

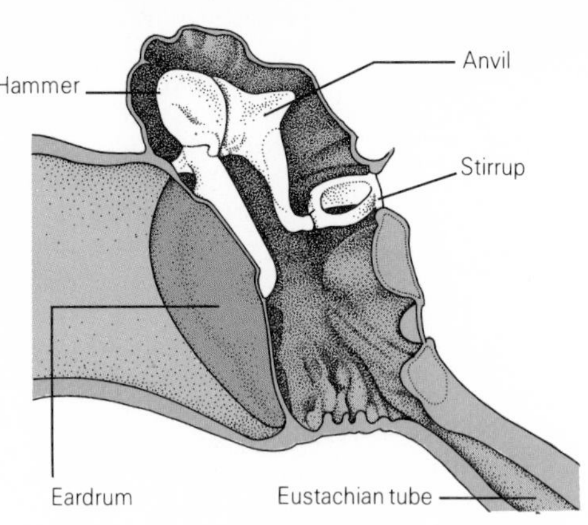

Otosclerosis

An abnormal growth of spongy bone can occur at the entrance to the inner ear and immobilize the base of the stirrup, a tiny bone through which sound waves pass into the inner ear. As a result, the stirrup cannot transmit some or all of the sound waves that enter the ear. This causes conductive hearing loss (see p.355) in that ear. In about 80 percent of all cases of otosclerosis both of the ears are affected, either simultaneously or one after the other. Often this is an inherited disorder that is passed through a family from one generation to another.

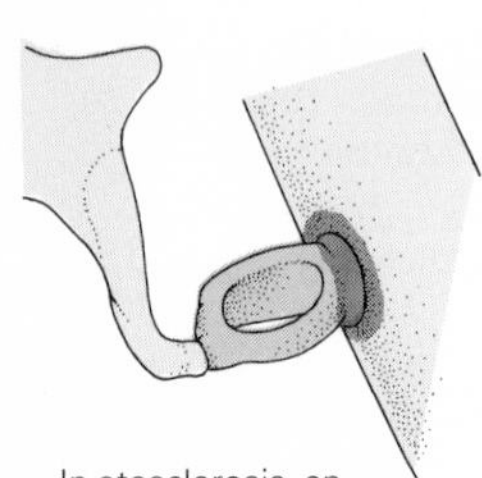

In otosclerosis, an abnormal growth prevents the stirrup from moving. This causes conductive hearing loss.

What are the symptoms?
Without treatment, otosclerosis usually leads to a slow loss of hearing, eventually resulting in a 60-decibel conductive loss so that you require a hearing aid to hear normal conversation. In a few cases, usually in children, the hearing loss progresses much faster. In some other cases the hearing loss stops well short of deafness.

At first, the affected person's voice sounds normal, unlike the abnormally loud voices of people with hearing loss from inner ear or nerve damage. As the disease progresses, some sensorineural hearing loss (see p.355) may occur. If this happens, it may cause noises in the ear and louder speech.

A woman with otosclerosis who becomes pregnant may find that her rate of hearing loss accelerates at the same time.

What are the risks?
The main risk is the danger associated with deafness, but this risk can be avoided if you have the disorder treated. Another risk is the emotional effect of the social isolation that sometimes occurs.

What should be done?
If your hearing deteriorates or you hear ringing in your ears, see your physician. He or she will examine your ears and give you simple hearing tests. You may have several special tests (see Box, Hearing loss and hearing aids, p.361) to confirm the diagnosis and help plan for a hearing aid or surgery.

What is the treatment?
The only treatment that will halt or cure otosclerosis is an operation called a stapedectomy, which improves hearing significantly in 90 percent of cases. However, about 1 percent or less of these operations result in total deafness in the affected ear. You and your physician should consider this risk carefully. Only one ear is operated on at a time, so that if the operation fails, you can still hear with the other ear. If the procedure is successful, the second ear may be operated on 6 months or a year after the first one. Physicians do not perform this surgery if you only have one good ear.

In a stapedectomy, the surgeon folds the eardrum out of the way, removes the diseased stirrup, and replaces it with a tiny metal substitute. The patient may feel dizzy for a short time after the operation, but usually does not have to stay in the hospital overnight. The eardrum heals on its own in 1 to 2 weeks. In another 2 to 3 weeks, the patient can usually return to normal activities.

In some cases, there is no immediate improvement in hearing after a stapedectomy because a blood clot occurs in the middle ear and the eardrum becomes swollen. Hearing improves about 2 to 4 weeks after the operation. Hearing usually improves as the clot disappears gradually.

Barotrauma

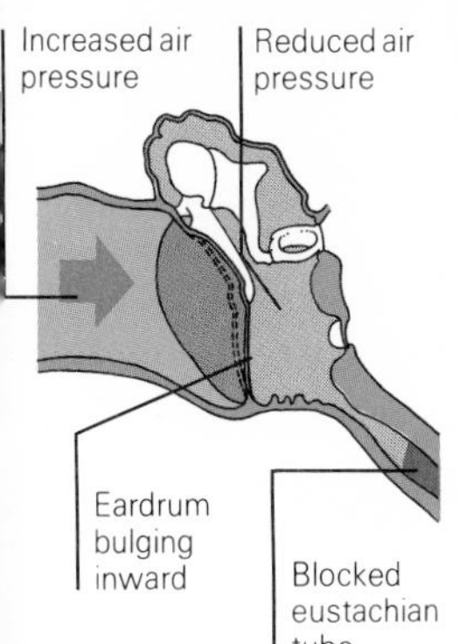

Normally, because of air passing through the eustachian tube, the air pressure in the middle ear is the same as the air pressure in the outer ear. If a severe imbalance occurs, the eardrum can be ruptured by the resulting air pressure. This is called barotrauma. The most common symptom of barotrauma is bleeding, but you don't see any blood. Instead a blood clot forms that blocks your hearing.

Barotrauma often occurs when someone who has a nose or throat infection travels in an airplane. Before takeoff, the airplane is depressurized, which lowers the air pressure in the cabin. Air pressure in the ear also falls.

During the descent, the cabin is repressurized. The resulting raised air pressure in the outer ear canal would normally be balanced by air moving back through the eustachian tube to the middle ear, but if the tube is badly blocked because of an infection, air cannot get through. This creates greater air pressure on the outer surface of the eardrum than there is on its inner surface, and barotrauma pushes the eardrum inward.

The symptoms of barotrauma are moderate to severe pain in the ear, a plugged feeling, and some degree of hearing loss. You may also hear noises and feel a little dizzy. All of these symptoms usually clear up on their own in 3 to 5 hours.

If you have a nose, sinus, or throat infection and you must travel by air, use a decongestant spray or oral medication. Suck candy or chew gum to encourage frequent swallowing. These measures usually keep the eustachian tube open. You can also breathe in, hold your nose, and then try to force air up your eustachian tube by gently blowing out while keeping your mouth closed.

If you have barotrauma, your physician may perforate your eardrum and remove any fluid from the middle ear to equalize the air pressure inside your ear. The eardrum will heal on its own in 1 to 2 weeks.

Ruptured eardrum

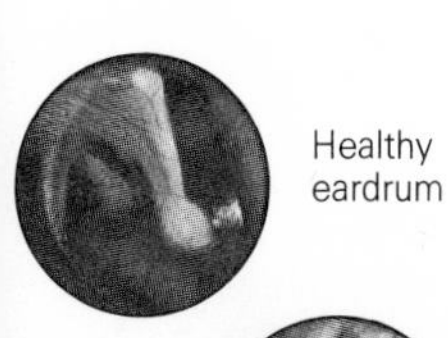

A healthy eardrum is almost transparent. But, when the eardrum ruptures, you may see the middle ear bones.

There are five common causes for ruptured eardrums: a sharp object put into the ear to relieve itching; an explosion; a severe middle ear infection; a slap over the ear; and an injury while water skiing or diving. A less frequent cause is a fractured skull.

What are the symptoms?

Some possible symptoms of a ruptured eardrum are pain in the ear (usually slight), partial loss of hearing, and slight discharge or bleeding from the ear. The symptoms usually last only a few hours.

What are the risks?

There is a risk that infection may enter the middle ear through the rupture. If you suspect that you have a ruptured eardrum, see your physician as soon as possible.

What is the treatment?

Self-help: To relieve pain caused by the rupture, cover the affected ear with a heating pad set on low and take aspirin.

Professional help: Your physician may prescribe an antibiotic and keep checking the ear until it heals. This usually takes 1 to 2 weeks. He or she may also place a temporary plastic patch over the eardrum. Any small perforation may be closed by your physician in a procedure performed in his or her office. If these measures are ineffective and your eardrum has not healed within 3 months, your physician may suggest surgery in which a tiny piece of tissue, sometimes taken from a vein, is grafted to the eardrum. This simple procedure usually solves the problem. Once a ruptured eardrum has healed, it usually leaves no problems, and hearing loss is minimal.

Acute infection of the middle ear

(acute otitis media)

Acute otitis media is a bacterial infection that usually follows a viral upper respiratory tract infection, such as a cold, flu, or measles, that inflames the cells lining the middle ear cavity. The disorder often develops when the virus infection is complicated by a bacterial infection of the middle ear. Infection may also enter through a ruptured eardrum (see previous article).

Middle ear infections often occur in children. More than half of all children have an infected middle ear at some time; repeated episodes of the problem often occur.

What are the symptoms?

A person with an acute middle ear infection usually has a feeling of fullness in the ear, sometimes followed by severe stabbing pain. This pain may be mild or may be severe enough to prevent sleep and many normal waking activities. Other symptoms are chills, fever, sweats, and hearing loss in the affected ear. If the infection is severe and is not treated, the pressure of pus within the middle ear may burst the eardrum. This produces a discharge of pus, sometimes with blood, that is accompanied by relief from the pain.

What are the risks?

If treatment is delayed too long, there is a danger that the problem may become chronic (see next article), or that the infection may spread to a portion of the bone behind the ear called the mastoid process.

What should be done?

See your physician for treatment of this condition as soon as possible.

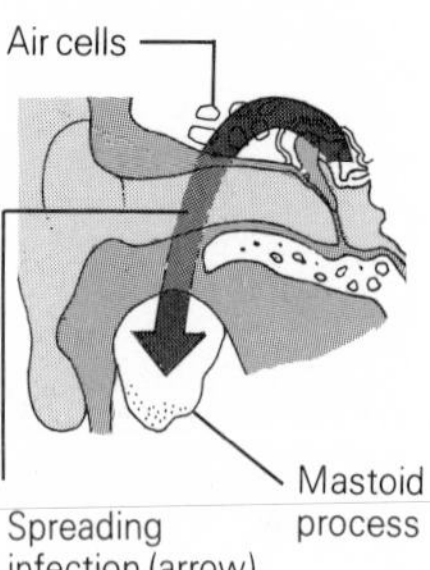

The spread of infection Infections of the middle ear can spread to the mastoid process. Antibiotic treatment may heal this infection.

What is the treatment?

Self-help: To provide some relief from pain, take aspirin and place a heating pad set on low against the ear. Do not sleep with the heating pad under you.

Professional help: Your physician may prescribe decongestant drugs and antibiotics to help unblock the eustachian tube and clear up the infection in the middle ear. The swelling of the eardrum, which is the gateway to the middle ear, subsides with the antibiotic treatment. Sometimes the eardrum will rupture and drain by itself while you are taking the antibiotics. It may take as long as 6 weeks for the infection to clear up completely, and a child with a middle ear infection should return to his or her physician in 6 weeks, if not sooner.

If a child has repeated infections of the middle ear, the adenoids (see p.724) may be acting as a reservoir of infection. In such cases, your physician may suggest that the child's adenoids be removed. Persistent sinusitis (see p.373) also often leads to middle ear infection.

Chronic infection of the middle ear

(chronic otitis media)

A chronic infection of the middle ear is much more serious than an acute infection. An acute infection flares up suddenly and often painfully, but usually causes little damage. A chronic infection is slow and relentless and can cause permanent damage. Chronic infection of the middle ear is often the result of an untreated ear infection in childhood. Either the infection never completely clears up, so that some of the organisms that caused it remain in the ear, or it eventually clears up but leaves a site in the middle ear that is particularly susceptible to infection. Pus produced continually from the chronic infection often damages, scars, or destroys the small bones of the middle ear.

What are the symptoms?

Grayish or yellowish pus, often with odor, seeps from the ear periodically. You may have some hearing loss, depending on how long the infection has been present.

What are the risks?

In the rare cases of unsuccessful treatment for chronic infection of the middle ear, the bones of the ear may become damaged, or scar tissue may fuse the bones together so that they can no longer transmit sound. This can cause permanent deafness. Chronic draining ear infections are always associated with a perforation or a cholesteatoma (see p.362).

What should be done?

See your physician, who will probably examine your ears with an otoscope and arrange for a CT scan of your head to find out if the infection has spread. Only then can your physician determine if you need surgery. In the early 1980s many children with chronic infections had surgery in which pus was removed through a cut in the eardrum and a tube inserted for drainage; this surgery is usually not recommended today because of the risk of further infections.

What is the treatment?

Self-help: Keep your ear dry and clean. Wipe away any discharge with cotton.

Professional help: Your physician will probably clean your ear and prescribe drops containing an antibiotic, a corticosteroid, and an antibacterial drug.

He or she may then recommend an operation to remove the remaining infection and restore any lost hearing. The surgeon removes infected tissue in the middle ear and mastoid area, and either mends the tiny bones in the middle ear or replaces them with plastic substitutes. Then the eroded eardrum, which usually cannot heal naturally because of the scar tissue built up by repeated damage, is repaired by a tissue graft. In 70 percent of cases, the middle ear can be rebuilt and some hearing is restored.

Hearing loss and hearing aids

Do you have difficulty hearing?

Hearing loss is not a disease. It is a symptom of some underlying disorder. Some hearing loss is common as you get older (see Aging and the senses, p.771), but if you are under 50 and have difficulty hearing, you should see a physician, preferably an otolaryngologist (ear specialist), who will examine your ears. The ear specialist may then give you a simple hearing test or have an audiologist do more sophisticated testing.

Audiometry

This test takes place in a soundproof room. The first part of the test measures how well you hear sounds conducted through the air. You listen through earphones, with one ear at a time, to sound frequencies that range from low tones to high ones. For each frequency, the sound starts at an inaudible level, then increases in loudness until you can just hear it. That level is known as your threshold for that frequency.

The second part of the test measures how well you can hear sounds conducted through the bones of your head. The procedure is the same as in the first part of the test, but this time you wear special earphones that vibrate against your head. Your thresholds in both tests are recorded on a graph called an audiogram. In general, the first part of the test gauges your overall hearing, and the second part differentiates whether any hearing loss you have is conductive or sensorineural (p.355).

Impedance testing

In a healthy ear, the air pressure is the same inside and outside the eardrum. This allows the eardrum to vibrate freely when sound waves hit it. The vibrations pass through the ear so that we hear, and they also reflect back into the air. Too much or too little air pressure on the inner side of the eardrum makes the eardrum too stiff to conduct and reflect sounds properly.

Impedance testing measures the ability of your eardrum to reflect sound waves. This indicates how well your eardrum passes the sound waves into the ear. The tester puts a probe covered with a soundproof material such as cork into your outer ear canal, and seals up the entrance to the ear. A transmitter in the probe aims sounds at the eardrum. A receiver in the probe measures the reflections while air pumped through the probe changes the air pressure in the canal rapidly from high to low. Tympanometry detects fluid in the middle ear, perforation of the eardrum, and disorders of the tiny sound-conducting bones of the middle ear.

Brainstem auditory evoked responses

This is a computerized hearing test that measures electrical responses in the brainstem in reaction to sounds. It facilitates testing of otherwise untestable patients such as infants and is helpful in ruling out acoustic neuromas.

Hearing aids

Most hearing aids increase the volume of sound electrically, through a device that usually fits unobtrusively in the ear. The apparatus contains a tiny microphone that transforms sounds into electrical signals, an amplifier that increases the strength of the signals, and an earphone that turns the signals into louder sounds. A battery provides electrical power. The battery lasts a week or 2.

It is important to choose both the right kind of hearing aid, and one that fits you properly. If you need a hearing aid, your physician will probably refer you to an audiologist or a hearing aid dealer for a hearing aid evaluation. In this test, you will try different kinds of hearing aids. You should tell your physician or ear specialist immediately if you notice any change in your hearing between your regular checkups, even after you get a hearing aid.

Behind-the-ear aid

The microphone, amplifier, and tiny battery are contained in a small, light, plastic case worn behind the ear. The earphone fits into your ear canal and seals it up so that no amplified sound is lost. The earphone is connected to the rest of the device by a short tube. The aid can be attached to the earpiece of your glasses.

In-the-ear aid

This type of hearing aid, which is most frequently prescribed, is so small that the microphone, amplifier, and battery are housed in a light plastic case worn inside the ear. The aid is molded to seal your ear canal so that no amplified sound is lost. It is less awkward to put in your ear, and the volume is easily adjusted.

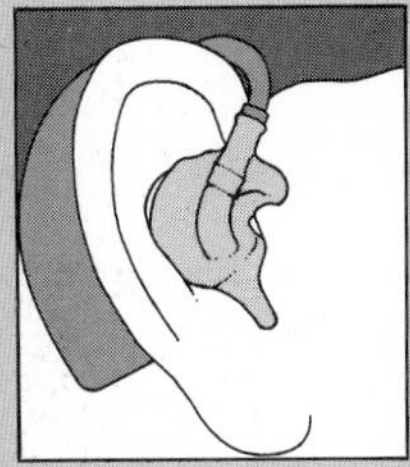

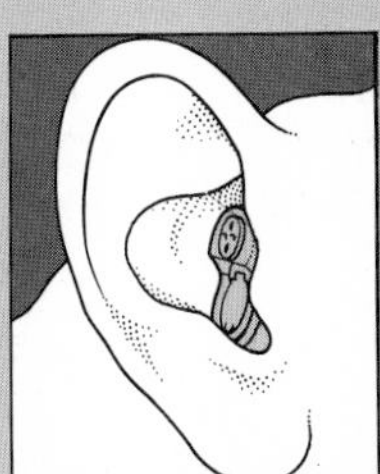

Cochlear implants and sensorineural hearing loss

A few children are born with total sensorineural hearing loss, and some children and adults develop the condition as a result of damage to the inner ear. However, if the auditory nerve is intact, it is sometimes possible to boost hearing by inserting a cochlear implant inside the inner ear.

In this operation, a special signal processor is implanted in the cochlea; electrodes (very thin wires) are also implanted to connect the processor to the auditory nerve. The other principal components—a power source and microphone—are worn on the body.

The device works by the microphone converting sound into electrical signals, which are then transmitted to the signal processor. The signal processor converts the signals into electrical impulses that travel along the electrodes and directly stimulate the auditory nerve, which carries the impulses to the brain's hearing center.

Thousands of people throughout the world have received cochlear implants. The results are improving steadily, but the hearing that is achieved is still a long way from normal.

Cholesteatoma

A cholesteatoma is a growth of the skin of the eardrum into the middle ear. This skin forms a pocket that fills up with dead cells shed by the eardrum, roughly forming a ball. Physicians think that a cholesteatoma is caused by repeated middle ear infections. The ball becomes infected and produces pus. This erodes the bone that lines the cavity and damages the delicate bones in the middle ear.

What are the symptoms?

Mild to moderately severe loss of conductive hearing is a common symptom of this disorder. Sometimes pus seeps from the ear. Headache, earache, weakness of the facial muscles, and dizziness are also commonly occurring symptoms of cholesteatoma.

What are the risks?

If the cholesteatoma is not treated effectively, it can eat away the roof of the middle ear cavity. This sometimes causes facial nerve paralysis, vertigo, profound sensorineural hearing loss, epidural abscess (see p.292) or meningitis (see p.290). An abscess can also form behind the ear.

What should be done?

If you have any of the symptoms described, especially if you had a history of ear trouble as a child, see your physician. If he or she suspects that you have a cholesteatoma, you will probably be referred to an ear, nose, and throat specialist (an otolaryngologist) for an examination and probably a hearing test (see previous page).

If the cholesteatoma is small or in an early stage, it is sometimes possible to remove it and thoroughly clean out the middle ear cavity in an operation.

If the cholesteatoma is large or in a later stage, damage to the middle ear may be extensive. In that case, removing the cholesteatoma becomes more complicated, involving an operation to rebuild the hearing structures and repair the broken eardrum.

In about 20 percent of cases of cholesteatoma, the condition recurs. The otolaryngologist will probably check your ears at least once a year to make sure you are not having a recurrence.

If your hearing is badly damaged, a hearing aid may help (see previous page).

Implantable bone conduction hearing device

An implantable device is available for people who have disease that narrows the ear canal or those who are born with a small channel and who have hearing problems; such people cannot wear a standard hearing aid.

With local or brief general anesthesia, an incision is made into the scalp behind the ear. A hole is drilled into the outer table of the skull and a small metal magnet is screwed into the hole. The metal vibrates when stimulated by an electric current. The current is produced when sound waves are converted to electric impulses via a microphone worn by the person. Complications are uncommon.

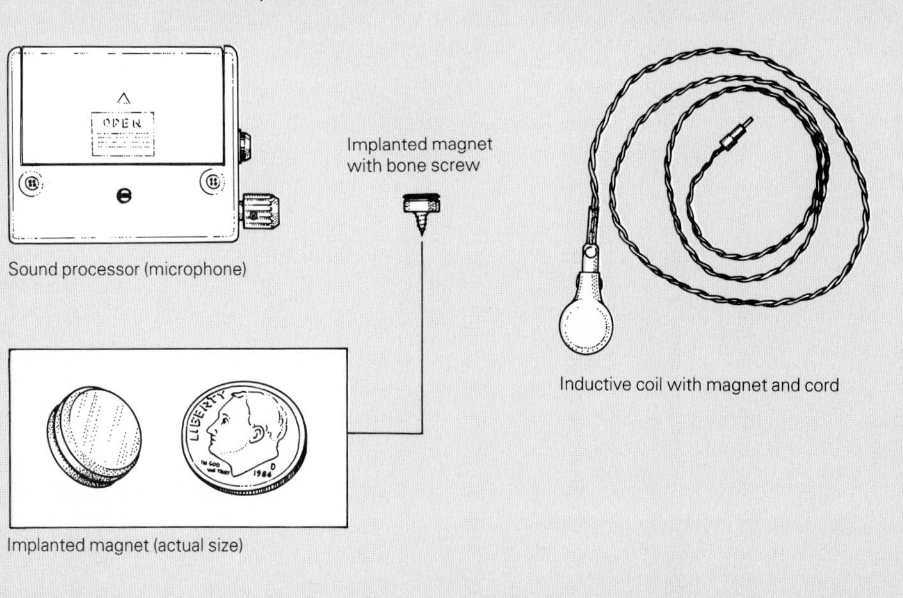

Sound processor (microphone)

Implanted magnet with bone screw

Inductive coil with magnet and cord

Implanted magnet (actual size)

The inner ear

Disorders of the inner ear affect two extremely sensitive structures: the cochlea, which transforms sound vibrations into electrical signals for transmission to the brain along the auditory nerve, and the labyrinth, which affects balance. If either of these structures is damaged, repair is impossible, because they are far too delicate for surgery. One result is often sensorineural hearing loss, which is caused by damage to either the cochlea or the auditory nerve. This type of hearing loss is usually permanent, because it can seldom be treated or cured (see p.355).

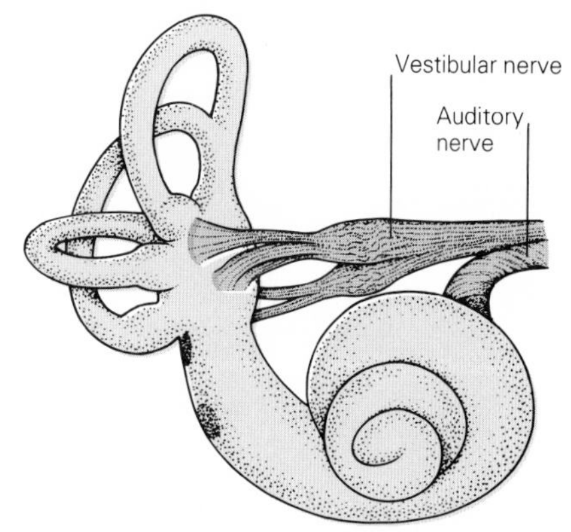

Meniere's disease

In Meniere's disease there is an increase in the amount of fluid in the labyrinth, the part of the ear that is involved in balance. This increases pressure in the inner ear, which distorts, and sometimes ruptures, the membrane of the labyrinth wall. This disturbs your sense of balance. For a detailed description of how the labyrinth helps maintain your balance, read How the ear works (see p.355). The cochlea, which is next to the labyrinth, may also be damaged by the pressure. The damage caused by this disease may impair your hearing.

The disease affects one ear, and then, about half of the time, it also affects the other ear. The cause of Meniere's disease is unknown, and the disorder is rare.

What are the symptoms?

Symptoms may flare up periodically. These episodes vary in frequency from every few days to every few weeks to every few years and last from 20 minutes to several hours. Symptoms include vertigo, or dizziness; nausea and vomiting; ringing in the ear; and muffled, distorted hearing, especially of low tones. Hearing is almost always affected during the episodes. Sometimes you feel pressure in the affected ear before or during an episode. The episodes usually become less severe, but some hearing loss and noises in the ear may persist between episodes. Finally, severe episodes may return, and if they do they may become increasingly serious.

What are the risks?

In most people, the disorder is mild and clears up by itself. In others the episodes may stop after a few years but the person will have some hearing loss. In a few severe cases complete deafness eventually occurs either in one or both ears.

What should be done?

If you have the symptoms described, see your physician, or an ear, nose, and throat specialist (otolaryngologist) immediately.

The first test he or she performs may be audiometry (see Hearing loss and hearing aids, p.361). If the result is unclear, it may be repeated after you prepare yourself by not drinking any liquids or by taking a diuretic, which promotes fluid loss. Either method is thought to reduce pressure in the labyrinth by reducing the amount of fluid in it. If the repeat test shows that your hearing has improved by a specific amount, you probably have Meniere's disease.

If the results are still not clear from the second test, or if your physician needs more information, you may need to have a test in which the ear is flooded with water at different temperatures. After each flooding, you experience a whirling sensation that makes your eyes flicker. How your eyes flicker is an indication of whether or not the labyrinth is diseased. Your physician will also rule out the possibility of a tumor of an auditory nerve inside the skull.

What is the treatment?

Self-help: Lie still when you are having an episode. This should considerably ease the symptoms. Cut down generally on your intake of fluids and salt. This should reduce the frequency and severity of attacks.

Professional help: In most cases, your physician will prescribe medication such as meclizine to control nausea and vomiting. He or she may also prescribe a diuretic to prevent excess fluid accumulation in the labyrinth and to try to prevent further episodes.

If, despite treatment, there is enough fluid in the labyrinth to damage it, or if you are incapacitated by the symptoms of the disorder, you may need surgery. In one possible operation, a surgeon drills a hole through the bone of your middle ear into the labyrinth to release the excess fluid. In about 70 percent of cases such an operation cures the vertigo at least temporarily and prevents further loss of hearing in the affected ear. In some cases the operation improves hearing. However, the disease usually returns after a year or more.

If the disease is severe enough to cause vertigo that is seriously disabling, cutting the vestibular nerve (which is crucial to balance) or, less commonly, destroying the labyrinth by surgery may be necessary.

Labyrinthitis

In labyrinthitis, the labyrinth, a group of fluid-filled chambers that controls balance, becomes infected. The infection usually results from a virus that inflames it.

What are the symptoms?
The main symptom is vertigo, or dizziness. You feel off balance; everything seems to be spinning. If you move your head, even slightly, the vertigo gets worse. In some cases, there is extreme nausea and vomiting.

What are the risks?
Although labyrinthitis can be very debilitating, it is not a dangerous condition when cared for properly. The symptoms are often so distressing that most people who have it seek professional help.

What should be done?
If you have severe vertigo, have someone help you get to your physician's office as soon as possible. Your physician will try to determine whether the vertigo has some cause other than labyrinthitis.

What is the treatment?
You will probably have to rest quietly in bed for several days. Your physician may prescribe medication to combat the nausea, vomiting, and vertigo (dizziness), and to decrease nerve cell activity in the part of the brainstem that receives impulses from the vestibular nerve. The symptoms of labyrinthitis are frightening, but they usually disappear. Most cases of labyrinthitis clear up completely, within 1 to 3 weeks.

Noise damage to hearing

Prolonged exposure to noise at or above 90 decibels (see Sound and noise levels, next page), especially if the noise is high-pitched, can damage the sensitive hair cells lining the cochlea, the innermost part of the ear. This may cause partial to severe hearing loss. Some occupations that are particularly hazardous to unprotected ears are heavy construction, driving a tractor, and working around very noisy equipment. Exposure to loud rock music over long periods of time also endangers your hearing. Listening to a personal stereo at too high a volume may also put you at risk.

What should be done?
Brief exposure to loud noise may cause a temporary hearing loss, but sensorineural hearing loss (see p.355) that is caused by damage to the cochlea is irreversible. Therefore, prevention is crucial. Regulate the volume of your personal stereo so that it is inaudible to other people; higher volume than this may be damaging to your ears. If you are exposed to loud noise at work, wear appropriate ear protectors. Ear muffs that are designed for this purpose are the most effective. They resemble earphones and almost totally insulate the ears from noise. If the person wearing the ear muffs needs to communicate with coworkers, as on the flight deck of an aircraft carrier, a small microphone and earphones can be added to the ear muffs. The second most effective type of protectors are ear plugs made of foam, plastic, wax, or rubber.

If you work in very noisy conditions, your employer should test your hearing at regular intervals; if not, have your physician test your hearing. If you detect loss of hearing early, you can take steps to prevent further damage to your ears. If you think that the noise level where you work is too high, you can contact the person responsible for safety in your plant or your union representative. You can also contact the local office of the Occupational Safety and Health Administration (OSHA) or the local health department and file a complaint. See also the box Sound and noise levels, p.365.

Sound and noise levels

What are sound and noise?

Sound is a series of air pressure waves, or alternate peaks of high pressure and valleys of low pressure, traveling through the atmosphere. Noise is a term people use to describe a variety of loud sounds, usually of different pitch, or frequency, that they find unpleasant.

Loud sound and noise

The loudness of sound or noise is measured in units called decibels by a decibel meter. Sounds that are softer than 10 decibels are very difficult for the human ear to hear, and sounds that are at least 120 decibels are usually painful. A sound loud enough to cause pain can damage your ears, often permanently. You should quickly eliminate the sound or get away from it to prevent damage to your ears. Exposure to noise that is loud enough to cause prolonged ringing in your ears may cause lasting damage to the sensitive hearing structures. There are recommended time limits on levels of exposure to high-decibel sound (see diagram).

If you are regularly exposed to noise levels above about 90 decibels, you may be in danger of hearing loss (see previous article for more information).

MAXIMUM NOISE EXPOSURE ALLOWED ON JOB BY LAW, IN HOURS PER DAY

Decibels	Hours
90	8
92	6
95	4
97	3
100	2
102	1½
105	1
110	½
115	¼ or less

Note: A small increase on the decibel scale results in a much louder sound because sound pressure doubles with an increase of 6 decibels. To most people, a rock concert that registers 100 decibels on a decibel meter sounds much more than twice as loud as a rushing stream that registers 50 decibels.

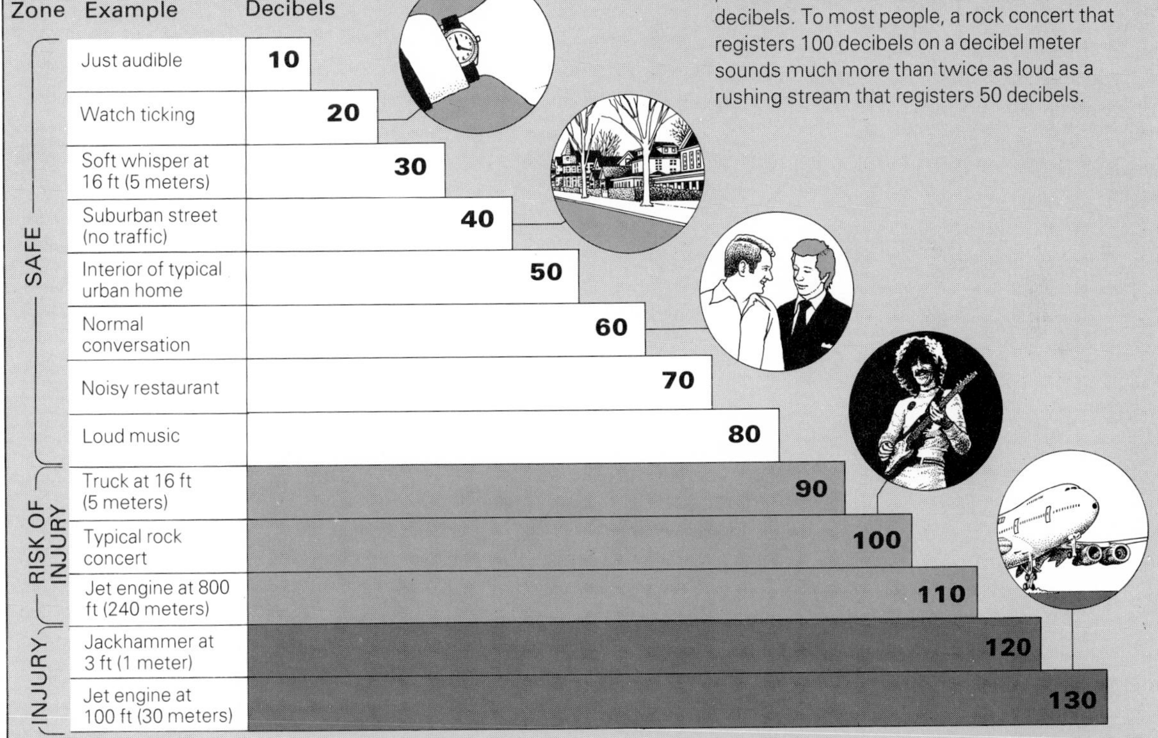
Zone
Example
Decibels
SAFE
RISK OF INJURY
INJURY
Just audible
10
Watch ticking
20
Soft whisper at 16 ft (5 meters)
30
Suburban street (no traffic)
40
Interior of typical urban home
50
Normal conversation
60
Noisy restaurant
70
Loud music
80
Truck at 16 ft (5 meters)
90
Typical rock concert
100
Jet engine at 800 ft (240 meters)
110
Jackhammer at 3 ft (1 meter)
120
Jet engine at 100 ft (30 meters)
130

Disorders of the respiratory system

Introduction

Your respiratory system enables you to breathe to supply your body with oxygen and to get rid of carbon dioxide, a waste product of energy production. The center of the respiratory system is the lungs, in which the oxygen in the air you breathe is exchanged for carbon dioxide from your blood. The channel that carries the air in and out of your lungs is called the respiratory tract. It includes the nose, throat, and trachea (or windpipe). Deep in the chest the trachea divides into two main tubes, which are called bronchi. Each one goes into one lung, where it divides into progressively smaller air passages that are called bronchioles. At the tip of each bronchiole are clusters of balloon-like structures called alveoli. There are about 300 million of these alveoli in each lung. They can be likened to a bunch of grapes. The vital exchange of oxygen for carbon dioxide occurs through minute blood vessels in the thin walls of the alveoli.

You use several muscles to suck air into your lungs. The diaphragm, a dome-shaped muscular sheet attached to the lower ribs, divides the chest cavity from the abdomen. When the diaphragm contracts, along with other muscles between the ribs, a mild vacuum is created around your lungs. This causes them to expand and suck air into the respiratory tract. When the muscles relax, the lungs contract, forcing the air back out. If this mechanism works well, you hardly notice that you are breathing. However, a number of things can go wrong with the lungs or other parts of the respiratory tract.

The articles in this section are arranged in three groups. Each group concentrates on disorders that affect one area of the respiratory system. The first group deals with problems that affect the nasal cavity and the sinuses, or air spaces above and behind the nose. The second group of articles deals with disorders of the throat. These include problems of both the larynx, or voice box, which is located at the top of the trachea, and the pharynx, the funnel that leads from the nasal cavity and the back of the mouth down to where the esophagus, which carries food and water to the stomach, separates from the trachea. The third group of articles deals with common diseases of the trachea, lungs, and breathing mechanism.

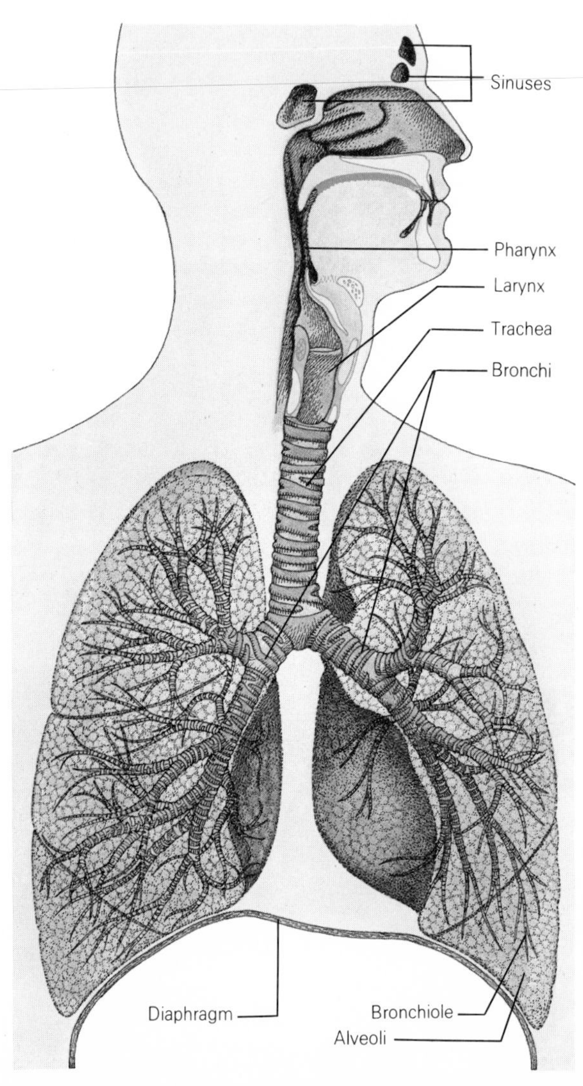

Details of the respiratory system

How you breathe

Air you breathe in through your nose is warmed by small blood vessels very close to the surface of the nasal cavity and moistened before it passes into the lungs. In addition, tiny hairs that line the nose provide a filtering system to clean the air by keeping foreign bodies such as dust particles from getting into your lungs.

When you breathe in, your diaphragm, which is dome shaped when relaxed, is pulled flat. At the same time, muscles between your ribs contract and pull your rib cage upward and outward. These movements increase the volume of your chest so that your lungs expand and air is sucked into them. The stronger the muscle action, the more air enters your lungs. Your rate of breathing in and out is determined mainly by the amount of carbon dioxide that must be expelled from your bloodstream.

When you breathe out, your chest muscles and diaphragm relax. This makes your rib cage sink and your lungs, which are very elastic, contract and squeeze out air. The air that you breathe out still contains some oxygen. Cardiopulmonary resuscitation (CPR) is effective in restoring breathing in an emergency precisely because the person performing CPR breathes oxygen into the victim.

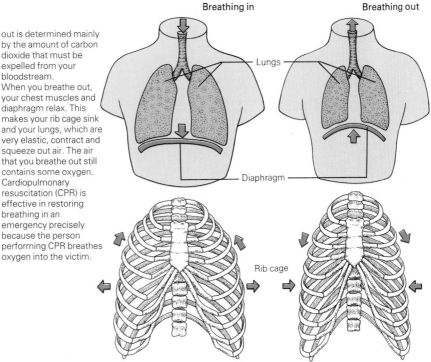

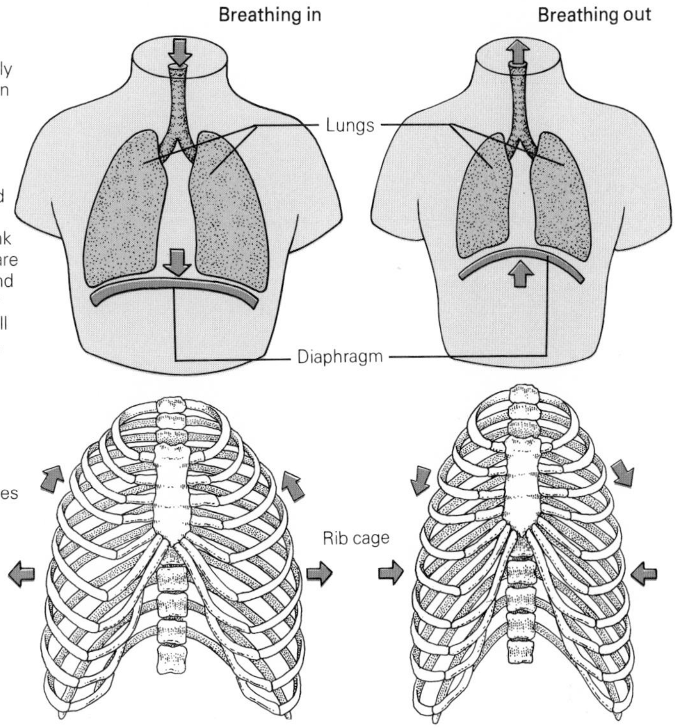

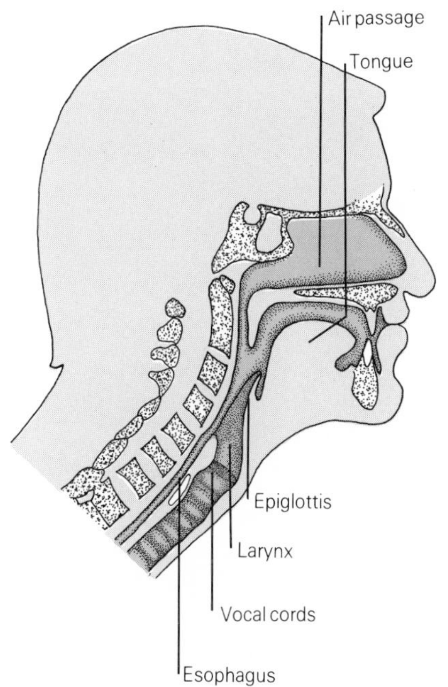

The pleura

Each lung is surrounded by a thin membranous covering called the pleura. This is folded back on itself to form a double layer all around each lung. There is a tiny space between the layers that contains a small amount of fluid. The inner layer is attached to the lung and the outer layer is attached to the rib cage. The pleura serve as a cover for the lungs and the inner surface of the rib cage and diaphragm. When you breathe in and your rib cage lifts up and out, your lungs are pulled up and out at the same time.

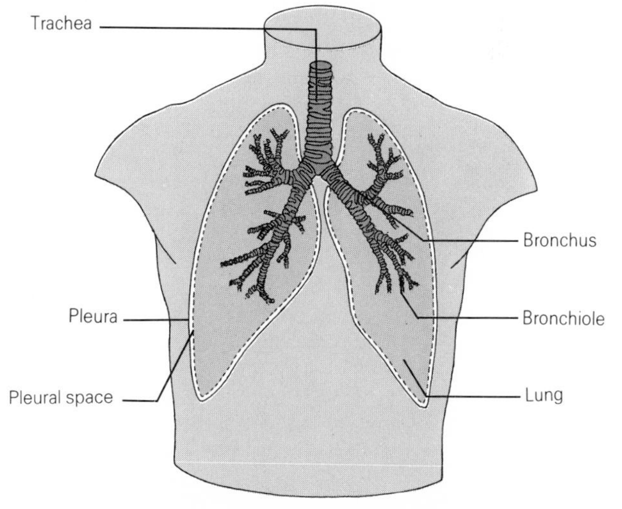

The nose

The nose is the main entrance to your respiratory system. It is lined with a mucous membrane that contains many tiny blood vessels close to the surface. The front of the nose also has protective hairs. The nasal lining filters, moistens, and warms the air you breathe as it goes through the nasal passage toward your throat and lungs. The nasal passage runs along the top of the palate, or the shelf separating the nose from the mouth, and turns down to join the passage from the mouth to the throat.

The nasal passage is not a simple tube. A series of baffles called turbinates makes the passage winding rather than straight. Also, in several places, the nasal passage opens into sinuses, which are pairs of air-filled cavities in the bones of the skull. Nasal infections, which are discussed in the following articles, sometimes spread into the sinuses as well as into the rest of the respiratory system.

The nose is also the organ of smell, and you may not be able to smell anything if a disorder "stuffs up" your nose. However, permanent loss of smell is rare.

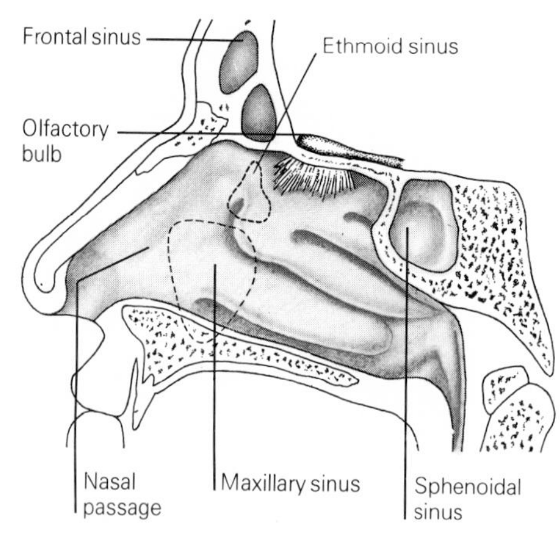

A cross section of the nose
The nasal passage is linked to 4 pairs of sinuses or air-filled cavities in the skull. The sensitive hair-like endings of the olfactory nerves project into the nasal passage. They detect odors in the air and pass the information to the olfactory bulb and on into the brain.

Colds

Medical myths

You can avoid colds by taking vitamins regularly.

Wrong. Despite various research studies, there is no clear evidence that large doses of any vitamin, including vitamin C, will prevent or cure colds.

Wet feet or exposure to drafts will almost certainly bring on a cold.

Wrong. There is no scientific evidence to support this widely held assumption.

The disease we call the common cold is really a minor illness that results from infection by any one of almost 200 different viruses. Usually a common, or head, cold is confined to the nose and throat, and sometimes the larynx (see Laryngitis, p.377) and the lungs (see Acute bronchitis, p.379, and Pneumonia, p.384). These viral infections sometimes are followed by more serious bacterial infections of the throat, lungs, or ears.

All of us get colds. Most people have their first cold during their first year of life. Most children are extremely susceptible to nasal viral infection between the ages of 1 and 3. Then they gradually become immune to many common viruses. The frequency of colds increases again during early school years, because the school environment contains new types of viruses. Also, schoolchildren may be careless about covering their mouths when they sneeze. Most people acquire more immunity as they grow older and catch fewer and less severe colds. Young adults may have 2 or 3 colds per year; elderly adults may have only one or none. (For more information about colds in infants, see recurrent colds in children, p.727).

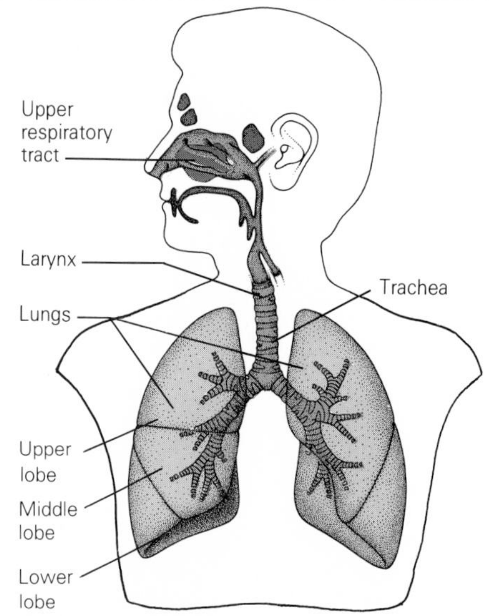

Where the common cold strikes
A cold can affect almost any part of the respiratory system. Sneezing and a runny nose mean that the upper respiratory tract is affected. The infection may also irritate the trachea and cause a cough or irritate the larynx, which makes your voice hoarse. Occasionally the lungs become infected, resulting in pneumonia.

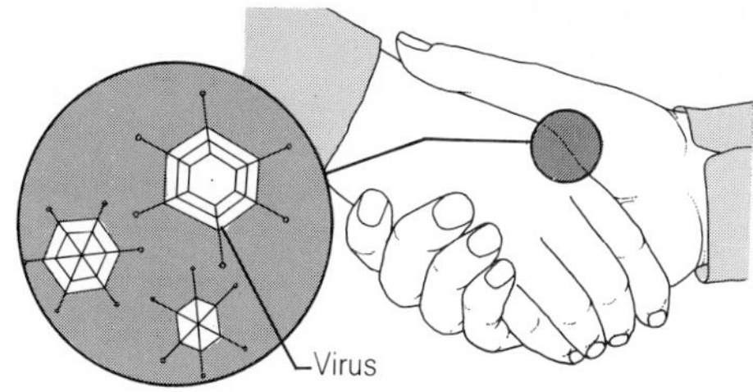

Spreading colds
Many people believe colds spread only through the air, but hand-to-hand contact is another possibility. If you have a cold, you may hold your hand in front of your mouth when you cough or sneeze and may then pass on the virus by hand.

What are the symptoms?

To some extent the symptoms depend on which virus is responsible for the cold. Major symptoms include runny nose, sneezing, watering eyes, sore throat, hoarseness, and coughing. At first, the nasal discharge is usually rather watery if there has been secondary infection with bacteria. Then it becomes thick and greenish-yellow. You may also have a headache and slight fever. This rise in temperature may cause shivering and chills. However, a very high temperature and general body pains are more likely to be symptoms of influenza, or flu (see p.597).

Every person, regardless of age or sex, gets an occasional cold. Nobody is sure how colds are spread. The major way seems to be through direct contact with other people who have colds. Also, coughs and sneezes spray the viruses into the air. Colds occur far less frequently in isolated communities, where everyone soon becomes immune to the viruses that are in circulation.

What are the risks?

An ordinary cold often clears up in 3 to 4 days. Even with a bacterial infection, a head cold should not last longer than a week. But because the respiratory tract is a series of spaces connected by passages, secondary infections can spread from your nose and throat to your middle ear, sinuses, larynx, trachea, or lungs, and can lead to serious respiratory disorders.

What should be done?

Anyone with a cold should stay home. This precaution is mainly so that you do not pass on your cold to other people, but it also gives you the chance to rest and recuperate. Consult your physician if the cold lasts more than 10 days, if there are symptoms that suggest that the infection has spread beyond the nose and throat, or if you often get bronchitis or ear infections. Some symptoms should send you to your physician promptly. They include earache, pain in the face or forehead, a temperature above 102°F (39°C), and a combination of persistent hoarseness or sore throat, shortness of breath and wheeziness, and a dry, painful cough. To help prevent serious respiratory infections, an annual flu shot is important for infants under age 1, people over 65, and people with chronic respiratory tract diseases (see Influenza, p.597).

What is the treatment?

Self-help: There is no effective drug treatment for a common cold. But some advice is worth following. Stay at home, in a warm (but not overheated) room, and increase the moisture in the air with some type of vaporizer or humidifier. Drink plenty of fluids, and take an aspirin or two to relieve any aches and pains and help you sleep. Over-the-counter cold medications, cough syrups, and nasal sprays may also give you temporary relief from your symptoms, but you should use them only in moderation.

Professional help: Your physician generally will not prescribe antibiotics, since viruses do

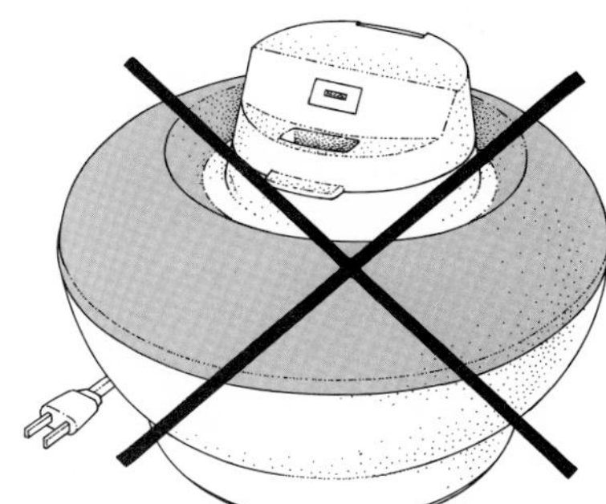

Vaporizers
Vaporizers moisturize the air in a room to help you recover from a cold. The benefit of using steam vaporizers is questionable. These devices pose an electrical fire hazard along with the risk of possible scalding if the steaming hot water is accidentally spilled.

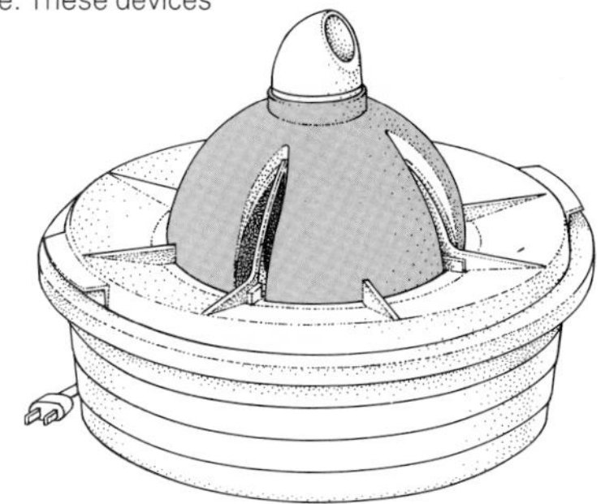

The cool vaporizer (above) breaks water into tiny droplets and sprays them into the air of the room without using heat. It is useful in winter.

Self-help for a stuffy or runny nose

Many of the illnesses discussed on these pages cause a nasal discharge. Although some of the illnesses—especially the common cold—cannot be cured, the nasal discomfort they cause can be eased considerably by using the self-help advice on this page. In addition, always remember that the lining of the nasal passageways is fragile and has many tiny blood vessels just below the surface; be careful not to blow your nose too hard and cause a nosebleed.

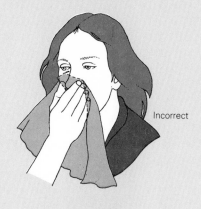

Steam inhalation
You can boost the relative humidity in your home by using a central or room humidifier. This keeps your mucous membranes from becoming excessively dry, so you can blow out accumulated mucus. This is especially important in cold climates, in which you are heating your indoor air. Maintaining fluid in the body by drinking ample amounts of liquid is most important. Over-the-counter preparations sold to be added to the steaming water have not been shown to be effective.

Nasal decongestants
Nasal decongestants are intended to shrink and dry out the swollen, mucus-producing tissue inside the nose and sinuses, and liquify the remaining mucus so you can blow your nose and obtain relief. They are available as tablets, sprays, or drops. Never exceed the maximum dose advised on the label; overuse of drops or sprays can lead to a "rebound" reaction, in which the tissues respond to the drug in the decongestant by producing even more mucus than before.

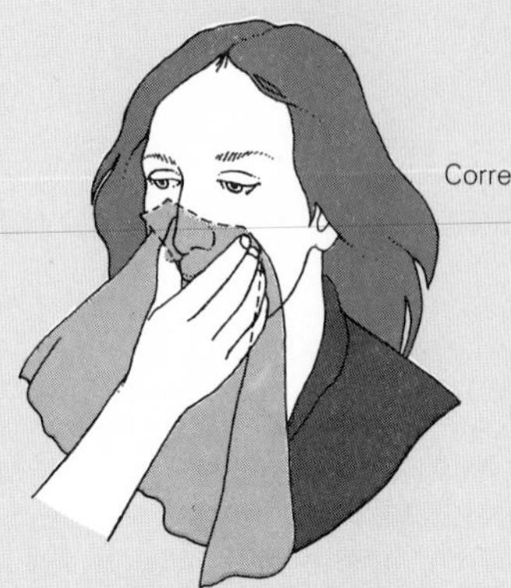

Blowing your nose
Blow gently into a disposable tissue or a clean handkerchief. Clear your nostrils one at a time, keeping the other one closed by pressing on that side of the nose. One common error (above, right) is to press both nostrils almost closed as you blow. This not only prevents you from clearing your nose thoroughly, but also may allow infection to spread to your ears.

not respond to them. An antibiotic might actually make matters worse by producing side effects such as diarrhea. Nasal inhalation of interferons (drugs made in a genetics laboratory but based on one of the body's natural defense mechanisms) has been shown to speed recovery from colds, but the treatment is of no practical value because interferon is very expensive and can provoke symptoms that are very unpleasant. If you have recurrent attacks of sinusitis, bronchitis, or frequent ear infections, however, you should see a physician at the first sign of a head cold since your cold may present special problems. Your physician can explain how a cold affects your individual situation and recommend appropriate treatment. He or she may prescribe antibiotics or other drugs.

Allergic rhinitis

(including hay fever)

Allergic rhinitis, commonly called hay fever when it occurs seasonally, is similar to asthma (see p.381) except in one respect. In asthma, an airborne substance causes an allergic, or hypersensitive, reaction in your lungs and chest. In allergic rhinitis, the reaction occurs in your eyes, nose, and throat. Exposure to an airborne irritant (called an allergen) triggers the release of histamine, a body chemical. Histamine causes inflammation and fluid production in the fragile lining of the nasal passage, the sinuses, and the eyelids and surface layer of the eyes.

Since allergy-based diseases such as asthma, contact dermatitis (see Eczema and dermatitis, p.269), and allergic rhinitis often affect many members of the same family, the cause is partly genetic.

If you have allergic rhinitis, you react to specific allergens. For example, you may be sensitive to grass pollen, which is abundant in early summer, to tree pollen, which is in the air in spring, to ragweed, which blooms in the late summer, and to dusts or molds in the fall. Hay fever is a type of allergic rhinitis that is caused by ragweed pollen.

In addition to pollen, almost any airborne substance derived from a living organism can cause allergic rhinitis, including any traces of animal skin, hair, and feathers. You may also be allergic to house dust, or more precisely, to the tiny mites that infest the dust.

There are two types of allergic rhinitis, seasonal and perennial. Seasonal allergic rhinitis only bothers you part of the year because it is an allergy to a substance that is not in the air year round. Perennial allergic rhinitis occurs year round because it is caused by exposure to airborne allergens that may be present at any time.

What are the symptoms?

If you have allergic rhinitis, you sneeze frequently, your nose runs, and your eyes are red, itchy, and watery. If you rub your eyes, it makes them worse. Itchy skin, dry throat, and wheezing can also occur. If you have hay fever, the symptoms are most severe when there is a lot of pollen in the air. To varying degrees among individuals, the symptoms of allergic rhinitis last from early July to the middle of September.

Because airborne allergens are generally too small to see, it is difficult to predict when you may have an attack. For example, if you are allergic to cat dander (small flakes of animal skin or hair), you may start to sneeze when you enter an empty room, because invisible traces of hair and shed skin from a recent feline occupant are still in the air.

Allergic rhinitis is very common. Although there is a widespread belief that allergic rhinitis is a childhood disorder that you outgrow in your late teens or early 20s, this is not necessarily so. You can develop the disorder at any age and later recover. However, you are particularly susceptible if you are under 40 and have another allergic condition such as asthma or dermatitis, or if other family members have similar disorders. Many people react to more than one allergen, and some people have both seasonal and perennial episodes of allergic rhinitis.

What are the risks?

This disorder does not usually endanger your general health.

What should be done?

If you find that allergic rhinitis interferes with your daily life, see your physician, who will probably first ask questions to find out how serious the problem is for you. He or she may advise you against desensitization or oral corticosteroid medication treatment, because of the possible side effects. If you do not know what causes your allergic rhinitis, your physician may suggest skin tests to find out which specific allergens make you react. Your physician scratches the skin on your forearm and places drops of liquid that contain a common allergen on the same spot. If the skin under any of the drops turns red and starts to itch, you are allergic to the allergen in that particular drop.

What is the treatment?

Self-help: If you get hay fever regularly, stay indoors as much as possible during the hay fever season, especially when the news media report a high pollen count. Pollen counts are generally higher in the morning;

Substances that trigger allergic rhinitis

Pollen
Pollen from certain plants may trigger an allergy episode. Symptoms appear whenever the plant or plants to which you are allergic bloom and produce pollen.

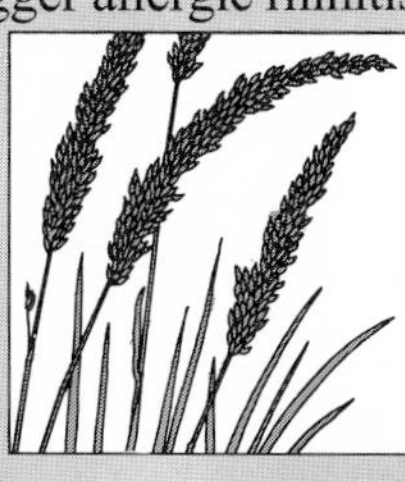

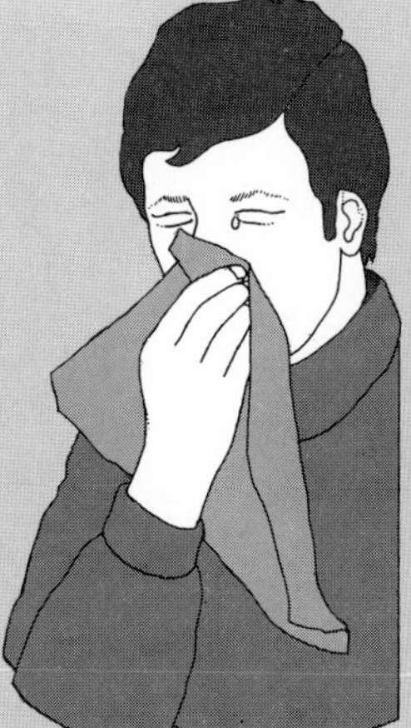

Mites in house dust
House-dust mites are found in almost every home. If anyone in your family is allergic to these mites, be sure to wash your sheets and pillow cases frequently and keep your house as free of dust as is possible.

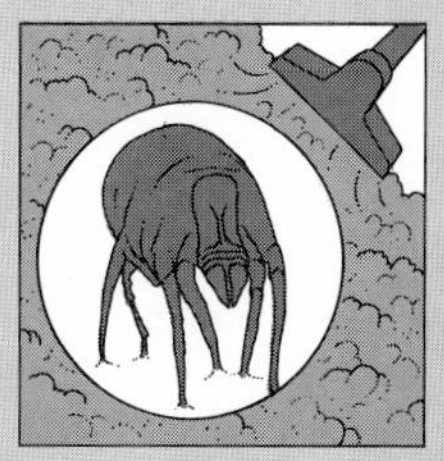

Animal hair
People think they are allergic to animal hair but are not. They are affected by dander, the tiny skin flakes that the animal sheds and that often cling to the hairs.

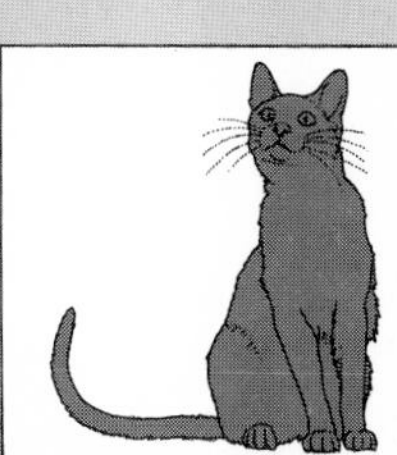

Feathers
An allergy to feathers is relatively easy to deal with. Avoid products that are stuffed with feathers or down, such as some jackets, coats, sleeping bags, and pillows. Also, you will not be able to keep pet birds.

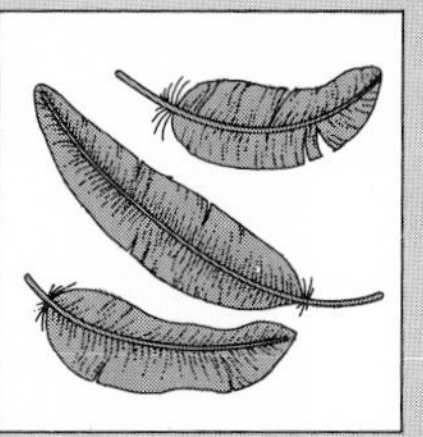

it's a good idea to stay home then, if possible. You should avoid wearing contact lenses when the pollen count is high, because they can increase eye irritation. Resist the temptation to rub your eyes. If your allergic rhinitis is perennial rather than seasonal, try to find out what you are allergic to, and take steps to avoid it or minimize your exposure to it. It's important to keep your house clean and free of dust and mold. Physical exercise, in addition to its many other benefits, helps keep your nasal passages open. Self-help recommendations for people who have asthma (see p.382) also apply to people who have allergic rhinitis.

Whether your condition is seasonal or perennial, there are many drugs that ease the symptoms of allergic rhinitis, including a large number of nonprescription medications. The most commonly used drugs are antihistamines, which are generally effective for both preventing and stopping episodes. To be fully effective, antihistamines must be taken regularly, often for several days at a time. Some common side effects from antihistamines are drowsiness and dryness in the nose and throat. The side effects may be more annoying than the allergic rhinitis itself. Since antihistamines often make you sleepy, you should never take them if you intend to drive a motor vehicle or to operate machinery within the next few hours.

For quick temporary relief from a stuffy nose, you can use either nonprescription decongestant nose drops or nasal sprays, which can ease symptoms within minutes. However, do not use such medicines often or for more than a few days in a row. They eventually aggravate the symptoms they are supposed to suppress, and you may become dependent on them.

Professional help: If your hay fever causes you only minor irritation, over-the-counter remedies may be the only treatment you require. If, however, your symptoms are severe and persistent, ask your physician for more effective treatment. This may take the form of preventive therapy with an inhaled (cromolyn sodium) drug that blocks the action of the histamine-releasing cells in your nose. Or your physician may prescribe the antihistamines terfenadine or astemizole or corticosteroid nasal sprays, any of which can be used for months or years (unlike nonprescription nasal sprays, which, as mentioned above, may be used safely only for a few days at a time).

These treatments are so effective that desensitization is used less frequently than it once was. Desensitization is based on identifying the specific substance or substances that cause your symptoms and then giving a series of injections of minute quantities of this substance in gradually increasing dosages to stop your reactions. However, desensitization is not always successful and may need to be repeated for a number of seasons; very occasionally it may provoke a dangerous reaction. Before you decide to have desensitization treatment for your allergies, you should consider the possibility that it may not work for you and discuss the risks and benefits with your physician (see Allergies, p.754).

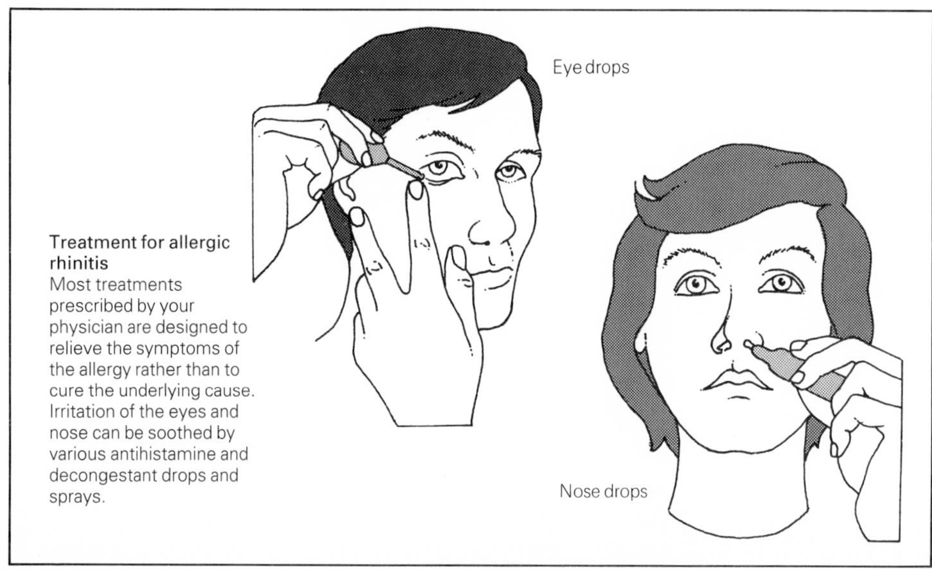

Treatment for allergic rhinitis
Most treatments prescribed by your physician are designed to relieve the symptoms of the allergy rather than to cure the underlying cause. Irritation of the eyes and nose can be soothed by various antihistamine and decongestant drops and sprays.

Sinusitis

The sinuses are air spaces in the bones around your nose. Sinusitis is an inflammation of the mucous membranes of the sinuses that fill the sinus cavities with pus and mucus. It is caused by bacterial or viral infection. The frontal sinuses, which are in the forehead just above the eyes, and the maxillary sinuses, which are behind the cheek bones, are the ones that are commonly infected.

Sinusitis occurs when a virus infection closes or partially closes the nasal cavity, resulting in an inability to drain and an infection by bacteria already in the sinuses. This probably only occurs in people who are born with either a narrowed sinus opening or, more commonly, with allergic rhinitis (see p.370) or other types of rhinitis.

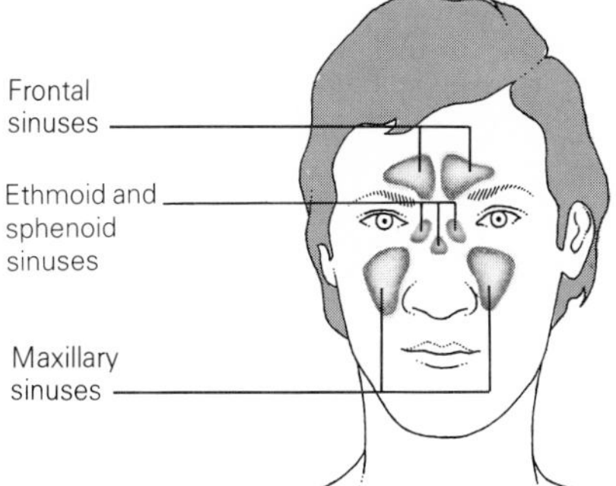

Headache over one or both eyes indicates that your frontal sinuses are inflamed. Your cheeks may hurt if your maxillary sinuses are affected, but this is less common.

Examining the sinuses by CT scan
If you suffer from persistent sinusitis, your physician may arrange for a CT scan (bottom) of your sinuses to help diagnose your problem. The healthy air-filled sinuses show up (right) as dark patches surrounded by gray areas of bone. The right maxillary sinus contains a polyp (gray circle).

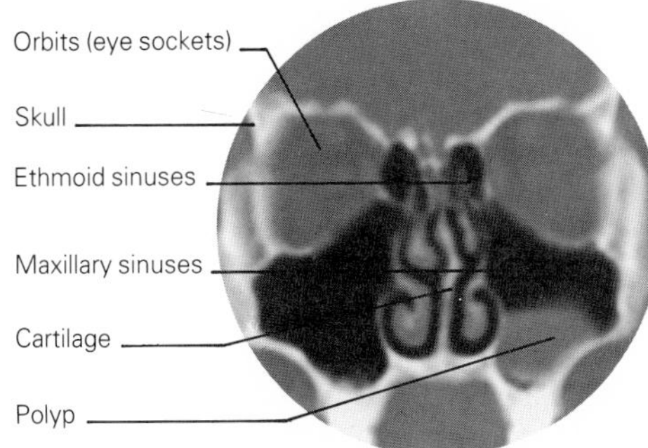

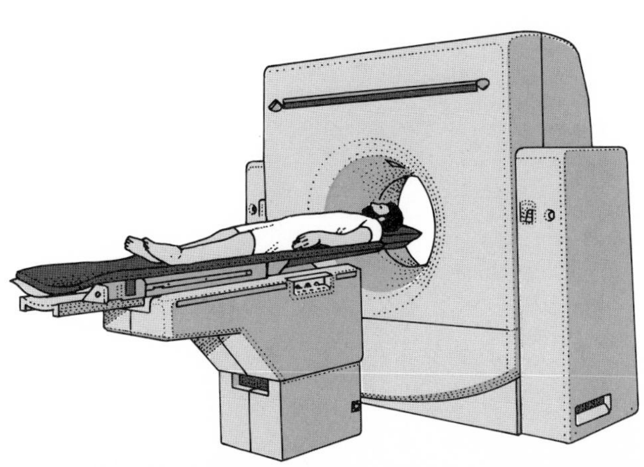

What are the symptoms?
After the first few days of a cold, the blockage in your nose may get worse and the greenish discharge may increase. Later, because the passages between the nose and the sinuses also become blocked, the discharge may stop, leaving you more stuffed up than ever. You have to breathe through your mouth, your speech becomes nasal, you may have bad breath, and you feel generally ill. If the frontal sinuses are affected, you may have a headache over one or both eyes. The headache is worse when you wake up in the morning, or when you bend your head down and forward. The undersurface of your forehead just above the eyes may feel tender.

If the maxillary sinuses are affected, one or both of your cheeks may hurt. You may feel as if you have a toothache in your upper jaw. Occasionally, sinusitis may follow dental treatment, because infection can spread from the roots of your tooth into one of your sinuses (see Tooth abscess, p.473). When ethmoid sinuses are involved, your lower eyelid may be swollen, especially when you wake in the morning.

Sinusitis is fairly common, but some people never get it, while others, particularly smokers, get it every time they have a cold. Others may get sinusitis by jumping into water feet first without holding their noses. Damage to your nasal bones, or even a foreign body caught in your nostril, may make you more susceptible to infection and, thus, bring on an episode. The ethmoid and sphenoid sinuses (deeper in the nose) are frequently infected first, and the infection spreads to the maxillary and frontal sinuses.

What are the risks?
The risks of sinusitis are minimal if it is treated with antibiotics. Before the availability of antibiotics, the infection sometimes spread through the mucous membrane of the sinuses into the bones and even to the meninges (three membranous layers that protect the brain and spinal cord) or the brain. Such serious complications of sinusitis happen infrequently today.

What should be done?
Try the self-help measures recommended below. If the symptoms persist after 3 or 4 days, consult your physician. He or she will listen to your symptoms and examine you; for particularly difficult or severe cases, he or she may order a CT scan.

What is the treatment?

Self-help: Stay indoors, in a room with a steady temperature. Add moisture to the air with a vaporizer or humidifier. Blow your nose gently with tissues. Drink plenty of fluids and use nasal decongestant drops or spray. Also, it may help to keep your head elevated; try using extra pillows or a foam wedge at night while you sleep.

Professional help: Your physician may prescribe an antibiotic and also suggest that you use oral decongestant medication, nose drops, or a nasal spray. Decongestants shrink the swollen mucous membrane, which widens the respiratory airways. For sinusitis, however, decongestants should be used only as prescribed by your physician. If decongestant drops or sprays are used incorrectly, they can aggravate the condition, doing more harm than good.

Further treatment for your sinusitis will probably be unnecessary; however, if the sinusitis persists, your physician may recommend that you bathe your sinuses with a nonprescription saline mist spray three times a day in each nostril.

Nasal polyps

A growth that forms on the mucous membrane that lines the nose and protrudes into the nasal cavity is known as a nasal polyp. Polyps are caused by overproduction of mucus in the cells of the membrane. This can be caused by a condition such as allergic rhinitis (see p.370). These polyps are harmless, but a big one or several little ones can obstruct your nasal passages, make breathing difficult, and impair your sense of smell. If the opening between the nasal cavity and one of the sinuses is blocked by a polyp, infection may result, and you may have headaches or pain in your face.

What should be done?

If your nose is gradually becoming blocked, you may have nasal polyps. You may be able to see them in a mirror by shining a light up your nostrils. They look like pearly gray lumps. However, polyps are often at the back of the nose, where they can be seen only with a special instrument. Nasal polyps are usually discovered by your physician during an examination of your nose. Corticosteroid nasal sprays may shrink the polyps and relieve symptoms; otherwise the way to treat nasal polyps is to remove them. Your physician may refer you to a specialist for surgery. Sometimes you need to take oral corticosteroid medication for a few days at the start of the treatment for polyps.

People with nasal polyps are often allergic to aspirin and should take acetaminophen for the relief of headaches and any other minor pains associated with the polyps.

Examining the nose
To examine the inside of your nose, your physician may separate your nostrils with a special instrument, a nasal speculum, which looks like a pair of small tongs.

Deviated septum

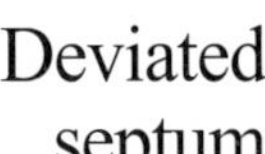

If the nasal septum, or the wall between the nostrils, is very crooked, it makes the air passage narrow on one side. This obstruction can make breathing somewhat difficult, because the flow of air through the narrower passage may become blocked. Substantial deviation of the septum is rare. It usually happens because of an injury, and the outside of the nose can look straight. There are no significant symptoms. The septum can be straightened by surgery if the deviation is annoying. Whatever the complaint that prompts the surgery, it may not be improved following the operation. Most people who have a deviated septum simply live with it.

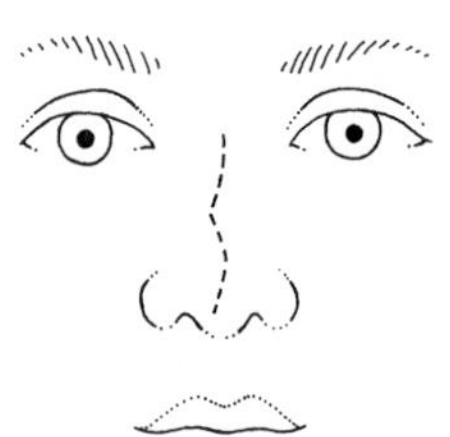

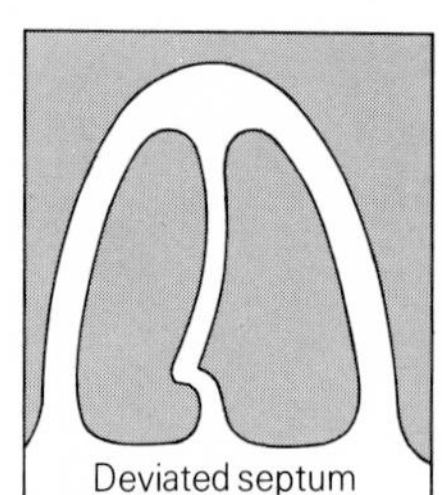

Straightening a deviated septum
The operation used to straighten a deviated septum involves removing the bent or excess cartilage. The surgery is usually done only if there are problems with breathing.

Anosmia

Anosmia is the medical term for a loss of the sense of smell and taste that persists even when there is no obvious cause, such as a head cold. Usually it clears up on its own. Most frequently, anosmia follows a cold or other virus infection. It may be a symptom of a tumor of the brain (see p.301), but this is very rare. It may also occur because of a skull fracture. This may happen because such an injury sometimes damages the olfactory nerves, which carry smell sensations from the nose to the brain.

What should be done?
If you have lost your sense of smell or taste, consult your physician. If there is no sign of abnormality in your nose, your physician may refer you to a neurologist for some diagnostic tests. The loss of smell may be temporary or permanent. If you smoke, your physician will recommend that you stop.

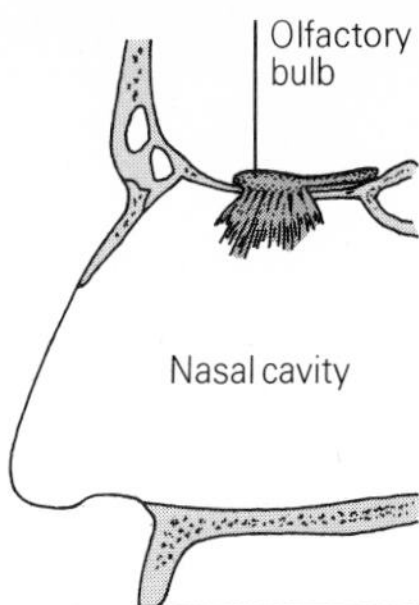

The position of the olfactory nerves
Olfactory nerves, which are fibers located at the top of the nose below the olfactory bulb, convert smells into nerve impulses, which travel to the bulb and from there to other parts of the brain.

Nosebleed

When your nose begins to bleed, it is usually sudden and from only one nostril. In most cases of nosebleed, unless the nose has been injured, there is no apparent explanation for the bleeding. One relatively common cause is a cold or other infection, which causes crusting that can damage the sensitive membrane that lines the nose. Nosebleeds are seldom cause for concern, since they are unlikely to be a symptom of any other disorder. A generalized bleeding disorder such as thrombocytopenia (see p.456) could cause nosebleeds, but in such cases there is usually a considerable amount of bleeding at other locations in your body, such as from the gums or under the skin.

What is the treatment?
Self-help: Follow the instructions with the illustration "stopping a nosebleed" in this article. Once the bleeding has stopped and 12 hours have passed, remember to blow your nose very gently so you will not dislodge the blood clot that has stopped the bleeding.
Professional help: If bleeding continues, consult your physician or, if necessary, go to a hospital emergency department. Your physician will probably pack a strip of gauze into the bleeding nostril and tell you to leave it in for several hours. The purpose of the gauze packing is not only to absorb the blood and stop its dripping from the nose, but also to apply pressure to the ruptured blood vessels. If the bleeding persists or keeps recurring, the bleeding area may have to be closed by means of chemicals, heat treatment, or laser. Despite appearances, however, little blood is lost through nosebleeds.

Older people especially may have posterior epistaxis, which is bleeding in the back of the nose. With posterior epistaxis, you swallow blood but may not see blood when you blow your nose. People with this condition may require deeper packing with gauze, hospitalization, and, occasionally, surgery.

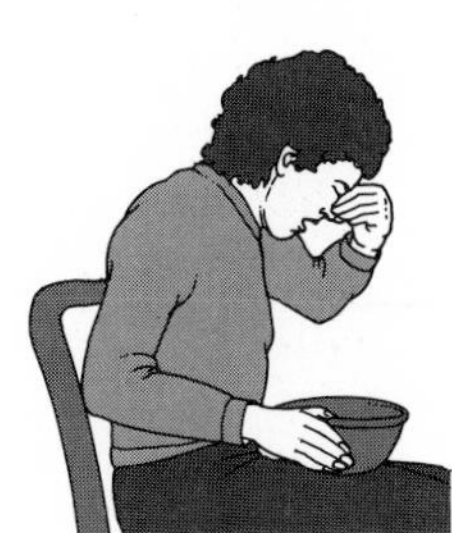

Sit with your head forward

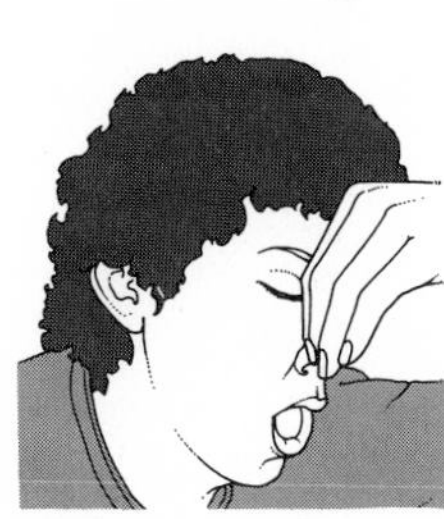

Pinch the fleshy part of your nose

Stopping a nosebleed
If you have a nosebleed, sit down and lean over with your head forward. Press together both sides of your nose between your thumb and finger, and breathe through your mouth. Hold it for about 5 minutes so that a blood clot forms and seals the damaged blood vessels. Do not blow your nose for 12 hours after the bleeding has stopped, so you will avoid dislodging the blood clot. If the bleeding has not stopped after about 20 minutes, go to your physician.

The throat

The throat, also known as the pharynx, is part of a multipurpose funnel leading from the back of the nose and mouth down to both the trachea, or windpipe, and the esophagus. When you breathe, air passes through your throat into the trachea on its way in and out of the lungs. When you swallow, chewed food lubricated with saliva moves down the throat into the esophagus on its way to the stomach.

When you speak, you use your larynx, or voice box, which is located in the throat at the top of the trachea. Air passing over the vocal cords, which are stretched flaps of tissue in the larynx, makes them vibrate and produce the relatively broad range of sounds that your mouth shapes into speech.

Like the rest of the respiratory system, the throat is affected mainly by infection, which often spreads up, down, or in both directions to involve the entire system. Although a sore throat may be caused by a streptococcal infection (see p.600), it is seldom a disorder in its own right.

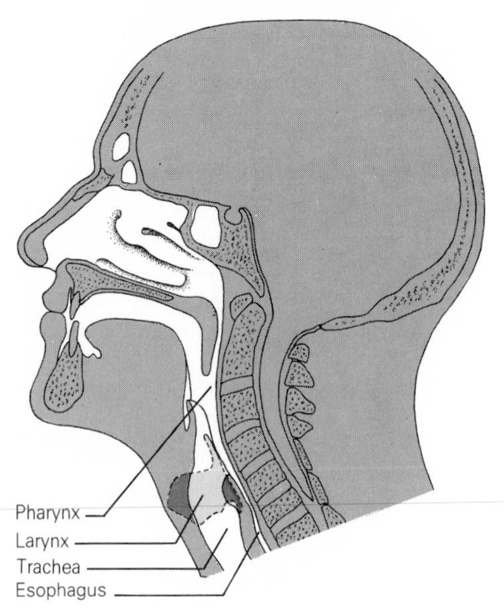

Pharyngitis

The pharynx is the part of the throat between the tonsils and the larynx, or voice box. Pharyngitis is acute inflammation of the pharynx. It is similar to acute inflammation of the tonsils, or tonsillitis (see next article). Both diseases are caused by the same bacteria and viruses, but pharyngitis tends to be less severe than tonsillitis. Some physicians refer to both conditions as acute sore throat. Pharyngitis is sometimes the first symptom of a generalized illness such as acute mononucleosis (see p.601) or influenza, or a symptom resulting from infection caused by a low white blood cell count triggered by some medications.

What are the symptoms?

If you have pharyngitis, your throat is very sore, you have trouble swallowing, and you may feel feverish. As in tonsillitis, your throat is red and raw.

Chronic throat pain is usually the result of gastroesophageal reflux (a cause of heartburn), chronic postnasal drip, mouth breathing, chronic sinusitis, overuse of throat muscles, or any inflammation of the tonsils. Smoking and drinking alcohol probably intensify throat pain caused by the conditions noted above.

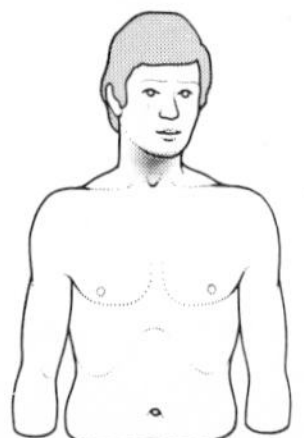

A sore throat
Although the sore throat of pharyngitis is rarely serious, it can be painful and make it difficult to breathe, swallow, or talk.

What is the treatment?

Self-help: If you have pharyngitis, do not smoke. Minimize your difficulty swallowing by switching to a mostly liquid diet for a short time. Nonprescription lozenges and mouthwashes can temporarily relieve the symptoms and discomfort caused by acute pharyngitis. Gargling with salt water may also help. Aspirin or an aspirin substitute recommended by your physician may ease general aches and pains caused by the inflammation. If your sore throat persists for more than a few days, consult your physician.

Professional help: For a severe episode, your physician may do a throat culture and then prescribe an antibiotic, often in oral form. For chronic pharyngitis he or she will probably try to find and treat the primary cause.

Tonsillitis

Tonsillitis, or acute inflammation of the tonsils, is primarily a children's disease (see p.723). It occurs occasionally in adults, and the early symptoms are very similar to those of a cold.

Look at your throat if you feel ill and have a sore throat, if it hurts to swallow, if pain in your ears could be coming from your throat, or if you have a headache, chills, and fever. Pus may be present on your tonsils if they appear red and inflamed and seem larger than usual. Another common symptom is swelling and tenderness of the glands near the infected area. Check the glands in your neck and under your jaw.

What should be done?

Stay in bed and rest for a couple of days. Take one or two aspirins every 4 hours, and drink plenty of liquids. Consult your physician if your sore throat and fever last for more than 48 hours, or if you are having any of the symptoms noted above.

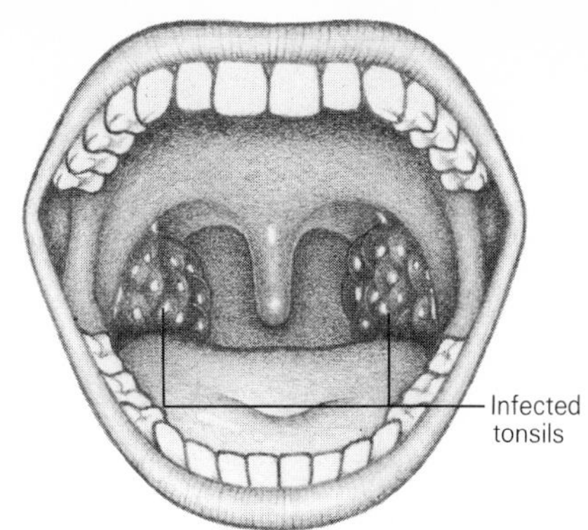

The tonsils
The tonsils are glandular swellings at either side of the throat that are vulnerable to invasion by viruses and bacteria. The resulting infection and inflammation is known as acute tonsillitis.

Laryngitis

Laryngitis is usually caused by viral or bacterial infection of the larynx, or voice box. The larynx is at the top of the trachea, or windpipe. The infection causes inflammation and swelling of the mucous membrane of the larynx, including the vocal cords. In children, because the opening of the larynx is narrow, the swollen membrane sometimes interferes with breathing (see Croup and stridor, p.725). Laryngitis is caused by irritation of the larynx from gastroesophageal reflux (a cause of heartburn), habits such as clearing your throat frequently, tobacco smoke, alcohol, or excessive shouting, talking, or singing.

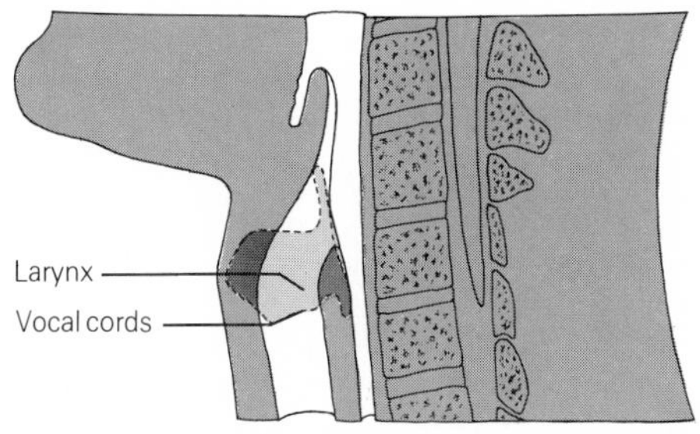

What happens in laryngitis
An infection of the upper respiratory tract may affect the vocal cords, and they may become inflamed. When you speak, air passes over the swollen cords, and the sounds are distorted. This causes the hoarseness of laryngitis.

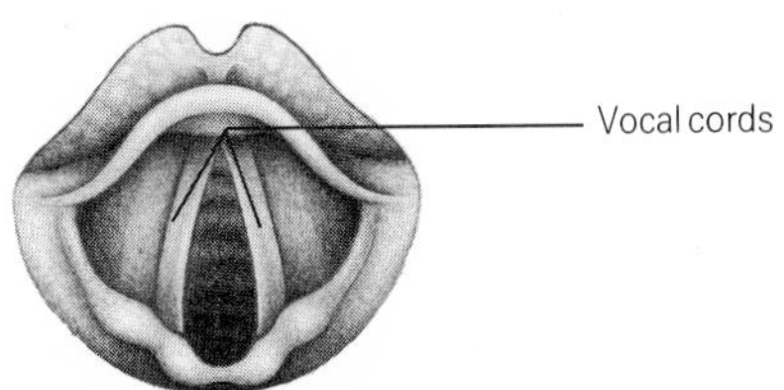

The main symptom is hoarseness, which may lead to loss of voice in 2 or 3 days. Speaking may even become painful. There may be fever or other symptoms that are associated with influenza, or flu (see p.597). Most people recover in a few days.

What are the risks?

Uncomplicated bouts of laryngitis are not dangerous. The main risk is that a condition similar to laryngitis is one symptom of tumors in the larynx (see next article).

What should be done?

Rest your voice and drink plenty of liquids while you are hoarse. You should talk softly, but do not whisper, because whispering is hard on the voice. Also, do not take aspirin for laryngitis while you are hoarse. It may lead to bleeding into the vocal cords and possible permanent hoarseness. If hoarseness persists for more than a week, consult your physician, who may ask you questions about your general health and examine your throat. If there is no inflammation, you do not have laryngitis, and you may have a polyp or tumor on your larynx.

Tumors of the larynx

The two most common benign growths (unlikely to spread) are papillomas and vocal cord polyps or nodules. Papillomas are caused by a virus, are usually multiple, and can cause hoarseness and difficulty in breathing. They are found more often in children, tend to recur after surgery, and may require multiple operations. Polyps and nodules may be on one side or (more often) both sides and are usually the result of vocal overuse. They can cause hoarseness but do not cause breathing difficulties. They usually go away or stop causing symptoms with voice retraining therapy; but some tumors, especially those that are on one side only, require surgery. Malignant tumors (likely to spread and threaten life) occur most often in heavy smokers.

What are the symptoms?

Hoarseness is usually the only symptom of a tumor of the larynx. There are no flulike symptoms as in laryngitis (see previous article). If the tumor is malignant, and has a chance to grow, it may eventually make swallowing difficult, and you may have an increasingly obvious lump in your neck.

Hoarseness that is not caused by cancer may be intermittent, but hoarseness from cancer is continuous and gets worse. Since it is not painful and comes on slowly, you may scarcely notice it during its early stages.

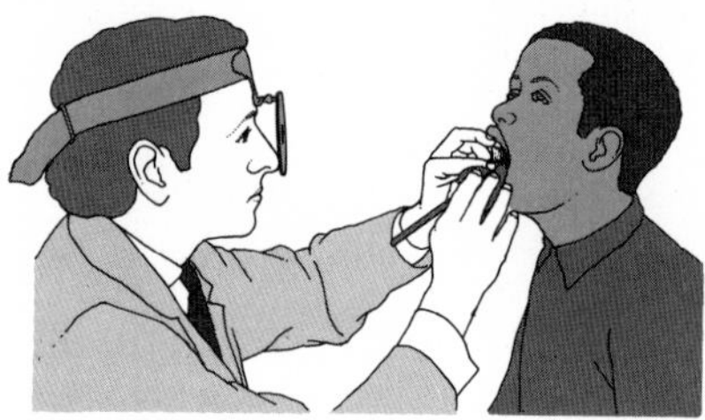

Examining the larynx
To examine your larynx, your physician uses a system of mirrors. Light is reflected from a physician's head mirror, which is basically a mirror with a hole in it for the doctor to look through. Another small mirror attached to a long handle is held at the back of your throat. It reflects the light into your larynx and a view of the larynx back to your physician.

What are the risks?

Although neither type of tumor of the larynx is very common, malignant tumors are slightly more common than benign ones. The American Cancer Society estimates that more than 12,000 people died from cancer of the larynx in a recent year; about 10,000 of the total were men.

If you ignore slowly increasing hoarseness, and if that hoarseness is caused by a malignant tumor, it may be too late to treat the cancer successfully. Cancer of the larynx can almost always be cured if it is diagnosed early. If the cancer is not discovered until a later stage, it can either spread to other parts of the throat or get into the bloodstream and produce metastases, or secondary cancers, elsewhere in your body.

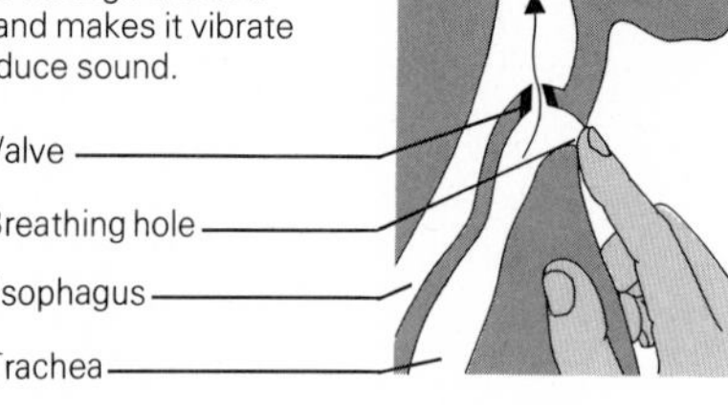

Speaking without your larynx
You may have surgery to create a breathing hole in your throat and to make a valve from your own esophageal tissue. This replaces your vocal cords. When you want to speak, you place a finger over the hole. Air from your lungs passes through the new valve and makes it vibrate to produce sound.

What should be done?

Do not ignore unexpected vocal changes. If you are hoarse for more than a week, or if hoarseness recurs, consult your physician. If your throat shows no signs of the inflammation that accompanies laryngitis, your physician may refer you to an ear, nose, and throat specialist, who will examine your larynx (*left*). If there are signs of any growth, the specialist will probably perform an examination with an endoscope (viewing tube) and a biopsy (sampling of tissue), to determine if your growth is malignant.

What is the treatment?

Self-help: No self-help is possible.

Professional help: Benign growths, whether papillomas or polyps, can usually be removed in an operation performed under general anesthesia, which allows your physician to use an operating microscope and provides a better opportunity to feel the tissues. Malignant tumors discovered early can be successfully treated either by radiation therapy or by partial removal of the larynx. No matter which method is used, all or part of your voice is usually preserved. Advanced cancers usually require removal of the entire larynx. Even in such cases, chances for a cure are good. If your entire larynx is removed, there are several methods by which you may regain your speech. With the help of a speech therapist, you may learn how to use your esophagus as a substitute for the larynx. Or you may learn to use a special electromechanical device that generates sounds that you modulate with your tongue and teeth to produce speech. In some cases a valve may be implanted between the trachea and esophagus (*above*). This enables you to divert air from the lungs into the esophagus, where you can produce the sounds for speech.

The lungs and chest

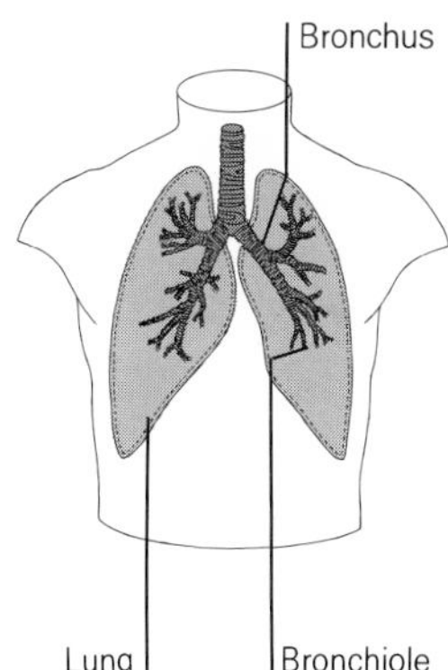

Your body needs a constant supply of oxygen to stay alive. It also needs to dispose of carbon dioxide, one waste product of metabolism. In your lungs oxygen from the air you breathe is transferred to your blood and carbon dioxide is released from the blood. The blood transports the oxygen to all parts of your body. The carbon dioxide is exhaled. The heart pumps blood that has less oxygen and lots of carbon dioxide in it back to the lungs through the pulmonary arteries to get more oxygen and release carbon dioxide.

The bronchus, or main airway that leads into each lung, divides into smaller and smaller airways called bronchioles. Each bronchiole ends in a cluster of tiny air sacs called alveoli. Each alveolus contains several small capillaries (minute blood vessels). The walls of those capillaries are thin enough to allow oxygen and carbon dioxide to move between the air and the blood. There are millions of alveoli in each lung.

Your lungs are especially vulnerable to particles in the air. Viruses and bacteria that cause disorders like pneumonia (see p.384); irritants such as tobacco smoke, which can cause lung cancer (see p.392); and, in some people, airborne allergens, which cause asthma (see p.381) or farmer's lung (see p.391), can all interfere with lung function.

Acute bronchitis

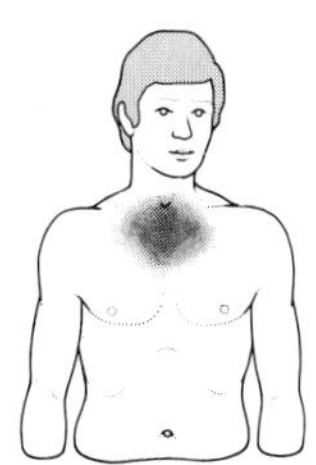

Inflammation of the mucous membrane that lines the bronchi, or main air passages of the lungs, is called bronchitis. If you have a respiratory infection, you may develop acute bronchitis, since the disorder is caused when the viruses that cause colds (see p.368) and pharyngitis (see p.376) spread into the bronchi. If you have a healthy heart and healthy lungs, bronchitis usually clears up in a few days. In chronic bronchitis (see next article), prolonged, recurrent episodes cause gradual deterioration of the lungs.

What are the symptoms?

The main symptom of bronchitis is a deep cough that brings up grayish or yellowish phlegm, or sputum, from your lungs. Other symptoms are breathlessness, wheezing, and a fever. You may also have pain in the upper chest, which gets worse when you cough.

Air pollution
Bronchitis occurs more often in areas with severe air pollution.

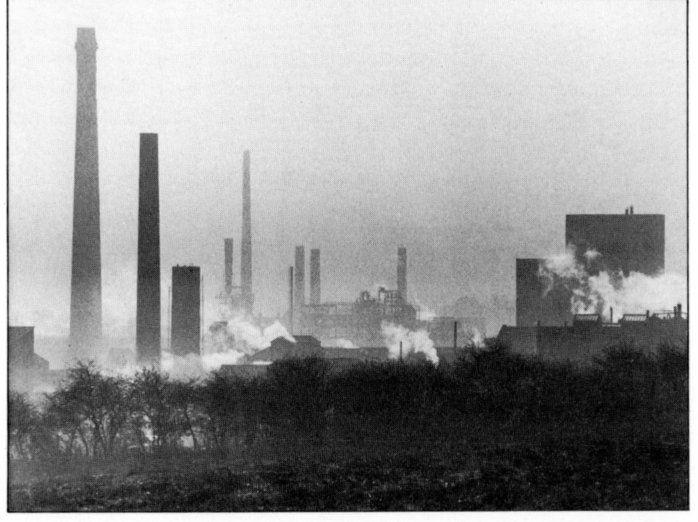

What are the risks?

Virtually everyone has an occasional episode of acute bronchitis. If you do not smoke cigarettes and you do not have chronic lung or heart trouble, you may have it once every few years. If you smoke, have a chest disorder such as asthma (see p.381) or bronchiectasis (see p.389), or live in an area where the air is very polluted, you are likely to get the disease more often. If your lungs are congested because of heart failure (see p.408), you may also be particularly susceptible to acute bronchitis.

If you are a nonsmoker who is otherwise healthy, there are few risks from acute bronchitis. If you are susceptible to bronchitis for any of the reasons mentioned above, you may have repeated episodes. These can damage the lining of the bronchi, impairing your ability to clear mucus from your air passages and leading to chronic bronchitis.

What should be done?

Do not ignore repeated bouts of acute bronchitis. Consult your physician. If you have not had bronchitis before, or if this is your first episode in several years, follow the self-help procedures suggested below.

What is the treatment?

Self-help: If you have a fever, take aspirin 3 or 4 times a day to bring your temperature down. Take an over-the-counter cough medicine recommended by your physician, and follow the instructions on the label, to help soothe your cough. Stay home, not necessarily in bed but in a warm room. Use a vaporizer or a humidifier to moisten the air in your home. This may help to clear your nasal passages and bronchi. This simple treatment is usually all that is needed. Call your physician if you become breathless, if you cough up blood, if you have a temperature above 101° F (38.5° C), or if you do not feel better in 48 hours.

Professional help: Because acute bronchitis is usually a virus infection, no specific treatment is possible. However, it is possible to relieve the symptoms. If your breathing is wheezy, your physician may prescribe a bronchodilator drug, which is usually taken via an inhaler. If your chest is sore from repeated episodes of coughing or if your cough is dry, your physician may prescribe a cough suppressant. If your sputum becomes greenish-yellow, which indicates that you probably have a secondary bacterial infection, your physician may prescribe an antibiotic. Some physicians prescribe antibiotics in the early stages of the disease in an effort to prevent any secondary bacterial infection from occurring.

Chronic bronchitis

An episode of acute bronchitis (see previous article) that fails to heal leads to chronic bronchitis, in which the inflammation persists and gets worse. In its early stages, chronic bronchitis has few symptoms. However, it is dangerous, because repeated infections of the bronchi and bronchioles thicken the lining of these tubes. This causes them to narrow and become obstructed by the secretion of too much mucus and by excessive contraction of the muscles in their walls.

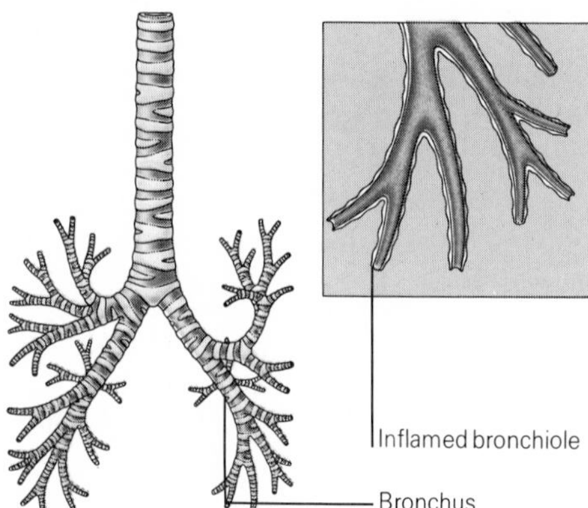

Some risks of chronic bronchitis
Repeated infections of the bronchi and bronchioles damage the linings of these passages and leave the lungs susceptible to further infection. If the infection spreads to the alveoli (not shown), it can cause pneumonia.

What are the symptoms?

The first symptom of chronic bronchitis is a morning cough that brings up phlegm, or sputum. Smokers may regard the cough, if they notice it at all, as a "normal" smoker's cough. Over the years the amount of phlegm gradually increases, and the coughing continues all day. Breathlessness and wheezing become increasingly troublesome.

In the early stages of chronic bronchitis, only bad colds or influenza cause flare-ups. In the later stages, every minor head cold can bring on a severe episode. Many people have several flare-ups every winter. One definition of chronic bronchitis is a recurrent cough with phlegm production that occurs on most days during at least 3 months a year, usually in winter, for at least 2 consecutive years.

In the last stages of the disease, coughing, breathlessness, and wheezing occur, usually on a nearly continuous basis.

What are the risks?

If you smoke, you are more likely to get chronic bronchitis than if you are a nonsmoker. Children of heavy smokers may be affected by cigarette smoke too. As infants they seem to be particularly susceptible to acute bronchitis and pneumonia (see p.384), and these disorders increase the risk of chronic bronchitis. Children of smokers are also more prone to lung cancer. Because air pollution can trigger both lung cancer and chronic bronchitis, these diseases are also more common in industrialized countries and in urban areas than in developing countries and rural areas.

If you have chronic bronchitis and do not obtain treatment for it in its early stages, there are several risks involved, including death. Usually, the disease has an established cyclical pattern of bronchial infection, which damages your lungs, and in turn leads to an increase in your vulnerability to further infection. If the infection eventually spreads into the alveoli, or air sacs at the ends of the bronchioles in the lungs, you may contract pneumonia (see p.384) and emphysema (see p.383). Chronic bronchitis may also lead to pulmonary hypertension (see p.447) and right-sided heart failure (see p.408). Also, your entire respiratory system could fail, which is a medical emergency (see Injuries and emergencies, p.834).

Some people who have chronic bronchitis gradually become blue around the lips and in the rest of the face because they are not getting enough oxygen. They may eventually experience respiratory failure because their lungs cannot supply their bodies with enough oxygen. Others develop lung cancer (see p.392), not because chronic bronchitis causes cancer, but because smoking is a cause of both diseases. If you have chronic bronchitis and you start to notice a marked increase in breathlessness and a change in the nature of your cough, these symptoms may be the first signs of cancer.

What should be done?

If you have a morning cough with phlegm and if you smoke, you have even more reason to stop smoking. If the symptoms persist, consult your physician, who will probably consider such factors as your smoking and where you live and work before making any recommendations. If necessary, your physician will recommend some diagnostic tests, which may include a chest X ray and pulmonary function tests.

What is the treatment?

Self-help: If you have chronic bronchitis, stop smoking and avoid smoky environments. Stay away from people who have colds. A cold, which is a minor illness to a person with healthy lungs, may cause an episode of bronchitis for you. If you work or live in a polluted environment, you should consider changing jobs or moving. If you move, try to select not only a cleaner environment, but also a warmer, drier one. You are running a risk if you spend your winters in a cold, damp place. However, don't make a permanent move without trying the location for a while to see if you feel better in a new climate.

Professional help: Treatment depends on how far the disorder has progressed before you consult your physician. If you are already suffering from breathlessness, your physician will probably prescribe an aerosol inhaler. Use it 3 or 4 times a day to relax the muscles of your bronchi. This will widen the airways in your lungs. If you are having a bad episode of infection and coughing up phlegm, your physician may prescribe an antibiotic. If you are having a serious attack, your physician may hospitalize you for treatment with intravenous antibiotics.

Your physician may prescribe small doses of an antibiotic for a period of several weeks or even months to prevent bacterial infection, or advise you to take a full dose only at the first sign of a flare-up of bronchitis. There is no consensus among physicians about the best way to treat chronic bronchitis. Although antibiotics are not effective against a virus infection, they are often prescribed even when a virus rather than a bacterium causes an episode. This is because a virus infection may increase the chance of a secondary bacterial infection in the lungs.

Asthma

Asthma is a chronic condition marked by periodic attacks of wheezing and difficulty breathing, especially in expelling air. The cause of asthma attacks is partial obstruction of the bronchi and bronchioles resulting from spasm of the muscles in the bronchial walls. With bronchitis you have constant coughing until you recover, but with asthma, attacks come and go and there are wide variations in the degree of obstruction at different times. Asthma cannot be cured, but an attack can be relieved and often prevented by treatment. If asthma attacks are not treated, they may gradually subside on their own.

Most asthma is triggered by an allergy to such substances as pollen; skin particles (dander) from cats or dogs; minuscule mites in house dust; some foodstuffs, such as eggs or milk or a food additive such as flavoring, dye, or preservative. Some attacks start for no apparent reason. Attacks can also be caused by infections (especially of the respiratory tract), medications, inhaled irritants, vigorous exercise, and stress.

What are the symptoms?

The main symptoms of asthma are difficulty breathing, a painless tightness in the chest, coughing, and varying amounts of wheezing. At times, the wheezing is audible only with a stethoscope, but sometimes it is loud enough to hear across a crowded room. In severe cases, breathing becomes so difficult that it may cause sweating, an increased pulse rate, and severe anxiety. In very severe attacks the face and lips may turn blue because of the diminishing supply of oxygen in the body.

What are the risks?

Asthma is a fairly common condition in school-age children. Most children outgrow it, and no more than 2 or 3 percent of the adult population has asthma.

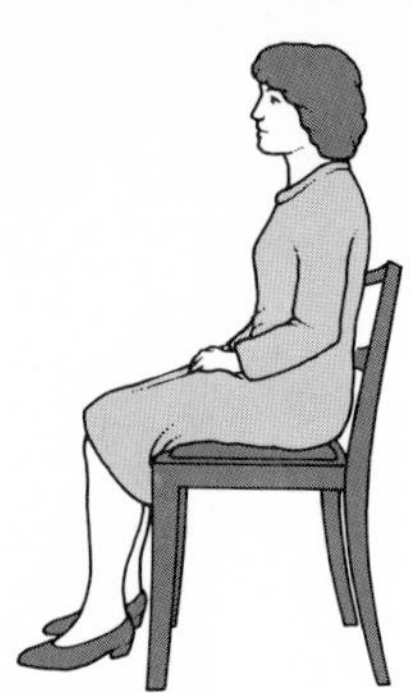

Stay quiet to stop an asthma attack
When an asthma attack begins, you may feel better if you sit quietly in an undisturbed setting.

A succession of severe asthma attacks can be very disabling. Each year several thousand people die during an attack. However, many of these people are older and have other illnesses too. Today, because many treatments have been developed, there is little risk of lasting disability or death for people who take their asthma seriously and consult a physician about it.

What should be done?

If you have asthma, there are some steps you can take to control asthma attacks. Learn about your disease, follow the self-help measures recommended below, and see your physician whenever you have a severe and persistent period of breathlessness. Asthma is an illness that you and your physician can work together to control. You can never be sure that the symptoms you have at home will be the same as they are when your physician examines you, so try hard to give a clear description of what happened both before and during the attack.

What is the treatment?

Self-help: Because asthma is most often caused by an external irritant—a substance to which you have developed a sensitivity—your first step in controlling the disease is to try to identify the irritant that bothers you. Skin tests (p.754) may help identify substances to which you are allergic, but you can do much of the detective work yourself. Do you have your asthma attacks mainly at one time of the year, and do you also have hay fever? If so, your allergens are probably pollen grains. Do your asthma attacks occur more often on certain days of the week than on others? This might suggest a link with dusts at work, such as flour in a bakery, or a substance you come in contact with only when you pursue a hobby, such as flowers in a greenhouse, or with some stressful situations, such as regular visits to a hospital. Is your asthma worse in one room of your house than another? You may be allergic to mites in house dust, especially in bedrooms, or to feathers or dander (skin particles) from a pet. An electrostatic precipitator (clean-air machine) may be used to clear allergens from closed spaces.

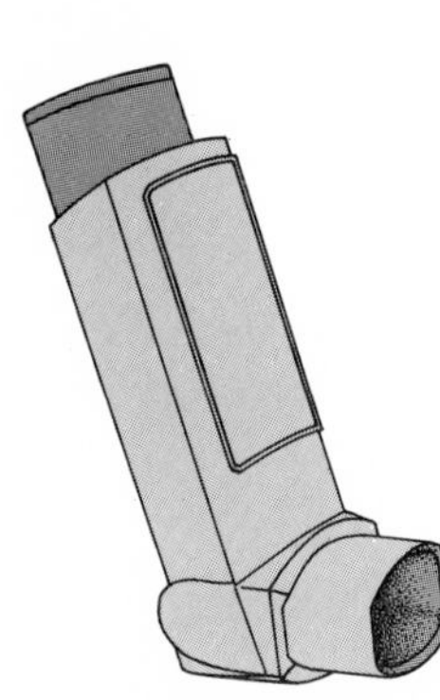

The aerosol inhalant
Aerosol inhalants are prescribed to relieve symptoms of asthma attacks. You breathe out, with your open mouth around the mouthpiece. Then, as you breathe in, you press the top down, so that a fine spray of the drug is released and is drawn into your lungs with the inhaled air.

Another possibility is an allergy to a drug, a food, or a drink. Aspirin, shellfish, and eggs are some common examples.

Keep a detailed record of the frequency and severity of your asthma attacks. Also, keep track of how often the asthma attacks coincide with times when you are exposed to suspected allergens.

Once you have identified an allergen, the best treatment for your asthma is to avoid exposure to that substance. This is relatively simple if the substance you are allergic to is a particular food or a domestic animal. However, if the allergen is a substance all around us such as grass pollen, you can only take precautions such as staying away from the country in midsummer. You will have to work in cooperation with your physician to try to control most of your symptoms.

Even if you cannot identify your allergen, you may have fewer attacks if you reduce the amount of dust in your house. Replace feather pillows and fiber-filled mattresses with those filled with nonallergic material. Use a vacuum cleaner to remove dust from crevices, and eliminate rugs or carpets or choose types that can be kept dust-free. Be aware, too, that other factors such as some forms of exercise or psychological stresses can bring on attacks.

Professional help: Once the diagnosis of asthma has been made, much can be done for you. The accuracy of your description of symptoms and probable allergens may help your physician make the diagnosis without allergy tests. In the past few years the methods for treating asthma have improved enormously with the introduction of new drugs, which can be taken as pills, liquid, or inhalants. Bronchodilator aerosols can be used on a regular basis to prevent attacks and as needed to abort an asthma attack that has already started.

Inhalation has the advantage of bringing the drug directly to the site of the obstruction in the lungs. Many bronchodilators are packaged in small aerosol containers with a mouthpiece, enabling you to inhale a measured dose of the drug when necessary. Some people with asthma have learned to use home nebulizers; these devices mix the drug with a fine mist of water vapor, which is the ideal form for inhalation deep into the lungs.

If no pill, liquid, or inhalant succeeds in relieving the symptoms of a severe case of asthma, a bronchodilator drug may be injected into the bloodstream. This method almost always works. One group of drugs, corticosteroids, is effective not only in preventing asthma attacks but also in relieving the symptoms once an attack of asthma is under way.

If your asthma attacks are caused by an allergy to grass pollen or some other inhaled dust, it may be possible to desensitize your lungs to the responsible allergen with a series of injections. If you suspect that the cause may be something you eat or drink, you should consult your physician. He or she will

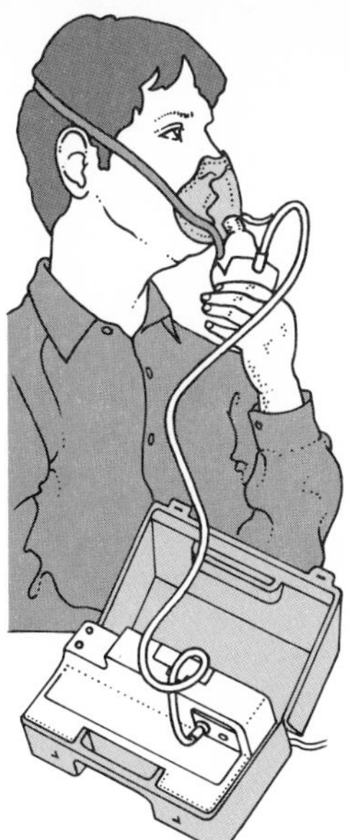

The asthma nebulizer
Asthma nebulizers are used to treat severe attacks in the hospital or at home. A measured dose of drugs is mixed with water in a reservoir, and either air or oxygen is blown through the fluid to produce a fine mist, which is inhaled through a face mask.

help you decide whether to begin a search for substances that may trigger an allergy or simply to rely on the control of symptoms with the highly effective drugs now available.

Despite the success of drug treatment, an asthma attack is sometimes severe enough to require hospitalization, for three reasons. First, you may be given drug treatment with a nebulizer (few patients have this equipment at home, and nebulizers used in hospitals are often more effective than home models). Second, if you are hospitalized, you can be given muscle-relaxant drugs and connected to a ventilator. This treatment eliminates muscle spasms in the air passages inside the lungs. And because the ventilator does the work of breathing, your chest muscles can relax and your respiratory system has a chance to recover. Third, the presence of nursing and medical staff 24 hours a day may relieve your anxiety about being unable to breathe.

What to do for an acute attack

A sudden, acute attack of asthma can be frightening for you and your family. In most cases your physician will have prescribed an inhalant of a bronchodilator or corticosteroid drug. If one dose does not relieve your wheezing, you can repeat it in 30 minutes if a second dose was prescribed by your physician. However, you should not use the inhalant again if the second dose proves to be ineffective. An overdose may be dangerous. Call your physician immediately; do not hesitate to call because, even with today's drugs, severe, prolonged asthma attacks may be life threatening.

Members of the family of a person with asthma are often alarmed when the person has a severe attack, but they may feel helpless because they do not know what to do about it. Here are some actions the family can take in such a situation:

1. Get the drugs and inhaling equipment together on a table, and note the time the person with asthma takes the first dose of any medications that the physician has prescribed for emergencies.

2. Help the person with asthma find the position that is most comfortable for him or her. Usually the best position is sitting up, leaning slightly forward, and resting on the elbows or arms. Plenty of fresh air is also important.

3. Don't gather around the person in a worried group. This only raises the level of anxiety for the person with asthma. Someone who is calm and level-headed should stay with the person. If possible, everyone else should quietly leave the room.

4. Keep on hand the telephone number of the physician who treats the person with asthma and call him or her promptly. If you call and the physician is not in, be ready to take the person, quickly but calmly, to the nearest hospital emergency department.

Emphysema

In emphysema, the lungs become less and less efficient because of progressive damage to the millions of alveoli, or air sacs, at the ends of the bronchioles in the lungs. Oxygen and carbon dioxide exchange takes place in the walls of the alveoli. Healthy lungs have an elastic, spongy texture, so they contract and expand fully. If the alveoli become stretched or rupture, the elasticity of the lungs is gradually destroyed. This type of damage occurs when the alveoli are constantly subjected to higher pressure than normal. This happens to people who have a long-standing lung disease. Certain conditions, such as chronic bronchitis (see p.380) or asthma (see previous article), for example, cause narrowing of the lung airways. The labored breathing and increased pressure caused by spasms weaken and may ultimately damage the walls of the alveoli.

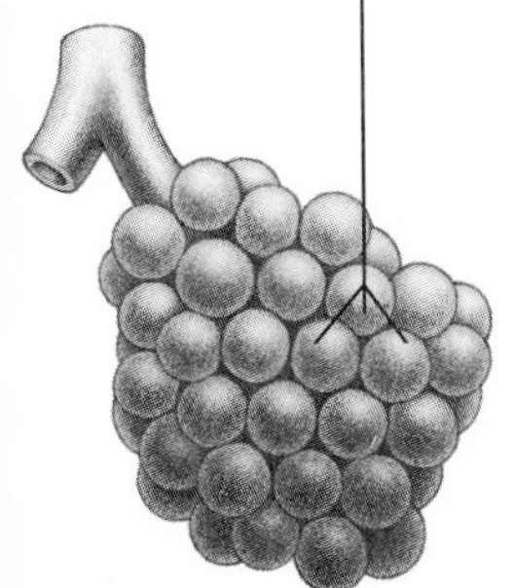

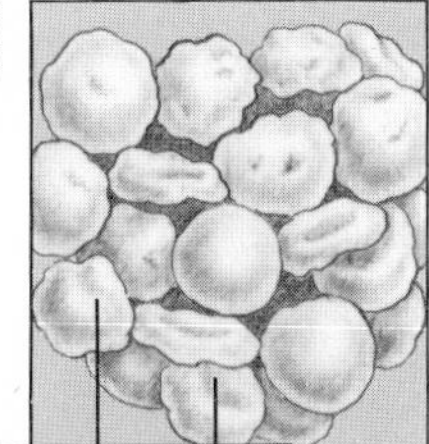

What happens in emphysema
Damaged alveoli (air sacs in the lungs) may burst and merge to make fewer but larger alveoli. This causes reduction in the lung's surface area. Less oxygen is able to travel through the walls of the alveoli and into the bloodstream.

What are the symptoms?

The main symptom of emphysema is shortness of breath, which is likely to get worse gradually over a period of years. If you have emphysema, your chest may become distended into a barrel-like shape. If you also wheeze, cough, and bring up phlegm, these are symptoms of bronchitis and asthma, which frequently coexist with emphysema.

What are the risks?

Emphysema is much more common in men than in women, and your chances of having it increase if you smoke and/or live in an area where the air is polluted. Some people are particularly susceptible to emphysema because of an inherited defect in a factor in the blood serum that protects the lung tissue in case of an infection. Without that factor infections that otherwise are successfully controlled by the body's defenses cause a loss of lung tissue. If your job requires exceptionally forceful use of lung power, you may also be highly susceptible. Some examples of such professions are glass blowing and playing a wind musical instrument. If you have increasing shortness of breath, you risk death from eventual respiratory failure. Emphysema also makes you more susceptible to chest infections such as pneumonia that can be life threatening. There is also a risk of a pneumothorax (see p.388). In addition, since blood cannot flow freely over the surfaces of the damaged alveoli, the resulting strain on the right side of the heart, which pumps blood to the lungs, can lead to heart failure (see p.408).

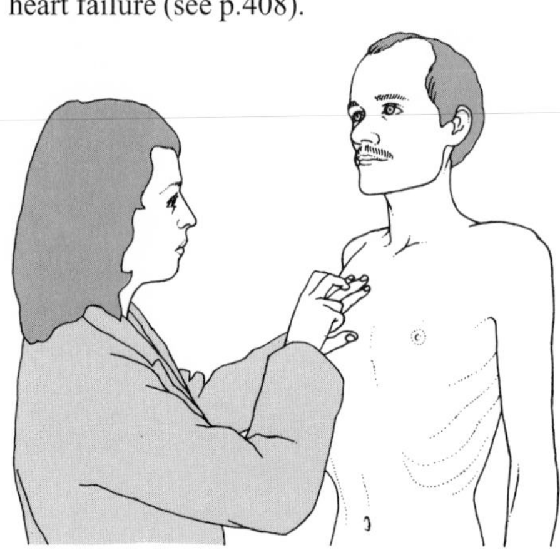

Percussing the chest
Because emphysema patients have enlarged air sacs in their lungs, a physician can diagnose the condition by percussing the chest. Your physician places two fingers on your chest and taps them with the fingers of the other hand. The enlarged alveoli produce a hollower sound than normal alveoli.

What should be done?
If you are experiencing breathlessness, you should consult your physician. In the initial examination, your physician will probably percuss, or finger tap, your chest, and listen to it with a stethoscope. He or she may also ask you to have a chest X ray and to blow hard into a flow meter or spirometer, machines that measure your breathing capacity. Additional breathing tests called pulmonary function tests may also be necessary.

What is the treatment?
Self-help: If you smoke, stop. Avoid places with polluted air. Keep away from people who have coughs or colds. Exercise moderately but regularly in fresh, clean air.
Professional help: Physicians can relieve the symptoms and delay the progress of emphysema, but they cannot cure it. If you have bronchitis along with emphysema, you may be advised to inhale bronchodilator drugs, which widen the airways and help prevent further damage to the alveoli. Because bronchitis and lung infections of any kind aggravate emphysema, the best way to help control the disease is to prevent respiratory infection so your physician may prescribe antibiotics.

Very few patients with very severe cases of emphysema have been successfully treated with a heart-and-lung transplant. Although a lung transplant is usually all that is required to treat emphysema, for technical reasons the heart and lungs are frequently transplanted together (see Transplants, p.432).

Pneumonia

(pneumonitis)

Pneumonia, also called pneumonitis, is not a specific disease. Rather, it is a general term for several kinds of inflammation that can occur in the lungs. Pneumonia is usually caused by a bacterial or a viral infection, but it can also be caused by chemical damage to the lungs from inhaling a poisonous gas. The pneumonia, or lung inflammation, can be anything from a complication of an upper respiratory tract infection to a life-threatening illness.

The symptoms, the treatment, the impact, and the outcome of pneumonia depend on the cause, the general health of the person concerned, and on other factors such as the effectiveness of drug treatments. For instance, viral pneumonia does not respond to treatment with antibiotics. See the table that accompanies this article for a comparison of the causes and symptoms of some of the most common types of pneumonia.

The many varieties of pneumonia have led to many popular and medical descriptive terms. If you are told that you have "double" pneumonia, it means that both your lungs are affected. If your pneumonia is caused by bacterialike microbes called *Mycoplasma*, you may be said to have "atypical" pneumonia. "Bronchopneumonia" consists of patchy inflammation of the alveoli of one or both lungs, and "lobar" pneumonia affects the entire volume of one or more lobes of the lung. Inflammation may involve lung tissue between the walls of the alveoli. This is called "interstitial" pneumonia.

What are the symptoms?
No single symptom is characteristic of all types of pneumonia. You should consider the possibility of pneumonia, however, if you already have a respiratory illness with symptoms such as a cough and fever, and you

become short of breath with little or no activity. Additional symptoms to watch for besides coughing and a fever are chills, sweating, chest pains, cyanosis (a bluish tinge to the lips and skin under your nails), blood in the phlegm, and, occasionally, mental confusion or delirium. The larger the lung area that is affected, the more severe will be the symptoms you experience.

How quickly the symptoms begin and which symptoms are most prominent varies with the cause of the infection. An especially virulent strain of the influenza virus can cause a pneumonia that can kill a weakened person within 24 hours. In a healthy young adult pneumonia resulting from a mild respiratory infection may cause symptoms that are no worse than those of a severe cold.

What are the risks?

In the US, about 15 people out of 1,000 have pneumonia each year. The disorder is often the final complication of some other debilitating disease, and this is why many people who get pneumonia die of it. Anyone whose resistance is already low is very susceptible to pneumonia, so for people who are dying of heart failure, cancer, stroke, or emphysema, the actual cause of death is often pneumonia. In anyone who is semiconscious and bedridden for a period of time, infection of the lungs is an extremely common occurrence. This is because under such conditions the normal coughing reflex that keeps the lungs clear of mucus and stagnant fluid is reduced, or possibly even absent.

People are also much more likely to get pneumonia if they are very young (under 2) or very old (over 75), if they have a chronic chest disease such as asthma (see p.381) or some other chronic illness that reduces the body's resistance to infections, or if they are heavy smokers or drinkers.

Pneumonia is a common illness in people whose immune systems have been reduced in efficiency. Such people include (1) those who have had an organ transplant and have been given immunosuppressive drugs to prevent rejection of the transplant (see Transplants, p.432); (2) people who have leukemia, Hodgkin's disease, or some other form of cancer and who are being treated with corticosteroid drugs or anticancer drugs, because these medications all suppress the

COMMON KINDS OF PNEUMONIA

Cause	Onset of symptoms	Temperature	Other possible symptoms
Pneumococcus bacterium	Abrupt (within hours of infection)	Up to 104°F (40°C) or above	Chills, chest pain, blue tinge of lips and under nails, and, later, a cough with rust-colored sputum
Influenza virus	Abrupt (within hours of infection)	104°F (40°C) or above	Severe dry cough, blue tinge of lips and under nails
Cytomegalovirus	Gradual (over several days)	About 101°F (38.3°C)	Dry cough, lethargy in the afternoon
Other viruses	4 to 5 days after infection	About 101°F (38.3°C)	Dry cough, tiredness
Mycoplasma (bacteriumlike)	3 to 4 days after infection	About 101°F (38.3°C)	Dry irritating cough, headache
Legionnaire's disease bacterium	2 to 10 days after infection	Up to 104°F (40°C) or above	Nausea, vomiting, chills, muscle aches, headache, bloodstained sputum, chest pain
Pneumocystis carinii (a protozoan)	Abrupt or gradual (over several weeks) in AIDS patients, kidney transplant patients, or others with impaired immune systems	About 104°F (40 °C)	Rapid breathing,cough, shortness of breath

body's immune system; (3) people with certain chronic diseases (such as rheumatoid arthritis) who are taking corticosteroids or similar drugs; and (4) people infected with HIV (human immunodeficiency virus) or who have AIDS (acquired immune deficiency syndrome), whose immune systems have already been impaired by the disease.

In all these cases, pneumonia may be caused by microorganisms (such as the cytomegalovirus or *Pneumocystis carinii*) that usually affect people whose immune systems are already weakened. These "opportunistic" infections often have a slow, subtle onset so that at first the affected person may simply feel listless, lack energy, and may possibly have a slight fever and a dry cough. Later, the more usual symptoms of pneumonia develop—shortness of breath, chest pain, and fever, for example. The diagnosis of these less common types of pneumonia depends on laboratory tests, including (for *Pneumocystis carinii* pneumonia) a transbronchial lung biopsy, in which a specimen of lung tissue is removed through a bronchoscope (a viewing tube). However, biopsy is no longer always needed to diagnose this kind of pneumonia since techniques for finding the organism in the sputum have become increasingly accurate.

Because pneumonia varies so much, no generalizations can be made about its outcome. In older, weak, or debilitated people, the main risk is death. Any type of pneumonia may lead to pleurisy (see next article) or empyema (see p.390). However, in healthy adults influenza and other virus pneumonias can be, but are rarely, fatal. Bacterial pneumonia can be virulent but at least is a type of pneumonia that can be treated with antibiotic drugs. With increasing age or chronic illness, the chances of surviving even a mild case of pneumonia are reduced. So it's important to seek treatment promptly for respiratory illness if you are older or have a chronic disease.

What should be done?

Even if you have some of the symptoms usually associated with pneumonia, do not assume that you have it. Assume instead that you have a cold or other infection of the respiratory tract, and take care of yourself accordingly. Consult your physician immediately, however, if you become short of breath unexpectedly, if your chest hurts when you breathe, or if you cough up blood-stained sputum. Your physician will probably listen to your chest through a stethoscope, percuss (finger tap) your chest, and ask you questions about the onset of symptoms and your smoking habits. It may be possible for your physician to make a firm diagnosis of pneumonia, and even of the type of pneumonia, based on such an examination. However, more tests such as a chest X ray and laboratory examination of both blood and phlegm samples may be necessary.

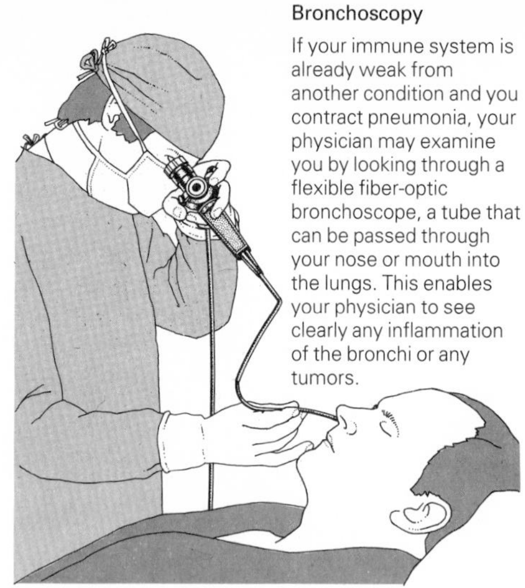

Bronchoscopy

If your immune system is already weak from another condition and you contract pneumonia, your physician may examine you by looking through a flexible fiber-optic bronchoscope, a tube that can be passed through your nose or mouth into the lungs. This enables your physician to see clearly any inflammation of the bronchi or any tumors.

What is the treatment?

Self-help: None is possible.

Professional help: The best treatment may be simply a combination of keeping warm, drinking lots of liquids, and taking soothing cough medicines and antibiotics. However, professional supervision and observation may be desirable during the early stages of pneumonia, especially if there is some doubt about the precise cause and extent of the inflammation. If your physician suspects certain types of pneumonia that can suddenly become severe in a matter of hours, he or she may recommend hospitalization.

Antibiotic medications may be given orally or by injection. There is a wide variety of antibiotics, and your physician will choose one based largely on the probable cause of your illness. Laboratory tests of your blood and sputum should indicate which microorganism is causing your infection. Your physician will also need to know if you are allergic to any antibiotics.

Painkillers such as aspirin help to relieve chest pain. If you are very breathless and your skin looks blue, you are probably in need of oxygen, which is supplied with a face mask or a tube in your nose. If you have problems with your lungs despite all attempts at treatment, your physician may recommend bronchoscopy to exclude other causes such as lung cancer or a foreign object, or to obtain samples of secretions (such as mucus) for additional laboratory study.

A healthy young person should recover completely from pneumonia within 2 to 3 weeks. Even in cases of viral pneumonia, the chances of serious complications developing are minimal, since antibiotics can prevent secondary bacterial infection.

Following recovery, you may still feel very tired and have a persistent cough for a long time after the infection is gone. A heavy cigarette smoker, or someone who is chronically ill, may need many months to recover from pneumonia.

Pleurisy and pleural effusion

When you breathe normally, your lungs and rib cage expand and contract easily and rhythmically. Each lung is enclosed in a moist, smooth membrane called a pleura. The outer layer of the pleura lines the rib cage. Between the two thin layers is a virtually imperceptible space, which is called the pleural space. If either of your pleura becomes inflamed and roughened because of an infection, this seriously and painfully impedes the movement of the layers, and you have pleurisy, or pleuritis.

Pleurisy is actually a symptom of an underlying disease rather than a disease in itself. The pleura may become inflamed as a complication of pneumonia (see previous article), tuberculosis (see p.602), pneumothorax (see next article), or a chest injury. Inflammation of the pleura sometimes creates a further complication by allowing fluid, which may be clear or contain pus, to seep into the pleural space. This condition is called pleural effusion.

Pleural effusion can also occur as a complication of a generalized disease such as rheumatoid arthritis (see p.589), a liver or kidney disorder, or heart failure (see p.408). Cancer cells that are spreading across the surface of the pleura from a tumor in the lungs, breast, or ovaries can also sometimes cause pleural effusion.

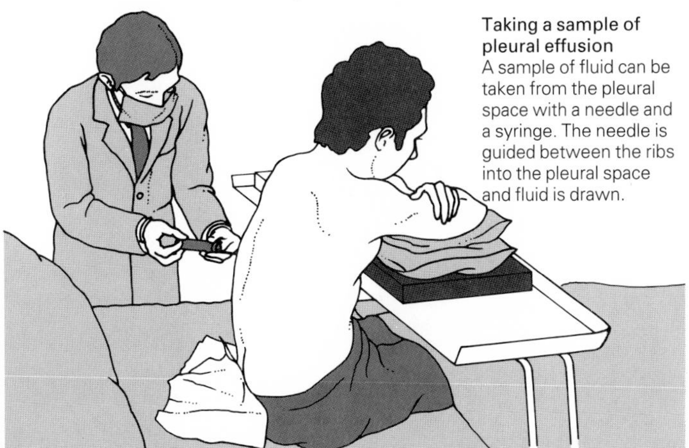

Taking a sample of pleural effusion
A sample of fluid can be taken from the pleural space with a needle and a syringe. The needle is guided between the ribs into the pleural space and fluid is drawn.

What are the symptoms?

If you have pleurisy, it hurts to breathe deeply, cough, or sneeze. You may also have severe, but one-sided, continuous chest pain. These symptoms are accompanied by others that are associated with the underlying disorder. The pain may ease when pleural effusion follows the onset of pleurisy, because the accumulating fluid may prevent the roughened or inflamed layers of the pleura from rubbing against each other.

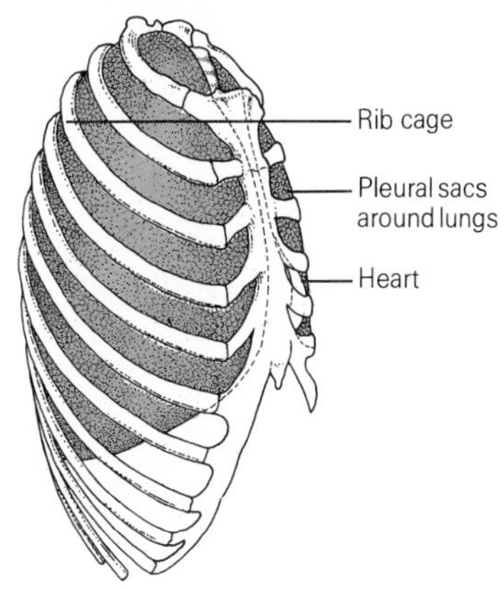

What are the risks?

In most cases the risks of pleurisy are the same as the risks associated with the underlying cause. Advanced pleural effusion can compress the lungs and cause severe breathlessness. Pleural effusion may also lead to empyema (see p.390).

What should be done?

Consult your physician if breathing becomes painful, you seem unusually short of breath, and either or both of these symptoms is accompanied by a fever, no matter how slight. After questioning you about your symptoms and previous illness, your physician will probably listen to your chest with a stethoscope and will percuss, or finger tap, your chest while listening for typical sounds (friction rub) made by irritated pleura and pleural effusion. You may need a chest X ray to help verify that you have an effusion and determine what has caused the pleurisy.

If you have pleural effusion, one way to diagnose the cause is to analyze the fluid, so a sample of fluid may be taken from the pleural space with a needle and syringe.

What is the treatment?

Because pleurisy and pleural effusion are symptoms of other disorders, the only way to cure them is to treat the underlying disease. Meanwhile, to ease the chest pains, your physician may recommend that you use a nonprescription painkiller such as aspirin.

Pneumothorax

A pneumothorax occurs when air gets into the pleural space between the two layers of the pleura, a membrane that surrounds each lung. Part of the lung, sometimes the entire lung, collapses, and the air is squeezed out. A pneumothorax may be caused by a chest injury; more commonly, it is caused by air escaping into the pleura from a ruptured blister on the surface of the lung. A small pneumothorax often simply disappears on its own. But sometimes enough air enters the pleural space to cause large portions of the lung to collapse.

What are the symptoms?

The major symptoms of a pneumothorax are breathlessness and chest pain, generally on the affected side, but sometimes at the side of the neck adjacent to the shoulder. The pain is usually sudden and sharp, though it may be little more than a sensation of discomfort. You may also have a feeling of tightness across your chest. The severity of the symptoms depends on the volume of the compressed lung and on your general health.

If you are young and in good health, you may have slight pain and little difficulty in breathing, even if you have a fairly large pneumothorax and a large portion of your lung collapses.

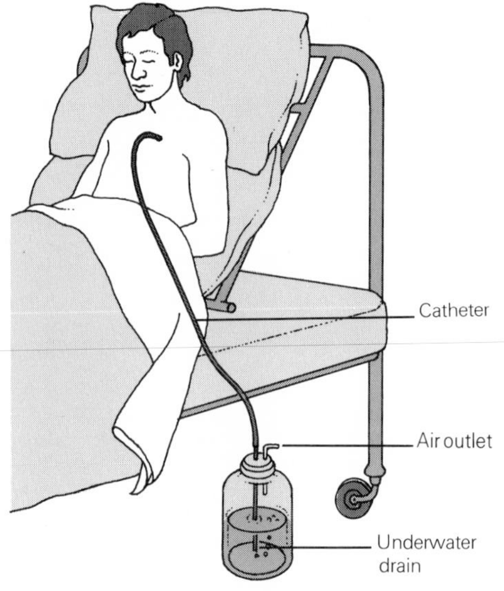

Treatment
To remove air from the pleural space a tube is inserted into the pleural space. As you breathe out and pleural volume decreases, air is squeezed out through the tube. An underwater drain and a seal on the drain ensure that the air travels only away from the pleural space.

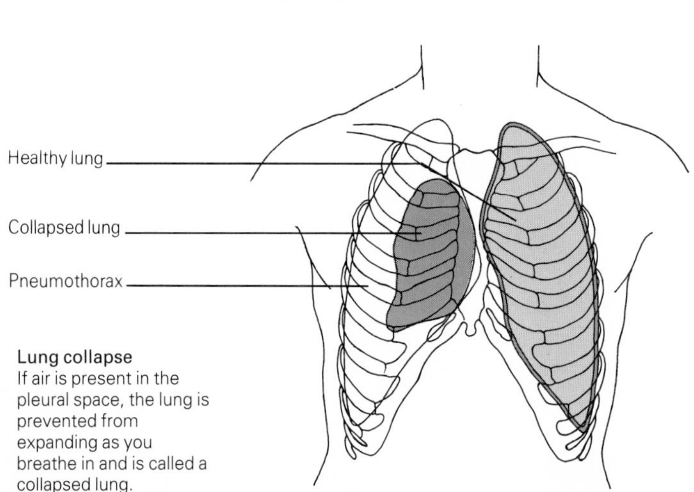

Lung collapse
If air is present in the pleural space, the lung is prevented from expanding as you breathe in and is called a collapsed lung.

If you are a middle-aged or older person and have emphysema, a small pneumothorax can be very painful and cause extreme difficulty in breathing.

What are the risks?

Pneumothorax is relatively rare. It occurs primarily in otherwise healthy young men, for no apparent reason, and in middle-aged or older men and women whose lungs have already been damaged by asthma, chronic bronchitis, emphysema, lung abscess, or tuberculosis.

How serious a pneumothorax is depends on how the air is getting into the pleura. Often a small pneumothorax is not serious and heals by itself. But if there is a tear in the pleural membrane that covers the lung that allows the pneumothorax to get larger, you will become increasingly breathless and have increasing pain as more and more of the lung collapses. If the disorder remains untreated, death from respiratory failure can follow.

What should be done?

If you suspect that you have this condition, consult your physician immediately. An examination of your chest can reveal a large pneumothorax, but your physician may need a chest X ray to find a small one. In any case, even if there is only a suspicion of a pneumothorax, you will probably be admitted to a hospital for observation and tests.

What is the treatment?

The treatment depends on the size of the pneumothorax and the condition of your lungs. If the pneumothorax is very small, the leak may seal itself off and you will need only a few days of bed rest to make sure that the air in the pleural space is gone and that the collapsed portion of the lung has regained its elasticity and is full of air again. However, if the extent of lung collapse is larger, then it is usually necessary to suck the air out of the pleural space with a tube known as a catheter, which is inserted between the ribs and into the pleural space. If the air leak persists, even with a catheter in the pleural space, surgery may be needed to close the leak.

Bronchiectasis

Bronchiectasis is the distortion and enlargement of one or more of the bronchi, or main air passages into the lungs, often as a result of frequent infections in childhood. The disorder takes years to develop. It leads to impaired drainage of the fluid that is normally secreted by bronchial cells. This fluid may then remain in the lungs where it becomes stagnant. The stagnant fluid can lead to further infection.

What are the symptoms?

The main symptom of bronchiectasis is a frequent cough that brings up large quantities of green or yellow phlegm, or sputum, which sometimes contains spots of blood. The quantity of phlegm generally increases when you change position. This is especially true when you lie down at night or when you arise in the morning.

If you have bronchiectasis, you are susceptible to repeated infections of the lung when you catch a cold.

What are the risks?

Bronchiectasis is rare today because many childhood infections that caused the disorder, such as sinusitis and the chest infections that often followed measles or whooping cough, now can be prevented by immunization or effectively treated with antibiotics. Similarly, tuberculosis, a disease that also damages the bronchi, has become rare. Even people who have bronchiectasis can usually lead active lives if they take antibiotics at the first signs of infection.

What should be done?

If you repeatedly cough up large amounts of green or yellow phlegm, consult your physician, who will probably listen to your chest with a stethoscope. He or she may also want you to have a chest X ray, a CT scan, and a bronchoscopy, a procedure in which your physician examines your lungs by looking into an instrument attached to a tube passed down your throat via your nose or mouth. The results of these tests will help your physician make a diagnosis.

What is the treatment?

Self-help: If you have bronchiectasis, make a special effort to avoid getting colds and sore throats. Do not smoke, and stay out of dusty or contaminated locations. If the lower part of your lung is infected, as it probably is if you have bronchiectasis, your physician may recommend a self-help technique called postural drainage to help get rid of bronchial secretions. In this technique, you place yourself so that the bronchus leading to the affected lobe of your lung is pointing down. The fluid then drains out, and you can cough it up. Lying on a bed with your head and chest hanging over the edge for 5 to 10 minutes twice a day can help your lungs drain. Having another person gently clap your back and the sides of your chest may loosen phlegm.

Professional help: At the first sign of bronchiectasis your physician will probably prescribe an antibiotic and instruct you to take the entire prescription even if the infection seems to clear up. If your condition is very localized, if a lot of blood is mixed with the phlegm, or if you have repeated episodes of pneumonia in the same portion of your lung, your physician may advise you to have the affected part of the lung removed. Such surgery is seldom necessary for this condition. However, surgery may cure bronchiectasis only if the involved segment of bronchus can be removed.

Lung abscess

An abscess, or a contained infectious area, in the lung usually results from one of two conditions. It may be a complication of some type of pneumonia (see p.384), or it may be caused by inhaling material, such as food or a fragment of a tooth, while you are either conscious or unconscious. You might inhale such a fragment while under an anesthetic, knocked out by a head injury, or drunk. Abscesses associated with pneumonia are very rare because antibiotics usually prevent such complications. Lung abscesses occur most often among people who are suffering from malnutrition.

The main symptoms are alternating chills and fever. You may also have chest pain and a cough that brings up thick phlegm that contains pus and blood. A chest X ray will help your physician locate the site of the abscess, and tests of the phlegm will identify what has caused the abscess. You should recover completely if you take the prescribed antibiotics. If the abscess is chronic and thick-walled, it might be necessary to drain or remove it surgically.

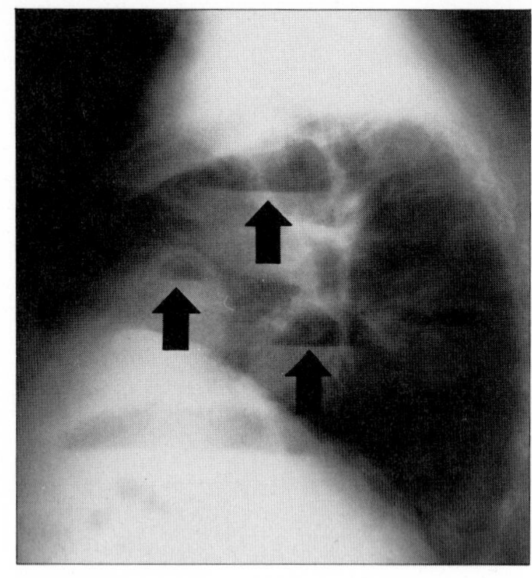

X-ray diagnosis of a lung abscess
An abscess in the lung is at least partially filled with fluid. The fluid-filled area shows up on an X ray as a pale patch surrounded by a dark, air-filled area.

Empyema

Empyema means an accumulation of pus in any body cavity. The term is generally used to refer to an infected pleural effusion (see p.387). In pleural effusion, fluid seeps into the space between the two layers of the pleura, the membrane that surrounds the lung and also covers the inner surface of the chest cavity. In empyema, this fluid has thickened into pus. This may be a complication of a lung disease such as pneumonia (see p.384) or of an abdominal infection that crosses the diaphragm and spreads into the chest. There are no special symptoms of empyema, and the diagnosis is based on an examination of a sample of the fluid taken from the pleural space. This fluid is removed from the space with a needle and syringe.

Empyema has become rare since the introduction of antibiotics. Most people who develop it are already being treated for some underlying disorder. The appropriate treatment and prospects for full recovery from this condition depend on what the underlying disorder is.

Pneumoconiosis

(and other dust diseases)

Pneumoconiosis is lung disease that occurs as a result of the inhalation of metallic or mineral dusts. The term refers to an occupational disease resulting from long-term exposure to dusts. If you have been inhaling such particles continuously for many years, little patches of scar tissue may have formed in one or both of your lungs. If the scar tissue caused by the reaction to the particles has made your lungs less flexible, you have some type of pneumoconiosis. A common form of the disorder in this country is appropriately named coal miner's pneumoconiosis, or black lung disease. Silicosis is another form of pneumoconiosis. It affects workers in quarries and foundries, stone masons, metal grinders, and miners who drill rock. Others who may also be susceptible to pneumoconiosis are people who work with aluminum, asbestos, beryllium, and talc. People who work with cotton, sugar cane, grain dust, wood dust, and various synthetic fibers may develop reactive airway disease (a form of asthma).

It usually takes about 10 years from first exposure before a dust disease becomes apparent. Coal miner's pneumoconiosis (anthracosis) sometimes takes up to 25 years to develop fully.

What are the symptoms?

Breathlessness from exertion is the dominant symptom of pneumoconiosis. In silicosis the symptoms usually become progressively worse, and there may be other symptoms associated with tuberculosis of the lungs (see p.602). In all types of dust disease there is usually a cough with phlegm, or sputum, similar to the cough in chronic bronchitis (see p.380). The phlegm of coal miners with pneumoconiosis is often black.

What should be done?

If you are exposed to dust regularly at work, find out what the dust is and if it carries some risk of pneumoconiosis. Check with your employee safety committee, management, union, or company physician. If you work under these conditions and have chest complaints, see your physician, who will probably want to see a chest X ray and results from pulmonary function tests to find out if you are severely affected. If you are working in dusty, unventilated conditions, it may be advisable to change jobs, if possible. Workers' compensation and other laws are available to help workers stricken with these diseases. However, it is important to find out about your state's eligibility requirements for compensation and treatment programs.

If you smoke, give it up. If you have a potentially serious case of pneumoconiosis, you are more likely to develop other disorders or diseases that are caused by or intensified by tobacco smoke, including lung cancer (see p.392).

What is the treatment?

Only a few types of pneumoconiosis can be treated, usually with corticosteroid drugs. However, the best treatment is prevention and avoiding unventilated, dusty work areas.

Farmer's lung

Farmer's lung is caused by frequent exposure to a fungus that grows in moldy hay or grain. It affects only people who have become allergic to the fungus from earlier exposure. The allergy causes lung inflammation that narrows the air passages and thickens the alveoli walls. A similar allergic reaction to certain kinds of fungus occurs among workers who deal with malt, mushrooms, sugar cane, and several other plant substances. Another similar disorder affects people who handle animals in laboratories and pigeon breeders or others who have frequent contact with birds.

What are the symptoms?

The main symptom of farmer's lung is breathlessness. This becomes a problem a few hours after you are exposed to the fungus. It generally goes away after another few hours. The breathlessness is usually accompanied by a dry cough. Since you may also have symptoms such as fever, chills, and headache, you may mistake farmer's lung for persistent, recurring influenza or may even think that it is asthma. A clue to the diagnosis is that symptoms recur repeatedly after you are in the barn or wherever the contaminated hay or grain is located.

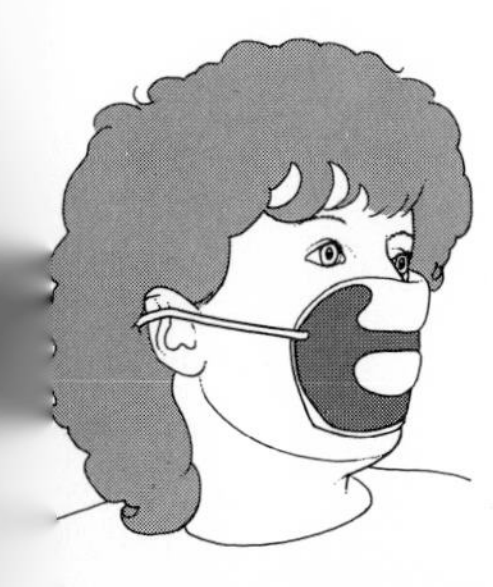

Avoiding farmer's lung
This is the most simple, least expensive dust mask. It has limited effectiveness. Highly sensitive, heavily exposed people may need more sophisticated types of protection, such as cartridge or cannister masks.

What are the risks?

Farmer's lung and similar allergic reactions are rare, since only a small proportion of the people who are in constant contact with the fungi are susceptible to the disorder.

If you do have recurring symptoms, and you are repeatedly exposed to the fungus, your condition will probably get worse over time. Whenever there is longstanding, untreated inflammation of the lungs, the elastic lung tissue is replaced by stiff scar tissue. The result of lung inflammation that goes untreated is permanent scarring, progressive breathlessness, and potentially fatal respiratory failure and heart failure (see p.408).

What should be done?

Consult your physician if you have repeated episodes of breathlessness. If you are frequently exposed to any substance that can cause farmer's lung, be sure to tell your physician. You will probably need to have a chest X ray and some blood tests so that your physician can establish the nature and extent of the disease.

What is the treatment?

Self-help: Avoid further exposure to the fungus. Otherwise, wear a protective mask over your nose and mouth whenever you may be exposed to the substance. If possible, you may need to find another job that does not expose you to the fungus.

Professional help: If you have had farmer's lung for some time, it may be much more difficult to treat than it is in earlier stages. The most effective treatment for farmer's lung may be corticosteroid drugs.

Lung cancer

(bronchogenic carcinoma)

Although there are several kinds of lung cancer, only one, bronchogenic carcinoma, is common, and it is almost always caused by lung damage from cigarette smoking.

Inhaled tobacco smoke damages the cells that line the bronchi. Many scientists believe that the damaged cells (called dysplasia) represent an early stage of cancer. Some of these cells may gradually form a wartlike tumor, which is the starting point of bronchogenic carcinoma. As the tumor grows, it spreads into the lungs from the bronchi. The cancer cells often get into the bloodstream and are carried to the brain, liver, bone, and skin, where they establish metastases, or secondary cancers.

What are the symptoms?

The first symptom of bronchogenic carcinoma is usually a cough, which is most often an increase in what the person considers a "normal" smoker's cough. The disease is closely associated with chronic bronchitis (see p.380). More than half the people who develop lung cancer have had bronchitis for years. Along with the cough there is generally some phlegm, which may be bloodstained. You may also be a little breathless and you may have chest pains. They are either sharp pains that become sharper when you take a deep breath, or dull and persistent pains. You may sometimes wheeze.

Sometimes the first symptoms of lung cancer originate from other organs to which the cancer has already spread. Bronchogenic carcinoma spreads in about one out of eight cases, and in those cases the secondary cancer may alert your physician that the primary cancer is in the lung. The symptoms of the secondary cancer depend on where the cancer cells have settled. If they are in your brain, you may have headaches, feel confused, have an epileptic seizure, or have other symptoms. In the bones the symptoms are pain, swelling, or even fracture. If the cancer is in your skin, cystlike swellings appear. If it is in your liver the symptoms may be fatigue, weight loss, and jaundice.

What are the risks?

Bronchogenic carcinoma is the most common form of cancer in the US. It affects more men than women, probably because lung cancer takes a long time to develop, and smoking has been more common among men than women. There has recently been a drop in the incidence of the disease among men and a rise in the incidence among women. This may be because men are smoking less but smoking by women has been on the rise.

Your chances of getting the disease vary according to how much you smoke. If you have never smoked, it is very unlikely that you will get bronchogenic carcinoma. Light smokers are ten times as susceptible as nonsmokers, and heavy smokers are 25 times as susceptible. As soon as you stop smoking, the risk starts to decrease. After 15 or more years of nonsmoking, you have about the same chance of getting bronchogenic cancer as do lifelong nonsmokers.

If lung cancer is discovered early, either as soon as the symptoms develop or by chance, the affected portion of the lung can some-

OPERATION:

Lung removal

(pneumonectomy or lobectomy)

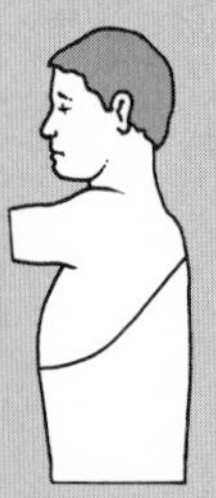
Site of incision

Pneumonectomy is an operation to remove a lung. If a lobe of a lung is removed, it is called a lobectomy. If the tumor is small it may be removed with a wedge of lung tissue. Surgery is performed to treat lung cancer when the disease is diagnosed at an early stage and there is a good chance for a cure. Occasionally it is performed for tuberculosis, bronchiectasis, or lung abscess.

During the operation You receive a general anesthetic. The surgeon makes an incision around the rib cage on the affected side along the line of a lower rib. One rib is usually removed and the affected lung or part of the lung is removed through the gap. The operation usually takes between 1 and 3 hours.

After the operation You will spend a couple of days in the intensive-care unit. While there, you will receive some nutrients and drugs intravenously, and at least one drainage tube will drain the incision. You may have to breathe through an oxygen mask. You can help your own recovery best by coughing frequently to bring up any secretions.

Convalescence You will need to convalesce for several months after you leave the hospital, as you gradually recover. You will be strongly advised to quit smoking for life.

times be removed by a surgeon. About one fourth of patients treated surgically survive for 5 years or longer, but for many people, the disease is already too far advanced for treatment by surgery by the time a lung cancer is found.

Smokers increase their risk of contracting not only cancer, but also several other life-threatening diseases that are associated with the smoking habit. These diseases include coronary artery disease (see p.400), stroke (see p.285), chronic bronchitis (see p.380), and emphysema (see p.383).

What should be done?

To avoid bronchogenic carcinoma, stop smoking now (see How to quit smoking, p.51). A tumor takes years to develop, and if you remove the cause, the process may slow down or even stop. If you are experiencing symptoms such as increasingly severe smoker's cough, chest pains, and blood in the phlegm, you should see your physician, who will probably listen to your chest with a stethoscope and arrange for a chest X ray. If the X ray shows signs of a possible cancer or if your physician suspects you have cancer, you may be referred to a chest specialist, who may use a bronchoscope to look for cancerous growths in your bronchi. You may need a CT scan.

Medical myth

There is no point in quitting smoking if you have smoked for years. If you are going to get lung cancer, it can no longer be avoided.

Wrong. There is firm evidence that people who have smoked heavily for many years improve their chances of avoiding lung cancer by quitting.

What is the treatment?

Self-help: No self-help is possible, except for quitting smoking.

Professional help: Surgical removal of the cancer is the best possible treatment for bronchogenic carcinoma, but in many cases the cancer turns out to be too advanced or other health problems (heart disease, reduced breathing capacity due to chronic bronchitis or emphysema) prevent surgical removal. Radiation therapy sometimes slows down the progress of the cancer and may relieve the symptoms for months or in some cases years.

Another possibility is treatment with cytotoxic drugs (chemotherapy). These drugs kill cancer cells while doing little damage to normal cells. Drug treatment for bronchogenic carcinoma is similar to methods that have proved effective in cancers such as Hodgkin's disease (see p.464) and leukemia (see p.457). One or more courses of treatment may be necessary, each lasting several weeks. The side effects of the drugs are very unpleasant, but most people who undergo chemotherapy find their symptoms are relieved and the progress of the disease halted. The remission that follows treatment with drugs may last months or sometimes several years, but a permanent cure of bronchogenic carcinoma is rare.

Which treatment is most appropriate for you depends on the extent of the disease, the results of the biopsy (laboratory examination of a piece of the tumor), and your general health. Discuss the possibilities with your physician. Although a diagnosis of lung cancer is very serious, it is possible to treat it and sometimes to cure it.

Deaths caused by lung cancer

Lung cancer was a rare disease in the US before cigarette smoking became a popular habit. Since records of deaths from lung cancer have been kept, the numbers rose steadily and steeply for men until only a few years ago. The number of women who died of lung cancer rose only slightly between 1900 and 1940, but in the last 50 years there has been a large increase. This is because more women have decided to smoke cigarettes in the years since World War II. In a recent year in the US, the survival rate for people diagnosed with lung cancer 5 years before was 15 percent.

Interstitial fibrosis

Interstitial fibrosis is also called diffuse interstitial fibrosis or pulmonary fibrosis. The function of the lungs is impaired by an accumulation of fibrous matter that thickens the walls of the alveoli. The alveoli are tiny air sacs at the ends of the bronchioles. In the walls of these tiny sacs the oxygen we need to live is taken from breathed air by the blood. Here, too, the blood releases the waste gas carbon dioxide to the lung to be exhaled. Interstitial fibrosis is a rare, serious disorder. Its cause is unknown.

What are the symptoms?

Interstitial fibrosis may be either acute or chronic. In the acute form of this condition,

Clubbed fingers
Deformed fingers are a symptom of chronic lung disease. Your cuticles seem to disappear and your fingernails curve around the ends of your fingers. The ends of your toes may be similarly affected. The reason for this deformity is not yet known.

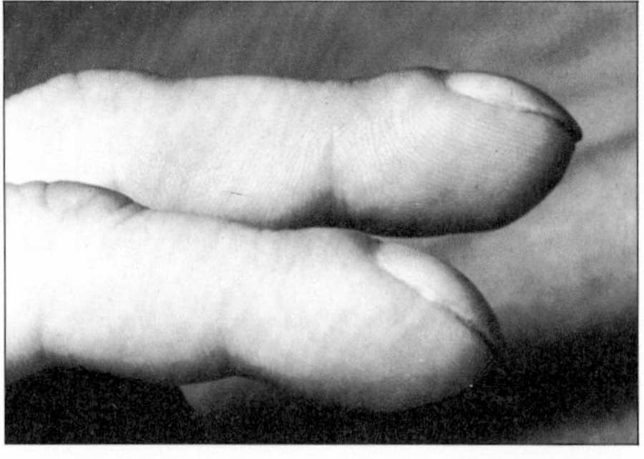

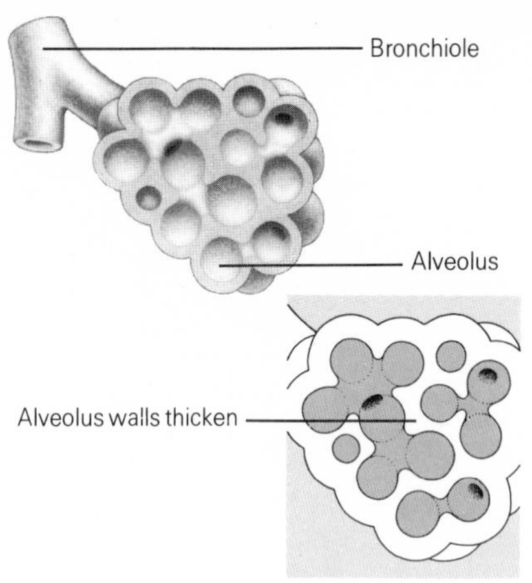

Fibrous tissue in the alveoli walls
Very rarely, fibrous tissue can develop in the walls of the alveoli and reduce both their size and their potential for getting oxygen into the bloodstream. This tissue also affects the elasticity of the lungs, so that they expand and contract with less efficiency.

the major symptom is increasingly severe shortness of breath, with coughing. The progress of the disease is so rapid that most people who get it die within a year. The chronic form of the condition is more common. It starts in middle age, and the symptoms develop much more slowly. Another symptom that is found with chronic interstitial fibrosis is clubbing, a deformity of the fingertips that also occurs in a number of other chronic lung and heart diseases.

What is the treatment?

Treatment with corticosteroid drugs may relieve the symptoms. Both acute and chronic forms of this condition end in respiratory failure and, ultimately, in death.

Pulmonary edema

Pulmonary edema is an acute, dramatic, and sometimes life-threatening symptom of heart failure (see p.408). The edema, or swollen tissue, results from inefficient pumping action of the left side of the heart. This causes the blood in the pulmonary veins, which bring oxygenated blood to the heart from the lungs, to become dammed up. This raises the pressure in these and other blood vessels in the lungs. As a result, fluid seeps from the blood vessels into the alveoli, the saclike parts of the lungs where oxygen and carbon dioxide are exchanged, and the spaces between them. This accumulation of fluid stiffens the lungs, making it very difficult to breathe and interfering with the normal uptake of oxygen in the lung. If you have this problem, you suddenly become breathless. This is called an episode of pulmonary edema. It sometimes happens to someone who has heart disease and is not aware of it.

What are the symptoms?

An episode of pulmonary edema consists of breathlessness that becomes progressively worse over a few hours. This often occurs in the early morning. You may have a frightening sense of needing to fight for breath. The breathlessness is generally accompanied by a cough, which is dry and tickling in the early stages, but which may eventually bring up bloodstained, frothy phlegm, or sputum. In a severe episode your skin may look blue because there is not enough oxygen in your blood.

What should be done?

If you have an episode of pulmonary edema, you may already be under treatment for heart failure. At the first sign of sudden severe breathlessness, contact your physician immediately. You will probably need to get to a hospital promptly. Oxygen is often necessary, and therefore an ambulance or medically equipped emergency vehicle may be needed. This is an emergency that will respond to treatment, but delay may be fatal. Your blood pressure will be taken and your chest examined with a stethoscope. Chest pain in addition to breathlessness may indicate that you are also having a myocardial infarction, or heart attack (see p.406).

What is the treatment?
Self-help: Try to keep calm. Sit up in a chair to make breathing easier.
Professional help: The main objective is to relieve breathlessness as quickly as possible. This is done best in a hospital intensive-care unit, where you receive oxygen and where an electrocardiogram monitors your heart rate and rhythm. Your physician may prescribe one of several drugs, which can be injected directly into a vein to act quickly. Morphine is used to slow and deepen breathing. A diuretic will help drain fluid from your lungs and open up filled air spaces in the lungs. Vasodilators are used to expand arteries and veins, reducing the workload of the heart. If you are not taking digitalis, your physician may start you on it to strengthen the pumping action of your heart. If the episode of pulmonary edema has been triggered by a chest infection, your physician may also prescribe an antibiotic.

If pulmonary edema is treated rapidly and efficiently, and if your episode has not been brought on by a heart attack, your stay in the hospital may be brief. Several tests of heart function and efficiency may be performed. Your physician will probably continue to treat you for heart failure in order to prevent further complications.

Adult respiratory distress syndrome

Adult respiratory distress syndrome is rapidly developing and extensive injury to the lung resulting from injury, infection, or in rare cases, some types of allergies. It is life threatening and has been given its name because it resembles a similar disease previously identified in infants.

What are the symptoms?
This disease rarely develops in otherwise healthy people, except for those who have been severely injured (such as in an automobile accident). Therefore, people with adult respiratory distress syndrome usually have symptoms and signs of an underlying disease. If you have adult respiratory distress syndrome you will experience severe respiratory distress with significant shortness of breath and a rapid, shallow breathing pattern. Your skin color looks gray and your lips have a purple tinge. Your physician will order a blood test, which will show that the amount of oxygen in your blood is markedly reduced. Even when you breathe in high concentrations of oxygen, the blood oxygen level increases to only a limited degree. Extensive, large fluffy spots throughout both lungs can be seen on a chest X ray.

What is the treatment?
Adult respiratory distress syndrome is a very serious, life-threatening condition and requires treatment in a hospital intensive-care unit. In addition to oxygen, you may need some form of mechanical assistance to breathe. If the syndrome occurs with an infection, antibiotics are essential. While your physician provides intravenous fluids needed to maintain blood pressure and kidney and heart functions, he or she monitors you to avoid giving you too much fluid, which would then accumulate in your lungs.

Sarcoidosis

This is a disease more common among young black adults, in which multiple, tiny patches of inflammation suddenly appear in one or several parts of the body, frequently in the lungs. The word sarcoid should not be confused with sarcoma (which is a type of cancerous tumor). The inflamed tissues of sarcoidosis are not a kind of tumor. They are also not caused by an infection. Nobody knows why sarcoidosis occurs, or why it clears up, as it usually does, on its own.

Sometimes symptoms include fever and pain in the joints. Often there are no symptoms. When there are symptoms, they depend on which tissues or organs of your body are affected. For example, if your lungs are affected by sarcoidosis, you may have some shortness of breath.

Other tissues and organs that may be affected include the skin, lungs, lymph glands, liver, spleen, eyes, and the bones in the hands and feet.

What should be done?
A chest X ray almost always confirms or disproves suspected sarcoidosis. Several laboratory tests can help confirm the diagnosis and help provide an assessment of the causes and outcome of the disease. Most people with sarcoidosis will not require treatment, and the condition will generally disappear in 2 to 3 years. If your condition does not improve after several months, your physician may prescribe a corticosteroid drug, which seems to relieve some of the symptoms of sarcoidosis of the lungs.

Disorders of the heart and circulation

Introduction

Your blood is your body's transport system. Its main function is to carry nutrients and oxygen, which provide raw materials and energy to the tissues of your body. The blood also carries waste away from the tissues and helps maintain body temperature. To do these vital jobs, your blood must circulate continuously.

Your heart is the moving force of the circulatory system. Its steady beating pumps at least five quarts of blood through a full circuit of your body every minute. The heart consists of two pumps side by side. The pump on the right side moves blood to your lungs, where waste gases such as carbon dioxide are removed and oxygen is added. Freshly oxygenated blood returns to the pump on the left side, which moves it out into the rest of your body. Blood flows away from the heart, either to the lungs or to the rest of the body, through blood vessels called arteries. These branch many times, and the branches become smaller, forming blood vessels called arterioles. These, too, become smaller and smaller and branch repeatedly until they become very tiny vessels called capillaries. Capillaries are very thin walled—only about 1 cell thick—so small that they are only about the width of a red blood cell. As your blood passes through the many miles of capillaries, it delivers nutrients and oxygen to the tissues and picks up wastes. As the blood moves on through the capillaries, the blood vessels gradually become larger and eventually become veins. The veins carry the blood through organs such as the kidneys and liver, which remove the wastes, and back to your heart. Then the cycle begins again.

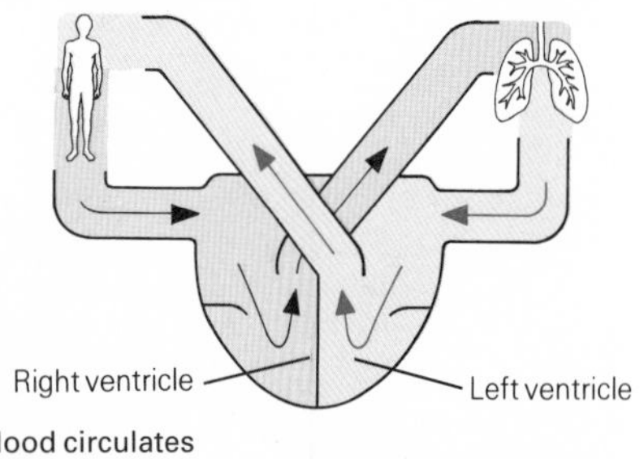

How blood circulates
The heart pumps blood through the body. Deoxygenated, or "used," blood (gray) has made a full circuit of the body and is pumped from the right ventricle into the lungs. There it exchanges carbon dioxide for oxygen. The newly oxygenated blood (brown) enters the left side of the heart, and the circuit is completed as the blood is then pumped out of the left ventricle to all body tissues.

Disorders of the heart and circulation are many and varied. Only the most common ones are covered in this chapter. Congenital, or inborn, heart disorders are covered elsewhere (see p.702). One disorder that has become especially common in recent years is coronary artery disease, which is caused by atherosclerosis, a thickening of the inside lining of the blood vessels. Atherosclerosis has complex, multiple causes not yet fully understood. Among the factors known to increase the likelihood of this condition developing are cigarette smoking, high blood pressure, obesity, lack of exercise, and excessive fat in the diet, leading to an increase in blood cholesterol level.

If you are healthy, the two sides of your heart beat synchronously and regularly. In some disorders the beats become irregular or abnormally fast or slow. These disorders of rhythm, called arrhythmias, can usually be corrected by drugs or by attaching a pacemaker (see p.420) to your heart to regulate your heartbeat.

Your heart contains one-way valves to ensure that the blood flows in one direction only. If your valves either do not open fully or close completely, you have valvular heart disease. Damaged valves can be repaired or replaced. Finally, even if the heart is sound, damaged blood vessels can cause disorders.

Treatment of heart and circulation disorders has improved significantly in the past 30 years, largely because of improved surgical techniques. In too many cases, however, the first symptom of serious trouble is permanent disability or even sudden death. Since several kinds of circulatory system diseases probably can be prevented, physicians are increasing their emphasis on prevention and a healthy life-style.

The heart and blood vessels

The heart

The heart is a muscular bag made up of two pumps, each divided into two compartments linked by valves. The largest compartment is the left ventricle, which pumps freshly oxygenated blood through the aorta to all parts of the body. The blood then returns to the heart, entering the right atrium through two large channels (the superior and inferior venae cavae). From the right atrium the blood passes through the tricuspid valve into the right ventricle. It is then pumped through the pulmonary artery into the lungs, where it receives oxygen and gets rid of carbon dioxide. This oxygenated blood flows back to the left atrium of the heart via the pulmonary veins. From the left atrium it passes through the mitral valve into the left ventricle.

Superior vena cava
Aorta
Pulmonary artery
Pulmonary veins
Inferior vena cava
Left ventricle
Tricuspid valve
Aortic valve
Right atrium
Mitral valve
Pulmonary valve
Right ventricle
Left atrium

Blood vessels

Blood vessels that lead to and from the heart carry blood to all parts of the body. For a detailed illustration of how the blood circulates, see p.396.

Arteries
Arteries carry blood away from the heart. The walls of the arteries need to be strong, because blood is pumped through them under pressure from the heart. Arteries have three layers: a fibrous outer coating, a middle layer of strong muscle and tough elastic tissue, and a membranous inner lining.

Capillaries
Capillaries are tiny, very thin-walled extensions of the smallest arteries. They carry blood to the cells of the body. Oxygen and other nutrients in the blood penetrate the capillary walls (arrows) to reach body tissues, while waste matter is taken up to be carried to veins that take it to breakdown and disposal points.

Veins
Veins run parallel to the arteries and return blood to the heart. Since the blood they carry is under much less pressure than that in the arteries, veins have thinner, less elastic, less muscular walls. Compression of the walls by ordinary muscle activity squeezes the blood back to the heart. Valves in the veins (bottom left) keep blood from flowing in the wrong direction. The veins have three layers a fibrous outer coating, a thin layer of muscle, and a membranous inner lining.

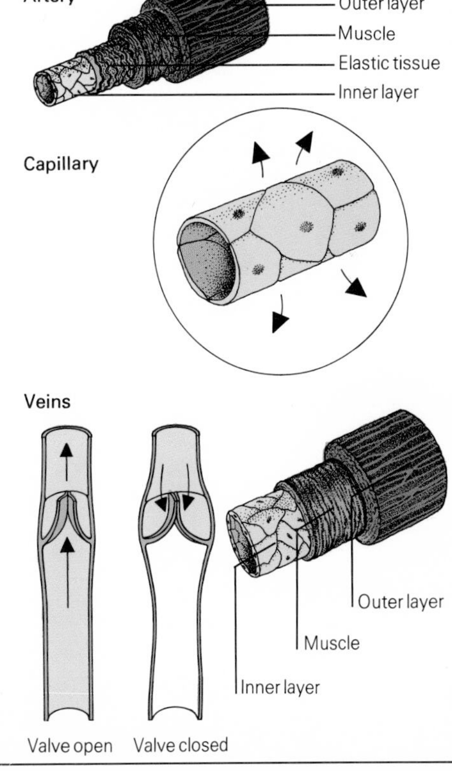

Major disorders

Heart disease accounts for almost one third of all deaths in Western countries, and most of these deaths result from coronary artery disease and hypertension (high blood pressure). Coronary artery disease is caused by atherosclerosis, a thickening of the inside lining of the blood vessels that is linked with fatty substances, including cholesterol, in the blood. These disorders and their complications, including shock, heart failure, angina, and heart attack, are discussed in the opening pages of this chapter.

Atherosclerosis

Your arteries are the vessels that carry blood from the heart to the rest of your body. If you are healthy, your arteries have walls that are muscular, smooth inside, and elastic enough to accommodate extreme variations in blood pressure, so that blood passes through freely. Sometimes, though, fatty streaks appear on the inner walls of arteries. These streaks may start at stress points, such as where an artery branches or where the wall is slightly damaged. A deposit of this fat is known as atheroma. Plaque, which is a large mass of atheroma, usually begins when cholesterol infiltrates the lining of the vessel. The body attempts to repair the damage with connective tissue, which thickens the vessel wall and narrows the passageway through which blood can flow. As more cholesterol is deposited, the vessel wall becomes even thicker and blood flow is further constricted. The name of the disorder, atherosclerosis, means literally "hardening from atheroma." Atherosclerosis is an important contributory factor in arteriosclerosis (see Hardening of the arteries, p.435). It is also the cause of coronary artery disease (see next article).

Atherosclerosis is common in the US and most other developed countries of the world. The frequency with which it occurs differs from one country to another, but in general atherosclerosis increases as the diet contains greater amounts of cholesterol and saturated fat. Even children may be affected.

Your chances of having the disease are highest if you have higher than normal levels of cholesterol in your blood, if you are a man of any age or a woman who is past the menopause, if you smoke, and if you have a condition such as diabetes (see p.558), kidney failure (see p.550), or high blood pressure (see p.411). (For further details on those who are at risk from atherosclerosis, see Coronary artery disease, next article.) The severity of atherosclerosis increases with age.

Atheroma formation
An atheroma, or patch of fatty tissue that damages arterial walls, tends to form at the point at which an artery branches and the flow of blood is naturally disturbed. As atheroma increases, atherosclerosis develops.

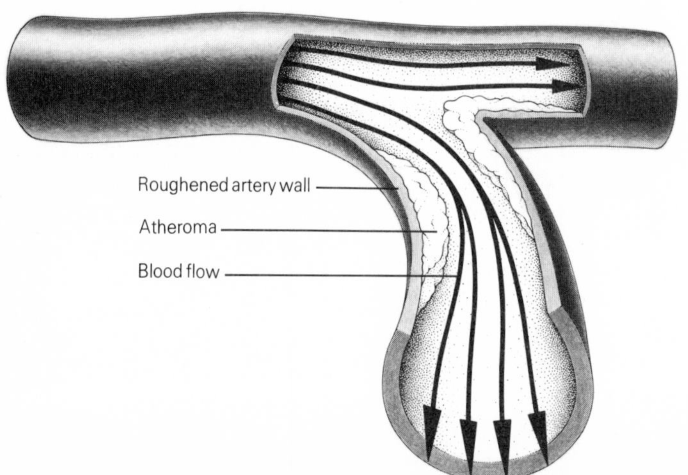

What are the symptoms?

There are rarely any noticeable symptoms of atherosclerosis until after it causes extensive damage. When you finally see symptoms, generally after several years, it is because a particular part of your body is being deprived of blood. Therefore, the symptoms depend on which part is affected. You may merely have cramps in your legs during exercise, or you may have a stroke (see p.285), kidney failure (see p.550), angina (see p.403), or a heart attack (see p.406).

What are the risks?

The ill effects of atherosclerosis may not become apparent to you for a time. Many parts of your body are supplied with blood not only by a particular artery and its branches, but also by minor branches of neighboring arteries. These branches may not be affected even though the major supply channel is badly damaged. As the supply of blood from the major artery decreases, other arteries can sometimes compensate by enlarging, which allows the total blood supply to that area of your body to remain almost constant. Even when the disorder affects body tissues that rely on a single artery for their blood supply, the channel can often be narrowed considerably without any apparent ill effects. This is possible because the normal supply of blood to a tissue is usually more than it actually needs to remain healthy—a built-in system of protection.

Preventing heart disease

Despite substantial reduction in chronic disabling disease from coronary heart disease, it remains the biggest killer of middle-aged and older men and women in the US and other developed countries. Research studies have greatly improved our understanding of atherosclerosis and the underlying disease process. It is now known that (1) the disease begins early in life, as early as the teens in many cases; (2) a person rarely experiences symptoms until the disease is advanced; in around one third of cases he or she dies shortly after the first symptom appears; and (3) advanced disease is very difficult to reverse; once a heart attack has occurred, the heart muscle that has been replaced by scar tissue is not reparable. Clearly, the best strategy to defeat coronary heart disease is prevention, rather than waiting for symptoms to appear.

Know your risk factors

Current advice on prevention is based on the painstaking unravelling of the multiple causes of atherosclerosis, many of which are still not fully understood. Physicians do know that it occurs earlier in life and most severely in people who have all or most of the identified risk factors. The three most important risk factors are:

- Smoking, especially inhaling cigarette smoke;
- High blood pressure;
- High blood cholesterol;

Other risk factors are less well established, such as:

- Lack of exercise;
- Obesity;
- Family history;
- Other diseases such as diabetes

The two risk factors easiest to modify without a physician's help are smoking and exercise. With increased public knowlege of the dangers of smoking, smoking has become steadily less socially acceptable. Few health-conscious people now smoke at all, since they know that it increases their risk not only of heart disease and lung cancer but also of other cancers (cervix, bladder, larynx, and tongue). Smoking accelerates the aging of the skin and the lungs, and smokers are less physically fit at all ages. Quitting is not easy.

Exercising regularly, like quitting smoking, has many benefits and no drawbacks. It helps keep your weight in the optimum range, helps maintain the strength of bones and muscles, and enhances mental and physical well-being. To develop cardiopulmonary fitness and possibly to protect yourself against coronary heart disease, you must exercise regularly, at least three times a week for at least 20 minutes each time. You do not need to exercise vigorously. Ask your physician to recommend some exercises.

Everyone should know what his or her blood pressure and blood cholesterol levels are, and what the results mean. If your blood pressure is consistently raised (see p.411), your physician will recommend treatment; you may have to lose weight, reduce your salt intake, and exercise regularly. If medications are needed, drugs to lower blood pressure have few side effects and do not restrict normal activities.

Cholesterol

The issue of high cholesterol diet and heart disease in those without known coronary artery disease is more controversial. However, experts agree that the typical American diet contains too much fat, especially saturated (dairy and animal) fat. On an average, Americans get about 40 percent of their calories from fat; people would be healthier, have a lower risk of heart disease, and have fewer cancers if they cut their fat intake to 20 to 30 percent (see p.32 in the introduction). Once the coronary artery disease is evident (by the development of angina or a heart attack), lowering cholesterol levels may decrease the progression of the disease.

Reducing your cholesterol intake is especially important if you have any of the other risk factors listed above.

There is less agreement on what level of cholesterol is high enough to warrant treatment. Levels below 200 mg/dL are considered normal. In the US around one fourth of middle-aged men and women have total cholesterol levels above 240 mg/dL. If your cholesterol is in this range, have the test repeated for confirmation, and if the results differ, repeat the test until you get a consistent answer. If your cholesterol level is consistently high, you will need further evaluation, including a breakdown of the components of your total blood cholesterol (see p.33). If your total cholesterol is above 240 mg/dL and most of the excess consists of the high-density lipoprotein (HDL), the "good" cholesterol portion of the cholesterol, then you may not need treatment. If you do require further treatment, discuss this in detail with your physician. Your treatment will probably be based on a rigorous low-fat, low-cholesterol diet and, if needed, cholesterol-lowering drugs.

If your total cholesterol is between 200 and 240 mg/dL, your physician will probably recommend a change in diet alone. However, each individual is evaluated in the light of other risk factors such as smoking habits, high blood pressure, family history, life-style, or diabetes.

Thus, atherosclerosis may do you little or no apparent harm for many years. However, in addition to reducing gradually the flow in the artery, atherosclerosis can cause other problems. At times, the smooth covering over the plaque can crack, exposing the blood in the vessel to the fatty material of the plaque. This causes sudden and complete obstruction of the vessel, markedly decreasing blood flow through it. If this happens in the coronary arteries, which supply blood to the heart, you have coronary artery disease. If the cerebral arteries, which supply the brain, are affected, you may have a stroke (see p.285). Other possible consequences of the disorder are gangrene in an arm or leg (see p.447) or kidney damage, which leads in many cases to chronic kidney failure (see p.551).

What should be done?

Do not wait for symptoms to develop before doing something about atherosclerosis. As explained above, by the time symptoms appear, the disease has produced dire consequences. The time to begin using the self-help measures recommended below is now, before these symptoms develop. Self-help measures may help prevent or slow down the onset of atherosclerosis.

Research studies suggest that a fatty streak on the lining of an artery can disappear through diet changes and medication but that little can be done about an established plaque, or large, hard mass of cholesterol. Vigorous treatment of atherosclerosis can reduce the likelihood of both strokes and heart attacks, but few people are prepared to accept such treatment while they are free of symptoms and feel in good health. This is not to suggest that you should ask your physician for immediate tests to show whether you already have atherosclerosis and how advanced it is. Such tests are complicated and expensive, and they involve some risks. Self-help measures are enough for almost everyone.

You should consult your physician, however, if you have 2 or 3 close relatives with heart or circulatory disorders, if you know that some of your close relatives have high levels of cholesterol in the blood, or if you have diabetes. Your physician will suggest a blood cholesterol test and a blood pressure check. If you have high blood pressure or cholesterol, talk to your physician about options for treatment. Other tests that your physician may perform to help confirm a diagnosis of coronary artery disease are an electrocardiogram (ECG), an ECG during exercise (stress test), a radioisotope injection during exercise, and, if necessary, an arteriogram.

Professional help: Talk to your physician if you require treatment for high blood pressure or elevated cholesterol (see box on Prevention, p.399). He or she may ask you to make return visits for regular monitoring of your response to changes in your diet and drug treatment.

Coronary artery disease

(coronary atherosclerosis, ischemic heart disease, coronary heart disease)

To keep itself healthy and functioning, your heart muscle requires a constant flow of oxygen- and nutrient-rich blood, which is only indirectly related to the blood required to fill the heart's chambers. Blood reaches your heart through two main coronary arteries, and a branching network of smaller blood vessels over the surface of the heart muscle nourishes it.

Fatty deposits, or atheroma, can form in your arteries, and this narrowing of the passageways is part of a condition that is called atherosclerosis (see p.398). If your coronary arteries become narrowed, they can fail to provide your heart with enough oxygen and other nutrients. Also, the blood that flows through the arteries may form a clot, or thrombus, which can block an artery. In response to any physical or psychological stress, your heart beats faster and your blood pressure goes up. Your heart requires increased oxygen and nutrients, but severely narrowed or blocked coronary arteries cannot cope. The resulting discrepancy between demand and supply causes angina, or heart pain (see next article). If the blood flow to part of your heart muscle is suddenly reduced by a clot in one of your coronary arteries, you will have a heart attack (see p.406).

What are the symptoms?

Often there are no symptoms of coronary artery disease, especially in the early stages. For recognizable symptoms that ultimately occur, read the articles on angina (see next article) and heart attack (see p.406).

What are the risks?

Coronary artery disease is common in the US and other developed countries, where it accounts for 30 percent of all deaths. More men than women are affected. The incidence of the disease is much lower in developing countries. Here are some additional facts that can help you determine whether you are likely to have coronary artery disease.

1. More young men than young women have coronary artery disease, but the risk to women increases after menopause, and women over 65 are almost as susceptible to the disorder as are men.
2. If you smoke cigarettes, you are at least twice as susceptible as a nonsmoker. Deaths from the disorder in the 35 to 45 age group are five times more common in smokers.
3. There is an increased risk if you have high blood pressure or diabetes. Males with diabetes are twice as susceptible as other men, and females with diabetes are five times as susceptible as other women.
4. Coronary artery disease seems to run in families. You are more at risk if several of your close relatives have had it.
5. If you are overweight, you are more at risk than a person of normal weight.
6. If you have a sedentary job you may be more susceptible than people whose work includes some hard physical labor.
7. If you are a woman over 35 who takes birth control pills and also smokes cigarettes, you are at increased risk of having coronary artery disease.

If you have coronary artery disease, and the disease is not treated, your arteries may become increasingly blocked. With sudden development of a clot, the blood supply to your heart may be so reduced that you have a heart attack, which could be fatal. However, even after a major attack you may recover partially or fully, depending on the extent of muscle damage. Sometimes, however, the heart muscle is damaged to such an extent that pumping action is weakened. This causes heart failure (see p.408).

Many people live for years with coronary artery disease and have no trouble. Others may be forced to modify their activities because of recurrent attacks of angina. Many of these people can also lead relatively active lives as long as they keep the disease under control and take medication that helps restore the balance between demand for oxygen and nutrients and the ability of the narrowed or obstructed coronary artery to meet this demand. Some people must live a much more restricted life, being careful to avoid even slight physical or emotional stress. Yet, if they can adjust emotionally, even people with severe disease can be comfortable.

What should be done?

Coronary artery disease is much more easily prevented than it is treated—see Prevention, p.399. For advice on what to do if you experience either of the main symptoms of coronary artery disease, read the articles on

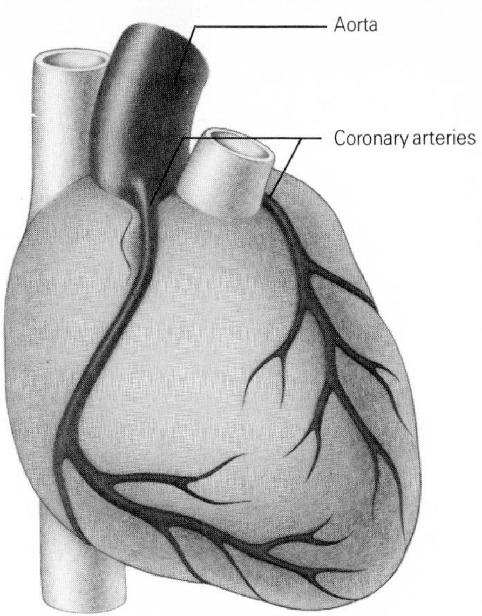

The coronary arteries
Some of the freshly oxygenated blood that is pumped out of the aorta flows into two coronary arteries. These arteries form a branching network over the surface of the heart and supply the heart muscle with the nutrient-rich blood it needs to function.

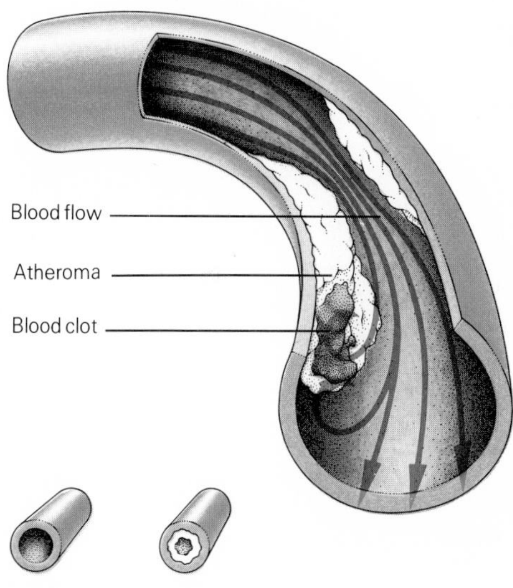

A blood clot forms in the arteries
An atheroma, or patch of fatty deposit, forms in a spot where the flow of blood is naturally disrupted. It roughens the arterial wall and causes increasing turbulence in blood flow. This can trigger the formation of a clot that may grow and block the artery.

angina (see next article) and heart attack (see p.406). If you are worried that you may be at risk, start taking preventive measures. Too often, sudden death is the first sign of the disease. The following recommendations for self-help are useful if you already have heart trouble, or if you want to improve your chances of avoiding it in the future.

If you want to check the state of your heart, see your physician, who, after examining you, may decide to order some of the tests mentioned in the article on angina. You should also have your blood pressure checked whenever you visit your physician (see High blood pressure, p.411).

What is the treatment?

Self-help: If you have symptoms, you can still benefit from the preventive measures explained in the box on Prevention (p.399). Attention to diet, blood pressure, smoking, and exercise will all bring dividends in terms of slowing the progress of the disease and improving your general health.

Professional help: Your physician will arrange for tests to be done (see below) to evaluate the seriousness of your coronary artery disease and the state of your general health. He or she will then discuss with you a treatment program designed to reduce your risks of having a heart attack or other symptoms of coronary artery disease.

This treatment program will have three components: prevention, drugs, and surgery.

For prevention your physician will treat your blood pressure or your blood cholesterol if either is too high (see Prevention box p.399) and give you advice on diet, exercise, and losing weight if necessary. He or she may recommend that you take a small dose of aspirin daily or every other day to make your blood platelets less sticky and reduce the likelihood of your having a heart attack. He or she may also prescribe other drugs to reduce this risk.

Drug treatment to relieve symptoms of coronary artery disease (see the next article on Angina and the article on Heart attack,

Tests for coronary heart disease

The electrocardiogram (ECG) measures the changes in electrical activity of the heart muscle with every beat. When combined with exercise in a stress test, it is useful in diagnosing coronary heart disease resulting from atherosclerosis. These changes are detected by means of electrodes attached to the arms and legs, and the front of the chest. The heart's electrical activity is either displayed on a screen or recorded as a trace on paper.

The ECG tracing from a normal, healthy heart has a characteristic shape, or waveform. Any irregularity in the heart rhythm or damage to the heart muscle shows up on the ECG trace as deviations from the normal wave form.

Recent technical advances have made the ECG an even more useful test for heart disease. You can wear a portable version while engaging in your everyday activities instead of spending time in the physician's office or in the hospital. For example, if your physician believes that your symptoms (such as chest pain or blackouts) may be caused by narrowing of the coronary arteries or by periodic irregularities of the heartbeat, he or she may ask you to wear a portable ECG monitor for a 24-hour test period, during which you follow your usual daily routine while the machine continually monitors your heart's activity. This technique of ambulatory ECG monitoring can reveal episodic heartbeat irregularities or show evidence of coronary artery disease that would not be revealed by ECG testing in the physician's office.

If you are suffering from attacks of chest pain that could be from angina (see next article) but the ECG done at rest is normal, you may be asked to undergo an exercise stress test, which as mentioned above is an ECG while performing controlled exercise. First, a calculation is made of your maximum heart rate based on your sex and age. Then you are connected to the ECG machine and you exercise (by pedalling an exercise bicycle or walking on a treadmill) until your heart is beating steadily at the calculated rate. This method often reveals characteristic changes in the ECG pattern in people with narrowing of the coronary arteries. The exercise ECG is also widely used to test people who have recently recovered from a heart attack as a first step in assessing the state of the heart's blood supply.

Other tests that may be used include radioisotope scanning (at rest and with exercise), echocardiography (see Glossary), and magnetic resonance imaging, all of which provide information about the blood flow and the extent of damage (if any) to the heart muscle. In people who cannot exercise because of arthritis, arterial disease in the legs, or orthopedic problems, the coronary blood flow can be increased by use of a vasodilating drug, which, along with radioisotope scanning, can give the same information about blood flow to the heart and the extent of damage to the heart muscle as exercise with radioisotope scanning. Depending on the results of these tests, your physician may recommend that you also have a coronary angiogram, in which a special dye is injected into the coronary arteries so that they are clearly outlined in X-ray photographs. This technique provides the most reliable information about any narrowing or blocking of the coronary arteries, but it does cause some discomfort and carries a risk of complications. It is usually not performed unless surgery or balloon angioplasty is being considered.

p.406) may include nitrates, beta-blockers, calcium channel blockers, and angiotensin converting enzyme (ACE) inhibitors, all of which reduce the workload of the heart muscle, and some of which also help improve the blood flow through the coronary arteries and reduce the risk of dangerous irregularities in the heart rhythm. Your physician monitors your response to the medication you are taking and may want to repeat some of the tests of heart function periodically or if your symptoms get worse.

Surgery for coronary artery disease may take the form either of the relatively minor operation called transluminal (balloon) angioplasty, or of the major procedure of coronary artery bypass grafting (see p.404).

In cases where the symptoms suggest that a blood clot has blocked a coronary artery within the previous 4 to 6 hours, the physician may attempt to restore the blood flow to normal by injecting a clot-dissolving (thrombolytic) drug into the coronary artery or, more commonly, into a vein in your arm.

Despite these substantial advances in treatment, many people still die of coronary artery disease, usually within an hour or so of the appearance of symptoms. Most cardiologists now agree that the way to reduce coronary artery disease fatalities is to emphasize the importance of prevention—especially persuading people not to smoke cigarettes and to detect and lower an elevated cholesterol level—and in education about the early symptoms of a heart attack. Anyone who develops a crushing pain in the center of the chest, accompanied by difficulty breathing, sweating, or feeling faint, may be having a heart attack and needs immediate emergency treatment.

Angina

(angina pectoris)

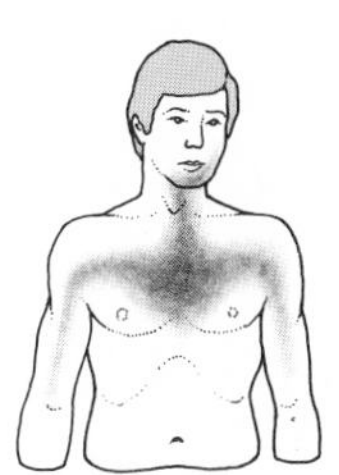

Site of the pain

Angina pectoris is not a disease in its own right. It is the name for pain that occurs when the muscular wall of the heart becomes temporarily short of oxygen. Normally, the coronary arteries that supply blood to the heart can cope with an increased demand, but this ability is restricted if you have coronary artery disease (see previous article). Some other less common causes of angina are aortic stenosis (see p.427), anemia (see p.450), and hyperthyroidism (see p.565). If you have a condition that restricts the supply of oxygen to your heart, the supply may be adequate for some activities but become inadequate if there is an increased demand for oxygen, as occurs when you exercise, are subjected to extremes of temperature, or become highly emotional. When the oxygen requirement falls, the pain usually disappears.

What are the symptoms?

The main symptom of angina is pain in the center of your chest. The pain can spread to your throat and upper jaw, your back, and your arms (almost always the left one). Angina is a dull, heavy, constricting or pressure-like pain that characteristically appears when you are active and fades when you stop activity and rest. Less commonly, the pain may occur only in your arms, wrists, or neck, but you can recognize it as angina if you know that it occurs whenever you are abnormally active or excited and disappears when you calm down. Additional symptoms that often accompany the pain of an attack of angina include difficulty breathing, sweating, nausea, and dizziness.

Angina is a common condition. In men it usually occurs after age 30 and it is nearly always caused by coronary artery disease. Angina tends to begin later in life for women except among women over 35 who smoke and also use oral contraceptive pills. The risk of coronary artery disease also increases after a woman goes through menopause.

What are the risks?

Since angina is a symptom rather than a disease, the risks are basically those of the condition that causes it. The heart may become so deprived of oxygen that there is a risk of heart attack (see next article). The angina may occur more readily as time goes by, and it may last longer. You may find that you have to become less and less active to avoid the pain.

What should be done?

If you think you are having attacks of angina, see your physician. Accurate diagnosis is essential. The discomfort could be related to other problems such as a spasm of the esophagus (food pipe) and may not be angina at all. With accurate diagnosis your physician can prescribe medication to help relieve the discomfort and determine what treatment might be necessary. Consult your physician at once if the pain of angina lasts longer than 5 minutes after you stop exercising, if your attacks of chest pain are increasing rapidly in frequency, length, or severity, or if the angina comes on at rest and without emotional or physical stress. These are all signs that the condition may be deteriorating.

OPERATIONS:

Transluminal (balloon) angioplasty and coronary artery bypass

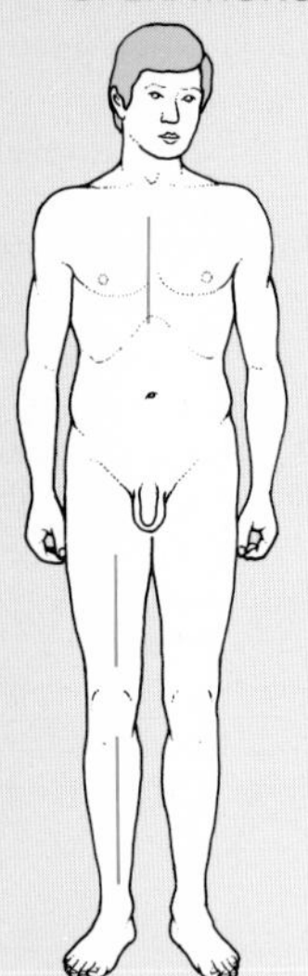
Sites of incisions in a coronary artery bypass operation

Coronary artery bypass graft operations are performed in cases of coronary artery disease in which the narrowing or blockages are multiple or involve the left main coronary artery. Angioplasty is performed on one, two, or occasionally three sites in the coronary arteries except the left main artery. Transluminal (balloon) angioplasty is described below. Research is being done with laser and other instruments (called atherectomy devices) that vaporize or pulverize and remove the atherosclerotic plaque. Coronary angiography (see p.405) helps your physician determine the extent and severity of your condition and decide whether transluminal (balloon) angioplasty (a relatively minor operation) or coronary bypass surgery (a major surgical procedure) is most appropriate in your particular case.

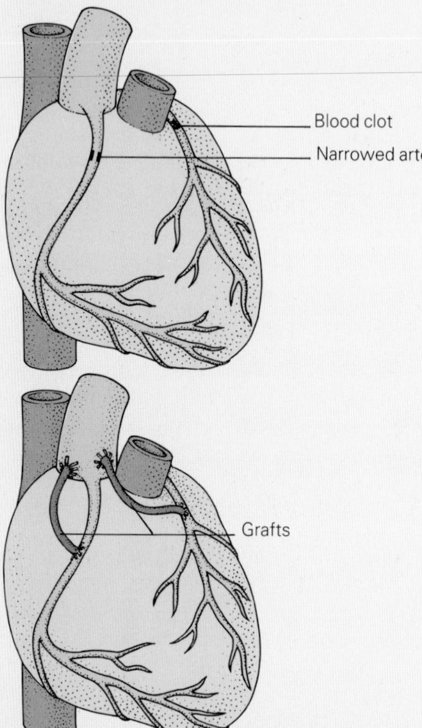

During the operation Transluminal (balloon) angioplasty restores normal blood flow by stretching the narrowed section of artery from the inside. The cardiologist inserts a long, fine tube (catheter) into an artery in your arm or leg and threads it in—following its progress by means of X rays to ensure that it goes to the right place—until it reaches the coronary artery. The catheter carries a tough plastic balloon, which is positioned in the narrowed section of artery and then inflated under pressure. The balloon stretches the artery and cracks the plaques, thus enlarging the width of the channel of the artery. As the lining heals, further debris is removed, and the artery widens even more. Two or three narrowed sections may be treated in a single session. The operation is usually performed under a local anesthetic and takes about 45 minutes. Many arteries treated in this way become narrowed again because a clot may form on the injured plaque or the damage to the wall may stimulate excessive thickening of the artery lining.

If the narrowed or blocked sections of coronary artery are critically located or too extensive for angioplasty (or if angioplasty has been used but has failed to restore the blood flow to normal), the alternative surgical treatment is a coronary bypass operation. This requires stopping the heart; your circulation and breathing are taken over by a heart-lung machine, which ensures that your brain and other vital organs receive an adequate supply of oxygenated blood. An incision is made in one or both of your legs and a length of vein is removed. Meanwhile, another incision is made down the center of your chest and your rib cage is opened to expose your heart. The surgeon then uses the vein from your leg to make one or more grafts to bypass the blockages in the coronary artery and so restore the blood flow to normal. Sometimes a small artery from the chest wall or abdomen is used as a graft instead.

After the operation You may spend a few days in an intensive-care unit, where your heartbeat and respiration will be constantly monitored. You will receive fluid and blood through intravenous drips. Surgical drains through tubes will be placed in your chest. You may need to breathe oxygen or be placed on respirator.

Convalescence As you recover, ask your physician about exercise, life-style changes, and when you may return to your routine.

Long-term prospects Research shows that coronary artery bypass grafting can extend one's lifespan if the coronary artery disease affects three vessels or the left main artery, especially if there is already a decreased ability of the heart to contract forcefully. Furthermore, the operation is also highly effective in relieving angina. However, research also shows that less severe coronary artery disease may be treated just as effectively with drugs that lower blood pressure and combat the bad effects on muscle of an increased demand for oxygen.

Medical myth

If you have angina, you must avoid exercise and lead the life of an invalid.

Wrong. Regular exercise is good for you, as long as you keep it within the limits imposed by the disorder. Experience and guidance from your physician will tell you how much you can do without pain. Also, do not be afraid to have sexual intercourse.

After closely examining you, your physician may order a blood test for hyperthyroidism, anemia, or some other possible cause contributing to chest pain. You may need a separate blood test to determine the level of lipids, or fats, in your blood. You may also need to have blood and urine tests to determine if you have diabetes, since diabetics are particularly susceptible to coronary artery disease. Tests that may also be required in order to obtain an accurate diagnosis include a chest X ray, an electrocardiogram (ECG), an exercise stress test (see Tests for coronary heart disease, p.402), and a coronary angiogram (sometimes called an arteriogram, see below).

Among other tests that may be done are radioisotope scans of the heart, which enable the physician to assess the adequacy of blood flow to the heart muscle, and ultrasound scanning (echocardiography), which shows the movement of the heart wall muscle with every heartbeat. Research continues with positron emission tomography (PET), which may be used to evaluate whether a segment of heart muscle remains unscarred and will benefit from bypass surgery or angioplasty. In general, extensive testing is recommended only for patients who are considered candidates for and who are willing to undergo transluminal (balloon) angioplasty or surgery, if it should prove to be necessary.

What is the treatment?

Self-help: Although prevention is the most effective strategy (see the box on prevention p.399), people who already have angina can still benefit from the measures described here. If you smoke, you should quit. If your cholesterol level is elevated, you should lower it by proper dieting and/or lipid-lowering medication. If your blood pressure is elevated, get it down. Exercise is also beneficial for people with angina, though you should consult your physician about the best type of exercise and how much to exert yourself. Do not use your angina as an excuse to become inactive.

Professional help: Once the cause of your angina is confirmed, your physician will decide whether medical or surgical treatment is best. The angina will disappear or decrease if the treatment succeeds. When coronary artery damage is not severe, angina can be

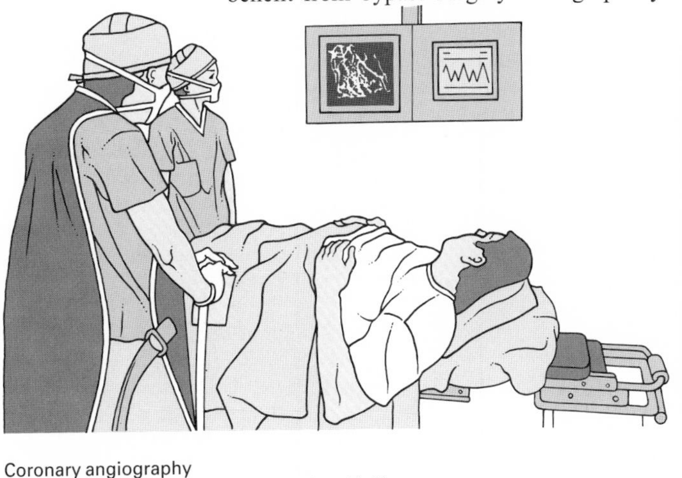

Coronary angiography

A coronary angiogram (sometimes called an arteriogram) is done to identify where a coronary artery is narrowed or blocked. You will be sedated but conscious during the procedure. It involves injecting a contrast agent, which shows up on an X ray, into a coronary artery. A narrow tube (catheter) is inserted into an accessible artery, usually in the arm or groin, and then threaded up to the heart and into a coronary artery. To do this, the physician is guided by a picture on an X-ray screen. The special contrast agent is injected through the catheter. X-ray movies are taken of the heart while the dye travels through the coronary artery and its branches.

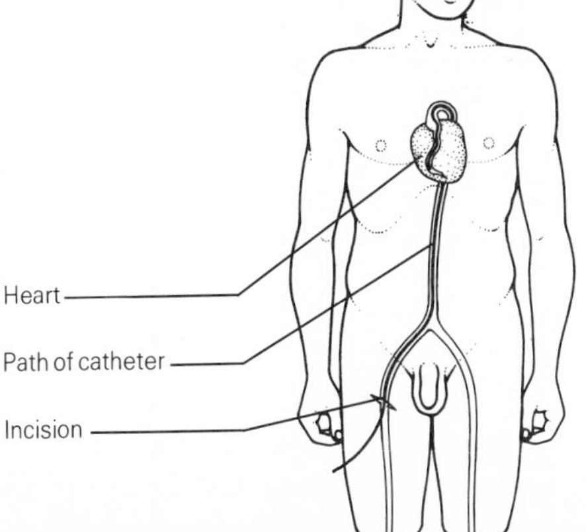

What the X ray shows

The heart is visible as a shadowy outline on the X-ray screen. The coronary artery and its branches show up as white lines while the contrast agent flows through them. A narrowing of a line indicates the presence of plaque. Where a line stops abruptly, that part of the artery is completely blocked by atheroma or a blood clot.

treated with drugs, weight loss, and giving up smoking. However, coronary artery disease cannot be "cured," and your physician will concentrate on preventing it from getting worse and on easing the discomfort and restrictions that are being caused by the angina itself.

Of the many drugs that effectively control or prevent angina, the most commonly prescribed one is nitroglycerine, sometimes known as "nitro." Most people with angina who take nitroglycerine are pleasantly surprised at how fast it usually works. In most cases it is literally only a matter of seconds between the time the tablet is put under the tongue and the relief of pain. If your physician prescribes this drug, make sure to refill your prescription frequently, because nitroglycerine tablets can lose their potency after only a few weeks, especially if the container is not sealed tightly. Your physician will probably instruct you to dissolve a tablet under your tongue the moment an angina attack starts. Or if you know that some activity such as climbing stairs always brings on your angina, you can usually prevent the episode by taking a tablet shortly before you begin the activity, rather than waiting for the pain to occur. If you are under any amount of psychological stress, try to minimize it. Your physician may prescribe nitroglycerine in the form of a slow-release patch that you wear on your chest.

A side effect of the nitroglycerine is that it may cause headaches. After you have taken nitroglycerine for a week or two, there is frequently less of a tendency to develop headaches. In any event, the headaches are usually mild and not reason enough to discontinue the treatment. If you get severe headaches from taking a whole tablet, your physician may suggest that you put only part of a tablet under your tongue.

Among other drugs used for controlling angina are the beta-blockers and the calcium channel blockers. Both of these drugs reduce the oxygen needs of the heart, reduce the heart rate, and lower blood pressure. They also reduce the likelihood of dangerous heart-rhythm irregularities.

Today's treatment for angina is very effective, but the powerful drugs prescribed must be taken exactly as directed, and you may need to consult your physician about unpleasant side effects they may produce, such as dizziness or lack of energy.

If your angina cannot be controlled by medication, your physician may recommend angioplasty or surgery. For example, if your angina is associated with aortic stenosis (p.427), replacement of the defective valve with a substitute will relieve your symptoms dramatically. If your angina is from coronary artery disease, transluminal (balloon) angioplasty or coronary artery bypass grafting (see p.404) should improve the blood flow to the heart and so remove the cause of your angina.

What are the long-term prospects?

The death rate of all patients with coronary artery disease is about 3 to 4 percent per year. The risk is greater if the efficiency of the heart is diminished. The degree to which your life needs to change depends on your determination to cooperate, the severity of the problem, and your response to treatment.

Heart attack

(coronary thrombosis, myocardial infarction)

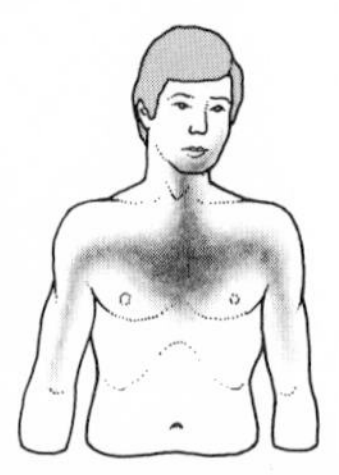
Site of the pain

The most common type of heart attack is caused by a thrombosis, or blockage, of one of the coronary arteries by a thrombus, or blood clot. This cuts off the blood supply to the region of the heart muscle served by the artery, damaging or killing the deprived tissue. Heart attack generally occurs only if your coronary arteries are already narrowed by coronary artery disease (see p.400). If the infarct, or damaged area of the heart, is small, does not cause a rapid ineffective heart rhythm, and does not impair the electrical conducting system that regulates heartbeat, the attack should not be fatal and you will have a good chance of recovery.

What are the symptoms?

The main symptom of a heart attack is usually a crushing pain in the center of your chest. The pain may also appear in the neck, jaw, arms, and upper abdomen. A heart attack can come on gradually, preceded by a few weeks of angina (see previous article), but it can also happen without any warning. The pain may vary in degree from a feeling of tightness in the chest to an agonizing, vise-like sensation. The pain may be continuous, or it may last for only a few minutes, then fade away, and then return. It may come on during exercise or emotional stress or at rest. Unlike the pain of angina, the pain of a heart attack does not go away after the exercise or stress ceases.

Other possible symptoms of heart attack are dizziness, shortness of breath, sweating, chills, nausea, and fainting. In a few instances, mainly in older people, there are few if any symptoms. This condition, known as a silent infarct, can be confirmed only by electrocardiographic and blood enzyme tests.

In the US there are more deaths from heart disease than from any other disorder. Heart attack is the most common cause of these deaths, but for every fatal heart attack there are at least 2 nonfatal ones. For most of this century the death rate from heart attack increased steadily in Western countries, but the rise stopped and began declining in the US in the late 1960s and is now also slowing down in Europe. Some physicians attribute this improvement to a greater emphasis on preventive changes in life-style (see p.399).

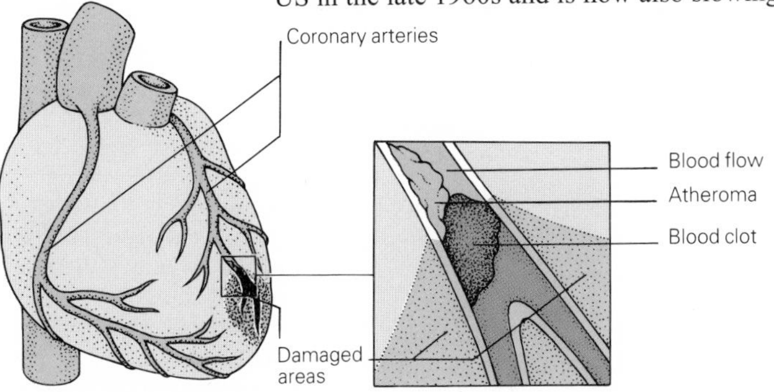

Heart attack
An artery is more likely to be blocked by a blood clot (a condition known as thrombosis) if atheroma has already built up within its walls. A blood clot in a coronary artery can cut off the blood supply and cause a heart attack.

What are the risks?

Two out of three people who have a heart attack recover, but the attack may be fatal if it inteferes with the electrical impulses that regulate your heartbeat or if it severely damages your heart muscle. Most deaths from heart attack occur within 2 hours of the onset of symptoms. About 10 percent of patients admitted to hospitals with heart attacks go into shock (see p.839), which can also be fatal. Heart failure (see next article) may also develop.

After a heart attack, a thrombus, or clot, may form inside one of the four chambers of the heart. If the thrombus becomes detached (it is then called an embolus) and is swept into the circulation, it can travel and cause damage elsewhere in the body. Fortunately, this occurs in only about 5 percent of cases.

Damage caused by heart attack may weaken and stretch one of the walls of the heart chambers. The resultant aneurysm, or bulging, can lead to complications such as heart failure. There is the added risk that bed rest may cause thrombosis (blood clots) in the veins, especially in the legs.

What should be done?

A heart attack is a medical emergency. If you or someone you know has the symptoms, call an ambulance or your physician, who may want to meet you at the hospital emergency room where, if the diagnosis is confirmed, therapy with thrombolytic drugs (which dissolve blood clots) can be started if the

After a heart attack

If you have just left the hospital after recovering from a heart attack, the most important thing to remember is that you are not an invalid. A damaged heart can heal.

After you have left the hospital, your physician may arrange for tests to evaluate the extent of any underlying coronary artery disease if they had not already been done before you left the hospital. These tests will include electrocardiograms (ECGs) at rest and during exercise (see Box, p.402), with or without some type of heart scan, and possibly also coronary angiography (see p.405) or echocardiography. The purpose of the tests is to determine accurately the amount of damage to the heart muscle caused by the attack, and whether or not there are any narrowed or blocked sections in the coronary arteries that might benefit from a coronary artery bypass graft or transluminal (balloon) angioplasty.

The results of the tests might indicate to your physician that you seem to have made a full recovery and require no further treatment; or that you should have long-term drug treatment to reduce strain on your heart, improve its efficiency, and prevent irregularities in its rhythm. If you find resuming your activities difficult but your physician has assured you that you are well, it is possible that anxiety is holding you back. Whatever your job was before the attack, you will probably be able to return to it. There is no evidence that taking a less responsible job or working part-time will help your health, if your doctor says that such a change is not necessary. However, you can make changes in your life that most physicians believe will reduce your risks of further heart attacks, as follows:

- Avoid sexual intercourse for about 6 weeks after your attack (ask your physician for advice), but do not be afraid to resume your sex life thereafter.
- Do not smoke.
- Keep your weight down to normal (see p.35) and eat a low-fat, low-cholesterol diet.
- Exercise regularly. There is some evidence that regular exercise reduces the likelihood of further attacks. Ask your physician to recommend exercises that you can perform alone or as part of a group in a setting where counseling and monitoring are available. You need to find a physical activity you enjoy and gradually increase both the amount of exercise and the vigor of your exertions each day. Ideally, you should spend 20 minutes a day doing an activity that raises your heart rate above 100 beats a minute.

onset of symptoms was no more than 4 to 6 hours earlier. Local practice will vary as to whether the thrombolytic drug is started in the hospital's emergency department or the intensive-care unit if one is available. What is vitally important, however, is that no time is lost in starting the drug once the diagnosis of a heart attack is established. While waiting for assistance, keep the person who is having the attack warm and calm. If the affected person loses consciousness (see Cardiac arrest, p.416), do not give up. If someone with emergency training in cardiopulmonary resuscitation (CPR) is present, he or she should take the person's pulse, and if there is none, give him or her CPR (see Injuries and emergencies, p.836.)

If you have had a heart attack, you may be put in an intensive-care or coronary-care unit of a hospital. You will need to undergo a number of diagnostic tests, including an electrocardiogram (ECG). Several ECG recordings may be needed. In coronary-care units the ECG is continuously monitored. Blood enzyme tests will be done at intervals to assess damage to your heart muscle. Continuous monitoring of important vital signs will be started, and you will be carefully watched for the possible development of any complications of the attack.

What is the treatment?

Self-help: None is possible.

Professional help: The most effective treatment for a heart attack is to dissolve the blood clot that caused it, but this is possible only within a few hours of the start of a heart attack, which is why it is vital to treat any possible heart attack as an emergency. Once the person's diagnosis is confirmed by electrocardiography and possibly other tests, a clot-dissolving (thrombolytic) drug is given, usually by injection into a vein. As mentioned earlier, this is most effective within 4 to 6 hours of the onset of the attack. Further tests will be performed, including possibly coronary angiography (p.405), to assess whether this treatment has been successful. If the coronary artery is still blocked, an attempt may be made to reopen the artery by transluminal (balloon) angioplasty (see p.404). If the opened artery is narrowed, and there is evidence of continued oxygen deprivation to the heart muscle, transluminal (balloon) angioplasty may be performed again a few days later.

To decide which of these treatments may be appropriate, your physician considers your general health, your age, and various other complicating factors. Meanwhile, you will continue to receive conventional treatment with painkillers, aspirin to interfere with platelet stickiness, and possibly also with anticoagulants to help reduce the risk of blood clots reforming in the coronary arteries or forming in the veins (see Deep vein thrombosis, p.445).

If your attack is a minor one, without complications, you may be allowed out of bed after 48 hours. Even if the attack is more serious, you will probably be permitted to use a bedside commode or portable toilet almost as soon as treatment begins, since physicians think that some mobility reduces the risk of abnormal blood clotting. Prior to discharge, a stress (exercise) electrocardiogram may be done to assess whether there is still a lack of oxygen supply to the heart muscle, as well as how much exercise may be desirable and whether you are a candidate for a cardiac rehabilitation exercise program.

What are the long-term prospects?

If you are reading this after having had a heart attack, the outlook is good. Mortality figures vary according to age and type of attack, but most deaths from heart attack occur within minutes or hours of the attack. This is why it is important to call for help immediately. If you show no sign of heart failure or disturbances of heart rhythm 6 hours after the pain disappears, you have an excellent chance of full recovery. If you are alive 1 month after even a severe attack, you have about a 70 to 80 percent chance of surviving for 5 years. After a heart attack you are naturally very concerned about your health and might be temporarily depressed. For advice on how to continue on with life after a heart attack, see the box on page 407.

Heart failure

(and congestive heart failure)

In heart failure, the pumping action of your heart becomes inefficient, for one of several reasons: because your heart muscle is weakened by disease, it has been weakened by a mechanical fault in the valves that control the flow of blood, it has to work too hard because of high blood pressure, or it has to pump an overload of blood. Heart failure does not mean that your heart stops pumping, as in cardiac arrest; it means that it is not working effectively.

Heart failure usually affects both sides of the heart; however, in some cases it affects only one side.

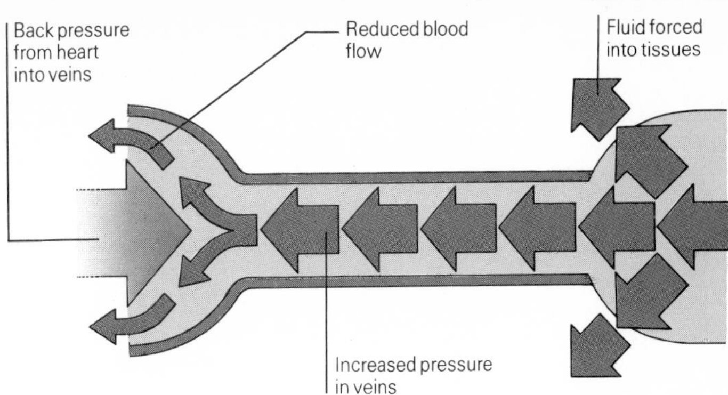

Heart failure forces fluid into tissues
When the heart fails, it is unable to maintain its normal output of blood. This, in turn, means that it can take in less blood from the vessels leading to it. These fill with a backlog of blood. The amount of blood is increased because the kidneys retain salt and water. The pressure then forces fluid into surrounding tissues.

If your heart cannot pump out a normal volume of blood sufficient to meet your body's demands, blood accumulates in the veins leading to it. The body interprets what is happening as a lack of blood supply to the organs, and to compensate, the kidneys begin to retain salt and water, thus increasing the volume of blood. This increased volume of blood stretches the ventricles and increases the output of the heart, thus increasing the blood flow to the organs. In left-sided heart failure the blood accumulates in the veins that carry blood from the lungs, increasing the blood pressure in the capillaries of the lungs. As a result, the lungs become swollen and congested with fluid. The fluid then passes from blood vessels into lung tissues (see Pulmonary edema, p.394). In right-sided heart failure blood accumulates in the veins that lead to the heart from other parts of the body. The affected parts, most obviously the legs, then become waterlogged.

The "congestion" in the organs produced by this heart failure gives the name congestive heart failure to this condition. At times the major problem is not that the heart fails to put out enough blood but that resistance builds up in the organs against the blood flow. The pressure it takes to fill the heart rises enough to cause an increase in capillary pressure, which in turn causes congestion in the lungs.

Despite its name, heart failure is not necessarily an immediately life-threatening disease. The outcome depends on the seriousness of the underlying disorder and whether you get treatment promptly.

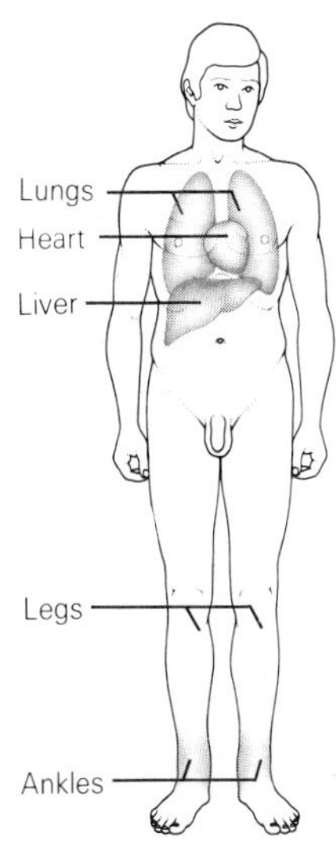

The effects of heart failure
Many parts of your body may be affected by heart failure. In left-sided failure, your lungs become congested. In right-sided failure, your liver, legs, ankles, and a number of other parts of the body that accumulate fluid easily may be affected.

What are the symptoms?

Left-sided heart failure: The main symptom is breathlessness. At first you may feel breathless only after exercising, but this symptom becomes more and more apparent, especially in the evenings when you are tired. Because it may be hard to breathe when you lie down, you may need to sleep with several pillows under your head or even sitting up. Severe attacks of breathlessness can awaken you from sleep and may become so bad that you want to go outside to breathe fresh air. Difficult breathing may be accompanied by wheezing, which can be mistaken for asthma. Bad attacks usually last no more than an hour, but the experience can be very disturbing.

Sometimes the lungs become so congested that you may hear a bubbling sound when you breathe. You may also have chest pain and frothy, blood-flecked sputum, or phlegm. The fluid in your lungs decreases your resistance to infection; pneumonia (see p.384), for example, is a common complication of left-sided heart failure.

Right-sided heart failure: The most common symptom is fatigue, but this is a sign of so many illnesses that on its own it is not conclusive. A more reliable symptom is the swelling of the lowest part of your body from accumulation of fluid. If you are up and around, your ankles may swell. If you are bedridden, the swelling will be the most noticeable in the lower part of your back. Internal organs such as the liver can also become swollen, and this can cause abdominal pain. In addition, weight gain results from accumulation of fluid.

With congestive heart failure you are likely to have symptoms of both left-sided and right-sided heart failure. In addition, you may also lose your appetite and experience considerable confusion.

What are the risks?

Untreated heart failure imposes a strain on your entire system that can be fatal. If heart failure is successfully treated, the main risks are those caused by the underlying disorder.

What should be done?

If you have symptoms of heart failure, see your physician, who will perform a physical examination. Diagnostic tests may include a chest X ray to look for lung problems and to check your heart size and an echocardiogram to look for valve disease, evaluate individual heart chamber size and function, and look for other diseases. An electrocardiogram (ECG) may help determine the type of heart problem, and other tests may be necessary.

What is the treatment?

Self-help: Get plenty of rest to conserve energy. Although you should reduce your physical activities, do not become bedridden. A favorite armchair is better than a bed. An incident of heart failure does not mean you must lead a restricted life indefinitely. Treatment of heart failure and the underlying condition may eventually allow you to resume your normal activities.

Even while you are resting, keep your legs in motion by frequently shifting your position or relaxing and contracting your leg muscles. This helps because your circulation is sluggish after you have heart failure, and your blood tends to clot, especially in your legs and pelvis. The pumping action of your leg muscles helps move the blood along.

You should also substantially restrict your daily intake of sodium, because it leads to fluid retention in the body.

Professional help: Apart from treating the underlying cause, your physician can prescribe drugs that relieve your symptoms. Among these are diuretics, which cause you to pass more urine than usual and thus lower the fluid content of your body. It is usually best to take a diuretic in the morning, because most people find it more convenient to urinate frequently during the day than to disturb their sleep at night.

Other medications commonly used in heart failure include vasodilators, such as angiotensin converting enzyme (ACE) inhibitors and digitalis preparations (usually digoxin). Digitalis slows the heart rate while increasing the strength of the heartbeat and the output of the heart. ACE inhibitors dilate both small arteries and veins. They also counteract some of the substances produced by the kidney that increase salt retention and cause excessive constriction of small arteries. ACE inhibitors reduce the workload on the heart and thus relieve symptoms; treatment with these drugs substantially prolongs survival in many cases. These are powerful drugs, and you and your physician may need to spend some time adjusting the dosage before reaching an optimum. Such drug treatment is often so successful that you want to stop taking your medication. This would be a serious mistake; follow your physician's instructions exactly.

If you must have a long period of bed rest, you may also need to take an anticoagulant, a drug that keeps blood from clotting. If your physician prescribes an anticoagulant, your blood must be tested at intervals to make sure the dose is correct. An overdose of such drugs can cause bleeding into the intestines, skin, brain, or other organs of the body.

Acute, or sudden, heart failure, with extremely severe breathlessness, is a medical emergency. If this occurs, go to a hospital, where oxygen can be administered and medications are injected to help relieve the symptoms quickly.

What are the long-term prospects?

With drug treatment your symptoms of breathlessness and swelling should subside. If you carefully follow a low-sodium diet and take your medications regularly, you can probably expect many years of nearly normal life ahead of you. If heart failure reaches a point where it no longer responds to rest, diet, and drugs, however, the only remaining possibilities are a heart transplant (see Transplants, p.432) or the use of an artificial, mechanical heart. Heart transplantation is now a proven, effective procedure with a high success rate. About 85 to 95 percent of people who have the surgery are alive 1 year later; 70 to 80 percent are alive 5 years later. Without the surgery, half would die within 6 months. However, a heart transplant operation requires a skilled team of surgeons and other specialists, and a shortage of donor hearts limits the transplant option.

As yet, replacement of a diseased heart by a man-made mechanical substitute remains a holding action prior to a transplant.

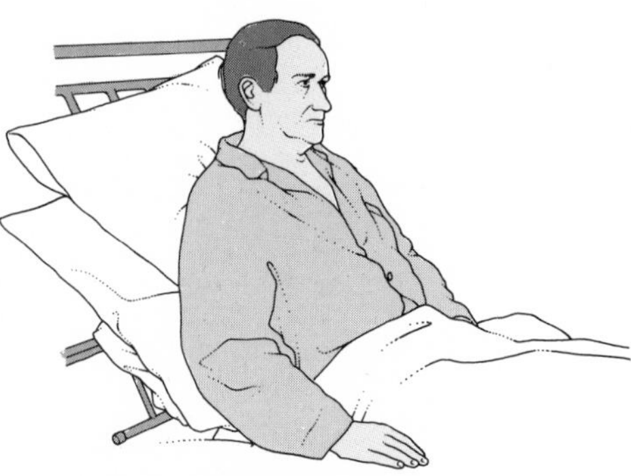

Coping with breathlessness
If you have left-sided heart failure, you may find it difficult to breathe when you lie down. To ease this, prop yourself up with several pillows.

High blood pressure

(hypertension)

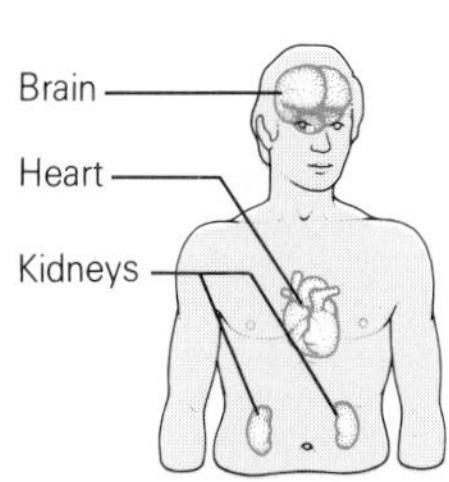

Organs affected by high blood pressure
Untreated high blood pressure can lead to heart failure or kidney failure. It can also affect vessels in the brain, causing a stroke.

As your heart pumps blood through your arteries, the force of the blood flow exerts pressure on the arterial walls, just as air pumped into a tire exerts pressure on its lining and surface. And just as too much air pressure is bad for the life of a tire, so too much blood pressure eventually damages your arteries. If your heart pumps blood through your circulatory system most of the day with a force that is much greater than necessary to maintain a steady flow, you have hypertension, or high blood pressure that never returns to normal range. This puts your whole circulatory system under a strain that may ultimately cause great problems.

Blood pressure varies from person to person and even in different parts of your body. For example, it is higher in your legs than in your arms. For the sake of convenience, it is usually measured in one of the large arteries of one or both arms (see p.412). Two types of pressure, systolic and diastolic, are measured. Systolic pressure is the peak pressure at the moment when your heart contracts and pumps out the blood into the arteries. Diastolic pressure is the lowest pressure in the arteries just before the next contraction of the heart. Therefore, the systolic figure, which represents the moment of greatest pressure, is always higher than the diastolic figure. If someone tells you that your blood pressure is 120 over 80, this means that your systolic pressure is 120 millimeters of mercury (mm Hg), and your diastolic is 80 mm Hg. Those figures are within the normal range for a healthy young adult. (See also Postural hypotension, p.448.)

Whether you have high blood pressure depends largely on medical judgment of your individual case. For instance, if you are over 65, and your blood pressure reading is 140/90, your physician may consider this to be normal pressure for you, since blood pressure tends to rise slightly with age. But when you are in a relatively calm emotional and physical condition and your blood pressure exceeds 150/100, there is cause for concern. Even if only one of the two figures is high, especially the diastolic (lower) figure, you may have high blood pressure.

There are actually two types of high blood pressure, essential hypertension and secondary hypertension. In essential hypertension, you have high blood pressure for no reason that the physician can determine. In secondary hypertension, the cause of the disorder has been identified by your physician. Some possible causes are kidney disease, hormonal disorders such as Cushing's syndrome (see p.563) and aldosteronism (see p.564), and changes in the body produced by taking oral contraceptives (see p.650) or becoming pregnant (see p.670).

About 95 percent of people with hypertension have essential hypertension. A tendency toward essential hypertension seems to run in families. In other words, blood pressure appears to be influenced by heredity along with your health habits. It also seems likely that people who are overweight when they are young are more apt to have high blood pressure in middle age than their lean contemporaries, and that there is a link in some people between high blood pressure and high sodium intake. If you are hypertensive and overweight, you may be able to lower your blood pressure by reducing your weight and the amount of sodium that you consume in your diet.

In most cases of hypertension, the blood pressure continues to rise over a number of years unless it is treated. Occasionally, however, an exceedingly high blood pressure develops very quickly. This dangerous condition, which can result from either essential or secondary hypertension, is known as malignant hypertension. Untreated malignant hypertension is followed rapidly by stroke, kidney, and/or heart failure.

What are the symptoms?

High blood pressure is almost always a symptomless disease. If you have hypertension, you may feel fine, without the slightest indication of physical problems. Such symptoms as severe headaches, palpitations, shortness of breath, and a feeling of ill health usually occur only when some damage has already taken place from the hypertension in your retinas, brain, heart, or kidneys. So it is risky to wait for treatment until symptoms develop.

You should always consider that you may have high blood pressure, especially if you are over 40, if there is a history of hypertension in your family, and if you are overweight. Be sure to have your blood pressure checked every time you have any reason to visit a health care facility.

High blood pressure is extremely common, especially in the US. One study suggests that more than one in 10 Americans is hypertensive. The incidence rises steeply with age and appears to be twice as high among African Americans as among whites. The study also indicates that women are only about half to three fourths as likely to have high blood pressure as men. Malignant hypertension is rare, but it requires rapid diagnosis and treatment.

Testing blood pressure

The meter

In the most common type of meter for measuring blood pressure (illustrated below) the reading appears on a compact, round dial. However, because the earliest method of measuring blood pressure involved the use of a mercury-filled glass column, blood pressure is usually expressed as millimeters of mercury.

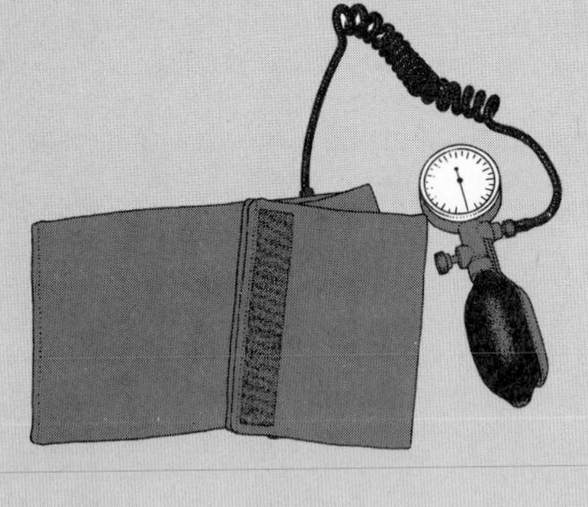

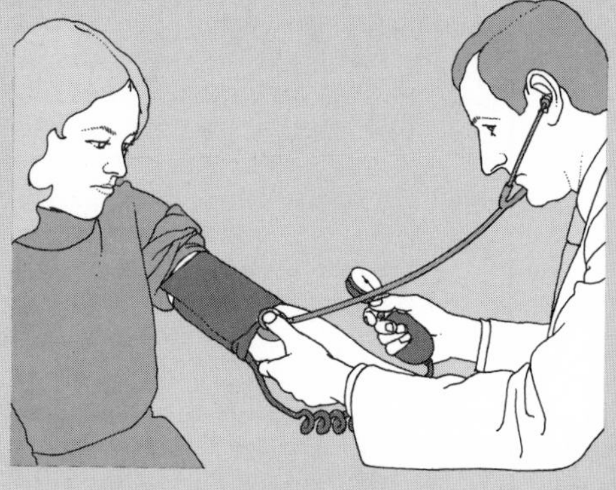

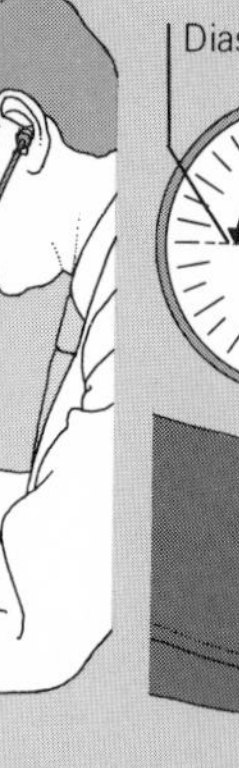

Measuring blood pressure

The tester wraps a soft, rubbery cuff around your upper arm and inflates it until it is tight enough to stop the flow of blood. The cuff is gradually deflated until the tester, listening through a stethoscope, can hear blood forcing its way through the main artery in your arm. A reading is taken of this maximum amount of pressure, which is called systolic. The cuff is then deflated to a point where blood flows steadily through the now-open artery. A second reading, of the diastolic pressure, is then taken. Depending on several factors, if either reading is too high you may have high blood pressure. The same principles apply to the automatic digital readout units available for home use today.

What are the risks?

Even mild hypertension may lower your life expectancy if you do not get treatment for it. If you have untreated severe high blood pressure, the disorder may shorten your life considerably. In particular there are major risks to the heart and brain in such cases. Untreated malignant hypertension can be fatal within 6 months.

The reason high blood pressure is dangerous is that increased pressure in the circulatory system forces your heart to work harder to keep your blood moving. This extra work can damage the inner lining of your coronary arteries. Over the years fatty tissue called atheroma is likely to form where damage has occurred, and your coronary arteries may become narrowed or close completely. The result may be a heart attack. If you have hypertension, you are six times more likely to develop heart failure than someone who has normal blood pressure.

Moreover, if you have high blood pressure, your chances of having a stroke (see p.285) are four times greater than they would be if your blood pressure were normal. This is because increased blood pressure can lead to the formation of atheroma in the arteries that supply the brain with blood and result in hemorrhage from weakened vessels.

Your kidneys may also be damaged, significantly so if you have malignant hypertension. Kidney damage (see Chronic kidney failure, p.551) also leads to a further rise in blood pressure. The brain, eyes, and other organs also can be affected by damage to or bleeding from the blood vessels that supply them with needed oxygen and nutrients.

High blood pressure during pregnancy (see p.670) should be treated. If it is allowed to persist, high blood pressure can interfere with the supply of nutrients and oxygen to the fetus through the placenta.

What should be done?

Have your blood pressure checked once a year and remember what your blood pressure was. If your doctor fails to tell you the value, ask him or her to tell you. If you are taking oral contraceptives or estrogen, or if you are pregnant, you should have your blood pressure checked more frequently. Never pass up the opportunity to have your blood pressure checked. Many health, community, and work organizations sponsor free blood pressure screening programs.

Even if you show signs of high blood pressure during a first examination, your physician may want to test your pressure a couple of times before treating you. Because exertion, excitement, or some other physical or psychological factor can result in a momentarily elevated reading, it is preferable not to make an immediate diagnosis. In a second examination the physician will probably perform a careful and complete physical examination. He or she will spend a few minutes looking into your eyes with an ophthalmoscope, because the blood vessels on your retina are the only blood vessels that the physician can see without elaborate equipment, and their condition often gives valuable information about the effects of abnormally high blood pressure.

Further investigation will depend on your age and whether your physician needs to check if you have essential or secondary hypertension. You may need a chest X ray, an echocardiogram (see Glossary), and an electrocardiogram (ECG), to determine whether your heart is enlarged. The ECG also records any previous damage to the heart muscle. Your physician will arrange blood and urine tests to see if you have kidney trouble. Your physician may also recommend an intravenous pyelogram (IVP), a test in which dye is injected into your body and your kidneys are examined by X ray.

What is the treatment?

Self-help: When the primary cause is treated successfully, secondary hypertension is generally eliminated. If the primary cause cannot be cleared up, treatment is usually the same as it is for essential hypertension, which can be controlled but not cured.

In many cases, changes in your weight, diet, and life-style can lead to satisfactory lowering of the blood pressure without the use of drugs. Here are some suggestions of how to change your life-style.

Assessing the condition of blood vessels
Blood vessels on your retina can be examined easily by a physician with an ophthalmoscope. The vessels in the eye are particularly sensitive to the long-term effects of untreated high blood pressure and are a good index of how severe your disease is.

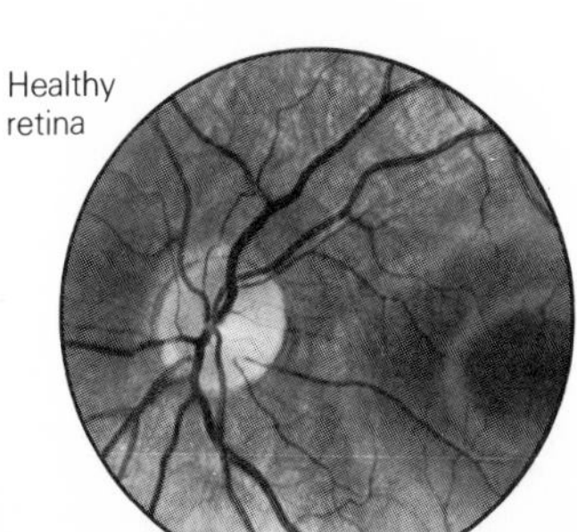

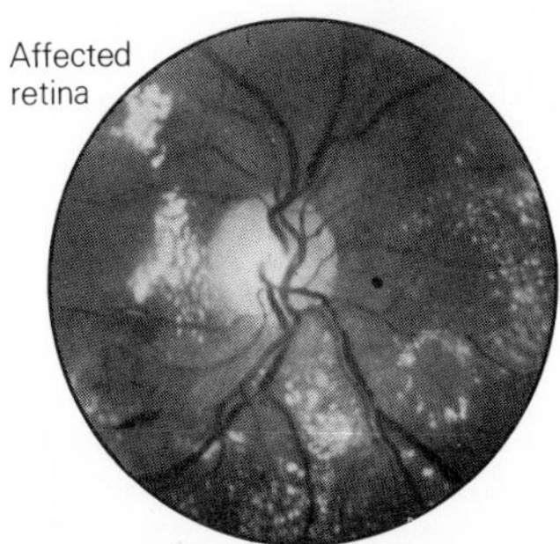

1. If you smoke, quit. Cigarette smoking is not a cause of hypertension, but people who have hypertension and who smoke have a greater risk of developing complications. Furthermore, there *is* a link between smoking and coronary artery disease. Because the chances of heart trouble are increased by both cigarettes and high blood pressure, by giving up smoking you can reduce the risk instead of increasing it.

2. If you are overweight, choose a sensible weight loss diet (see p.34), stick to it until you reach an appropriate weight for your age, sex, and height, and then try to maintain the weight. Again, there is no firm evidence that hypertension is controlled by weight reduction alone, but we do know that trim people have high blood pressure less often than those who are overweight, and trim people are less likely to get certain serious diseases that are linked with hypertension.

3. Do not add salt to your food, and give up sodium-rich foods.

4. Try to make your work schedule and recreation less demanding, and learn to sidestep crises. Some studies indicate that a person who is always pressing ahead to the next objective, talks rather than listens, and constantly looks at his or her watch—the so-called "Type A" personality—is at greater risk of coronary artery disease.

5. Try to avoid using alcohol. Alcohol consumption can increase blood pressure and can interact with blood pressure medications. Some people maintain that small quantities of alcohol help to lower blood pressure. There is no convincing evidence that this is true.

6. Very mild hypertension can often be treated without drugs, by exercise, weight reduction, decreased sodium intake, and relaxation techniques such as meditation. Before trying any form of relaxation therapy, consult your physician.

Professional help: If self-help does not lower your blood pressure to a normal range, you need drug treatment. The drugs used to treat high blood pressure must always be administered under the supervision of a physician. Since all of these drugs may have side effects, continue your self-help measures; in general, the lower the dose you need of these drugs, the less chance you have of experiencing the side effects.

Since essential hypertension is usually a symptomless disease, you may be tempted to stop taking the drugs because you do not feel ill. Because high blood pressure cannot be cured, you will probably have to go on taking regular doses of medication for the rest of your life. Most of these drugs produce side effects, some tolerable (if the benefit justifies it); others are unpleasant or downright threatening. With the substantial number of drugs available, your physician should be able to find a drug or drugs that are safe, effective, and acceptable to you.

For all these reasons your physician will not put you on drugs without being satisfied that you really need the treatment.

Your physician will base the decision on a number of considerations, such as your age, general state of health, and sex (women appear to be less susceptible than men to the complications that result from hypertension). When the decision on which medications to try has been made, it is important that you and your physician agree to the treatments and that you follow his or her instructions carefully and completely.

A diuretic medication to help reduce your blood pressure expels fluid from your body, thus lowering the volume of the blood. Diuretics make you urinate frequently, so it is a good idea to take them in the morning rather than at bedtime. Some diuretics also cause you to lose potassium. In some cases, you must replace this nutrient by taking supplements prescribed by your physician or by eating foods that are rich in potassium, such as oranges, bananas, or other fruits.

Several other types of drugs are used to control high blood pressure, including beta-blockers, calcium channel blockers, and angiotensin converting enzyme (ACE) inhibitors. These drugs not only lower blood pressure, but also reduce the strain on the heart and help prevent irregularities in its rhythm. They generally produce few side effects when taken in low dosages. If you do experience unpleasant side effects you should consult your physician, who may prescribe a different type of drug.

Medical myth

High blood pressure is exclusively a disease of executives and other people with very demanding jobs.

Wrong. There is no apparent correlation between type of job and susceptibility to hypertension. People from all walks of life have this disorder.

What are the long-term prospects?

If you have high blood pressure but you control it carefully, you will avoid nearly all risk of heart failure and considerably reduce the likelihood of stroke and kidney failure. The effect of control on the chance of having a coronary thrombosis, or heart attack, is less clear-cut, because many other factors are involved, and the damage to the coronary circulation that is caused by high blood pressure is irreversible. Since your heart works under less strain when you lower your blood pressure, you may be less likely to suffer a heart attack than you were before treatment for the disorder brought your symptoms under control.

Generally, the outlook is good if you have hypertension and you are being treated for it successfully. Regular visits to your physician and careful attention to your physician's instructions regarding medication, diet, and life-style are an important part of effective treatment for this disorder.

Shock

Shock is defined as a condition in which the flow of blood throughout the body suddenly becomes inadequate, and vital parts, deprived of oxygen, drastically reduce function, at least briefly. The systolic blood pressure usually falls below 80 or 90 millimeters of mercury (mm Hg). This usually happens for one of three reasons. One is that your heart fails to pump out a sufficient supply of blood; this is called cardiogenic shock. The second possible reason for shock is loss of blood or some other body fluid, to the point where there is not enough blood in your body to maintain pressure. This is called hypovolemic shock, and it can be the result of an injury, a disorder that causes blood loss or hemorrhage, a perforated ulcer (see p.501), a bad burn, or prolonged diarrhea. The third possible cause of shock is when the diameter of your small blood vessels becomes so large that your blood pressure drops and you become relatively short of blood. Called anaphylactic, or septic, shock, this may result from a severe allergic reaction or infection.

If shock develops, your body enters a dangerous downward spiral. Lack of blood flowing to the brain deprives it of oxygen. As the brain is affected, the blood vessels become overdilated and unresponsive because the nervous system cannot control blood vessel diameter as it normally does. In a spiral of events, the blood pressure then drops even further because your blood vessels are enlarged. Once caught in this downward spiral, your body cannot recover without medical intervention.

What are the symptoms?

The symptoms of shock include sweating, faintness, nausea, panting, rapid pulse rate, and pale, cold, moist skin. Blood pressure falls to dangerously low levels, resulting in inadequate blood flow to the kidneys so that the kidneys stop producing urine (see Postural hypotension, p.448). As the blood supply to the brain falls, the person in shock becomes drowsy and confused and may also lose consciousness.

Shock and circulation

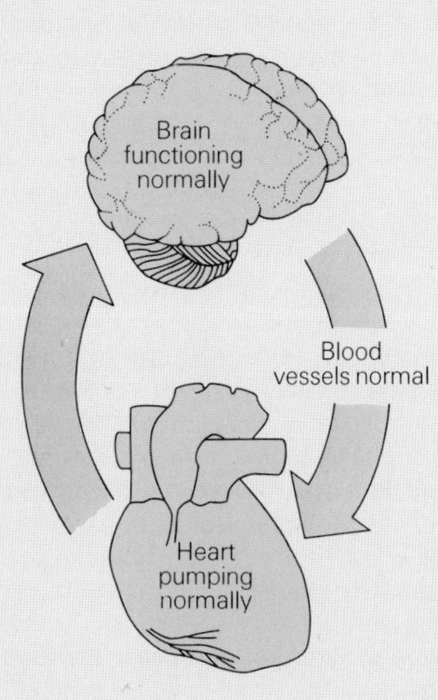

A person is in shock when blood pressure drops and body tissues and organs receive an inadequate supply of blood. The brain first tries to compensate by constricting the blood vessels in nonessential areas of the body such as the skin. You turn pale and your heart rate speeds up to compensate. However, if the pressure remains low, the brain can do nothing more to help. Muscles in the blood vessel walls relax and blood pressure drops even further. If this condition is not treated, the body's vital organs quickly die from lack of oxygen.

Poor blood supply to brain and nervous system

Blood vessels are affected and dilate (widen)

Brain and other organs begin to die

Loss of blood or dilation (widening) of small blood vessels with drop in blood pressure

SHOCK blood vessels widen with further drop in blood flow to brain, kidneys, and heart

DEATH

If shock is unsuccessfully treated, heart begins to fail

Heart pumping normally

START HERE

What are the risks?

Apart from accident victims, the people most likely to go into shock are those with internal bleeding from any cause, severe blood poisoning (see p.452), coronary artery disease that can lead to heart attack (see p.406), severe heart failure, acute obstruction of the pulmonary arteries from an embolism (pulmonary embolism), massive pericardial effusion (see Acute pericarditis, p.430), or a severe attack of asthma (see p.381).

Untreated shock eventually leads to death because the body cannot recover naturally on its own. Since the brain can function for only a few minutes without oxygen, prolonged shock can cause brain damage even if you otherwise recover. The kidneys are also affected quickly by lack of blood. Acute kidney failure (see p.550) can cause death even if recovery procedures begin within minutes. Hemodialysis (a method of purifying the blood to treat kidney failure) is then sometimes used. The chances for recovery from hypovolemic shock are fairly good if emergency replacement of fluid or blood is started immediately. Other types of shock, however, are more likely to be fatal.

What should be done?

If someone is in shock call 911 or call for an ambulance to get the person to an emergency department immediately. For advice on what to do while waiting for emergency assistance, read about shock in Injuries and emergencies (see p.839).

As soon as possible, the person in shock will be hospitalized, probably in an intensive-care unit. Here there is special equipment to monitor the person's cardiovascular health. The heart monitor gives a continuous picture of the heartbeat. This information is vital to evaluate the patient's condition and control treatment. The main tasks of the physician are, first, to stabilize the patient's shock; second, to assess how severe it is; third, to identify the cause; and fourth, to assess the response to treatment.

What is the treatment?

In most cases the first goal of treatment is to restore blood pressure to normal, so that body organs get enough oxygen to stay alive. To achieve this, fluids including blood may be infused through a plastic tube inserted into a vein, and drugs may be used to strengthen the heartbeat and raise blood pressure. If the brain is not damaged, it responds by regaining control of blood vessel tone and diameter. The output of urine is monitored to help detect the possibility of kidney failure.

When emergency procedures have restored the person's blood pressure to nearly normal levels, treatment for the underlying condition causing the symptoms can begin. The physician's choice of treatment will depend on the severity and cause of the condition. For example, an operation may be performed to repair a bleeding ulcer, or high doses of antibiotics may be injected directly into the bloodstream to combat a severe infection. The prospects for recovery depend partly on the underlying cause of the condition and partly on how promptly emergency treatment was received.

Heart rate and rhythm

The muscles of the heart must contract in unison for the heart to function effectively as a pump. Your heart has four chambers: the left and right atria on the top; and the left and right ventricles on the bottom. Valves between these chambers keep the blood moving between them in the proper direction, and electrical impulses from a group of cells in the right atrium help control the frequency and regularity of the muscle contractions. These electrical impulses flow swiftly along specialized muscles that act like nerve pathways; they branch out in all directions in all four chambers of the heart. If some portion of this complex conducting system goes wrong, the regular rhythm of your heartbeat is disturbed. An isolated irregular heartbeat is called an ectopic beat (see p.418). More persistent irregularities of the heartbeat are called cardiac arrhythmias.

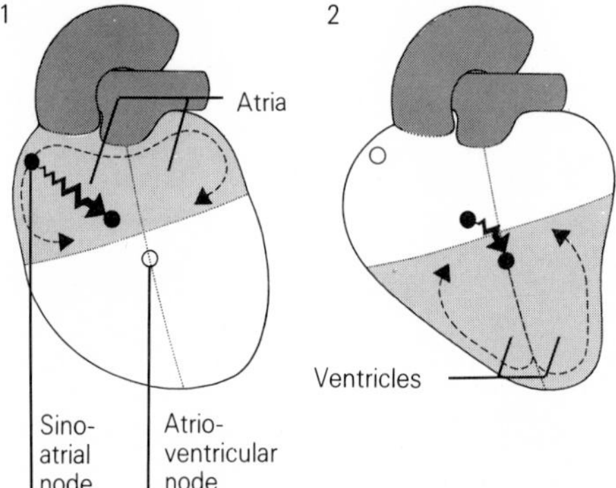

The electrical impulse that initiates a heartbeat originates at the sino-atrial node, passes through the atria walls to the atrioventricular node, and is relayed to the ventricles.

For practical purposes arrhythmias are divided into the tachycardias, in which the heartbeat at rest is faster than 100 beats a minute, and the bradycardias, in which the heart rate is below 60 beats a minute. Both kinds of arrhythmias may be regular or irregular. An arrhythmia may be persistent or may alternate with periods in which the heart rhythm is normal. Any sudden very rapid or very slow arrhythmia may cause fainting or dizziness resulting from a reduction in the blood flow to the brain.

Atrial flutter and atrial fibrillation are two types of arrhythmia affecting the upper chambers of the heart.

The first stage in the assessment of anyone who seems to have an arrhythmia is to investigate the pattern of the heartbeat by performing an electrocardiogram (ECG), a test that shows the electrical activity in the heart muscle and the pattern of heart rate and rhythm. If the arrhythmia seems to be intermittent it may be necessary to record the ECG for 24 hours using a portable ECG (Holter) monitor.

Sometimes the person is placed on a table that is rotated from horizontal to vertical while an ECG is performed. Other tests used to diagnose the cause of an arrhythmia include the cardiac catheterization procedure. (see illustration on p.427).

The principal arrhythmias and their treatment are described in the following group of articles.

Cardiac arrest

(including ventricular tachycardia and ventricular fibrillation)

Cardiac arrest occurs when there is no effective mechanical heartbeat. This can occur when there is a very rapid ventricular tachycardia (rapid ineffective heartbeat whose originating impulse is in the ventricle), ventricular fibrillation (a totally disorganized, ineffective quivering attempt by the ventricles to beat), or cardiac asystole (cessation of heartbeat). When cardiac arrest occurs and your heart cannot beat effectively, your brain no longer gets the blood it needs to function, and you lose consciousness immediately. Cardiac arrest in someone who seems to be in good health usually results from an unsuspected case of coronary artery disease (see p.400). Cardiac arrest can start with a fast ventricular tachycardia and degenerate into ventricular fibrillation.

What should be done?
It is possible to recover from cardiac arrest if the heartbeat and circulation can be restored by cardiac massage within a few minutes. (If cardiac arrest occurs when you are alone, it is fatal.) A person trained in cardiopulmonary resuscitation (CPR) can help revive someone whose heart has stopped until he or she can be taken to the hospital. If the heartbeat has stopped, immediate CPR can stimulate the heart and restore the normal heartbeat. If ventricular tachycardia or fibrillation occurs, CPR can keep the brain alive until electrical defibrillation restores the normal heartbeat. To refresh yourself on CPR, read the section on Injuries and emergencies (see p.836) before an emergency occurs. Whether you are trained in CPR or not, have someone call for an ambulance immediately when a person around you suffers cardiac arrest. If you are the lone rescuer, call 911 first and then begin CPR procedures.

A device may be implanted in persons who have recurring bouts of ventricular tachycardia that does not respond to treatment with drugs. The device, an implantable cardioverter and defibrillator (an apparatus that briefly passes an electric current through your heart), senses the onset of the abnormal rhythm and automatically provides a potentially lifesaving shock. Some implantable cardioverters and defibrillators also function as heart pacemakers (see p.420).

The prospects for recovery from cardiac arrest are good if emergency treatment is given promptly and the circulation is kept going until the person reaches the hospital. If the cardiac arrest is caused by ventricular fibrillation, the person's heartbeat can often be restored with a defibrillator. If emergency treatment is delayed, the damage done to the heart and brain may prove fatal.

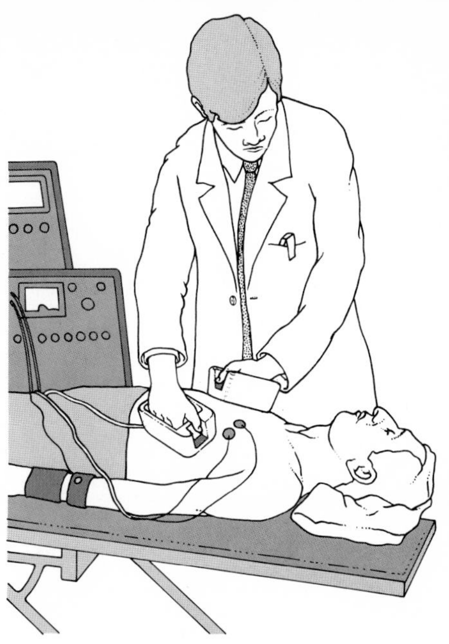

Using a defibrillator to restart the heart
A defibrillator sends an electrical shock to the heart via two metal plates placed on the chest wall. The shock discharges all the heart cells at the same time and permits the heart's normal pacemaker to restart the heart.

Atrial fibrillation and flutter

If you have atrial fibrillation, the muscles in the two atria, or upper chambers of the heart, electrically fire at a rate of 400 to 600 pulsations a minute. This is much too fast for all the impulses to get through the atrioventricular node to the ventricles, the two lower chambers of the heart. Only 120 to 180 impulses per muscle reach the ventricles. Thus the ventricular rate is rapid and the rhythm irregular. Atrial fibrillation reduces the efficiency of the heart as a pump, because the speeded up atrial contractions are uncoordinated and push out too little blood. The action of the upper and lower chambers of the heart is not coordinated and, as a result, the ventricles have a shorter filling period.

Atrial flutter is similar to fibrillation, except that in atrial flutter the muscles contract more regularly and at a somewhat slower rate (up to about 300 beats a minute). Both fibrillation and flutter tend to come and go, with periods of normal heart rhythm between episodes.

Atrial fibrillation and flutter usually occur as a consequence of coronary artery disease (see p.400), or of heart disease brought on by rheumatic fever (see p.422). The fibrillation or flutter can also be caused by an overactive thyroid gland, a high fever, or an alcoholic binge. Any disease that causes heart failure and enlargement of the right or left atria can cause atrial flutter or fibrillation. In about 10 percent of cases, especially among older people, there is no obvious cause.

What are the symptoms?
Often there are no symptoms. The most common symptom is palpitations (awareness

of your heartbeat). If you have atrial fibrillation, you may also experience some dizziness, occasional episodes of angina (see p.403), and fainting spells. You may also develop some or all of the symptoms of heart failure (see p.408).

What are the risks?

One danger of atrial fibrillation or flutter is an increased risk of embolism, which is a blood clot that forms in either atrium and travels through the circulatory system to a point where its size prevents it from going any farther. The damage caused by an embolism depends on its size and location. (See also Stroke, p.285.)

Another possible risk is heart failure (see p.408). Normally, even though the atria are not functioning well, the ventricles alone can cope with the task of pumping blood. However, if the ventricles are not pumping efficiently, and if the ventricular rate is excessively fast for a long time, heart failure may develop with atrial fibrillation, especially if the ventricles are also diseased.

What should be done?

If you have symptoms associated with either of these disorders, consult your physician, who will suggest an electrocardiogram (ECG) and other tests. Since atrial fibrillation or any other arrhythmia often comes and goes, you may need to have a continuous ECG recording for 24 to 48 hours with a portable (Holter) monitor.

What is the treatment?

Self-help: None is available.

Professional help: Treatment largely depends on the cause of the disorder. Digitalis is frequently prescribed to help improve the efficiency of the heart by slowing ventricular contractions, because your circulation depends on efficient pumping by your ventricles. Drugs called beta-blockers are used to improve the efficiency of the ventricles by slowing the impulses from the atrial nodes. Anti-arrhythmic drugs can help return the heart rhythm to normal. Your physician may also prescribe an anticoagulant drug to prevent an embolism.

If your heart is basically healthy, or if the underlying cause of atrial fibrillation is being treated and atrial flutter or fibrillation persists, your physician may consider a treatment called cardioversion. This consists of an electric shock administered to your heart while you are under mild anesthesia. This treatment frequently restores a normal rhythm to your heart.

Ectopic heartbeats

The word "ectopic" comes from a Greek word meaning "out of place." Ectopic heartbeats are early beats in an otherwise steady pulsation. If you feel as though your heart has missed a beat, or gained an extra beat, you are experiencing this common and usually minor disorder. Do not worry about it. Usually, the condition is harmless, especially if there is no underlying heart disease, and does not require treatment.

If you are bothered by an occasional irregular heartbeat and you are not comforted by your physician's reassurances, he or she may prescribe a drug for the condition. Frequent incidents of ectopic heartbeat are often associated with excessive use of tobacco, alcohol, or caffeine. If you use these substances, quit smoking and cut down on alcohol and coffee along with other caffeine-containing beverages.

Heart block

(atrioventricular block)

Your heart rate usually is controlled by a natural pacemaker, which consists of a group of specialized cells in the wall of the right atrium, or upper right chamber of the four heart chambers. This pacemaker transmits electrical impulses over the two atria, and ultimately to the ventricles. These impulses cause the rhythmic contractions of heart muscle that we call heartbeats. If the natural pacemaker functions too slowly and too irregularly (the sick sinus syndrome), episodes of dizziness, confusion, or fatigue may result. Similar symptoms may be due to heart block, which occurs when the system that conducts the electrical impulses throughout the heart muscles fails, either partially or completely. Then the beating of the atria, or the upper half of your heart, is not coordinated with the beating of the ventricles, or the lower half of your heart. Heart block is more common as you age.

In first-degree heart block the impulse simply takes longer to go from the atrium to the ventricle. This does not affect the heart rate and causes no symptoms. In second-degree block some of the atrial impulses fail to get through to the ventricles, and your pulse becomes irregular. Symptoms may or may not occur. In the disorder known as third-degree heart block (complete heart block) the impulses are not conducted, and the ventricles go on beating slowly, independent of the pacemaker and the atria.

Normally your heart rate, the pulse you can feel in your arms, quickens to cope with exertion or emotion. But during heart block this can no longer happen. As a result, your heart pumps too little oxygenated blood to your brain and other parts of your body at times when a greater supply is needed.

Heart block can occur for no obvious reason, but it is often associated with coronary artery disease or heart attack (see p.406). An overdose of the drug digitalis can also cause a heart block condition.

What are the symptoms?

There are often no symptoms of first- or second-degree heart block. If you do not exercise much and do not experience emotional stress, you may never know you have first- or second-degree heart block. The most severe symptoms occur with third-degree (complete) heart block, also called Stokes-Adams attacks, including sudden loss of consciousness, which is often accompanied by seizures or strokes. Such attacks can occur if the ventricles are beating without any control from the pacemaker cells and either slow down drastically or miss beats for a few seconds, not pumping enough blood to keep the brain functioning normally. On the other hand, third-degree heart block sometimes produces symptoms similar to those of heart failure (see p.408).

What are the risks?

Since more older people have been screened for abnormalities of the heart's pacemaker and conducting system, physicians have learned that minor degrees of the sick sinus syndrome and heart block are more common than previously thought. As a result of treatment with pacemakers, many older people have been restored to health. The more severe forms of heart block once had a poor outcome, with 50 percent of patients with third-degree block dead within a year of its diagnosis. But now, with implanted pacemakers, the outlook is much improved.

What should be done?

Any older person who has episodes of dizziness, weakness, or confusion should consult a physician promptly. These symptoms have many possible causes, but if you have heart block, early treatment of the condition may be lifesaving.

What is the treatment?

If the heart's electrical timing system is the cause of your symptoms, your physician may recommend the insertion of an artificial pacemaker (see next page).

Paroxysmal atrial tachycardia

If you are a healthy adult, your heart beats 60 to 100 times a minute, and rises to about 160 a minute during periods of exertion. If you have an attack, or paroxysm, of atrial tachycardia, your heartbeat suddenly speeds up to a rate of 160 or more beats a minute. An attack of paroxysmal atrial tachycardia can last for a minute or for several days.

What are the symptoms?

The main symptom of this disorder is palpitations (awareness of your heartbeat). You suddenly become aware of your rapid heartbeat, and you may become anxious. Some people who have paroxysmal atrial tachycardia say it is accompanied by a premonition of impending death. Additional symptoms of the disorder may include breathlessness, fainting spells, chest pain, and abnormally frequent urination.

What are the risks?

Despite any anxiety or fear that it causes, paroxysmal atrial tachycardia is not usually a serious disorder. There is a risk of congestive heart failure (see p.408) if the heartbeat is extremely rapid, but there is usually no danger to your health.

What should be done?

When you get a pounding feeling in your chest that characterizes paroxysmal atrial tachycardia, you may be alarmed, especially if this is your first attack. Although there is little cause for concern, you should see your physician if the symptoms last for more than a few minutes. It is difficult to make a diagnosis from your description of your symptoms alone, and it is easier to diagnose the problem if your physician can examine you during an attack.

If you are young to middle aged, with no history of heart trouble, atrial tachycardia is unlikely to be serious. Try to relax, and practice the self-help measures suggested below. However, if you get recurrent attacks, worry, and become exhausted, seek help. After examining you, your physician may order other tests including an electrocardiogram (ECG) or an ambulatory ECG with a portable (Holter) monitor if the tachycardia comes and goes.

What is the treatment?

Self-help: When an attack occurs, note whether the rhythm is regular and count the pulse (the number of heartbeats in 1 minute) so you can report this to your physician. Heart rate can be slowed by certain nerve impulses, which can be induced in several ways. Hold your breath for a while, or take a slow drink of water, or bathe your face in cold water. If none of these measures works, it may help if you hold your nostrils closed and try to blow through your nose hard enough to make your eardrums "pop." Strong stimulation of the vagus nerve, which slows the heart rate, occurs if you induce vomiting by tickling the back of your throat.

If you have had an attack of paroxysmal atrial tachycardia, you may take some preventive measures against further episodes. Cigarettes, alcohol, tea, and coffee may all increase your susceptibility. Try to stop smoking and cut down on alcohol and caffeine. There also seems to be a link between anxiety and atrial tachycardia, but it is unclear whether the anxiety is a cause of or an effect of the disorder.

Professional help: Your physician may massage the carotid artery in your neck to try to slow down your heart. If your attack warrants further treatment, your physician may give you an injection of a drug that helps slow a rapid heartbeat. In extreme cases of paroxysmal atrial tachycardia, your physician may advise you to have cardioversion, a procedure in which an electric shock is administered to your heart directly, while you are under a mild anesthetic.

As preventive treatment, your physician may prescribe drugs that decrease the excitability of the heart muscle. These drugs help keep your heart from speeding up.

Pacemakers

A pacemaker is a device that provides an artificial, regular electrical impulse to replace an irregular or absent natural impulse in your heart. It is used to treat disorders such as second- or third-degree heart block. An electrode is placed in contact with your heart wall, usually through a thin tube guided into your circulatory system via a neck or arm vein. This electrode is connected to a small generating unit powered by a battery with a life span of 8 to 10 years, depending on the type of battery.

Today's pacemakers are designed to monitor the heart rate and rhythm and to respond to abnormalities as they occur. A "demand" pacemaker takes over for the heart if the rate becomes too slow. Many pacemakers detect atrial impulses and ventricular impulses and can pace one or both if needed. Some automatic implantable cardioverters, which detect life-threatening arrhythmias and restore the normal rhythm by generating an electric shock that is administered at exactly the right time in the heart cycle, can also serve as pacemakers.

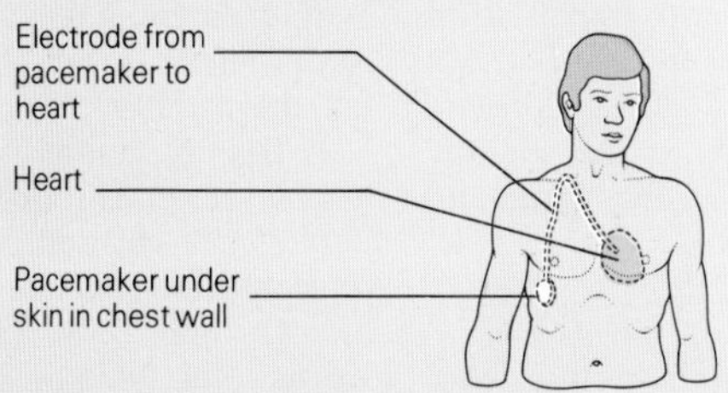

Positioning a pacemaker
The pacemaker wire is guided to your heart along a vein that runs close to your collar bone. If the pacemaker is permanent, the physician will insert it under the skin on your chest wall.

Many pacemakers can vary the heart rate according to the body's needs, so that the rate generated is faster during exercise than it is during periods of sleep.

If a pacemaker is required for only a short time, such as after a heart attack temporarily disturbs your heart rhythm, you can wear the generating unit of the pacemaker on a belt. Otherwise it is implanted under your skin, usually in the loose tissues of your chest wall just under your collar bone. If you have a pacemaker, your physician needs to examine you periodically to make sure the device is working well. A battery that is low on power can be replaced quickly and easily. Periodic evaluation by telephone using special equipment is also performed.

Modern pacemakers are remarkably resistant to outside interference. If you have a pacemaker, however, you should stay away from powerful radio or radar transmitters, and avoid going through security devices at airports, stores, and libraries. Some models can be influenced by electromagnetic impulses from microwave ovens, electric shavers, MRI scanners, and similar devices. If you undergo surgery, your surgeon may also need to take certain precautions since some forms of surgery use diathermy (electrical heat) units for controlling bleeding that can adversely affect the function of your pacemaker.

Heart valve diseases

The heart has four valves. The mitral valve controls the flow of blood from the left atrium (the left one of two chambers in the top of the heart) into the left ventricle (the left one of two chambers in the bottom of the heart). The tricuspid valve is the equivalent of the mitral valve on the right side. The pulmonary valve controls the exit from the right ventricle into the pulmonary artery, which carries blood into the lungs. The aortic valve controls the output of blood from the left ventricle into the aorta, the artery through which blood flows to the body. Inflammation of a valve or other changes such as scarring can ultimately cause stenosis or incompetence. Stenosis is a thickening of the valve, which narrows its opening. Incompetence is a distortion of the valve, which prevents it from closing fully.

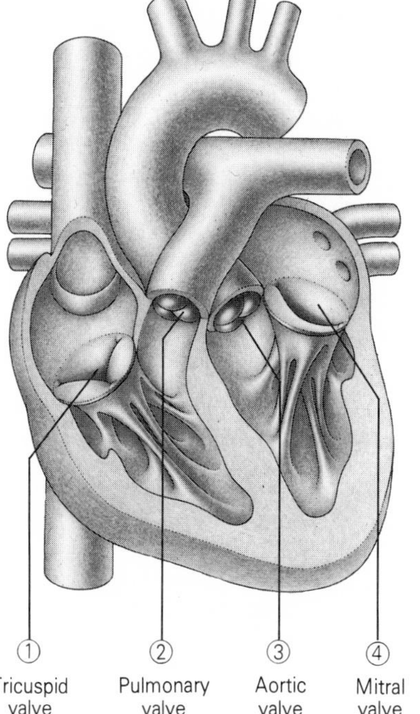

How the valves work
With each heartbeat the ventricles contract and force the blood out of the heart. The aortic and pulmonary valves open to let the blood out. Between heartbeats the ventricles relax and the aortic and pulmonary valves close. The mitral and tricuspid valves then open to allow blood to flow into the heart from the veins. The constant and regular repetition of this cycle keeps the blood flowing throughout your body.

Blood out

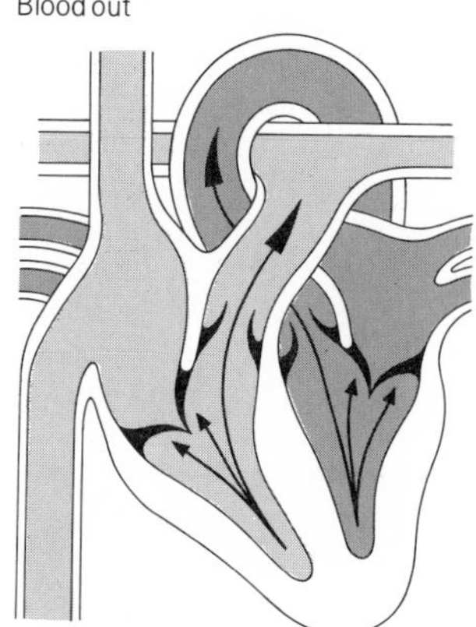

Valves ② and ③ open
Blood pumped out of heart to lungs and body tissues

Blood in

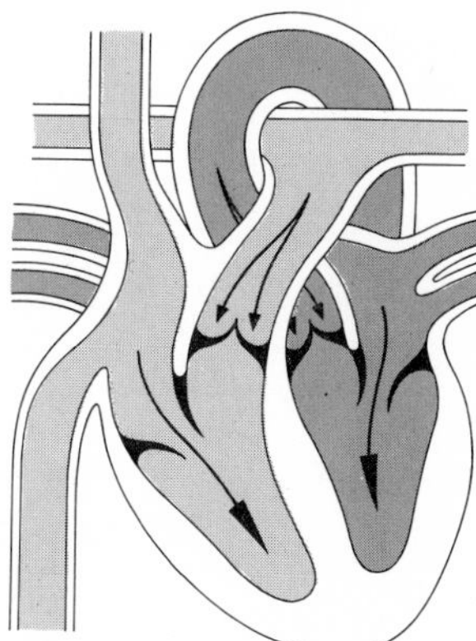

Valves ① and ④ open
Blood passes into the heart from the body tissues and the lungs

What can go wrong
When a valve does not open wide enough, the heart must generate more pressure to pump through an adequate supply of blood. When a valve does not close completely, some of the blood that has flowed through it leaks back into the heart, which must pump it out again. Both conditions increase the heart's work load and can lead to thickening of the heart muscle and ultimately to heart failure.

Normal opening

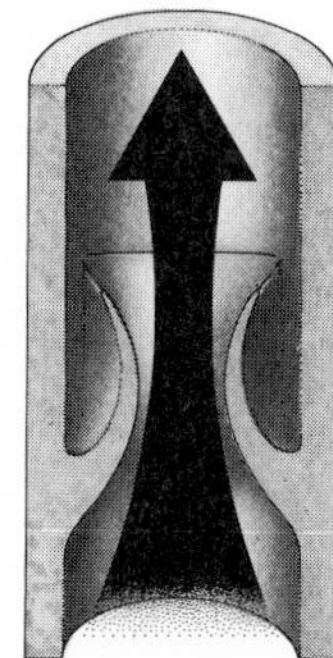

Inadequate opening (stenosis)

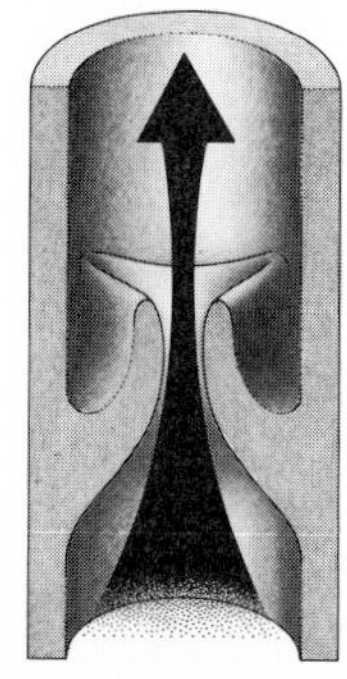

Normal closing

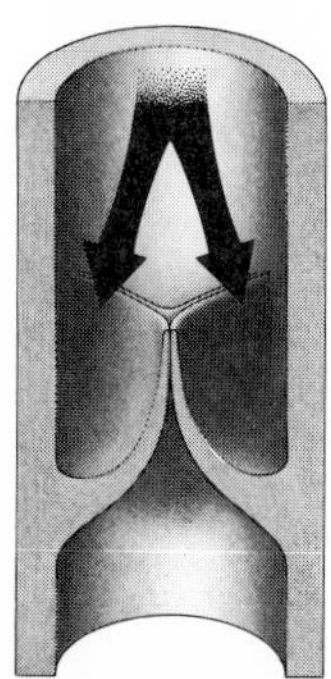

Inadequate closing (incompetence)

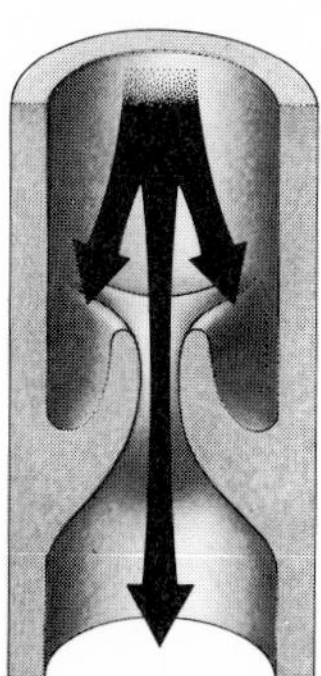

Rheumatic fever

Rheumatic fever is a disorder that affects several parts of the body, including the heart. It is included here because its most significant consequence may be some type of valvular heart disease.

Rheumatic fever had virtually disappeared from the US in the late 1960s and 1970s, but it reappeared in a few outbreaks in the late 1980s and clearly has not been eradicated. It remains a major health problem in developing countries. It usually begins with a throat infection caused by certain strains of *Streptococcus* bacteria and is followed by general illness, the main symptoms of which are fever; inflamed, aching, and swollen joints; a characteristic rash; and sometimes inflammation of, and damage to, various body tissues. If the heart is involved, all heart tissues, including the pericardium, which is a membranous bag that encloses the heart, can be affected. But the heart valves are most often involved, and damage to the valves is the only permanent result of rheumatic fever.

What are the symptoms?

Rheumatic fever usually begins with a sore throat that seems to clear up quickly, but you begin to feel tired and feverish about 3 weeks later. Other symptoms depend on which organ or organs are most severely affected. Inflammation of the heart may not produce any obvious symptoms. Inflamed joints, however, are easier to recognize. The disorder usually affects the knees and ankles, but it may extend to the fingers, wrists, and shoulders. Symptoms include swollen, tender, hot, red, and extremely painful joints. The same joint on both sides is usually involved, and the pain and swelling migrate from one set of joints to another. If the person has repeated infections with a beta strain of *Streptococcus*, rheumatic fever may recur.

What are the risks?

Rheumatic fever is a less threatening disease than in the past because recurrences can now be prevented by treatment with penicillin, but over half of all people with the disorder still develop valvular heart disease. The severity of the heart trouble is often related to the number of episodes of rheumatic fever. There is also a risk of heart failure (see p.408) as the result of a very severe infection.

What are the long-term prospects?

Once an episode of rheumatic fever is over, there are few if any symptoms. The joints generally heal completely. The chance of damaged heart valves remains, especially in someone who has had more than one episode. Sometimes this heart damage may not become evident for years.

Infective endocarditis

(including bacterial endocarditis)

The endocardium is the inner lining of the heart muscle. It also covers the heart valves. If the endocardium is damaged (for example, by mitral incompetence, see p.424), then bacteria or occasionally fungi may infect the damaged area. As the organisms multiply, they damage the area further, and some of them may move through the circulatory system to other parts of the body. They can form infected emboli, which can block small arteries and prevent blood from reaching tissues supplied by those arteries (see Arterial embolism, p.438). But it is the heart valves that are primarily affected by bacterial endocarditis. As the valves are gradually destroyed by the multiplying bacteria, heart failure (see p.408) is apt to develop.

What are the symptoms?

No single symptom signals this disease. There is usually some fever, but your temperature will rarely exceed 102°F (about 39°C). In addition, you may have sudden chills (especially when the bacteria spread throughout your bloodstream), headaches, aching joints, fatigue, and loss of appetite. If the valves have been affected, eventually some or all of the symptoms of heart failure may appear too.

Other symptoms depend on the location of each embolus. You may have painful lumps in the tips of your fingers or small bruises behind your nails. It is common for emboli to lodge in the brain, and this may cause weakness on one side of your body or loss of your vision (see Transient ischemic attack, p.287). Emboli from bacterial endocarditis can lodge in any part of your body, sometimes forming small abscesses.

Although exact figures are not available, infective endocarditis is rare, especially among children and older people. But it occurs commonly in people who use intravenous drugs. Most cases of the disease occur in people between ages 15 and 60.

What are the risks?

Most people who develop infective endocarditis have underlying valvular disease. In the past this resulted from rheumatic fever, but now other valve problems such as mitral valve prolapse (see p.426), congenital valvular lesions, and heart valve replacements (see p.425) are common underlying conditions that may lead to endocarditis. Bacteria can enter the bloodstream during minor operations, tooth extractions (even teeth cleaning), endoscopy, or intravenous injection of illicit drugs using unsterilized, contaminated syringes and needles. People who are susceptible to bacterial endocarditis (primarily those who already have heart trouble) generally need to take prescribed antibiotics immediately before surgery or dental work or promptly when they develop boils or other skin infections. This precaution helps kill any bacteria that might otherwise get into the bloodstream and cause bacterial endocarditis.

If bacterial endocarditis is not discovered and treated within a few weeks of the initial infection, it can cause irreversible heart damage, which might necessitate surgery and valve replacement. Emboli may also do permanent damage to the brain and other parts of the body.

What should be done?
If you have many of the symptoms mentioned above, consult your physician immediately. The symptoms can be confused with a wide variety of problems, so be sure to tell your physician (especially if you are seeing him or her for the first time) that you have, or have had, heart valve disease or heart murmur, or any of the symptoms commonly associated with endocarditis.

If a diagnosis of bacterial endocarditis seems likely, your physician will admit you to a hospital. There samples of your blood will be tested to discover what kind of microorganism is causing your endocarditis and a Doppler ultrasound scan (see Glossary) will help determine both the location and severity of damage to the valve.

Bacterial endocarditis may also cause you to become anemic and to have kidney disease. These conditions will clear up when the infection is cured.

What is the treatment?
The treatment depends on which organism, either bacteria or fungi, is found in the blood sample. Your physician will choose an antibiotic to combat that microorganism. If your case of bacterial endocarditis is diagnosed and effectively treated within 6 weeks of the initial infection, you have a 90 percent chance of complete cure of the infection. The long-term results depend on which valve is injured and on the severity of the damage.

Mitral stenosis

Mitral stenosis occurs when the mitral valve, which is between the left atrium (the left one of the two upper heart chambers), and the left ventricle (the left one of the two lower heart chambers), becomes scarred, the leaflets (valve flaps) stick together, and the channel becomes abnormally narrow. In order to force blood through the narrow opening, the atrium enlarges and pressure inside the chamber gradually rises. This pressure is transmitted back through the pulmonary veins and capillaries to the lungs, which, over a period of years, makes them become congested. The higher the cardiac output (amount of blood pumped by the heart in a minute), the higher the pressure in the pulmonary vessels. To keep blood flowing through the lungs at a normal rate, the right ventricle must also pump more and more vigorously, and it too becomes enlarged.

What are the symptoms?
The main symptom of mitral stenosis is breathlessness, which is caused by congestion in the lungs. It is most apparent after exercise, but it can occur at night or whenever you are lying down. After going to sleep you may suddenly wake up with a feeling of being smothered that makes you sit up quickly. You may cough up small amounts of blood or blood-flecked frothy phlegm. You may become susceptible to wheezing and worsened breathing, which could be mistaken for an episode of bronchitis (see p.379).

As pressure builds up through the entire circulatory system, you may experience general fatigue, swollen ankles, and other symptoms that indicate right-sided heart failure (see p.408). If this happens, chest symptoms usually diminish because the heart failure and the decreased cardiac output relieve pressure on the lungs.

About 50 percent of people who have had rheumatic fever (see p.422) later develop heart disease. Almost 75 percent of these people have some degree of mitral stenosis. But because the number of cases of rheumatic fever has declined in recent years, mitral stenosis is much less common today than it was in the past.

What are the risks?
Breathlessness and general weakness can be disabling, especially if you are pregnant or if

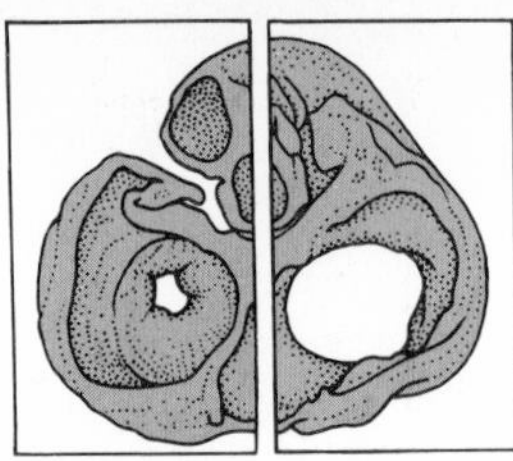

Mitral stenosis
The edges of the valve flaps are stuck together. Now only the tip of one finger can pass through the opening.

Healthy mitral valve
Looking through a healthy, opened mitral valve (2 fingers can normally pass through this channel).

Vertical cross section through valves
Normal blood flow through healthy mitral valve (below); restricted blood flow through valve with mitral stenosis (bottom).

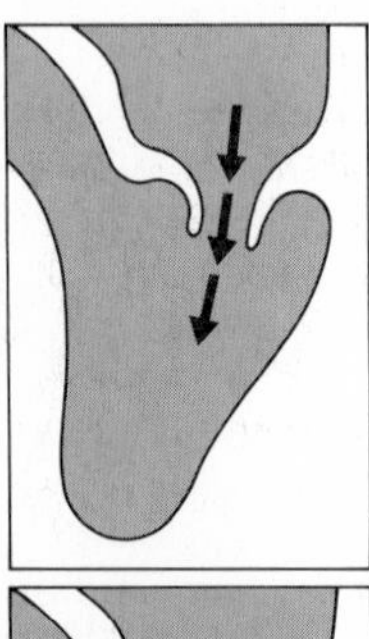

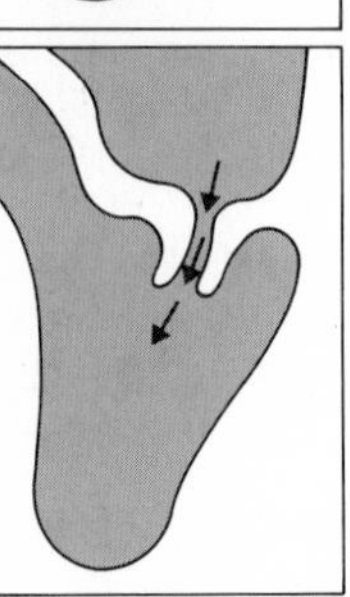

you have a chest infection, an overactive thyroid gland (see Hyperthyroidism, p.565) or any condition in which the cardiac output is increased. The main danger with mitral stenosis is of atrial fibrillation (see p.417), which often causes heart failure and formation of a clot in the left atrium with the risk of an embolus breaking away from your heart and causing blockage in a distant blood vessel, often in the brain.

What should be done?

Consult your physician if you have any of the symptoms mentioned above. Sometimes mitral stenosis is discovered by accident during a regular check up. After examining you, with special attention to your heart, your physician may be able to diagnose mitral stenosis by listening for a heart murmur (see p.702). If additional testing is needed, your physician may want you to have a chest X ray, an electrocardiogram (ECG), and possibly a Doppler echocardiogram. With ultrasound, the Doppler echocardiogram can measure the velocity of blood flow through the valve, and this allows your physician to calculate how much it has narrowed.

What is the treatment?

Self-help: None is possible. If you have no disabling symptoms, you can live an active life without any treatment for mitral stenosis. However, if you have this condition, you should always ask your physician for antibiotics before you have dental work or surgery to protect you from infective endocarditis (see p.422).

Professional help: If breathlessness is troubling you, your physician may prescribe a diuretic drug, which rids the body of excess fluid. However, diuretic drugs may also cause you to lose potassium. This mineral, which is essential to muscle contraction and maintaining a normal heart rhythm, must be replaced. Your physician may prescribe supplementary potassium.

If you have atrial fibrillation, it can usually be controlled by certain heart drugs and your physician may prescribe anticoagulants to prevent the formation of clots in the left atrium and resulting emboli.

If your mitral stenosis is so severe that it restricts your daily activities, your physician may advise you to have surgery. Surgery may also be necessary if you become pregnant and your symptoms worsen. The operation is called mitral valvotomy, in which the valve is repaired while the patient is on a heart-lung machine. The surgery involves widening the narrowed valve. Such an operation involves some risk, but if your health is otherwise good, the survival rate from the operation is 98 percent. In general the results are highly successful, and often the symptoms do not return for years. If your symptoms return, you may require a second valvotomy, or more often you may have to have your mitral valve replaced with an artificial one. About 80 percent of those who have had valve replacement operations have survived for at least 5 years. Recently, a technique that uses a balloon on a catheter has been developed; it has been successful in stretching open the stenotic mitral valve without surgery. The long-term results of this procedure have not yet been determined, and its use has not become widespread. Read the following article on mitral incompetence for more information about mitral valve replacement.

Mitral incompetence

If your heart's mitral valve does not close properly, the blood circulating through your heart may leak back into the left atrium (the left one of the two upper heart chambers) from the left ventricle (the left one of the two lower heart chambers). This is called mitral incompetence or mitral regurgitation. If you have this disorder, your heart has to work harder than usual, and the muscular heart wall enlarges in an attempt to cope with the additional work load. With the leak, the left atrium also enlarges. In the US the usual cause of mitral regurgitation is an abnormality of the mitral valve called mitral valve prolapse (see p.426). This disorder causes the valve to move abnormally back too far into the left atrium during contraction of the ventricles. The valve flaps therefore often fail to come together and the valve leaks. In developing countries rheumatic

OPERATION:

Heart valve replacement

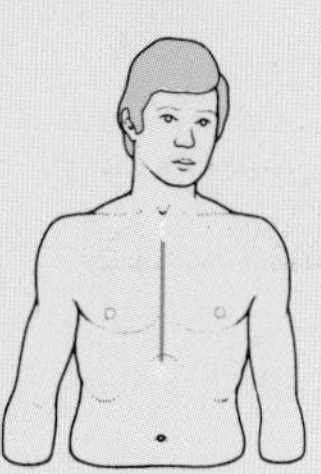

Site of the incision

A heart valve replacement operation is performed to replace damaged heart valves either with specially designed plastic and metal valves or with valves made from tissue, either of humans or other animals. One type incorporates a pig's aortic valve, which is sewn onto a frame.

During the operation You are under a general anesthetic and your circulation is taken over by a heart-lung machine. Your breathing is monitored by the anesthesiologist. An incision is made either along your breastbone or along the line of a lower rib on your left side. Your ribs are parted and your heart is opened. The damaged valve is removed. The new valve is then sewn into place with stitches. The operation takes from 2 to 4 hours.

After the operation You will spend the first few days in the intensive-care unit. One or two drainage tubes will be placed in your chest and attached to suction bottles. You will breathe oxygen through a tube leading into your nose and may need the help of a ventilator. Your bladder will be drained by a catheter. You will receive fluid and blood through intravenous drips and your heart and vital signs will be monitored constantly.

Choice of valve The type of valve most appropriate for you depends on factors such as your age and general health. Mechanical valves last a long time, but you will need to take anticoagulant drugs. Valves taken from animals or made from human tissues may need to be replaced after a period of years, but fewer people with such valves need to take anticoagulants than those with mechanical valves. The risk of complications is low with both types of valves.

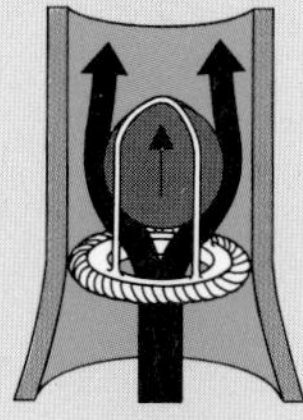

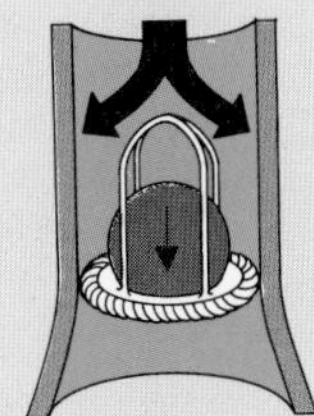

With a ball-and-cage heart valve, blood can flow in one direction (as it should) by forcing the ball away from the ring into the cage. If blood begins to flow in the opposite direction, it forces the ball firmly against the ring and closes the valve.

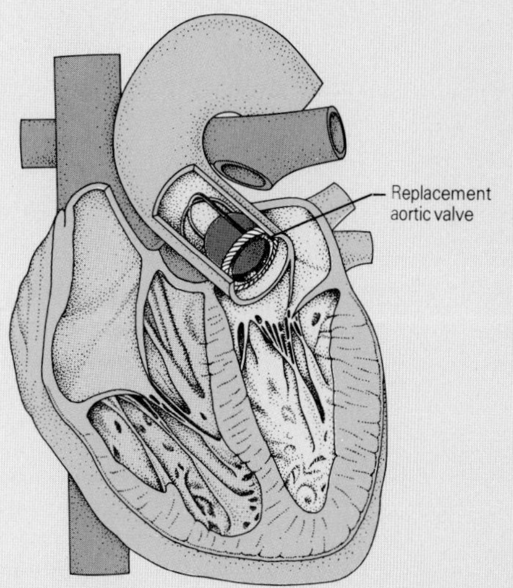

Types of valves
Replacement heart valves may be made of synthetic materials or of grafted tissue. The ball-and-cage and the newer St. Jude valves are made of plastic and metal; the tissue valve is made from animal or human tissue.

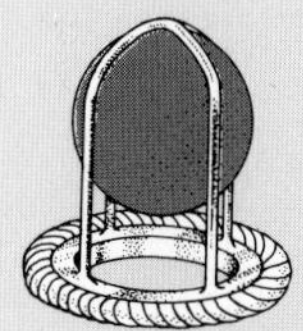

Ball-and-cage

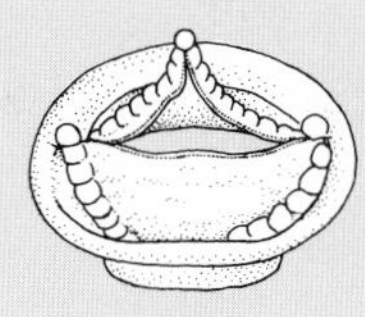

Tissue

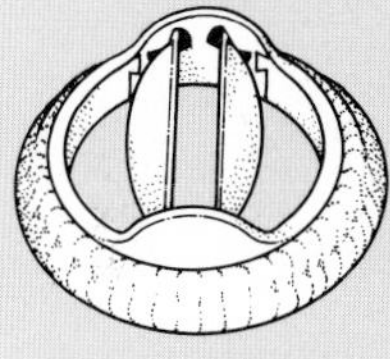

St. Jude

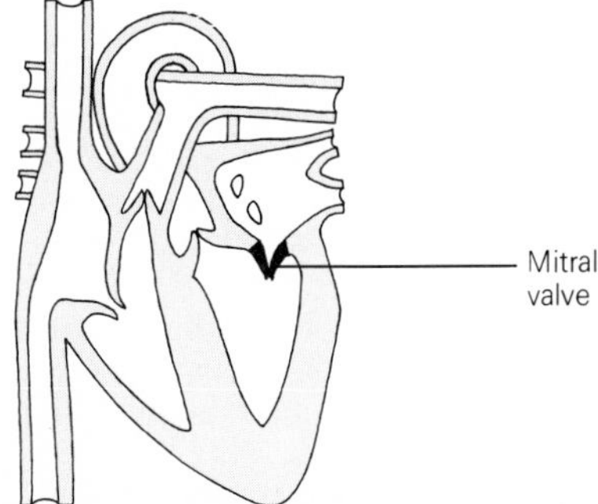

fever (see p.422) is usually the cause of the disorder, but mitral incompetence may be present from birth (see Congenital heart disorders, p.702). The condition may also result from infective endocarditis or another type of heart muscle disorder. Any disorder that causes the left ventricle to enlarge and dilate (widen) can cause mitral regurgitation.

What are the symptoms?

Often there are no apparent symptoms of mitral incompetence, but this disorder can lead to shortness of breath, fatigue, and other symptoms of congestive heart failure (see p.408). As the left atrium becomes enlarged, atrial fibrillation (see p.417) usually results.

Surgery is recommended when mitral valve prolapse progresses so the valve flaps cannot close and mitral incompetence is placing a strain on the efficiency of the heart valve. About 5 percent of the US population has mitral valve prolapse.

What are the risks?

The risks are similar to those of mitral stenosis. If the workload of the left ventricle is too great for too long, the ability of the left ventricular muscle to contract properly can fail permanently. If this occurs, even fixing the valve will not benefit you, so your physician will follow up on your condition to detect any signs of deterioration promptly and to recommend surgical repair or replacement of the valve. Infective endocarditis (see p.422) is a serious complication of mitral incompetence.

What should be done?

For detailed information read the previous article on mitral stenosis.

What is the treatment?

As with mitral stenosis, no treatment is likely to be required unless you have symptoms. If you have mitral incompetence, be sure to start antibiotic treatment before having your teeth cleaned or undergoing any kind of surgery. This is necessary to protect you against the risk of infective endocarditis.

Medical treatment for mitral incompetence is much the same as for mitral stenosis (see previous article). If the symptoms of mitral incompetence are severe, your physician may recommend surgery in order to have the incompetent valve repaired or replaced with an artificial one. Repair of the valve is preferable, but not all patients have a valve that can be repaired. Only careful evaluation before and at the time of surgery can determine this.

There are two possible types of replacement, a mechanical valve or a valve grafted from animal or human tissue. Your surgeon must decide which of these replacements is more appropriate for you. Mechanical replacements are efficient, but they cause clotting of blood, which is the basis for dangerous emboli (see Arterial embolism, p.438) that can travel from the heart to the brain or elsewhere in the body. Emboli can occur in 3 to 4 percent of patients every year. If you have a mechanical valve replacement, you will need to take an anticoagulant drug to guard against this complication. Anticoagulants must be considered with extra caution for anyone with a peptic ulcer that may bleed, or for anyone who is unable to have the blood tests necessary to monitor this treatment.

Mechanical valves can also cause hemolysis (a breakdown of red blood cells) because of the mechanical damage the valve causes to the blood by opening and closing. Tissue-graft valves involve much less risk of clotting, but they may be less durable.

If, at any time after the operation, you suddenly become short of breath, faint, or dizzy, or if your urine looks abnormally dark or your chest begins to ache, see your physician as soon as possible. Any of these symptoms may indicate a mechanical failure of the replacement valve.

Mitral valve prolapse

This is a common deformity of the mitral valve, located in the left side of the heart, that can produce mitral incompetence (see p.424), in which blood that has been pumped through the heart leaks back into the heart. Mitral valve prolapse causes a characteristic heart sound or heart murmur that your physician can hear through a stethoscope. Also known as "floppy valve syndrome," the condition affects up to 5 percent of the US population and is much more common in women.

The cause is not known in most cases, but there is some evidence that you can inherit a weakness in the connective tissue structure of the valve that permits it to bulge. Occasionally the prolapse results from rheumatic fever (see p.422), coronary heart disease, or cardiomyopathy (see p.430). Symptoms may include chest pain, irregular heartbeat, shortness of breath, and fatigue, but half the people with mitral valve prolapse have no symptoms.

Treatment is usually not required. However, if you have any condition affecting your mitral valve, you need to take antibiotic drugs before having dental work or any type of surgery to prevent infective endocarditis (see p.422). Occasionally, mitral valve prolapse may produce chest pain, arrhythmia (disturbance of heart rhythm), or a leakage of the valve sufficient to cause heart failure. These conditions may be treated with heart drugs (such as beta-blockers, diuretics, or digitalis) or heart valve surgery. Those needing surgery are usually over age 50.

Aortic stenosis

Aortic stenosis occurs when your aortic valve (the valve between the aorta and the left ventricle) becomes abnormally thick or the leaflets become stuck together, which narrows the opening. The aorta is the artery through which the left ventricle, one of the two lower heart chambers, pumps blood into the body. Thus, the narrowing decreases the quantity of blood that the heart can pump throughout the body. In an effort to squeeze more blood through the valve and keep the cardiac output (amount of blood pumped by the heart in a minute) normal, the left ventricle then develops a thickened muscular wall. This thicker, harder-working tissue requires more and more blood to supply it with the oxygen and nutrients it needs to work so hard. The blood squirting past the obstructed valve causes a sound called a heart murmur that your physician can hear.

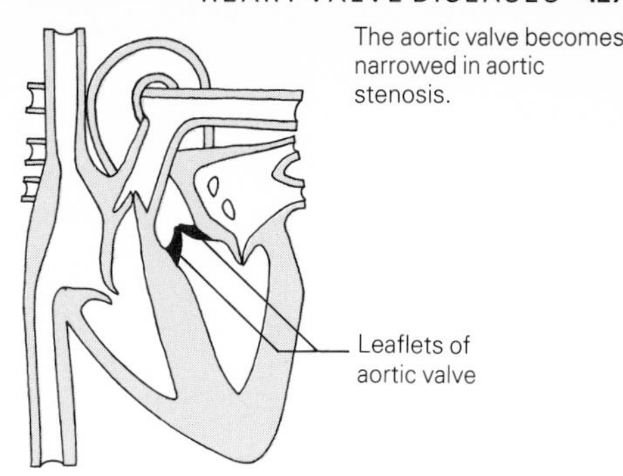

The aortic valve becomes narrowed in aortic stenosis.

What are the symptoms?

At first, aortic stenosis may produce no symptoms at all. As the condition worsens, you will begin to feel breathless after physical activity. You may then develop angina (see p.403) or dizzy spells, or you may faint when you exert yourself. Eventually your symptoms may be those of left-sided heart failure (see p.408).

There are three causes of aortic stenosis. The aortic valve can be malformed from birth (congenital aortic stenosis), can develop scarring and thickening as you age (degenerative or calcific aortic stenosis), or can be narrowed because of rheumatic fever. The chances of having aortic stenosis are three times greater for men than for women. The reasons for this difference are not known.

What are the risks?

Because of the increasing workload for the left ventricle, there is a shortage of blood supplied to the heart muscle that can cause angina, heart attack, ventricular fibrillation, and sudden death.

Once any of the symptoms mentioned above occurs, the risk of dying, even dying suddenly, increases significantly. About 50 percent of the people who have symptoms die within 3 years.

What should be done?

As with mitral stenosis (see p.423), you may first learn that you have aortic stenosis because your physician discovers it during a routine medical examination. If you have any of the symptoms of aortic stenosis, consult your physician immediately. A chest X ray may show whether or not your heart is enlarged. An electrocardiogram (ECG), a test of the heart's electrical system, can help your physician determine the source of the problem. The diagnosis can then be confirmed with a Doppler ultrasound scan (see Glossary). Cardiac catheterization and coronary arteriography are usually performed if surgery is being considered.

What is the treatment?

Self-help: If you know you have mild aortic stenosis, avoid strenuous activity. There is no reason, however, to become an invalid. Moderate exercise is still possible and in fact, desirable. For example, play golf and go for walks, but do not play racquetball or run for buses. Do not be afraid to have sexual intercourse, but let your partner be the more active one. Ask your physician to prescribe antibiotics for you before you have surgery or a tooth extraction to protect you from the risk of infective endocarditis (see p.422). And make sure that you have your heart examined yearly by your physician.

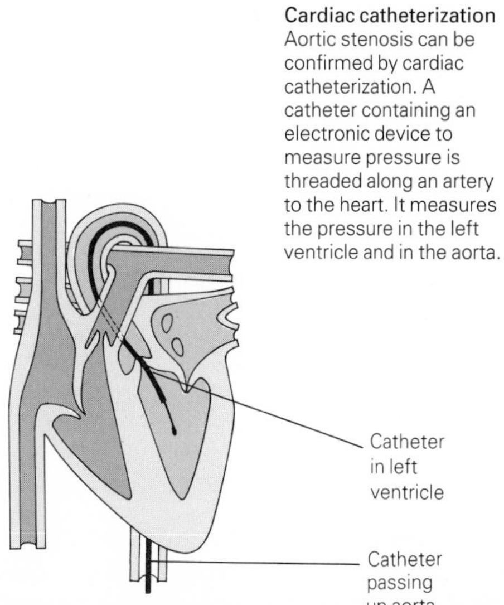

Cardiac catheterization
Aortic stenosis can be confirmed by cardiac catheterization. A catheter containing an electronic device to measure pressure is threaded along an artery to the heart. It measures the pressure in the left ventricle and in the aorta.

Professional help: The only treatment for aortic stenosis that is causing symptoms is surgery, and the most common form of surgery is valve replacement (see p.425). Decisions that must be made, the possible risks of the operation, and prospects for recovery are similar for all heart valve disorders. Balloon valvuloplasty (in which a catheter containing a balloon is passed through a blood vessel in an attempt to enlarge the valve opening) has been performed on people who are poor surgical candidates, but the results are not optimal and surgery, if possible, is preferable.

Aortic incompetence

If your aortic valve, the valve between your aorta and your left ventricle, does not close properly, you may develop aortic incompetence (also known as aortic regurgitation or aortic insufficiency). The aorta is the artery through which the left ventricle, the left one of the two lower heart chambers, pumps blood into the body. But if the aortic valve does not close properly, blood may leak back to the left ventricle. The abnormally leaking blood causes a sound that your physician can hear through a stethoscope. Congenital (from birth) abnormality of the valve is probably the most common reason for aortic incompetence, but other possibilities include infective endocarditis (see p.422), syphilis (see p.655), and stretching of the tissues supporting the aortic valve. If you have a severe case of aortic incompetence, your left ventricle will enlarge and its walls will thicken. This is your heart's response to the fact that the ventricle must work harder to pump blood through the aorta to the rest of the body. The large amount of blood that is pumped into the aorta, much of which leaks into the left ventricle, also causes the arteries to pulsate abnormally, which is a sign that tells physicians that the aortic competence is severe. Sometimes, too, the aortic valve can rupture because of damage from infective endocarditis, an infection of the inner lining of the heart muscle (see p.422).

What are the symptoms?

There are often no symptoms for years, but symptoms develop swiftly if the valve is suddenly ruptured or if the heart muscle decompensates (loses its effectiveness), resulting in breathlessness, along with all the other symptoms of congestive heart failure (see p.408).

What should be done?

Consult your physician if you have any of the symptoms of aortic incompetence. Examination and diagnostic tests are similar to those that are performed for other heart valve disorders. But in addition, blood tests may be included to find out whether you have had rheumatoid arthritis (see p.589), ankylosing spondylitis (see p.591), or syphilis (see p.655). Treatment is the same as it is for aortic stenosis (see previous article); surgery for valve replacement is required.

Tricuspid stenosis and incompetence

These disorders involve narrowing and leakage of the tricuspid valve of the heart. Tricuspid incompetence occurs whenever there is right ventricular failure, which enlarges and dilates (widens) the heart chambers. Tricuspid stenosis and incompetence generally occur together only in conjunction with other valvular disease caused by rheumatic fever, and account for less than 5 percent of all valvular heart diseases. They are more common in women than in men.

What are the symptoms?

The symptoms of these tricuspid disorders are much like those of right-sided congestive heart failure (see p.408).

What are the risks?

The symptoms of heart failure may gradually get worse. Fluid retention causes progressive swelling of the ankles and fluid in the abdomen. Congestion of the liver brings jaundice and liver abnormalities. Finally, you may become disabled by the disease. As with other heart valve diseases, tricuspid stenosis and incompetence pose an additional risk of infective endocarditis (p.422).

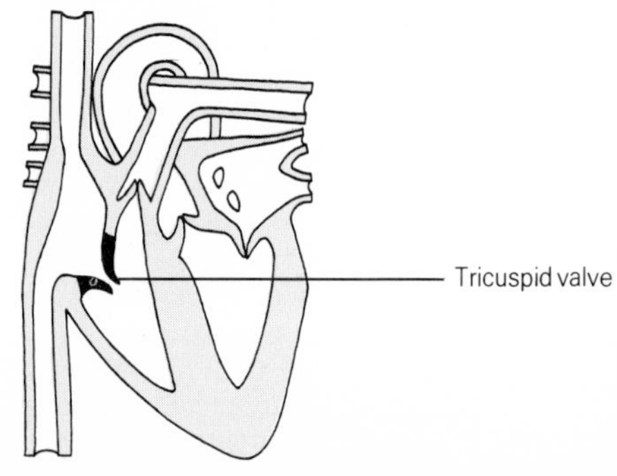

What is the treatment?
No treatment is required for mild cases. If treatment is necessary, it is similar to that for mitral stenosis (see p.423): your physician may prescribe a diuretic drug to reduce excess body fluid and other drugs to stimulate your heart's contractions. However, valvotomy, or widening of the valve, is rarely successful. A heart valve replacement (see p.425) may be necessary.

Pulmonary stenosis and incompetence

Pulmonary stenosis almost always results from congenital malformation of the valve (see p.704). Noncongenital pulmonary valve disorders, usually caused by rheumatic fever, are rare, comprising less than 2 percent of all heart valve disorders resulting from an earlier episode of rheumatic fever.

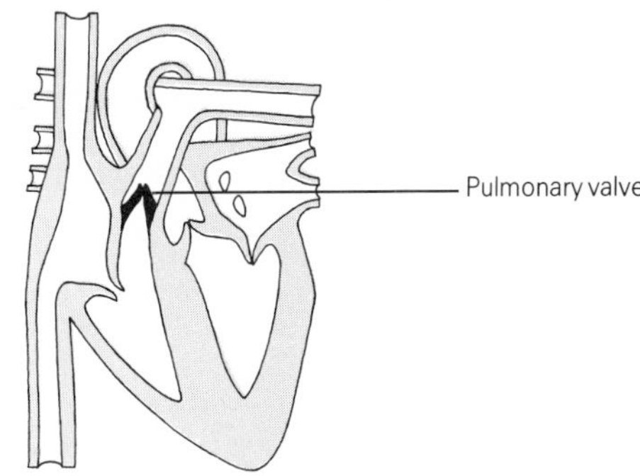

Pulmonary stenosis and incompetence may be discovered during a routine examination when your physician hears the heart murmur caused by the blood squirting past the obstructed valve. If the pulmonary valve is severely affected, your physician may advise you to have a pulmonary valvotomy operation (see Mitral stenosis, p.423).

However, pulmonary stenosis is effectively treated with balloon valvuloplasty (in which a catheter containing a balloon is passed through a blood vessel in an attempt to enlarge the vessel), and surgery is now rarely needed for this condition.

Heart muscle and pericardium

The walls of your heart are made of muscle that contracts rhythmically about 100,000 times a day. If your heart muscle becomes diseased, the force of your heartbeat decreases and this affects the circulation of blood. There are several forms of a heart muscle disorder known as cardiomyopathy. The tiny muscle fibers of the heart may be affected by a disease such as a virus infection, or by a toxin such as alcohol, or by an unknown cause. Over time, this weakens the contraction of the heart muscle, leading to widening of the ventricles and finally congestive heart failure. In some cases the disease is confined to the heart. In other cases the heart is only one of the organs that is affected. Cardiomyopathies are generally less common than most other types of heart disease. Certain kinds of cardiomyopathy can run in families. But most often the reason why a person develops cardiomyopathy is unknown and cannot be found even if your physician conducts multiple tests. The three most common kinds of cardiomyopathy are covered in this section. In addition, two disorders of the pericardium, which is the membranous bag that surrounds your heart, are discussed in the following articles.

Myocarditis

Myocarditis, or inflammation of the heart muscle, is a type of cardiomyopathy that occurs as a rare complication of one of several infectious diseases, usually caused by a virus. In mild cases, the only symptoms may be slight chest pain, shortness of breath, and rapid pulse. In more serious cases, such as those caused by diphtheria (see p.750), myocarditis can lead to heart failure (see p.408), complete heart block (see p.418), and death.

If, while treating you for the underlying disease, your physician thinks you may have myocarditis, you may need to have a chest X ray, an electrocardiogram (ECG), and an echocardiogram so that your physician can estimate the severity of your heart problem. Other possible diagnostic tests include a biopsy of the heart muscle itself. In a biopsy, a small amount of tissue is removed during a cardiac catheterization (see p.427) and closely examined under a microscope. The primary aim of treatment for myocarditis is to eliminate the underlying infection. In addition, you will be advised to rest completely. In some forms of myocarditis, treatment with corticosteroids and other drugs is believed to speed healing, although this theory still has not been proven.

Alcoholic and nutritional cardiomyopathy

Like any muscle, the heart muscle can be damaged by a poison. The most important form of such cardiomyopathy in the US is found among alcoholics (see Alcohol abuse, p.329). Heart specialists attribute the damage directly to the alcohol, which acts as a poison. Rarely, a lack of vitamin B_1, which is often deficient in an alcoholic's diet, may cause cardiomyopathy. In people who are not alcoholics, nutritional cardiomyopathy can also occur because of vitamin B_1 deficiency, but this is rare in the US.

The symptoms of alcoholic and nutritional cardiomyopathy vary greatly. You may simply have palpitations, which is increased awareness of your heartbeat, or irregular or very rapid heartbeat, and swollen hands and feet. Because the damage can cause disorders such as atrial fibrillation (see p.417) and heart failure (see p.408), you also may have the symptoms of those disorders.

Treatment usually consists of complete abstinence from alcohol. In rare instances of lack of vitamin B_1, proper diet or added vitamin B_1 may cure the disorder. If alcohol is entirely eliminated, about one third of patients experience improvement in their heart problem.

Hypertrophic cardiomyopathy

If for some reason there are defective cells in your heart muscle possibly as a result of a congenital (from birth) abnormality, the walls of your heart may thicken in an effort to compensate for the weakness. In severe cases the swollen walls may impede the flow of blood into and out of your heart, resulting in hypertrophic cardiomyopathy. The symptoms of this disorder include fatigue, chest pain, shortness of breath, and palpitations, which is increased awareness of your heartbeat. If you have any of these symptoms, see your physician, who may order diagnostic tests such as a chest X ray, an electrocardiogram (ECG), and an echocardiogram to help establish the diagnosis.

There is no treatment for hypertrophic cardiomyopathy, but the symptoms may be relieved by beta-blocker drugs, which help slow the heart rate, and diuretics, which help rid the body of excess fluid. Calcium channel blockers are an oral medication that has been useful in allowing the heart to fill more normally. If symptoms become severe, especially if there is obstruction of flow of blood out of the heart, surgical removal of some of the excess heart muscle can significantly decrease the symptoms. A number of people who have been in danger of fatal heart failure as a result of hypertrophic cardiomyopathy have had successful heart transplants (see p.432).

Acute pericarditis

Pericarditis is an inflammation of the pericardium, which is a membranous bag that surrounds your heart. When the pericardium becomes inflamed, fluid can collect in the space between it and the heart. This condition, which is called pericardial effusion, may cause further complications. In acute pericarditis, there is a severe episode of chest pain beneath the breastbone that comes on suddenly. The inflammation in acute pericarditis is usually caused by a viral infection, but it may also be caused by tuberculosis (see p.602), rheumatic fever (see p.422), diseases of the connective tissue such as systemic lupus erythematosus (see p.594), or chronic kidney failure (see p.551). Acute pericarditis can also follow either a heart attack (see p.406) or an injury to the chest, but these causes are uncommon.

Mild pericarditis is probably a common feature of many viral illnesses. But a case of pericarditis that is severe enough to cause a sharp pain is unusual.

What are the symptoms?

The main symptom of acute pericarditis is severe pain, which is usually located in the center of your chest. The pain may radiate to your left shoulder. Unlike the pain of angina (see p.403), this pain becomes worse if you breathe deeply, cough, or twist your body. You may also feel that you are short of breath. Frequently, if you have acute pericarditis you may also have a slight fever.

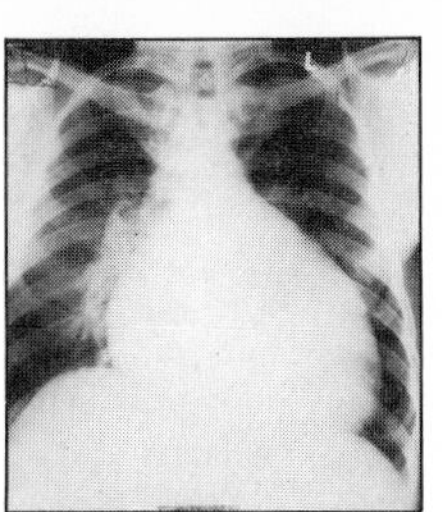

X ray of pericardial effusion
The fluid that collects around the heart (pericardial effusion) is opaque to X rays and makes the heart look much larger than normal.

What are the risks?
There is a slight risk that a pericardial effusion will grow rapidly enough to cause dangerous pressure on the heart. This interferes with the normal filling of the heart and can result in a severe decrease in cardiac output (the amount of blood pumped by the heart in a minute) and can even result in death. But generally pericarditis is not a serious disorder itself, although it can be associated with more serious illness.

What should be done?
Chest pain, especially if it is accompanied by difficulty in breathing, can be a symptom of several serious illnesses, including pneumonia (see p.384), pulmonary embolism (see p.446), and heart attack (see p.406). If the pain is severe and lasts for more than 10 to 15 minutes, consult your physician. After examining you, your physician will probably order diagnostic tests such as a chest X ray, an echocardiogram, an electrocardiogram (ECG), and/or blood tests. These tests will help determine whether you have pericarditis and, if so, what has caused the inflammation of the pericardium. Most cases of pericarditis, however, are caused by a virus, which may be evident only on blood tests.

What is the treatment?
Pericarditis caused by a viral infection usually clears up without treatment. If the pain is quite severe, nonsteroidal anti-inflammatory drugs such as aspirin, ibuprofen, or indomethacin can be effective painkillers. The inflammation subsides within 10 to 14 days and leaves no after-effects. In rare cases, such as when pericarditis occurs a few weeks after a heart attack, your physician may prescribe a corticosteroid drug to speed up healing. When acute pericarditis is the result of a connective-tissue disorder or metabolic disorder, the underlying disease must be treated. Your physician may insert a needle into your chest to remove some of the fluid either for diagnostic purposes or as treatment if a large pericardial effusion prevents your heart from filling normally.

Constrictive pericarditis

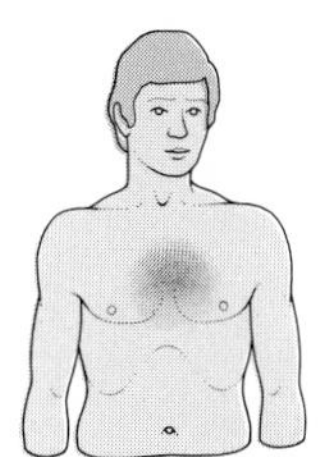

Site of the pain

When pericarditis, or inflammation of the membranous bag that surrounds the heart, results from a chronic infection such as tuberculosis (see p.602), or radiation therapy, the course of the illness is very different from that of acute pericarditis (see previous article). Constrictive pericarditis results from long-standing inflammation, frequently of unknown cause, which can thicken, scar, and contract the pericardium until it shrinks so much that the normal filling of the heart is restricted. Because tuberculosis is no longer widespread and the direction of X-ray beams is better controlled, constrictive pericarditis has become less of a problem today than it was in the past.

What are the symptoms?
The main symptom of constrictive pericarditis is that your legs and abdomen swell because fluid accumulates in those areas. Any or all of the other symptoms of right-sided heart failure (see p.408) may also develop from constrictive pericarditis.

In fact, without surgical treatment, right-sided heart failure is virtually inevitable, and becomes more and more severe.

What should be done?
Whatever the cause, you should consult your physician if you have any of the symptoms that indicate you might have right-sided heart failure. Recommended diagnostic tests will probably include a chest X ray, an echocardiogram (see Glossary), an electrocardiogram (ECG), and often other tests. A cardiac catheterization is sometimes necessary to measure pressure in the arteries and ventricles, to judge the thickness of the pericardium, and to rule out other diseases. Currently, magnetic resonance imaging (MRI) or CT scans are the best way to evaluate the thickness of the pericardium.

Also, skin and sputum tests will probably be necessary to check for tuberculosis.

What is the treatment?
No self-help or treatment by drugs is possible. But constrictive pericarditis can be treated by an operation that is called a pericardectomy. In this procedure, the surgeon carefully removes the thickened pericardium from the surface of your heart. You can expect significant relief of symptoms after removal of the pericardium.

Transplants

Surgery to replace some damaged body organs with healthy ones is now routine, and several thousand such operations are performed every year around the world. Healthy replacement organs come either from people who have consented (or whose surviving relatives have consented) to the medical use of parts of their body after death, or, in the case of organs such as the kidneys, which are paired, from living donors who are usually related to the person needing the transplant. Many state and national organizations provide organ donor cards for people who are willing to donate their vital organs.

Quick action is of critical importance. For instance, a kidney must be removed within 30 minutes of the donor's death and can be kept in storage for only a limited number of hours before transplantation.

What are the difficulties?

The major problem with organ transplantation is that the body's immune system treats a transplanted organ as if it were an invading organism and tries to destroy it through the action of white blood cells and antibodies. An ideal transplant organ has tissues identical to those of the organ it replaces. An organ transplant between identical twins, for example, involves no risk of rejection because the tissues of the twins are a perfect match and do not provoke a response from the body's immune system. Corneal transplants are another exception. They "take" easily because the cornea has no blood supply and therefore does not initiate the "foreign object" response. Donated organs are matched as closely as possible to the patient by tissue type, but a completely perfect match is impossible.

To prevent rejection of a transplanted organ, the body's immune response must be suppressed by treatment with immunosuppressive drugs.

Early immunosuppressive drugs had serious and dangerous side effects. Today, however, use of cyclosporine (a very potent immunosuppressive drug) is routine, and improved immunosuppressive drugs are being developed and tested.

In addition, better methods of preserving and transporting donor organs have also contributed to the greater success of organ transplants by making sure that the organs arrive quickly and in good condition. Increased publicity has resulted in greater public awareness of the need for donor organs, but far fewer organs are donated than are needed.

What are the long-term prospects?

Treatment with cyclosporine and, if necessary, corticosteroids and other immunosuppressive drugs, begins immediately after the transplant operation and must continue for the rest of the patient's life. Although these drugs have serious side effects, many transplant recipients find that their lives are not unduly restricted by this necessity, all else considered.

The chances of someone who has had an organ transplant being alive and well 2 years after the operation are now better than the chances of surviving for 2 years after an operation for lung or intestinal cancer. About 90 percent of the people who receive a heart transplant are alive 1 year after the surgery; 80 percent are alive 5 years after the operation. Many people who have had kidney transplants, and some heart and liver transplant recipients, have had rejection problems with their original transplants and have been given another transplant.

Kidney transplants

With sophisticated medical and surgical techniques, a kidney transplant is straightforward. It is also less risky than many other organ transplants. While rejection of a transplanted heart, liver, or lung may mean death, rejection of a kidney is not necessarily fatal because the patient can be kept alive with an artificial kidney machine, by dialysis (see Dialysis: the artificial kidney, p.551). A kidney transplant may be performed primarily to improve the quality of life of the patient, rather than as a life-saving necessity. Of the people who have had a kidney transplant, more than two thirds are alive 2 years after the operation, with the transplanted kidney still functioning normally, and another one sixth – whose transplants have been rejected – are able to go back onto dialysis until another kidney becomes available for transplantation.

Pancreas transplants

When a kidney transplant is performed on a person who has diabetes mellitus, it is becoming increasingly common to transplant a pancreas at the same time. Although the pancreas transplant is often less successful than the kidney transplant, physicians often think that the risk is worth the chance it gives the patient to become independent of insulin injections and to avoid the risk of destruction of the new kidney from the diabetes. A pancreas-only transplant is more risky, because it is not essential in order to save the person's life and it carries the combined risks of a major, technically difficult operation and drug therapy with strong immunosuppressive medications.

Heart transplants

Because the heart cannot yet be successfully replaced by a machine (the artificial hearts now available are still experimental and are not sufficiently developed to offer a feasible long-term alternative to a natural heart), surgeons usually suggest a transplant only when the patient's heart is near complete failure and the patient is near death. However, as a result of technical advances, heart transplants today are performed more frequently and are used to treat not only severe heart failure or coronary heart disease, but also cardiomyopathy, a condition in which the walls of the heart become thickened because of an internal fault in the heart muscle. Heart transplants now have a high success rate: of those people who have received a new heart, about 80 percent are still alive 5 years after the transplant operation.

Heart-and-lung transplants

Heart-and-lung transplants present several problems, the most pressing of which is the lack of potential donors with normally functioning lungs. Pulmonary changes and infections tend to occur very soon after death, and because it is difficult to preserve the heart and lung as a single unit, the donor must be near the recipient's hospital when the organs are removed so that they can be transplanted into the recipient immediately.

For a few people with serious lung disease—young adults with cystic fibrosis, for example—double-lung transplantation offers the only hope of a cure. For some people with advanced heart and lung disease caused by pulmonary hypertension, heart and double-lung transplantation is performed. Single-lung transplants are performed for people with advanced lung disease, including pulmonary fibrosis.

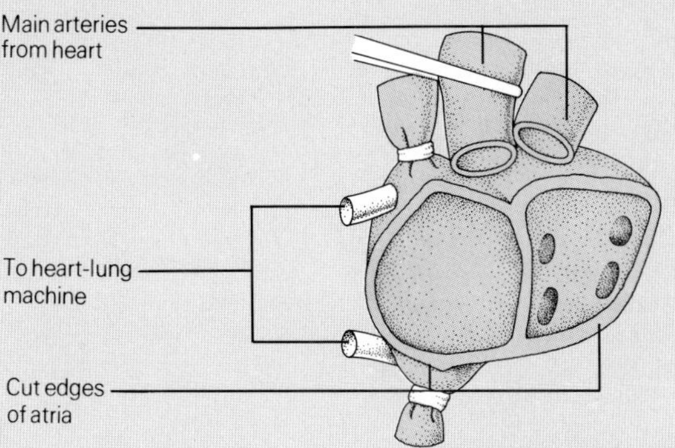

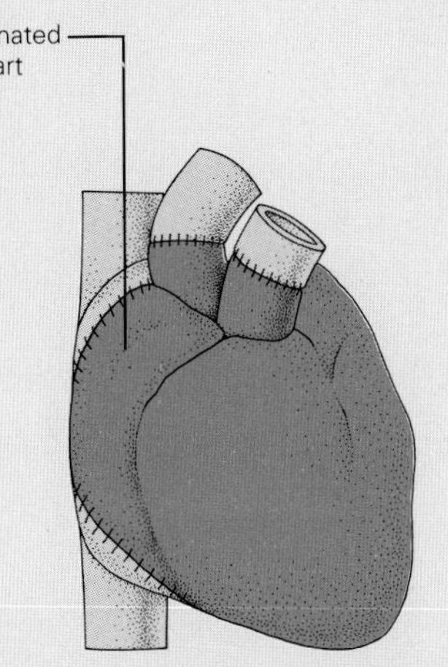

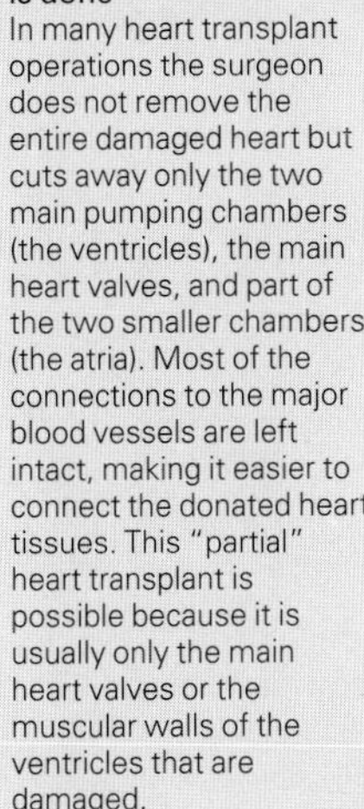

How a heart transplant is done

In many heart transplant operations the surgeon does not remove the entire damaged heart but cuts away only the two main pumping chambers (the ventricles), the main heart valves, and part of the two smaller chambers (the atria). Most of the connections to the major blood vessels are left intact, making it easier to connect the donated heart tissues. This "partial" heart transplant is possible because it is usually only the main heart valves or the muscular walls of the ventricles that are damaged.

Liver and intestine transplants

Transplantation of the liver and of sections of intestine are technically difficult operations, but liver transplantation is now routine. Transplants of small intestine are investigational but show promise.

Liver transplantation is performed on adults who have potentially fatal liver disease, especially some types of progressive cirrhosis, and on children with metabolic disorders or with congenital (from birth) abnormalities of the bile ducts. In both cases results tend to be better if the operation is done at an early stage of liver disease before the patient has become critically ill. The supply of donor organs is still too small for all patients who might benefit; in a handful of cases physicians have removed a segment of a mother's liver and transplanted it as a donor organ into her child. The survival rates after liver transplantation are now approaching those of heart transplantation.

People who have a major part of their small intestine removed must be fed intravenously for the rest of their lives. Transplantation of the small intestine, which is still an experimental procedure, offers the prospect of a return to a much more normal life-style. However, only a small number of operations have been performed, and just a few patients have survived for at least 1 year after the procedure.

Bone marrow transplants

Bone marrow transplantation is now a routine treatment for most forms of leukemia, Hodgkin's disease, other lymphomas, and other cancers, and is also being used increasingly to replace malfunctioning bone marrow in various noncancerous disorders, such as aplastic anemia, congenital (from birth) immune deficiencies, and thalassemia major (see p.454). The major problem associated with bone marrow transplants is the reverse of that presented by other organ transplants, in which the host tends to reject the implanted organ. With a bone marrow graft, some of the cells of the implanted marrow may attack the host cells, producing a condition known as "graft-versus-host disease."

Transplantation involves two stages: marrow is destroyed by radiation and drugs; then new marrow is injected into the bone. Ideally, this new marrow should come from a closely matched donor, such as a brother or sister. However, in some cases, instead of using marrow from a donor, so-called primitive cells are extracted from the recipient's blood and are infused into a vein; the healthy cells then find their way back to the marrow and multiply. Growth-stimulating factors derived by genetic engineering have greatly reduced the risk of infection and shortened recovery time by causing blood counts to return to near-normal levels more rapidly. Marrow that is nearly a perfect match can be used, but is more likely to cause graft-versus-host disease and other problems. To help prevent these problems, immuno-suppressive drug treatment with cyclosporine is started immediately after the operation.

Circulation

Your blood makes two separate circuits through your body, to and from its central pump, the heart. First the heart pumps blood freshly supplied with oxygen throughout your body. This is called the systemic circulation. Its purpose is to supply all your tissues with nutrients and pick up waste products before returning the blood to your heart. In the shorter of the two circuits, the pulmonary circulation, the "used" blood is pumped to your lungs for more oxygen; the carbon dioxide waste is discarded in the lungs. Then the blood is returned to the heart, and the cycle repeats itself.

The arteries that carry blood away from the heart have thick, muscular walls to restrain and absorb the peaks of blood pressure that occur each time your heart beats. The main artery, the aorta, has an internal diameter of about 1.25 in (30 mm). It branches into smaller arteries, then into tiny arterioles, and finally into microscopic capillaries, whose thin, porous walls permit easy exchange of nutrients and oxygen for waste products between the blood and the tissues. Gradually the capillaries merge to form venules, and the capillaries in turn merge to form soft-walled, flexible veins, which return oxygen-depleted blood to your heart.

Your blood does not flow at a constant rate to all parts of your body. The rate varies according to how much blood is needed by certain tissues at a given moment. For example, the uterus of a pregnant woman makes greater demands on the circulation than the uterus of a woman who is not pregnant. When you run, blood is diverted to your leg muscles at the expense of other tissues such as your abdominal organs. Therefore, you should not exercise right after a big meal because your abdominal organs need and get more blood at this time, to aid digestion. When you feel cold, less blood flows in vessels near the chilled skin, and more flows in deeper vessels, to conserve heat. This pattern is reversed so that you flush when you are overheated.

Your circulatory system is highly complex, and it can break down not only if the central pump malfunctions, but also if problems arise within the blood vessels. There can be a weakness in an artery wall, or the hardening of an artery that makes it unable to absorb increased blood pressure. Blood clots can form and cause blockages, and a variety of other disorders, some severe and some merely annoying, can affect your circulation. The most common of these conditions are described in the following group of articles.

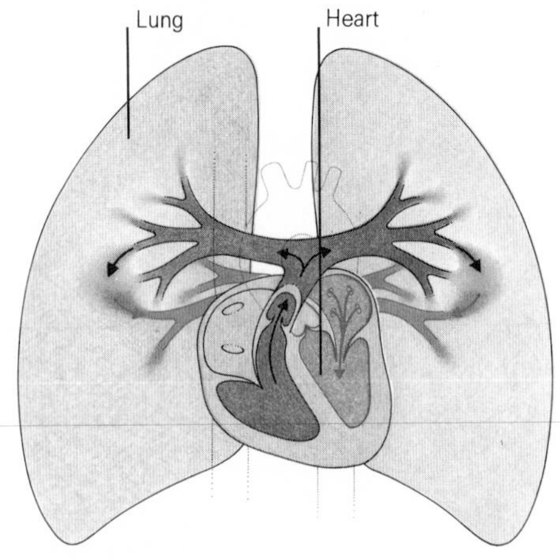

Pulmonary circulation
"Used" blood is pumped from the right venticle through the pulmonary artery into the lungs. Capillaries in the lungs surround tiny air sacs in which the blood absorbs oxygen and releases carbon dioxide. The capillaries merge to become pulmonary veins. These carry the freshly oxygenated blood into the left side of the heart.

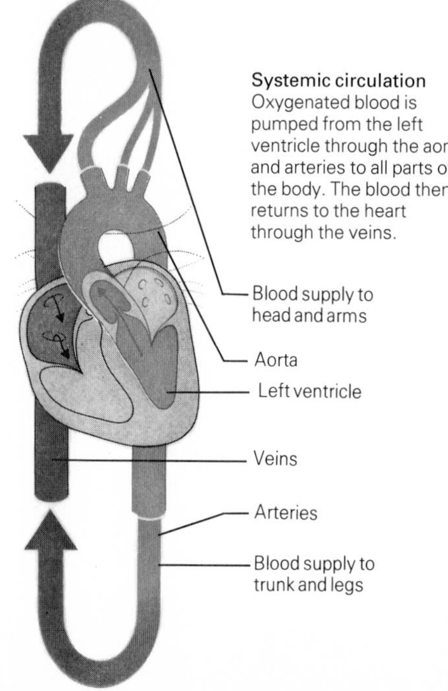

Systemic circulation
Oxygenated blood is pumped from the left ventricle through the aorta and arteries to all parts of the body. The blood then returns to the heart through the veins.

Hardening of the arteries

(arteriosclerosis)

Arteriosclerosis is the general term for hardening of the arteries. Atherosclerosis (see p.398) is a type of arteriosclerosis that primarily affects the inner lining of the artery. As people grow older, their arteries tend to harden, so that most adults have some degree of arteriosclerosis. Although gradual loss of elasticity in arterial walls is inevitable, the seriousness of arteriosclerosis is directly linked to how much you are affected by atherosclerosis, or fatty deposits in the lining of your blood vessels (see p.398). A combination of arterial aging and fatty deposits makes the arteries increasingly narrow and also stiffer—that is, less and less able to expand. These effects decrease the amount of blood that can pass through the arteries and increase the pressure in the arteries when the ventricle ejects its required volume of blood.

Arteriosclerosis can affect all major arteries, but more often the arteries in which the blood supply is seriously reduced are the smaller ones that carry blood to your brain, heart, and legs. At times arteriosclerosis weakens the wall of an artery so that it expands. Then it is called an aneurysm.

What are the symptoms?

Arteriosclerosis that impairs the flow of blood to your legs can cause pain, most often in your calves. You will probably feel pain only when you exercise your legs. The pain increases with activity and disappears with rest. In some cases instead of pain you feel severe fatigue or heaviness or tightness in the muscles. Again, this disappears quickly when you rest. Another possible symptom is pain in your toes or foot, which persists even when you are resting. This happens only with severe obstruction to blood flow. It tends to be worst at night; the best way to relieve it, at least in the early stages, is to dangle your legs over the edge of the bed. This causes more blood to flow into your toes.

At times an atherosclerotic fatty deposit in an artery becomes roughened and attracts platelets that clump together. These can be swept off downstream and cause temporary obstruction of the flow in small blood vessels. In sensitive areas, such as the brain, this causes numbness or an inability to move an arm or leg, or inability to speak, as with a stroke, but the problem clears up completely in a short while. These are called transient ischemic attacks (see p.287).

Much more dangerous is thrombosis, the formation of a blood clot in a blood vessel; it is more likely to cause a stroke (see p.285) if it occurs in a diseased artery.

What are the risks?

As with atherosclerosis (see p.398), the risks associated with arteriosclerosis depend on what part of your body is affected. Among possible serious complications are stroke (see p.285), coronary artery disease (see p.400), gangrene of an arm or leg (see p.447), aneurysm formation (see p.436), and kidney failure (see p.550).

Cigarette smokers are particularly at risk. The older you are, the more likely you are to be severely affected by arteriosclerosis. The disease seems to run in families, and its effects are likely to be more serious if you have anemia (see p.450), diabetes mellitus (see p.558), or heart failure (see p.408).

What should be done?

Start now on self-help measures to slow down the development of atherosclerosis, even if you have no symptoms.

If you think you have symptoms of arteriosclerosis, consult your physician, who, after examining you, may recommend that you have tests for blood cholesterol and diabetes. Other tests, such as an exercise (stress) electrocardiogram (ECG), may be performed to evaluate the condition of your coronary arteries.

What is the treatment?

Self-help: Recommendations in the article on atherosclerosis (see "What should be done?" p.400) are generally also applicable to arteriosclerosis.

It is particularly important to quit if you smoke cigarettes. In addition, if your legs are affected, try to keep them as warm and dry as possible. Exercise improves the blood circulation and efficiency of the muscles in people who have pain in the legs because of atherosclerosis. But the benefits of exercise last for only as long as you continue to work at it, so you should find a form of regular exercise you enjoy (see "Why exercise is good for you," p.20). Your physician will be able to recommend an appropriate exercise program.

It is extremely important to take excellent care of your feet and to avoid any injury. Also, when you cut your toenails, avoid cutting the skin; an open wound on the affected part of your body heals very slowly and is highly susceptible to infection and can permit gangrene to develop when you have arteriosclerosis, especially with diabetes.

Professional help: Your physician can also help you by treating other conditions such as anemia, diabetes, or heart failure that aggravate the effects of arteriosclerosis. Among medications sometimes prescribed by physicians for people with arteriosclerosis are vasodilator drugs, which widen your blood vessels, and anticoagulant or antithrombotic drugs, which help prevent the blood from clotting as readily as it normally would. If your physician prescribes any such drugs, you will probably need to take them on a long-term basis.

Depending on your age and the nature and severity of your symptoms, your physician will decide whether detailed testing is warranted. Tests are now available using Doppler techniques (see Ultrasound, p.260) to measure the location and extent of the narrowing of your arteries and the effects of narrowed arteries on blood flow. If one or more arteries are severely affected, surgery may be recommended. To evaluate the extent of obstruction if surgery is being considered, angiography will be performed. In this procedure, a contrast agent is injected through a catheter directly into the aorta and motion-picture X rays are taken. Bringing more blood to the heart may be accomplished with transluminal (balloon) angioplasty (see p.404), in which the narrowed section of artery is either stretched by a balloon catheter or "cleared" using a laser or a drilling instrument. Sometimes the best approach is to remove the blocked or narrowed section of artery and replace it with either a plastic artificial graft or with a section of vein taken from elsewhere in the body.

What are the long-term prospects?

Although arteriosclerosis is almost certain to become more severe as you grow older, symptoms such as the pain in your legs may subside. This lessening of symptoms occurs because your body compensates for the inadequate quantity of blood flowing through some arteries by developing alternate pathways and expanding circulation in other, healthier arteries that supply the same area. If you eat sensibly, do not smoke, and exercise regularly and moderately, you can often delay or even prevent complications from arteriosclerosis.

Aneurysms

An aneurysm is a permanent distention of an artery caused by a weakness in its wall. Aneurysms can form anywhere, but the most common and problematic sites are the arteries of the brain, and the aorta, the large major artery through which the heart pumps blood to the rest of the body. There are three basic reasons why an aneurysm might develop in one of your arteries:

1. There are three layers of tissue in your arterial walls. The supportive strength of your arteries is supplied by the muscular middle layer, and this layer may be congenitally (from birth) defective. The normal pressure of blood in the affected artery causes a balloonlike swelling, which is called a saccular aneurysm, to develop at that point. Aneurysms resulting from congenital defects are almost always found in arteries at the base of the brain. Because of their shape and because more than one of them are often clustered together, these aneurysms are known as berry aneurysms.

2. Inflammation, whatever the cause, may weaken an arterial wall. Most arterial inflammation is caused by disorders such as polyarteritis nodosa (see p.594), syphilis (see p.655), bacterial endocarditis (see p.422), or inflammatory disease of unknown origin called aortitis.

3. A portion of the muscular middle layer of an arterial wall may slowly degenerate as the result of a chronic condition such as arteriosclerosis (see p.435) or atherosclerosis (see p.398), and degeneration may be accelerated by high blood pressure (see p.411). An aneurysm caused by arteriosclerosis is likely to be a sausage-shaped swelling called a fusiform aneurysm that runs along a short length of the artery. High blood pressure can accelerate arteriosclerosis and is frequently associated with the formation of aneurysms. Increased pressure of blood in an artery, however, can stretch the wall in many different ways. It can even split the layers of the artery and force blood between them. This is called a dissecting aneurysm.

Outer layer
Layers of muscular and elastic tissue
Inner layer
Aneurysm

How an aneurysm forms
If part of the wall of an artery is damaged or weakened, the pressure of blood pulsating through it may cause that part of the wall to swell out like a balloon.

Aneurysms can burst, which leads to hemorrhage, or internal bleeding, at the site of the aneurysm and to a loss of blood supply

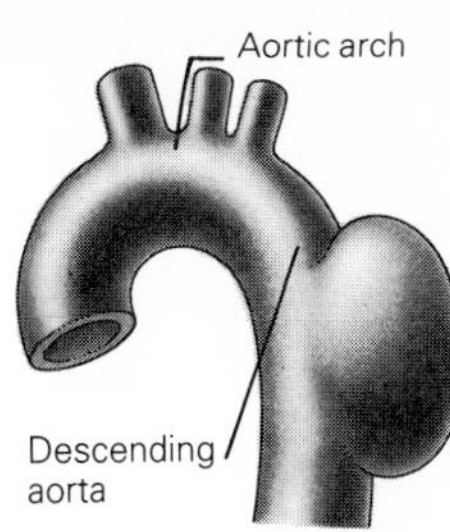

A saccular aneurysm develops when part of the muscular middle layer of the artery has been damaged.

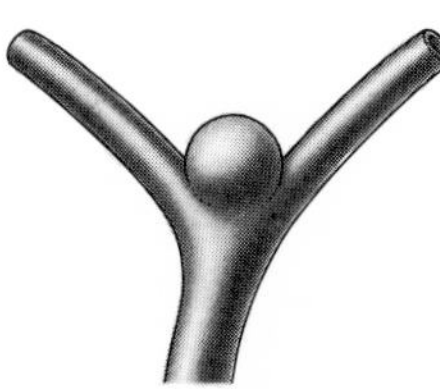

Berry aneurysms are found at the base of the brain, where an artery branches. A congenital defect causes them.

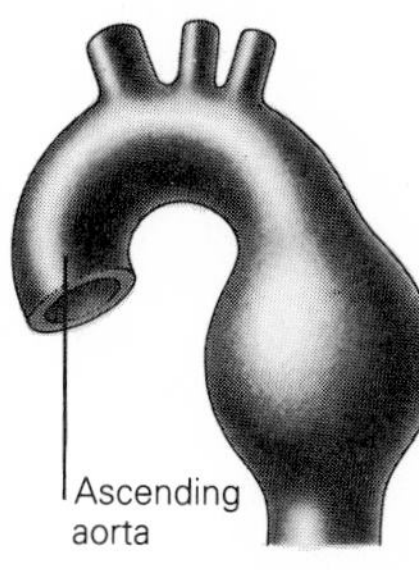

Fusiform aneurysms are formed when the arterial wall is weakened all the way around.

to certain tissues. Aneurysms can swell so much that they press on and damage neighboring organs, nerves, or other blood vessels. They also can disturb the flow of blood to such an extent that its turbulence causes dangerous clots to form.

What are the symptoms?

The symptoms of aneurysm vary according to the type, size, and location of the swelling. Berry aneurysms, at the base of the brain, usually cause no obvious symptoms until they burst. A sudden severe headache at the back of your head, or even unconsciousness, may be the first sign of this aneurysm (see also Subarachnoid hemorrhage, p.288).

If you have an aneurysm of the aorta, your symptoms will depend on these factors: what section of the aorta is affected and what structures the aneurysm presses on; and what type of aneurysm you have. Most commonly, saccular and fusiform aneurysms do not cause any symptoms. When they do, the most common symptoms of a saccular or fusiform aneurysm in the thoracic aorta, or the portion of that artery that passes through your chest, are chest pain, hoarseness, difficulty in swallowing, and a persistent cough that is not helped by cough medicine. If you have an acute dissecting aneurysm in the same area of your aorta, you are likely to have severe pain that can easily be mistaken for a heart attack (see p.406). In either case, you will not be able to see or feel the swelling on the surface of your chest, because your thoracic aorta is confined inside your rib cage.

A saccular or fusiform aneurysm in the abdominal portion of your aorta, if large enough, can often be seen as a pulsating lump. If the aneurysm is located toward your back, it may press on the bones of your spine and cause severe backache, especially if it is expanding or rupturing. Dissecting aneurysms that affect only the abdominal aorta are relatively rare. When they do occur, the main symptom is severe abdominal pain. Aneurysms in peripheral arteries of the arms and legs are uncommon and less hazardous, although aneurysms of the artery behind the knee can suddenly clot, resulting in gangrene of the leg (see Gangrene, p.447).

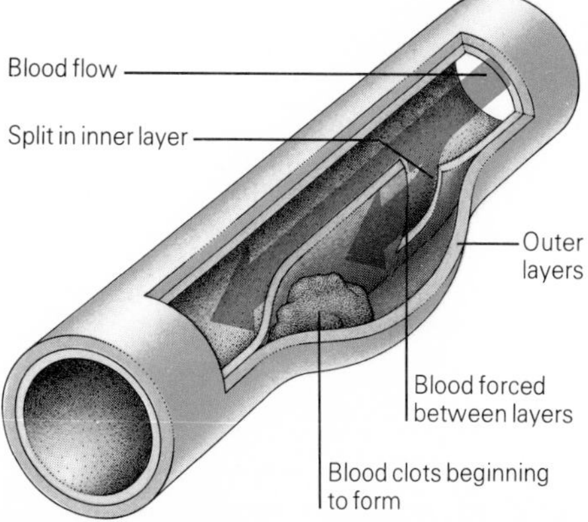

Dissecting aneurysms
High blood pressure may cause the inner and outer layers of an artery to split apart. Blood is then forced between the layers and causes the outer wall to stretch. The blood that is trapped between the layers tends to form a clot, which may fill the aneurysm and seal it off.

What are the risks?

The major risk of an aneurysm is that it may burst and cause a hemorrhage, allowing blood to flow into the surrounding area, and depriving tissues of oxygen and nutrients. The entire circulatory system may collapse if the leak drastically reduces the volume of blood. Without immediate medical help, a burst aneurysm in the aorta is fatal.

Even when it does not burst, an aneurysm of the aorta causes turbulence in the flow of blood that can cause the formation of a thrombus, or clot, with all the associated dangers. Emboli, which are parts of a blood clot that break away from the thrombus, can block smaller arteries such as those that supply the kidneys or other organs, and this can lead to permanent damage to these organs. An aneurysm of the ascending aorta may involve the ring at the base of the aorta, which stretches the aortic valve of the heart and causes aortic incompetence (see p.428).

More than 40 percent of all people who have a burst berry aneurysm die as a result.

What should be done?

You can do very little about berry aneurysms. However, if you have a severe, persistent headache and impaired vision, see your physician immediately. If you have any of the symptoms of an aneurysm of the aorta or if you develop an unexplainable lump anywhere on your body, especially on your abdomen, and particularly if it throbs, consult your physician immediately. Long before it causes symptoms, an aneurysm of the abdominal aorta may be detected by an ultrasound examination, or confirmed by ultrasound if your physician has found it during a physical examination. A small aneurysm may not require treatment. If you are in good physical condition, an elective operation on a large aneurysm or one that is increasing in size carries far less risk than an operation done as an emergency when the aneurysm has leaked or ruptured.

What is the treatment?

Self-help: The best ways to prevent aneurysms are to take steps to prevent or slow down atherosclerosis (see recommendations on p.399) and, if you have high blood pressure, to keep it under control (see p.411). If an aneurysm has already developed, there is no effective self-help.

Professional help: Surgery is the usual treatment for an aneurysm. Surgery for aneurysms of the aorta has become a routine procedure, although it remains a major one. Survival after elective operations on either the thoracic (chest) or the abdominal aortas is now better than 90 percent in people who are otherwise healthy, and the long-term results of these operations are excellent. For some berry aneurysms, instead of treatment by open surgery, the surgeon inserts a catheter and passes a blood-clotting substance to the aneurysm to stop the bleeding.

What are the long-term prospects?

About 30 percent of people with ruptured berry aneurysms die instantly, and about another 15 percent die from further bleeding within a few weeks. The outlook for long-term survival is excellent if you have a successful operation and live for 6 months after the first hemorrhage occurs.

Surgery for aneurysms of the thoracic aorta is at times impossible; in such cases the outlook is poor. With operable thoracic aneurysms there is an 80 to 90 percent chance of survival. Abdominal aneurysms are frequently a much less serious problem. In general, they need to be removed only if they are large or if they are growing.

Arterial embolism

An embolus lodges
An embolus carried along in the flow of blood in the arteries may lodge where the arteries branch or narrow. An area that depends on the blocked artery for blood supply will be damaged if the problem is not treated.

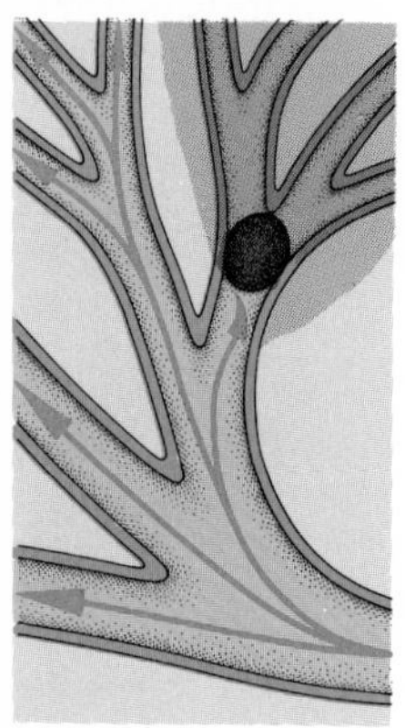

An embolus is a particle, usually a fragment of clotted blood or a piece of plaque (fatty deposit), that is carried along in your bloodstream. The embolus may be very small, but because arteries divide into successively smaller vessels—first arterioles, then capillaries—eventually the embolus will get stuck and create an embolism, or blockage, that prevents the tissues in the affected area from getting an adequate blood supply. The embolus may originate in your heart because of a heart attack (see p.406) or some other heart disorder. It may be a fragment of bacterial growth resulting from bacterial endocarditis (see p.422). In rare cases, an embolus may even consist of a tiny foreign object that entered an artery through a wound or a gas bubble that formed in your tissues as you experienced decompression sickness ("the bends").

The severity of an arterial embolism depends on its size and location. Some organs such as the brain, kidneys, and heart are most sensitive to a sudden decrease in blood supply. Other organs with multiple sources of blood supply can survive an embolism in one of the arteries and produce few symptoms. The parts of the body that are most commonly affected are the brain and legs. But arterial embolisms can occur anywhere at all in your body.

What are the symptoms?

A small embolism in an internal organ usually goes unnoticed unless it affects a large area or a very sensitive organ such as the heart or brain. An embolism may cause loss of function in part of the intestine, however, and cause the same symptoms as intestinal obstruction (see p.503). For the symptoms of cerebral embolisms, read the articles on stroke (see p.285) and transient ischemic attacks (see p.287). For the symptoms of embolism to the heart muscle, see the article on heart attack (see p.406). In other parts of the body, particularly the arms and legs, pain may be the earliest symptom. This is followed by a tingling or prickling sensation, and the affected area eventually becomes numb, weak, and cold. If the embolism is in an arm or leg, the skin is pale at first but later turns bluish from the slow blood flow that depletes the oxygen and leaves the bluish-colored oxygen-poor hemoglobin. Both legs may be affected if a large embolus blocks the aorta (the main artery from your heart to your trunk), where it divides in two. Such embolisms, which are called saddle embolisms, can cause severe pain in your abdomen, back, and legs.

What are the risks?

If one of your major arteries is blocked, the tissues it supplies with oxygen and nutrients will be damaged if the blockage is not treated promptly; gangrene (see p.447) will occur. In the brain the result of an embolism can be a fatal stroke. If you have blockage in your aorta, you have only a 50 percent chance of survival without surgery.

The more extensive and severe the symptoms, the more quickly you should consult your physician, who will probably make a swift diagnosis. You will need an arteriogram, an MRI, or a Doppler ultrasound before any surgery is performed.

What is the treatment?

Self-help: If the symptoms are in your arm or leg, you should keep the affected arm or leg cool and immobile until medical help arrives. This reduces the need for oxygen. Do not elevate the arm or leg because this will further reduce the blood flow into it. No self-help is possible for embolisms in any part of the body other than the arms and legs.

Professional help: An embolism in an arm or leg that is diagnosed within 3 or 4 hours may be treated by drugs, including anti-coagulants such as heparin and thrombolytic agents such as streptokinase or TPA (tissue plasminogen activator). The combination of anticoagulant and thrombolytic therapies encourages the body's natural processes to dissolve the blood clot and prevent further clots from forming.

If in a few more hours, in spite of drug treatment, a major artery remains blocked, surgery will be necessary to prevent gangrene (see p.447). The operation, called an embolectomy, involves inserting a tube into the artery and mechanically sucking the embolus out through it. If surgery is performed in time, complete recovery usually occurs.

Temporal arteritis

(cranial arteritis, giant-cell arteritis)

If any of your arteries are chronically inflamed, and if the inflammation causes thickening of their lining and a reduction in the amount of blood that they can carry, you have the disease known as arteritis. If the disease affects the aorta, then it is called aortitis. Temporal arteritis gets its name because the arteries chiefly affected are the two that run behind the temples in your scalp. These temporal arteries are branches of the carotid arteries, which supply blood to your head and brain.

Temporal arteritis affects mainly people over 55. Women are twice as susceptible to the condition as are men.

What are the symptoms?

The most common symptom of temporal arteritis is a dull, throbbing headache on one or both sides of your forehead. The artery that is the source of the headache may be swollen, red, and tender if you touch it. Among other possible symptoms are mild fever, loss of weight, loss of appetite, and a generalized muscular ache. Such muscle aches, however, are more characteristic of a similar disease called polymyalgia rheumatica (see p.595). A serious symptom is blurring of vision or temporary loss of eyesight in one eye.

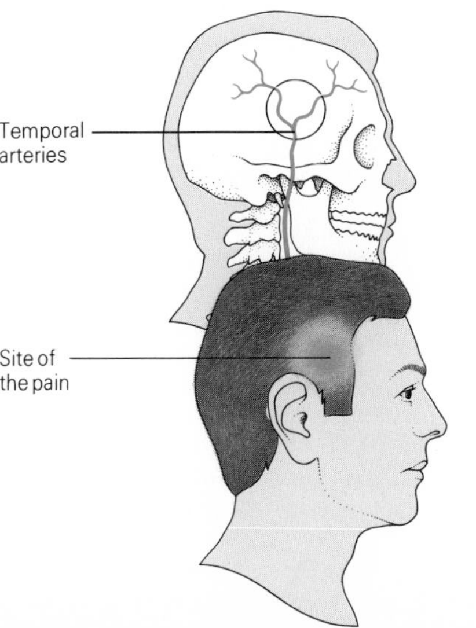

What are the risks?

In severe cases, temporal arteritis can cause a stroke (see p.285). But the disease more commonly affects the eyes. About half the people who have this disease have eye problems, which can lead to some loss of vision. Before today's drugs were available, about 30 percent of people with temporal arteritis became blind.

What should be done?

If you have persistent headaches from any cause, you should consult your physician. If your headaches are accompanied by other symptoms of temporal arteritis, and if you are over 55, your physician may evaluate you for temporal arteritis. A blood test will help indicate whether temporal arteritis is causing your symptoms.

Your physician may also decide to perform a biopsy, in which a small piece of one of your temporal arteries is removed for microscopic examination, to help make the diagnosis. This procedure can be performed using a local anesthetic. More than one biopsy may be necessary.

What is the treatment?

Self-help: None is available.

Professional help: Your physician will probably prescribe a corticosteroid drug, which you may need to take for a long time, hopefully in diminishing doses. Regular blood tests will show whether the corticosteroid is sufficiently suppressing the disease by reducing the inflammation of the affected arteries. There are several possible side effects of corticosteroids, but the most serious side effects are unlikely to occur from the dose of the drug usually required as maintenance treatment for temporal arteritis.

Once you start on the drug, however, you must continue to take it regularly until your physician agrees that you should stop. You should continue to see your physician as often as directed; as you respond to treatment he or she will gradually reduce the dose of the medication.

What are the long-term prospects?
If you see your physician promptly, and if the corticosteroid treatment is effective, you have a 75 percent chance of complete recovery. However, treatment for temporal arteritis is less likely to be successful if the disease is diagnosed at a later stage.

Frostbite

Frostbite is freezing of the skin and underlying body tissues. It occurs when part of your body is severely affected by temperatures well below freezing. The flow of blood to the affected area stops, and skin cells may be permanently damaged in severe cases. Any part of your body may be affected, but exposed parts such as your hands, feet, nose, and ears are most at risk. Frostbitten skin is hard, pale, cold, and numb. When the skin has thawed out, it becomes red and painful. Anyone subjected to several hours of extreme cold may become frostbitten, but people who have atherosclerosis (see p.398) or who are taking beta-blocker drugs, which decrease the flow of blood to the skin, are particularly susceptible to frostbite.

Medical myth

The best way to deal with frostbite is to rub the affected area with snow.

Wrong. Rapid rewarming is the right treatment. This should be done in warm water 104°F to 110°F (40°C to 44°C). For complete instructions, see Injuries and emergencies, p.841.

What should be done?
When you must go out in extreme cold, wear several layers of warm clothes under a waterproof, windproof outer garment. Make sure that your ears, hands, and feet (and nose, if possible) are protected. Remember that fatigue, drinking alcohol, and lack of oxygen resulting from high elevations can affect your judgment, which can cause you to disregard the feeling that you are too chilled and ought to go indoors.

Infants and children may lack the ability or knowledge to dress protectively enough to avoid frostbite. Parents should make sure their children are dressed adequately.

Frostbite must be treated promptly. Every minute of delay lessens your chances of recovery. Memorize the instructions for dealing with this problem (see Injuries and emergencies, p.841), especially if you will be in a remote area where medical help may not be available. If, after warming the frozen area, you do not fully recover, see your physician promptly. Avoid overheating the frostbitten area and getting a burn. Gangrene may occur with frostbite, in which case you may need to have the affected part amputated, especially if it is a finger or toe. If frostbite is treated quickly, however, it may have no long-term aftereffects.

Raynaud's disease

(and Raynaud's phenomenon)

This circulatory system disorder affects your fingers and occasionally your toes. It occurs when the small arteries that supply them with blood become extra-sensitive to cold and other factors that can produce narrowing and sudden spasm of the vessel. This reduces the flow of blood to the affected area. At first there is only a temporary spasm that can be eased by warmth, but the spasm may eventually recur more frequently. Lack of oxygenated blood makes the affected area of skin pale, often with a bluish tinge. When a temporary spasm ends, blood flows back into the skin, and the paleness disappears and is replaced by a flush.

The disease may also occur as a secondary effect of conditions other than cold. It is sometimes an occupational disorder of people who work with vibrating equipment such as chain saws or pneumatic drills. It can be caused by a disorder of the connective tissue such as scleroderma (see p.595), by pulmonary hypertension (see p.447), by an emotional disorder, or by a nerve disorder. And it can be caused by sensitivity to certain drugs that can affect the blood vessels. In all cases where it is secondary to another disorder, this condition is called Raynaud's phenomenon instead of Raynaud's disease. Both conditions are common, especially among women. Raynaud's disease nearly always begins in young adulthood, not when you are older.

What are the symptoms?
Change of color in the fingers or other affected areas is the main symptom. Normally the color changes from white to bluish to red at a rate that varies according to the temperature to which those areas are exposed. There is generally no pain, but there may be numbness or a feeling of "pins and needles" in the affected area.

Raynaud's disease worsens very gradually. Raynaud's phenomenon, on the other hand, may get worse quickly. In late stages of either

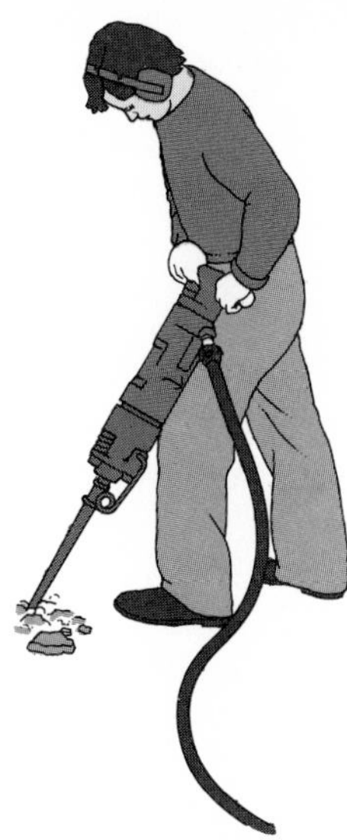

Regular use of high-vibration machinery such as pneumatic drills can damage the blood vessels and lead to Raynaud's disease.

disorder the affected tissue may shrink, and small ulcers may form on the tips of the fingers or toes as the tissues become damaged because they do not receive an adequate blood supply.

What are the risks?

Prolonged spasm of the arteries may result in gangrene (see p.447), but this is rare. More often the poor blood supply to muscles and nerves eventually weakens your fingers and diminishes your sense of touch.

What should be done?

If the self-help measures suggested below do not work, consult your physician, who will take a detailed history of your symptoms.

What is the treatment?

Self-help: Keep your hands and feet warm and dry. Wear loose-fitting gloves and socks and comfortable, roomy shoes. Keep your whole body warm because sometimes the spasm in the vessels is set off by the body itself becoming cold, even when your hands are protected. If you smoke, give it up, because cigarette smoking causes inadequate circulation to get worse. Moving to a warm climate is probably the best solution for the problem, but a move is not practical for everyone. Try, at least, to stay indoors during very cold weather.

Professional help: Medical treatment of Raynaud's disease is based on attempts to prompt your contracted arteries to expand. Even when your arterial walls have been permanently damaged, vasodilator drugs sometimes improve circulation. Calcium channel blocker drugs are the treatment of choice. Antiadrenergic drugs often relieve symptoms. Other vasodilators, such as sympatholytic drugs, have been helpful but side effects often limit their use.

Raynaud's disease is infrequently treated by an operation called a sympathectomy, in which the nerves that control contraction of the arteries are cut. Although this procedure often produces a dramatic improvement in the disorder, the results may be only temporary. In some cases there may not even be temporary improvement after surgery. Sympathectomy is more successful when the toes rather than the fingers are affected by the disorder. Most people learn to live with Raynaud's disease.

For Raynaud's phenomenon, the treatment is determined by the underlying cause of the condition.

Acrocyanosis

You have the condition known as acrocyanosis if your fingers, toes, wrists, hands, or feet look blue. The bluish tinge comes from the sudden spasm of tiny arteries that carry blood in the skin of your hands and feet, causing these parts to get less blood. As blood gives up more oxygen, the red pigment of the remaining red blood cells turns bluish-purple. This gives the skin its abnormal color.

Nobody knows why acrocyanosis develops. The condition is intensified by cold. It is present to an equal degree in both hands or both feet. It is not painful, but the affected hands or feet nearly always feel cold and may be sweaty. Acrocyanosis does not cause ulceration or other skin problems.

What should be done?

Do not be too concerned if you have acrocyanosis. It is fairly common, especially among women. It is not a sign of a major disorder, and it does not need treatment. To prevent acrocyanosis, protect your hands and feet from extreme cold.

Varicose veins

Varicose veins are veins under the skin that have become stretched and swollen. This disfiguring and sometimes painful condition usually occurs in the legs as a result of the strain imposed on the valves in the leg veins by our upright posture. It is through the veins that blood is returned to the heart from the tissues of the legs. Since the heart is not strong enough to pump the blood back unaided, it must be helped by the pumping action of your leg muscles.

Normally, blood is collected from leg tissues in a network of superficial veins (those on the surface of the muscles), which are connected to deep veins (those embedded in the muscles) through what are called perforating veins. When a muscle relaxes, the deep veins and perforating veins expand and suck blood in from the superficial veins. All deep veins and perforating veins have one-way valves that prevent blood from flowing back into superficial veins. So when the muscle contracts, blood is pumped up the deep veins toward the heart.

If, for some reason, possibly because of congenital (from birth) abnormalities, the valves of the perforating veins do not close, some blood may be pumped the wrong way, back into the superficial veins. They respond to the increased pressure by dilating and stretching. Thus, varicose veins are often visible because they lie just under the skin. Most people have varicose veins that are unsightly, but that do not cause serious symptoms. Even severe cases of varicose veins do not progress to circulatory problems, which most often occur after clotting in the deep veins. There appears to be a hereditary component in some people with severe varicose veins.

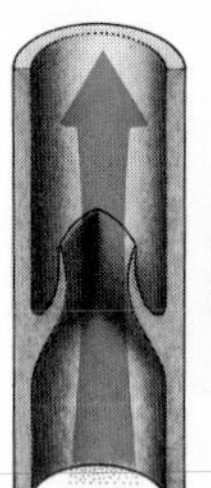

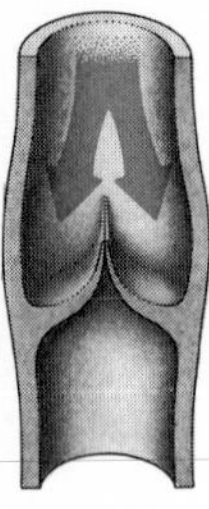

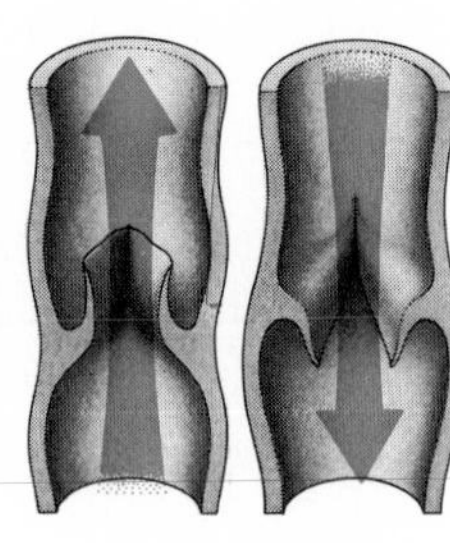

Normal vein

Varicose vein

Varicose veins occur when the valves in veins become damaged. This may occur because the veins are swollen as a result of extra pressure on them from standing or some other cause.

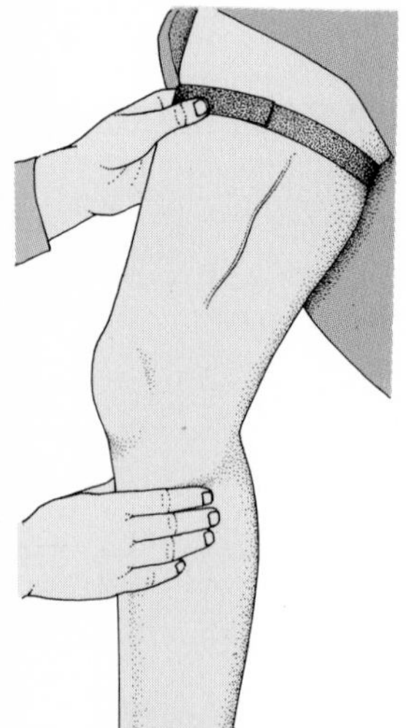

Finding the faulty valves
Your physician applies a tourniquet to your leg while you are lying down. The tourniquet should stop the flow of blood through the vein. But if a valve is damaged at that point, some blood will leak through when you stand, and the varicose vein stands out below the tourniquet. This is repeated at various points down your leg.

What are the symptoms?

The most common early symptom of varicose veins is the appearance of a prominent, bluish, swollen vein in your leg when you stand up. The most common site is either at the back of the calf or up the inside of the leg anywhere between your ankle and your groin. Varicose veins can also occur around your anus (see Hemorrhoids, p.520), in your vagina if you are pregnant (see p.669), or at the junction of your esophagus and stomach if you have advanced cirrhosis of the liver (see p.524).

A swollen leg vein may grow increasingly prominent. The vein may become tender to the touch, and the skin above it or at your ankle may begin to itch. Your whole leg may ache, especially if you stand for long periods, and you may find that your feet become swollen after a short period of standing and your shoes seem too tight by the end of the day. During pregnancy, varicose veins get worse because of the increased pressure in the abdomen.

Your symptoms will not worsen beyond this stage if you have only the superficial (surface) form of varicose veins, in which connecting or deep veins are not involved. But some people with varicose veins have a severe disturbed flow in the superficial, connecting, and deep veins, sometimes as a result of earlier clot formation in deep veins (deep vein thrombosis). These people find that the impaired circulation causes persistent leg swelling and a brownish discoloration of the skin, especially near the ankles. Injury may cause ulcers of the skin on the inner side of the lower leg and ankle. Rash (see Eczema and dermatitis, p.269) of the skin near the veins is another possible symptom.

What are the risks?

Varicose veins are usually annoying rather than disabling, but they occasionally have serious consequences. For example, a combination of the force of gravity and valve failure in perforating veins can give your tissues so little blood that the undernourished skin breaks down and an ulcer develops. Varicose ulcers (see p.276) do not heal as long as the veins associated with them remain under pressure.

Another risk, which is rare, is that bumping or cutting the skin over a varicose vein may cause bleeding from the swollen vein. This requires prompt pressure on the site and immediate medical attention. The greatest risk of varicose veins is inflammation of the wall of the vein. Blood tends to clot on the inflamed, roughened wall, and this can lead to thrombophlebitis (see p.444).

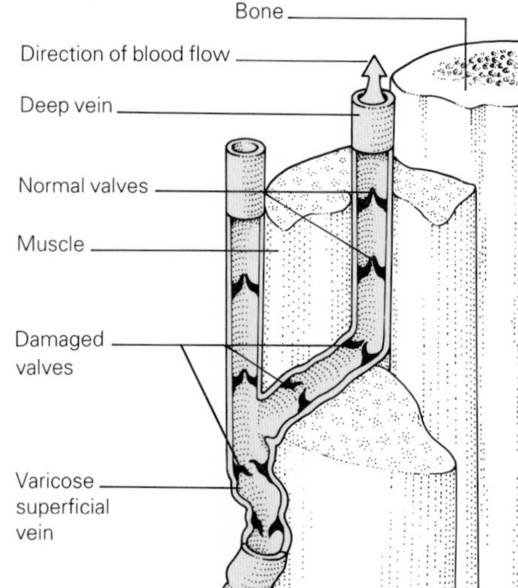

What should be done?

If you think you are susceptible to varicose veins because they run in your family, guard against them by adopting the self-help measures recommended below, especially if you are pregnant. If you already have varicose veins, the self-help measures will ease your symptoms and slow down the progress of the condition, but they will not

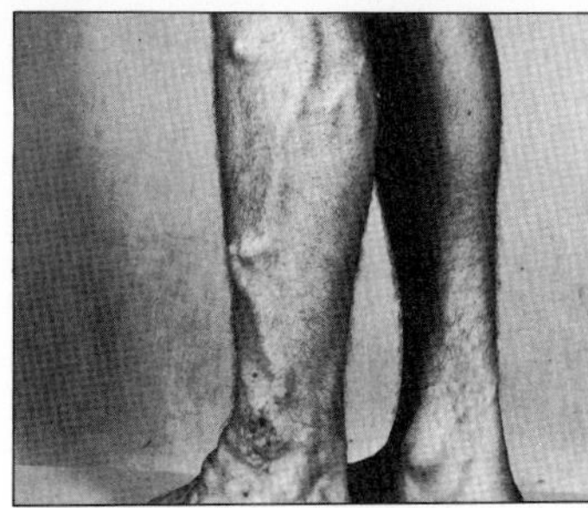

When valves in the veins do not close and are unable to support the column of blood that flows from the veins to the heart, the high pressure in the superficial veins results in stretching and twisting of the veins.

cure it. If your discomfort increases, consult your physician. He or she probably will not need special tests to confirm the diagnosis. A simple procedure involving the use of elastic tourniquets on your leg (see illustration) will usually show which of your perforating veins have damaged valves.

Small spider veins are very tiny visible veins under the skin of the thighs and legs. You may not like their appearance and opt for a cosmetic procedure in which a laser is used or a solution is injected into the veins to make them less visible. But this procedure is not medically necessary, may have side effects, and may not produce permanent results.

What is the treatment?

Self-help: If you are experiencing discomfort from varicose veins, try to stay off of your feet as much as possible. Whenever you can, sit with your legs raised. If your symptoms are very irritating, lie down or sit down as often as you can, with your legs raised above the level of your chest. This position ensures good drainage from your ankles and feet. Ask your physician if you need support stockings, which can be tailored to your measurements, and put them on before you get out of bed every day. Some people prefer elastic bandages, but before using them yourself, ask a nurse or physician to show you how to put them on properly. The bandages or stockings may be uncomfortable, especially in hot weather.

If you break your skin, and blood begins to flow from a varicose vein, lie down, raise the affected leg, and keep it raised. Do this promptly no matter where you are. The bleeding will immediately slow down, and you can control it by moderate pressure with a clean handkerchief. You should then get professional medical help to clean and bandage the wound.

Do not try to treat varicose ulcers or a rash on your leg yourself. And never scratch an itch caused by varicose veins because this can cause ulceration. See your physician for treatment. Be assured that varicose veins associated with pregnancy will subside within several weeks after childbirth.

OPERATION: **Varicose vein removal**

Varicose veins can be removed. The work of the veins is taken over by nearby veins.

During the operation You are usually under an epidural anesthesia (see p.682). Incisions about 2 inches long are made at the top of your inner thigh and at the ankle to reveal parts of the affected vein. Several very small cuts are also made down the leg where branches of the main vein go deeper into the leg. The branches are severed, then tied to stop them from bleeding. A flexible wire is passed from the ankle to the thigh through the main vein. A hook is attached to the wire at the upper end. As the wire is withdrawn, the hook pulls the vein from beneath the skin. At the same time the leg is bandaged tightly to prevent bleeding. The operation usually takes 30 minutes for each leg.

After the operation Your legs will remain bandaged for several weeks and you will later need to wear elastic bandages. This surgery may be performed on an outpatient basis or you may stay in the hospital overnight.

Convalescence Once you are at home you will probably be advised to walk up to several miles a day and always relax with your feet up. Your physician will encourage you to gradually increase your activity and return to work as soon as possible.

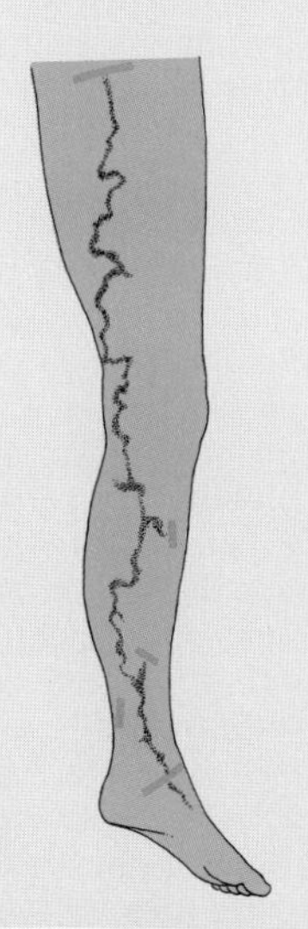

Sites of the incisions

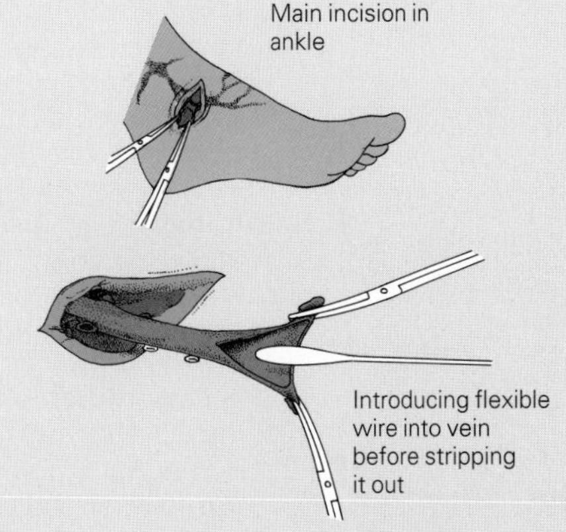

Professional help: Your physician can recommend support stockings or soothing dressings to relieve skin irritation. If you have both deep and superficial varicose veins, surgery is not recommended. Instead, your physician will recommend that you wear elastic bandages on your leg and avoid prolonged standing. But the most satisfactory treatment for uncomplicated varicose veins that produce symptoms is surgery. In the most common form of surgery, the affected veins are stripped from your leg. This procedure does not leave a noticeable scar, since a large section of vein can be removed through a tiny incision. The malfunctioning valves in the perforating veins are tied with thread to close them permanently. The remaining small veins rapidly enlarge to take over the function of collecting blood and channeling it to the deep veins.

As an alternative to traditional surgery, varicose veins can sometimes be treated by injection. A small amount of a sclerosing (corrosive) chemical is injected into the swollen veins. This makes the walls become inflamed and mat together, so that the veins stop carrying blood. If you have the injection treatment, it will probably be as an outpatient and involve only 2 or 3 visits to the physician. There are several drawbacks. The solution is very caustic, and if it is accidentally injected outside a vein the solution causes burns and scars. Injection is unlikely to succeed if the varicose vein is in your thigh. Therefore, many physicians recommend stripping the veins first. If there are minor recurrences later, they can usually be treated by injection.

After either treatment, you will have to wear support stockings or elastic bandages for about 6 weeks. You should walk as much as possible, and avoid standing or sitting with your legs hanging down.

Simple self-help
If you have varicose veins, wear support stockings or elastic bandages. If you use an elastic bandage, always wrap it from the foot upward. Don't wrap the bandage too tightly, or you'll do more harm than good. Also, try to sit with your feet propped up.

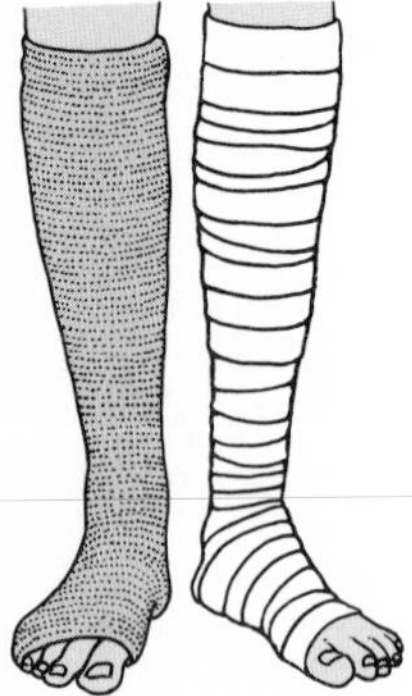

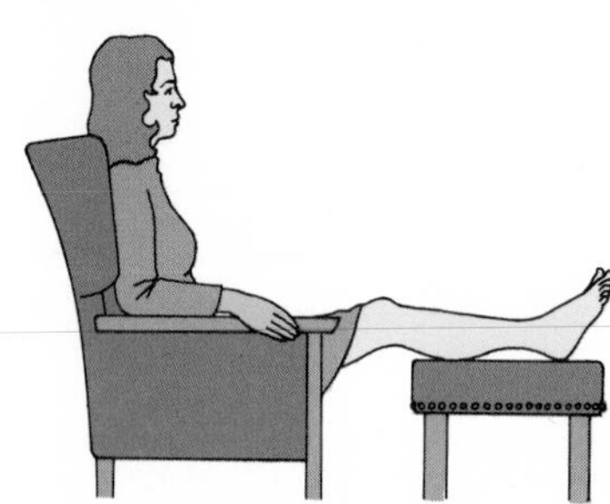

Thrombophlebitis

Phlebitis is inflammation of a vein, usually caused by infection or injury. When this happens, blood flow through the roughened, swollen vein may be slowed. Then thrombi, or blood clots, may develop and adhere to the wall of the inflamed vein. The resultant disorder is called thrombophlebitis, and it more commonly occurs in the surface veins of the legs, and sometimes in the arms.

Women are slightly more susceptible than men to the disorder. It is almost never a cause of death. You are more likely to get thrombophlebitis if you have varicose veins (see p.441) or, rarely, if you are undergoing medical treatment that involves piercing your veins with tubes or needles.

What are the symptoms?

The main symptoms of thrombophlebitis are pain, redness, tenderness, itching, and a hard, cordlike swelling under the skin along the length of the vein that is affected. If infection is present, you may also have a fever.

What are the risks?

If there is infection and it remains untreated, it can lead to blood poisoning or septicemia (see p.452). There is a very slight chance that blood clots may break off, but the real danger of thrombophlebitis is extension of the clot to a more vulnerable spot, such as a deeper vein (see Deep vein thrombosis, p.445), most likely in your leg or in the pelvic area. There the embolism becomes a danger.

What should be done?

Thrombophlebitis usually clears up in a week or two. Consult your physician, who will probably be able to diagnose your ailment without special tests.

What is the treatment?

Self-help: Take aspirin to ease the pain of thrombophlebitis. Follow the directions on the container. A nonprescription zinc oxide ointment should be effective in relieving any itching you have. Warm, moist packs are helpful along with elevation of the leg or arm.

Professional help: The inflammation and pain caused by thrombophlebitis may be relieved with a nonsteroidal anti-inflammatory drug such as ibuprofen. If you have an infection, your physician may prescribe an antibiotic drug and suggest that you rest in bed, elevate the affected leg, and apply warm, moist compresses. Your physician may also advise you to wrap the affected area with an elastic bandage. With treatment, thrombophlebitis nearly always clears up in a matter of 2 or 3 weeks.

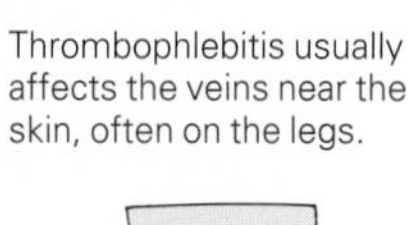

Thrombophlebitis usually affects the veins near the skin, often on the legs.

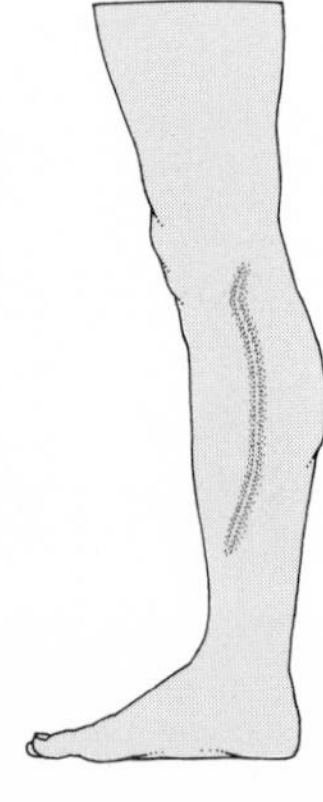

Deep vein thrombosis

(phlebothrombosis)

Thrombosis is the formation of a thrombus, or blood clot, which may partially or completely block a blood vessel. Thrombosis in a vein near the surface of the skin results in thrombophlebitis (see p.444). But if blood clots form in a deeper vein, the result is called deep vein thrombosis. There are many causes of deep vein thrombosis. Although the condition occurs most frequently in the legs and lower abdomen, it can occur anywhere in your body. There are two main circumstances that may lead to deep vein thrombosis—injury to the lining of the vein and sluggish blood flow. An unusual tendency of the blood to clot is a third cause, but this is rare.

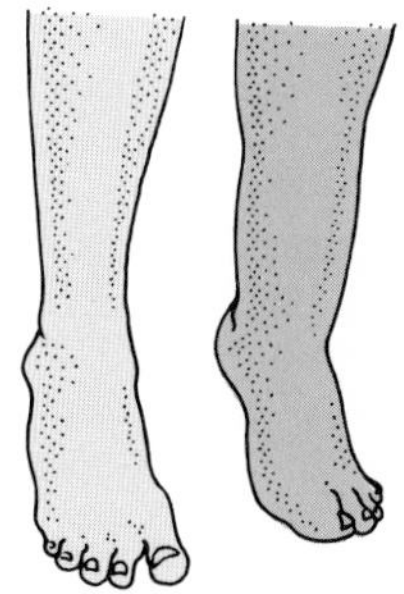

Thrombosis in the leg
The leg swells and becomes painful at the site of the blood clot, especially when you are walking.

Deep vein thrombosis is fairly unusual, but if you are older or overweight, or have had an injury to your pelvis or bones of your leg, you are particularly susceptible. The disorder may also affect people with blood that clots more easily than normal. This may result from a genetic (inherited) variation in blood clotting factors or from diseases such as disseminated lupus erythematosus (p.594) or polycythemia (p.460). It also may result from the use of estrogen, either in the form of birth control pills or as estrogen replacement therapy or treatment for cancer of the prostate. The condition often develops during periods of immobility, especially while you recover from surgery or an illness. It is also frequent when an arm or leg limb is immobilized in a cast to stabilize a broken bone. This is because at such times your blood flow has a tendency to become sluggish.

What are the symptoms?

The area drained by the vein, usually your calf or thigh, becomes swollen and painful as the normal flow of blood out of the leg is obstructed. This raises the pressure in your veins and capillaries. In your leg this causes edema, or swelling, that can remain indented if you press it with a finger. If the thrombosis is not in your leg, there may be no symptoms unless pieces of the clot break off, enter the blood, and cause an embolism (see Pulmonary embolism, next article). If the swelling is chronic, the skin may become brownish and may become easily injured, causing skin ulcers.

What should be done?

If you have symptoms of a deep vein thrombosis, see your physician. To locate a deep vein thrombosis in your leg, your physician may perform a Doppler ultrasound examination. Or your physician may perform venography, in which a contrast agent is injected into a vein in your foot and X rays are taken. Radioisotope scanning of the lungs is used if your physician suspects that any blood clots have been carried through the bloodstream to the lungs.

What is the treatment?

Self-help: If you are a woman smoker over 35 and you are taking oral contraceptives, ask your physician about alternative methods of birth control and stop smoking. The risks of thrombosis associated with birth control pills increase with age.

Professional help: If you are about to have surgery for another reason and your physician believes you are susceptible to deep vein thrombosis, you may be given injections of an anticoagulant drug either before or after the operation.

If you are bedridden, you will probably be encouraged to flex your leg muscles, wiggle your toes, and bend your ankles to keep your circulation active. If you are immobilized for a long period of time, your legs also may be mechanically elevated and put in plastic bags, which are alternately filled with air and deflated. The resultant pumping effect keeps your blood flowing normally.

If deep vein thrombosis has already occurred, and especially if blood clots have traveled to the lungs, you may be given treatment with thrombolytic drugs, which dissolve the clots, and with anticoagulants, which prevent the formation of more clots. Because these drugs can cause unwanted bleeding if you use them incorrectly, you must take them exactly as they are prescribed, usually for a period of several weeks.

Most clots are gradually absorbed into the bloodstream. Sometimes, surgery is necessary to remove blood clots. The only lasting cure for deep vein thrombosis, however, is to alter the factors that predispose you to thrombus formation.

Part of the clot in deep vein thrombosis may break off, forming an embolus. Swept into the circulation, the embolus could block circulation in the lungs.

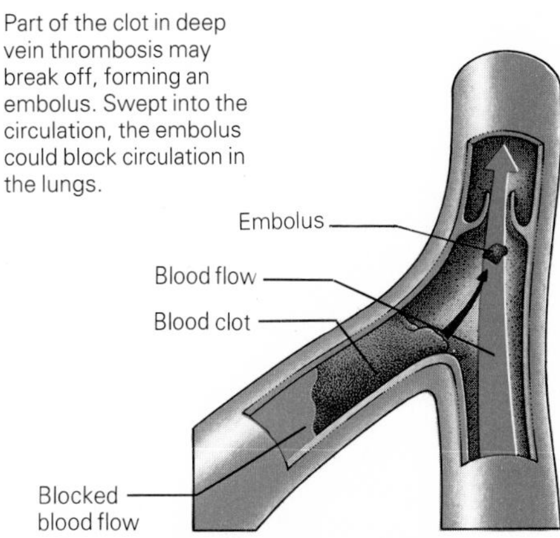

Pulmonary embolism

Pulmonary embolism nearly always occurs as a complication of deep vein thrombosis (see previous article). A blood clot detaches from the wall of a deep vein and moves into your bloodstream, through your heart, and along the pulmonary artery toward your lungs. If the loose clot, or embolus, is fairly large, it may become lodged in an artery inside your lungs, where it can block off the blood flow. If most of the pulmonary artery is obstructed the right ventricle suddenly must beat more forcibly, and very frequently right-sided heart failure occurs. This reduces the volume of freshly oxygenated blood that is returning to the left side of your heart, and if the volume of blood is reduced greatly, shock may occur (see p.414). Any such pulmonary embolism can be serious or even fatal.

In the US there are 650,000 cases of pulmonary embolism during an average year, and approximately 30 percent result in death. Pulmonary embolism affects three women for every two men, and people who are in bed recovering from operations are particularly at risk for the disorder. Massive pulmonary embolism, an episode in which most of the blood flow in the lungs is blocked off, is very serious. About one of every 10 cases results in sudden death within 1 hour.

What are the symptoms?

The symptoms depend on the size of the pulmonary embolus and its location in your lungs. Because your heart and body tissues do not get all the oxygen they need, you will almost always have some degree of breathlessness. You may also feel faint and have chest pain when you inhale. You may have a cough, bloody sputum, and cyanosis, or blueness, around your mouth. In some cases, a massive pulmonary embolism can cause collapse and death within minutes.

What are the risks?

Any blockage of the flow of blood into your lungs can lead to right-sided heart failure (see p.408). Your susceptibility to chest infection is increased by even a small pulmonary embolism, and if you have a massive pulmonary embolism, you can die from the collapse of your circulatory system.

What should be done?

Anything that predisposes you to deep vein thrombosis also increases your chances of having a pulmonary embolism. See your physician if you have any of the symptoms of either disorder, especially if you have recently been confined to bed.

Your physician will examine you and, if pulmonary embolism is suspected, will want a chest X ray and an electrocardiogram (ECG) to see if your heart, especially the right side, is under strain. To confirm the diagnosis a radioisotope lung scan may be ordered. If any doubt still exists, a pulmonary arteriogram will confirm the diagnosis.

If you collapse with suspected massive pulmonary embolism, you require immediate emergency treatment similar to the treatment of shock (see p.414).

What is the treatment?

Self-help: To prevent pulmonary embolism, follow the self-help advice of the article on deep vein thrombosis (see previous article). If the symptoms of an embolism occur, you must get professional help.

Professional help: You will need to be hospitalized for treatment with anticoagulant and thrombolytic drugs (see also Heart attack, p.406). Heparin, an anticoagulant, helps prevent more blood clots from forming in the lungs and veins. The drug is injected at 4- to 6-hour intervals either under the skin or directly into a vein. Thrombolytic drugs such as streptokinase or TPA (tissue plasminogen activator) help dissolve the blood clots in the lungs. The combination of thrombolytic and anticoagulant drug treatment carries the risk of internal bleeding, and careful monitoring of the blood coagulation factors is necessary.

Emergency treatment is required if the embolism is severe. Initial efforts will be made to control shock. If this is not successful within a short time the blockage can be removed surgically. This is a major operation performed under very risky conditions, and it must be done almost immediately after the embolism occurs.

What are the long-term prospects?

If you survive the critical first few days after an episode of massive pulmonary embolism, you stand a good chance of complete recovery. Chances are even better when the source of the blood clots that are moving

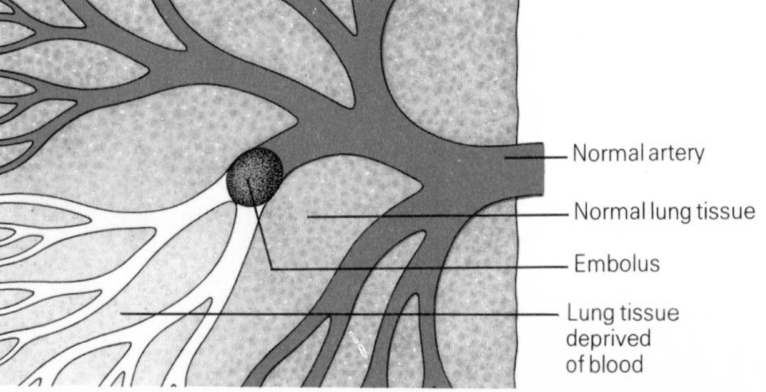

Embolism in the lung
An embolus, or loose blood clot from a vein, can travel to the lungs and block off vital blood flow.

through your bloodstream is found and treated. A less severe embolism may damage part of the lung, but you will almost always make a satisfactory recovery from this disorder if the embolisms are prevented from recurring. Your physician will prescribe an anticoagulant drug to help prevent more blood clots.

Gangrene

Gangrene is dead tissue. Its characteristic black color is a sign that the skin, and often underlying muscle and bone, are dead. There are two basic types of gangrene: dry and infected "wet" gangrene. Dry gangrene does not involve infection; it occurs when the flow of blood to certain tissues is stopped or reduced. This may be the result of arterial embolism (see previous article), poor circulation caused by diabetes (see p.558), or hardening of the arteries (see p.435). It may be caused by prolonged frostbite (see p.440). The oxygen-deprived area dies, but gangrene does not spread.

While the tissue is dying, it can be extremely painful. Once dead, it becomes numb and slowly turns black. A visible line separates the dead tissue from living tissue.

Infected "wet" gangrene may develop when an area of muscle and overlying skin is killed by toxins produced by bacteria known as *Clostridia*, which multiply in dead tissue. This is also known as gas gangrene, since the bacteria produce gas in the tissues. Infection with these bacteria is a possibility whenever a wound is contaminated, as may occur after gunshot wounds, traffic accidents, or other injuries that deprive muscle or skin of their blood supply. Surgeons can usually prevent this infected "wet" gangrene by careful wound hygiene. This involves removal of all the tissue with poor blood circulation and all contaminants. Sometimes, if gangrene is to be prevented, amputation of part of an arm or leg is unavoidable. The term "wet" gangrene is also used when dry gangrenous tissue becomes secondarily infected with organisms other than *Clostridia*.

What are the symptoms?

Dry gangrene may develop in the foot or leg of anyone with poor circulation. In the early stages, the limb is cold, and there is a dull, aching pain that increases with physical exertion. If the foot is painful or unusually pale, and you have poor circulation, consult your physician without delay. Pain is also the main symptom of infective gangrene. The area around the wound becomes red, swollen, extremely painful, and oozes pus. The wound may develop an unpleasant smell.

What should be done?

Dry gangrene may be avoided by measures that help to maintain circulation, such as not smoking. If you have diabetes, keep your diabetes under control. Take special care of your feet to prevent sores. You should wear shoes that fit well. If you think you may be getting dry gangrene, see your physician immediately for treatment. Infected "wet" gangrene is treated by antibiotics and prompt surgical attention.

What is the treatment?

The priorities in the treatment of any type of gangrene are removal of all dead skin, muscle, and bone (the breeding grounds for bacteria) and improvement of the circulation. When toes have become gangrenous they may fall off or be removed. To prevent infection from spreading to the remaining healthy toes, your physician may recommend that you soak your foot in an antiseptic solution, that you clean off any layer of pus that forms on a toe with gangrene, and that you elevate the affected foot as much as possible. The bacteria are treated with antibiotics. With prompt treatment the outlook for a case of gangrene is good, but major surgery, including amputation, may be necessary in some cases. Usually, some of the living tissue next to the dead, gangrenous tissue must also be removed.

Pulmonary hypertension

(cor pulmonale)

Pulmonary hypertension is elevated blood pressure in the lungs. This disorder of the circulation can be caused by any disease that blocks the flow of blood through the lungs. Among the common causes are congenital (from birth) heart disease, chronic bronchitis (see p.380), and emphysema (see p.383). People who live for many years at high altitudes are especially susceptible to pulmonary hypertension, but almost any lung disease can lead to this condition. When no underlying cause can be found, the disease is called primary pulmonary hypertension. Whatever the cause, the main result is increased pressure within the pulmonary arteries, which carry blood from your heart to your lungs. In time this leads to thickening of the arteries and narrowing of the arterial passageways, which further obstruct the flow of blood. In its effort to compensate for poor circulation, the right side of your heart becomes enlarged, and the extra work the heart must do can eventually cause right-sided heart failure (see p.409).

What are the symptoms?

Women are 5 times more likely than men to develop pulmonary hypertension. There are often no symptoms of this disease until the condition is advanced. Thereafter the main symptom is swollen ankles, usually noticeable only when your chest disorder is giving you problems. Your skin may have a bluish tinge because the blood contains less oxygen than it should. The low oxygen content of the blood stimulates the production of more red blood cells, a condition called polycythemia. When the red cell count becomes too great, the blood becomes thicker and harder to push through the small vessels of the lung, further increasing the pulmonary artery blood pressure and decreasing the cardiac output (amount of blood pumped by the heart in a minute). If you already experience breathlessness because of underlying lung disease, pulmonary hypertension is likely to make you even more breathless and you may also experience other symptoms of right-sided heart failure (see p.409).

The main risks are from the lung disease that causes pulmonary hypertension, but if heart failure develops, there is an added risk of complications such as the failure of your liver or your kidneys.

What should be done?

If you have a chest condition and notice that your ankles are swelling at times when the condition seems particularly severe, see your physician promptly.

What is the treatment?

Self-help: If you smoke, quit now.

Professional help: Heart failure caused by pulmonary hypertension can be relieved by bed rest and treatment with oxygen, which reduces spasm in your pulmonary arteries, and diuretics, which rid your body of excess fluid. Occasionally, vasodilating drugs can be effective in reducing the blood pressure in the pulmonary arteries. Further episodes are likely, though, unless the underlying disorder is treated. Treatment depends on the underlying disease. Your physician may prescribe prolonged daily home treatment with oxygen, which sometimes helps to lower pulmonary blood pressure.

If your pulmonary hypertension is caused by chronic lung disease, the goal of long-term treatment is to stop further deterioration of your lungs. Your physician may prescribe antibiotics and immunize you against influenza and the pneumococcus bacteria to help prevent acute chest infections.

People who have pulmonary hypertension and progressive heart and lung disease can be treated successfully by transplantation of the heart and lungs (see Transplants, p.432) or just the lungs if the heart has not been damaged. However, major surgery of this kind carries substantial risks and is only performed when all other treatment for the disorder has failed.

Postural hypotension

Chronic high blood pressure (see p.411) is a serious problem, but chronic lower-than-average blood pressure is not a serious problem. However, if your blood pressure drops suddenly from time to time, you may have problems. When you stand up abruptly from a sitting or lying position, your blood vessels, both small arteries and veins, have to contract to maintain normal blood pressure in the new posture. Normally this process occurs automatically by reflex action of your nervous system. If you have postural hypotension, however, the reflex action is defective. As a result, your blood pressure falls and the flow of blood to your brain is temporarily reduced when you suddenly change position to upright. This causes the alarming symptoms of dizziness or even brief loss of consciousness and fainting.

Postural hypotension may be caused by medications prescribed for high blood pressure, as a side effect or if the dosage is too high. Your physician may advise that you reduce the dose of the medication. Occasionally, postural hypotension may occur as a minor complication of pregnancy or certain other conditions such as diabetes (see p.558), hardening of the arteries (see p.435), or Addison's disease (see p.564).

What should be done?

If you have dizzy spells or feel faint when you stand up abruptly, make a habit of standing up slowly from a sitting or lying position. If you have frequent fainting spells, consult your physician, who will recommend tests to help determine the underlying cause of the problem.

Blood disorders

Introduction

Your blood has two basic parts: blood cells, which are also called blood corpuscles; and plasma, the fluid in which the blood cells are suspended. The disorders of the blood that are discussed in this section are principally concerned with the blood cells.

Most of the blood cells in your body are red blood cells. Their main function is to carry oxygen from the lungs to all parts of the body. Red blood cells contain a protein called hemoglobin, which combines with oxygen in the lungs and releases it to the tissues as the blood circulates through your body. The red blood cells also carry some of the waste product carbon dioxide from the tissues to the lungs so that it can be exhaled.

Your body also contains several kinds of white blood cells, which protect the body from infection. Most white blood cells are neutrophils, which attack and engulf bacteria. Another kind, the lymphocyte, recognizes foreign cells, other infectious agents, and other foreign substances and participates in the body's immune reaction against them. There are other varieties of white blood cells, but these two are the most common.

A third type of blood cell is the platelet. Platelets gather wherever a blood vessel is injured as the first stage in the blood-clotting process. Chemical substances in the plasma then assist the platelets in forming a blood clot that seals the wound.

Most blood cells are produced in the bone marrow. Although lymphocytes are produced in the bone marrow, they are also found in the lymph glands in the neck, armpits, groin, and many other parts of the body. The spleen and lymph glands, together with the channels and ducts connecting them, are called the lymphatic system. When red blood cells and platelets become old or defective they are filtered out of the bloodstream and broken down in the spleen, and also in the liver.

Disorders of the blood are grouped as follows: lack of hemoglobin, which causes anemia; disorders in clotting, which cause bleeding and bruising or excessive clotting; cancerous changes in the white cells, which cause leukemia and bone marrow conditions such as multiple myeloma; and disorders that affect the lymphatic system.

Basic parts of the blood

Blood can easily be separated into its different parts much like cream from milk. Red blood cells are heavier than white blood cells and platelets, which in turn are heavier than blood plasma.

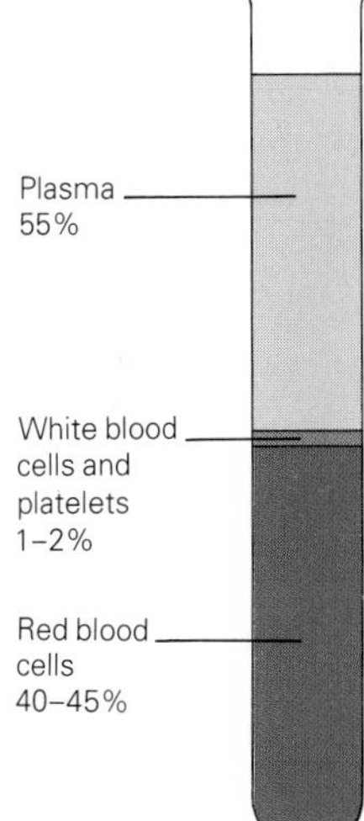

Plasma
Plasma is a yellowish fluid that contains minerals, antibodies, and blood-clotting factors.

White blood cells
White blood cells protect the body against infection by destroying bacteria and producing antibodies.

Platelets
Platelets help plug damaged blood vessel walls and form the first stage of a blood clot.

Red blood cells
Red blood cells normally account for about 40 to 45 percent of your blood; they contain a protein, hemoglobin, that carries oxygen throughout the body.

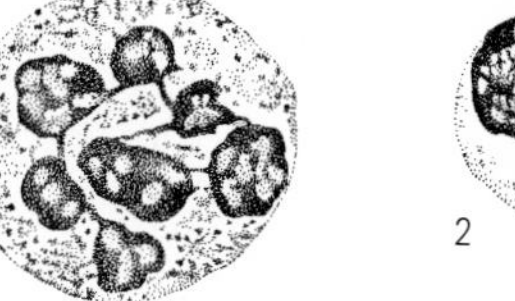

White blood cells
1. Neutrophil
2. Lymphocyte

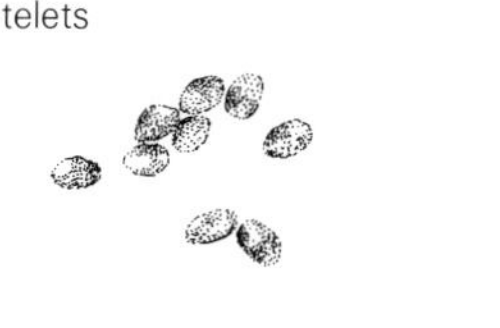

Platelets

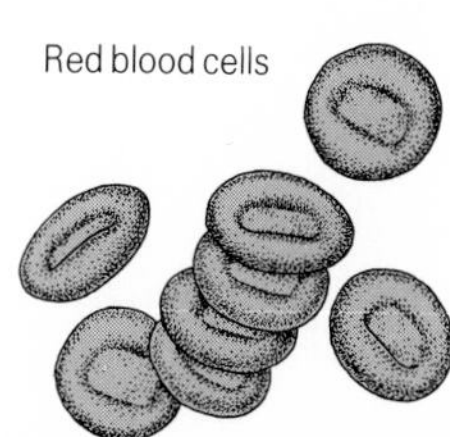

Red blood cells

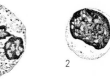

Anemia

The main component of red blood cells is the protein hemoglobin, which combines with oxygen in the lungs and carries it throughout your body; oxygen is then released to the tissues. Anemia is defined as a decrease in hemoglobin or in the number of red blood cells to below the normal level.

If you have anemia your blood is less effective in transporting oxygen from the lungs to the tissues, and carbon dioxide from the tissues to the lungs. When the anemia is moderately severe, symptoms and signs include pale skin, fatigue, weakness, fainting, breathlessness, and palpitations.

Anemia may be due to loss of blood from heavy menstrual periods, from internal bleeding caused by a peptic ulcer, or from hemorrhoids. A healthy person whose diet contains plenty of iron and vitamins can produce large amounts of new blood, but if your diet is inadequate, even small, persistent losses of blood may lead to anemia.

Blood loss leads to a particular type of anemia described in detail below (see Iron-deficiency anemia). Other causes of anemia include severe deficiencies of vitamin B_{12} or folic acid and various inherited abnormalities in the makeup of hemoglobin. In hemolytic anemia the red blood cells are destroyed more quickly than they normally would be. In addition, anemia is a characteristic of many chronic diseases in which red blood cell production is suppressed. For people with chronic kidney disease, the hormone erythropoietin, produced by genetic engineering, has helped treat anemia.

Iron-deficiency anemia

Iron is an essential component of hemoglobin, the protein in red blood cells. Insufficient iron in your body causes an inadequate production of hemoglobin and leads to iron-deficiency anemia.

Normally, extra iron is stored in your body and then used to produce hemoglobin in new red blood cells. Most of this iron is recovered as old red blood cells are destroyed. The small amount of iron lost from the body is replaced by iron absorbed from your diet. Some people have little or no iron stored in their bodies. If you are one of these people, you can stay healthy if you balance the iron you lose with iron absorbed from your diet. If you lose more iron than you are able to absorb, anemia develops. It is important to determine whether you have anemia or some more serious underlying disorder.

There are three general causes for inadequate amounts of stored iron. First, there may not be enough iron in your diet to replace the amount that is lost each day. This occurs mainly in young children (see Iron-deficiency anemia in children, p.728), pregnant women, and in people who, for one of several reasons, are eating restricted diets.

The second reason for iron deficiency is that the person's digestive system is unable to absorb iron, even though there may be enough iron contained in his or her diet. This occurs in certain disorders of the small intestine that affect absorption of nutrients, such as celiac disease.

The third reason for iron deficiency is that the stored iron may become depleted through excessive loss of blood. This is the most common cause. If blood is lost because of a temporary problem, reserves of iron will rebuild in time. Many women have heavy menstrual periods, which can gradually deplete their stored iron if they don't replenish their iron reserves through their diet. In other cases, blood loss may occur from the intestinal tract. This type of blood loss, in sufficient quantity, can produce bloody or black stools. However, if the blood loss is persistent but small there may be no sign of the bleeding. Some of the common causes of intestinal blood loss include the following: gastric erosion (see p.497), stomach ulcer and duodenal ulcer (see Peptic ulcer, p.500), cancer of the large intestine (see p.518), and hemorrhoids (see p.520).

What are the symptoms?

Symptoms are those characteristic of most forms of anemia. You may be weak, pale, tired, faint, and/or breathless. You may also have palpitations, or an increased awareness of your heartbeat that occurs when your heart tries to compensate for anemia by pumping blood at a faster rate.

What are the risks?

In general, iron-deficiency anemia is not life threatening. However, it does weaken your body's resistance to the effects of other illness or injury, especially if you lose large amounts of blood. It also produces additional stress on your heart and lungs.

What should be done?
If you have the symptoms listed above, see your physician. Do not attempt to treat the condition yourself. Your physician will look for any underlying disease that can be treated. He or she may test a sample of your blood to determine the cause of the anemia. Measurements of the blood iron level and vitamin B_{12} level are done, along with a test for blood in the stool. A bone marrow test may also be necessary. If bleeding is detected, other tests, such as upper and lower gastrointestinal endoscopy (examination with a viewing tube), may be needed.

What is the treatment?
Iron-deficiency anemia is treated by dealing with the cause of the depletion of stored iron. It is very important that any correctable cause be treated. Usually the iron deficiency itself can be treated with oral iron medication. This can cause indigestion or intestinal upsets, but should not if you take the medication right after you eat and do not take more than your physician has prescribed. The iron may darken your stools, which is normal. If you do have difficulty with the oral iron medication, your physician may give you iron by injecting it into a muscle or a vein. Ordinarily the anemia disappears after a few weeks of treatment. If the anemia is severe and threatens the function of your vital organs, your physician will arrange for a blood transfusion.

When your anemia has cleared up, your physician will usually suggest that you continue to take iron supplements for an additional few months to build up your stored iron. If the cause of the anemia was a poor diet, your physician can recommend changes in your diet that will help you prevent the problem from recurring.

The prospects for people with iron-deficiency anemia are generally excellent. In many cases, treatment of the underlying disorder eliminates the iron deficiency.

Anemia of chronic disease

This type of anemia is often a complication of other diseases. Disorders that may bring on this type of anemia include rheumatoid arthritis (see p.589), hepatitis (see p.523), and tuberculosis (see p.602).

The symptoms of anemia of chronic disease are the same as those for other forms of anemia, combined with the symptoms of the underlying disease.

People with chronic kidney failure usually acquire anemia because their damaged kidneys stop making the hormone erythropoietin, which regulates the production of red blood cells by the bone marrow. An artificial form of erythropoietin is now available, produced by genetic engineering, to treat those who have anemia caused by a deficiency of this hormone. The treatment produces a dramatic rise in the hemoglobin within a few days and an equally dramatic improvement in your general health.

Erythropoietin is not an effective treatment, however, in anemia resulting from other types of chronic disease. In such cases, treatment consists of blood transfusions or treatment of the underlying disease.

B_{12} deficiency anemia and folic acid deficiency

Red blood cell production takes place in the bone marrow, and depends primarily on two vitamins, vitamin B_{12} and folic acid. Your body absorbs these vitamins from certain foods (see Vitamin guide, p.534). If you do not get enough of either vitamin, red blood cell production falls. Also, those red cells that are formed are defective. The result is one of the following forms of anemia.

In the US, nearly everyone's diet has enough B_{12}. A deficiency can occur because your body cannot absorb it. In a healthy person the liver stores vitamin B_{12}. If you develop an inability to absorb B_{12}, your body will eventually use up the stored B_{12} and anemia will develop.

There are various reasons why some people cannot absorb B_{12}. Your body normally absorbs B_{12} from the lower small intestine. But before this can occur the vitamin must combine in the stomach with a special substance known as intrinsic factor, which is secreted by the stomach lining. In some people, the stomach lining stops secreting enough intrinsic factor. Without it, sufficient quantities of vitamin B_{12} cannot be absorbed by the body. This is the most common type of B_{12} deficiency, and it is called pernicious anemia.

If you have had some forms of digestive tract surgery, or if you have malabsorption from the intestines such as celiac disease, your body's ability to absorb B_{12} may be reduced, sometimes to the point where it cannot absorb the vitamin at all.

Folic acid deficiency usually results from inadequate amounts of the vitamin in the diet. Folic acid is generally supplied by green vegetables. Your body cannot store large amounts of this vitamin, so any deficiency shows up within a few weeks as a form of anemia called folic acid deficiency. If you have celiac disease (see p.509), you are also susceptible to folic acid deficiency because you cannot absorb sufficient amounts of folic acid, even if it is plentiful in your diet. Finally, some people have an increased requirement for folic acid, and they need more of the vitamin than an ordinary diet provides. Folic acid deficiency may occur with the long-term use of certain anti-bacterial, immunosuppressant, or potassium-sparing antihypertensive drugs.

Both types of anemia produce the symptoms associated with anemia in general, but B_{12} deficiency anemia is more serious because B_{12} is vital to the maintenance of the nervous system as well as to the production of red blood cells. Deficiency of B_{12} therefore damages the brain, the spinal cord, and the peripheral nerves, which causes symptoms that include dementia in older people and weakness and tingling in the arms or legs.

What are the symptoms?

The main symptoms of B_{12} and folic acid deficiency anemia are those of other anemias. They include paleness, fatigue, shortness of breath, and palpitations (awareness of the heartbeat), particularly if you exert yourself. In both disorders, your mouth and tongue may be sore, and your skin may become pale yellow. If the spinal cord is affected by B_{12} deficiency, you may not be able to walk normally or keep your balance, and you may feel continuous tingling in your hands and feet. You may also have memory loss, confusion, and depression.

Pernicious anemia, the most common type of B_{12} deficiency, is equally common in men and women, and rare before age 40. If you have a close relative who has pernicious anemia, you have a greater than average risk of contracting this type of anemia. Folic acid deficiency is somewhat more common than B_{12} deficiency. It often occurs in older people, who may not eat a well-balanced diet. It also occurs in pregnant women, who need extra supplies of the vitamin for the developing fetus. It is particularly common in cases of severe alcoholism, because alcoholics often do not eat properly.

What are the risks?

If you have B_{12} or folic acid deficiency anemia, and if it is treated promptly, you will probably recover completely. If you do not obtain prompt treatment for B_{12} deficiency anemia you risk permanent damage to your spinal cord and, to a lesser extent, irreversible intellectual impairment.

What should be done?

If you have symptoms of anemia, see your physician. If you have continuous tingling or other sensory disturbances in your hands and feet, or problems with movement, balance, or memory, see your physician immediately. Be sure to tell your physician if you have a close relative who has pernicious anemia. Blood tests can usually establish whether you have either of these vitamin deficiencies. If you do, the underlying cause usually can be determined only by further tests.

Blood poisoning

Blood poisoning, which is also called septicemia, is a life-threatening condition that is caused by the spread of bacterial infection or the toxins (poisons) made by bacteria in your bloodstream.

Even a minor infection such as a boil (see p.267) or a small contaminated wound releases some bacteria into your bloodstream. Many routine dental procedures, such as tooth extractions, also release bacteria into your blood. If you are healthy, your body destroys these automatically. Blood poisoning from bacteria, called bacteremia, produces fever, chills, fatigue, loss of appetite, and a general sick feeling. Antibiotic drugs can help your body's immune system in eliminating such an infection. A blood test may identify the infecting microorganism and antibiotic sensitivity studies can help your physician choose the proper antibiotic.

It is important to consult your physician for treatment of urinary tract infections, wound infections, and major burns because bacteria tend to invade the bloodstream in these conditions. Large numbers of bacteria and/or toxins in your blood may cause septic shock (see p.414). You may have severe chills and become pale, cold, and clammy, accompanied by a serious drop in blood pressure. Septic shock usually, but not always, begins from an infection in some part of your body. This is a very serious condition, and requires immediate medical attention.

What is the treatment?

Once your ability to absorb vitamin B_{12} through the digestive tract has been lost, it can never be regained. Treatment of pernicious anemia and other types of B_{12} deficiency consists of taking vitamin B_{12} for life. Most physicians prefer to give the vitamin by injection. However, an oral form of vitamin B_{12} is available. It is important that you do not stop your medication; if you do, your symptoms will ultimately return. Problems with walking and balancing may take months to improve. If these symptoms existed a long time before treatment began, they may never disappear completely.

Folic acid deficiency that is caused by an inadequate diet can be cleared up completely. At first, your physician may prescribe folic acid supplements. He or she will advise you on how to make sure that your diet contains adequate amounts of the vitamin (see p.534). If the deficiency is caused by a failure to absorb normal quantities of folic acid, or by an increased requirement for it, extra folic acid may be prescribed in oral form for an indefinite period.

Sickle cell anemia

In the inherited disease called sickle cell anemia, the red blood cells contain an abnormal hemoglobin, called hemoglobin S. If you have this disease, you have no normal hemoglobin in your red blood cells because you have inherited a sickle cell gene from each of your parents. This condition must be distinguished from sickle cell trait, in which you inherit only one sickle cell gene from one parent. Then you have red cells that contain half normal hemoglobin and half hemoglobin S, and your health is not impaired. Hemoglobin S causes red cells of persons with sickle cell anemia to become deformed in a sickle shape, especially in parts of the body where the amount of oxygen is relatively low. These abnormal blood cells do not flow smoothly through the capillaries, or smaller blood vessels. They may clog the vessels and prevent blood from reaching the tissues. This blockage causes anoxia, or lack of oxygen, which makes the sickling worse. Episodes of this kind are called sickle cell crises. They can be very painful and may be associated with hemolysis (destruction of red blood cells).

What are the symptoms?

If you have sickle cell anemia, you will have all the symptoms of anemia (see p.450). In addition, you may have occasional sickle cell crises, which produce episodes of pain in the bones and abdomen. You may also develop blood clots in the lungs, kidneys, brain, and most other organs. Leg ulcers and painful bone problems are also common.

How often crises occur varies from person to person. Crises are more likely to occur during infections and after an injury. They also occur with anesthesia and surgery if appropriate precautions are not taken.

Both sickle cell trait and sickle cell anemia occur almost exclusively in people of African descent and people from Italy, Greece, India, and the Middle East. About 1 in every 1,000 black Americans has sickle cell anemia.

What are the risks?

There is a risk of mild anemia from sickle cell trait, but a man and woman who both have the trait have a 25 percent chance of producing a child with sickle cell anemia (see also Genetic counseling, p.664).

What should be done?

If you or your child displays any of the symptoms described, see your physician, who will consider the possibility of sickle cell anemia, especially if you know that the disease runs in your family. Analysis of a blood sample will disclose whether the disease is present. Sickle cell anemia can be diagnosed during pregnancy by the genetic analysis of cells removed from the fetus by chorionic villus sampling (see p.684) between the sixth and eighth weeks of pregnancy, or amniocentesis later in the pregnancy. In some states all newborn infants are tested for sickle cell disease so that children with the disorder can be treated without delay.

What is the treatment?

There is no cure for sickle cell anemia, but the symptoms can be treated. Crises of acute pain are treated with painkillers, and you may have to be admitted to the hospital where you will be treated with oxygen and intravenous fluids. It is extremely important that you do everything possible to maintain good health, and that you obtain prompt treatment for infections, injuries, and other illnesses. Also, you should regularly see a physician who is thoroughly familiar with the disease. Special precautions are necessary before you have any surgery, including dental surgery. Also, you should not fly in an unpressurized airplane because that could result in a crisis.

Thalassemia

In this disorder an inherited defect prevents the formation of normal amounts of hemoglobin A, the type of hemoglobin found in the red blood cells of normal adults. As a partial compensation in people with thalassemia, the body produces hemoglobin F, a type of hemoglobin that is usually found only in fetuses and newborn babies. However, a majority of the red cells produced in this condition are destroyed, and those that remain can survive only a short time.

The full-blown form of the disorder, called thalassemia major, is also called beta thalassemia because it is caused by a beta form of hemoglobin. Thalassemia major occurs only if an infant inherits the defect from both parents (see p.752). It produces severe, usually fatal, anemia. When you inherit the defect from only one parent, you inherit the thalassemia trait. This rarely causes any symptoms or disability.

What are the symptoms?

The symptoms of the various forms of thalassemia are failure to grow, severe anemia, jaundice, chronic leg ulcers, a mongoloid appearance, delayed sexual development, and mental retardation.

What are the risks?

Thalassemia trait is several times more common than thalassemia major. Both forms of the disorder are relatively common in people from the Mediterranean area, the Middle East, and the Far East.

A child with thalassemia major needs repeated blood transfusions. This treatment eventually causes a buildup of iron in the body, which damages the liver and the heart. At one time, this led to death from liver or heart failure. A treatment now available makes it possible to remove the iron.

What should be done?

If your child has any of the symptoms described, see your physician, who will arrange for a blood test to confirm or reject the possibility of thalassemia. If you have any form of the disease in your family, even the trait, and you are considering having a child, see your physician about genetic counseling (see p.664) to estimate the risks.

Thalassemia can be diagnosed during pregnancy by analysis of cells removed from the fetus by chorionic villus sampling (see p.684) early in the pregnancy, or by amniocentesis later in the pregnancy.

Regular blood transfusions relieve the child's symptoms of anemia, and it is now possible to use only young red blood cells in the transfusions. These cells survive longer, and therefore the child does not need as many transfusions. Bone marrow transplant is recommended for very severe cases.

Hemolytic anemia

Hemolysis is a process in which your red blood cells are destroyed prematurely. When this occurs, your body attempts to compensate by producing new red blood cells. If destruction exceeds production, the resulting disorder is hemolytic anemia.

Hemolytic anemia may be hereditary (present at birth), or you may acquire it later in life. In the inherited types, hemolysis occurs because a specific enzyme needed by the red blood cells is deficient. Thus, your red blood cells become less able to protect themselves against adverse effects produced by a particular drug treatment or infection.

One type of acquired hemolytic anemia occurs when your body produces antibodies, substances that normally protect you from infections, that destroy the body's own red blood cells. Hemolysis may also occur when your body produces antibodies against red blood cells that you receive in a transfusion. Finally, red cells may also be destroyed after they are damaged by artificial heart valves, abnormal blood vessel walls, or toxins such as certain snakebite venoms.

The disease is rarely fatal, although some forms are difficult to treat.

What are the symptoms?

The main symptoms of hemolytic anemia are paleness, fatigue, breathlessness, and palpitations (awareness of your heartbeat), especially with exertion. Your skin may become pale yellow, and your urine may contain blood pigment and be darker than normal. If your red blood cells continue to be destroyed prematurely over many years, gallstones (see p.526) often result.

What is the treatment?

If you have the symptoms described, see your physician promptly. The principal treatment for some types of hemolytic anemia is a splenectomy, an operation to remove most of the spleen. Most red blood cells are destroyed by the spleen as they wear out. Removing most of the spleen can considerably improve hemolytic anemia but does not cure it.

Hemolytic anemia that is caused by drugs is treated by substituting other drugs.

Bleeding and bruising

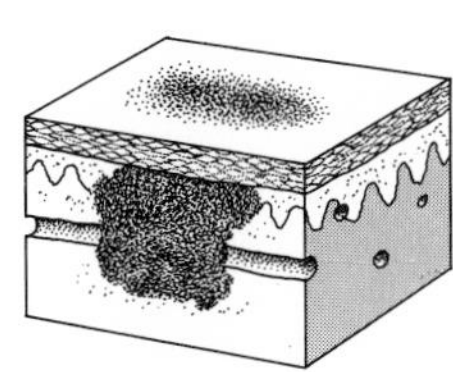

Bruises
Blood from an internal injury collects in surrounding tissue to form a bruise. Once the internal bleeding has stopped, white blood cells called monocytes help break down the leaked red blood cells.

Bleeding occurs when a blood vessel is damaged. If the vessel is internal, blood seeps into surrounding tissue, and a bruise forms. Where delicate blood vessels are near the surface of tissue, as they are in the nose, for example, a very slight injury or irritation may cause bleeding.

For most people, minor bleeding causes no harm because the body soon stops it, by means of three mechanisms that act together. The nearby blood vessels contract and restrict the flow of blood to the area of the wound. The platelets in the blood gather where the blood vessels are damaged and stick to the vessel walls and to each other to form a plug. In addition, interlacing strands of material called fibrin form in the damaged area. Blood cells are then trapped in the fibrin mesh and form a clot that seals the break and effectively stops the bleeding.

In most diseases in which bleeding occurs, one or more of the mechanisms that halt blood loss is not working properly. Bleeding from a cut, which should stop within 5 or 10 minutes, may continue for hours, possibly even for days. Minor injuries may cause extensive bleeding. There may be internal bleeding, and bleeding in the joints may produce acute pain and cause disabling damage. Two common bleeding disorders, hemophilia and thrombocytopenia, are discussed in this section.

Hemophilia

Hemophilia A is the best known of the bleeding diseases. Although it is the most common of these diseases, it is still rather rare. In this disorder, there is a substantial reduction in the amount of a protein called antihemophilic globulin, or factor VIII, in the blood. Factor VIII is vital to the clotting mechanism of the blood.

Because of the way hemophilia is inherited, generally only males have the disease, but it is passed from one generation to the next by female carriers. Female carriers may have decreased levels of factor VIII and increased bleeding problems. In the US about 1 male in 10,000 has hemophilia. In about 75 percent of cases, there is a family history of the disease. However, for the remaining 25 percent of cases, the person with hemophilia is the first of his line, probably because of a mutation, or spontaneous change, in the genes of that person's mother.

What are the symptoms?

Symptoms usually appear in childhood, as soon as the affected male child becomes active. He gets bruises on his knees and elbows after he crawls, and any cuts bleed for a long time. Internal bleeding caused by falls may cause large, deep bruises, which may make an arm or leg swollen and painful for several days. Repeated bleeding into joints and accumulation of scarred tissue produce stiff joints that limit the child's movement. There is a great deal of variation in the amount of bleeding from one person with hemophilia to another.

What are the risks?

Today the risks of being disabled or dying from hemophilia are greatly reduced because of effective treatment. However, a major injury is still particularly dangerous for anyone who has hemophilia. Also, if you have hemophilia, special precautions must be taken before you have any operation, even a tooth extraction.

What should be done?

Any member of a family with a history of hemophilia should seek genetic counseling (see p.664) before starting a family. Your physician or local public health organizations can tell you where to find such counseling. If you have a male child who shows the symptoms described, see your physician.

If you are an adult male and you notice that you bruise or bleed in a way that seems abnormal to you, you should also see your physician. He or she may refer you to a hematologist, or blood specialist.

If you or your child have hemophilia, you may be given a card that describes the disease. The person with hemophilia should carry the card at all times, so that if an injury occurs the appropriate treatment can begin without delay.

What is the treatment?

Self-help: If you have hemophilia, unless it is a very mild case, your physician will advise against activities that could cause even minor injury. This means that you must avoid most physical contact sports. Solitary exercise such as running or gymnastics may be recommended in moderation. Your physician will also advise that you not take aspirin or any drugs that contain aspirin, because it increases the chance of bleeding.

Professional help: Preventive treatment for hemophilia has become possible by regular transfusions of factor VIII, the clotting substance. People with hemophilia can be taught to give themselves transfusions by injection. In case of injury, any bleeding or bruising that occurs can be stopped by a further injection or transfusion of factor VIII. Such treatment may involve a short stay in the hospital. Today genetically engineered factor VIII is available that avoids the risk of infection with HIV (human immunodeficiency virus, which causes AIDS) from human-derived factor VIII.

What are the long-term prospects?

Hemophilia is almost always inherited, and so it is advisable for women who have a family history of the disorder and who plan to have children to consult a genetic counselor. It can be confirmed whether a woman is a carrier of the defective genes. Amniocentesis (p.684) or chorionic villus sampling (p.684) can also be performed to determine whether the fetus has hemophilia. These tests should be done in early pregnancy to help plan any possible treatment.

Thrombocytopenia

The blood cells known as platelets play a vital part in the mechanisms that stop bleeding. If you have thrombocytopenia, your blood contains considerably fewer than the normal number of platelets. As a result, you will bleed longer than is normal if you are injured or if you bleed for any reason.

Thrombocytopenia is usually caused when the body forms antibodies (normally protective proteins) that attack its own platelets. Healthy platelets are damaged and then removed from the bloodstream at a high rate. This type of thrombocytopenia is known as acute ITP, which stands for immune or idiopathic thrombocytopenic purpura. Its cause is unknown. Thrombocytopenia may also occur because of a drug you are taking for an unrelated purpose. This disorder occurs relatively often in people who are receiving radiation therapy or chemotherapy in treatment for some type of cancer.

Thrombocytopenia can occur as a result of leukemia (see next article), when abnormal white blood cells crowd out platelet-forming blood cells. Also, your platelet count can be reduced if you receive many blood transfusions in a short period of time, such as during surgery or when abnormal bleeding and clotting occur as a result of another disorder. Thrombocytopenia is often associated with Hodgkin's disease (see p.464) or systemic lupus erythematosus (see p.594).

What are the symptoms?

The main symptom of thrombocytopenia is a rash that consists of tiny, bright red, and dark red spots. These spots are actually minute areas of bleeding in your skin. The rash can appear on any part of your body, but it often begins on the legs and wherever your skin has been irritated. Nosebleeds and a tendency to bruise are also very common symptoms. Also, bleeding from cuts is prolonged, and major internal bleeding may occur when your platelet count is very low.

What should be done?

Consult your physician immediately if you notice the characteristic rash or any abnormal bleeding. Your physician will question you about any drugs you may be taking and will take a blood sample for laboratory analysis. The blood test will show the platelet level and may indicate whether the thrombocytopenia is a sign of another disease. Usually a bone marrow examination is required to determine if enough healthy platelets are being made in the bone marrow.

What is the treatment?

Your physician will probably stop most or all drugs you may be taking, because virtually any drug can produce thrombocytopenia. If the cause appears to be an antibody, your physician may prescribe a corticosteroid drug to decrease the destruction caused by antibodies. This will allow the level of platelets in your blood to rise. The disease often improves or disappears after several weeks. If it does not, your physician may advise you to have a splenectomy, an operation in which most of your spleen is removed. The spleen normally destroys worn-out red cells, but it can become enlarged and overactive. If this occurs, the spleen may also destroy platelets and prevent you from recovering quickly.

If you have thrombocytopenia caused by abnormal clotting or by underproduction of platelets by the bone marrow, your treatment will be determined by the type and severity of the underlying disorder.

Leukemia

Leukemia is a cancer of white blood cells. Normally the number of white blood cells that are produced equals the number that die as part of the natural cycle of cell growth in the body. This keeps the total number of white blood cells constant. In leukemia, abnormal white blood cells often multiply at an increased rate. It is also significant that the cancerous cells tend to live longer than normal white blood cells. Thus the number of abnormal cells increases, either gradually or rapidly, and this causes an overaccumulation of leukemic cells throughout the body. These cells often interfere with the functions of various organs. And, because the leukemic cells are abnormal, they do not cope effectively with infectious agents such as bacteria that normal white blood cells help to eliminate from the body.

There are two main types of leukemia, which affect different types of white blood cells. Lymphocytic leukemia is a malignancy of the cells from which lymphocytes originate (see p.449). Myelogenous (or granulocytic) leukemia is a cancer of the cells from which granulocytes originate. Both of these leukemias may be acute or chronic. Acute lymphocytic leukemia mainly affects children; for more information about that disease, see Leukemia in children, p.729.

Acute myelogenous leukemia

This disease, which is also called acute granulocytic leukemia, is caused by a malignant (likely to spread) change in cells that produce granulocytes, one of the types of white blood cells made in the bone marrow. The resulting leukemic granulocytes multiply and survive longer than normal cells. As their numbers gradually increase, the leukemic cells "pack," or fill up, the bone marrow and disrupt the production of normal white and red blood cells and platelets.

The number of leukemic granulocytes then begins to increase and they enter the bloodstream. Next they invade organs and tissues, particularly the spleen and liver. These organs may become very enlarged.

What are the symptoms?

The common symptoms of acute myelogenous leukemia are feelings of fatigue, infections, fever, lip and mouth ulcers, and a tendency to bruise and bleed easily.

The disease often occurs suddenly, with the symptoms becoming pronounced over 1 or 2 weeks. But, sometimes, the symptoms appear gradually over 2 months.

What are the risks?

If acute myelogenous leukemia is not treated, it can be rapidly fatal, sometimes within only a few weeks. Chemotherapy produces a remission that lasts about 1 year in about 50 percent of patients. More intensive prolonged chemotherapy increases the period of remission to about 1½ years in people who respond to it. About 20 percent of the people in this group are cured with this type of treatment. If a closely matched donor is available, bone marrow transplant with very high dose chemotherapy offers these patients a chance for a cure.

The main hazards of this form of leukemia are serious infection and bleeding (see Thrombocytopenia, previous page).

What should be done?

Anyone with the symptoms described should see a physician immediately. After examining you, the physician will probably arrange for you to have blood tests and usually a bone marrow biopsy. In a biopsy some of your bone marrow is removed by aspiration (a needle with a syringe draws the cells from your marrow), stained, and examined under a microscope for the presence of leukemic granulocytes.

What is the treatment?

As soon as diagnosis of this form of leukemia has been confirmed, you will be admitted to a hospital. Because the treatment is complicated and difficult, it should generally be performed by a physician who treats acute leukemia regularly. In the hospital, you will get transfusions of red blood cells and platelets when you need them. If you develop a fever or other evidence of infection, the infectious agent will be identified and antibiotics that are known to be effective against it may be given intravenously. Transfusions of healthy granulocytes may also be necessary. Platelet transfusions are usually provided to prevent bleeding as a result of thrombocytopenia (see p.456).

The results of this type of treatment have improved substantially with the use of bone marrow transplantation operations. A bone marrow transplant replaces diseased leukemic cells with healthy cells taken from the person during a remission or from a closely matched donor.

The first stage of treatment is the administration of chemotherapy (anticancer) drugs to try to eliminate the leukemic cells. A few weeks after this treatment starts, you should return to normal health. However, if you stop treatment at that point, this remission would be of only short duration and the disease would recur.

The next stage of this treatment is to find an appropriate bone marrow donor, whose tissue type should be a very close match to yours. A brother or sister is the most likely candidate for a donor; however, bone marrow registries will try to find an appropriate match elsewhere. The donor is anesthetized and some of his or her bone marrow is removed with a syringe from one of the pelvic bones. However, before you can receive the bone marrow transplant, you must receive massive doses of chemotherapy, either alone or with radiation, to destroy all leukemic cells at the same time. Your own bone marrow is completely destroyed by the strong treatment.

Immediately after the bone marrow transplant or chemotherapy the recipient's white blood cell count is virtually zero, and he or she has no resistance whatsoever to infection. As a result, the person is placed in isolation to prevent any possibility of infection. Once the new bone marrow begins to produce white cells in adequate quantities, isolation is no longer necessary because the patient will have regained his or her resistance to infection.

Medication derived from human protein is used to stimulate the rapid growth of white cells. Deaths from infection or hemorrhage sometimes occur after bone marrow transplants or chemotherapy.

Chronic lymphocytic leukemia

This disease begins when one or more lymphocytes, a type of white blood cell, become malignant (likely to spread). Instead of maturing and dying in the normal way, the leukemic blood cells multiply and produce more leukemic cells. After some time, the leukemic cells gradually crowd out normal white blood cells in the lymph glands and bone marrow, and this reduction in normal white cells reduces the ability of the remaining healthy cells to fight infections. The leukemic cells also overflow into the bloodstream, and from there into the spleen, the liver, and other parts of the body. As the number of leukemic cells in the bone marrow rises, they interfere increasingly with the ability of the marrow to produce other blood cells. This in turn leads to a number of problems, including anemia, susceptibility to a variety of infections, and bleeding.

What are the symptoms?

The disease often produces no symptoms for a while and is most often discovered by a blood test done for another purpose. In some cases, the first signs are enlarged lymph glands in the neck, armpits, or groin, or a feeling of fullness in the upper left abdomen because of an enlarged spleen. In other cases the first symptoms may be those caused by anemia (see p.450) or infection. In some cases, general ill health, loss of appetite and weight, fever, and sweating at night are the first indications of the disease.

What should be done?

Anyone who has some of the symptoms listed above should see a physician, who can arrange for a blood sample and other tests.

What is the treatment?

When the disease is in an early stage, you do not need any treatment, and only periodic checkups are necessary. Treatment is required, however, when symptoms or signs of the disease appear, such as significant increases in the size of your lymph glands, spleen, or liver; anemia; a low platelet count in your blood; or fever and weight loss.

Your physician will probably first use an anticancer drug that is usually effective in eliminating or reducing most symptoms. Your enlarged lymph glands and spleen will probably decrease in size. Your blood count will improve, and your symptoms will go away. If this drug does not work, or if it stops working after a period of successful treatment, you will probably be treated with a combination of other anticancer drugs and occasionally a corticosteroid. These often produce improvement again.

Many people with chronic lymphocytic leukemia live for several years without needing treatment. When treatment becomes necessary, it usually maintains the person in reasonable health for several years; indeed, many people with this form of leukemia actually die of other causes, such as a number of diseases that accompany old age.

Chronic granulocytic leukemia

Chronic granulocytic leukemia begins as a malignant (likely to spread) change in the bone marrow cells that produce granulocytes, a type of white blood cell. As a result of this change, the number of granulocytes in your blood rises excessively, often to between 20 and 40 times the normal level. The excessive granulocytes in the bone marrow may limit the production of red blood cells and platelets, so you may bleed more readily and become anemic. The accumulation of leukemic cells may cause enlargement of both your spleen and your liver.

What are the symptoms?

If you have chronic granulocytic leukemia, you feel ill, have little appetite, and lose weight. You may have a fever and sweat at night. In addition, if your spleen becomes enlarged, you have a sense of fullness in the left upper portion of the abdomen.

What are the risks?

If chronic granulocytic leukemia is not treated, it may be fatal within weeks or months. The disease usually responds very well to initial treatment. Early in the course of treatment your physician may recommend a bone marrow transplant to avoid a relapse in which the leukemia can suddenly turn into the quickly fatal acute form.

What should be done?

If you have several of the symptoms described, see your physician. Blood tests will either rule out the disease or indicate the need for further tests. To establish a clear diagnosis, you also need a bone marrow aspiration and biopsy, in which a small sample of marrow is removed.

What is the treatment?

Most people who have the disease can be treated as outpatients except when a transplant is performed. The basic treatment consists of anticancer drugs that usually restore bone marrow production to normal and clear up the symptoms. Some people need to take the medication regularly, while others require it only intermittently. Your physician will watch your condition and take blood tests. This is important because the dose of medication often needs to be adjusted, and too much of the drug decreases your blood count to dangerous levels.

The prognosis (outlook) for this condition has greatly improved in recent years, with treatment by very high dosage chemotherapy (and sometimes radiation), followed by a bone marrow transplant from a compatible donor. The donor is usually a sister or brother. The transplant carries risks along with the potential benefits.

Blood transfusion

If your blood level is deficient—as a result of disease or hemorrhage (especially blood loss during surgery or after an injury)—you may be given a blood transfusion to restore the blood to the correct level. A transfusion may consist of whole blood or of only the parts in which you are deficient—such as platelets if you have thrombocytopenia (see p.456).

Blood donors

Although research groups in the US and Japan are developing synthetic blood substitutes, at present the only source of blood and its products continues to be blood donors. The outbreak of AIDS (see p.465) has highlighted the importance of testing the blood of potential donors for HIV, which causes AIDS, or the organisms responsible for hepatitis, malaria, or syphilis.

To give blood, a donor visits a blood bank, where a blood test determines whether the donor has anemia. If he or she does not, about one pint of blood is removed from a vein with a needle. This procedure, which takes 10 to 20 minutes, is virtually painless and totally safe. Giving blood does not expose the donor to HIV or any other disease.

An alternative to using blood from donors is to use self-donation, in which units of blood are removed over a period of a few weeks before planned surgery. This blood may be stored and used during or after the operation; your bone marrow will replace the missing blood in the interim. This method is being used increasingly, because it presents no problems with blood matching or transmitting infection. Or you may select donors whose blood will be given to you in directed donations.

Blood groups and blood matching

There are four main blood groups, and a transfusion is safe and effective if the donor and the recipient are compatible.

The surface of each red blood cell is coated with a substance called an antigen. The antigens differ for the blood groups A, B, and AB. People with type O blood do not have A, B, or AB antigens and thus are able to donate blood to all other groups. There are also many other blood groups, including the Rhesus (Rh) factor, and M and N. The blood groups of donor blood are recorded on each unit of blood so that the appropriate blood type goes to a person needing a transfusion. Before any transfusion, small quantities of the recipient's and the donor's blood are mixed in the laboratory to ensure that they are in fact compatible. This test is essential to ensure the safety of every transfusion.

Bone marrow

The marrow inside your bones is an active tissue with a rich blood supply. Your bone marrow produces most of your blood cells, including all of the red cells and platelets and most of the white cells.

The blood that flows through the marrow moves the blood cells that the marrow produces into the bloodstream. In an adult, active blood-forming marrow is found only in the bones of the body's trunk. The bones of the arms and legs contain fatty, nonactive marrow, which can change to active, blood-forming marrow in adults if the body needs to produce more blood cells. In a healthy young child, all the bones have active blood-forming marrow.

This section includes diseases that affect the blood cells in bone marrow. These disorders may affect all types of blood cells, as in aplastic anemia and polycythemia, or may only affect one type of cell, as in multiple myeloma and agranulocytosis.

Polycythemia

Normally your body adjusts the production of blood cells in the bone marrow, so that the number of blood cells that are made equals the number that are destroyed. If you have polycythemia, the mechanism becomes faulty and your marrow produces far more blood cells than usual.

There are two main types of the disorder. The first, polycythemia vera, is an over-production of red blood cells, granulocytes, and platelets. The second type of polycythemia is known as secondary polycythemia. This type occurs as a result of an underlying cause such as a severe lung disease, certain kinds of congenital heart disease (see p.702), and living at high altitudes. These conditions can prevent the red blood cells from getting enough oxygen to pass on to the body's tissues, and the bone marrow responds by producing many more red blood cells. There is a third and less important type of the disorder, which is called stress polycythemia or pseudopolycythemia. In this condition, the number of red blood cells in a blood sample is high, but the cause is a decrease in the amount of plasma in the blood. This decrease usually results from smoking, but it can be caused by taking diuretic drugs or by becoming dehydrated.

Polycythemia vera is the most serious form of the disease, and it can be treated directly. Secondary polycythemia and stress polycythemia are treated by diagnosing and treating the underlying condition.

What are the symptoms?

The typical symptoms of polycythemia vera include recurrent headaches, dizziness, a feeling of fullness in the head, and a ruddy complexion. Sometimes there is severe itching, and hot baths make the itching worse. After examining you, your physician may find that you have an enlarged spleen.

What are the risks?

Although polycythemia vera cannot be cured, a remission can be achieved for several months or a year. Many people who have the disease live for many years. Possible complications from the disease include heart attack (see p.406), stroke (see p.285), deep vein thrombosis (see p.445), peripheral arterial thrombosis, bleeding, gout (see p.537), and myelogenous leukemia.

What should be done?

If you have the symptoms of polycythemia, see your physician. He or she will arrange for a blood test. Polycythemia is also diagnosed by measuring how many red blood cells you have. In this test, for example, a small amount of radioactive albumin and a small quantity of your red blood cells labeled with radioactive chromium are injected into a vein in one arm, and a blood sample is removed from your other arm about 30 minutes later. Then the volume of red blood cells and plasma in your bloodstream can be determined. A bone marrow aspiration (removal of cells through a needle) may be necessary to rule out the possibility of other disorders.

What is the treatment?

If you have polycythemia vera, you may be able to receive treatment as an outpatient. The first goal of treatment is to lower the number of red cells in your blood and thereby its viscosity (thickness); this will reduce the risk of thrombosis, or blockage from a clot. To do this, about a pint of blood is regularly taken from a vein in your arm. How often the blood is removed depends on how quickly the level of hemoglobin in your blood returns to abnormally high levels.

Drugs may be used to control the overproduction of blood cells. Depending on what drug your physician prescribes, you may take it by mouth for several weeks or it may be injected into a vein. Drug treatment may control the disease for up to several years. Some physicians may inject radioactive phosphorus in your arm for treatment. Treatment is repeated when the blood counts begin to increase again.

Multiple myeloma

The plasma cells are among the less common types of white blood cell in the bone marrow. They produce antibodies that help to destroy bacteria, viruses, and other infectious agents and foreign cells. In addition, they also produce antibodies in response to vaccination or immunization.

Normally, plasma cells make up only a small percentage of the cells in the marrow, but in multiple myeloma one plasma cell undergoes a malignant (likely to spread) change and begins to multiply excessively. This has three serious effects. First, it disrupts the production of red blood cells, platelets, and granulocytes and lymphocytes (types of white blood cell) in the marrow, which may lead to anemia (see p.450), thrombocytopenia (see p.456), and a reduction of granulocytes and lymphocytes in the blood. Second, the excess plasma cells cause painful destruction of bone. Third, the remaining normal plasma cells produce fewer antibodies, which reduces resistance to infection.

What are the symptoms?

The most common symptom of the disease is pain in your bones, particularly in the vertebrae. Other symptoms include weakness, easy fatigue, increased levels of calcium in the blood (due to bone loss), and increased susceptibility to infection.

What are the risks?

Myeloma is a rare disease, occurring in less than 4 of every 100,000 people in the US; however, its incidence may be increasing. Myeloma affects mainly people over 50 and is somewhat more common in men.

Myeloma cannot be cured, but if you have the disease, treatment may give you several years of fairly normal life, depending on how advanced the disease is. Recurrent infection is a common problem with this disease, and it can be serious. There is a risk of chronic kidney failure (see p.551), and bleeding is another common problem.

What should be done?

If you are over 50 and you have developed bone pain, especially in your back, see your physician. If you have multiple myeloma, laboratory analysis of blood and urine samples and X rays of the skeleton will usually detect it.

What is the treatment?

In the early stages of multiple myeloma, if there are no complications and if there is no anemia, no treatment is necessary. If the disease has become more advanced, an anticancer drug is used.

This treatment provides only a temporary remission but must be repeated. Because your resistance to infection remains low, antibiotics may be prescribed if you have any symptoms of an infection. Bone pain and complications caused by fracture can usually be relieved by radiation therapy.

Researchers are experimenting with very high dose chemotherapy and bone marrow transplantation or replacement of primitive stem cells (precursors of blood cells) obtained by plasmapheresis (see Glossary in this volume) from human blood. Several people who have had such treatment have had complete remissions.

Aplastic anemia

If you have aplastic anemia, your bone marrow's production of blood cells decreases. This causes a gradual or sudden reduction in the total number of cells in your bloodstream. In most cases the cause cannot be identified. Sometimes the cause can be tentatively traced to exposure to a toxic substance such as benzene, a drug taken for another disorder, or radiation. Most anticancer drugs produce similar changes in the bone marrow, but the condition usually improves when the drug is discontinued.

What are the symptoms?

There are three main groups of symptoms. The decrease in production of red blood cells causes the symptoms of anemia (see p.450). The decrease in production of granulocytes, a type of white blood cell, makes you more susceptible to infection. Finally, the decrease in platelet production (see Thrombocytopenia, p.456) leads to spontaneous bruising, red spots on the skin, and bleeding from the nose, mouth, and other sites.

What are the risks?

The main risks associated with aplastic anemia are infection and bleeding. Both may be severe enough to become life-threatening. Your condition may improve spontaneously or with treatment, but progressive failure of the bone marrow may also occur and make your condition worse.

What should be done?

If you develop any of the symptoms described, see your physician immediately. This is especially important if you are taking certain medications, working with certain chemicals (such as benzene), or working with radioactive materials.

Your physician will probably arrange for a blood test. If the test results show that aplastic anemia may be present, your physician may need to perform a bone marrow aspiration and biopsy, in which a small amount of bone marrow is removed through a needle and examined under a microscope. This examination should allow your physician to make a definite diagnosis.

What is the treatment?

In cases where the disease is associated with a drug that is being taken for another problem, your physician will stop the drug and find a substitute. If there is any suspicion of continuing exposure to a toxic compound in your work or home environment, you should remove yourself from contact with it.

Your physician will probably treat anemia and hemorrhage (bleeding) with blood transfusions, and treat infections with antibiotics. The antibiotics are usually given intravenously for best results.

If there is no improvement within a few weeks, medication will be prescribed to stimulate the functioning of the bone marrow. Granulocyte-stimulating factors (genetically engineered proteins) may be helpful.

If this treatment does not cause normal production of cells in your bone marrow, a bone marrow transplant may be recommended if you are otherwise healthy and have a donor with a matching tissue type. The donor marrow is injected into a vein and makes its way to your bone marrow, where (if the transplant is successful) it takes over the production of blood cells. Granulocyte-stimulating factors may be given after the graft to help the development of the donor marrow within the recipient's bone.

Agranulocytosis

The white blood cells known as neutrophils act as the body's first defense against infections. Normally the neutrophils are produced in the bone marrow and are then simply released into the bloodstream. In agranulocytosis, the neutrophils are not being made or are being suppressed in the bone marrow, and there is a severe reduction in the number of neutrophils that are circulating in the blood. The result of this is decreased resistance to infection.

This rare disease is most commonly caused by cancer chemotherapy. Infrequently it is caused by drugs being taken for other disorders. It can also be caused by a viral infection or by an antibody, which is a normally protective biochemical in your blood, that you develop against your own white blood cells. The disease may be the first sign of leukemia (see p.457) or aplastic anemia (see previous article).

What are the symptoms?

The characteristic symptom of the disease is susceptibility to infection. This is especially true in the mouth and throat, where ulcers and infection with sore throat often occur. Sometimes, if you have agranulocytosis, infections such as pneumonia (see p.384) progress unusually rapidly and are extremely severe, or even fatal.

What should be done?

If you have had one infection after another, see your physician, particularly if you are taking a prescription (or even a non-prescription) drug. Some drugs carry a risk of damaging bone marrow. Your physician may arrange for a blood test. If the results show that you may have agranulocytosis, he or she will confirm the diagnosis by performing a bone marrow aspiration and biopsy, in which a small amount of bone marrow is removed through a needle and examined.

What is the treatment?

The treatment is to wait for restoration of neutrophils and deal with complications, which may include hemorrhage (treated with red blood cell and platelet infusions) and infection (treated with antibiotics). Any offending drug will be discontinued immediately. If you know that a drug has caused this problem, tell your physician.

Lymphatic system

The lymphatic system consists of lymph glands, or nodes, that are found throughout your body, the small vessels called lymphatics that link them, and the spleen.

Lymphocytes, a type of white blood cell, are produced in bone marrow and the thymus and evolve into their adult form in the lymph glands. Lymphocytes recognize foreign cells, infectious agents, and other foreign substances and participate in your body's immune reaction against them. The glands also act as barriers to the spread of infection through the lymphatics, because they trap infectious agents. The lymph glands become swollen as they react to an infection.

The spleen is part of the lymphatic system. It is actually a large lymph gland and is located in the upper left part of the abdomen, behind the ribs.

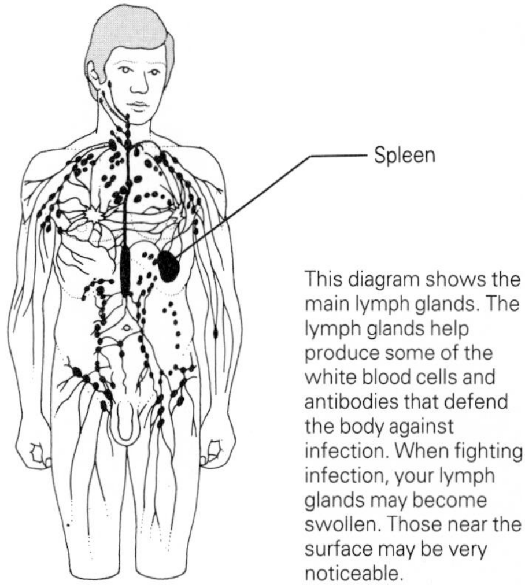

This diagram shows the main lymph glands. The lymph glands help produce some of the white blood cells and antibodies that defend the body against infection. When fighting infection, your lymph glands may become swollen. Those near the surface may be very noticeable.

Lymphomas

A lymphoma is a malignant tumor of the lymph glands. There are two general types of lymphomas. One is called Hodgkin's disease (see next page). The other is non-Hodgkin's lymphomas, which include lymphosarcoma. These are discussed below.

What are the symptoms?

The first symptom of non-Hodgkin's lymphomas is usually a swollen gland. This can occur anywhere in your body, but the first swollen glands commonly appear in your neck, armpit, or groin. Other possible symptoms include feeling generally ill, losing your appetite, losing weight without trying to do so, fever, and sweating at night.

What are the risks?

Lymphomas are a rare form of tumor. In a very slow-growing form, the disease may not need treatment for years and may even disappear on its own in some people for a time. In the aggressive (rapidly growing) form, the disease requires prompt treatment or is soon fatal.

What should be done?

If you have a swelling or lump that persists for no obvious reason for more than 2 weeks, see your physician. If the swelling is an enlarged lymph gland and there is no evidence that the swelling has been caused by an ordinary infection, your physician may take a blood sample and arrange for you to have the gland examined or removed. The blood test and an examination of the gland tissue will usually help your physician determine if you have a lymphoma and, if so, what type you have.

Treatment of lymphomas depends on the type of tumors you have and how many parts of the body are affected. Treatment also involves careful examination, including X rays and a CT, magnetic resonance imaging (MRI), or a gallium (radioactive isotope) scan. In some cases, a lymphangiogram may be performed to assess the number of affected glands and the location of the lymphomas. Generally a bone marrow aspiration and biopsy are performed to determine whether the marrow is affected.

Lymphomas and other types of cancer occur in people infected with HIV (human immunodeficiency virus), the virus that causes AIDS. Changes in lymphocytes (a type of white blood cell) may encourage tumors to form.

What is the treatment?

Standard treatment is chemotherapy (anticancer) drugs, which are likely to induce remission. For people who fail to respond, high-dose chemotherapy and bone marrow transplant (see Hodgkin's disease, next article) can be lifesaving. For treatment of AIDS, see p.465.

Hodgkin's disease

Hodgkin's disease, which occurs chiefly but not only in young people, produces swelling in the lymph glands, or nodes, and to that extent is similar to non-Hodgkin's lymphomas (see previous article). However, non-Hodgkin's lymphomas are believed to be caused by malignant (likely to spread) transformation of a lymphocyte, a type of white blood cell, while Hodgkin's disease is probably caused by transformation of another type of cell (a macrophage). Hodgkin's disease is much easier to cure than non-Hodgkin's lymphomas.

What are the symptoms?
The main symptom of Hodgkin's disease is persistent swollen glands, usually in the neck, armpit, or groin. Other possible symptoms include fever, sweating, fatigue, weakness, weight loss, and itching.

The response to treatment for Hodgkin's disease is very good. Therefore, it is vital that you tell your physician about any unexplained swellings promptly. Samples of your blood will probably be taken and a swollen gland will probably be removed for examination and diagnosis. If you have Hodgkin's disease, you will need tests to determine the extent of the disease. Tests include a bone marrow aspiration and biopsy, in which a small amount of bone marrow is removed and examined. Further tests, as for lymphoma, may include a chest X ray, an MRI (magnetic resonance imaging), CT, or gallium (radioactive isotope) scan, a lymphangiogram, and possibly a laparotomy (see p.513). The test results and the type of Hodgkin's disease you have will determine what treatment you need.

What is the treatment?
Radiation therapy is used to treat the disease if it is detected at a relatively early stage. Depending on the type of Hodgkin's disease you have, radiation therapy has an 80 to 90 percent success rate. Young people have an even higher survival rate. If the disease is at an advanced stage when it is discovered, you will be treated with one or more chemotherapy, or anticancer, drugs, sometimes in combination with radiation therapy. The treatment usually continues for about 6 months. High dose chemotherapy and bone marrow transplant are used for those who relapse or are resistant to treatment. Bone marrow transplant, which is necessary after your cells are destroyed by chemotherapy, may be from a donor's bone marrow, your own bone marrow extracted before chemotherapy, or replacement of primitive stem cells (precursors of blood cells) through plasmapheresis (see Glossary in this volume) of your blood.

Once treatment is completed, your progress is monitored by periodic checkups for several years.

Immunodeficiency

An immunodeficiency is the result of a weakening of your body's immune system. There are two general types of immunodeficiency. In one type of immunodeficiency, there is an inadequate production of antibodies (substances that protect your body from infectious diseases), in response to a previous infection or an immunization. This may affect only one type of antibody, or several types at once. Because of this immunodeficiency, your resistance to some kinds of infection, especially bacterial infection, is considerably decreased.

The second type of immunodeficiency results from disorders of, or decreased numbers of, the various kinds of lymphocytes. These are white blood cells from the bone marrow and the lymph glands. In this form of the disorder, the ability of the lymphocytes in your bloodstream to gather around and kill invading organisms is decreased. As a result, your resistance to infections caused by fungi, certain viruses, and the type of bacteria that causes tuberculosis is impaired. It is possible to have both general types of immunodeficiency at the same time.

There are many types of inherited defects of the immune system. If you are born with one of these, you are susceptible to certain types of infections. Many diseases also impair the functioning of the immune system. These diseases include the leukemias (see p.457), the lymphomas (see previous page) and Hodgkin's disease (see previous article), cancer in general, diabetes mellitus (see p.558), and uremia. Finally, some drugs that are used to treat a wide range of disorders, especially corticosteroid drugs and chemotherapy (anticancer) drugs, and also radiation therapy, can have a very negative effect on your immune system.

What is the treatment?
If your child has an inherited deficiency of antibody production, injections of antibodies taken from other people may be helpful. This treatment must be repeated for your child every few weeks. In another form of immune

deficiency, lymphocytes taken from the person are infected with a harmless virus linked to a normal gene for the enzyme that is defective. These "normalized" lymphocytes can then be returned by injection into a vein. This treatment is highly experimental but offers great promise. Bone marrow transplant, often from a brother, sister, parent, or other appropriate donor, has been successful in some people.

AIDS

(acquired immune deficiency syndrome)

AIDS, or acquired immune deficiency syndrome, is not one disease but a susceptibility to many diseases. AIDS is caused by the human immunodeficiency virus (HIV). The virus destroys one type of the body's white blood cells, which weakens the infected person's immune system, lowering his or her resistance to some infections and certain types of cancer. The virus is transmitted through infected blood, semen, or vaginal fluids. There is no cure for AIDS yet, but it is important to know that early treatment can prolong life.

HIV multiplies inside one type of white blood cell, the CD4 lymphocyte, or helper cell. When the virus penetrates one of these cells it takes over the nuclear material and uses it to make more virus particles. The cell then dies and the new virus particles are released into the bloodstream to infect more CD4 cells. Gradually the number of CD4 cells in the blood is reduced, and as this happens the infected person becomes more susceptible to various infections and cancers that occur more frequently in the presence of a weakened immune system, when conditions are favorable for their development. These "opportunistic" diseases are rarely found in people whose immune systems are functioning normally. Sudden occurrence of these rare diseases in large numbers of otherwise previously healthy young homosexual men in 1980 first drew widespread public attention to AIDS.

Scientists do not know where or how the first infections with HIV occurred. In the 1980s AIDS spread rapidly in the US, Europe, and Africa. By the 1990s more than 200,000 cases of AIDS had been reported in the US to the Centers for Disease Control and Prevention (CDC).

HIV infection is primarily sexually transmitted, but it may also be transmitted by infected blood and blood products. Therefore, HIV may be passed on by transfusion of infected blood or by sharing a contaminated hypodermic needle. HIV can also be transmitted by an infected woman to a fetus during pregnancy, or to an infant during childbirth or through infected breast milk. Initially, AIDS and HIV infection were most prevalent among—but not limited to—male homosexuals, male and female prostitutes, and intravenous drug users who shared needles. However, while the number of new AIDS cases among male homosexuals and drug users has begun to level off, the number of new AIDS cases among heterosexuals, particularly women and young adults and adolescents of both sexes, continues to rise. In the early 1980s many people with blood disorders such as hemophilia, who require repeated transfusion of blood products, became infected with HIV before blood banks began testing donated blood for the HIV antibody. Genetically engineered versions of blood products are now available to prevent HIV transmission, and a test to screen for the virus now ensures a safe blood supply for recipients of blood transfusions. AIDS is not spread through casual contact, such as working next to someone, sharing a towel or using the same toilet seat or drinking glass, or by hugging or shaking hands.

What are the symptoms?

When first infected with HIV many people have no symptoms, but others have a short, feverish illness similar to mononucleosis (see p.601) with a sore throat, fever, swollen glands, and rash. Occasionally, the virus causes symptoms of meningitis (see p.290). These symptoms clear up without treatment in a few weeks. Some people who have been infected with HIV have remained without symptoms for as long as 10 years, but by 10 years about 75 percent of infected people have developed at least some symptoms of HIV infection.

The most common first symptom is persistently swollen lymph glands, particularly at the back of the neck, under the arms, and in the groin. This condition is called persistent generalized lymphadenopathy; people with this disorder may remain in otherwise good health or they may go on to develop one or more other symptoms—fatigue, chills, fever, sweating at night, sudden weight loss (10 lb or more, without dieting), chronic diarrhea, dry cough, and *Candida* (thrush) infections of the mouth and esophagus. People infected with HIV may experience one or more of these symptoms for a prolonged period or they may rapidly develop AIDS.

You are diagnosed as having AIDS if an HIV antibody blood test indicates you are infected with HIV, you have a CD4 cell count below 200 (a normal count is around 1,000), and you have one or more complicating disorders, such as certain rare bacterial, viral, and fungal infections, including cytomegalovirus; a form of cancer called Kaposi's sarcoma; some types of lymphatic cancer; *Pneumocystis carinii* pneumonia (PCP); pulmonary tuberculosis; and invasive cervical cancer. Infection of the nervous system with HIV can cause progressive dementia. People with AIDS may also develop meningitis caused by *Cryptococcus* organisms or brain infections caused by *Toxoplasma* and fungi.

Because HIV infects people regardless of age (from infants to older people), sex (males and females), or sexual orientation (homosexuals, heterosexuals, and bisexuals), everyone is at risk.

What are the risks?

It is not yet known why some people infected with HIV become ill while others remain in apparent good health for years. Once the number of CD4 cells in the blood falls below 200, however, progression of the disease seems inevitable unless the infected person receives treatment. Survival time is significantly improved for most people with chemotherapy.

What should be done?

If you think you may be infected with HIV, see your physician, or call your local health department for referral to an HIV testing site in your area. There is a blood test to determine whether your body has developed antibodies to the virus. Someone with antibodies to HIV is said to be HIV-positive. A positive antibody test shows that you have acquired the virus and that you are infectious to other people. However, it does not mean that you will inevitably develop AIDS or any AIDS-related illness. Find out about counseling in your area, because a positive test result is likely to be very disturbing.

The chance of acquiring HIV from having unprotected sexual intercourse once with an infected person is small; repeated risky sexual encounters are more likely to lead to infection. In most instances, you become HIV-positive within 4 to 6 months after exposure to the virus.

What is the treatment?

Intense research efforts are continuing to find a cure for people who are HIV-positive or who have AIDS. A vaccine against HIV and possible curative drugs are being tested. Several treatments can slow the progress of the infection and combat the complications of AIDS and AIDs-related disorders.

Several antiviral drugs are currently used to slow the destruction of CD4 cells by HIV. The treatment of choice for slowing the multiplication of the virus is the drug zidovudine (AZT). It has been shown to delay development of full-blown AIDS in people who are HIV-positive but who have no symptoms. AZT also increases survival time for people who have full-blown AIDS. Some experts believe that the earlier treatment begins, the more effective it is likely to be in the long term.

Two other drugs are used to fight HIV infection. Didioxyinosine (ddI), which helps boost CD4 cell levels and slow their destruction, is used by people who cannot tolerate AZT or for whom it is no longer an effective treatment. Dideoxycytidine (ddC) is used only in combination with AZT. These drugs all have unpleasant and potentially dangerous side effects.

Meanwhile the infections and cancers that develop in people with AIDS can be treated, and some people with AIDS are also given preventive treatment against *Pneumocystis carinii* pneumonia (PCP). The combination of antiviral treatment and treatment of symptoms extends the life span of many people with HIV infection. However, the best treatment is still prevention (see box on "Safer" sex at left). For current information about HIV and AIDS, call the National AIDS Hotline at 800-342-AIDS.

"Safer" sex

To help prevent the transmission of HIV, follow these precautions:

- Avoid sex with a stranger or with someone who has multiple partners. Monogamy (having only one sex partner, who has only you for a sex partner) is best.
- Use a latex condom every time you have sex. Never reuse a condom.
- Use water-based spermicidal jellies (those containing nonoxynol-9) as lubricants during sex; evidence shows they have some antiviral effect.
- Oral sex, to be safer, requires a latex condom on the penis or a dental dam (a piece of latex) on the vagina; both are available without a prescription at drugstores.

Disorders of digestion and nutrition

Introduction

Your body needs a regular supply of nutrients to grow, to replace worn-out tissue, to form protein, and to supply energy for the thousands of chemical reactions occurring in your body all the time. These nutrients are extracted from the food you eat as it passes through the digestive system. This system consists of the digestive tract, which is essentially a tube running from the mouth to the anus, and the digestive glands, including the liver, gallbladder, and pancreas. The tract and glands work together as a system, to take in food and break it down so that the nutrients in it can be absorbed into the bloodstream.

The first part of the tract is the mouth, where the teeth tear and chew the food into small pieces and mix it with saliva. The saliva functions as a lubricant and contains an enzyme, or digestive aid, that breaks down starch.

The tongue moves the food around the mouth as it is chewed, and then forms it into a ball called a bolus for swallowing. Most people think of the tongue as useful only in its role in speech, but imagine yourself trying to chew and swallow a mouthful of food without having the help of your tongue.

The second section of the tract is the esophagus. When you swallow, food slips down this muscular 1½ ft tube and through a ring of muscles that relaxes to let it through into the third section of the tract, the stomach. Muscles in the stomach wall pummel the food into a pulp as digestive juices, formed in the stomach wall, start to break the food chemically into even smaller pieces. The half-digested food then passes through another ring of muscles and along a short tube, the duodenum, which is the first part of the small intestine. In the small intestine, further breakdown of food requires help from some other organs of the body.

Just beneath your liver lies the gallbladder, a pear-shaped sac about 3½ in (9 cm) long. Your gallbladder stores and concentrates a fluid called bile, which is produced by the liver and trickles into the gallbladder through a network of tiny tubes. Your gallbladder contracts and expels the bile, when it is needed, into your small intestine through an opening that is called the bile duct. The bile helps digest fats. Besides the bile, your pancreas releases digestive enzymes through a duct that joins the bile duct just before it enters your small intestine. Digestive enzymes are also formed and secreted by the cells that line the small intestine.

The food is pushed along the intestine by waves of contractions of the muscles in its wall. As this is happening, enzymes and other chemicals reduce the food to smaller and smaller pieces that can seep through the lining of the wall of the small intestine and be absorbed into the bloodstream.

Once in the blood, the nutrients reach the liver, where some are stored, some are assembled into more complex compounds, and along with other nutrients are transported to other parts of the body. These nutrients ultimately end up afloat in the liquid that surrounds each cell in your body. The cells use the nutrients as they need them, pulling them inside their cell membranes through a number of simple but effective mechanisms. Once inside the cell, the nutrients are sorted and broken down still further. Finally some nutrients are used to provide energy and others are used to make new tissues and other biological substances such as enzymes.

The next-to-last section of the tract is the large intestine (colon). Here, water is absorbed into your body from the indigestible remains of food. What is left becomes semisolid waste. The waste is expelled as stool through the anus, the end of the digestive tract.

Most disorders of the digestive tract affect only one section. Such disorders are grouped together, along with a general description of each part of the tract. Some disorders affect two or more sections of the tract, and these are also grouped together. Finally there is a group of articles describing disorders of nutrition related to the amount or type of food you eat or to the ability of your digestive system to absorb nutrients from the food.

Some nutritional disorders are rare, inherited diseases that require that you eat a special diet for the rest of your life. Others may be widespread in the general population. Obesity is a particularly good example of a common disorder. It is covered at length in this section along with other problems related to nutrition and metabolism.

The digestive system

The digestive system is divided into several sections, each of which has a vital part to play either in the breakdown and absorption of food or in the expulsion of waste matter. Digestive enzymes (biological substances that speed up chemical reactions) assist in the process of breaking down food into pieces small enough to pass through the wall of the small intestine and into the bloodstream.

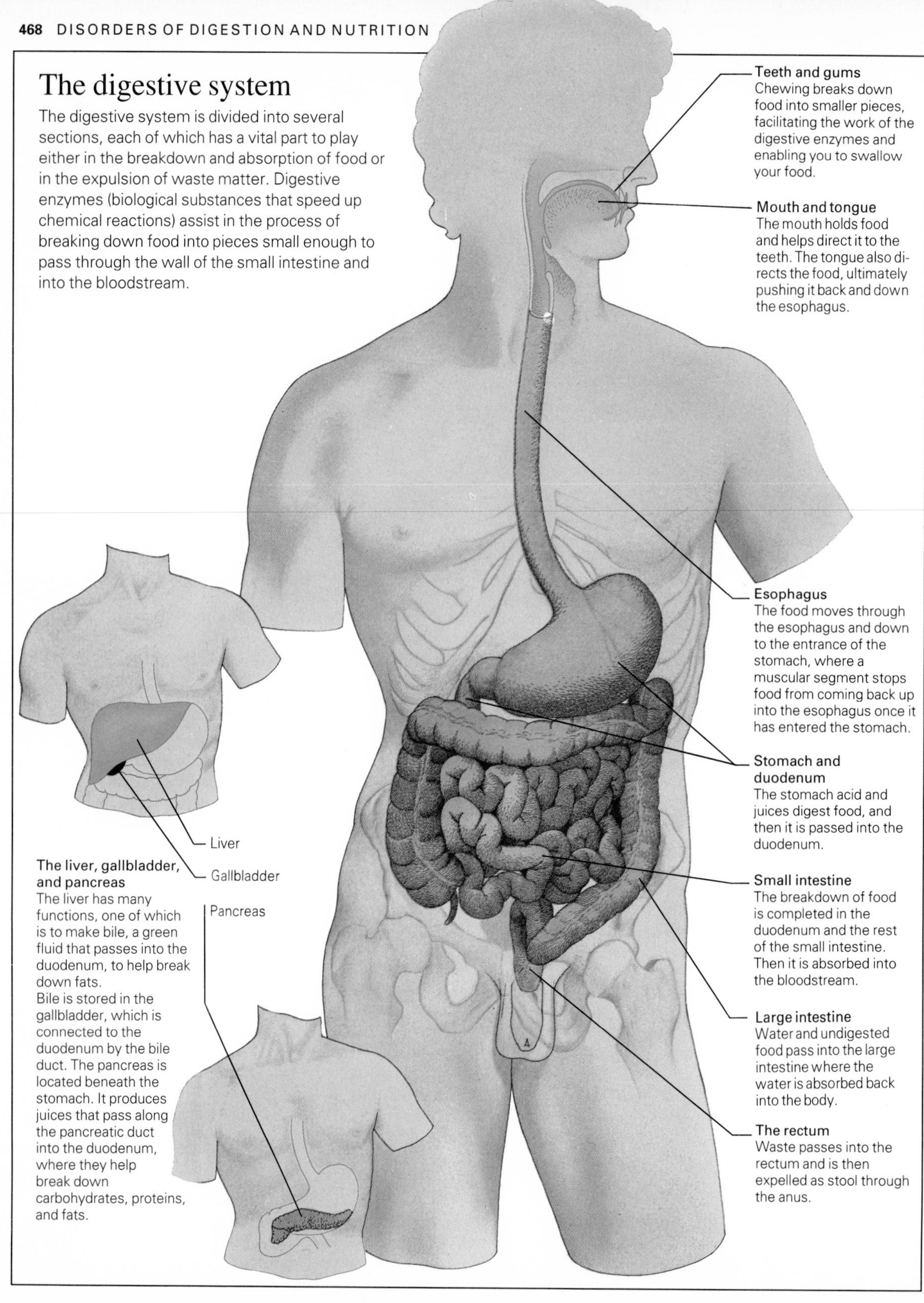

Teeth and gums
Chewing breaks down food into smaller pieces, facilitating the work of the digestive enzymes and enabling you to swallow your food.
Mouth and tongue
The mouth holds food and helps direct it to the teeth. The tongue also directs the food, ultimately pushing it back and down the esophagus.
Esophagus
The food moves through the esophagus and down to the entrance of the stomach, where a muscular segment stops food from coming back up into the esophagus once it has entered the stomach.
Stomach and duodenum
The stomach acid and juices digest food, and then it is passed into the duodenum.
Small intestine
The breakdown of food is completed in the duodenum and the rest of the small intestine. Then it is absorbed into the bloodstream.
Large intestine
Water and undigested food pass into the large intestine where the water is absorbed back into the body.
The rectum
Waste passes into the rectum and is then expelled as stool through the anus.
Liver
Gallbladder
Pancreas
The liver, gallbladder, and pancreas
The liver has many functions, one of which is to make bile, a green fluid that passes into the duodenum, to help break down fats.
Bile is stored in the gallbladder, which is connected to the duodenum by the bile duct. The pancreas is located beneath the stomach. It produces juices that pass along the pancreatic duct into the duodenum, where they help break down carbohydrates, proteins, and fats.

Teeth and gums

Your teeth break up the food you eat into pieces that can be easily swallowed and digested. Teeth also give shape to the face and help you speak clearly. Teeth are alive; the pulp at the heart of each tooth contains blood vessels and nerves that nourish the tooth and sense heat, cold, pressure, and pain. A hard substance called dentin surrounds the pulp. On the crown, the part of the tooth above the gum, the dentin is covered by enamel. The root of the tooth is covered by a sensitive bonelike material known as cementum. The gums fit tightly around the teeth, and the roots of the teeth fit into sockets in the jawbone. A shock-absorbent material, periodontal ligament, lines the socket of each tooth, to support the root and to prevent the skull and jawbone from being jarred.

Enamel is the hardest substance in your body, but acids produced by the action of bacteria on sugar and other simple carbohydrates can erode the enamel and cause tooth decay. If it is unchecked, decay progresses through the dentin and into the pulp, which may cause an abscess (infection) and eventually cause loss of the tooth.

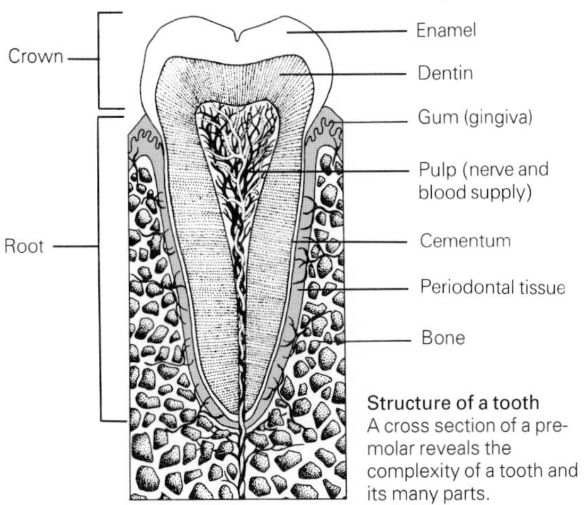

Structure of a tooth
A cross section of a premolar reveals the complexity of a tooth and its many parts.

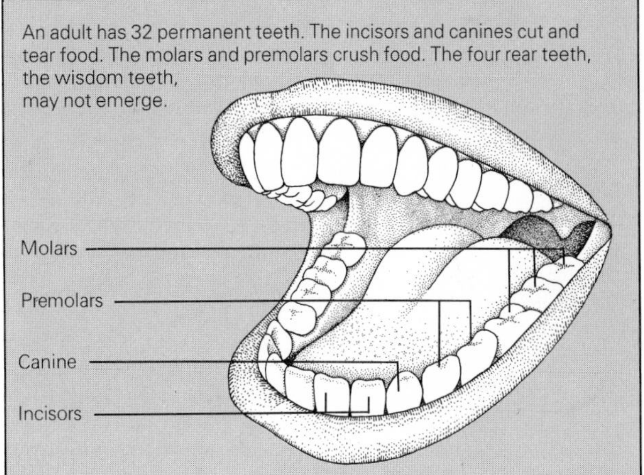

An adult has 32 permanent teeth. The incisors and canines cut and tear food. The molars and premolars crush food. The four rear teeth, the wisdom teeth, may not emerge.

Tooth decay

(dental caries)

If you pass the tip of your tongue over your teeth several hours after brushing them, you can feel patches of a slightly rough, sticky substance. This substance is called dental plaque. It consists of mucus, food particles, and bacteria, and forms mainly in two places: between the teeth and where the teeth meet the gums. Bacteria in the plaque break down the sugar in your food, and this process forms acid. The acid dissolves the calcium and phosphate in the tooth's enamel and forms a minute cavity. This is the beginning of tooth decay, or dental caries.

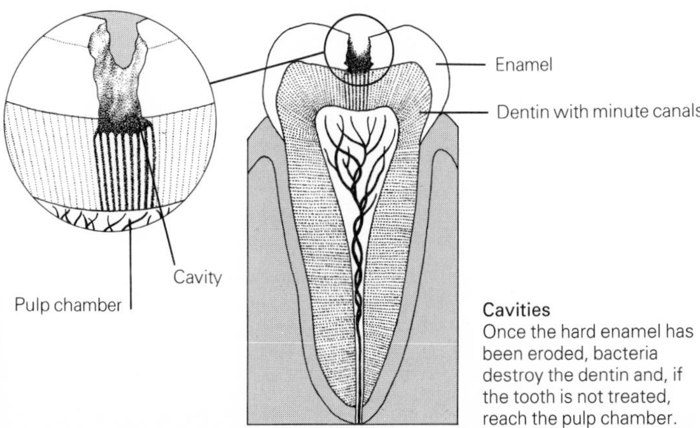

Cavities
Once the hard enamel has been eroded, bacteria destroy the dentin and, if the tooth is not treated, reach the pulp chamber.

If the decay is not treated, the acid destroys the enamel and damages the dentin beneath it. Dentin contains minute canals that lead to the pulp, and the bacteria eventually inflame the pulp. Your body responds by sending more white blood cells to the pulp to combat the bacteria. The blood vessels around the tooth enlarge to accommodate the extra blood and white cells. The enlarged vessels press on the nerves entering the tooth, causing toothache. The acid may also reach the nerves and contribute to pain, especially at the point in the decay process when decay reaches nerve

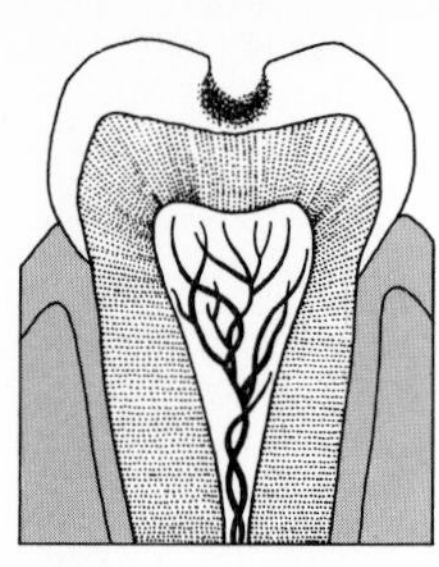
Acid causes decay of enamel

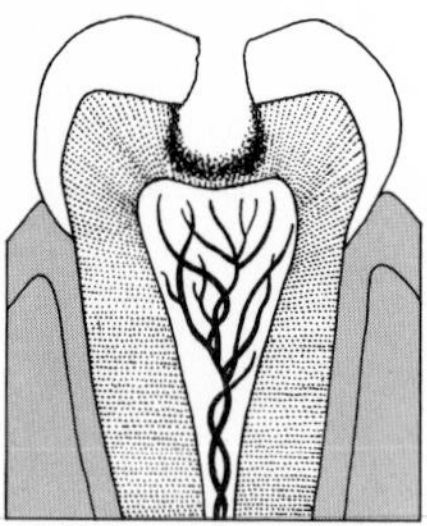
Acid eats into dentin

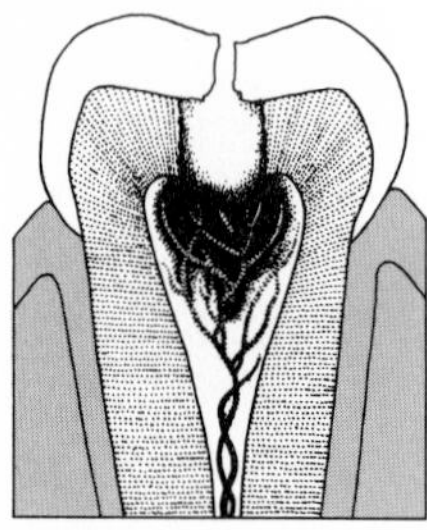
Pulp becomes inflamed

endings in the dentin. If a significant number of bacteria physically invade the pulp chambers, the nerve of the tooth usually dies, even though the white blood cells are fighting the infection (see Root canal treatment, next article). This ends the toothache, but may lead to an abscess (see p.473).

What are the symptoms?
In the early stages of tooth decay there are often no symptoms. In the later stages the main symptom may be a mild toothache when you eat something sweet, sour, hot, or cold. If the decay continues, you may have pain and an unpleasant taste in your mouth that is produced by stagnant food and bacteria that are packed into the cavity.

In the final stage of decay, the pulp of the tooth becomes inflamed. If this occurs, you may suffer persistent pain after eating sweet, sour, hot, or cold food. You may also have sharp, stabbing pains, sometimes in the jaw above or below the decayed tooth. It may be difficult to tell which tooth is hurting.

What are the risks?
Tooth decay generally presents no serious danger to health if it is caught and treated early. But there is a risk for people who have heart disease. If bacteria from an infected tooth enter the bloodstream, the disease may get worse (see Infective endocarditis, p.422). Also, if you have a clotting disorder such as hemophilia (see p.455), you should have a tooth extracted only after you have consulted your physician.

What should be done?
Keep tooth decay to a minimum by taking good care of your teeth (see next page). Brush and floss them thoroughly each day, reduce your sugar intake, limit snacks, use a fluoride toothpaste and mouthwash, drink fluoridated water, and visit your dentist regularly to have your teeth cleaned and examined. Allow X rays to be taken every year or two if your dentist recommends it.

If you have young children, do not allow them to go to sleep with a bottle of milk, juice, or other liquids that contain sugar. The liquid bathes the teeth, promoting tooth decay. Also, children probably should have annual fluoride applications starting at about age 3 to 4, even if your community's water supply is fluoridated.

Your dentist may recommend that you have a sealant applied to your teeth or your child's teeth, which may help prevent decay. The sealant is made of plastic and helps keep your teeth, particularly the molars, free of invasion by bacteria.

What is the treatment?
Self-help: Pain-relievers such as aspirin may help until you can get to your dentist. Prevention is the best treatment; see "Keeping your teeth and gums healthy" (next page).

Professional help: In the early stages of the disease, your dentist will usually clean and fill the cavity immediately. If the decay is too far advanced, the dentist may perform a root canal procedure (see next article). In rare cases, the dentist may extract the tooth.

Root canal treatment

(endodontics)

At the heart of every healthy tooth is the pulp, a living tissue that nourishes the tooth and makes it sensitive to heat, cold, pressure, and pain. When the pulp dies, professional treatment is needed to save the tooth.

The pulp may die after tooth decay (see previous article) has penetrated it, or sometimes after a blow to the tooth. Occasionally, pulp dies for no apparent reason. Pain and swelling may accompany diseased or damaged pulp. When pulp dies, there is no pain. You may not even know the pulp has died until your dentist tells you. Once dead pulp has been detected, it should be treated. There is a risk, especially after tooth decay, that bacteria from the dead pulp will seep out through the end of the root and cause an abscess (see p.473). This infection can spread throughout the body.

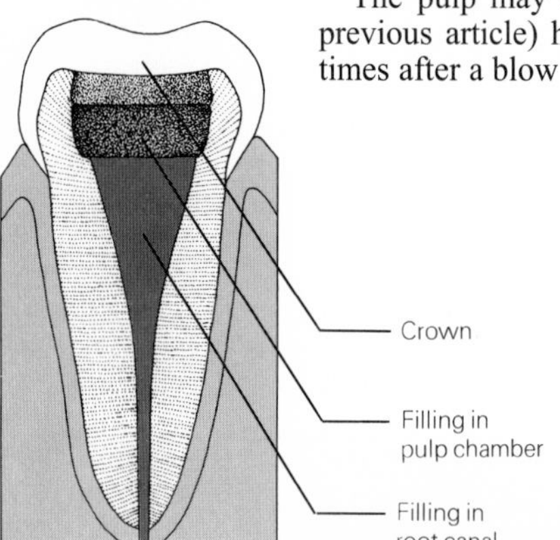

Root canal treatment
When the pulp becomes infected, an abscess usually forms. The tooth must be treated by cleaning out the root canal, destroying any bacteria, and then filling and sealing the canal and restoring the crown.

What is the treatment?
A tooth with dead pulp can continue to function efficiently, so there is usually no reason for it to be extracted unless it is too badly decayed. The dentist usually cleans out the tooth, disinfects it, and fills the pulp chamber and root canal. Then a crown is placed over the tooth to restore the tooth's structure, function, and appearance.

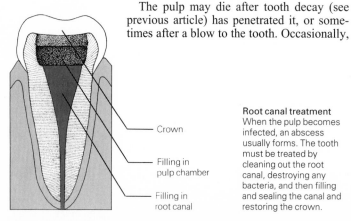

Keeping your teeth and gums healthy

Even if you try to keep sugar consumption to a minimum, it is virtually impossible to avoid tooth decay completely. However, you can keep decay to a minimum and keep your own teeth healthy for a lifetime by taking some simple steps.

1. Brush your teeth thoroughly at least twice a day. You should also use dental floss to remove food particles and plaque from places that you cannot reach with your brush, especially between teeth and near the gumline.

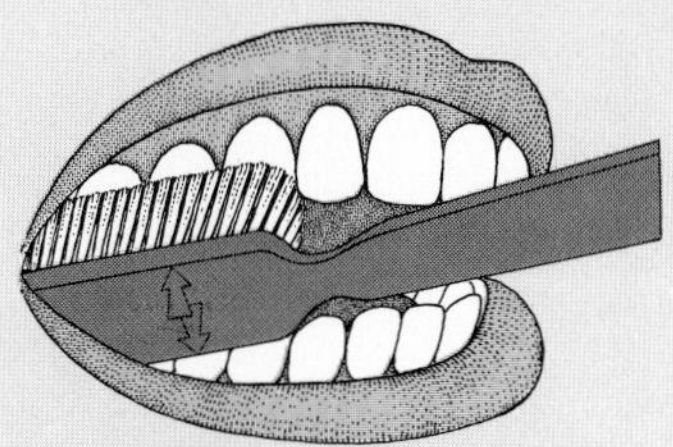

Your dentist or hygienist will show you how to brush your teeth and to use floss properly. As you brush, begin at the gums and move the brush toward the teeth. Gently massaging the gums with your toothbrush helps to maintain your gums' circulation and health.

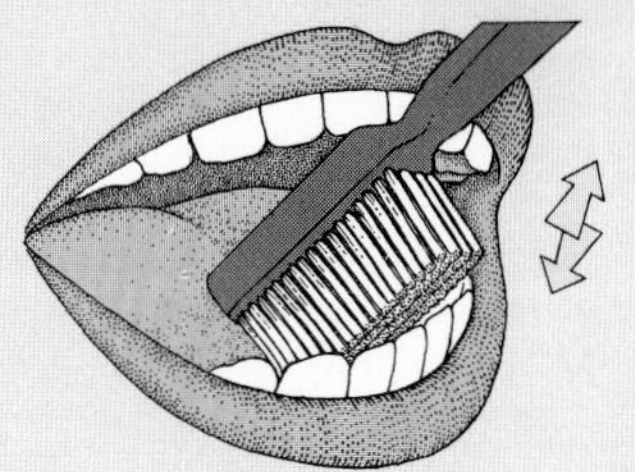

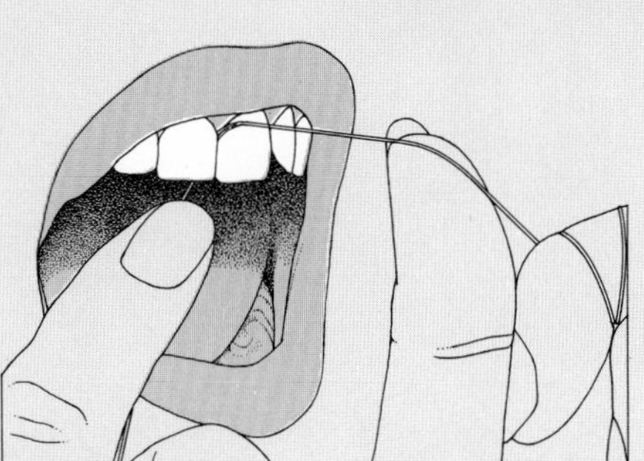

Using dental floss
Dental floss, waxed or unwaxed, is thread that you draw between your teeth to remove plaque and food particles. Be sure to floss every day. Take about 18 in (45 cm) of floss and wind most of it around the middle fingers of each hand, with about 1 in (2½ cm) of floss between your fingers. Draw the floss between the teeth and, with a gentle sawing action, rub the sides of each tooth. Use a clean area of floss for each tooth.

2. Reduce your sugar intake and eat a balanced diet. Candy, other sweet snacks, and refined carbohydrates between meals are especially harmful, because after you eat or drink them your teeth are attacked for about 20 minutes by acid. Try to eat sweet foods only during meals. Better still, cut them out altogether and finish meals with nuts or low-fat cheese rather than with ice cream or cake. Cheese is particularly effective in neutralizing acid formation.

3. Strengthen your tooth enamel with fluoride. The level of fluoride in the water should be between 0.7 and 1.2 parts per million, depending on the climate. Your dentist, local water authority, or public health department can tell you what the fluoride level is in your community's water supply. Also, children under 13 should have fluoride applied to their teeth every year, because their enamel is still forming. Your dentist will advise you on the use of fluoride mouthwash or tablets and may apply a fluoride gel to your teeth. In addition, the family should use a fluoride toothpaste.

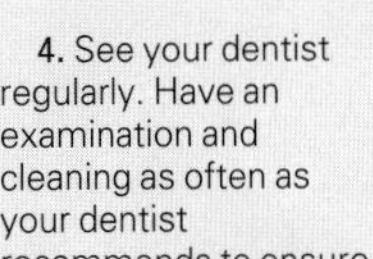

Fluoride tablets and solutions

Disclosing tablets
These tablets contain a dye that temporarily stains plaque. Remove the visible plaque with dental floss and a toothbrush.

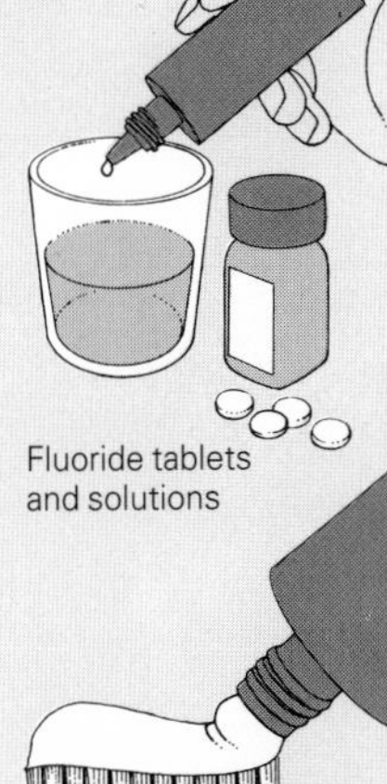

Fluoride toothpaste

4. See your dentist regularly. Have an examination and cleaning as often as your dentist recommends to ensure that any new cavity is filled before decay can spread and any gum disease is treated before it can become serious.

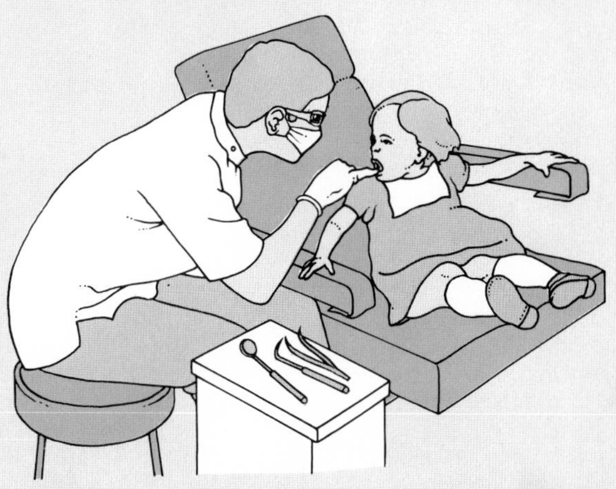

Going to the dentist

When should you go?

You should see your dentist regularly at least once a year or as often as he or she recommends. Regular examinations are necessary not only to minimize tooth decay, but also to check on the health of your whole mouth. A neglected mouth, besides being vulnerable to the various disorders described in this section, can create the risk of infections entering the bloodstream, which can endanger your general health. Dentures, like natural teeth, need to be checked regularly, and all dentures eventually wear down and need to be replaced. If you have a full set of dentures and have no problems with them, you still should see your dentist regularly for oral examinations.

What happens during the examination?

The dentist first examines your mouth for signs of any diseases that are not confined to the teeth. Red, puffy, or receding gums indicate gingivitis (see p.481) or periodontitis (see p.482). A white discoloration of the inside of the mouth may indicate that you have oral thrush (see p.484), leukoplakia (see p.485), or oral lichen planus (see p.485). The dentist then examines your teeth with a mirror and a needle-shaped probe, looking for any color changes that indicate decay or any crack that indicates the beginning of a cavity. Fillings are examined to see if any parts have been chipped off or if any fresh cavities are developing around the edge of a filling. If you have dentures, the dentist will check them for fit and examine their effects on the gums and remaining teeth.

Before the examination, the dentist or dental hygienist usually will ask about your general health. This is very important. It may have a direct bearing on your treatment. If, for example, you have some types of heart conditions and have a tooth extracted, or any other treatment that causes bleeding gums, you run the risk of contracting bacterial endocarditis (see Infective endocarditis, p.422). People with diabetes whose disease is not carefully controlled may become ill if they undergo stress in the dentist's chair. Also, if dental treatment of a person with diabetes requires a general anesthetic, the treatment may have to be performed in a hospital. People who have had some types of jaundice may be symptomless carriers of hepatitis (see p.523) and may need a blood test before the dentist can decide how to treat them. If you have an allergy, you may react dangerously to certain drugs, such as penicillin. If you are pregnant, the dentist will examine your gums with particular care, looking for signs of gingivitis. And if you are taking any medication, the dentist must be careful to avoid possible harmful reactions between it and any drug the dentist decides to give you.

Why are X rays taken?

Every year or two, "bite-wing" X rays are taken to check for oral conditions that cannot be detected during a visual examination. A full set of mouth X rays or a panoramic X ray should be taken every 3 to 5 years. X rays are also taken of endodontically treated teeth (see Root canal treatment, p.470) to check for an abscess (see p.473) at the tip of the root. They may also be used to check the growth of your wisdom teeth (see p.478), or to show how much bone is supporting the teeth if you have periodontal disease (see Gingivitis, p.481, and Periodontitis, p.482).

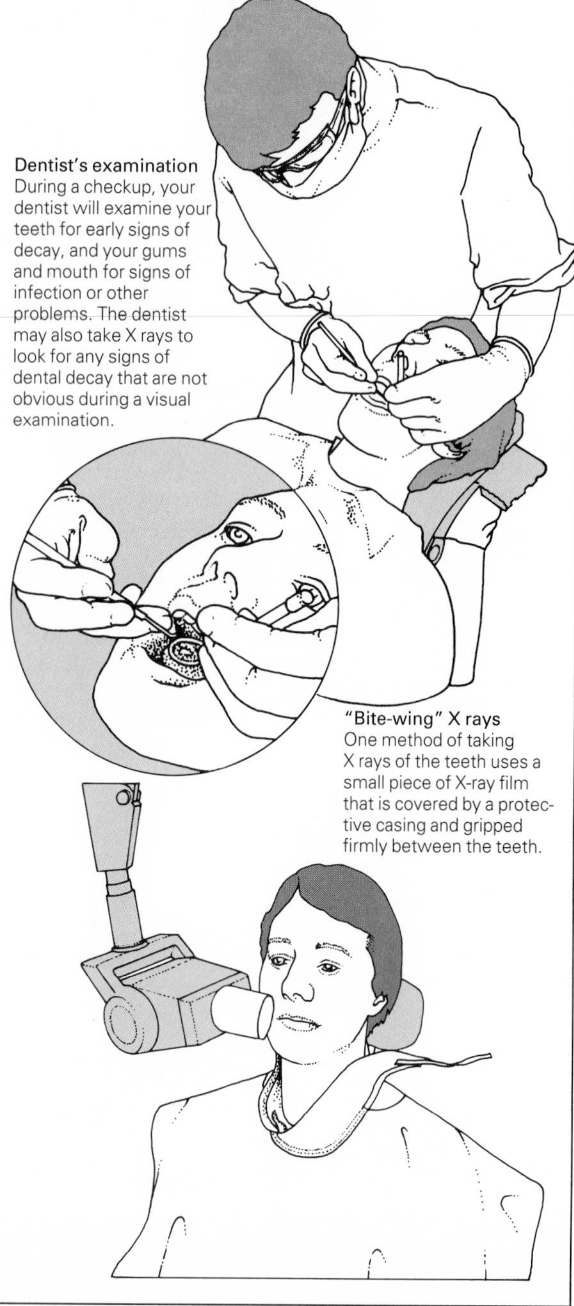

Dentist's examination
During a checkup, your dentist will examine your teeth for early signs of decay, and your gums and mouth for signs of infection or other problems. The dentist may also take X rays to look for any signs of dental decay that are not obvious during a visual examination.

"Bite-wing" X rays
One method of taking X rays of the teeth uses a small piece of X-ray film that is covered by a protective casing and gripped firmly between the teeth.

Tooth abscess

A tooth abscess is a pus-filled sac in the tissue around the tip of the tooth's root, which is embedded in the jawbone. The abscess usually forms when a tooth is decaying (see p.469) or its pulp dies (see Root canal treatment, p.470), or when the gums have receded severely. A tooth's dead pulp, together with invading bacteria, can infect the surrounding tissue. Even when a tooth has received root canal treatment (see p.470), bacteria occasionally remain in the tissue around the base of the roots of the tooth and cause an abscess to form.

If the abscess is not treated, it may damage the jawbone until it has eroded a small canal, or sinus, through the bone and its overlying gum. Just before the canal reaches the surface of the gum, it can form a swelling. The swelling may remain for weeks, but in some cases the abscess bursts, leaving a drainage channel called a fistula. In these cases, foul-tasting pus drains into the mouth and there is sudden relief of pain. But this bursting allows the infection to spread throughout the body, where it can cause fatigue and lowered resistance to disease.

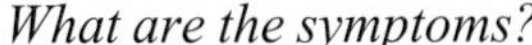

Anyone who does not visit the dentist regularly and has untreated decay is likely to have a tooth abscess at some time. The pulp of untreated decayed teeth will die, and a dead pulp eventually causes abscesses.

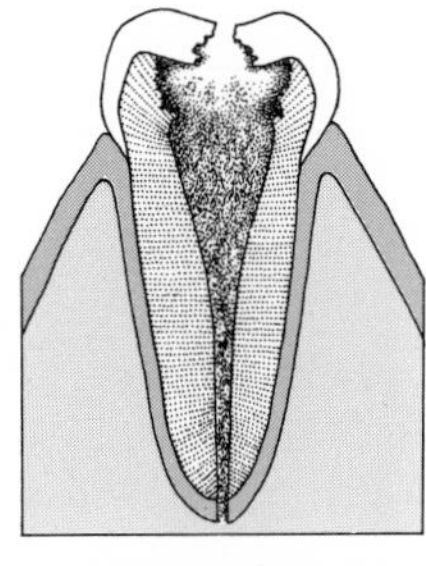

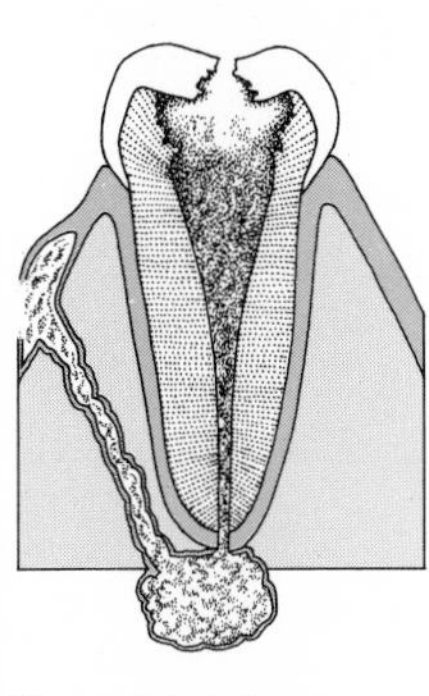

How a fistula forms
If tooth decay is not treated, the pulp may become infected. Pus may begin to form. Pus in the base of the tooth may develop into an abscess and seep out through the root of the tooth. The infection may then injure the jawbone and erode a channel called a sinus. It emerges in the gum and causes a painful swelling called a fistula.

What are the symptoms?

The abscessed tooth aches persistently or throbs and usually is extremely painful when you bite or chew. The glands in your neck may swell and become tender and, if the abscess spreads, the affected side of your face may become swollen. Often you will also have a fever and feel ill in general.

What are the risks?

If the abscess is not treated by a dentist or physician, there is a risk that the spreading infection could cause generalized blood poisoning (see p.452) or affect the adjacent bones. If the dead pulp and bacteria in the tooth are not removed by a dentist, the infection will continue.

What should be done?

See your dentist immediately if the swelling is spreading into your face or neck. If your dentist is not available, call your physician, who may prescribe an antibiotic. Then see your dentist as soon as you can.

What is the treatment?

Self-help: Take aspirin to help relieve the pain. Rinse your mouth every hour with warm salt water, to speed the bursting of the abscess and help bring relief of pain and healing of the abscess. When the abscess bursts, wash away the pus with an extra rinse. See your dentist for treatment of the abscess as soon as possible.

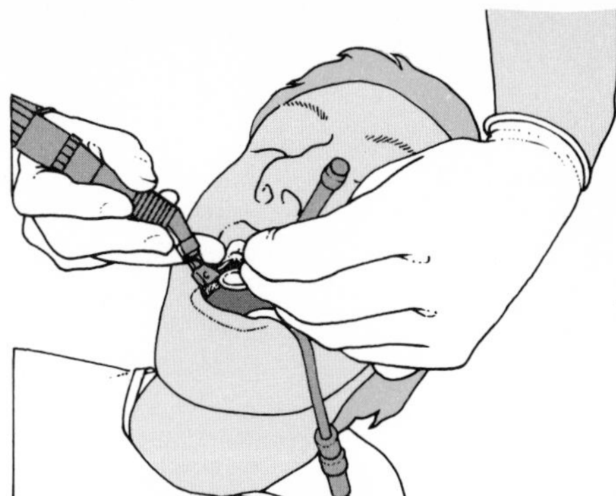

Treating an abscess
Your dentist may try to save an abscessed tooth by drilling a small hole through the crown to release the pus. The dentist can then clean out the pulp chamber and root canals, disinfect it, and put in a temporary filling. Later, he or she will put in a permanent filling.

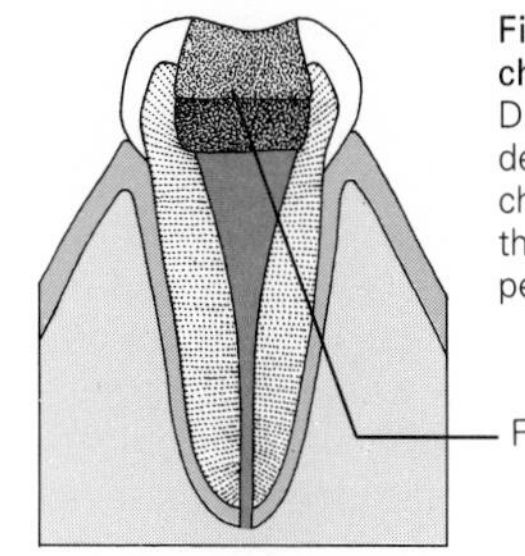

Filling the pulp chamber and canals
During a later visit your dentist will fill the pulp chamber, root canals, and the drilled hole with a permanent filling.

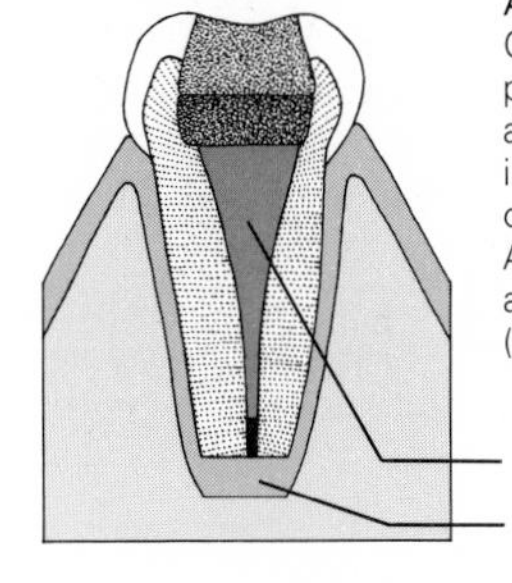

Apicoectomy
Occasionally a dentist will perform an apicoectomy, an operation in which the infected tissue at the base of the tooth is removed. An apicoectomy is used after root canal treatment (see p.470).

Professional help: The dentist may extract a thoroughly infected back tooth or a primary tooth. To save a tooth, the dentist drills a small hole through the crown and into the pulp chamber. If the abscess has not yet burst, the drilled hole releases the pressurized pus, and this relieves the pain. The dentist cleans out and disinfects the pulp chamber and root canals. At a later visit, if the infection has cleared up, the dentist will put a permanent filling in the pulp chamber, root canals, and the drilled hole. About 6 months later, the dentist will probably take X rays of the area to make sure that new bone and tissue are growing into the cavity left by the abscess. If the new growth is occurring, no further treatment is probably required.

In a few cases of abscessed teeth, the abscess does not clear up, and a small infected area remains at the tip of the root even after endodontic treatment. Antibiotics cannot clear up the infection permanently, and to treat persistent bacteria, your dentist may refer you to an oral surgeon or an endodontist. The oral surgeon may perform an apicoectomy, a procedure used after you have already had a root canal but still have problems with that tooth. Using a local anesthetic, the oral surgeon makes a small cut through it, drills away the bone that covers the tip of the root, and removes the infected tissue. In rare cases this may fail to clear up the trouble, and the tooth must be extracted (see Going to the dentist, p.472). The tooth then is best replaced with a bridge.

Discolored teeth

Teeth may become discolored, which is different from the slight yellowing that occurs with age, for a variety of reasons. Smoking can cause brown staining of tooth surfaces. Certain foods and beverages (for example, coffee) also cause staining. The death of the pulp of a tooth (see Root canal treatment, p.470) can turn it gray. Certain drugs, if they are taken in large doses or at critical times during childhood, can cause faulty, discolored enamel to form. Severe attacks of certain childhood infections, such as whooping cough and measles, can produce patches of discoloration on the teeth. And extremely excessive amounts of natural fluoride in the water, as found in some parts of the world, can cause fluorosis, or white or brown markings in the teeth. This is not a problem, however, in areas where a controlled amount of fluoride is added to the water to reduce the incidence of tooth decay.

What is the treatment?

If the discoloration is just on the surface, your dentist or dental hygienist will clean the tooth or teeth with a rotary polisher and polishing paste. Deeper discoloration can be treated by bonding a tough white porcelain or plastic crown to the tooth or by attaching a synthetic veneer. If an endodontically treated tooth is brittle, the crown may be ground down to a post that anchors a new artificial crown (see Going to the dentist, p.472).

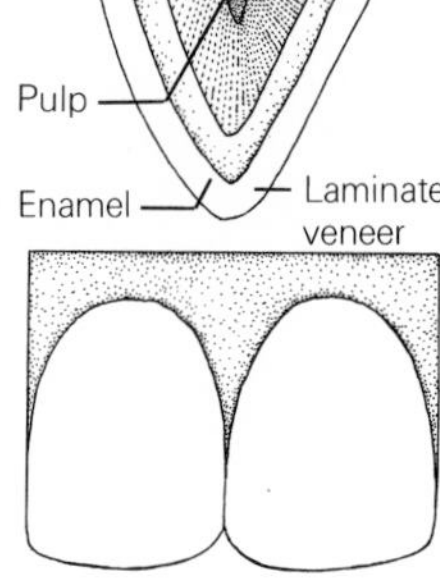

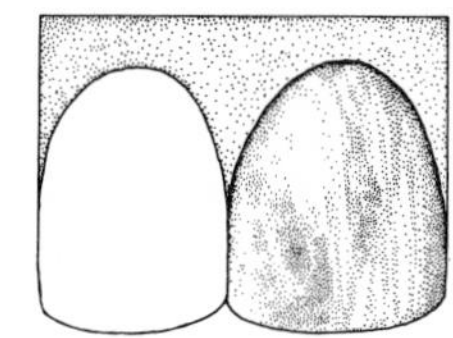

One possible treatment for a discolored tooth is to cover it with a veneer, a material such as porcelain or acrylic resin that closely resembles the color of the teeth. The veneer is applied to the tooth in thin layers.

Orthodontia

Orthodontia refers to treatment of problems in the position of your teeth. The ideal set of teeth are straight, regularly spaced with neither overlap nor gaps, and exactly the right size for the jaws. The occlusion, or the relationship of the upper and lower teeth when the mouth is closed, is such that the upper teeth slightly overlap the lower teeth, and the points (cusps) of the molars mesh with the spaces between opposing teeth. Few

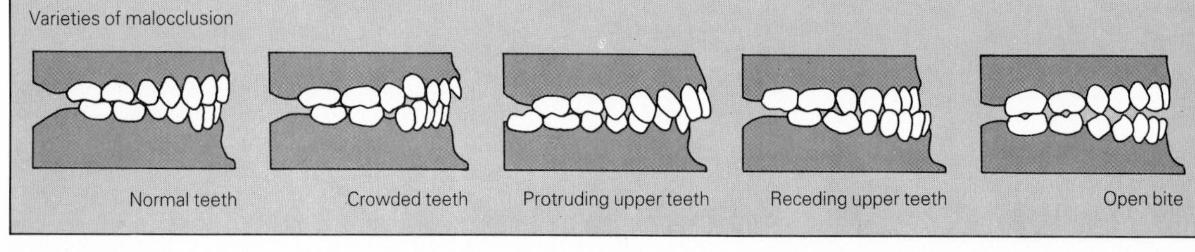

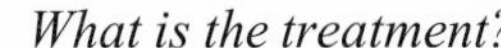

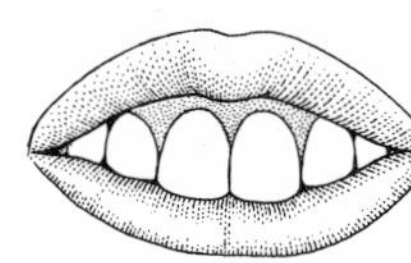

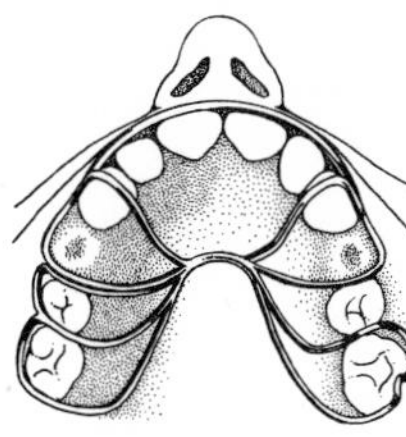

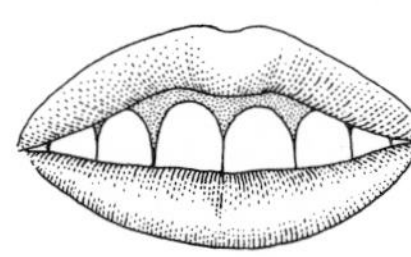

Crowding can produce front teeth that protrude so much that the mouth cannot be closed normally (top). A plate can gently pull back these teeth, and premolars may be removed to make room (center). The result is not only cosmetically more desirable (bottom), but also allows normal movement of the teeth and jaw.

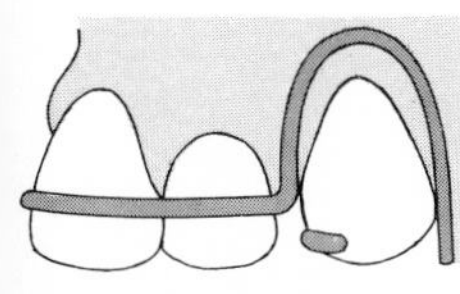

Retainer plate in position
This is a simple device that holds the teeth in their new position.

people have perfectly aligned teeth, however. One reason for this is that you inherit different characteristics from each of your parents, and sometimes the two sets of characteristics do not match. For example, your teeth may be too big for your jaws. If so, they can develop only by sloping backward or forward, by turning, or by overlapping their neighbors. If your teeth are too small for your jaws, there will be some gaps between your teeth. If your lower jaw is smaller than your upper jaw and your lips are also small, the teeth in your upper jaw may protrude. Or, your permanent upper front teeth may bite just behind the lower teeth. These are all examples of a faulty bite, or malocclusion. Also, the position of the back teeth may prevent the front teeth from meeting properly (this is known as an open bite).

Heredity is not the only cause of irregularity of teeth. Crowding is sometimes the result of loss of primary teeth ("baby teeth") through decay. For example, when primary molars are lost prematurely, the permanent molars move forward in the jaw to fill the gaps. Then, when the permanent premolars and canines appear, between the ages of 10 and 12, they are crowded out of the natural arch of the teeth. In some cases, some permanent teeth fail to appear at all (see Missing teeth, next article).

In mild cases of crowding, there is an increased risk of dental decay and gum disease, because it is more difficult to keep crowded teeth clean. In rare cases, when the crowding is severe, it can sometimes cause dental disease, difficulty in chewing food comfortably, and sometimes concern over the appearance of the teeth.

Many teenagers can benefit from treatment of crowded teeth. Such treatment can help them keep their teeth and gums clean.

What should be done?

If you are an adult with a minor problem such as a few crowded or twisted teeth, your dentist will probably tell you that the problem can be corrected by a specialist, if you are willing to spend the time and money. If the problem is severe, and may cause damage to or loss of your permanent teeth, you should have the problem corrected.

If your children are developing crowded or malocclued teeth, ask your dentist when to begin to correct the condition. Orthodontic treatment usually is most effective during childhood and early adolescence, when the teeth and jaws are both still growing and developing. Also, the texture of the bone facilitates tooth movement at this time.

What is the treatment?

If you are an adult and have a minor problem, your dentist may extract some teeth and/or fit you with braces to correct the crowding or malocclusion. More adults than ever before are choosing to wear braces, and there is no need to feel self-conscious about them.

If, as an adult, you have severely crowded or maloccluded teeth, or if your jaw protrudes or recedes, it is possible to have corrective surgery. An oral surgeon can reposition or remove pieces of the jawbone and some teeth. Another possible treatment is to have crowns and bridges made (see p.476 and p.477) to help correct the problem.

In the case of children, your dentist may be able to treat minor crowding, but for major treatment the child is usually referred to an orthodontist, who specializes in correcting irregularly positioned teeth.

The orthodontist will use X rays to check that all the adult teeth have formed and are likely to emerge. In most cases, the orthodontist will make plaster casts of the teeth and the jaw. If crowding seems likely, one possible treatment is to create a space by extracting a neighboring tooth that has already appeared. Generally, the treatment for irregularly positioned teeth is to wear braces over a period of months. Braces are anchored by fitting them around several teeth, or by attaching wires to bands that are placed around each tooth. A newer technique involves bonding metal or plastic brackets directly onto the teeth, and using wires to gently pressure teeth into the correct position.

Fixed braces are often used when a child's upper incisors protrude and the canines are prominent and crowded. Some premolars may be extracted first. Then braces can be fitted to move the canines into the correct position and later refitted to pull back the upper incisors and prevent a gap between them and the canines. Such treatment starts around the age of 12 and lasts for 18 to 30 months. The child makes visits to the orthodontist every 3 to 6 weeks to have the braces adjusted. The final part of the treatment, after braces are removed, is to fit a retainer to hold all the teeth in their new positions. The retainer is worn for several months to make sure that the surrounding tissue has enough time to stabilize.

Braces and retainers can trap plaque, the sticky substance that forms on teeth from food particles, mucus, and bacteria. Plaque can cause tooth decay and gum disease, so you must clean both your teeth and braces thoroughly after every meal. You should also avoid snacking between meals.

What are the types of dental treatment?

Cleaning and polishing If any of your teeth are covered by calculus, which is a chalky mineralized deposit that can trap plaque, it will be removed by probelike instruments, ultrasonic units, or other mechanical implements called scalers. Because they must be used near the base of the tooth, scalers may cause the gums to bleed slightly.

After scaling, the teeth are polished, because a smooth surface slows down the deposit of calculus.

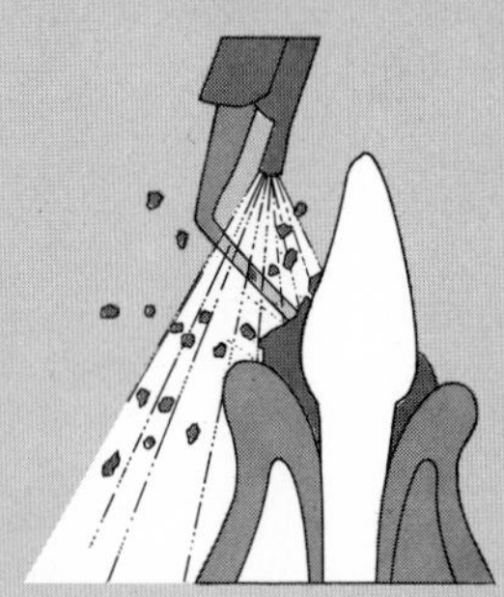

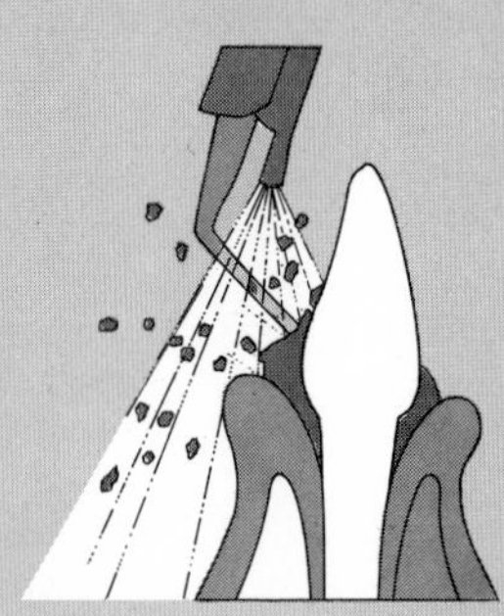

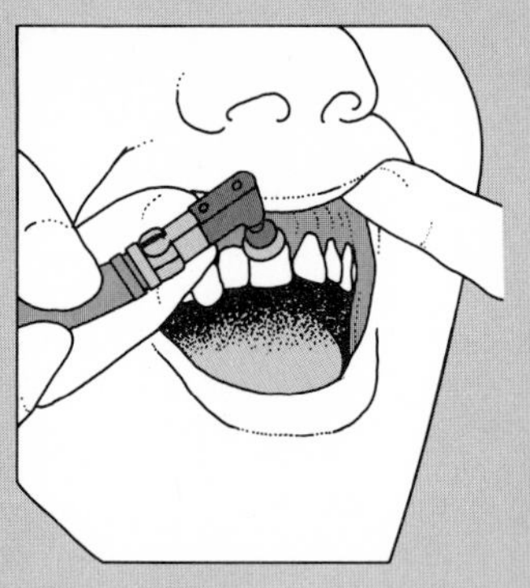

Filling When a tooth is partly decayed or chipped, the dentist replaces the damaged area with a filling. White fillings often are used on front teeth. Silver amalgam, a mixture of silver, tin, and mercury, is generally used on back teeth. If the treatment is likely to cause discomfort, the dentist will inject your gum with a local anesthetic. The dentist removes any decayed area and shapes the hole to retain the filling securely. If a front tooth is chipped, the dentist roughens the surface and bonds the filling to it. Laminate veneers or bonded resins also may be used. After having a local anesthetic, be careful to avoid biting your lip or tongue while it is still numb.

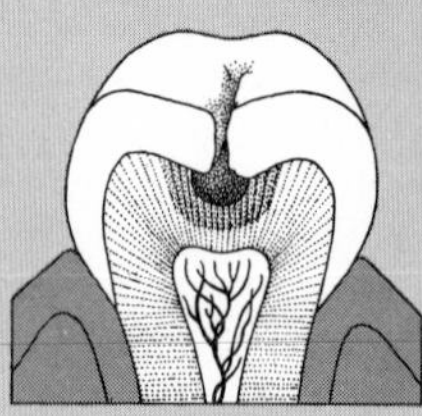

The dentist fills a tooth if the enamel has been damaged. This procedure is performed because bacteria can destroy the dentin inside the tooth and, if not checked, then attack the pulp.

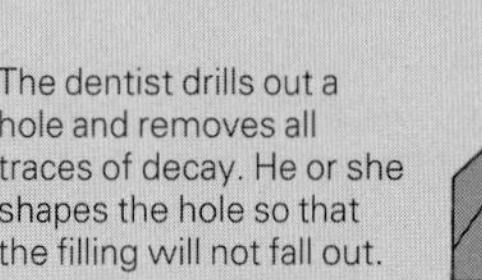

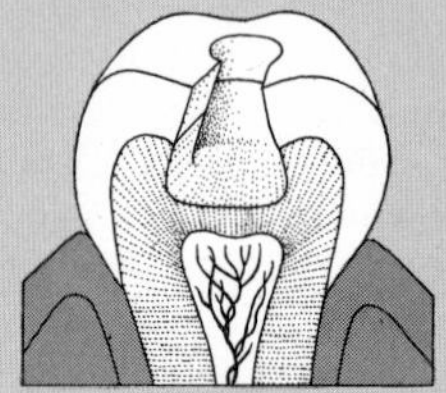

The dentist drills out a hole and removes all traces of decay. He or she shapes the hole so that the filling will not fall out.

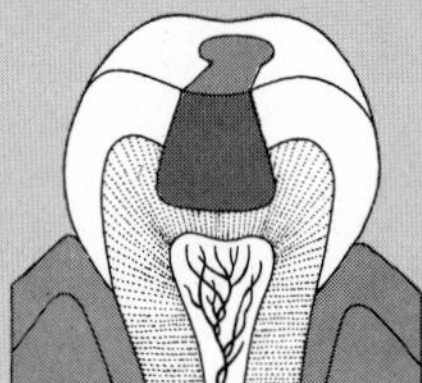

The hole is filled with a mixture of silver, tin, and mercury. If a filling will be easily visible, the tooth may be filled with a white filling made of quartz in a plastic resin.

Crowns When a tooth is severely decayed, broken, or brittle, the dentist usually makes an artificial crown for it if the base of the tooth and the roots are sound. Generally, a white porcelain crown is fitted on a tooth that can be seen. On back teeth, gold or a less-expensive alloy is used. Porcelain that is fused to metal can also be used for crowns for back teeth. The treatment usually requires two visits—the first one to prepare the tooth and the second one to put on the crown. Between visits a temporary crown may be worn.

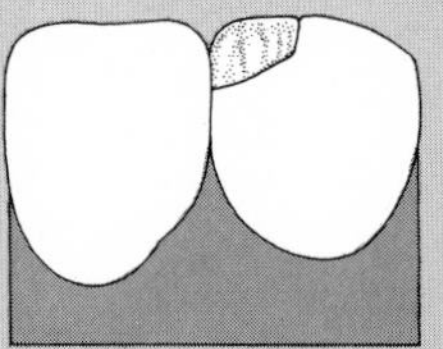

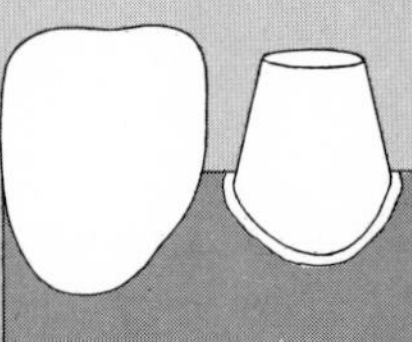

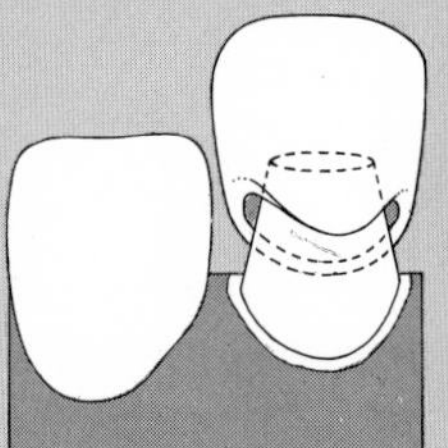

A broken, cracked, or heavily filled tooth can be repaired with a crown. The remaining part of the tooth is shaped to receive the crown.

The crown, a hollow shell, is fitted over the old tooth and cemented on.

Fitting a post crown

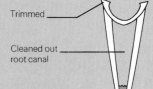

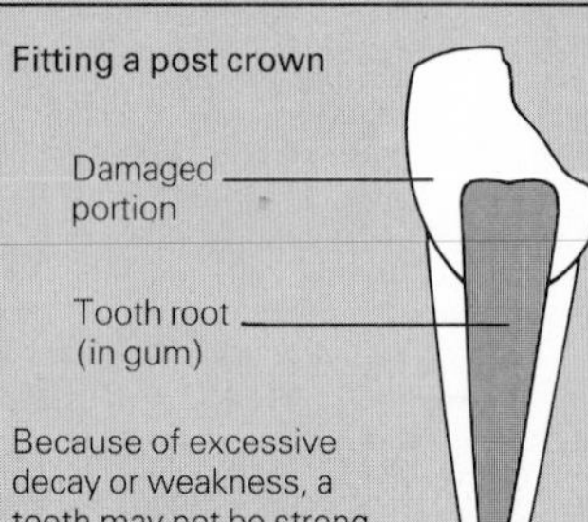

Because of excessive decay or weakness, a tooth may not be strong enough to hold a crown. A metal post can be inserted into the tooth to make it stronger.

The tooth is trimmed down to the gum and the pulp is removed from the root canal, which is then sealed with an antiseptic filling material. The post is then fitted into the root.

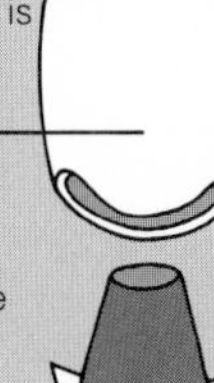

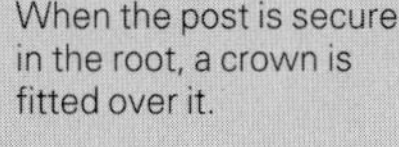

When the post is secure in the root, a crown is fitted over it.

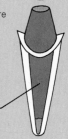

Bridges If you have a gap or gaps of up to about four teeth, flanked by sound natural teeth, you may need a bridge, an artificial tooth or teeth to bridge the gap. A bridge helps prevent remaining teeth from shifting or tipping out of place. The dentist will prepare your natural teeth for crowning, then cement into place the bridge and the crowns, to which the bridge is attached. There should be enough of a gap left between the base of the bridge and the gum ridge so that you can clean the area properly. Bridges at the front of the mouth are made of an alloy faced with porcelain. There are also resin-bonded bridges for front teeth. Those at the back are usually made of gold or other less-expensive alloys. Putting in a bridge normally requires three or four visits to the dentist.

Extractions There are several reasons for extracting a tooth. It may be too decayed or badly broken to be saved by root canal therapy or crowning, or it may be causing crowding or malocclusion (see Orthodontia, p.474). It may be loose because of advanced gum disease, or it may be preventing another tooth from erupting above the gum. Before most extractions, the dentist injects a local anesthetic to numb the tooth and gum. A general anesthetic or injection of a sedative may be used for a young child, to extract badly impacted wisdom teeth (see p.478), to extract several teeth at once, or for extremely nervous patients. After an extraction you must not do anything that might dislodge the clot that forms on the wound. If the socket bleeds persistently, bite on a clean, tightly folded handkerchief or a gauze pad, as a compress. Keep it in place for half an hour by clenching your teeth.

Dentures To replace many missing teeth, a partial denture is required. A full denture replaces all your natural teeth. Dentures are made of tough plastic or of metal and plastic.

Full dentures stay in place by resting on the gum ridges and by suction in the case of upper dentures. On a partial denture, the baseplate (artificial gums) often has clasps that fit around natural teeth to help keep the denture in place.

Fitting a denture usually requires several visits. The dentist takes impressions of the gums, and the relationship between the upper and lower jaws is recorded. You and your dentist also discuss the size and color of your dentures. In most cases, the dentist makes a preliminary denture, and makes any necessary adjustments with this preliminary model. After the final denture is made, the dentist fits and adjusts it so that you bite evenly.

Replacing a missing tooth
If all of a tooth is missing, the gap can be filled by building a bridge.

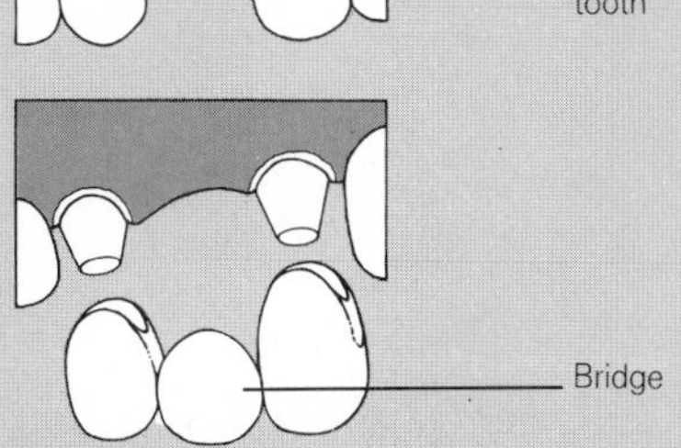

The two teeth on either side of the gap are shaped so that they can anchor the bridge.

The bridge is cemented to the two shaped teeth so that they hold the replacement in position.

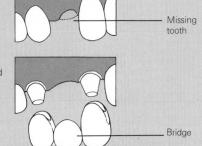

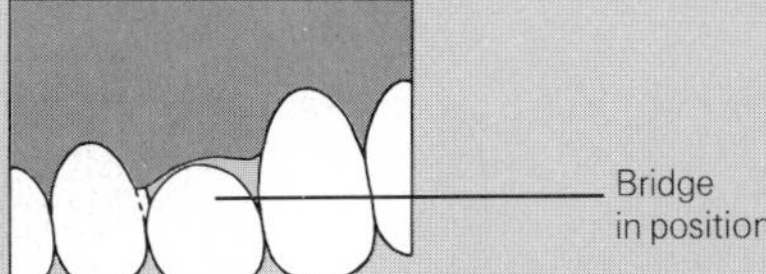

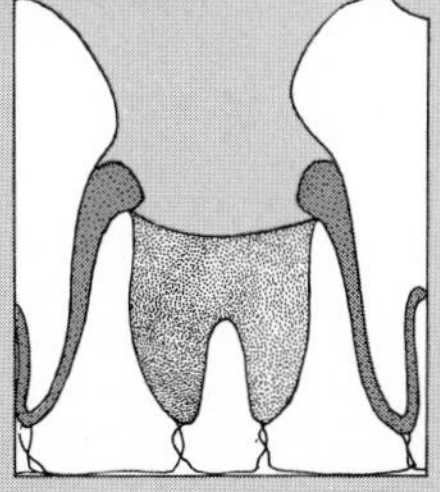

After a tooth extraction
When a tooth is pulled, a blood clot usually forms in the socket.

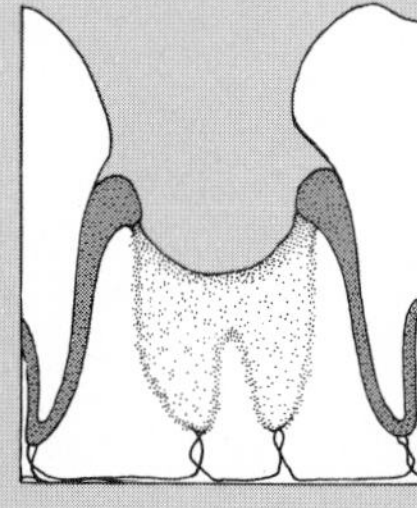

Sometimes the blood clot breaks down. This leaves what is called a dry socket.

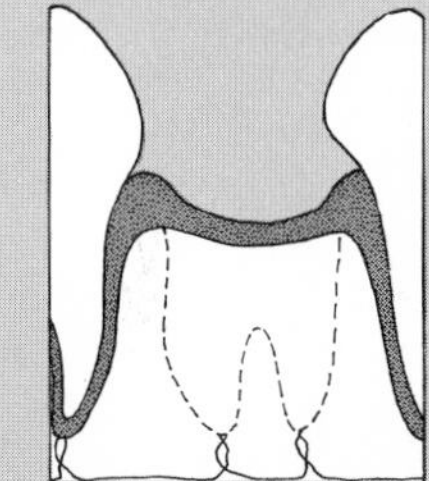

Eventually new bone grows into the gap and is covered by tissue.

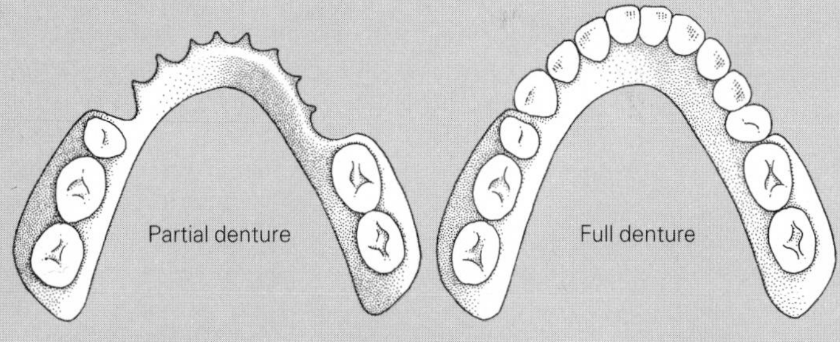

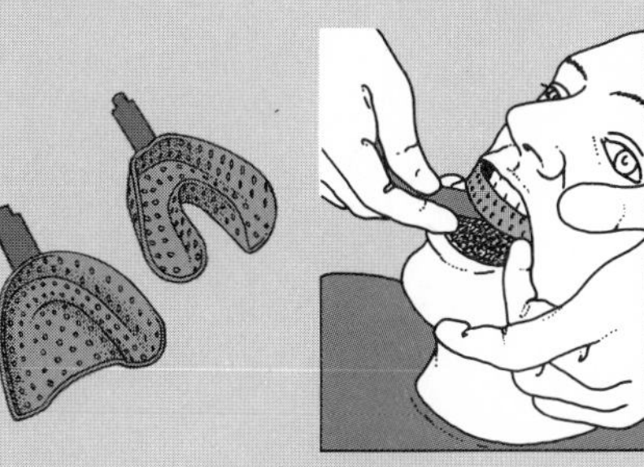

The trays (right) are filled with a puttylike substance to take impressions of your gums. The one with a recess is used for the lower jaw, the other for the upper jaw.

Missing teeth

Permanent teeth that are missing from a child's mouth after loss of the first teeth can cause dental problems in later life unless steps are taken to prevent it.

Adult teeth may be missing for one of three reasons. The most common reason is that the teeth have been lost through early decay or an accident. Molars and premolars (see p.469) are most susceptible to early decay because they have natural grooves that can trap bacteria. Another reason is that the teeth have failed to develop. This happens most commonly with the upper teeth, the incisors, the premolars (see p.469), and the third molars. Finally, they may be impacted, which means they cannot erupt through the gum.

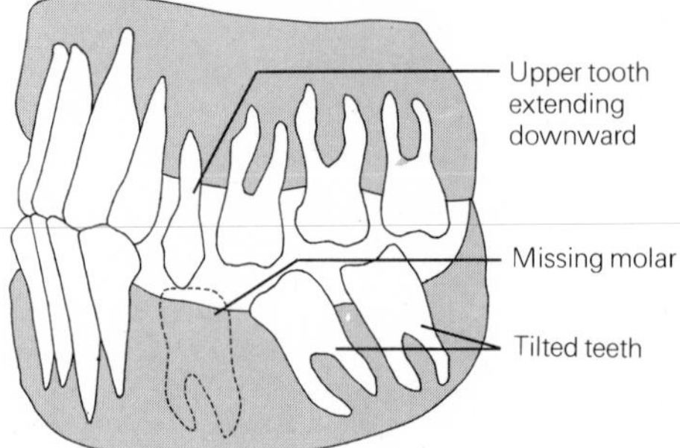

Problems caused by a missing molar
The tooth above a missing molar descends to fill the gap and the teeth around the gap tilt. Chewing becomes difficult and, because cleaning is also difficult, decay and gum disease are likely.

This can cause a number of problems. Some of the teeth that most commonly are impacted are the upper canines, premolars, and wisdom teeth, or third molars (see next article).

Even if a child loses only one molar through an accident or tooth decay, it can cause problems later. One is that the molar in the jaw opposite the space has too much room to grow into. When you chew, your jaw moves from side to side as well as up and down, and if a molar fits into a space in the row of teeth above or below it, it interferes with the sideways motion of your jaw. The dentist usually extracts such a molar or grinds its cusps down, because this condition can prevent you from chewing food properly.

Another common problem is that the teeth on either side of the missing molar begin to tilt in the gum because they do not receive the usual supporting pressure.

Other teeth naturally tend to tip toward the spaces left by missing teeth. To do so, they may emerge too much from the gum or grow at an angle. This can produce maloccluded teeth, or a faulty bite (see previous article). Then, when you bite or chew, teeth do not come together correctly, which places stress on the teeth and jaw. The stress occasionally causes temporomandibular joint disorders, which may involve pain in the joints of the jaw. Other problems caused by malocclusion include wear of some teeth and difficulties with the muscles of the face.

A more common risk of teeth growing into gaps at an angle is that cleaning these areas may be difficult. Plaque may build up in hard-to-reach spaces and lead to tooth decay (see p.469) and periodontal disease (see Gingivitis, p.481, and Periodontitis, p.482).

What should be done?

If you think that your child has a missing primary (baby) or permanent tooth, take the child to the dentist. If you have had teeth missing since childhood and you have any of the problems described above, discuss your situation with your dentist.

What is the treatment?

Your dentist may choose to restore your occlusion by inserting a permanent prosthesis (false tooth) by bridgework, or by making a partial denture that you can remove. (See Going to the dentist, p.472). Your dentist may also refer you to an orthodontist, a dentist who specializes in treating irregularly positioned teeth. To treat any pain in the jaw caused by malocclusion, your dentist may either fit a bite-plane over your upper teeth and gums or grind down the high spots in your teeth in order to correct the bite.

Problems with wisdom teeth

(third molars)

The last teeth in the back are the third molars, also known as wisdom teeth. The four wisdom teeth usually appear between ages 17 and 21, but in some people one or more of them never emerge. Lack of wisdom teeth is nothing to worry about, unless the teeth are impacted (blocked under the gum) or causing problems. In fact, it may be an advantage, since wisdom teeth often cause problems as they emerge. Even when they form normally, wisdom teeth are difficult to clean, and therefore decay more readily than other teeth.

Sometimes a wisdom tooth emerges at an angle. The space between the wisdom tooth and the next tooth can trap plaque and food particles and cause dental problems. Often a wisdom tooth fails to emerge properly because it becomes impacted, sometimes by the tooth next to it. This can also cause dental problems. The gum forms a pocket around an impacted tooth in which plaque and food tend to collect. Bacteria can eventually produce an infection, called pericoronitis, around the impacted tooth.

If one of your wisdom teeth simply fails to appear, you probably will not have any symptoms. If it erupts at an angle and forms a pocket that attracts plaque and food particles, you may have bad breath and possibly an unpleasant taste in your mouth.

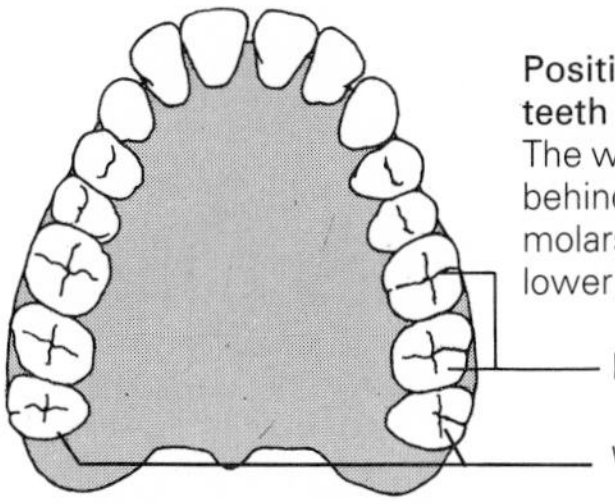

The main symptoms of pericoronitis are pain when you bite on the tooth or the gum partially covering the tooth, and an unpleasant taste. You will probably also have redness and swelling of the gum around the tooth. If you have any of these symptoms, see your dentist or physician as soon as possible.

Position of wisdom teeth
The wisdom teeth are behind the first two molars in both upper and lower jaws.

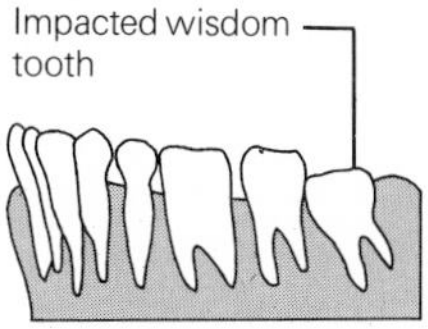

Molars

Wisdom teeth

Impacted wisdom tooth
An impacted wisdom tooth is one that is blocked when it grows at an angle against the adjacent tooth. The problem usually is solved by removing the wisdom tooth itself.

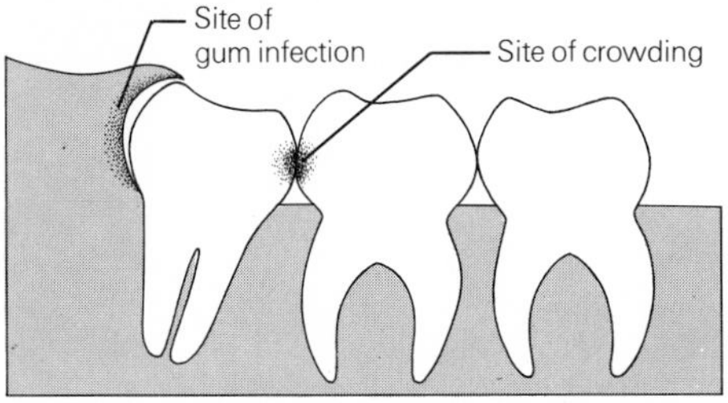

Impacted wisdom tooth

Site of gum infection

Site of crowding

Gum infection
If an impacted wisdom tooth has partially emerged, food and bacteria can become trapped under the gum flap and cause decay, bad breath, and gum disease.

What is the treatment?

Self-help: You can obtain temporary relief from the pain by taking aspirin or rinsing the area around the tooth with warm salt water.

Professional help: Your dentist or physician may prescribe an antibiotic to clear up the infection, and will probably advise you to continue to rinse with warm salt water to keep the area clean and relieve the pain. However, the antibiotic usually offers only temporary relief, and the long-term solution to the problem is to drain the infection, which usually requires having the wisdom tooth extracted soon after the infection has subsided. Your dentist will take X rays to determine the position of the tooth. If the tooth lies at a difficult angle, or if the other wisdom teeth are similarly affected, you may be referred to an oral surgeon for extraction. This requires either a local anesthetic or a sedative.

Denture problems

Most dentures, or false teeth, look natural and fit well, but no denture is as efficient and comfortable as your own teeth. With natural teeth, the stresses of biting and chewing are absorbed by the teeth, the roots of the teeth, and the special shock-absorbent material, called the periodontal ligament, that lines the tooth sockets in the jawbone. With dentures, the stresses are absorbed in unnatural ways. The most critical of these is the pressure that the baseplate, or false gums, places on the ridges of the natural gums, especially if the dentures are worn both day and night. This pressure can cause inflammation of the gums and, eventually, can lead to mouth ulcers and also to degeneration of the jawbone underneath the gum tissue.

The base of a partial denture also places an abnormal sideways load on the natural teeth that are used to anchor the denture base. Partial dentures, especially poorly fitted ones, have another disadvantage. They trap plaque and food particles, which can cause decay in the remaining teeth (see p.469) and may lead to gingivitis (see next article) or even periodontitis (see p.482). The fungus that causes oral thrush (see p.484) can also lead to a painful mouth condition, especially if you have been taking antibiotic medication.

What are the symptoms?

The early symptoms of excessive pressure on the ridges of the gums are pain when the dentures are in place, especially when you are eating, and either white and patchy or red and inflamed gums. If the inflammation persists, the gums may become deep red and soft and may bleed easily—after you rub them with your toothbrush, for example. A mouth ulcer (see p.483) may form on any spot where your denture rubs your gums. After a denture has been worn for many years, hard, pale pads called dental granulomas may form at the main pressure points, especially near the edges of the denture.

Further symptoms arise when the gums and jawbone shrink, which inevitably occurs after a few years of continuous pressure even if the denture has caused no other problems. (Note also that bone shrinks naturally after tooth loss, not only when dentures are worn.) When this happens, you must close your

Biting and chewing with dentures
With the loss of your teeth you lose periodontal tissue, a shock-absorbent material that lines the sockets of the jaw bones. Dentures can press against your gums, leading to soreness, inflammation, and mouth ulcers. Regular visits to the dentist and proper denture care will minimize your problems.

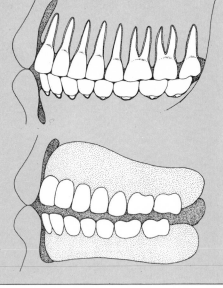

Taking care of your dentures
Always remove your dentures at night and keep them in a glass of water mixed with a cleansing agent, so that they do not dry out and warp.

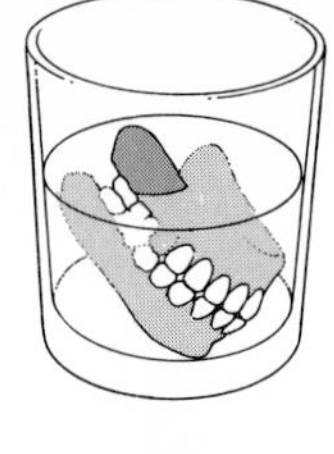

Clean your dentures daily and make sure that all food and plaque are removed. Your dentist or hygienist will show you the best method.

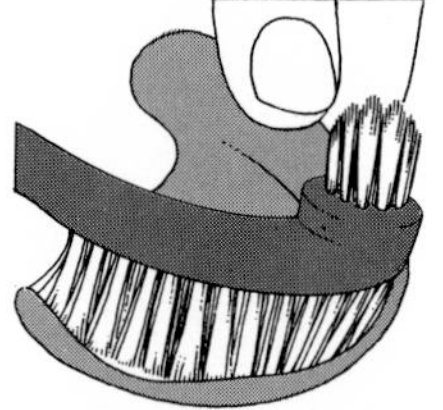

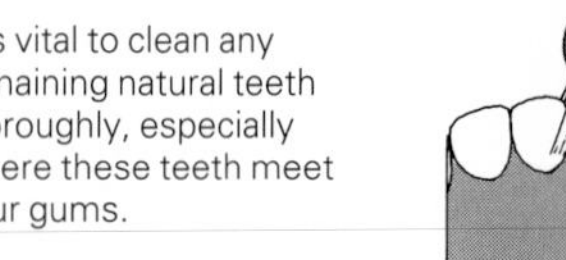

It is vital to clean any remaining natural teeth thoroughly, especially where these teeth meet your gums.

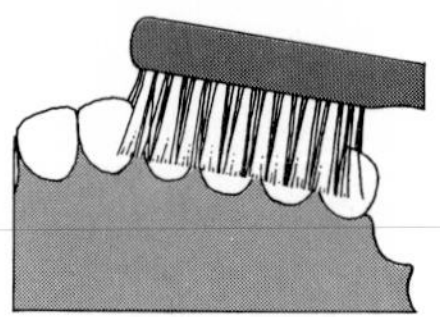

mouth further to bite properly, and even further if your dentures are worn down. The common symptoms of gum and jawbone shrinkage are loose dentures, sunken cheeks, and a protruding lower jaw. You may have pain in the jawbone joints from the extra movement needed to bite.

What are the risks?

A long-term risk for anyone who has problems with dentures is that your jawbone and gums will slowly shrink after most or all of your teeth have been removed. Because of this, the movement and appearance of your mouth may change a great deal. Also, chronic irritation from friction, inflammation, and pressure can lead to infection or sometimes to cancerous changes in the gums.

What should be done?

If you have full dentures, have your dentist check the way they fit and any effect they may be having on your gums. Your general oral health should be checked by a dentist at least once a year. If you have a partial denture or a bridge, see your dentist regularly (see p.472), to make sure the partial or bridge fits properly and to safeguard your natural teeth and the general health of your mouth. If you have pain, sores, or bleeding in your mouth, consult your dentist immediately.

What is the treatment?

Self-help: Always remove your dentures at night, to give your gum tissues a regular rest period, and to allow you to adequately clean your mouth and dentures. When not in the mouth, many dentures must be kept in a glass of water or they warp when they dry out. Partial dentures often feel a little tight when you insert them in the morning, but this is normal and the feeling quickly disappears. Thoroughly clean your dentures daily, according to your dentist's or hygienist's instructions, and clean your natural teeth and gums thoroughly, especially around the base of the teeth. If you wear dentures and have a sore mouth, keep your dentures scrupulously clean and soak them overnight in a cleaning solution designed for this purpose. Also, you should clean and massage your gums with a finger, damp cloth, or soft brush.

Professional help: The useful life of dentures varies, depending on the condition of your gums and jawbone, the denture material, and how well the dentures fit. When your dentures become worn or your gums and jawbone shrink, your dentist will make new dentures. Or if your dentures are not too worn, the dentist can sometimes adapt the existing denture baseplate to the new shape of your gums.

To clear up inflamed gums, your dentist may prescribe an antifungal agent and teach you how to take better care of your gums and dentures to avoid future problems. Some people have major problems coping with dentures and never really adapt to them. It may also become difficult to adapt to new dentures as you grow older.

Gingivitis

Gingivitis is an early stage of periodontal (gum) disease. It is caused by plaque, a sticky deposit of bacteria, mucus, and food particles that forms at the base of the teeth. It may also be caused by a vitamin deficiency, by certain medications, and by some glandular disorders and blood diseases.

Researchers think that irritation from plaque causes the gums to become inflamed and swollen. As the edge of the gum swells, a pocket forms between the gum and a tooth. This becomes a trap for more plaque, the gum swells even more, and the pocket deepens. If the condition is not treated, it may develop into periodontitis (see next article).

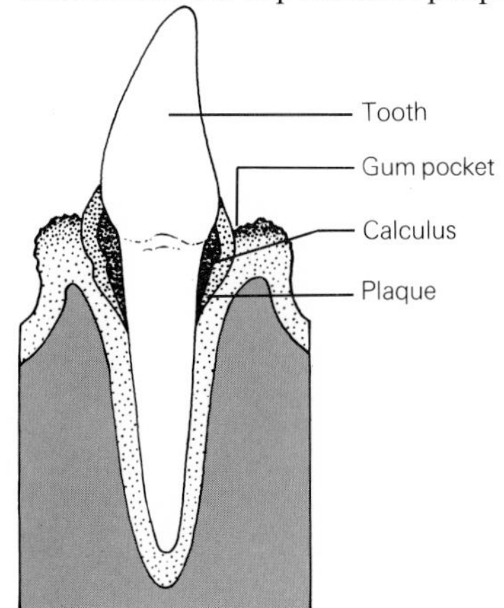

Avoiding gingivitis
If plaque builds up, bacteria in its deeper layers die and then mineralize and harden to calculus. Proper brushing and flossing and regular care by your dentist prevent calculus formation and the gingivitis it causes.

Gingivitis is quite common in adults. Pregnant women and people with diabetes are particularly susceptible because of changes in hormone levels. The disorder is less common in healthy children.

What are the symptoms?

Healthy gums are pale pink or brown (there are racial differences in coloration of gums), firm, and look speckled. In gingivitis, your gums become red, soft, shiny, and swollen. They bleed easily, even from gentle brushing. Unless it is stopped, gingivitis can eventually lead to serious gum and bone disease (see Periodontitis, next article).

What should be done?

Only mild gingivitis is likely to develop if you keep your teeth and gums clean and have regular dental care. If you have not taken care of your teeth and gingivitis has developed, see a dentist as soon as possible.

What is the treatment?

Self-help: Brush your teeth thoroughly at least twice a day and after meals, if possible, and use dental floss at least once a day, to remove all plaque. To see how successfully you are cleaning, use a disclosing tablet occasionally (see Box, p.471).

Professional help: In serious cases of gingivitis your dentist may prescribe an antibacterial mouthwash after removing any plaque and calculus (a hard, chalky deposit that traps plaque) from the base of your teeth. Calculus is removed with a scaler (see Going to the dentist, p.472). Some people develop calculus despite careful tooth care, and need to have their teeth cleaned professionally every few months.

Most cases of gingivitis respond to treatment, and the gums return to normal. It is then up to you to keep your teeth and gums clean to avoid recurrence of the disease.

Neglect and gum disease
Inadequate brushing allows plaque build-up, which promotes gum disease. Your gums become inflamed and sore and stay that way until the plaque is removed. If this is not done, the disease progresses, and eventually teeth may have to be extracted.

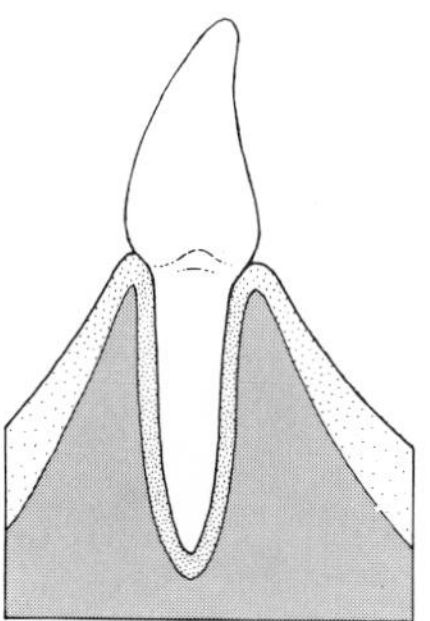

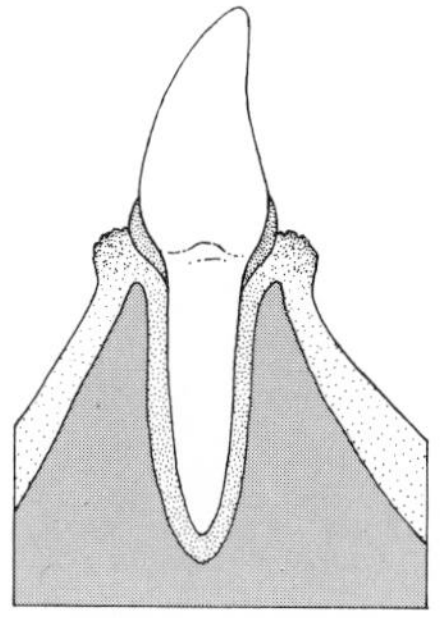

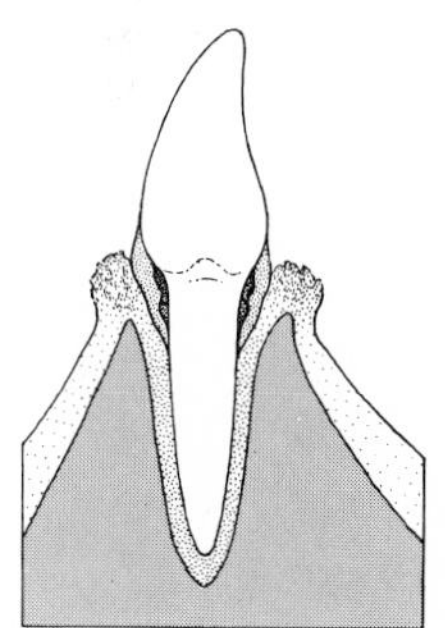

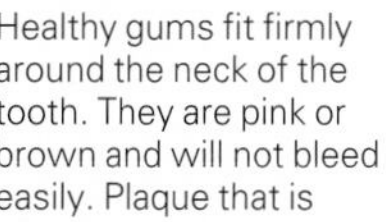
Healthy gums fit firmly around the neck of the tooth. They are pink or brown and will not bleed easily. Plaque that is allowed to build up between the teeth and the gums can cause painful inflammation. It eventually finds its way to some of the bone and fibers that anchor the tooth. Bacteria in the plaque can do severe damage.

Periodontitis

Periodontitis is the end result of gingivitis (see previous article) that has been treated too late or not at all. In gingivitis, plaque, a sticky deposit of bacteria, mucus, and food particles, collects in pockets between swollen gums and the base of your teeth. The bacteria in the plaque may, over a period of years, cause destruction of the bone that surrounds and supports your teeth. Eventually, the bony sockets can become so eroded that the teeth become loose and must be extracted.

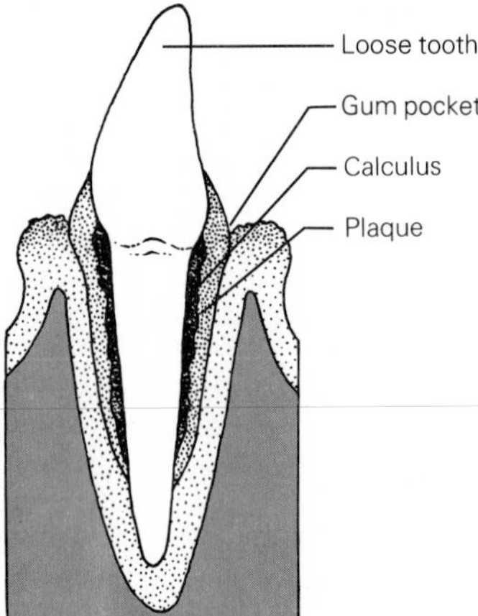

Damage caused by gum disease
The bacteria in unchecked plaque destroys the bone and tissue that surround and anchor the tooth. They also form calculus, which can pry the gum away from the tooth. Both processes can loosen and ultimately make it necessary to extract the tooth.

What are the symptoms?
The pockets between gums and teeth gradually deepen and the plaque in the pockets may cause an unpleasant taste and bad breath. As the disease progresses, the teeth may loosen in their sockets. More and more cementum, the sensitive tissue that covers the root of the tooth, is exposed, and it aches when you eat very hot, very cold, or sweet food. Sometimes an abscess (p.473) forms deep inside a pocket and its accompanying infection destroys more bone.

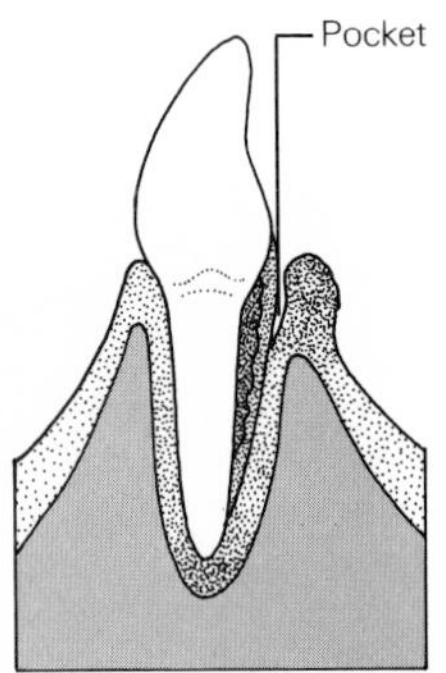

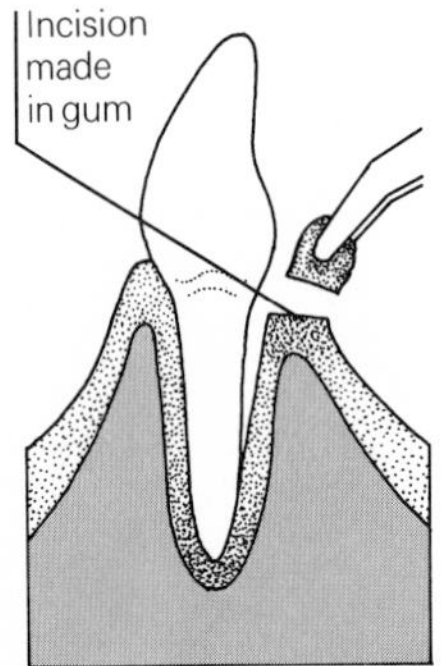

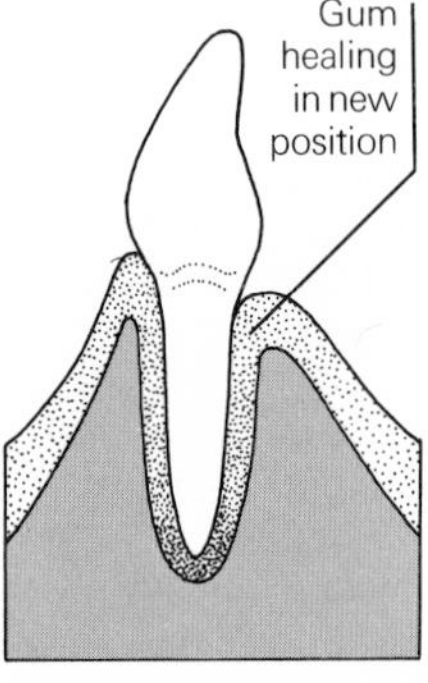

Treatment of periodontitis
Plaque and calculus building up between tooth and gum form a deep pocket between them. In treatment, the pocket is cleaned and the soft-tissue wall of the pocket is removed. Severe cases require surgery on the gum.

What are the risks?
Adults lose more teeth from periodontal disease than from dental decay. The problem is common among young adults, and the likelihood of having it increases with age.

If you have periodontitis, you may need to have all your teeth extracted. They will have to be replaced with dentures, which are never as satisfactory as your natural teeth.

What should be done?
The disease often can be halted before it reaches an advanced stage. See a dentist as soon as you notice any of the symptoms of periodontitis described above. To find out how advanced the disease is, the dentist usually measures the depth of the pockets and takes X rays to determine the condition of the underlying bone. This is an important factor in how the dentist will treat the problem.

What is the treatment?
Self-help: Follow the measures described in Keeping your teeth and gums healthy (see p.471). Pay special attention to cleaning your gums and the base of your teeth.
Professional help: If the disease is at an early stage, your dentist can help keep it under control by treating any dental disorders that encourage plaque to form or allow it to persist, such as crowded or crooked teeth (see Orthodontia, p.474). Your role in controlling plaque is to clean your teeth thoroughly (see Keeping your teeth and gums healthy, p.471).

If the pockets have become very deep, periodontal surgery may be required. A gingivectomy is a minor operation performed in the office by a dental specialist, in which the soft tissue wall of the pocket is removed. If your bone has been damaged, minor surgery may be required to reshape the gum and bone. After the surgery, the gumline is covered with a protective coating called a periodontal pack, which should stay in place for 1 to 2 weeks until the gum heals. The coating usually does not prevent normal eating and drinking. If you have any problems, call your dentist or specialist.

Cementum (which covers the roots) that has been worn away can be replaced by synthetic material bonded to the tooth. Particularly sensitive cementum can be protected with a layer of sodium fluoride, or your dentist may prescribe a toothpaste that also provides protection. Very loose teeth can be anchored. Ask your dentist about possible procedures for this.

Mouth and tongue

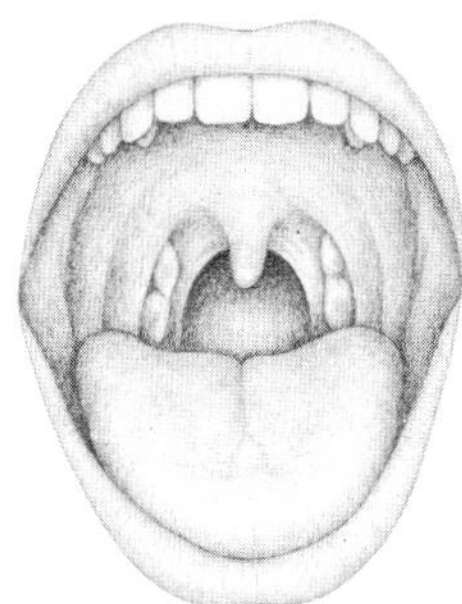

The mouth
The mouth is the first part of the digestive tract. The teeth crush the food so that enzymes can break it down, while saliva lubricates it, to make it easier to swallow.

The inside of your mouth is covered by a delicate lining of mucous membrane. It is kept moist and lubricated by saliva, which is produced in three pairs of salivary glands in your mouth. These are the sublingual glands, which are located under your tongue, the submandibular glands, which are in the floor of your mouth, and the parotid glands, which are above the angles of your jaw.

Your tongue has a complex system of muscles that enables it to move food around as you chew and then to mold chewed food into a ball for swallowing. The surface of your tongue is covered with hairlike projections that are called papillae, and groups of tastebuds are clustered around them. The tastebuds can distinguish four main types of flavor: sweet, salty, sour, and bitter. It is to these tastebuds, along with your sense of smell, that you are indebted for the pleasure of a fine meal. More important, it is often your tastebuds that warn you if you eat food that has spoiled.

Changes in the shape of your mouth, lips, and tongue enable you to form a variety of sounds produced by the vocal cords, including those that are necessary for speech.

The majority of disorders that affect your mouth and tongue are not serious and are relatively simple to treat. However, because it is possible for malignant (likely to spread) tumors to form there, consult your physician or dentist about any condition of the mouth or tongue that persists for more than 10 days. Read the articles on salivary gland tumors and tumors of the mouth and tongue in the following pages. If you think you have a tumor, see a physician as quickly as possible.

Canker sores

(and other mouth ulcers)

See p.256,
Visual aids to diagnosis, 64.

A canker sore, or aphthous ulcer, is a break in the lining of the mouth that uncovers the sensitive tissue beneath. All sores in your mouth look very much the same, but they vary considerably in cause and seriousness. The two most common and painful types of ulcers are canker sores, which tend to occur when you are under stress, run down, or ill, and traumatic ulcers, which result from an injury to the mouth's lining. Canker sores are not infectious or contagious. Traumatic ulcers may be caused by a toothbrush, a rough denture, or hot food.

Some canker sores are caused by infection by a virus. A virus that commonly causes sores in your mouth is herpes simplex (see Cold sores, next article). This virus causes blisters that eventually turn into ulcers. Rarely, a sore may be the first sign of a tumor of the mouth (see p.487), or the sign of a more generalized disease such as anemia (see p.450) or leukemia (see p.457).

Canker sores are very common. They occur most often in adolescents and young adults, and more often in women (especially just before a menstrual period).

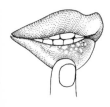

Canker sores
One type of mouth sore may appear in clusters on the lower lip. These ulcers are white and may be very painful.

What are the symptoms?

You usually first become aware of a mouth ulcer when you eat something spicy or acidic that makes it sting. You can usually see canker sores in a mirror as pale yellow spots with red borders. Canker sores are small, measuring about 1/10 in (2 to 3 mm) across. They usually occur singly but may appear in clusters on the sides of your mouth or gum, and last for 5 to 10 days. A traumatic ulcer is usually a larger, solitary sore, and lasts for a week or more. When a traumatic ulcer is caused by a rough tooth or denture, it heals only after the cause has been remedied.

What should be done?

The vast majority of canker sores do not indicate any major health problem and usually heal by themselves. But if a sore fails to heal within 10 days, or if sores keep recurring, see your physician to find out if the ulcers are caused by a more serious underlying condition. Your physician may want to have blood tests taken, and you may also have to undergo a biopsy of the sore. In a biopsy, part of the canker sore is removed under a local anesthetic, so that it can be examined microscopically. The results of these tests will show whether the canker sore signifies the presence of a serious disorder. If you think that a jagged tooth or a rough denture is causing traumatic ulcers, consult your dentist as soon as possible.

What is the treatment?

Self-help: You can buy nonprescription applications and lozenges that soothe and protect the exposed tissue in a sore. These preparations relieve the pain while healing takes place. Antiseptic mouthwashes or rinsing your mouth with warm salt water may also provide temporary relief.

To minimize any discomfort, avoid consuming spicy or acidic foods or drinks. You should avoid hot food or drinks as well.

Professional help: To deal with persistent canker sores, your physician may prescribe a mouth rinse or an ointment containing a corticosteroid drug.

Cold sores

(Herpes simplex)

See p.246, **Visual aids to diagnosis, 24.**

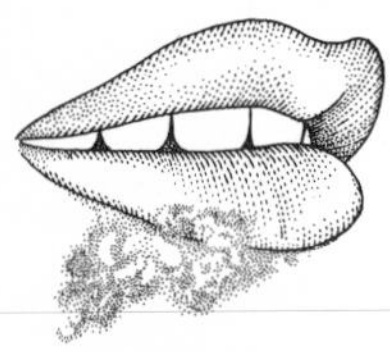

Most cold sores appear around the mouth. Tingling and numbness may precede or follow their appearance.

Herpes simplex is a virus that causes blisters to form on your lips and on the inside of your mouth. These blisters, called cold sores, develop into painful ulcers. Your gums become swollen and deep red, and often the tongue becomes furred. You may have a fever and feel ill. The older you are, the more severe the infection. A young child's initial bout may be so mild that it passes unnoticed.

After the infection has cleared up, the virus lies dormant indefinitely. Later, another infection (usually a cold), exposure to sunshine, a period of stress, or hormonal changes (pregnancy or menstruation, for example) reactivate the virus. This change causes a blister that bursts and forms an encrusted cold sore on the edge of the lip or somewhere else near the mouth.

Herpes simplex infection of the mouth is very common and seems to present no serious risks to your general health. The main danger involved is that, during an infection, if you touch the ulcers and then your eye, it could cause a herpetic corneal ulcer (see p.342) to form on that eye.

What is the treatment?

Mild cases of the infection need no treatment. If the infection is reactivated, consult your physician before the blisters are fully formed. At this stage of the infection, he or she may prescribe an antiviral drug called acyclovir that reduces the rate at which the virus multiplies. Treatment with acyclovir is especially useful when a person's natural defenses are impaired—as a result of treatment for a serious disorder such as leukemia, or in a person with HIV infection or AIDS, for example. If sores develop, applying ice to them often brings rapid relief.

Temporomandibular joint syndrome

Temporomandibular joint syndrome, which is also known as TMJ or myofascial pain-dysfunction syndrome, is a disorder that affects the joints at either side of the jaw (the temporomandibular joints). In this disorder, the joints and the jaw muscles are painful and it may be difficult to fully open the jaw. In some cases, pain extends to the ear, or even as far as the shoulder.

Most people who have spasmodic pain in the jaw muscles have temporomandibular joint syndrome. The cause of the condition is usually unclear, and X rays and laboratory tests performed on people with this syndrome often reveal no abnormality.

What is the treatment?

If you have pain in your jaw muscles, consult your physician or dentist. Treatment to relieve the painful spasms may include heat therapy, injections or sprays of local anesthetics, and use of analgesics (pain-relievers) such as aspirin or ibuprofen. Avoid hard foods or foods that are high in fiber.

Oral thrush

Oral thrush is an outbreak of the fungus *Candida albicans*, one of the many microbes that are usually present in small numbers in your mouth. Growth of this fungus is usually prevented by bacteria in the mouth. However, if your natural resistance to infection is low because of illness (including AIDS and other disorders associated with HIV infection), or if antibiotics or inhaled corticosteroids have upset the natural balance among the microbes in your mouth, this fungus may multiply out of control. This leads to sore patches in your mouth. Sometimes it can cause similar sore areas to form in your throat as well. The patches are creamy-yellow and slightly raised. If they are rubbed off when you eat or as you brush your teeth, they leave a painful raw area. The fungus can also cause denture problems (see p.479).

Many people have oral thrush at some time in their lives. It is most prevalent in very young children, older people, and people who are chronically ill or malnourished. The fungus can infect a woman's vagina and cause vaginal irritation and discharge (see Vaginal yeast infection, p.645).

If you have the symptoms described for oral thrush, see your physician for treatment.

What is the treatment?
Your physician will examine you and may take a sample of a patch for analysis, or perhaps arrange for you to have blood tests to rule out the possibility of any serious underlying disease, such as diabetes mellitus (see p.558). Meanwhile, the thrush may be treated with a topical antifungal agent and by practicing improved oral hygiene techniques. Oral thrush in itself is not serious and is quickly cleared up with antifungal treatment, but it does have a tendency to recur.

Leukoplakia

In leukoplakia, a part of the soft, delicate lining of your mouth or tongue thickens and hardens. This usually occurs to protect an area made sore by the repeated rubbing of a rough tooth or denture. Alternatively, it may be caused by a protective reaction to the irritation of inhaled tobacco smoke, in which case it is known as smoker's keratosis. However, irritation from smokeless tobacco (such as chewing tobacco) can also cause leukoplakia.

The patch, which develops over a period of weeks, is white or gray and may be any size. At first it causes no discomfort, but later it feels rough and stiff, and in advanced cases, where ulceration, fissuring, or malignant (likely to spread) degeneration has occurred, it may be sensitive to hot or spicy foods.

Anyone can develop leukoplakia, but it is most common in older men. If you develop the symptoms described, see your dentist or your physician. Certain forms of leukoplakia are precancerous.

What is the treatment?
The treatment is to deal with the source of irritation that caused the patch to form. A rough tooth or denture may have to be smoothed or adjusted. In the case of smoker's keratosis, you will be advised to give up tobacco. This is usually all that is needed to make the patch disappear.

If the patch has not gone away within 2 weeks, your physician will arrange for a biopsy of the patch, in which a small sample of it is removed and examined. This is necessary because about 5 percent of such patches are malignant (see p.487).

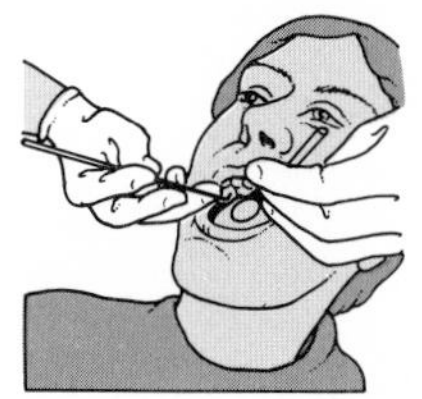

Taking a biopsy
Your dentist or your physician may remove a small piece of tissue from your mouth to help diagnose leukoplakia.

Oral lichen planus

In oral lichen planus, changes occur in the lining of your mouth that often cause minor discomfort—although there are usually no symptoms in the keratotic form of lichen planus, in which there is thickening and hardening of the mouth lining.

Oral lichen planus usually starts as a number of small, pale pimples that gradually join to form a fine, white, lacy network of slightly raised tissue. In other cases the disorder takes the form of shiny, red, slightly raised patches. The changes usually occur on the inside of your cheeks and the sides of your tongue.

The symptoms may include a sore mouth and dry, metallic taste, or there may be no noticeable symptoms.

The cause of oral lichen planus is unclear. It can be brought on by emotional stress, by patches or irritation in the mouth such as those that are caused by ill-fitting dentures (see Denture problems, p.479), or by an immunologic disorder.

Oral lichen planus is a rare disorder that can affect any adult but occurs most often in middle-aged and older women. Half of those who get oral lichen planus also have lichen planus on the skin (see p.278).

What should be done?
If they occur, symptoms of oral lichen planus appear rather suddenly. If you have any color or texture changes inside your mouth that do not clear up within 10 days, see your physician or dentist as soon as possible. In general, oral lichen planus is a chronic, recurrent condition that can be managed but not cured. An outbreak of the disorder usually lasts about 9 months, but in some rare cases, may last for several years.

One form of lichen planus that causes only skin changes may spontaneously disappear or may recur only during times of emotional stress; thus, it need not be treated. However, any possible sources of irritation should be treated; for example, poorly fitted dentures should be fitted properly and a rough tooth restoration should be smoothed. For painful forms of lichen planus, a topical agent or oral medication may be prescribed.

Salivary gland infections

A salivary gland usually becomes infected and swollen as a result of mumps (see p.748). However, such an infection can also be caused by bacteria, especially if you are run-down or dehydrated or if one of your glands has been damaged by salivary duct stones (see next article). When it is infected, the salivary gland becomes swollen and painful, and the lymph glands in your neck beneath the angle of your jaw may also feel enlarged and tender. Avoid spicy foods and citrus fruits because they will increase the pain and swelling. Pus from the infected gland trickles into your mouth and tastes bitter or foul. Sometimes an infection persists, and this may cause so much scarring in the gland that it may cease to function. If you have any swelling in your mouth, under your chin, or around your jaw, with or without fever, consult your physician or dentist.

What is the treatment?

Your physician will probably treat an infection of the salivary glands with an antibiotic, if the problem seems to be caused by bacteria. He or she may use probes in your mouth to attempt to dilate (widen) the ducts. If the infection is persistent, you may be sent to a radiologist for a sialogram (X ray of the salivary gland), provided you are not in a period of acute infection. A CT scan (see p.261) is most often used today. If the gland has been irreversibly damaged, you will probably be advised to have it removed. Your other salivary glands will compensate for the one that you have lost.

Salivary duct stones

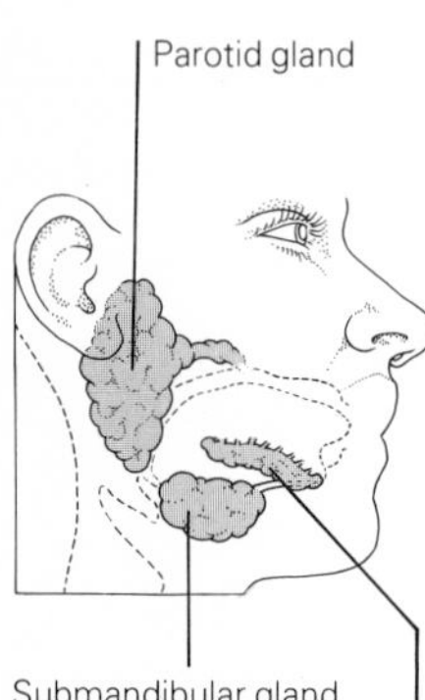

A stone, or tiny hard particle, forms in the duct of a salivary gland when chemicals and salts in the saliva encrust a minute bit of solid material or mucus in the duct. The stone partially blocks the duct, and most of the large quantity of saliva produced when you eat cannot pass the stone so that the gland becomes swollen. The submandibular salivary glands, in the floor of your mouth, are the most susceptible of your salivary glands to this uncommon disorder. Middle-aged and older people are most frequently affected by salivary duct stones.

What should be done?

If you have any swelling under your chin or behind or under the angle of your jaw, particularly while eating, and especially if it is painful, see your physician. He or she may arrange for an X ray (see p.258) to be taken of your mouth. If the cause is still not clear, you may have a sialogram (X ray of the salivary gland). In some cases, ultrasound testing or a CT scan may also be performed to help in the diagnosis of stones in your ducts.

What is the treatment?

If you have a salivary duct stone, it can usually be removed under local anesthetic. If it recurs, a permanent opening can be cut along the duct so that saliva can drain into your mouth almost directly from the gland. Then the possibility of further stones and subsequent scarring of the duct is avoided.

If a stone is inside the salivary gland itself, the gland may be surgically removed. This procedure is particularly advisable when frequent infections occur.

Salivary gland tumors

Most salivary gland tumors form in one of two parotid glands, which are located above the angle of your jaw. Most of these tumors are benign (unlikely to spread). Some salivary gland tumors recur at their original site or nearby. They generally develop slowly over several years, and gradually cause the gland to swell and remain swollen. There are no other symptoms. However, there is a very small risk that the growth may be, or may become, malignant (likely to spread).

If one or more of your salivary glands is swollen and possibly painful, or if you have any pain or discomfort in your mouth, see your physician or dentist. He or she may recommend a biopsy (a procedure in which a small sample of tissue is removed for examination), which can help diagnose a tumor. An MRI (see p.262) or CT scan (see p.261) can make a clear image of a salivary gland tumor.

What is the treatment?

If you do have a tumor in your salivary gland, you will probably be advised to have it removed surgically. If the tumor is found to be malignant, radiation therapy after the surgery is usually recommended.

In operations on the parotid gland, there is a risk of damage to an adjacent nerve that controls the movements of your lower face. Branches of the facial nerve may be cut or injured when other salivary glands are removed. However, surgery can usually repair such damage if it occurs.

Tumors of the mouth and tongue

Tumors can occur anywhere in or on your mouth, except on the teeth. There are two types of tumors, benign and malignant. The causes of both of these types are unknown. A benign tumor is usually a slow-growing lump that does not spread to surrounding areas and threaten life. A malignant (likely to spread) tumor of the tongue may grow within a few months, while those in other parts of the mouth spread over several years. (See also Salivary gland tumors, previous article.)

What are the symptoms?

Benign tumors of the mouth usually occur singly. Such a tumor starts as a small, pale lump, which then grows slowly over several years. If it grows larger than ⅓ in (about 10 mm) across, it may cause fitting problems with dentures, and even slight distortion of the face. A benign tumor on your tongue may rupture and bleed extensively. Benign tumors are rarely painful.

A malignant tumor also may begin as a single, small, pale lump, but then usually turns into an ulcer with a hard, raised rim and a fragile center that bleeds easily. The ulcer grows and erodes the surrounding area of your mouth. If the ulcer spreads over your tongue, the cancerous cells make the tongue muscles stiff and fixed, which then results in difficulty in eating, swallowing, and speaking. Malignant tumors are not usually painful until they grow in size and reach an advanced stage.

What are the risks?

Malignant tumors of the mouth are very rare generally, and they are extremely rare in people under 40. They are more common among heavy smokers, drinkers, and tobacco chewers. Malignant tumors are most common among people over 60. Tumors of the tongue and lip occur more frequently in men. Benign tumors of the mouth seem to be about as rare as malignant tumors.

Benign tumors usually do not present a risk. Malignant tumors carry the risk of metastasizing, or spreading, to other parts of your body. The later that a malignant tumor anywhere in your body is diagnosed and treated, the more likely it is that the cancer will become life-threatening.

What should be done?

Consult your physician at once if you have any lump, ulcer, or unexplained color change in your mouth that does not clear up within 10 days, or if your dentures do not fit well any more, or if your tongue has become stiff and difficult to control.

If you have a tumor, a small sample will be removed for a biopsy, a procedure that is done in a few minutes with local anesthesia. Treatment will depend on whether the tumor is benign or malignant.

What is the treatment?

Most benign tumors cause no problems. However, you should have your physician or dentist check them every 6 to 12 months to make sure there has been no change. Large benign tumors on the lips can be removed surgically, and your natural features can usually be restored by plastic surgery (see p.279). Special dentures can restore the natural appearance of your gums.

The treatment for malignant tumors and the success of the treatment depend on the stage the disease has reached by the time the problem is diagnosed and the treatment is begun. If this is an early stage and the tumor has not spread, it is removed surgically. If the tumor has spread, radiation therapy is often used, with or without surgery. Cases that are diagnosed and treated in an early stage are usually completely cured.

Tongue problems

The upper surface of the tongue is covered by papillae, or tiny hairlike projections of tissue. Groups of taste buds are clustered around the papillae. Normally, the papillae are pink and velvety and are crossed by fissures. These fissures expose the deep-red muscular body of the tongue beneath. But in some people various alterations take place in the normal color and texture of the surface of the tongue. Most such tongue problems are not serious and need no treatment. If, however, you have any tongue problem that persists for more than 10 days, you should consult your physician promptly.

Glossitis and geographic tongue

Glossitis is a treatable inflammation of the tongue in which the papillae no longer form properly and no longer cover the body of the tongue. Geographic tongue is a similar disorder, but it differs from glossitis in that it occurs in patches that come and go, and there is no known cause or treatment for it. In both disorders, the exposed surface of your tongue becomes smooth and dark red, with raised margins, and often feels sore, especially if you eat spicy foods.

Glossitis can have many causes, including infection, injury, nutritional deficiency, and

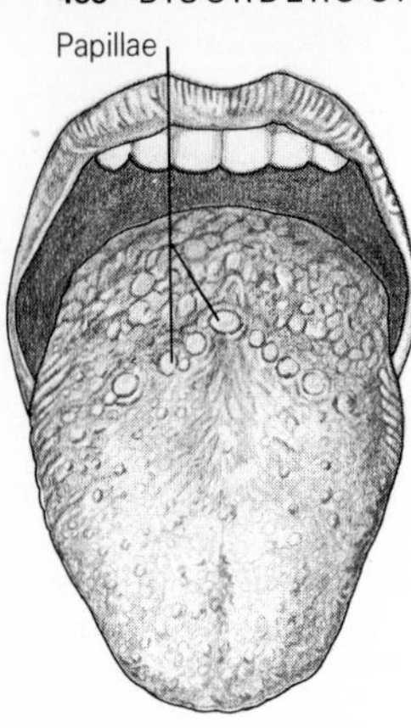

The tongue
The tongue is covered with circular papillae. Taste buds are scattered among them.

allergic reactions. If you have the symptoms described for glossitis, see your physician. If you have an underlying disorder, treating it will also clear up the glossitis. If there is no underlying cause of the inflammation, there is no need for treatment.

Your physician may prescribe an antiseptic mouthwash. If you avoid hot or spicy foods or drinks, alcohol, and tobacco, you may help relieve the soreness caused by glossitis or geographic tongue.

Discolored and fissured tongue

Your tongue may become discolored for any of several reasons, but this is usually not a problem. Some people have tongues that are fissured, or creased, more deeply or extensively than usual. Pieces of food, coffee, and tea accumulate in the fissures or on the papillae and may make your tongue appear to be black or dark brown. The discoloration may also be caused by fungal infections such as oral thrush (see p.484), by smoking, or by taking antibiotics. Sometimes the papillae become long and hairlike. Neither the fissures, the hairlike papillae, nor the discoloration is serious. To restore your tongue to normal, brush it gently twice a day with a toothbrush if it does not hurt to do so. Dip the toothbrush first into an antiseptic mouthwash. Also, any generalized disorders should be treated as well.

One type of discoloration, called furred tongue, may occur when you are ill with a viral infection, especially when you have a fever. You may notice a whitish or yellowish furry coating on the surface of your tongue. Your tongue usually returns to normal as soon as the illness clears up. No treatment is needed for furred tongue.

Esophagus

The esophagus is the muscular tube that runs from the back of your throat through your neck and chest to your stomach. As you swallow, the back of your tongue pushes a ball of food into the esophagus. The soft palate closes off the passage to your nose, and the epiglottis, a flap at the top of the windpipe, closes so that food cannot get into your trachea, or lower windpipe, and then into your lungs. Rhythmic contractions of the esophageal muscles move the food down through the chest into the base of the esophagus, where a segment of the muscle at the entrance to your stomach relaxes to let the food pass through.

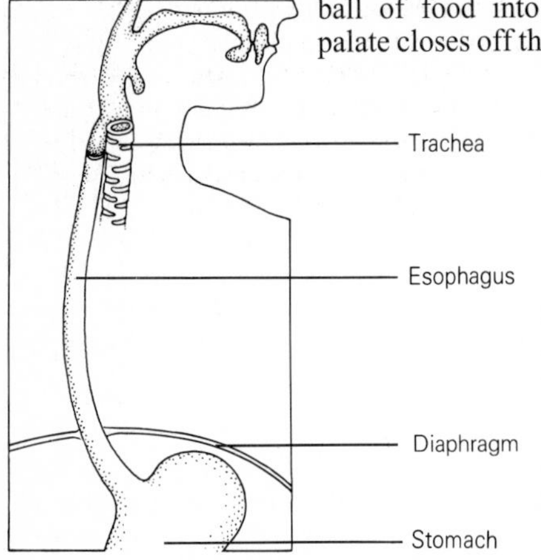

Swallowing
When you swallow, the top of the trachea temporarily closes so that food will move into the esophagus. Muscle contractions then move the food along the esophagus and into the stomach.

Difficult swallowing is called dysphagia; painful swallowing is called odontophagia. They are not diseases, but are symptoms of nearly all diseases of the esophagus. And since both are the major symptom of a malignant (likely to spread) growth in your esophagus, always consult your physician immediately if you begin to have trouble swallowing. Chances of having a serious disorder are slight, but if you do have a serious condition, an early diagnosis is essential for effective treatment.

Reflux esophagitis, heartburn, and hiatal hernia

Food and drink that you swallow pass through an opening controlled by the muscles at the junction of the esophagus and the stomach. If this opening leaks for any reason, stomach acid may back up into the lower esophagus, where it may cause inflammation and eventually, in severe cases, ulceration. This process is called reflux esophagitis and its main symptoms are increasing pain in the lower part of the sternum (breastbone) and heartburn. Heartburn is a burning sensation in the upper abdomen that may result from muscle spasm.

The esophageal opening into the stomach is controlled by esophageal muscles and by the sheets of muscle in the diaphragm, which

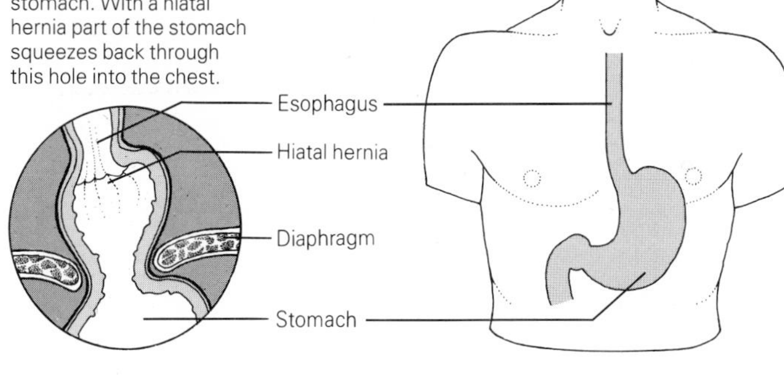

A hiatal hernia
The stomach is below the diaphragm. The esophagus passes through a hole in the diaphragm and enters the stomach. With a hiatal hernia part of the stomach squeezes back through this hole into the chest.

separates your chest from your abdomen. If control of this opening (hiatus) becomes weakened, acid reflux may occur, especially if your stomach is very full and you are lying flat, bending over, or stooping. In some cases the weakened hiatus allows part of the upper stomach to protrude into the chest; this condition is called a hiatal hernia. Some people have hiatal hernias but are not troubled by any pain or heartburn; some people have symptoms of reflux esophagitis but do not have hiatal hernias.

What are the symptoms?

The main symptom, if any, is usually a painful burning sensation in your chest. It occurs with some predictable regularity when the stomach is overly full, with changes in position, or when the abdomen is full, such as during pregnancy (see Heartburn during pregnancy, p.668). If you bend forward or lie down, stomach acid can more easily flow into the esophagus. Heartburn is often particularly common at night when you lie down after a heavy meal. It takes 2 hours for food to move through your stomach after you eat, so don't go to bed until at least 2 hours after dinner.

Another symptom is regurgitation of acid fluid into your throat. Belching is common.

What are the risks?

Hiatal hernia is common, especially among overweight, older people. But again, everyone with hiatal hernia does not experience heartburn. Hiatal hernia is not in itself a severe or dangerous ailment. But persistent acid reflux, no matter what causes it, can lead to inflammation or ulceration of the esophagus. Inflammation can lead to scarring and narrowing of the esophagus (see p.491). In rare cases, esophageal ulcers bleed, which may cause anemia (see p.450).

What should be done?

If the symptoms are troublesome, your physician may recommend an endoscopy (see p.264) and tests to measure changes in pressure that occur during swallowing, and changes in acidity that occur during the day.

What is the treatment?

Self-help: If you are overweight, one of the most effective self-help measures is to lose weight (see Obesity, p.530). Avoid stooping, lying down, or bending over, particularly after a meal. Do not wear tight girdles or belts. Raise the head of your bed about 4 to 6 inches by standing the legs on books or bricks, to reduce acid reflux at night. Avoid liqueurs, sweet drinks, syrups, or honey, which aggravate the symptoms. And do not smoke, since smoking encourages the production of stomach acid. Try taking a nonprescription antacid at least an hour before meals and at bedtime. Be sure to follow the directions on the label. These preparations neutralize stomach acid.

The symptoms of hiatal hernia can often be relieved by not overfilling your stomach, so eat several small meals each day instead of two or three large ones. Doing this will also help neutralize stomach acid.

Professional help: If taking nonprescription antacids is ineffective, your physician may prescribe a drug to block the formation of acid in the stomach. He or she may also prescribe a medication that increases the speed with which food passes through the stomach and into the intestines.

The above measures usually prevent acid reflux and relieve the pain and heartburn. If your symptoms persist, if you have a documented hiatal hernia, if severe inflammation of the esophagus occurs, and if complications develop, your physician may recommend surgery to repair the hernia.

Cancer of the esophagus

In this disorder, cells in the lining of the esophagus start to multiply rapidly and form a tumor that is likely to grow and spread to other parts of the body. The tumor eventually causes narrowing and constriction of the passageway to your stomach. As with other types of cancer, the cause is unknown, though cancer of the esophagus has been linked with prolonged exposure to irritants such as tobacco smoke and alcohol.

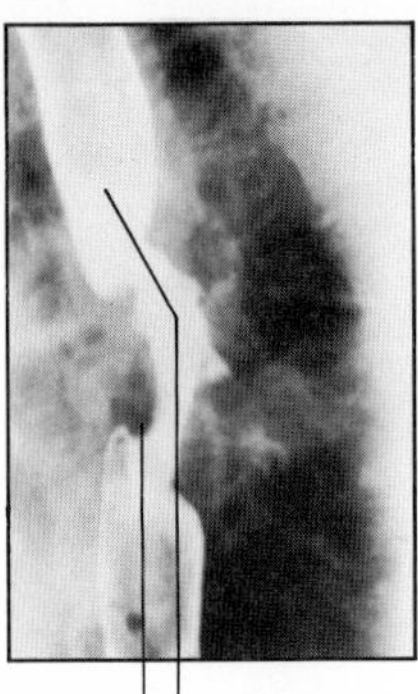

An X ray reveals a cancerous growth narrowing the esophagus.

What are the symptoms?
The main symptom is difficulty or pain when swallowing that worsens. At first only solids are hard to swallow, but then liquids also become a problem. An additional symptom is rapid, progressive weight loss. Occasionally, you may regurgitate bloody mucus also.

What are the risks?
Cancer of the esophagus is rare. Men are about twice as susceptible as women, and the risk seems to be greatest for heavy smokers and drinkers who are 50 to 60 years old.

If the condition is detected in an early stage, there is a chance for successful treatment. Otherwise, the cancer can spread swiftly, blocking the esophagus and also spreading to vital neighboring organs. Less than 10 percent of those who have cancer of the esophagus survive for 5 or more years after the condition is discovered.

What should be done?
If you experience difficult or painful swallowing, see your physician right away. Even though the chance of a cancerous tumor is slight, your physician will probably suggest diagnostic tests, including a barium swallow X ray, a thorough examination of the esophagus by endoscopy, and a biopsy, in which a sample of tissue is removed for examination under a microscope.

If you have cancer of the esophagus, the usual treatment is surgery. Radiation therapy may also be used to destroy cancer cells or to slow down the progress of the disease. Some cancers of the esophagus respond to chemotherapy (anticancer drugs).

Achalasia

When you swallow food, it is guided down the esophagus by rhythmic contractions of the muscles in its wall. When food reaches the entrance to the stomach, the muscle segment there relaxes and permits the food to pass. In the rare disorder known as achalasia, the nerves that control the muscles of the lower end of your esophagus become defective, and the muscle at this site is no longer able to relax, preventing food from leaving the esophagus. In time the contractions in the body of the esophagus become irregular and uncoordinated.

What are the symptoms?
The main symptom of achalasia is the regurgitation of food you have eaten a day or so before. Because food accumulates in the esophagus and there may be discomfort or pain in your chest, you are likely to have an unpleasant taste in your mouth and bad breath. At first, only solid food will be hard to swallow, but eventually you will have difficulty swallowing liquids also.

As achalasia worsens, the esophagus is never properly emptied, and there is always a chance that you might inhale food particles while you sleep. These can cause chest infections such as pneumonia (see p.384). Because most of your food does not pass into the intestines to be absorbed, you may also lose weight and show signs of malnutrition.

What should be done?
If you suspect you have achalasia, consult your physician, who will probably arrange to examine the esophagus by endoscopy. A barium swallow X ray may also be used to confirm the diagnosis. One form of treatment for achalasia involves passing a slender rubber bag down the esophagus and filling the bag with water or air in order to stretch the muscles at the bottom. This procedure allows food to pass into your stomach more easily. This relieves the problem for variable periods of time (6 months to several years) and can be repeated as often as necessary. An operation called a cardiomyotomy, in which some of the muscles at the stomach entrance are cut to open the passageway for food, is effective for some people but carries the risk of reflux esophagitis (see p.488).

Pharyngeal pouch

A pharyngeal pouch is a bulge or sac that develops at the pharynx, which is in the back of the throat just at the top of the esophagus. This rare disorder occurs most often in older men. It usually happens because the muscles become uncoordinated during swallowing, enabling the muscle bundles to spread apart and allowing the lining to push through and form the bulge. Food enters the bulge during swallowing; the bulge then stretches downward to form a baglike pouch. The pouch gradually grows bigger, and it becomes increasingly difficult to swallow. The pouch itself may show up as a swelling at the side of your neck. Regurgitation of fluid or undigested food into your mouth may occur. An irritating cough and a metallic taste in your mouth may also develop.

Pharynx
Pharyngeal pouch
Trachea
Esophagus

The main risk of a pharyngeal pouch is that fluid from the pouch may enter your lungs while you sleep and cause pneumonia.

What should be done?

Consult your physician if you have any difficulty in swallowing. He or she will usually be able to diagnose pharyngeal pouch from a physical examination and a description of your symptoms. However, a barium swallow X ray may be needed to confirm this diagnosis. Some people are able to learn to get the pouch to empty down the esophagus by kneading it with their fingers against the neck. Treatment is determined by your ability to help the pouch to empty and to maintain your weight; if this cannot be done and the pouch continues to expand, your physician will recommend surgical removal of the pouch.

Diffuse spasm of the esophagus

This is a rare condition for which there is no known cause. However, stress is often associated with the condition. It consists of irregular, repeated spasms of the muscles of the esophageal wall, which can cause chest pains and difficulty in swallowing. Diffuse spasm of the esophagus develops gradually, with intermittent attacks over a period of years. To help relieve the spasms, a calcium channel blocker drug may be prescribed.

Stricture of the esophagus

This is a rare disorder that occurs as a result of an accumulation of scar tissue in the esophagus, often caused by persistent acid reflux (see Reflux esophagitis, heartburn, and hiatal hernia, p.488). The scarred portions of the esophagus gradually constrict (narrow) the passageway for food. The result is difficulty in swallowing. Consult your physician immediately if you have this symptom.

The usual treatment for stricture is to enlarge the passageway with either a water-filled rubber bag (see Achalasia, previous page) or a flexible metal rod called a bougie. This procedure, which is done while you are sedated, must be repeated every few months. Surgery to remove the scar tissue may become necessary if enlarging the passageway becomes too difficult.

Infections of the digestive tract

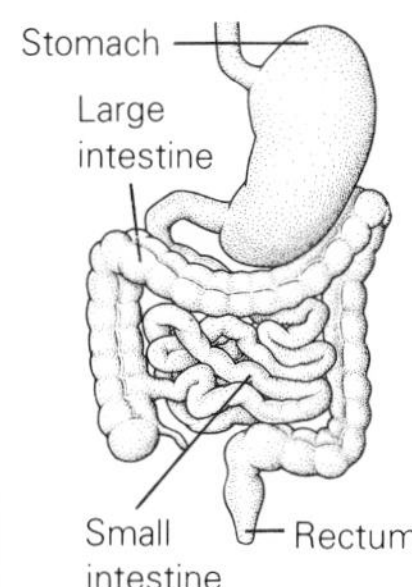

An infection of the digestive, or gastrointestinal, tract occurs when certain infectious agents, such as viruses or bacteria, multiply rapidly in your stomach and/or intestines. This causes disorders of various kinds and varying severity.

The intestines normally contain bacteria that are harmless. In fact, some of them are essential to the formation of some vitamins and are, therefore, desirable. The presence of such organisms is not considered an infection; this term is generally used only to describe the presence of large numbers of organisms that cause disease. The unchecked multiplication of such agents brings on a number of symptoms such as vomiting and diarrhea, along with symptoms of more generalized illness if the infectious organisms or their toxins (poisons) ultimately enter your bloodstream.

Gastroenteritis

Gastroenteritis refers to an irritation and inflammation of the digestive tract that causes upset stomach and intestines. It is most commonly caused by a virus infection, easily passed from one person to another without direct personal contact or the consumption of food or drink. Such infections are the most common cause of the 24- or 36-hour attacks of vomiting and/or diarrhea that are often called intestinal or stomach flu.

Gastroenteritis can also be caused by eating or drinking contaminated food or water. A different kind of food poisoning can occur if you eat something that contains a toxic substance, such as a nonedible mushroom or a rhubarb leaf. Such kinds of food poisoning are not caused by infection, but they are capable of bringing on attacks of gastroenteritis that can be very serious (see Box, p.495). Eggs, milk products, and shellfish have also been known to affect people who are sensitive to them.

Another possible cause of gastroenteritis is a change in the natural bacterial population of the digestive tract. If you have an illness that weakens you, or if you suddenly make drastic changes in your diet (for example, when you visit another country), the balance of bacteria in your digestive tract may become disturbed so that certain bacterial strains become stronger at the expense of others, and this can cause an upset stomach and intestines. Antibiotic drugs often have a similar effect by acting selectively and disrupting the bacterial equilibrium in your intestines, permitting unchecked growth of bacteria that secrete fungus yeast toxins (poisons).

What are the symptoms?

The symptoms of gastroenteritis range from a mild attack of nausea followed by diarrhea, which happens to nearly everybody at some time, to a severe illness. You may have one or two bouts of vomiting and some soft stools that hardly interfere with your routine. Or you may vomit repeatedly and have recurrent attacks of watery diarrhea with abdominal pains and cramps, fever, and extreme weakness. Occasionally, an extreme case of gastroenteritis lasts so long that it disables you, but usually the symptoms go away within 24 to 48 hours.

What are the risks?

Gastroenteritis is a very common ailment, and most people get their first attack early in life (see Gastroenteritis in infants, p.695).

Risks depend on the type and number of infectious agents, the amount and strength of the tainted food substances that you have eaten, and your age and general health. The danger of severe illness is greatest for newborn babies, infants less than about 18 months old, and chronically ill older people. Continuing diarrhea causes dehydration and loss of certain crucial body salts, which upsets body chemistry and, if unchecked, can lead to shock (see p.414). In a normally healthy person a bout of vomiting and diarrhea is no more significant than a common cold. But if there is also severe and persistent pain in the abdomen (not just an occasional cramp), the symptoms may be caused by some other abdominal disorder.

What should be done?

If the self-help measures recommended below do not relieve, or at least greatly improve, the symptoms within 2 or, at most, 3 days, consult your physician. After examining you, your physician may send a sample of your stools to a laboratory for analysis. More probably, your diagnosis will be confirmed by your answers to questions about what you have eaten and whether other family members or associates are ill, your physician's observations of the state of your health, and any information he or she may have about a local epidemic of this disorder.

Analysis of your stools may be necessary, however, if diarrhea is prolonged, to make sure that your gastroenteritis is not caused by a serious intestinal infection.

What is the treatment?

Self-help: If you have an attack of gastroenteritis, stay at home, rest, and after you have stopped vomiting, drink plenty of fluids until the attack subsides. The safest and most easily tolerated fluid is an oral rehydration solution, a mixture of water, salts, and glucose. The solution is available over the counter as a powder concentrate, or you can make a solution at home (see p.839). If you have diarrhea you should drink some of the fluid at half-hour intervals until you pass pale-colored urine; an adult with severe diarrhea may need to drink a few quarts (liters) of the solution in a day before this occurs. Once the diarrhea begins to ease, increase the kinds of fluids you drink to include unsweetened fruit juices, tea, clear broth or bouillon, and then add flavored gelatin, cooked cereal, and other bland, soft foods. After about 2 or 3 days of this routine you should be able to resume your diet.

Over-the-counter antidiarrhea medicines may relieve symptoms, but remember that they are not an alternative to the fluid replacement essential for treating diarrhea. Antibiotics should be used only on the advice of your physician. Gastroenteritis is often caused by poor hygiene and is easily passed on to others. Avoid restaurants where there is any hint of poor sanitation. Be sure that you wash your hands thoroughly after you use the toilet and also before you touch food.

Professional help: There is no specific treatment for viral gastroenteritis. If the diagnosis is clear and your nausea and diarrhea are relatively mild, your physician will probably advise you to continue the self-help measures recommended above. If your vomiting is severe, your physician may prescribe an antiemetic drug in suppository form or by injection. Diarrhea is sometimes treated with other medications such as narcotic-type drugs or antispasmodic drugs that slow down intestinal activity and may relieve cramping. Any such treatment is usually stopped as soon as the intestines begin to function normally.

If your vomiting and diarrhea are so severe that you become dehydrated, and especially if you also have a chronic disease such as diabetes mellitus (see p.558) or kidney problems (see p.540), your physician may admit you to the hospital so that fluid can be replaced intravenously and your blood chemistry can be restored to a proper balance.

Salmonellosis

Although the bacteria known as *Salmonella* are often present in the bodies of farm animals, these animals seldom appear to be ill. People who eat *Salmonella*-infected meat or eggs, however, may get salmonellosis, which is an infection similar to gastroenteritis (see previous article), but which has some additional unpleasant symptoms.

One cause of infection is failure to thaw food sufficiently before it is cooked, so that it does not cook all the way through. Also, sometimes meat is not frozen immediately after an animal is slaughtered. Any delay permits a small number of bacteria to multiply, and the meat becomes infected. *Salmonella* bacteria are not killed by freezing and even fresh, apparently safe, meats can contain them. However, the bacteria are killed by thorough cooking.

Salmonellosis often occurs as an epidemic if a number of people eat the same contaminated food. But you need not eat infected food to get salmonellosis. The bacteria can also spread from person to person on the fingers of anyone who handles infected foods or by the use of contaminated kitchen utensils. (See Box on food poisoning, p.495.) Finally, it is possible to carry the bacteria in your intestines even after you recover from the infection. So it is important that you wash your hands carefully before you handle food.

Food that can cause salmonellosis

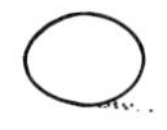

Raw or improperly cooked eggs

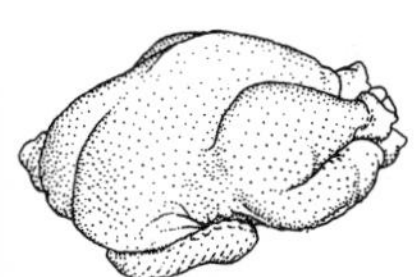

Insufficiently thawed poultry

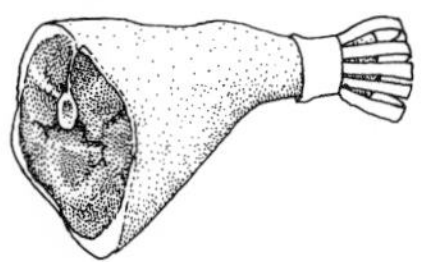

Improperly cooked meat

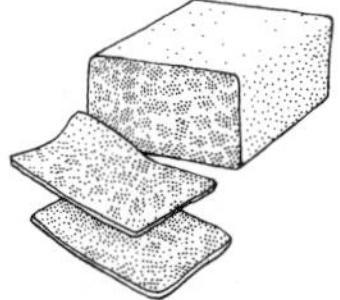

Cooked meat poorly reheated

What are the symptoms?

The main symptom is diarrhea. It is often accompanied by abdominal cramps, vomiting, fever, and chills. Occasionally there is blood in the stools. The type and degree of diarrhea varies. You may have only one or two loose bowel movements a day, or you may have a severe attack of watery diarrhea every 10 to 15 minutes. If this continues for a few hours, it can eventually cause total prostration and collapse. A mild attack of salmonellosis that clears up quickly on its own can easily be mistaken for a simple attack of gastroenteritis.

What are the risks?

Children under age 6 are the most likely to get the disease. Apart from an occasional epidemic, salmonellosis is not specifically identified, since the stools of most people with gastroenteritis are not sent to a laboratory for analysis. Nobody, therefore, knows how many cases of salmonellosis are erroneously diagnosed as gastroenteritis.

If the *Salmonella* bacteria spread from your digestive tract into your bloodstream, they may settle in the organs such as the liver, kidneys, gallbladder, or heart, or in the joints, and cause inflammation or perhaps an abscess. This seldom happens, however. Most *Salmonella* infections are mild and do not require treatment. In a severe attack of salmonellosis, the excessive loss of body fluid that results from repeated bouts of diarrhea can cause death from dehydration if the disease is not treated.

What should be done?

If you have diarrhea that lasts for more than 2 or 3 days, or if you have a combination of fever, chills, abdominal pain, diarrhea, and vomiting, consult your physician (see also Gastroenteritis, previous article).

What is the treatment?

If *Salmonella* infection spreads from the digestive tract, treatment depends on the resulting disorder. Treatment for the disease itself usually includes an antibiotic. Complete recovery can be expected.

Very rarely, after the diarrhea has gone and you are completely recovered, a few *Salmonella* organisms may still remain in your digestive tract and may be excreted occasionally in stools. Nothing can be done about this, and it seldom continues for more than 3 months. It is a problem, however, because it poses a continuing risk of spreading infection.

Bacillary dysentery

This is a fairly rare disease in developed countries, but epidemics of it may occur in densely populated areas with poor sanitation. It is possible to get it while traveling in such an area. It is caused by *Shigella* bacillus, a bacterium that invades the lining of the large intestine, and it is spread from person to person in unhygienic conditons, especially from food handlers to those eating the contaminated food. The main symptoms of bacillary dysentery are abdominal cramps, fever, and diarrhea, which are similar to those of gastroenteritis (see p.491), but the diarrhea may contain blood and pus if you have bacillary dysentery.

Preventive measures and treatment for this disease are much the same as they are for most other gastrointestinal infections (see Salmonellosis, previous article). However, if the symptoms become severe, your physician may prescribe antibiotics in combination with measures to restore body fluids.

Amebic dysentery

Amebic dysentery, which is caused by a microscopic single-celled organism, is more common in developing countries where there is poor sanitation. The main symptom is cramping diarrhea, which may be bloody and may persist for a few weeks if not treated. After the diarrhea subsides, it may recur from time to time. Occasionally the organisms spread from the digestive tract into the bloodstream and settle in the liver, where they form abscesses (pus-filled sacs). This infection is sometimes caught while traveling, most often in a developing country. It is spread by contaminated water and lack of sanitation among food handlers.

What is the treatment?

If your physician suspects that you have amebic dysentery, samples of your stool will probably be needed for analysis, and a blood test may also be performed.

Treatment involves taking specific anti-amebic drugs, usually for up to 3 weeks. After diarrhea has ceased, your physician will ask you to come in monthly with stool samples to be examined until no infecting organisms are found for 2 or 3 months in a row. Meanwhile, be careful to wash your hands thoroughly after you use the toilet to avoid reinfection or spreading the infection. Thorough cooking destroys the organisms.

Typhoid fever

Typhoid fever is an infectious disease spread under unsanitary conditions either from person to person or through contaminated food or water. Some people carry typhoid-causing bacteria in their bodies and infect others after they get over the disease or without getting the disease themselves. The symptoms of typhoid fever begin suddenly with headache, loss of appetite, and vomiting. These are followed by persistent fever of around 104°F (40°C), chills, increasing weakness, diarrhea (usually bloody), and often delirium. Early in the disease, you may have a pink abdominal rash, which then fades. Recovery takes 2 or 3 weeks if there are no complications. But typhoid fever can be a life-threatening disease because there may be very dangerous complications along with it, such as extensive gastrointestinal bleeding or rupture of the intestines.

Active immunization is effective in preventing this disease. Typhoid fever is rare in the US. Nearly all cases can be traced to recent travel or residence in a developing country, although the disease is still reported occasionally from rural areas of the US. If you are in such an area, or have recently returned, and if you have the symptoms described above, see a physician without delay. If typhoid fever is suspected, you will be admitted to a hospital isolation unit for diagnosis and treatment. You need to take antibiotics for about 2 weeks. It may take several more weeks before your digestive tract is free of infectious bacteria, and you do not have to worry about transmitting the infection. To make sure that you are free of typhoid bacteria, you are asked to bring in a stool sample monthly for 3 months—longer if you are a food handler.

Cholera

Cholera is a disease caused by bacteria that damage the intestinal lining and cause such severe diarrhea that up to 4 gallons (about 15 liters) of fluid per day are lost. The bacteria spread through polluted water, shellfish, or raw fruits and vegetables in places where sanitation is poor. This disease almost never appears in developed nations, and when it does, it can be traced to visits to or residence in developing countries. However, every year the US Public Health Service reports a few cases of choleralike illness caused by contamination of American shellfish with bacteria related to the cholera bacillus. The symptoms of the disease are abdominal pain and severe diarrhea. Bowel movements of people with cholera resemble murky water and may be passed almost continuously. You become extremely thirsty, have no fever, but you vomit intermittently without feeling nauseated. You may also have muscle cramps. If dehydration is not treated at once, cholera may quickly cause death.

If you are abroad or have just returned and have extremely watery, continuous diarrhea that does not improve within a couple of hours, get medical help immediately. The main treatment is to prevent or treat dehydration by replacing body fluids, usually by oral rehydration. You drink a mixture of salts, glucose, and water, which is quickly absorbed into your bloodstream, every few minutes until your body chemistry is restored to normal. Treatment with antibiotics is also helpful. Hospitalization may be necessary if you require intravenous fluids.

Food poisoning

The term food poisoning is commonly used to mean any illness with vomiting, diarrhea, and abdominal pain that is caused by food or liquids (including water) contaminated by infectious organisms or their toxins (poisons). It is a hazard especially associated with the precooking and reheating of foods that have been prepared without observing sanitation requirements. The most common types of food poisoning are described below.

Staphylococcal food poisoning comes from eating food contaminated with the toxin of *Staphylococcus* bacteria. It can cause gastroenteritis (see p.491), an acute bout of vomiting, abdominal cramps, and sometimes diarrhea. Symptoms usually develop within 1 to 6 hours of eating infected food such as potato salad or chicken salad, or other food prepared with mayonnaise, that has been standing at room temperature. In most otherwise healthy people, the illness goes away without specific treatment.

Outbreaks of this type of food poisoning are usually caused by food that has been contaminated during or after cooking, often from an infected cut or boil on the food handler's skin, and allowed to remain warm (not refrigerated) for several hours before it is eaten. Preventive measures include scrupulous hand washing by food handlers, rapid cooling of cooked foods before refrigeration, and immediate and thorough reheating of cold items.

Salmonella infections (other than typhoid) come from eating food—especially poultry, meat, and eggs—contaminated with the bacteria (see p.493). *Campylobacter* is another common cause of bacterial food poisoning; it may contaminate unpasteurized milk and dairy products or water supplies.

Listeria are bacteria that are widespread in soil and in the stools of animals, and they are common contaminants of foods such as soft cheeses. In contrast to most other bacteria they can multiply at temperatures close to freezing and so may grow in food stored in a refrigerator. Prolonged storage of foods such as whipped cream cakes in restaurant refrigerated cases that are allowed to fluctuate in temperature may lead to contamination with *Listeria*. *Listeria* rarely causes serious illness in healthy people, but the bacteria are a threat to pregnant women and their fetuses, to older people, and to anyone with lowered natural resistance to infections. Such people may develop symptoms including diarrhea and occasionally more serious disorders such as meningitis (see p.290).

Botulism is a rare but often fatal food poisoning caused by a *Clostridium* bacterium that produces a toxin in food that is preserved or smoked, but not cooked to 212°F (100°C). Home-preserved vegetables and canned fruit and fish products have been sources of botulism outbreaks. Symptoms include abdominal pain, vomiting, blurring of vision, muscle weakness, and eventual paralysis, since the toxin interferes with motor nerve function. Hospitalization is required. Injecting an antitoxin may reverse the muscle paralysis from the original toxin. The sooner the diagnosis is made and treatment started, the better the outlook.

Precautions

In your own kitchen: Be sure all frozen food and especially frozen poultry has thawed completely or has been defrosted in the microwave oven before cooking. Wash carefully with soap and very hot water all knives, other utensils, cutting boards, and other surfaces used for the preparation of uncooked meat, fish, and poultry. Do not allow cooked food to sit out to cool; food being stored or kept for the next meal should be either hot or very cold. Don't keep returning to the refrigerator leftovers that have been put on the table several times. Check the freshness seals on all containers of canned and bottled foods to be sure they are still intact before opening. If a jar's lid is leaking, or if air escapes from a can as you open it, do not eat the contents. And if you are sick—especially if you have diarrhea or an infected sore on your hand or finger—get someone else to prepare the food. If you have any concerns about the storage or preparation of food at a restaurant, notify your state or local public health department.

In the home, make sure that all family members routinely wash their hands with soap and water after using the toilet and that they wash them again immediately before food preparation and consumption.

Stomach and duodenum

The stomach stores and processes food. In the stomach, the bulk of a chewed meal is transformed into a slow trickle of pulp. Inside the stomach, rhythmical contractions of powerful muscles in the stomach wall crush and pulverize the food repeatedly, and the chemical action of acid and enzymes, made in the stomach lining, breaks it down further. All this activity continues only while food remains in your stomach. In an empty stomach there is little muscular activity and virtually no release of acid or enzymes.

The processed food trickles out of the stomach through a muscle segment, the pyloric sphincter, and into the duodenum, the uppermost and shortest section of the small intestine. In the duodenum, a tube about 10 in (25 cm) long, bile and more enzymes are secreted and further digest the pulp before it passes into the rest of the small intestine. It takes at least 3 to 5 hours for the contents of a meal to reach the lower parts of the small intestine and leave the stomach and duodenum empty. Because the chemicals of the stomach are very strong, overproduction or faulty production of them can cause damage to the mucous membrane that lines the stomach and duodenum. Also, in some people this membrane is easily irritated by certain drugs or fluids. In most cases irritation causes only the familiar symptoms of indigestion or gastritis. But sometimes the action of powerful stomach chemicals can lead to a more serious disorder such as an erosion of the membrane or an ulcer in either the stomach or the duodenum.

The stomach and duodenum
Food is both stored and partially digested in the stomach. It then moves into the duodenum where further digestion takes place.

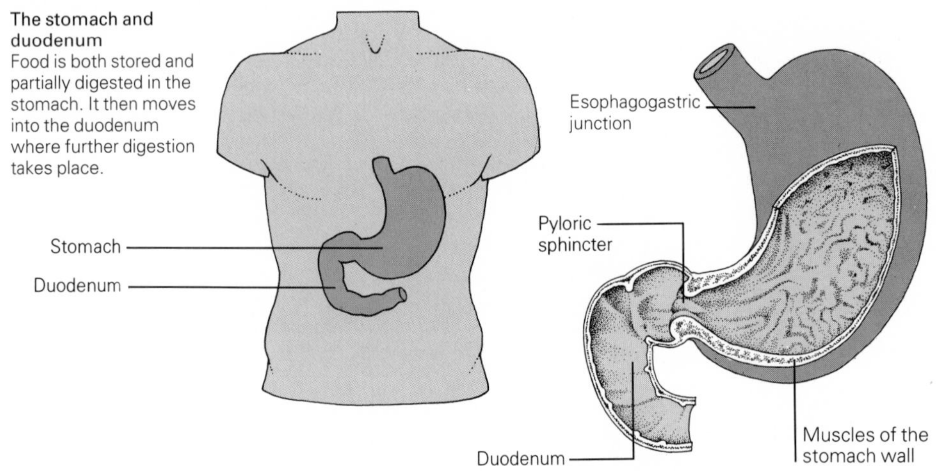

Indigestion
(dyspepsia)

Indigestion is a term used to describe any discomfort in the upper abdomen. If you have indigestion, you may feel a sense of discomfort or distension in your abdomen, or a sharp, dull, or gnawing pain in your lower chest. You may complain of heartburn, nausea, or the sour taste of acid fluid in your mouth. You may need to belch frequently. You may describe "butterflies" in your stomach and have more than one symptom.

What are the risks?

Some people get one or more of the symptoms of indigestion after eating particular foods such as cabbage, beans, onions, or cucumbers, or eating highly seasoned or fried foods, or drinking wine, after-dinner liqueurs, or carbonated drinks. Others suffer if they eat too fast or have an especially rich or big meal, or use syrup or honey. Still others get indigestion whenever they are anxious, nervous, or depressed. Pregnant women are very susceptible to indigestion, as are heavy smokers, people who are constipated, or overweight people.

Indigestion is troublesome, but it is not dangerous in itself. Many people have indigestion on and off throughout their lives without further complications, possibly because they repeatedly eat too quickly or eat foods known to disagree with them. There is always a chance, however, that the symptoms may be caused by a serious illness. You probably know how your stomach behaves in given situations, and you either use nonprescription remedies for indigestion whenever it occurs or try to prevent it by avoiding the things that cause it. Perhaps you take an occasional calculated risk by eating or drinking unwisely (for you) simply because the temporary pleasure outweighs the near certainty of later discomfort. There are usually no serious risks in such behavior. What you should watch out for, however, is a change in the symptoms. If the intensity or timing of your symptoms is different, if they come on spontaneously, or if they become more frequent, something other than your familiar indigestion may be causing them. You may have a peptic ulcer (see p.500), a gallbladder disorder (see Cholecystitis, p.528), a duodenal ulcer (see p.500), a liver disorder (see p.522), or even, very rarely, stomach cancer (see p.498).

What should be done?

Learn to recognize your symptoms and deal with them by using the self-help methods below. If the pattern of symptoms changes, consult your physician right away. Always seek medical advice if you notice any persistent loss of appetite or weight, or if your familiar attacks of indigestion become more frequent or more severe or start without an obvious cause. In such cases your physician will probably arrange for diagnostic tests that usually include endoscopy, and barium X rays of the stomach and duodenum. Other possible tests include an ultrasound (see p.260) of the gallbladder, blood tests, stool samples, and samples of digestive juices from your stomach.

What is the treatment?

Self-help: Avoid food or drink that causes your indigestion. Adjust your eating and drinking habits to your stomach's idiosyncrasies. Do not smoke. Avoid aspirin, which may cause stomach bleeding; use acetaminophen if you need a painkiller. Try to avoid losing your temper or becoming overexcited, especially during meals. Do not eat too quickly or gulp down your food. Try to relax for half an hour after a meal. Some people find that commercially available antacid preparations help relieve the symptoms of heartburn. For additional self-help suggestions, see the Gastritis article below.

Professional help: Your physician's first task is to find out whether your indigestion is caused by an underlying disease. The more accurately you can describe your symptoms and their relationship to food, drink, and stress and strain, the easier it will be for your physician to determine the probable cause. Recent advances in imaging techniques, especially the availability of endoscopy, ultrasound, and CT scanners, have made an accurate diagnosis possible in most patients with a chronic digestive disorder. New treatments have also been developed; your physician will probably be able to provide advice and prescription medications for the condition that is causing your symptoms.

Gastritis and gastric erosion

Gastritis is a misused and misunderstood term that literally means inflammation of the stomach lining (mucous membrane). It may appropriately be used for bacterial and viral infection or the inflammation and ulceration caused by drugs (such as large doses of aspirin, ibuprofen, and other nonsteroidal anti-inflammatory drugs), alcohol, or certain anticancer drugs. The very similar discomfort frequently caused by heavy smoking, overeating, or eating highly seasoned or fried food is called gastritis by many people but is instead a form of indigestion. One type of gastritis has been associated with *Helicobacter pylori*, a bacterium implicated as a cause of some peptic ulcers (see p. 500).

A gastric erosion is a very superficial raw area in the mucous membrane that lines the stomach. It is usually caused by certain drugs that can irritate the stomach lining when taken by mouth. The nonsteroidal anti-inflammatory drugs, including aspirin, used for the treatment of arthritis and other musculoskeletal problems may cause gastric erosions. Corticosteroid drugs used in the treatment of asthma and other disorders such as temporal arteritis may also cause gastric erosions or an ulcer. Similar stomach lesions may develop in people recovering from injuries or severe burns and also in people under prolonged emotional stress.

What are the symptoms?

The symptoms of infectious gastritis are similar to those of gastroenteritis (see p.491) but are predominantly nausea, vomiting, and discomfort in your upper abdomen. If the disorder is caused by smoking or excessive drinking or eating, or by irritation from a drug, the symptoms will resemble those of severe indigestion with or without nausea and vomiting (see previous article).

The main and sometimes the only symptom of a gastric erosion is bleeding of the affected area. If you vomit, there may be blood in your vomit; it may be red but is more likely to be smelly and a dark mahogany color because it is partly digested. Blood may appear in your stools. If the bleeding is substantial, the stools will look like a very foul, inky black ooze. If the bleeding is gradual you may be completely unaware of it, but you will eventually become anemic.

What are the risks?

Nearly everyone has an occasional relatively mild attack of gastritis. Such occasional attacks are most unlikely to be any danger to your health, but if you have recurrent severe attacks with pain and vomiting you should consult your physician.

Gastric erosions are not common and those severe enough to cause bloody vomiting are rare; but if you take aspirin or other anti-arthritis drugs regularly you substantially increase the risk of developing one.

If persistent internal bleeding is not detected and treated you will become anemic. There is also a slight risk of sudden severe bleeding, which will be vomited as red blood and/or passed as black stools. To minimize the risks many physicians recommend that their patients with arthritis use an enteric-coated aspirin that usually will not dissolve until it has passed out of the stomach. New antiarthritis drugs have been developed that seem to be less irritating to the stomach, but they are only for rheumatoid arthritis, and not for other forms.

If you are taking a painkiller or a drug for arthritis regularly, consult your physician immediately if you have any of the following symptoms: bloody vomiting, feeling abnormally fatigued, persistent indigestion, or black stools. If your physician definitely finds that you have bled from your stomach or duodenum but that you must continue to take these drugs, he or she may prescribe a drug that blocks gastric acid secretion or protects the stomach lining.

What should be done?

If you have repeated attacks of gastritis, you probably smoke, eat, or drink too much or carelessly. There are many good reasons for quitting smoking and giving up alcohol, especially if they cause symptoms such as stomachache. Try to eat regular meals on a consistent schedule. If you have an attack, follow the self-help ideas suggested below, but see your physician without delay if you have symptoms that suggest a gastric erosion.

If you have recurrent attacks of gastritis or symptoms of an erosion, your physician will probably recommend an endoscopy to examine the inside of your esophagus and stomach to look for any erosions and to exclude the possibility of an ulcer or cancer.

What is the treatment?

Self-help: If you are vomiting, eat nothing until the nausea and vomiting subside. Then take frequent small amounts of nonalcoholic liquids, preferably milk, water, or weak tea. After 24 hours begin to eat, but select only foods that you know agree with you and eat only a little at a time. If you have abdominal pain or discomfort, take an antacid. If you have repeated attacks, stop drinking alcohol, smoking, and eating any foods that you know are a problem for you for a month. If this works, the rest is up to you.

Professional help: To control some of your symptoms, your physician will probably prescribe an antacid. If the vomiting is severe you may be given suppositories or an injection of an antiemetic drug.

If you have gastritis or a gastric erosion caused by a drug, your physician may advise a change in medication. He or she may also suggest that you take your doses of anti-arthritis drug with food and regular doses of an antacid or acid-supressing drug. If there is no serious underlying disease and if you avoid taking the drug that has irritated your stomach, the gastric erosion should not recur.

Cancer of the stomach

A stomach cancer may first express itself with the symptoms of a peptic ulcer (see p.500). This does not mean that if you have a peptic ulcer it will inevitably lead to cancer. But it means that some cases of cancer of the stomach include an ulcer.

As in all cancers, the cells may spread to other parts of the body such as the lungs, the bones, or the liver. There are sometimes no symptoms at all until the disease has already spread too widely to be stopped.

What are the symptoms?

The first symptoms are easy to ignore. They are vague indigestion, with discomfort after eating, combined with loss of appetite. Only fairly late in the disease do symptoms such as severe pain in the upper abdomen, loss of weight, and frequent vomiting develop. Indications of prolonged bleeding from the cancer such as anemia (see p.450) and bloody vomit and stool are also symptoms that appear in the later inoperable stages.

What are the risks?

Cancer of the stomach has become significantly less common in the US over the past 40 years. It is twice as common in men as in women, and the chances of getting it increase with age.

If when a stomach cancer is discovered it is too far advanced to be removed, treatment cannot cure it, but anticancer drugs may help temporarily alleviate the symptoms.

What should be done?

If you develop symptoms of indigestion (see p.496) for the first time in your life, or if your usual indigestion changes in character, consult your physician without delay. If there is any suspicion of stomach cancer or if ulcers continue or recur, your physician will probably arrange for you to have an endoscopy and a barium X ray. A small piece of tissue may be removed from your stomach or the suspicious area may be scrubbed with a tiny brush to obtain some cells for analysis under a microscope.

What is the treatment?

Surgical treatment of early stomach cancer gives good results, because all of the affected region can be removed.

If the tumor is more advanced, an operation may still be recommended to relieve the symptoms and prevent imminent obstruction. Treatment with chemotherapy (anticancer drugs) and radiation therapy to provide temporary relief of symptoms may also be recommended in some cases.

OPERATION:

Stomach removal

(gastrectomy)

An operation to remove part of the stomach is called a partial gastrectomy. Surgery to remove the entire stomach is called a total gastrectomy. They are performed when ulcers fail to heal despite treatment, when an ulcer bleeds uncontrollably or perforates (breaks through the stomach wall), or for cancer of the stomach. Deaths during the surgery for total removal of the stomach, or shortly after, are not uncommon; survivors of the surgery face many adjustments to daily living, including difficulty maintaining body weight. But the adjustments are minor when the alternative, death from cancer, is the only other option.

A partial gastrectomy is performed for noncancerous stomach and duodenal ulcers and for stomach cancers that are located low in the stomach near its connection with the duodenum. Before the operation your stomach is emptied by a tube that is passed into your nose and down your esophagus. The tube remains in your stomach during and after the operation.

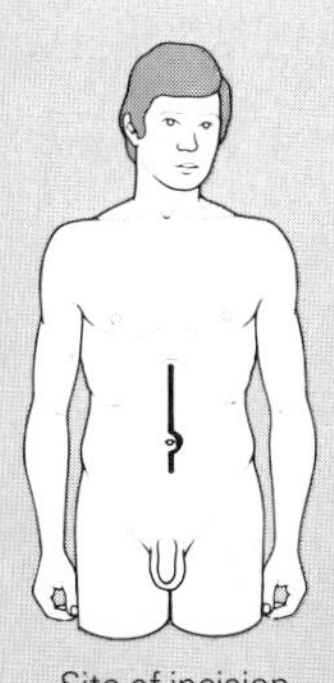

Site of incision

During the operation You are given a general anesthetic and the surgeon makes an incision in the upper abdomen and removes part or all of the stomach; he or she then sews together the remaining edges to maintain a passageway for food. A stomach removal operation usually takes about 2 to 4 hours.

After the operation You will be fed intravenously, and tubes will drain off excess fluid from your stomach and urinary bladder. After a few days your digestive tract usually recovers sufficiently for you to slowly resume eating and drinking.

Convalescence Your physician may prescribe drugs to control side effects such as nausea and diarrhea. Eating small, frequent meals is often advised. Most patients make a full recovery in 1 to 2 months.

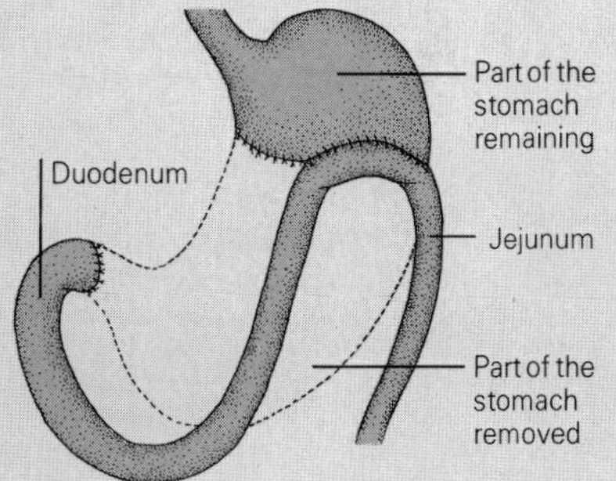

In one form of partial gastrectomy (illustrated), the remaining part of the stomach is attached to the jejunum, an area of the small intestine between the duodenum and the ileum. In another method, the duodenum is reattached to the remnant of stomach.

Peptic ulcer

Peptic ulcer is the term used to describe a disruption in the lining (mucous membrane) of the lower esophagus, the stomach, or the duodenum, or rarely of the small intestine. The areas involved are bathed by acid and digestive enzymes formed in gastric glands in the wall of the stomach. The main types of peptic ulcers are often called gastric and duodenal ulcers. The two have somewhat different symptoms, but the underlying disease process is essentially the same and, unlike erosions (see Gastritis and gastric erosion, p.497), the ulcers may penetrate or even perforate the wall of the stomach.

The digestive juices secreted by the stomach are strongly acidic and they dissolve protein, yet they do not digest the stomach lining. This is because the stomach lining is protected by a layer of mucus and bicarbonate also secreted by glands in the stomach wall. Although the cause of peptic ulcers is not yet completely understood, recent research may provide an explanation for some people with peptic ulcer. Bacteria called *Helicobacter pylori* are found in the stomachs of a large percentage of adults, and the bacteria may damage the protective mucous covering of the stomach or duodenum so that the acid and enzymes can attack the lining. This theory, not yet proven, explains some cases of peptic ulcers. In such cases elimination of the *Helicobacter* leads to at least temporary healing of the ulcer. *Helicobacter* bacteria are resistant to most of the antibiotic drugs used individually, so researchers have been trying to develop a satisfactory combination of antibiotics with bismuth powder. In other cases the main factor seems to be formation of excess quantities of acid by the stomach.

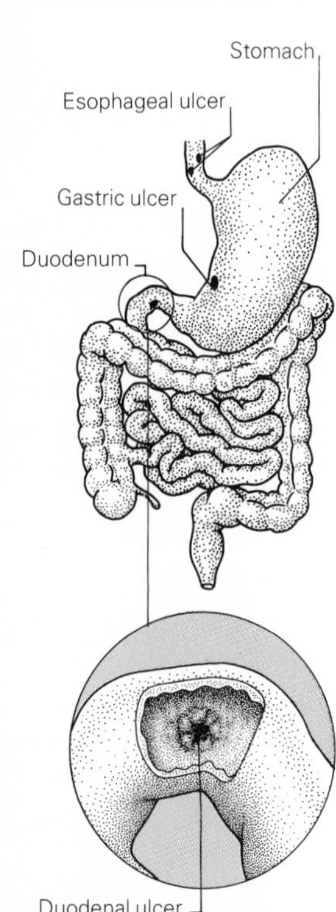

The exact cause of a peptic ulcer is not known. In part it results from acid digesting the mucous membrane. Types of peptic ulcers include gastric (stomach); duodenal (in the intestine); and esophageal (on the esophagus).

A gastric ulcer may vary in size from ⅕ in to 3 in (5 mm to 75 mm), and the main symptom is a burning, gnawing pain usually felt in the uppermost part of the abdomen and occasionally spreading to the lower part of the chest. The pain is almost always briefly relieved by food or antacids. Typically, the pain occurs one-half to 2 hours after meals. Attacks of ulcer pain come and go, weeks of pain alternating with pain-free periods of variable length. Other possible symptoms of a gastric ulcer are nausea—paradoxically relieved by food, antacids, or vomiting—loss of appetite, and weight loss.

A duodenal ulcer is usually less than ½ in (about 12 mm) wide, but variable in size, in the lining of the duodenum, the first part of the small intestine. Typically, the pain is confined to a spot in the uppermost abdomen, but in some cases the pain may be felt mainly in the back between the tips of the shoulder blades. The pain often resembles a constant hunger pain and comes on usually 2 to 3 hours after a meal and at 1 to 3 AM. It can generally be relieved by food, milk, or an antacid. Vomiting, if it occurs, usually relieves the pain temporarily. Loss of weight is unusual unless vomiting or pyloric stenosis (see following article) is present. People with peptic ulcers do not have symptoms that fit exactly into either of these categories; however, there is a rhythmic pattern to the pain characterized by the sequence: pain, food, relief, pain. Your physician will take a history of your symptoms and, if you have that particular cycle of eating and pain, probably diagnose peptic ulcer. The diagnosis can be confirmed by endoscopy, and the management of all peptic ulcers follows the same principles.

What are the risks?

Probably one in five men and one in ten women have a peptic ulcer at some time in their lives—although, for reasons unknown, the frequency of such ulcers seems to be declining. Stomach ulcers are about equally common in the two sexes; more men than women get duodenal ulcers, although this, too, seems to be changing. Peptic ulcers occur more often in people who smoke, those who consume alcohol heavily, and those who consume large amounts of painkillers such as aspirin, ibuprofen, and other nonsteroidal anti-inflammatory drugs.

Dark stools

Internal bleeding does not always cause obvious symptoms such as vomiting blood or fainting. Bleeding may be so minimal that there is no obvious change in the appearance of the stools, and tests are required to detect the blood. Often there are no symptoms when minimal bleeding occurs. If you are bleeding internally and the blood passes through the intestines fairly slowly, it will be partly digested and become dark mahogany or even jet black in color. This partly digested blood, or melena, makes the stool loose, sticky, and foul-smelling. If you begin to pass black, sticky stools, consult your physician immediately. Internal bleeding of this kind may be a sign of a gastric erosion (see Gastritis and gastric erosion, p.497), a peptic ulcer, a stomach cancer, or other disorders of the esophagus, stomach, or intestines. It should always be treated as an emergency.

The main risk from peptic ulcers is bleeding. Severe bleeding is not common but it may be life-threatening; such bleeding may cause you to vomit blood or have black, tarry stools. Another risk, although it is very small, is that the ulcer may erode completely through the wall of the stomach or duodenum. This is called perforation and will cause peritonitis (see p.503). Surgery must be performed promptly. Perforation is much more common with duodenal ulcers than with gastric ulcers. Duodenal ulcers do not become cancerous.

What should be done?
If your symptoms suggest that you have a peptic ulcer, try the self-help procedures below. If pain persists for more than a week or two, consult your physician. To determine if you have an ulcer and where it is, your physician will arrange for you to have an endoscopy that may be followed by an upper gastrointestinal barium X ray. Biopsy specimens may be taken during endoscopy, and tests of stomach acidity (samples are taken through a tube passed down into your stomach for measurement of amount and type of acid), blood tests, and tests on your stools may also be required. Even if you think that your symptoms are a recurring ulcer, it is wise to contact your physician.

What is the treatment?
Self-help: You should avoid taking aspirin because it may make your stomach bleed. Use acetaminophen instead for minor pains. If you smoke or drink alcohol in any form, stop. Eat small meals four, five, or six times a day, and try to relax for a short while after each meal. If you have pain between meals take an antacid in a dose recommended by the manufacturer or your physician to relieve it. Spend as much time as possible in nonstressful activities. If after 2 weeks of self-treatment you are still having pain or other symptoms, consult your physician.
Professional help: Your physician will probably supplement the self-help methods described above by prescribing medication. Drugs may be used to reduce the amount of acid being formed in the stomach or to coat the ulcer with a protective layer. Most ulcers heal within 3 to 6 weeks with treatment.

Once healing is complete, you should not smoke or drink alcohol or use excessive quantities of aspirin, ibuprofen, or other nonsteroidal anti-inflammatory drugs, to reduce the likelihood of the ulcer recurring. If your symptoms recur, you will need another course of treatment and your physician may recommend that after the ulcer heals you continue to take a low dose of one of the acid-reducing drugs.

Surgery is seldom necessary and is usually performed only when an ulcer fails to respond to treatment or when complications occur. The general goal of surgery is to reduce the acid-producing capacity of the stomach and ensure an adequate outlet from the stomach by cutting the nerves responsible for controlling acid production (vagotomy). Vagotomy is usually combined with a simple

Swallowed object (foreign body)

Normally, air goes down your windpipe into your lungs, and food goes down your esophagus into your stomach. If solid matter is accidentally "breathed in," it may get stuck in your throat and cause choking, or it may slip into your respiratory tract and obstruct or partially obstruct it. If this happens, immediate first aid is essential (see Injuries and emergencies, p.835).

Most foreign bodies that go down through the esophagus—even, amazingly enough, sharp and awkwardly shaped ones—are carried through the digestive tract and excreted without trouble. Consult your physician if you have swallowed anything sharp (like a fish bone or needle) or bigger than about ¼ in (6 mm) in diameter.

If you find it difficult to swallow, or have abdominal pain, you may need to have your digestive tract X rayed. This almost always allows your physician to locate and identify the foreign body, and if it is within reach, it can be removed with an endoscope with a special attachment. Surgery is usually required to remove an object that is large, firmly stuck, and/or pointed.

Vomiting blood

Vomiting can be simply a sign of excesses in eating or drinking alcohol. But you should never disregard blood in your vomit. It could indicate a serious disorder such as bleeding from a tear in the esophagus or a peptic ulcer (see p.500).

Fresh blood is recognizable as such. It is bright red and may occur as streaks in the vomit or may be virtually the only substance you bring up. On the other hand, blood that stays in the stomach for some time is turned brownish-black by stomach acid and may look like coffee grounds.

Consult your physician without delay if you suspect there is blood in your vomit. If you have blood in your vomit and, in addition, your skin is cold, you are sweating, and you feel weak and dizzy when you stand, go to a hospital immediately.

surgical widening of the stomach outlet (pyloroplasty). The vagotomy may be total or selective; that is, the surgeon will divide all of the nerve trunks, or only those most concerned with acid production.

Sometimes the vagotomy is performed with a partial gastrectomy, an operation in which the surgeon cuts away the portion of the stomach that contains the areas that secrete stomach acid (see Box, p.499). However, there are undesirable aftereffects to gastric surgery such as feeling faint, drowsiness, or sweating soon after eating; diarrhea and weight loss; anemia; or vitamin D deficiency (see p.534). These aftereffects generally subside in time.

Pyloric stenosis

(pyloric obstruction)

Pyloric stenosis is a rare disorder that occurs when the outlet from the stomach to the duodenum, which is called the pylorus, becomes partly or completely blocked. This usually happens as a result of scarring and deformity of the outlet from a chronic peptic ulcer (see p.500), but occasionally it is caused by cancer of the stomach (see p.498). Whatever the underlying cause, the disorder prevents your stomach from emptying normally. This produces an uncomfortable, distended abdomen, copious vomiting, and foul-smelling gas that you belch up.

If the pylorus becomes totally blocked, repeated vomiting may eventually result in loss of weight, dehydration (loss of body fluid), malnutrition, and a dangerous disturbance in the body's chemical balance. (For Congenital pyloric stenosis in infants, a different disorder, see p.706.)

What should be done?

If you are a long-term ulcer sufferer and repeatedly vomit fluid or food, consult your physician. If your physician suspects pyloric stenosis, you may need to have endoscopy.

If an ulcer is causing the problem, it may respond to treatment with drainage of all stomach contents via a tube passed into the stomach through the nose to permit any ulcer swelling to subside. If the scarring is from repeated ulcers, is too extensive, or is a result of cancer, surgery will be necessary (see Stomach removal, p.499).

Generalized abdominal problems

The intestines are a section of the digestive tract extending from the beginning of the duodenum to the anus. They consist of a long, thin, coiled tube called the small intestine that leads to a shorter, wider tube called the colon. The colon leads into a final, short tube called the rectum. The colon and rectum together are often referred to as the large intestine.

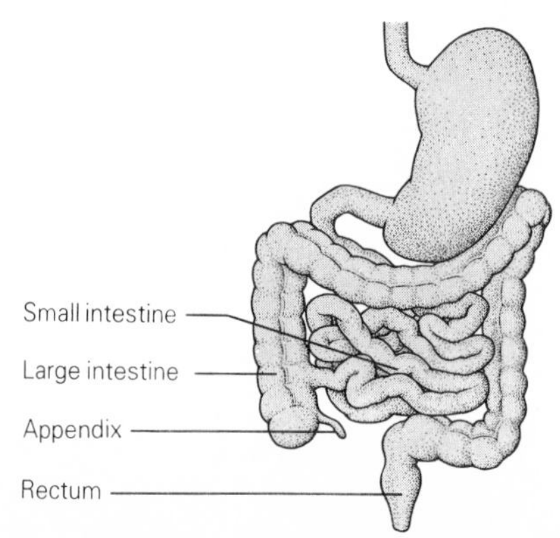

The intestines
The intestines are made up of the small intestine, the appendix, and the large intestine (colon and rectum). They form a long coil that fits into the abdominal cavity. Nutrients from food are absorbed by the lining of the small intestine. Waste moves through the large intestine and out of the body.

Food passes from the stomach into the duodenum and the rest of the small intestine, where it is further broken down by various digestive juices. As the food travels along the small intestine, propelled by rhythmic muscular contractions (called peristalsis), nutrients are absorbed from the food through the thin intestinal walls. As it passes into the colon, most of the remaining fluid is removed. What remains is a mixture of undigested and indigestible material, largely vegetable fibers ("roughage"), along with bacteria, mucus, bile pigments, and dead cells from the lining of the digestive tract. This waste material combines to make up the feces, or stools, which pass into the rectum and remain there until they are excreted through the anus in a bowel movement. The entire digestive process from mouth to anus usually takes from 24 to 72 hours.

Also included in this section is peritonitis, a serious disease that affects the peritoneum, the thin membrane that lines the abdominal cavity and encloses many abdominal organs, including all the intestines.

Peritonitis

Peritonitis is inflammation of the peritoneum, a two-layered membrane that lines the abdominal cavity and also covers the stomach, intestines, and other abdominal organs. This condition almost always results from an underlying disease. It may occur as a complication of a disorder in which your digestive tract is inflamed or ruptured, such as a peptic ulcer (see p.500), diverticulitis (see p.515), or appendicitis (see p.512). It may also develop as a complication of certain problems of the fallopian tubes. Another possible cause of peritonitis is infection from an injury that pierces the abdominal wall. Finally, peritonitis may also occur as a complication of abdominal surgery.

What are the symptoms?

The symptoms vary depending on the source of inflammation or infection, but there is always severe abdominal pain. It is most severe near the site where the problem began. For example, it is worst in the upper mid-right side of the abdomen if it is caused by a ruptured peptic ulcer. The pain increases when you move. You may be nauseated and vomit, and you will almost surely have a fever. After 2 or 3 hours your abdomen may become distended (inflated) as the pain becomes less severe and less localized. This lessening of your pain does not indicate that you are getting better. In fact, it is just the opposite; it is a very ominous sign that calls for emergency treatment immediately.

What are the risks?

If treatment for a ruptured duodenal ulcer, appendicitis, or an abdominal injury is delayed, peritonitis almost always develops. If peritonitis is not treated the risks are potentially catastrophic, including prolonged illness or death. You can become dehydrated or lose a dangerous amount of fluid and chemicals from repeated vomiting. Decrease of severe pain and paralysis of your intestines (see Ileus, p.504) indicates that death will follow unless you get emergency medical treatment immediately.

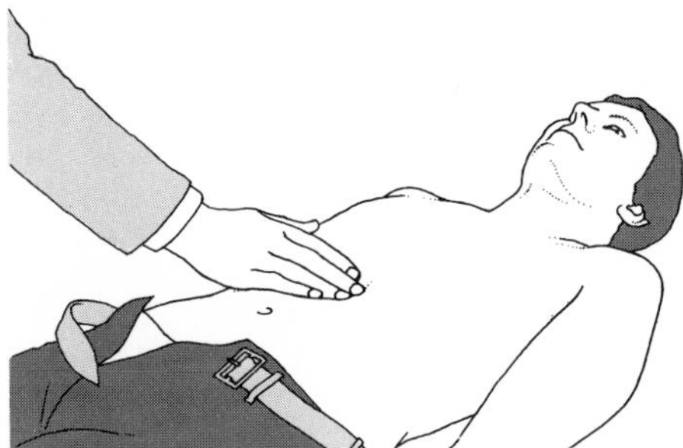

"Does this hurt?" Your physician will palpate, or gently press, your abdomen, if peritonitis is suspected. The characteristic hardness and pain can often be detected during such an examination.

What should be done?

Peritonitis is a life-threatening disorder. Have someone call your physician and an ambulance immediately if there is any possibility of peritonitis. To establish the underlying cause of your pain, your physician will question you and press on your abdomen in several places to pinpoint the inflamed area. To aid in diagnosis, you may also be given tests such as blood tests, X rays, and the insertion of a needle into the abdominal cavity to determine what fluid, such as blood or pus, might be present (see also Laparotomy and acute abdomen, p.513).

What is the treatment?

Prompt surgery to correct the underlying cause of peritoneal inflammation is usually the only possible treatment if a portion of the intestinal tract has ruptured. After you reach the hospital, the fluid contents and air in your stomach and intestines will be removed through a long tube passed down through your nose or mouth. To treat any infection and to strengthen you for the operation if you are weak and dehydrated, you may be given antibiotics, along with nutrients and fluids, intravenously. Your abdomen will then be opened, and the diseased organ that is the source of the trouble (such as a dead segment of intestine) will be removed or repaired (as in the case of a perforated ulcer). Segments of soft rubber will be placed in your abdominal cavity and brought to the surface to facilitate continued drainage of peritoneal fluid. Prospects for full recovery are excellent if treatment is started promptly. With the help of the many antibiotics available now, few people today die of peritonitis.

Intestinal obstruction

An intestinal obstruction is a partial or complete blockage of your intestines that makes it impossible for the digestive process to run its full course. Any one of several factors can cause a mechanical intestinal obstruction. The most common causes include a blockage of the intestine by an adhesion, or a band of tissue, that is usually caused by a prior operation or a prior inflammatory disease. However, the intestines can also be blocked by a growth such as cancer of the colon (see Cancer of the large intestine, p.518) or by a strangulated hernia (see p.505). Sometimes part of a healthy intestine can become knotted or twisted, a condition known as volvulus. Rarely, the cause of an intestinal obstruction is an indigestible object such as an accumulation of a hardened mass of a bulk laxative in a narrow area of the intestine.

What are the symptoms?

Symptoms depend on the location of the obstruction and on whether it is complete or partial. An obstruction in the small intestine causes cramplike pains in the middle of your abdomen, along with increasingly frequent bouts of vomiting. If vomiting temporarily relieves the cramping, the obstruction is probably partial. If the blockage is in your large intestine you may vomit very little or not at all. With a partial obstruction of the large intestine, the intense cramping pain is temporarily relieved by the passage of a rush of gas and loose stool. Complete blockage anywhere in the digestive tract results in distention of the intestine above the site of obstruction, and no stool or gas is passed.

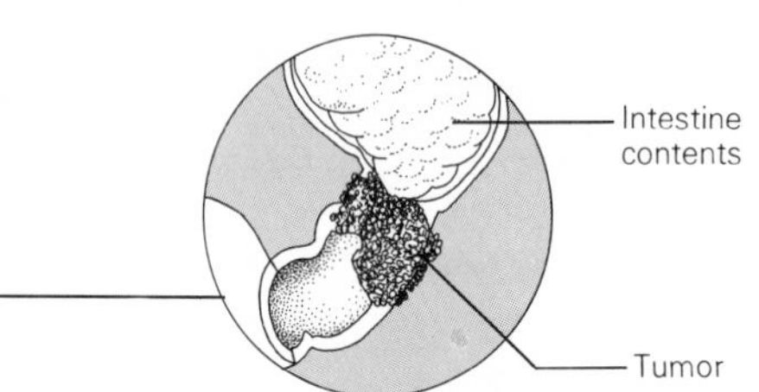

Blockage by a tumor
Part of this intestine has become completely blocked by a cancerous tumor, so that the intestinal contents are prevented from passing down into the rectum.

What are the risks?

Intestinal obstruction is fairly common. If it is possible for your physician to diagnose and treat the cause of the obstruction before blockage becomes complete, emergency surgery can be avoided. Any disruption of the normal functioning of the intestines can lead to their paralysis (see Ileus, next article). Persistent vomiting can cause dehydration and, eventually, shock (see p.414). If the blockage is not relieved, there is also a danger that the intestine will rupture and cause peritonitis (see previous article).

What should be done?

If you have symptoms of intestinal obstruction, call your physician and an ambulance immediately. Your physician may suspect intestinal obstruction after he or she examines your abdomen and you have given him or her a clear description of your symptoms. You will be admitted to a hospital so that the cause and exact site of the obstruction can be identified. You will probably be given intravenous fluids to prevent dehydration and shock, and the fluid contents and air in your digestive tract will probably be removed by passing a long tube down through your mouth. If your symptoms do not subside in a day or two with this treatment, an operation called a laparotomy (see p.513) is sometimes necessary to locate and remove the cause of the obstruction.

What is the treatment?

Surgery to relieve the blockage is done at the same time as the laparotomy. If the source of the trouble is a volvulus, the surgeon may be able to untwist the intestine in a way that will prevent the problem from recurring. Often, however, the preferred procedure is to cut out the small part of the intestine that has become twisted and rejoin the severed ends.

Prospects for full recovery are excellent after surgery if the underlying disorder has been effectively treated.

Ileus

Ileus is a serious disorder in which the intestines become paralyzed, causing disruption of normal digestive processes. This disorder can be caused by other disorders such as intestinal obstruction (see previous article) or a perforated ulcer (see Peptic ulcer, p.500), or by abdominal surgery.

Gas distends (inflates) your intestines and abdomen. The swollen abdomen presses on your chest and impairs your breathing. You are unable to pass gas or stool. Also, you may develop a fever and may repeatedly vomit foul-smelling liquid. In the beginning of an attack of ileus there is a persistent pain in your abdomen. Although the pain may soon disappear, relief from pain does not mean the condition has improved, and it may be fatal unless the underlying cause is successfully treated. Ileus can often be treated with decompression, which is the process of letting out some of the air that is inflating the area. Decompression is accomplished by passing a long tube through the stomach and into the intestine to suck out the intestinal contents (see previous article) and by treating the underlying disorder.

Some degree of ileus follows many abdominal operations and is routinely dealt with after surgery. In other cases, treatment depends on the underlying disorder. For example, when the condition arises from a serious disorder such as a perforated ulcer, you are likely to be extremely ill and in need of immediate treatment.

Carcinoids

(and the carcinoid syndrome)

A carcinoid is a rare type of tumor in the wall of the intestines. Although the growths are malignant (likely to spread), they develop so slowly that at least half of the people who have them never know they have a malignant tumor. If they are discovered at all, the growths are usually found during a diagnostic test or surgery for some other, unrelated disorder. The growths can become large enough, however, that they cause intestinal obstruction (see p.503).

In about 10 percent of all cases, carcinoid cells spread through the bloodstream to the liver, where they multiply and form hormone-producing tumors (see p.557) that have widespread effects on the body. The result is a characteristic group of symptoms called the carcinoid syndrome.

What are the symptoms?

The main symptom of the carcinoid syndrome is flushing of the skin on your head and neck, which is triggered by some activity such as exercising or drinking alcohol. It looks like a blush, but it lasts up to several hours because it is caused by the abnormal secretion of a hormone that causes skin changes. Other probable symptoms include puffy and watery eyes; explosive diarrhea, often with abdominal cramps; wheezing and other symptoms of asthma (see p.381); and the symptoms of heart failure (see p.408), including breathlessness.

If you have these symptoms, your physician may arrange for you to have blood and urine tests to identify the hormone secreted by the carcinoid, imaging including CT scans, and endoscopy.

What is the treatment?

If carcinoids are discovered in their early stages, the growths can often be surgically removed, but surgery does not cure the carcinoid syndrome. Treatment is aimed at easing symptoms. Medication may be prescribed to try to reduce the frequency and length of flushing attacks and to control diarrhea. Asthma is relieved by bronchodilators. A chemotherapy (anticancer) drug may be used to slow the progress of the disease.

Hernias

A hernia is a bulge or protrusion of soft tissue that forces its way through or between muscles. Normally, body muscles are taut and firm. They press on various tissues and organs, helping to restrain them and keep them in the correct position within your body. However, muscles sometimes become weak or slack, because of a strain or a congenital weakness, for example. When this occurs the organs inside the abdominal cavity are able to force their way through the weak point in the muscle and create a hernia.

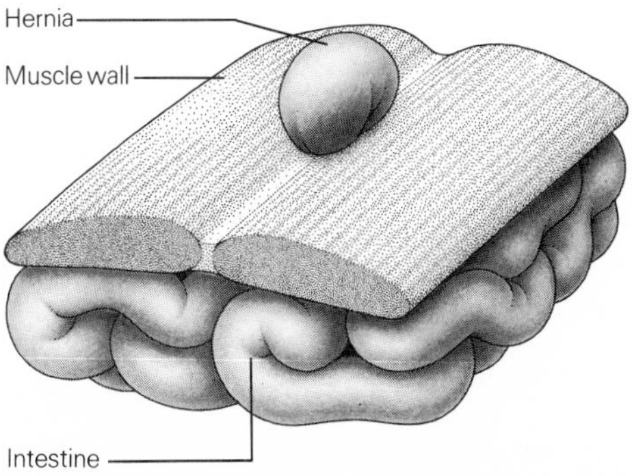

Hernia

Muscle wall

Intestine

A hernia is a bulge of soft tissue that protrudes through a weak point in a muscle wall. Injury and lack of use of the muscle are possible causes of a weak point. The hernia usually occurs because of increased pressure on soft tissue beneath the muscle wall.

Where do hernias occur?

Hernias can occur in many parts of the body, but they are most common in the abdominal wall. The abdominal wall is made up of flat sheets of muscle that cover and protect the abdominal organs: the stomach, intestines, liver, kidneys, and reproductive organs. Normally, these abdominal organs are held in by the firm muscles of the abdominal wall, even when the pressure inside rises, as it does when you cough, lift a heavy object, or strain to pass urine or move your bowels. But if a weak point occurs in the wall, pressure inside the abdomen forces the muscles to part at that point. Some portion of the abdominal contents, often the fatty apron (omentum) that covers the intestines, is pushed through the muscles and becomes a visible bulge or sac, a hernia.

One common hernia is a hiatal hernia. This type of hernia occurs in the sheet of muscle called the diaphragm, which separates the chest from the abdomen. Hiatal hernia can be a cause of reflux esophagitis (see p.488). Several other hernias, all of which occur in the abdominal wall, are shown on the next two pages, along with their causes, symptoms, and treatments.

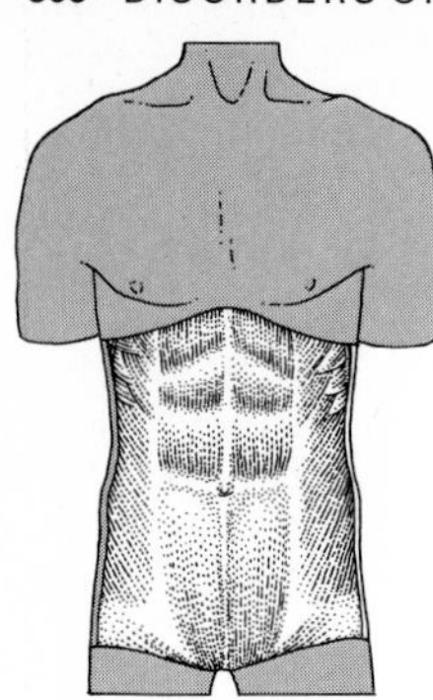

The abdominal wall is a large, layered sheet of muscles at the front and the sides of the abdomen. It keeps the abdominal organs firmly in place.

What are the symptoms?

Usually, the only symptom of a hernia is a bulge or swelling. The bulge usually appears slowly over several weeks, but occasionally it forms suddenly, such as during the strain of lifting a heavy weight. You may have a feeling of heaviness or tenderness and aching at the site of the hernia, especially if you have been on your feet for a long time.

Most hernias can simply be pushed back through the muscle opening into place. Such hernias are said to be reducible. However, these hernias sooner or later bulge out again, either on their own or with some form of straining. If a hernia cannot be replaced it is called irreducible.

What are the risks?

If a hernia contains intestine, the contents of the intestine may be prevented from moving through. This is called an obstructed hernia. If you have a hernia that becomes obstructed, you will have increasing abdominal pain, nausea, and vomiting.

Strangulation occurs when the blood supply to the loop of intestine inside the hernia is cut off. An obstructed hernia or strangulated hernia needs immediate attention. If the condition is not treated, the strangulation will result in gangrene of the bowel.

What should be done?

If you suspect you have a hernia, see your physician. A careful physical examination should confirm the diagnosis of a hernia, and your physician will discuss the various methods of treatment with you.

In general, surgery is the best treatment for a hernia. Your physician may advise you to wear a supportive truss until you have the operation; this is usually only a temporary measure. However, if a truss keeps your hernia under control, you can wear it indefinitely if you are unable to have an operation. Most hernias tend to slowly get worse, not better, and the dangers of obstruction and strangulation are present until the hernia is repaired. An obstructed or strangulated hernia often requires an emergency operation.

Hernias are repaired by pushing the protruding tissue back into place and tightening or sewing together the loose muscles. You must follow your physician's advice while you recover from the surgery, because of the risk of recurrence.

OPERATION:

Hernia repair

(herniorrhaphy)

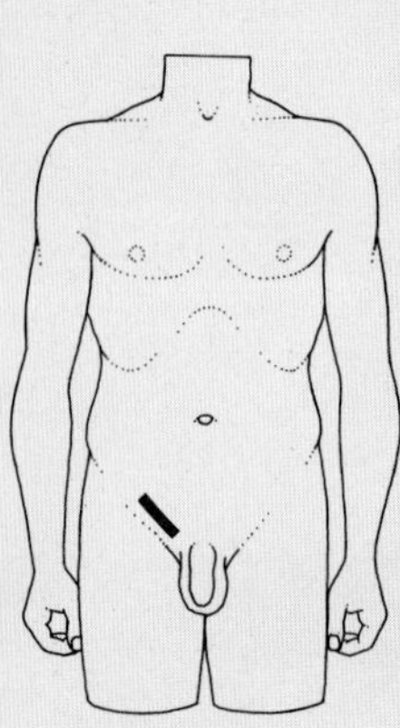

Site of incision for inguinal hernia

In a hernia repair operation, the bulge of soft tissue that has come through a weakened muscle or tissue layer is corrected surgically.

During the operation Depending on the position and severity of your hernia, you will be given either a local or a general anesthetic. A small incision is made over the hernia, and the bulging tissue is pushed back into place. The muscles or tissues are then sewn firmly together. A plastic mesh or sheet is sometimes used to reinforce a weak muscle or a muscle that has been replaced by scar tissue from previous repair operations. The operation usually takes less than an hour.

After the operation You will be encouraged to get out of bed the day of the operation. Many surgeons perform these operations in a hospital outpatient surgery unit, and you may be able to go home the same day. The area of the repair will be painful, so you may need to take painkillers. A hernia in the abdomen may require extensive surgery.

Convalescence You should be able to return to work and continue with your normal activities within a few days, but you will probably be advised not to lift any heavy objects for up to 8 weeks.

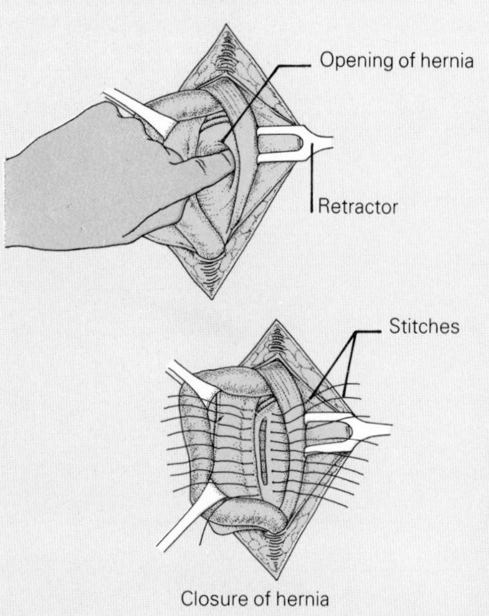

Closure of hernia

Different types of hernias

This illustration shows the most common types of hernias, along with the specific symptoms and treatments for each.

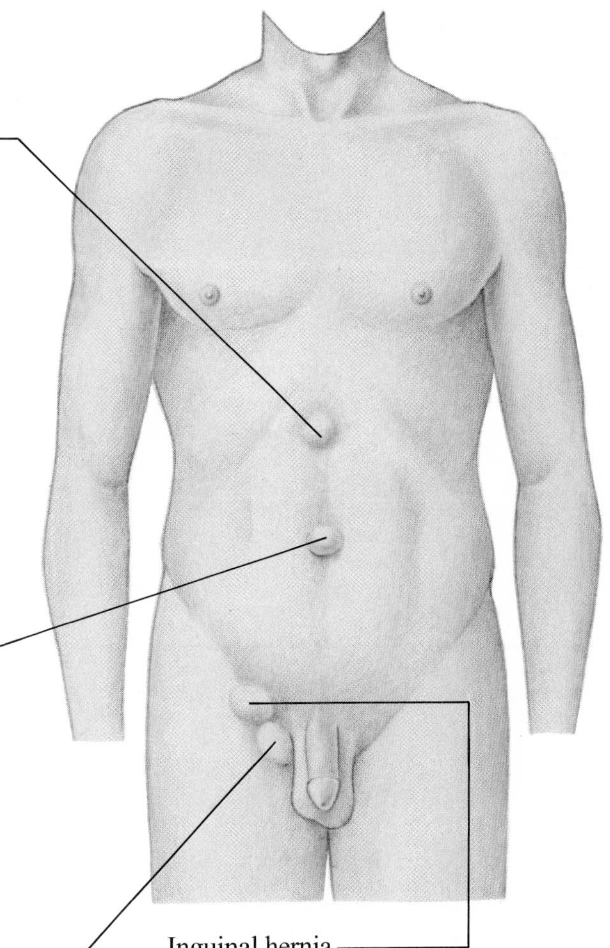

Epigastric hernia

Epigastric hernia occurs when a weak point in the fibrous tissue that joins the central abdominal muscles allows protrusion of a small piece of the fatty apron that covers the intestines. It occurs somewhere on the line between the navel and the breastbone. Epigastric hernia is more common in men than in women.
Symptoms: The hernia is usually small, but may be sore and tender.
Risks: Pain and strangulation are possibilities. The bulge is unlikely to be life-threatening if the hernia contains only fat.
Treatment: If the hernia causes no problems, it may not be treated. Otherwise surgery will repair the defect. Convalescence from surgery takes 1 to 2 weeks.

Paraumbilical hernia

Paraumbilical hernia occurs when a weakness develops in the abdominal wall muscles around the navel, but the soft bulge of the hernia appears to be at the navel. It occurs more often in women than in men.
Symptoms: The hernia may not cause any painful symptoms, or it may be tender or occasionally painful.
Risks: It may become trapped and/or strangulated.
Treatment: An abdominal binder or girdle often keeps the hernia from coming out. Your physician may recommend surgery to tighten the abdominal wall muscles, or sew them together at the site of the hernia. Convalescence from this surgery takes 1 to 2 weeks.

Femoral hernia

Femoral hernia occurs in a similar but slightly lower position than inguinal hernia. It is often difficult to detect in a physical examination. The condition is most common in overweight women who have had a large number of children.
Symptoms: This hernia often causes no noticeable symptoms, and many femoral hernias go unnoticed unless they become obstructed or strangulated.
Risks: Because the hole through which a femoral hernia protrudes is small, the risks of obstruction and strangulation are high.
Treatment: The same as for inguinal hernia.

Inguinal hernia

Inguinal hernia appears as a bulge in the groin. There are two types. In direct inguinal hernia the abdominal organs push aside weak abdominal-wall muscles that cover the groin. Indirect inguinal hernia protrudes down the inguinal canal, a tube through which a testicle descends from the abdomen to the scrotum, usually just before birth (see also Undescended testicles, p.739).
Symptoms: The hernia may cause no symptoms, or a heaviness in the groin that is more noticeable after standing.
Risks: Obstruction and strangulation of the hernia are possible.
Treatment: A truss can be worn by those unable to have an operation. An operation is performed to remove the hernia sac and shorten or sew together the weak muscles. Depending on the size of the hernia, you can usually return to normal activity in 1 to 2 weeks, but avoid heavy lifting for 6 to 8 weeks.

Umbilical hernia

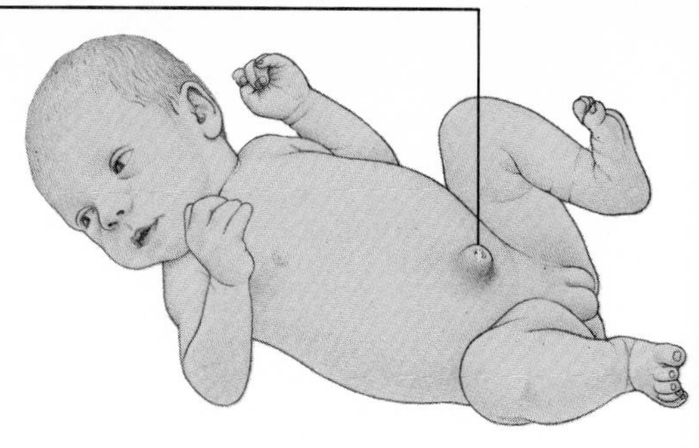

Umbilical hernia appears as a soft bulge of tissue around the navel of a newborn. It occurs when the abdominal wall is not fully developed.

Symptoms: The hernia is unlikely to cause the child any discomfort. It is most visible to the caregiver when the child cries.

Risks: Because the opening is wide, there is virtually no risk of strangulation or obstruction.

Treatment: Most of these hernias heal naturally in a few years. Large umbilical hernias or persistent cases can be treated surgically. It takes the child 1 to 2 weeks to recover from the operation.

Incisional hernia

Incisional hernia is an occasional result of abdominal surgery. The cut abdominal wall muscles and fibrous layers sometimes do not heal properly, and the intestines may bulge through this weak point. If you are overweight and you remain inactive after an abdominal operation you are most likely to develop an incisional hernia. Incisional hernias also affect older people or very thin, weak people. Wound infections and broken stitches can also cause defects in the abdominal muscle wall, resulting in incisional hernias.

Symptoms: Large incisional hernias can cause abdominal pain.

Risks: Strangulation and obstruction are uncommon.

Treatment: Sometimes a corset controls the problem, but more surgery may be a permanent solution. Because of the nature of this type of hernia, however, it sometimes recurs.

Small intestine

The small intestine is a tube about 1½ in (35 mm) in diameter and about 16 ft (5 m) long. It runs on a convoluted path from the stomach to the colon and is the main site where nutrients are digested and absorbed into the bloodstream.

In the small intestine the process of breaking down food into small particles, already begun in the stomach, continues. This process is aided by the secretion of additional enzymes and digestive juices from the pancreas, gallbladder, and the small intestine wall. Once food particles are dissolved into their smallest units, they pass through the thin lining of the intestine into the bloodstream or, in the case of fats, into the lymphatic vessels (lacteals) in the small intestine before they enter the bloodstream later. To make sure that as much food as possible is absorbed, the inside surface of the small intestine wall is covered with tiny fingerlike projections called villi. These projections provide a very large surface area inside the small intestine for the material to pass through.

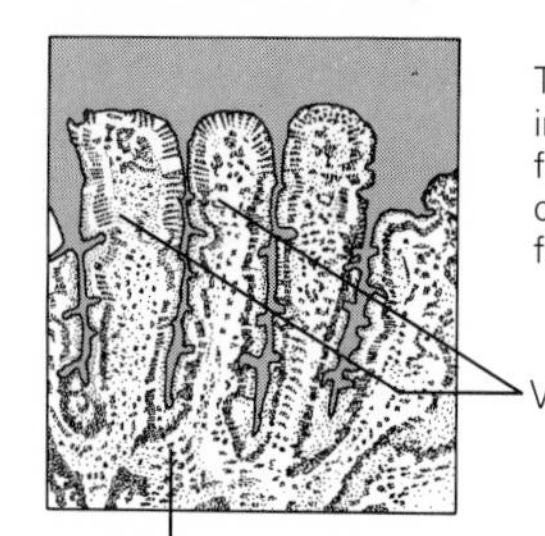

The inside of the small intestine is lined with fingerlike projections called villi, through which food is absorbed.

Crohn's disease

(regional ileitis)

Crohn's disease is a chronic, or long-term, recurring inflammation of part of the digestive tract. The part most commonly affected is the final section of the small intestine, although patchy inflammation can occur anywhere at all in the large or small intestine. The cause of the disease is unknown. It may occur more often in some families. It begins with inflammation that ultimately spreads to involve the full thickness of the intestinal wall and which also sometimes affects more than one part of the digestive system. Some of the affected segments of intestine heal, but they may leave scar tissue that thickens intestinal walls and narrows the passageway.

What are the symptoms?

Crohn's disease usually appears as periodic attacks of cramps, abdominal pain, diarrhea, and a general sense of feeling ill. You may also have a fever, loss of appetite, and weight loss. Attacks tend to begin when you are in your 20s and to recur, sometimes every several months, sometimes not for a number of years, for the rest of your life. In about one-fourth of all cases of Crohn's disease, the symptoms only appear once or twice, and the disease does not recur.

What are the risks?

Crohn's disease has been a rare disorder, but it is gradually becoming more common. There are about twice as many cases of it today as there were 30 years ago.

If Crohn's disease continues for years, it causes a gradual deterioration of bowel functioning. There is a risk of poor absorption of nutrients, with the associated loss of appetite and weight (see Malabsorption, p.511), or of intestinal obstruction (see p.503). Inflammation and scarring as well as the surgical removal of segments of bowel gradually reduce the amount of absorbing surface. Sometimes tiny channels burrow through the inflamed intestinal wall, and leak, and cause peritonitis (see p.503). In other cases localized abscesses burrow through the wall of an adjacent section of intestine, establishing an artificial bypass (fistula). Major bleeding from the intestine is rare. There is also a slight chance that Crohn's disease can increase the susceptibility to cancer of the intestine.

What should be done?

If your symptoms suggest the possibility of Crohn's disease, consult your physician. After examining you, he or she will probably want X rays of your digestive tract, for which you will need a barium upper gastrointestinal examination and a barium enema. You may also have to undergo endoscopy (an examination with a viewing tube) in order to locate inflamed areas. Samples of your blood and stool will be taken for examination.

What is the treatment?

Self-help: Follow your physician's advice about diet and both physical and emotional rest during an attack. You may need to reduce your activities and avoid stress.

Professional help: In most cases treatment with diet, rest, and drugs eases attacks of Crohn's disease. Among the drugs used are analgesics, antispasmodics, antidiarrheals, vitamin supplements, and one or more drugs to reduce inflammation. Your physician may also recommend that you eat certain foods and avoid eating some others and may suggest that you modify your daily routine to relieve tension, which may affect your nervous and digestive systems.

To guard against further attacks, long-term treatment with corticosteroids may be prescribed, alone or with immunosuppressant drugs that permit smaller doses of corticosteroids to be taken. However, long-term corticosteroid use involves considerable risks such as acquiring diabetes. Another drug that helps guard against further attacks, especially if your colon is affected, is a medication derived from the antibacterial drug sulfasalazine. Initial high doses of all these drugs may be decreased gradually.

Surgery for this recurring disease is used to treat the complications mentioned above; repeated extensive surgery itself can cause the person to be malnourished. An ileostomy (see Box, p.518) is not considered a solution to Crohn's disease that has spread to the large intestine because the disease sometimes recurs at the ileostomy. An ileostomy is sometimes performed as a temporary measure to relieve an obstruction or life-threatening widening of the colon. In some instances surgery can provide dramatic although temporary improvement.

Celiac disease in adults

In celiac disease, the lining of your small intestine reacts adversely to gluten, a protein found in wheat and other grains. The person needs to avoid not only bread made from wheat, but also food products such as pasta and beer that contain hidden gluten. Celiac disease rarely appears for the first time in adulthood; it almost always shows up in infancy. (See the children's section, p.690.)

In those rare cases in which celiac disease appears for the first time in an adult, the symptoms are abdominal pain and swelling, diarrhea, fatty yellow stools, weight loss, and lack of energy. Anemia, osteoporosis, and vitamin and mineral deficiency are likely to occur. If you have symptoms, see your physician. Diagnosis and treatment are basically the same for adults and children.

Tumors of the small intestine

Like growths in any part of the body, tumors of the small intestine can be benign (unlikely to spread) or malignant (likely to spread and threaten life). Most are benign and symptom-free, and these tumors usually remain undetected unless they are found through tests or treatment for some other disorder. But in about 1 of 10 cases, the growths are malignant. Very rarely they are of a type known as carcinoids (see p.505).

What are the symptoms?

Tumors in the small intestine may cause the symptoms of anemia (paleness, tiredness, and palpitations on exertion) if they ooze blood minimally but steadily and, occasionally if bleeding intensifies, black or bloody stools. A tumor occasionally grows large enough to produce abdominal pain and intestinal obstruction (p.503).

What are the risks?

Tumors of the small intestine are extremely rare, comprising fewer than 5 percent of all digestive tract tumors. If you have Crohn's disease (see previous page) or celiac disease (see previous article), your chance of developing malignancy of the small intestine is slightly greater than normal.

There is the risk of intestinal obstruction (see p.503) from any large growth. A malignant tumor is life-threatening unless it is discovered and treated at an early stage, so the main risk is that the absent or vague symptoms of cancerous tumors of the small intestine may be ignored until it is too late for effective treatment.

What should be done?

There are no "sure fire" clues to alert you to tumors of the small intestine. They grow silently until they bleed or cause an obstruction, or, when they have spread to distant sites, they may cause such symptoms as significant weight loss and weakness. Most of these tumors are discovered during tests for the above-mentioned symptoms or coincidentally during tests peformed for other problems. A barium X ray of the small intestine will help reveal any tumors.

What is the treatment?

Once they have been detected, tumors of the small intestine are usually removed surgically. Sometimes when malignant growths are discovered they are either too numerous or too widespread for cure. However, surgery is still performed to prevent obstruction or hemorrhage. Corticosteroid drugs, chemotherapy, and radiation therapy, either one at a time or in combination, are prescribed to help keep them under control.

Constipation and diarrhea

There is no "normal" pattern for bowel movements. Most people have about one formed stool a day, but some people have as many as three a day and others as few as three bowel movements a week. In general, the more frequent the bowel actions the softer and looser the stools. Consider yourself constipated only if your usual pattern changes and you begin to have irregular, unusually infrequent, and /or hard, dry movements. Similarly, you have diarrhea only if you have unusually frequent (four or more a day) and particularly loose bowel movements.

Constipation and diarrhea usually are symptoms of disorders that may be serious but often are not. Some people do not have regular bowel movements largely because they overuse laxatives, which may lead to bowel inactivity. This is because the laxatives can over-empty the bowel, prompting the user to take another laxative until a cycle is established. Other people lose their normal awareness of the need to have a bowel movement because they ignore the urge and rationalize that they are "too busy" to take time out for a few minutes in the bathroom. Other factors that influence the consistency of the stool or how long it takes to move through the intestine include diet, especially a low-roughage diet with inadequate fluid intake; the use of certain medicines, especially cough suppressants; hemorrhoids or an anal fissure, which can inhibit straining to have a bowel movement through fear of pain; or a disorder such as severe depression, in which intake of food is reduced and activity limited. Diarrhea can be brought on by a number of different factors, including stress, over-consumption of alcohol, medicines such as certain antacids or antibiotics, specific food sensitivities, fat intolerance, or lactase insufficiency (see p.733).

If constipation persists for more than 2 weeks or diarrhea for more than 48 hours, or if you notice any blood or other unusual change in the way you have your bowel movements, always talk to your physician. Your problem is unlikely to be serious, but have your physician evaluate it, to be sure.

Meckel's diverticulum

In Meckel's diverticulum, a pouch forms near the lower end of the small intestine. The disorder is congenital (present at birth). The pouch is a significant problem only when it becomes inflamed or is the site of bleeding. About 1 person in 50 has such a pouch, but most of these pouches do not cause any trouble. More men than women get this disorder. Sometimes misplaced stomach lining grows in the diverticulum, secretes hydrochloric acid, and ulcerates, causing severe bleeding from the rectum (the blood is maroon in color) and sometimes preceded by pain. Special radionuclide scans are used to pinpoint the Meckel's diverticulum as the cause of bleeding.

Inflammation of the diverticulum may cause abdominal pain, vomiting, and fever, and may be initially diagnosed as appendicitis (see next page), which may then rupture and cause an abscess or widespread peritonitis (see p.503). Sometimes there is an initial diagnosis of a perforated duodenal ulcer (see p.500), which causes severe pain and peritonitis. The initial treatment in such conditions is to open up the abdomen (see Laparotomy and acute abdomen, p.513). Unless a diagnosis was made beforehand, the surgeon then discovers the Meckel's diverticulum and removes it. This course of treatment, along with the treatment for peritonitis, if necessary, cures the condition.

Malabsorption

Many diseases and conditions can cause an abnormality of the structure of your small intestine or a deficiency or absence of the chemicals and enzymes within it that assist the digestive process. As a result, certain elements of your diet may not be fully absorbed. This is called malabsorption. Damage to the intestine may be due to your body's reaction to one element in your diet such as gluten (see Celiac disease, p.509). In a disease called lactase deficiency, one digestive enzyme (lactase) is missing, which causes an inability to digest lactose, the form of sugar present in milk (see Lactose intolerance, p.733). In other cases, large areas of the inner surface of the small intestine that normally absorb nutrients are destroyed by scars resulting from Crohn's disease (see p.508), or large sections of diseased small intestine are removed. Either condition reduces the capacity of the intestinal wall to absorb nutrients.

Malabsorption may cause iron-deficiency anemia (see p.450), vitamin B_{12} deficiency anemia (see p.451), and vitamin D deficiency (see p.532). Malabsorption may occur as a complication of diabetes mellitus (see p.558), cystic fibrosis (see p.732), or pancreatitis (see p.528). In some cases, malabsorption develops after digestive tract surgery.

Flattened villi
Flattened villi are usually found in cases of malabsorption. Such flattening reduces the amount of surface available for absorption of nutrients.

What are the symptoms?

The most common symptoms are rumbling and gurgling, abdominal bloating, and generally loose, yellowish-gray, greasy-looking stools that have a peculiarly strong odor and tend to float because of a high fat content. Over many months, unchecked malabsorption leads to loss of weight and energy, breathlessness, anemia, and other symptoms of vitamin or mineral deficiency such as a sore tongue, prickling sensations and numbness in the arms and legs, muscle cramps, and bone pain (see Vitamin and mineral deficiency, p.532).

What are the risks?

Prolonged malabsorption of nutrients can cause emaciation or death from starvation.

What should be done?

If you have reason to believe that you have malabsorption, and especially if you have yellow-gray stools that look greasy, soft, and bulky, consult your physician. After giving you a physical examination, he or she will probably want several blood tests to evaluate your nutritional deficiency and establish a cause for the malabsorption. Laboratory analysis of stool samples may also be done. A long tube with a capsule at its end may be passed through your mouth and into your small intestine to obtain a biopsy specimen of the lining (mucous membrane) to determine whether it is healthy.

Once malabsorption has been diagnosed, your physician's main task is to determine the underlying cause and treat that disorder. Your physician may prescribe a high-protein, high-calorie, low-fat diet with vitamin and mineral supplements. This type of treatment may partially relieve symptoms.

Large intestine

The large intestine, a tube about 2 in (5 cm) in diameter and about 5 ft (1.5 m) long, consists of two main sections: the colon and the rectum. The small intestine opens into a pouch-like chamber called the cecum, which is the first part of the colon. The rest of the colon then runs up the right side of the abdomen, across under the rib cage, and down the left side, forming a frame for the twists and turns of the small intestine. The rectum is a short tube about 5 in (12 cm) long that leads downward from the end of the colon to the anus. Fluid and various mineral salts from the intestinal contents are absorbed into the bloodstream through the wall of the colon; indigestible solids are compacted and moved toward the rectum, where waste is stored until it is released through the anus in the form of stools.

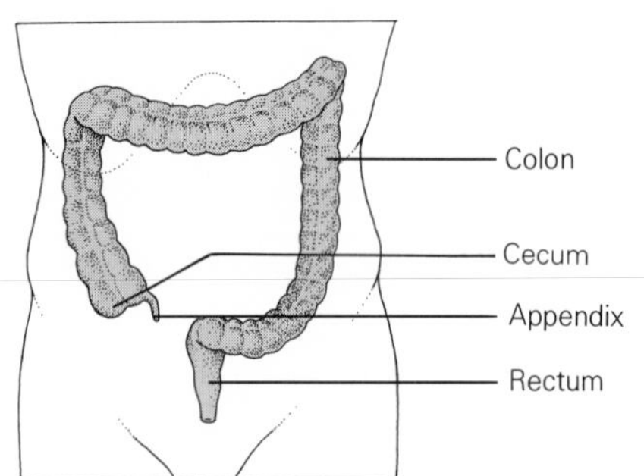

The large intestine
Undigested food in liquid form flows from the small intestine into the large intestine, where most of the water content is absorbed back into the body. The semisolid waste that remains moves down into the rectum and is excreted in a bowel movement.

The large intestine can develop problems for several reasons. It is particularly subject to inflammation because of infection, and it is more susceptible than other sections of the digestive tract to tumors and polyps. Also, the large intestine appears to be adversely affected by the type of diet many Americans eat, which is often too high in fat and low in fiber. The evidence for this is that colon and rectal disorders such as diverticulosis and tumors are far more common in the US than they are in Africa and Asia, where a higher fiber, lower fat diet is common.

Appendicitis

The appendix is a thin, worm-shaped pouch, about 3½ in (9 cm) long, that projects out from the first part of the colon (cecum). In humans the appendix is small and seems to have no function in digestion. It is significant, however, because it can become diseased.

In the condition known as appendicitis, a piece of stool or food may plug the channel of the appendix; it becomes swollen and inflamed and fills with pus.

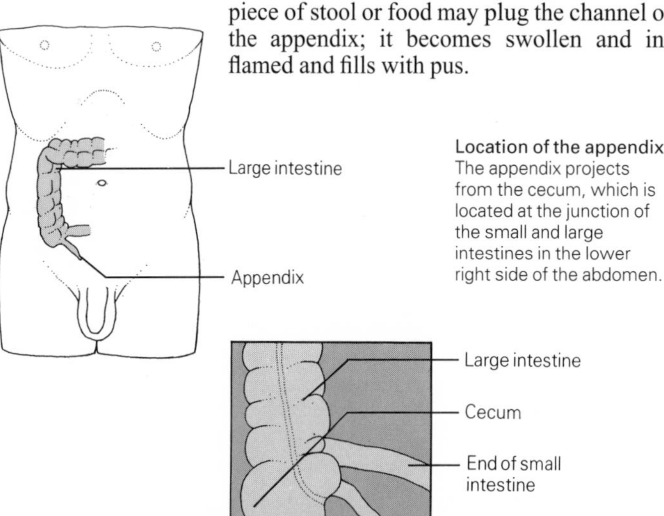

Location of the appendix
The appendix projects from the cecum, which is located at the junction of the small and large intestines in the lower right side of the abdomen.

What are the symptoms?

The main symptom is severe abdominal pain that usually starts as vague discomfort around the navel, but becomes sharper and more localized during the course of a few hours. You will probably feel pain and tenderness in a small spot in the lower right-hand part of your abdomen (the site of the inflamed appendix). Even slight pressure on the spot will increase the pain. You also feel feverish and nauseated and may vomit. You will lose your appetite, and just before the pain begins, you may recall you had not had a bowel movement for the previous day or two. However, a few people experience diarrhea instead of constipation.

What are the risks?

Every year, about 1 person in 500 has an attack of appendicitis. Anyone may be affected, but the disease is rare among children under 2 years old.

If you need surgery and it is delayed, there is a chance that the swollen appendix will rupture. When this happens, the contents are released into the abdomen and this usually causes peritonitis (see p.503). But it is possible that the omentum, an apron of tissue that covers the intestines, will envelop the

OPERATION:

Appendix removal

(appendectomy)

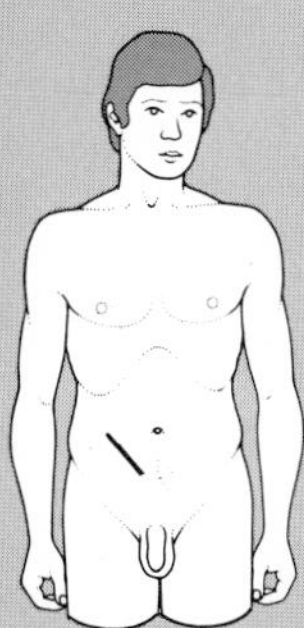

Site of incision

If the diagnosis of acute appendicitis is clear-cut, the surgeon will remove the appendix. Most often, this operation is performed through an incision a few inches long; sometimes a laparotomy is required, in which a larger incision is made (see Box below). Recently, surgeons have in some cases removed an appendix through a laparoscope. First, a viewing device is passed into the abdomen through a tiny "keyhole" incision. Instruments are passed into the abdomen through separate, small incisions, and the appendix is cut away and removed through the laparoscope, usually with no damage to other organs or to the muscles of the abdominal wall. Although recovery depends somewhat on the type of procedure that is performed, you will be able to resume eating and drinking within 24 hours of the operation and be ready to leave the hospital within a few days.

Convalescence You will probably be back to normal a couple of weeks after leaving the hospital. Lack of an appendix has no known effect on your health in the future.

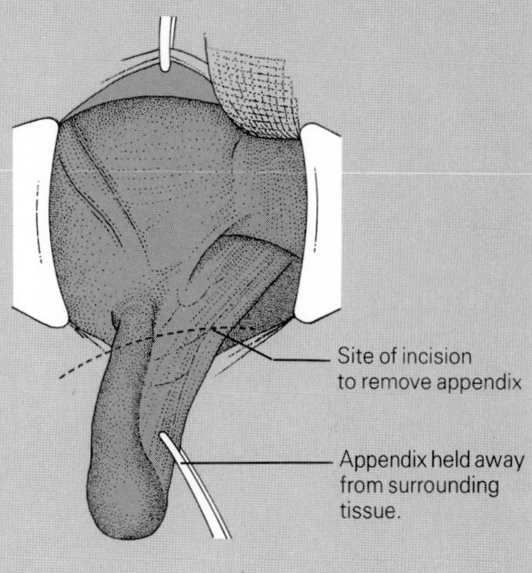

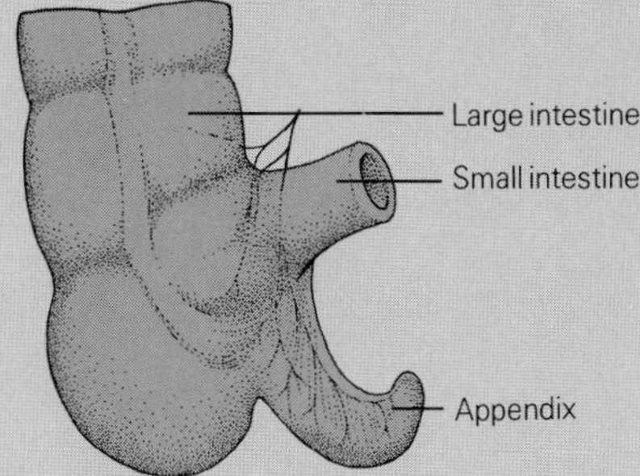

In its normal location (top right) the appendix is curved toward surrounding tissue. It is held away from the tissue (bottom right) during an appendectomy.

Laparotomy and acute abdomen

If your intestines and the inner lining of your abdominal cavity become inflamed (see Peritonitis, p.503), the result is pain, vomiting, abdominal distention, and fever. As the inflammation worsens, these symptoms become more noticeable, and the muscles of your abdominal wall often become rigid, so that your abdomen feels hard and boardlike. The symptoms are similar whether your inflammation is caused by a perforated duodenal ulcer (see p.500), an inflamed appendix (see previous page), acute Crohn's disease (see p.508), an inflamed diverticulum (see Diverticular disease, p.515), or bleeding into the abdominal cavity from an abdominal injury. If you have the above symptoms, do not delay. Call your physician and get to a hospital immediately; this is an emergency.

When no definite diagnosis can be made immediately, your physician may use "acute abdomen" as a working diagnosis. After your physician examines you, in most instances the correct diagnosis will be evident. However, if your physician is uncertain about the diagnosis and if he or she finds that your condition is deteriorating, the best course of action may then be for a surgeon to "take a look inside" in an operation called an exploratory laparotomy.

Laparotomy is an operation in which the surgeon opens the abdomen and looks for an unknown source of infection or disease. The operation is not always performed as an emergency. For example, if you have Hodgkin's disease or if you have had a fever for several weeks that is undiagnosed even after extensive testing, you may need to have a laparotomy. However, with ultrasound, CT, and MRI scans, the need for exploratory surgery has decreased.

Once your abdomen is open, the surgeon will deal with the disease he or she finds, such as ruptured ulcer, ovarian cyst, ectopic pregnancy, or a previously undiscovered cancer.

inflamed appendix, enclose the area, and prevent the spread of infection. When infection is confined in this way, the result is an abscess surrounding the appendix.

What should be done?

If you have a pain in your abdomen along with the other symptoms of appendicitis, consult your physician without delay. Do not take a laxative. It can cause an inflamed appendix to burst. Your physician will question you about your symptoms and will carefully examine your abdomen to test for the location and severity of the pain.

If the physician decides that you probably have appendicitis, you will be admitted to a hospital promptly. If your symptoms and the results of your physician's examination and any tests point clearly to appendicitis, you will have surgery immediately. If a diagnosis is not clear, you may undergo additional diagnostic procedures such as imaging procedures. As time passes you will be reexamined frequently to evaluate whether you definitely have appendicitis or are getting over what caused the attack. An exploratory operation called a laparotomy may be performed immediately (see Laparotomy and acute abdomen, p.513).

What is the treatment?

The treatment for acute appendicitis is swift removal of the affected organ. The operation, known as an appendectomy, is straightforward and there are few risks associated with it. Usually, the appendectomy can be performed as soon as a laparotomy has established the cause of the problem.

If diagnostic tests such as an abdominal ultrasound or a laparotomy show that your appendix is abscessed, then it is less likely that your appendix will have to be removed immediately. If the omentum is adhering to the inflamed organ the operation is more difficult. You will probably receive large doses of antibiotics to reduce the infection, and the abscess may be drained. You may be allowed to go home after a couple of days, although the antibiotics may be continued for a few weeks. Because appendicitis is likely to flare up again after 6 weeks or so, you will be readmitted to the hospital to have your appendix removed, but only when further tests show that the abscess has subsided.

Irritable colon

(spastic colon, mucous colitis, irritable bowel syndrome)

Irritable colon is one form of irritable bowel syndrome, which may include a number of symptoms attributed to various changes in or disorders of any organ of the gastrointestinal tract, which includes the esophagus, stomach, and small and large intestines. The symptoms are usually caused by altered function of the involuntary muscles in these organs and often mimic those caused by disease. The symptoms are brought on or aggravated by tension and strain and, often, a poor diet. The symptoms can be greatly intensified by your anxiety over the cause of the pain.

Irritable colon is a possibility when there is abdominal discomfort, which may be located anywhere along the course of the colon (see illustration, p.512), a change in your bowel habits (constipation or diarrhea), tension and strain in your life, and the absence of any active disease after diagnostic tests and a physical examination are performed.

Normally, the contents of the intestine are propelled along by coordinated waves of muscular contraction (peristalsis). Once a day, usually but not always, after breakfast the stools are propelled into the rectum. A stretch is put on the wall of the rectum, which we interpret as the need to have a bowel movement. If we heed this urge the lower bowel is usually emptied, and the stools are soft but formed. In irritable colon, the waves of muscular contraction are uncoordinated, and this conditon interferes with the progress of stool through the intestines and with your normal pattern of bowel movement.

Irritable colon is one of the most common gastrointestinal disorders. It is also one of the least understood. It is twice as common in women as in men and mostly begins in early adult life. It is not life-threatening.

What are the symptoms?

The symptoms of irritable colon may resemble those of any other gastrointestinal disorder. You may need to move your bowels several times a day and the stools you pass may be hard, soft, or fluid. Other possible symptoms may include attacks of nausea, cramping abdominal pain, abdominal distention, rumbling and gurgling, excess passage of gas, and a sensation that the rectum is never completely emptied. The symptoms vary. For example, the main symptom in some people is abdominal pain, while in others it is diarrhea or alternating bouts of constipation and diarrhea.

What should be done?

Because some of the symptoms are similar to those of cancer of the colon (see Cancer of the large intestine, p.518), ulcerative colitis (see p.516), and Crohn's disease (see p.508), all of which are potentially dangerous, you should consult your physician.

A series of tests such as imaging procedures, sigmoidoscopy, and examination of samples of stool for traces of blood or infectious agents may be performed.

What is the treatment?

Irritable colon is a difficult problem for both you and your physician because it is not clear what causes the disorder and as yet there is no complete cure for it. Several factors are known to make the symptoms of irritable colon worse, however, and you can take steps to prevent aggravation of your symptoms.

Self-help: Travel, changes in your occupation, emotional stress and pressures, and diet can all influence the severity of your symptoms. Therefore, you may be able to identify certain situations and substances that can then be avoided. For example, you should keep a diary of everything that you eat and drink and try to identify particular foods such as cabbage, beans, pork, and fried or highly seasoned foods, and drinks such as liqueurs or carbonated beverages that seem to cause your problems. Smoking often intensifies symptoms. People with constipation or those with alternating constipation and diarrhea may find that a high-fiber diet such as the one recommended for diverticular disease (see next article) dramatically relieves symptoms. However, people who have looser stools and excessive gas may have better results with a relatively bland diet. It is a good idea to ask your physician for advice about possible stress reduction techniques, in addition to changes in your diet.

Professional help: Your physician is likely to recommend a combination of self-help measures, as described above, and treatment that is aimed at restoring to normal the muscular contractions of your intestines. If your stools have been hard and irregular, your physician will probably prescribe a high-fiber diet that includes cooked or canned fruits and vegetables (including prunes and spinach), unrefined cereal products or whole-grain breads and cereals, and 8 to 10 glasses of liquids (water, skim milk, or prune juice) daily. He or she will also instruct you in correct and healthy toilet habits, including the use of glycerine suppositories, a 3-ounce oil-retention enema at bedtime, or the infrequent use of an 8-ounce tap water enema. You may not need any laxatives if you follow the program above.

If, however, your main symptom is diarrhea or abdominal pain, your physician may prescribe antispasmodic drugs and mild sedatives or tranquilizers. He or she will also teach you to avoid all or most of the fiber and laxativelike foods in your diet until your diarrhea is controlled.

Diverticular disease

(diverticulosis and diverticulitis)

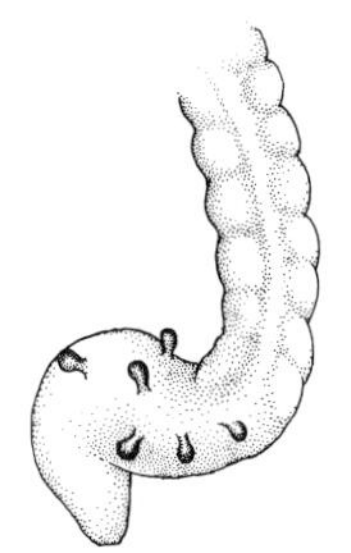

In diverticulosis, small pouches form in the wall of the colon and project into the abdominal cavity.

Small, saclike swellings called diverticula (singular: diverticulum) sometimes develop in the walls of the lowest part of your colon. Diverticula also may develop, although less frequently, in any other location along the gastrointestinal tract, including the throat (see Pharyngeal pouch, p.490), esophagus, stomach, duodenum, small intestine, and colon. Many older people develop diverticula without ever knowing it. This symptom-free, or almost symptom-free, diverticular disease is called diverticulosis. Occasionally, however, one or more of the diverticula become inflamed and cause the diverticular disease known as diverticulitis.

There seems to be some connection between diverticular disease and the low-fiber diet that many people eat in the US. Diverticulitis rarely occurs in Africa and Asia, where more fiber is consumed.

What are the symptoms?

If you have diverticulosis, you may have no symptoms at all, or you may have symptoms like those of an irritable colon (see previous article), including cramping pains and sometimes tenderness in the left side of your abdomen. The cramps may be temporarily relieved when you pass gas or move your bowels. Your stools are often small, round, and hard and you may have occasional attacks of diarrhea. Sometimes diverticula bleed, which causes you to pass red blood in some of your stools.

If you get diverticulitis, you will have severe abdominal pain, often cramping, then becoming more constant, in the lower left part of your abdomen. You may feel nauseated and have a fever. The abdominal pain is aggravated if you push on the sore spot. In some people diverticulitis flares up and then causes disabling pain within a few hours. In other people the symptoms may be mild for several days and then become severe.

What are the risks?

Only a small minority of those with diverticulosis ever develop the symptoms of diverticulitis but, left untreated, this can lead to serious complications, such as the formation of an abscess in or around the colon. If the abscess perforates the intestine, peritonitis (see p.503) can develop, which may cause death without immediate treatment.

What should be done?

Always consult your physician promptly if your bowel movement pattern changes persistently for 2 or 3 weeks or more, or if you have a persistent pain in your lower abdomen. After examining you, your physician may arrange for tests of your blood and samples of your stools, a flexible sigmoidoscopy of your lower bowel, and a barium enema, to make sure that cancer of the large intestine (see p.518), which may have similar symptoms, is not causing your problem.

What is the treatment?

Self-help: It may be possible to prevent the formation of diverticula by modifying your diet. Eat whole-grain breads, oatmeal or bran cereals, and plenty of fibrous fruits and vegetables. Be sure to drink plenty of liquids, too. Many individuals with mild symptoms of diverticulosis have found that the symptoms disappear within 7 to 14 days of beginning such a diet. A high-fiber diet of this kind can, however, cause some distention (inflation) of your abdomen, and you may pass some gas, which often subsides with time. It may be necessary to adjust the amount of fiber in your diet until you find out how much you need. Nonprescription preparations that add bulk to your stools may also be helpful. However, make a point of drinking ample amounts of water with these preparations. If diverticulitis develops and no self-help measures are effective, call your physician.

Professional help: If you have diverticulitis, you may be admitted to a hospital. If your abdomen is distended and you are not passing gas or stool, the contents of your stomach and intestine will be sucked out through a long tube. You will not be allowed to eat or drink at first, and may be given intravenous fluids. This will allow the inflammation to subside. You will receive injections of antibiotics and, if necessary, painkillers. After a few days, when your pain, fever, and abdominal distention have subsided and you are once again passing gas, you will gradually be allowed to eat and drink again.

If, however, the abdominal distention does not subside, this indicates that the channel through the colon is obstructed. A temporary colostomy (see p.518) will be performed if the obstruction is still extensive. The colostomy will be closed and the involved colon removed in about 6 to 12 weeks, when the inflammation has subsided. If the diverticulitis is confined to a small area at the time of surgery, the involved section of the bowel may be removed without the need for a colostomy. Such surgery may require a few days' stay in the hospital.

The prospects of full recovery from even a severe attack of diverticulitis are excellent; however, it may recur.

A cross section of the colon reveals the two forms of diverticular disease, diverticulosis and diverticulitis.

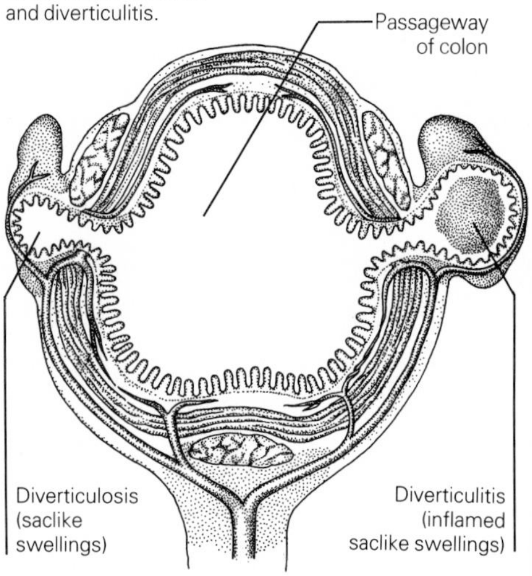

Ulcerative colitis

(inflammatory bowel disease, Crohn's colitis)

Ulcerative colitis is a long-term condition in which raw, inflamed areas called ulcers develop in the lining of the large intestine. These may first appear in the rectum and may gradually spread upward into the lower colon. In many cases the entire large intestine may become involved. No one knows what causes it, but in some cases it mimics Crohn's disease (see p.508). The two conditions have many features in common and are sometimes referred to as "inflammatory bowel disease." Ulcerative colitis is a rare condition. It is more common in women and is most likely to occur in young adults.

What are the symptoms?

Symptoms usually recur periodically for a number of years. You may have an attack of ulcerative colitis with hemorrhaging without any warning, or it may appear with small amounts of rectal bleeding. The most constant sign of the disease is bloody stools. The stool may be formed and covered with blood and mucus when the colitis is confined to the rectum (ulcerative proctitis), or it may be liquid and appear as if it were blood only. With diarrhea there are lower abdominal cramps, and with infection of the ulcerated bowel you have fever, chills, and sweats.

What are the risks?

The first attack is often the worst attack. In any severe attack there is a danger that you may lose large amounts of blood or the bowel may balloon out to several times its usual size and threaten to rupture. Surgery is often mandatory. However, the later attacks are usually not so severe. If you have had extensive ulcerative colitis for 10 years or longer, you are more likely to get cancer of the large intestine (see next page) than someone who has never had the disease.

What should be done?

If you have an attack of diarrhea, with blood, pus, and mucus in it, or just bloody formed stools, consult your physician. If tests of samples of blood and stool show no evidence of infection by bacteria or parasites, the most common cause of such symptoms, the next step is to arrange for endoscopy.

If you are having cramping and severe diarrhea or bleeding profusely, you will be hospitalized and these tests will be performed promptly. Your rectum and large intestine may be examined by sigmoidoscopy and sometimes by colonoscopy. A biopsy specimen from the intestinal wall will probably be taken during one of these tests. You may also have an air contrast barium enema and lower gastrointestinal X-ray examination. However, this test may be postponed until you are stronger.

What is the treatment?

Self-help: The most significant step you can take is to get as much physical and emotional rest as is possible. Your disease can be controlled with rest, diet, and medication.

This disease sometimes occurs after a bout of diarrhea provoked by certain antibiotics or from intestinal parasites acquired during a trip to a developing country. Be aware of these risks if you have ulcerative colitis.

Professional help: The main drugs used to treat ulcerative colitis are anti-inflammatory agents including corticosteroids and sulfasalazine, as well as its non-sulfa-containing salicylate derivatives. In some cases immunosuppressants are prescribed. Such drugs are almost always taken orally. In some cases corticosteroids are given by enema.

Treatment for a severe attack of ulcerative colitis is generally performed in the hospital initially. You may get mild sedation and receive large doses of drugs that require careful monitoring. If you have lost a lot of blood, you may be given transfusions.

Once the acute attack has been controlled, you will be sent home for further rest and convalescence. Your physician will prescribe long-term treatment, usually with smaller, gradually decreasing doses of the drugs mentioned above, to prevent recurrent attacks. If the disease does recur, if you develop complications that cannot be controlled, and if your general health deteriorates, your physician may advise removal of the colon, an operation called total colectomy, with a permanent ileostomy (see Box, next page). This operation usually produces a dramatic improvement.

Benign tumors of the large intestine

(including polyps)

Some tumors of the large intestine are malignant, or likely to spread and threaten life (see Cancer of the large intestine, next article). But benign growths, which are unlikely to spread, are much more common in this part of your body. They occur singly or in groups. Most of them are small, grape-shaped growths called polyps, although an occasional benign tumor can grow large enough to create an intestinal obstruction (see p.503). Since some benign tumors can become malignant, polyps over ½ in (12 mm) in diameter are removed.

Many people have symptom-free tumors that are discovered only as a result of endoscopy or a lower gastrointestinal X-ray examination performed for another reason. Sometimes benign tumors are discovered in the course of fecal occult blood tests, which are performed on stool samples to look for cancers that might be oozing small amounts of hidden blood. Polyps are frequently both diagnosed and removed by means of colonoscopy. Polyps are not usually removed with a flexible sigmoidoscope unless preparations for a full colonoscopy have been made (which includes drinking a sterilized laxative solution that empties the intestine not only of stools but also of explosive methane gas). If this is not feasible in your case, you may need a laparotomy (see Box, p.513) to remove the tumors.

Cancer of the large intestine

(cancer of the colon, cancer of the rectum)

Cancer of the large intestine, which is made up of the colon and rectum, occurs most often in the lowest part, in or near the rectum. As cancerous cells multiply, the normally smooth intestinal lining roughens, enlarges, and hardens, until it develops into an ulcerated area that bleeds easily or into a constriction that hinders bowel movement. If it is allowed to progress, the disease spreads through the intestinal wall to adjacent abdominal organs. It may also enter the bloodstream and spread to the liver and other parts of the body. The cause of the disease is not known, but it occurs at a greater rate in countries where a highly refined, low-fiber diet is common.

What are the symptoms?

There are several possible symptoms, depending on the site of the cancer and how far it has developed. One symptom that should not be ignored if it lasts for more than a week or two is a change in your usual bowel habits. Persistent, inexplicable, abnormal, newly developed constipation or diarrhea (see p.510) may be early warning signs. Bloody stools also should always be reported to your physician. Never ignore this symptom or assume that it is merely caused by hemorrhoids (see p.520).

There may also be vague indications of rumbling and gurgling, bloating, and discomfort, along with tenderness in the lower part of the abdomen. Sometimes the major symptom is simply a lump somewhere in the abdomen, in the bowel, or in the liver to which the cancer has spread. And sometimes there are no symptoms at all until the cancer causes an intestinal obstruction (see p.503) or until the intestine ruptures and causes peritonitis (see p.503).

What are the risks?

Cancer of the large intestine is the third most common type of cancer. Only lung cancer and breast cancer are more common. Men

---

OPERATION:

Intestinal resection with colostomy or ileostomy

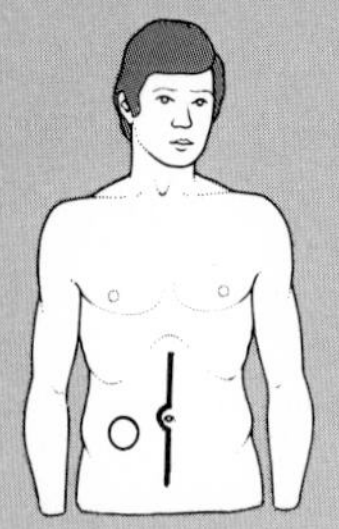

Incision site (line) and position of stoma (circle) in ileostomy.

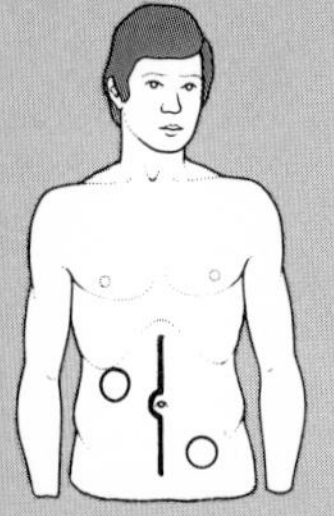

Colostomy incision (line) and possible stoma positions (circles).

In the treatment of certain digestive diseases such as cancer of the large intestine, diverticulitis, and ulcerative colitis, it may be necessary to have an intestinal resection (removal of all or part of the intestine). If possible the two cut ends are sewn together to maintain a passageway for stools. When this is not feasible, an opening called a stoma is made in the abdominal wall, through which stools can pass into a bag. This operation is called a colostomy when the colon opens through the stoma, and an ileostomy when the lower part of the small intestine (the ileum) opens through the stoma.

Before the operation, providing it is not done as an emergency, you will probably be given drugs to reduce the numbers of the natural population of bacteria and other organisms in your intestines.

During the operation You are given a general anesthetic, and through an incision made by the surgeon in the abdominal wall, the diseased part of the digestive tract is identified, the tumor is located, and is then removed. The upper end of the tract is joined to the lower end. If the intestinal channel cannot be preserved all the way to the anus, the remaining end of the intestine is stitched into a separate incision in the stomach wall to form the stoma.

After the operation You will receive nutrients intravenously, and fluid will be drained from your abdomen. Within 2 to 3 days you will start consuming a special diet and begin to pass waste materials and gases into the bag.

Convalescence You will be counseled by nurses who are experts in stoma care and equipment. Gradually, you will become adept at emptying and cleaning the bag. People with colostomies can eventually return to an almost normal bowel routine, sometimes needing to empty their bag only once a day. Sometimes bowel control becomes so good that the wearer needs only a pad over the stoma for most of the day. Those with ileostomies usually need to keep the bag in place all the time, although some surgeons modify the small intestine just inside the abdominal wall (to create a pouch reservoir) and create a form of valve at the stoma so the person can empty his or her ileostomy at will. This is called a continent ileostomy.

and women are equally susceptible to cancer of the large intestine, which is most prevalent among people over 40, especially among those who are in their 60s and 70s. Also, about 1 of every 20 people who have had ulcerative colitis for more than 10 years (see p.516) eventually has cancer of the colon.

Because most cancers of the large intestine develop and spread slowly, you have a good chance of complete cure if the disease is diagnosed early. If the malignancy has already spread to the liver, however, the outlook is less favorable, but further surgery and chemotherapy are available.

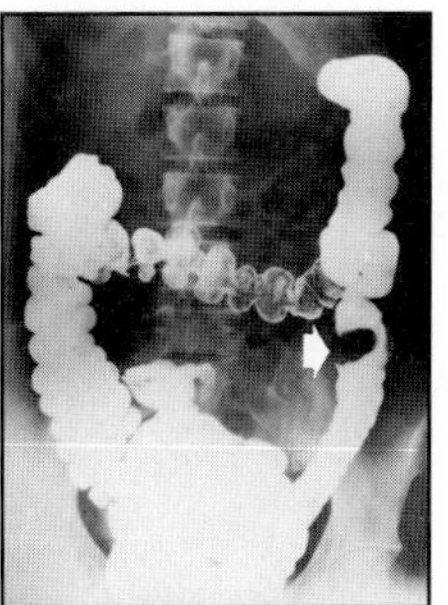

Cancer of the large intestine appears on an X ray as a dark mass (arrow) on the inner wall of the colon.

What should be done?

Research is continuing into the most effective way of screening for cancer of the large intestine in healthy people. Currently, most physicians recommend that tests on the stools for traces of blood (fecal occult blood tests) and a rectal examination should be included in the regular physical checkups of both men and women after age 50. If you have any of the symptoms mentioned above, consult your physician, who will examine you carefully and will insert a rubber-gloved finger into your rectum to check for a rectal growth. You may also need to provide stool samples for laboratory tests, and you may need to undergo other procedures such as an air contrast barium enema. Your physician may want you to have a proctosigmoidoscopy (an examination of the rectum and sigmoid colon by means of a flexible instrument fitted with a light) or possibly a colonoscopy (an endoscopy of the entire colon) if blood is found in your stool.

What is the treatment?

Surgery is the best treatment for cancer of the large intestine if it has not progressed too far. If it is confined to your colon, the growth is removed along with a nearby section of healthy colon. The two ends of the colon are then sewn together. If the cancer is very low in the rectum, a colostomy (see Box, p.518) may be necessary; however, with newer methods of stapling the ends of the intestine together, many colostomies can be avoided.

Survival of people with colon cancer has been enhanced when chemotherapy with drugs such as levamisole is used near the time of the surgery. Radiation therapy is used for some people who have rectal cancer that is inoperable or recurrent.

What are the long-term prospects?

Most people who have operations for cancer of the large intestine survive in good health for 5 years or longer. Annual screening for people over age 50 with flexible sigmoidoscopy improves survival time for many.

The anus

The anus is a canal 1½ in (4 cm) long. It leads from the rectum, down through a ring of muscles called the anal sphincter, to the anal opening, through which solid wastes are eliminated as stools. If you are healthy and past early childhood, you normally control the anal sphincter and the time for moving your bowels. The anus is relatively simple in its structure and function, so generally not much can go wrong. The only common anal disorder is hemorrhoids.

One reason that so many people have hemorrhoids may be the large amounts of highly refined, low-fiber foods in the typical American diet. Waste products of such nonfibrous foods form small, dry, hard stools that can stretch and even tear the sphincter walls as they pass through. And because they do not pass easily, nearly every such dry bowel movement requires enough straining potentially to damage the anus. Another reason for the prevalence of hemorrhoids is that many people worry unnecessarily about their bowel movements and work too hard, sitting too long on the toilet, forcing their sphincter muscles and increasing the pressure in the veins of the anus. Our normal upright posture is thought to contribute to the problem by increasing the pressure in the hemorrhoidal veins.

Hemorrhoids

Hemorrhoids are varicose veins (see p.441) in your anus. The affected veins lie just under the mucous membrane that lines the lowest part of the rectum and the anus. They become swollen because of repeatedly increased pressure within them, usually as a result of persistent straining as you move your bowels. Hemorrhoids often appear during pregnancy and immediately after delivery but usually subside in several weeks (see Varicose veins during pregnancy, p.669). Many people who are obese (see p.530) also have them, as do almost all people with advanced cirrhosis of the liver. If you have hemorrhoids, the swollen, twisted veins in your anus are thin-walled and easily ruptured by the passage of a hard stool. An internal hemorrhoid is one near the beginning of the anal canal. If the bulging vein is farther down, virtually at the anal opening, it is considered external.

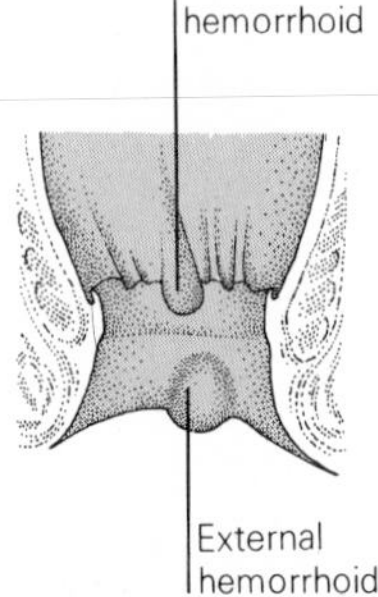

An internal hemorrhoid forms inside the lower part of the rectum and may not be visible from the outside. An external hemorrhoid forms at or just inside the anus and may become visible if it prolapses (protrudes) through the opening of the anus.

External hemorrhoids sometimes protrude outside the anus. This may happen only as you move your bowels, after which the vein springs back into place. Thrombosis may also occur, in which the blood in the hemorrhoid clots; this causes considerable pain.

What are the symptoms?

Bleeding is the main, and often the only, symptom. In addition, bowel movements may become increasingly painful to the extent that you hold back your bowel movements. This results in the stool remaining in the rectum, where more water is absorbed, which causes a cycle of harder, drier stools, more pain, and more bleeding. Protruding hemorrhoids often produce a mucous discharge and itching around the anus. If there is thrombosis in a hemorrhoidal vein, you may also have severe pain.

What are the risks?

Hemorrhoids are very common; most people have occasional bleeding from them. Serious trouble is less common. Hemorrhoids alone are not dangerous, though they can be annoying and painful. The risk is that you may assume bleeding is from hemorrhoids when it could be caused by cancer of the rectum or colon (see Cancer of the large intestine, p.518), especially if you are over 40. That is why you should always see your physician at the first sign of anal bleeding.

What should be done?

Consult your physician if you detect signs of anal bleeding. He or she may examine your anus with a rubber-gloved finger and look at the area through a proctoscope. To exclude the possibility of cancer, you may also need a barium enema and flexible sigmoidoscopy or even colonoscopy.

What is the treatment?

Self-help: To produce soft, easily passed stools, eat plenty of fruit, vegetables, bran cereals, and whole-grain bread. You should also drink plenty of water and other liquids, including prune juice, if needed. If you already have hemorrhoids, wash yourself thoroughly but gently after every bowel movement by using soft, moist paper and dry yourself very carefully afterward. Paper

OPERATION:

Removing hemorrhoids

(hemorrhoidectomy and ligation)

There are several different methods for removing painful or bleeding hemorrhoids. The traditional method, used less frequently today, is to cut them out by stretching then cutting each one at its base. You may need to take painkillers for the first few bowel movements following the operation.

Some clinics advertise the removal of hemorrhoids with a laser. The laser serves as a cutting device that seals blood vessels as it cuts. Heat probes applied to the hemorrhoid are also used to destroy the vessel.

Another more common method of removing hemorrhoids is to place a tight rubber band over the base of each one, obstructing its blood flow, so that it withers painlessly over a few days. This process, called ligation, can be done during a brief visit to the physician's office or a hospital outpatient clinic and usually does not require a local anesthetic.

pads impregnated with soothing oils are available over the counter to be used with toilet paper. If you have protruding hemorrhoids, tuck them back in with your finger after every bowel movement to avoid abrasion and irritation. A diet as discussed above and good hygiene will generally control hemorrhoids and may clear up a mild case. To soothe inflamed hemorrhoids use nonprescription rectal suppositories containing hydrocortisone, local anesthetics, and astringents. Always follow the directions on the package. For a painful attack stay in bed. An ice compress may relieve the swelling. Soaking in a warm bath a couple of times a day may also help. If pain persists for more than 24 hours, see your physician.

Professional help: If a thrombosed (clotted) hemorrhoid causes extreme pain, your physician may remove the clot. A local anesthetic may be used. A physician will usually suggest that you use soothing or painkilling ointments or suppositories that contain corticosteroid drugs. Some suppositories also contain a local anesthetic. Additional measures, if constipation persists, include a high-fiber diet with lots of fluids, attention to proper toilet habits (see Constipation and diarrhea, p.510), and, if necessary, a bulk laxative with even more fluids.

If your hemorrhoids do not heal, additional treatment may be necessary. One possible procedure is to destroy the hemorrhoids by cryosurgery, which involves freezing the affected tissue. Another treatment is to inject a special chemical that shrinks internal hemorrhoids. Occasionally, the swollen veins are removed surgically with a procedure called a hemorrhoidectomy. It is a relatively simple operation (see previous page).

Pruritus ani

(anal itching)

Itching around the anus is common, particularly in children and older people. In children the cause may be pinworms (see p.751), especially if the itching is worse at night. In adults, anal itching may be caused by hemorrhoids (see previous article), which prevent the anal canal from fully closing, allowing a bit of mucus to seep onto the skin around the anus, irritating it and causing itching. But more often there is no obvious cause. Itching tends to become more prevalent with age as the skin becomes drier and less elastic.

Anal itching can usually be relieved by careful hygiene. After a bowel movement clean the skin around the anus thoroughly with a moist tissue or paper treated with lubricants. You should not use soap as this may dry the skin and aggravate the itching. A warm bath or shower (without using soap) before bed should reduce the likelihood of itching during the night.

Anal fissure

A fissure is an elongated ulcer that extends upward into the anal canal from the anal opening. When you have a bowel movement, irritation of the ulcer causes spasm (tightening) of the sphincter, which causes severe pain and sometimes bleeding. This rare condition, which occurs most often in women, can sometimes be cured with the use of a high-fiber diet, plenty of fluid, and good toilet habits (see Constipation and diarrhea, p.510). Warm baths after painful bowel movements often help to reduce painful spasms.

If the fissure is persistent or recurs, however, you may need to have a minor operation on the anus to dilate (widen) the anal sphincter muscle and to remove the fissure. The surgery stops spasms, pain, and bleeding, and healing occurs rapidly.

Anal fistula

A spreading abscess within the anus can erode the tissue and cause the rare condition known as anal fistula. The fistula is a tiny tube that leads directly from the anal canal to a tiny hole in the skin near the anal opening. A continual discharge of watery pus through this small hole irritates the skin and may cause discomfort and itching. Sometimes, too, the underlying abscess is painful. There is a very slight possibility that an anal fistula indicates the presence of Crohn's disease (see p.508), ulcerative colitis (see p.516), or cancer of the large intestine (see p.518). If you consult your physician about this problem, you may need diagnostic X rays of the intestines and endoscopy.

The usual treatment, once your physician is certain that you do not have Crohn's disease, is a minor operation to remove the fistula and drain the abscess. A fistula caused by inflammatory bowel disease often heals when the disorder is brought under control.

Liver, gallbladder, and pancreas

The liver, gallbladder, and pancreas, together with the digestive tract, make up the digestive system. The liver is the largest single internal organ. It fills the upper-right-hand part of the abdomen behind the lower ribs. The liver has a crucial and complex role in regulating the composition of the blood and also plays a large part in many other body processes. Aging red blood cells, which contain the oxygen-carrying protein hemoglobin, are broken down in the spleen and to some extent in the liver. The hemoglobin is converted into another substance, bilirubin. A fluid called bile that contains bilirubin and various other substances (among them bile salts and cholesterol) trickles through tiny tubes to the gallbladder, a collecting bag that nestles against the undersurface of the liver (where water is absorbed and the bile stored). When you eat, the gallbladder empties the bile along the bile duct into the duodenum, the first part of the small intestine. Bile, a waste product, also plays an important role in digestion by helping to counteract stomach acid and by aiding in the digestion of fats.

The pancreas lies just behind the lower part of the stomach. It has two distinct functions, one of which is to make certain hormones, including insulin (see Diabetes mellitus, p.558). Its other function is to make enzymes, or digestive juices, that flow down the pancreatic duct and into the duodenum, where they break food down into molecules that are small enough to be used by and absorbed into the body.

Liver and stomach (front view)

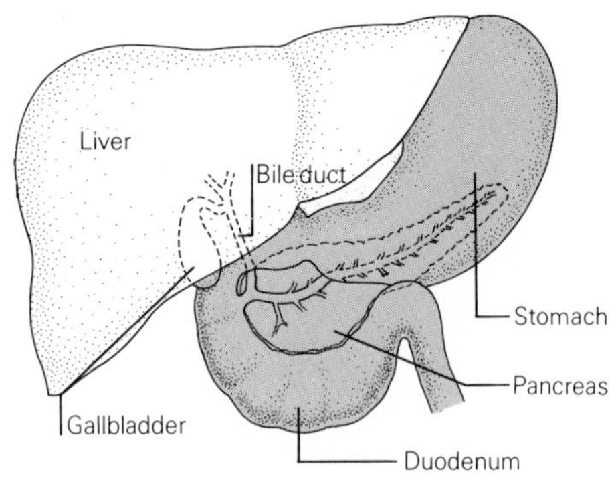

Closer view with liver omitted

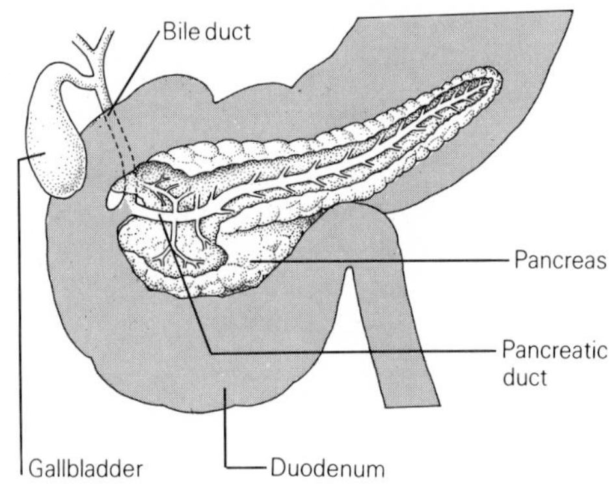

Jaundice

See p.252, **Visual aids to diagnosis, 47.**

Jaundice is a condition that discolors the skin and the whites of the eyes with a yellow pigment. The condition is caused by an excess of bilirubin in the bloodstream. Bilirubin is a by-product of the breakdown of aging red blood cells. The liver filters bilirubin from the bloodstream and excretes it into the bile ducts, which carry it to the gallbladder, and from there the bilirubin eventually flows into the small intestine. Most of the bilirubin is then broken down by bacteria normally present in your intestine, and the bilirubin is eliminated from the body as pigmented compounds in stools.

Looking at the whites of the eyes may help diagnose jaundice.

Jaundice most frequently results from liver diseases, including viral infections such as hepatitis (see next articles), cirrhosis (see p.524), and cancers that spread to the liver. Drug reactions can also cause it. Another possible cause is obstruction of the bile ducts. This can prevent bilirubin from entering the intestines, which creates pressure in the liver. This can happen with gallstones (see p.526) and pancreatic tumors (see Cancer of the pancreas, p.529). Jaundice also occurs in hemolytic anemia (see p.454), in which many red blood cells are destroyed and bilirubin is released into the bloodstream. In that case, the liver functions normally, but it is unable to remove bilirubin from the blood rapidly enough. This causes jaundice.

What should be done?

If you notice the symptoms above, consult your physician immediately. Treatment will depend on the underlying disorder. Once the cause is treated and brought under control or cured, the jaundice should disappear.

Acute hepatitis

Acute hepatitis is a sudden inflammation of the liver caused by one of several viruses, including the three viruses called A, B, and C, but a few attacks of hepatitis seem to be caused by yet other viruses. The viruses cause diseases with many characteristics in common, such as jaundice, pale stools, dark urine, loss of energy, loss of appetite, and fever; but there are also substantial differences in the way the diseases are transmitted and in their outlook.

Hepatitis A is spread from person to person by poor personal hygiene or when water or food is contaminated by sewage. The disease is very common in developing countries with inadequate systems of sanitation. The early symptoms of the disease are similar to other virus infections, with muscle and joint aching, fever, headache, and weakness, but the most prominent symptoms are loss of appetite and nausea. In some cases the illness disappears with no further symptoms or signs, but more often jaundice develops after a few days. Usually the hepatitis clears up without treatment in 2 to 8 weeks, but the recovery period may be prolonged by lack of energy and motivation for another period of weeks or months. In a very few cases the hepatitis may rapidly progress to cause liver failure and death.

Both hepatitis B and hepatitis C are spread from person to person by two main routes: contact with infected blood and heterosexual or homosexual activities. Outbreaks caused by contaminated water supplies have been reported on rare occasions. Until the mid-1980s these forms of hepatitis were commonly transmitted by blood transfusion and by treatment of patients with blood products (such as factor VIII for hemophilia), but this risk has now been almost eliminated by testing of blood donors and the use of genetic engineering to make safe blood products. Infection still occurs commonly, however, among drug addicts who share needles, and it may be transmitted by tattooists and acupuncturists who fail to sterilize their equipment. Hepatitis B and hepatitis C are also an occupational risk for physicians, nurses, and health care workers who come into frequent contact with blood.

Hepatitis B (and to a lesser extent hepatitis C) is a common sexually transmitted disease, and along with other such diseases occurs frequently in prostitutes and in male homosexuals with many partners. Hepatitis B, and probably hepatitis C, may be transmitted from a pregnant woman to her fetus; this is a serious problem in developing countries.

The blood of someone infected with either hepatitis B or C is highly infectious both during the incubation period (6 to 12 weeks, sometimes much longer, between the time you are infected and the time that symptoms appear) and after the illness has seemingly cleared up. Some people become lifelong carriers of these viruses.

The risk of progressive, life-threatening, chronic active hepatitis is greater in those infected with hepatitis B and C. People with hepatitis C are also more likely to develop chronic liver disease eventually.

What is the risk?

Blood banks now routinely use screening tests for the two types of hepatitis transmitted by blood, and the risk of contracting hepatitis from blood transfusion is declining. A vaccine against hepatitis B is available for people at high risk, such as physicians and nurses. Hepatitis A remains a risk for people traveling to remote areas of developing countries; if you are planning such a trip you should talk to your physician beforehand. A blood test can be done to determine whether you are immune; if you are not, immunization with gamma-globulin gives protection from hepatitis A for a few months.

What should be done?

If your physician suspects that you have virus hepatitis, he or she will ask you about risk factors, examine you, and then take a blood sample for laboratory testing. It is important to determine which virus is responsible, and the extent of damage to the function of your liver, to evaluate the potential severity of the illness. Blood tests may be repeated at regular intervals to monitor any damage to the liver. To help reduce the risk of getting hepatitis through sexual contact, see the box on "Safer sex," p.466.

What is the treatment?

Until you hear the results of your blood tests, you will not know which hepatitis virus is responsible, and you should assume that your stools and all your body fluids are infectious. If you are recovering at home, you should flush stools from any bedpan use directly down the toilet, sterilize the bedpan, and wash your hands scrupulously. An infected person may, however, share a bathroom with the rest of the family. Any soiled clothing or bed linen should be laundered in hot water with a detergent and bleach. Toilets and floors should be cleaned thoroughly and often with hot water and a disinfectant.

If your symptoms are mild, your physician will probably recommend that you stay home for several weeks, eat a high-protein, high-carbohydrate diet, and get plenty of rest. You should not drink alcohol. If your symptoms are more severe or if laboratory tests indicate that you have liver damage, you may be admitted to a hospital, possibly for a needle biopsy of the liver and for treatment. This may include corticosteroid drugs or antiviral agents such as interferon.

Chronic hepatitis

Anyone who has had an attack of acute hepatitis (see previous article) may develop chronic hepatitis. The risk appears to be highest with hepatitis C, with up to 50 percent of those who have the acute form developing chronic hepatitis C; the risk is less with hepatitis B. Many people, however, develop chronic hepatitis without any obvious acute hepatitis. It may be caused by other less common causes of liver inflammation or by reactions to drugs, including isoniazid, which is used to treat tuberculosis.

Chronic hepatitis is classified into two main types, chronic persistent hepatitis and chronic active hepatitis. In both diseases, the body responds with an immune response that may damage the cells in the liver. In chronic persistent hepatitis progression of the illness is slow, and the patient usually remains in good health and is unlikely to develop cirrhosis (see next article). Chronic active hepatitis is a less predictable disease. In a number of cases there is a steady, progressive destruction of the liver cells that leads to cirrhosis. In some people the disease comes and goes at times in response to treatment. In other cases, however, the disease responds well to treatment, and the symptoms of the disease clear up.

The severity of chronic active hepatitis varies from case to case. Some people have no symptoms of the disease for long periods but occasionally have episodes of jaundice, joint pains, nausea, fever, and loss of appetite. Uncommonly, people with chronic hepatitis B may have acute flare-ups caused by yet another hepatitis virus, the Delta virus, which affects only those already infected with hepatitis B. Others have no symptoms despite having mild liver inflammation for many years. For them, the disorder can be detected only by blood tests.

What should be done?

Your physician will consider that you have a form of chronic hepatitis if your health remains poor after an acute attack of jaundice and the results from your liver function blood tests remain abnormal. The condition may also be discovered during laboratory tests for vague symptoms such as loss of energy and poor appetite. Once the diagnosis is made, your physician is likely to recommend a liver biopsy (a procedure in which a small amount of tissue is removed for microscopic examination) so that he or she can assess the nature and the severity of the inflammation and plan your treatment.

Depending on your general health and the results of the biopsy, your physician may be able to reassure you that the disease is likely to clear up without treatment. Or, to prevent cirrhosis of the liver from developing, your physician may prescribe an immunosuppressive drug such as azathioprine or an antiviral agent such as interferon.

Most people who have chronic active hepatitis recover within 1 to 3 years. Those who do not recover develop cirrhosis of the liver (see next article).

Cirrhosis of the liver

Cirrhosis is a chronic disease that causes slow deterioration of the liver. Damage to the liver from one of many causes changes its structure by replacing its functioning cells with scar tissue; the liver becomes less able to carry out its many functions.

The most common cause of the disease in the US is alcohol addiction (see p.329). Malnutrition, hepatitis (see previous articles), parasites, toxic chemicals, drug reaction, and congestive heart failure (see p.408) are some other possible causes of the disease.

What are the symptoms?

In the very early stages, while there are still plenty of healthy liver cells, symptoms are absent or mild. As the disease progresses, however, loss of appetite, weight loss, nausea, vomiting, general loss of your sense of well-being, weakness, indigestion, and abdominal distention all become increasingly pronounced. There is a tendency to bleed and bruise easily. Small, red, spidery marks called spider nevi may appear on your face, arms, and upper part of the trunk.

In the later stages, jaundice (see p.522) may occur. Men may lose interest in sex, their breasts enlarge, and they become impotent. Women usually stop having periods (see Absence of periods, p.624). Eventually, liver failure may develop. Fluid retention in the abdomen and ankles, irritability, and an inability to concentrate are the most common symptoms. Memory is impaired and the hands tremble noticeably. Confusion and drowsiness occur and increase, leading to coma as the condition worsens. Life-threatening bleeding from enlarged veins in the esophagus may also occur.

What are the risks?

When cirrhosis develops as a complication of chronic active hepatitis (see previous article), the outlook for recovery is poor. By contrast, a heavy drinker who develops signs of early cirrhosis has excellent prospects for recovery if he or she stops drinking permanently and follows medical advice.

The disease progresses at different rates depending on your circumstances. If your disease is detected at an early stage, you can slow its progress by following the treatment carefully. If you do not give up alcohol, however, the disease will almost surely cause liver failure. Cirrhosis of the liver also increases the risk of severe bleeding in the digestive tract. If this happens it is usually difficult to control and may cause fatal hemorrhage from the blood loss or from liver failure that is set in motion by the bleeding. Very rarely, a tumor develops in the liver as a result of cirrhosis (see next page).

What should be done?

Consult your physician if you think you have cirrhosis; this is a distinct possibility if you consume alcohol heavily and regularly or if you have chronic hepatitis from any cause. A physical examination is often sufficient for a diagnosis, although you may have to have blood tests and a liver biopsy, in which a small portion of the liver is removed and examined to assess the extent of the damage. If you have an alcohol addiction, talk to your physician about whether your liver damage can still be reversed if you stop drinking.

What is the treatment?

Self-help: Whatever the underlying cause of cirrhosis, it is vital to stop drinking alcohol immediately. If your cirrhosis is due to alcohol and you stop drinking, you should be able to lead a relatively active life. If you continue to drink, the disease will certainly get worse. Your liver will remain particularly sensitive to alcohol, so any future drinking should be considered virtually suicidal.

If you suspect that you may be addicted to alcohol, see your physician as soon as possible and discuss the matter frankly. There are several ways of treating alcoholism, but until you admit your problem and deal with it, nobody else can help. Inaction and denial can cost you your life.

Do not take any nonprescription drugs or medication without your physician's approval. Try to follow a well-balanced, nutritious diet that contains adequate protein and plenty of carbohydrates and vitamins, but is also low in salt (sodium).

Professional help: Your physician can prescribe drugs to relieve the symptoms of cirrhosis, but they will not reverse the course of the disease. Diuretics reduce the fluid in your body, and antacids may relieve abdominal discomfort. To guard against malnutrition, your physician may recommend vitamin supplements. Depending on the cause of the cirrhosis, corticosteroids or other immunosuppressive drugs may also be prescribed. If you vomit blood (see p.501), you may need blood transfusions and surgery.

Hospitalization is necessary for the complications of extreme fluid accumulation or gastrointestinal bleeding, or if you go into a coma. Otherwise treatment is directed toward relief of symptoms.

The prospects for a person in the last stages of cirrhosis or liver destruction from certain poisons or toxins have improved dramatically as a result of some recent advances in liver transplants (see p.433). A person who has cirrhosis as a complication of chronic active hepatitis (see previous article) or a disorder known as primary biliary cirrhosis may be restored to an active life by a successful liver transplant. A transplant is recommended less often for a person who has advanced cirrhosis caused by alcohol, since the alcohol may also have damaged the heart, brain, and other organs. However, successful transplants have been reported in people who stop drinking alcohol permanently.

Tumors of the liver

Like tumors elsewhere in the body, liver tumors may be benign (unlikely to spread) or malignant (likely to spread). Benign tumors are extremely rare. If they are discovered, benign liver tumors can usually be removed safely and completely.

There are two types of malignant tumors. The majority are metastases, or cancers that have spread from other parts of the body through the bloodstream to the liver. About one third of all cancers spread to the liver in this way, and in some cases it is the symptoms of the secondary liver cancer that finally draw attention to a primary cancer elsewhere. Cancer may start in the liver (primary liver cancer), but this is very rare and is often associated with prior infection with the hepatitis B or C virus.

What are the symptoms?

The symptoms may be only those from the primary cancer, most often cancer of the breast, lung, or gastrointestinal tract. As liver cancer develops, it causes further loss of weight and appetite, abdominal discomfort, weakness, and fatigue. Jaundice (see p.522) may appear in the late stages.

What should be done?

Consult your physician. The outlook is poor once cancer has spread to the liver. Surgical removal of a primary tumor or a single metastasis, or even a liver transplant (see p.433), may be performed. Or, for a tumor that has metastasized from the colon and is confined to the liver, anticancer drugs may be an effective treatment.

Gallstones

Stones of varying composition sometimes form in the gallbladder, the reservoir in which bile collects. Bile is in part a waste product that flows from the liver to the gallbladder. From there it is excreted into the intestines, where it combats stomach acid to some degree and aids in fat digestion.

Bile is rich in cholesterol, which is excreted by the liver. Bile also contains bilirubin, a substance that is formed by the breakdown of hemoglobin (see Basic parts of the blood, p.449) from old red blood cells. Sometimes if the balance of these dissolved substances is upset, a tiny solid particle forms in the gallbladder. The particle may grow and become a gallstone as more cholesterol or, rarely, bilirubin builds up around it. Some people may have only one gallstone; other people may have several.

What are the symptoms?

Between one third and one half of people with gallstones do not experience any symptoms. However, some gallstones flow out of the liver with the bile and may get stuck in the bile duct. If this happens the result is biliary colic, an intense pain either in the right side or center of your upper abdomen, which may radiate around the ribs or through to your back. Over a period of a few hours the pain builds to a peak and then fades. It makes you feel very nauseated and causes you to vomit.

Biliary colic is a result of the gallbladder and muscle of the bile duct clamping down and trying unsuccessfully to empty the stone into the intestines. If the stone falls back into the gallbladder, or is forced along the bile duct into the intestines, the blockage that had been causing the problem is no longer there and the pain quickly ceases.

A more common problem develops when a stone blocks the cystic duct and inflammation develops in the gallbladder (see Acute cholecystitis, next article).

What are the risks?

Some 20 million people in the US have gallstones. About 1 million new cases develop each year. Autopsy studies show that 80 percent of all people who reach 90 years of age have gallstones when they die.

If a gallstone remains lodged in your bile duct for any length of time, it may block the exit for bile and cause obstructive jaundice (see Jaundice, p.522).

If the exit for bile is blocked, another risk is inflammation and infection of the bile ducts extending into the liver as the dammed-up

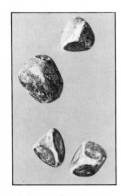

Gallstones form in different shapes and sizes. They may be large and smooth or small, sharp, and crystalline.

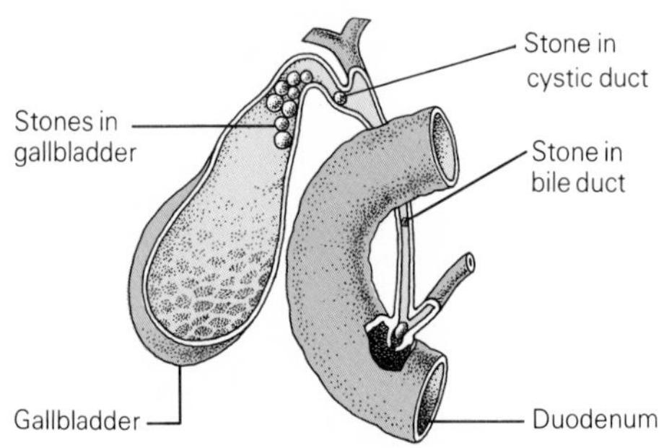

Gallstone sites
Gallstones may remain in the gallbladder or pass uninterrupted through the bile duct into the duodenum. In either case you will probably have no symptoms. Problems arise if the gallstones are trapped in a bile duct.

OPERATION:

Gallbladder removal by laparoscopy

Removal of the gallbladder is one of many operations that today can be performed by remote control through a small "keyhole" incision that leaves only a tiny scar. Having evaluated the number and location of the gallstones by ultrasound and X-ray investigations, your surgeon inserts a laparoscope into the abdomen. This narrow tube carries an optical system that transmits a clear image of the abdominal contents onto a video monitor. Tiny precision instruments passed down a channel in the laparoscope or through separate tiny abdominal incisions are used to remove any gallstones and the air in the gallbladder, to remove the now deflated gallbladder, and to tie off the cystic duct that connects it to the main bile duct and also to the blood vessels.

During the operation you are under a general anesthetic. The procedure takes less than an hour, and afterward you will have only a small dressing over the incisions. You usually are able to go home that day. But major complications can result from this procedure.

Clipping the cystic duct

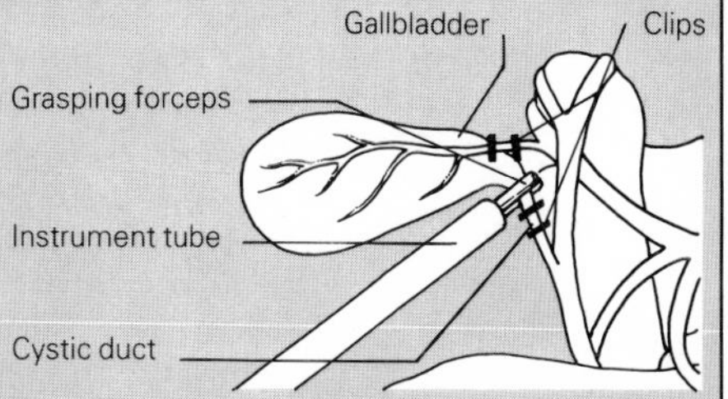

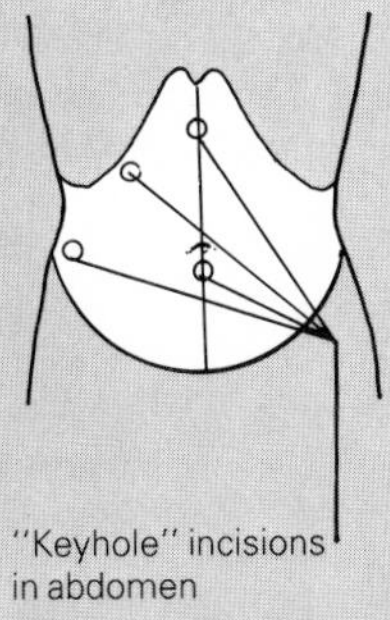

Inside the upper abdomen

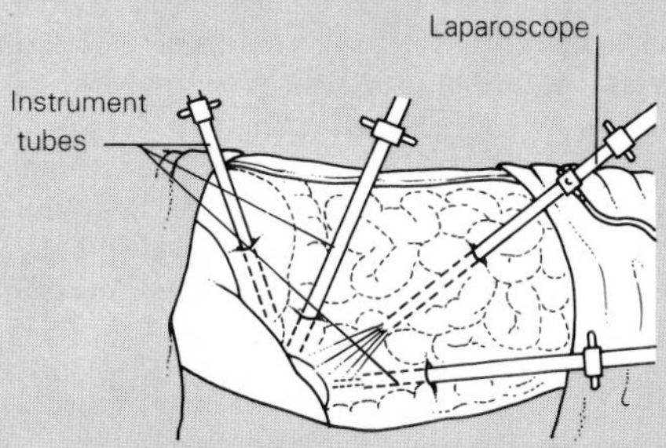

Removing the gallbladder

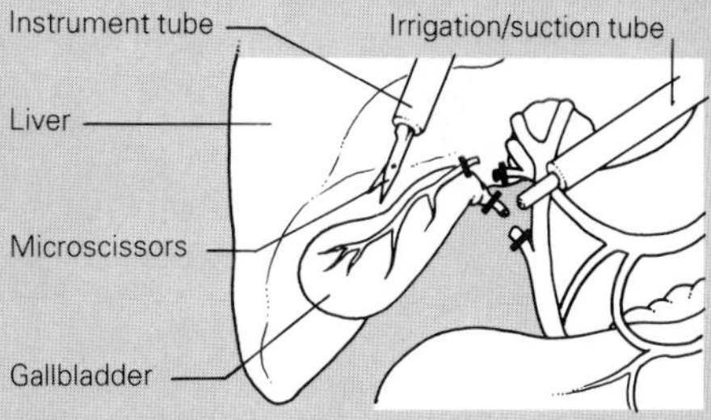

bile becomes stagnant. This requires immediate treatment including intravenous antibiotics and often surgery to remove any stone stuck in the bile ducts.

If you have gallstones, you are also susceptible to acute pancreatitis (see next page). This is because the pancreatic duct drains into the bile duct and it, too, may be blocked by a gallstone.

What should be done?

If you have a severe pain resembling biliary colic, consult your physician immediately or go directly to the hospital emergency department, where you will be examined and questioned about the pain. If gallstones are suspected to be the cause, the physician will probably take blood samples for analysis and an ultrasound scan will be performed.

What is the treatment?

Self-help: If biliary colic develops, call your physician and go to bed. Do not eat or drink.

Professional help: To relieve the colic initially, your physician may inject a strong painkiller. But if tests show you have gallstones in your bile duct, your physician will recommend that you have them removed. The stones may be removed using a laparoscope (see Box, above). In very ill people the stones may be removed via a laparotomy (see p.513) and incision into the bile duct, followed by removal of the gallbladder. The stone or stones may also be pulverized by means of extracorporeal sound wave lithotripsy (see next article). In another procedure, an incision is made into the circular muscle that guards the opening of the bile and pancreatic ducts into the duodenum with tiny instruments passed through an endoscope. Then the stones are grasped or pulled through in a tiny basket or (if numerous) allowed to pass through the new enlarged opening. Your surgeon will discuss with you the safest and most effective procedure for your condition.

Cholecystitis

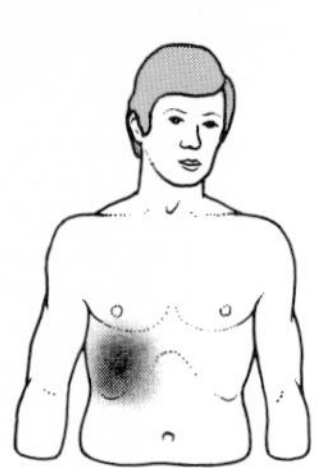

Site of the pain

In cholecystitis, the gallbladder becomes inflamed and swollen. This is usually a result of a gallstone that is lodged in the cystic duct (see previous article), blocking the flow of bile from the gallbladder into the intestine. Rarely, the inflammation is caused by an infection that is spreading upward into the gallbladder from the intestine.

The symptoms of cholecystitis itself are preceded by severe pain in the upper part of your abdomen, usually on the right-hand side, which may spread around your right rib cage to the tip of your shoulder blades. This is called biliary colic (see Gallstones, previous article). As cholecystitis develops, your temperature rises, and nausea and vomiting follow. If the condition is not treated you may develop jaundice (see p.522).

Three fourths of the people who have this disorder have had previous gallbladder problems. If, as happens in rare cases, the gallbladder swells so much that it bursts, a severe form of peritonitis (see p.503) may develop; this is a medical emergency.

If you suspect cholecystitis, especially if you already have gallbladder problems, consult your physician immediately.

You may be admitted to a hospital and given an intravenous drip to provide you with nutrition and fluid. You may not be allowed to eat or drink for a few days. You may be given painkillers and antibiotics by injection or intravenously. Tests may be performed to determine whether gallstones are present (see previous article). If you have had cholecystitis, you will be advised to have your gallbladder removed. In severe cases of cholecystitis, this may be done within a day or two after you are admitted to the hospital, but some surgeons prefer that you wait until after the inflammation has subsided.

The traditional cholecystectomy surgery involves a long surgical incision on the right side of the upper abdomen to allow the surgeon access to the gallbladder, which is removed along with the small duct connecting it to the bile duct. The operation is a safe and effective procedure; it provides a final treatment, and the stones will not recur. The disadvantages are that cholecystectomy is a major operation carrying a small but unavoidable risk of complications, including death, especially in older people.

Laparoscopic cholecystectomy is the treatment of choice (see Box, p.527). It requires at most an overnight stay in the hospital and is often performed in an outpatient surgical facility. The patient can return to work in 2 to 7 days, there is a tiny scar, and the procedure is as safe as traditional open surgery but is much less debilitating.

Gallstones may also be dissolved by long-term treatment with drugs, but this method has several disadvantages. You may need to take drugs for 1 to 2 years before the stones disappear completely, the drugs work in only half the cases, and even after the stones have gone, there is a high risk that they will recur once treatment is stopped. Furthermore, the medications cause side effects, especially diarrhea, in some people.

Yet another approach is for the stones to be pulverized by lithotripsy, or shock waves that pass through the skin. This method is appropriate for people with single small stones or stones in the bile duct. The combination of lithotripsy and stone-dissolving drugs is currently being evaluated.

Differences of opinion exist among physicians regarding the treatment of so-called silent gallstones—those found by accident during the investigation of other disorders. Many people have gallstones for years without any symptoms. You and your physician need to balance the risks associated with surgery now against future gallstone problems or the very remote possibility of gallbladder cancer.

Acute pancreatitis

In this infrequent disease, the pancreas suddenly becomes inflamed. About half the people who develop acute pancreatitis already have gallstones. Other causes are excessive use of alcohol and, less commonly, certain drugs, a penetrating duodenal ulcer (see p.500), hyperparathyroidism (see p.569), or an abdominal injury. It can also be a complication of mumps (see p.748).

What are the symptoms?

The main symptom is agonizing pain in the center of your upper abdomen. It often begins 12 to 24 hours after a large meal or a heavy bout of drinking. The pain seems to bore through to the back and is accompanied by vomiting. In severe cases you become very ill and feverish, have bruise marks on your abdomen from internal bleeding around the pancreas, and may even have the symptoms of shock (see p.414).

The main danger of an attack of acute pancreatitis is that shock, which can cause death, will develop. There is a long-term risk that acute pancreatitis may lead to chronic pancreatitis (see next article). However, the majority of people who have their first episode recover completely. Cystlike blisters (pseudocysts) sometimes form on the pancreas after an attack. If they cause symptoms they may require surgery.

What is the treatment?

If you have the symptoms mentioned above, you will be admitted to a hospital as soon as possible. Your physician's first task will be to establish the diagnosis by taking X rays and blood samples. Analysis of the blood samples for certain levels of pancreatic enzymes and other body chemicals often reveals the presence of the disease.

You will probably take painkillers and injections of drugs to reduce some of the pancreatic juices. Shock is treated with intravenous fluids. Antibiotics may be necessary. As you recover, you will gradually be able to eat and drink, but should never drink alcohol again. This is vital to prevent chronic pancreatitis. After further convalescence, an ultrasound scan is performed to look for gallstones, which your physician may then want to remove (see p.527).

Chronic pancreatitis

Chronic pancreatitis is a disease of the pancreas that develops over the course of several years. It sometimes follows recurrent attacks of acute pancreatitis (see previous article), usually associated with gallstones (see p.526) or alcohol abuse (see p.329). In such cases, you do not recover fully between attacks. Gradually the damaged pancreas loses its ability to supply its digestive juices and hormones.

What are the symptoms?

Pain is the main symptom, although in 1 in 10 cases there is no pain at all. It is a dull, cramping, boring pain that is aggravated by food and alcohol and is relieved when you sit up and lean forward. As the disease progresses the bouts of pain occur more frequently and last longer. Some people have indigestion between attacks. Additional symptoms may include mild jaundice (see p.522) and loss of weight. In severe cases a copious, yellow, bulky diarrhea and malabsorption (see p.511) may develop. In addition, the pancreas may become unable to make the hormone insulin, so diabetes mellitus (see p.558) may develop.

If you have these symptoms, consult your physician. Never ignore attacks of abdominal pain (see Laparotomy and acute abdomen, p.513). Your physician will recommend tests to determine the status of the problem. These include blood tests such as a glucose tolerance test for diabetes (see p.560), an endoscopy, and perhaps an ultrasound or a CT scan of your pancreas.

What is the treatment?

Self-help: Once you are diagnosed with chronic pancreatitis, stop drinking alcohol completely and adhere strictly to the diet that is suggested by your physician.

Professional help: Your physician may prescribe one of several painkilling drugs if your pain is particularly severe. There is a risk of addiction from the long-term use of narcotic painkillers. You may also need to take digestive enzyme medication with each meal to help you digest your food, because your damaged pancreas can no longer manufacture these enzymes. If you stop drinking alcohol permanently, stick rigidly to your diet, and take the pancreatic enzymes, your chances of long-term improvement are good.

In some cases, abdominal pain may become unbearable. You may be advised to have damaged pancreatic tissue removed, or the nerves that transmit the pain cut.

Cancer of the pancreas

A cancerous tumor in the pancreas can cause a number of symptoms, depending on which part of the pancreas (head, tail, or body) is affected. The main symptoms are loss of appetite, weight loss, nausea, vomiting, jaundice (see p.522), and abdominal pain. The pain, which often occurs when the cancer affects the body and tail of the pancreas, usually is in the upper abdomen, but may spread to the back. Cancer of the head of the pancreas often causes no symptoms until the tumor is incurable. The symptoms are as described above except that it causes no pain. If you have the symptoms described above, consult your physician immediately. There are several possible causes, including gallstones (see p.526). If cancer is suspected, tests may include blood tests, a CT scan, and an endoscopic examination of the pancreas.

If the cancer is detected early, surgery to remove part or all of the pancreas may provide a cure. Anticancer drugs and radiation therapy may also be used. If the cancer is detected late, the outlook is poor.

Nutrition and metabolism

Metabolism is a general term for the chemical processes in your body that change air, food, and other materials into the substances your body needs to function. Although metabolism is the same for all of us in general terms, in detail it is somewhat individual. For example, the chemical balance in your body and the rate of your metabolism differ from those of other people. These individual differences are determined in large part by the genes you inherit from your parents.

In general, there are two types of metabolic disorders that relate to the digestive system. One type includes problems caused by eating and drinking the wrong amounts of food for you. This is the more common of the two types, and you can help to eliminate the problems by changing your diet. The second type of metabolic disorder is genetic—that is, inherited from your family. These disorders generally cannot be cured. However, their symptoms often can be controlled when you modify your diet or your life-style (including getting more exercise).

There is some overlap between these two types of metabolic problems. For example, most people who have obesity can reduce their weight by eating less and exercising more. Other factors such as cultural patterns of eating and emotional issues may influence your weight loss. There are a few rare individuals who inherit specific diseases that predispose them to becoming obese and then staying obese, but this is rare.

Other disorders of nutrition can be caused by a lack of vitamins and minerals in your diet. Vitamins and minerals play an essential role in healthy metabolism, and therefore they are a part of good nutrition. Vitamin and mineral deficiencies are also considered to be nutritional disorders.

This section deals first with obesity and vitamin and mineral deficiency, both of which are related to digestion and nutrition. This section also covers inherited metabolic disorders including porphyria, hyperlipoproteinemia, and gout, all of which can be affected by your diet.

Obesity

Obesity is a disorder in which you are at least 20 percent over your normal body weight. Obesity always involves a high proportion of body fat in relation to muscle and bone. Your body needs food as a source of energy to maintain body temperature and to fuel chemical and physical functions. Food also provides raw materials for building and repairing body tissues.

Food requirements vary, even among individuals of the same height, build, age, and sex. The basic needs of most active people are about 2,000 calories a day for women and 2,500 for men. However, a professional athlete or a manual laborer may need 4,000 calories or more on days he or she is active.

Only 1 percent of people with obesity have a hormonal problem that is a cause of their weight problem. If you eat more than you need for the energy you expend, your body stores the surplus as fat. If the amount of fat becomes excessive, you are obese. About one in every five men and almost one in every three women in the US are obese.

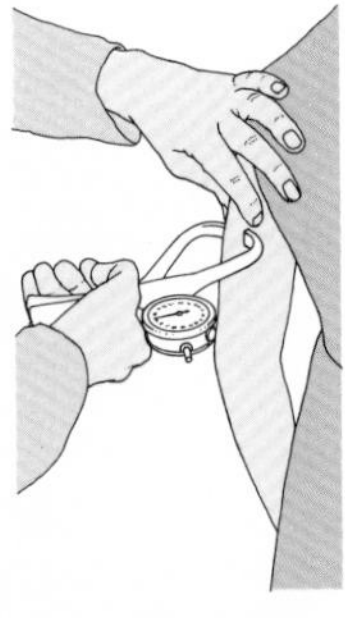

Measuring obesity
Skin calipers measure the thickness of skin, which indicates the degree of obesity.

What are the symptoms?

The most obvious symptom of obesity is an increase in weight. Not all people who put on weight are necessarily obese. For instance, a pregnant woman or anyone who begins to exercise after being sedentary gains weight for other reasons. But an increased amount of fat in the body tissues is the most common reason for weight gain. Obesity is associated with a wide range of serious disorders with many other symptoms.

What are the risks?

Statistics compiled by insurance companies and health organizations indicate that obesity is associated with increases in illness and death from diabetes mellitus (see p.558), stroke (see p.285), coronary artery disease (see p.400), and kidney and gallbladder disorders. The more overweight you are, the stronger this association becomes. The statistics suggest that if you are more than 40 percent overweight you are twice as likely to die of coronary artery disease as a person who is not overweight. If you are 20 to 30 percent overweight, you may be three times more likely than a person who is not overweight to die of diabetes. The risks seem higher when the excess weight is concentrated around the waist, and the ratio of the waist to the hip measurement is sometimes used to measure

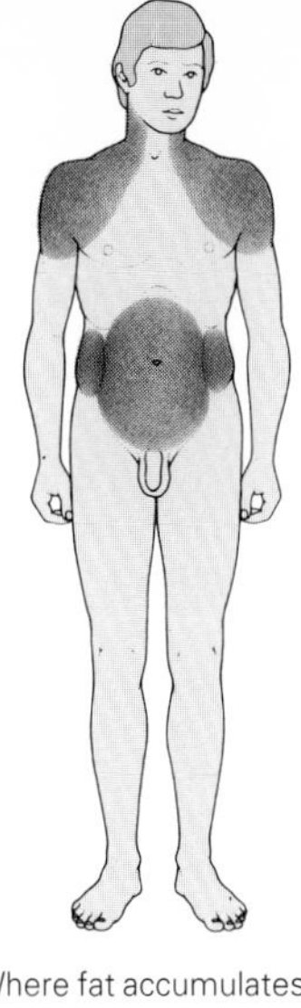

Where fat accumulates on men

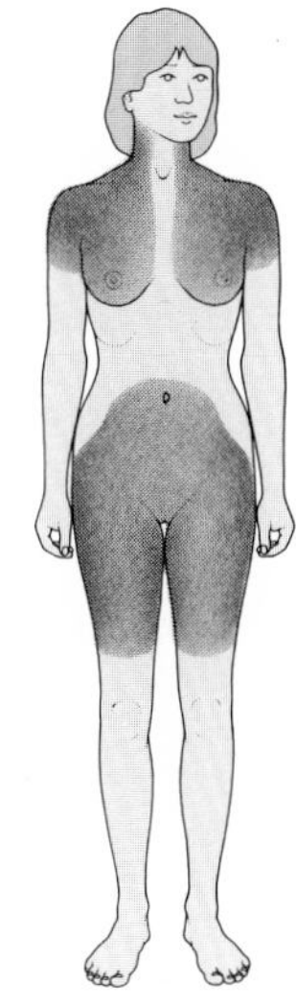

Where fat accumulates on women

this risk. People with a high waist-to-hip ratio are at greater risk than those whose excess fat is distributed in the hip area.

Obesity also contributes to high blood pressure (see p.411), which is itself a risk factor in both heart disease and stroke. If you have high blood pressure, you can reduce your blood pressure simply by losing weight.

Similarly, symptoms of diabetes (see p.558) sometimes develop in people with a family tendency as a direct consequence of obesity and disappear when excess weight is lost. Finally, very obese people who have surgery have more surgical and anesthetic complications than do people who are not obese. Childbirth may also be more risky for both woman and child.

What should be done?

Many people can cope with obesity themselves. To lose weight and keep it off, follow the self-help measures recommended below. Consult your physician if you are very obese and find it difficult to lose weight through a balanced diet and moderate, regular exercise. If you find that you cannot control your eating at all, you may need special help, such as psychological treatment.

What is the treatment?

Self-help: If you are overweight, it is because you consume more calories than you use. This may occur for one or more reasons, psychological as well as physical. In order to lose weight, you must help your body use up more calories than you consume. In other words, you must create an energy deficit. There are two ways that you can do this. First, change your diet; second, exercise more.

Crash diets, including very-low-calorie liquid diets, or a few days at a health spa seldom work if your goal is to lose weight permanently. If you lose weight that is mostly body water, the weight returns when you go back to your usual routines. Diets that are overly restrictive may compromise your intake of vital nutrients. These diets and strenuous exercise programs are not feasible for most people on a lifelong basis. Only 10 percent of people with obesity on highly restrictive programs successfully maintain their weight loss on a long-term basis.

So do not try to achieve massive weight losses in a few days, weeks, or even months. You should try to lose about 1½ to 2 pounds per week. Use a food and exercise program that gives you an energy deficit of around 750 calories a day. This will help you lose about 1½ lb (¾ kg) of fatty tissue a week. When you plan your diet, make sure that it is

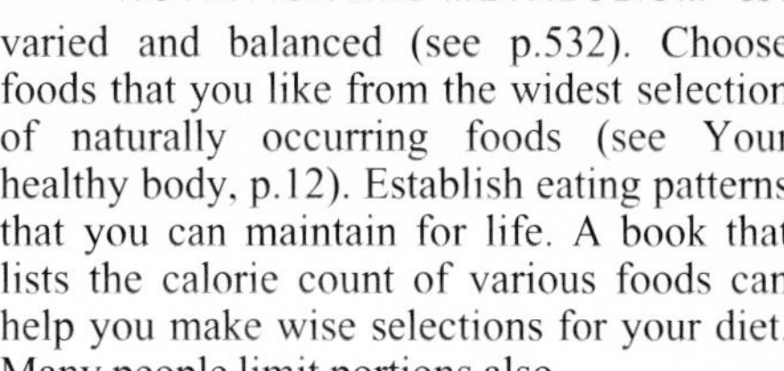

varied and balanced (see p.532). Choose foods that you like from the widest selection of naturally occurring foods (see Your healthy body, p.12). Establish eating patterns that you can maintain for life. A book that lists the calorie count of various foods can help you make wise selections for your diet. Many people limit portions also.

Many people are overweight because they eat almost unconsciously, even when they are not hungry, and hardly notice what they pop into their mouths. Dietitians and behavioral therapists have found that such people are greatly helped by following simple rules that turn eating into a formal ritual. If you need to lose weight, it may help you to follow these rules. Never eat between meals; or eat frequent low-calorie meals so that you are not hungry and tempted to snack. Eat with a knife, fork, and spoon, and never swallow a mouthful of food without pausing to chew it slowly and thoroughly.

To use exercise effectively in your weight-reduction program, go slowly but steadily. An hour of sustained moderate bicycle riding will burn about 400 calories, or more than half of a day's target energy deficit.

Some studies show that moderate exercise in sedentary people reduces appetite and might improve the efficiency of your metabolism so that you are able to burn calories more readily.

Finally, many overweight people find it easier to follow a sensible diet and exercise program if they do not have to do it alone. You may decide to join a weight-loss group. This can be a positive step, since it formalizes your intention to lose weight and also puts you in touch with people who share your weight-loss goal.

If your reasonable efforts to lose weight do not succeed, you may be one of the few people who have a metabolism that does not allow them to lose weight on diets that normally would work for others. Also, keep in mind that once you have lost some excess weight, your body adapts to a lower calorie intake by reducing its basic energy requirement, so you won't lose more weight unless you further reduce your calorie intake or increase the amount of exercise. If your weight has stabilized but you are still trying to lose weight, consult your physician.

Professional help: There are antiobesity drugs, but many physicians prefer not to prescribe them because certain ones can have major adverse effects such as addiction, paranoia, and high blood pressure. Moreover, most people with obesity do not have a problem specifically with excess appetite.

Many simply eat whether they are hungry or not. Their physicians may advise them to try a support group such as Weight Watchers or, if necessary, may recommend that they seek psychological help.

For people who cannot lose weight in any other way and are extraordinarily obese, physicians sometimes try more drastic forms of treatment. For example, your jaws can be wired together so that you cannot open your mouth to eat. The wiring may be kept in place for 6 to 12 weeks, during which you drink liquids through a straw, causing a dramatic loss of weight. This treatment is very uncomfortable and also has major drawbacks beyond the obvious ones associated with such an experience. Most important, the treatment does not help you change your eating habits, so you are very likely to regain the weight when your jaws are unwired and you begin to eat solid foods again. Also, infections and dental decay can occur because your teeth cannot be cleaned properly.

Over the years surgeons have tried a number of more complex and very risky procedures that may be recommended when obesity becomes life-threatening. Surgery may be performed to bypass part of the intestine. However, surgeons have become increasingly reluctant to bypass most of the absorbing surface of the small intestine or to attempt major surgery in very obese patients because the long-term results are so often poor. In the late 1980s many patients were treated by a plastic balloon inserted into the stomach. This procedure reduced the size of the stomach and produced a feeling of fullness. However, use of the balloon was suspended after highly serious complications developed in some people.

Another approach is for the excess fat to be cut away or sucked out from beneath the skin using the technique of liposuction by a cosmetic surgeon. Sometimes surgery is performed to staple the stomach to reduce its size so that you feel hungry less often. A gastric bypass is a similar procedure in which the surgeon bypasses your stomach to direct the food into your small intestine. The stapling procedure, with its own drawbacks (including the possibility of the stomach stretching and tearing away from the staples), is probably the best choice among these procedures. But there is a risk of major complications from each of these procedures; any surgery performed on very obese people carries a substantial risk, and you may not achieve the appearance you were hoping for. And in each instance you still need to modify your eating habits in the future.

Vitamin and mineral deficiency

Your body needs food for energy and for creating and repairing tissues. It also needs a variety of complex compounds that provide neither fuel nor structural material but are essential for smooth running. Vitamins are such compounds. Although your body can manufacture limited amounts of some vitamins, notably vitamin D and niacin, most of these compounds must be obtained from the foods you eat.

Minerals are also vital for good health. Like vitamins, minerals also ensure that your body functions properly. Your body needs small but regular supplies of minerals. These include sodium and potassium (although dietary deficiencies of these elements are virtually unknown), calcium, phosphorus, and magnesium. In addition, you require much smaller quantities of minerals known as trace elements; these include iron, iodine, zinc, copper, chromium, and selenium. The table on p.533 shows the essential minerals and outlines the roles they play in health.

The functions of some vitamins and minerals are not yet fully understood, but they are all known to be involved in basic metabolic activities. Vitamin D plays a role in controlling the absorption and excretion of calcium and in the concentration of calcium in bone, which is needed for strong bones and for the functioning of nerves and muscles. Iron is important in delivering oxygen to body tissues to provide energy and in protecting against infection. A lack of any vitamin or mineral can lead to many disorders. If the deficiency is severe or prolonged, the resulting disease can be disabling or even fatal.

Vitamin deficiency is uncommon in the US, and when it occurs it is usually caused by prolonged faulty eating habits, alcoholism, or gastrointestinal disorders (such as removal of parts of the stomach or small intestine, see p.499, or malabsorption, see p.511). Vitamin deficiency diseases that were once common now seldom occur because many foods are fortified with vitamins, and nourishing foods are available year-round. Mineral deficiency is most likely to occur if you follow a diet extremely restricted in calories or in the types of food you eat. Vitamin and mineral supplements are overpromoted; food can meet your needs best and most economically. Naturally occurring foods also provide the

MINERAL	MAJOR SOURCES	IMPORTANCE	SYMPTOMS OR EFFECTS OF A DEFICIENCY
Potassium	Low-fat milk, green leafy vegetables, dried fruits, nuts, beans, fish, potatoes.	Nerve function, muscle activity.	Muscle weakness, nausea, irregular heart rhythms, loss of appetite, constipation, lethargy.
Sodium	Low-fat dairy products, canned soups, tomato juice, pickles, bread, cereals, olives, table salt.	Nerve function, muscle contraction, maintains body fluid balance.	Rarely seen. Muscle cramping, nausea, lethargy, weakness, dizziness.
Calcium	Low-fat dairy products, green leafy vegetables, eggs, dried peas and beans, nuts, seeds, tofu.	Bone and tooth formation, blood clotting, nerve function, muscle contraction.	May relate to loss of bone density with age (osteoporosis), muscle cramping.
Magnesium	Dark green vegetables, nuts, shellfish, whole-grain cereals, low-fat dairy products, dried fruits.	Nerve function, muscle contraction, storage and release of energy.	Muscle tremors, muscle spasms, muscle weakness, growth failure.
Phosphorus	Low-fat dairy products, lean red meat, fish, poultry, eggs, peanuts, whole-grain products, dried peas and beans.	Bone and tooth formation, energy production.	Not common. Occur primarily in association with various diseases.
Iron	Liver, lean red meat, whole-grain or enriched breads and cereals, rice, pasta, nuts, broccoli, spinach.	Health of red blood cells (production of hemoglobin). Delivers oxygen to body tissues to provide energy.	Tiredness, pale skin, infections, sore mouth, nail changes, anemia.
Zinc	Seafood, lean red meat, nuts, eggs, whole-grain cereals, beans, poultry.	Growth, healthy skin, wound healing, energy production.	Poor wound healing, increased susceptibility to infection, poor growth and delayed sexual development in children.
Manganese	Green vegetables, tea, nuts, rice, oats, beans.	Bone structure, assists in carbohydrate metabolism.	None reported.
Fluorine	Seafood, tea, coffee, soybeans, fluoridated drinking water.	Bone and tooth formation.	Tooth decay.
Copper	Liver, shellfish, mushrooms, peas, beans, nuts, whole-grain cereals and breads, dried fruits, grapes.	Helps incorporate iron into hemoglobin, bone structure.	Not common. Anemia, fragile bones.
Chromium	Lean red meat, seafood, low-fat cheese, whole-grain breads and cereals, fruits, vegetables.	Helps the body use carbohydrates.	Increased blood sugar.
Selenium	Seafood, lean red meat, whole-grain cereals, low-fat milk.	Protects cells and tissues from damage.	None reported.
Iodine	Saltwater fish, shellfish, iodized table salt, low-fat dairy products.	Health of thyroid gland (hormone production).	Enlarged thyroid gland (goiter).

VITAMIN	MAJOR SOURCES	IMPORTANCE
A (retinol)	Liver, fortified low-fat dairy products, dark green leafy vegetables, carrots, eggs, cantaloupes, oranges, apricots, fortified soft margarine.	Essential for vision, particularly at night, for growth, for development o bones, for reproduction, and for healthy skin, hair, and mucous membranes.
B_1 (thiamine)	Pork, whole-grain and enriched breads and cereals, peas, eggs, potatoes, fish, low-fat dairy products.	Assists the functioning of nervous system and muscles, including hear muscle. Helps the body use glucose
B_2 (riboflavin)	Liver, kidney, low-fat milk, low-fat cheese, green leafy vegetables, eggs, lean meats, whole-grain and enriched breads and cereals, nuts, peas, beans.	Helps break down food to provide energy. Maintains healthy skin and mucous membranes.
B_3 (niacin)	Fish, lean meat, poultry, whole-grain and enriched breads and cereals, eggs, peanuts, low-fat milk, low-fat cheese, peas, beans, potatoes.	Helps break down food to provide energy. Maintains healthy skin.
B_6 (pyridoxine)	Most foods, especially those rich in other B vitamins, poultry, fish, whole-grain breads and cereals, bananas, peas, beans, liver, eggs, low-fat dairy products.	Assists the body in using protein. Essential for hemoglobin formatior Helps regulate function of nervous system cells. Maintains healthy ski
B_{12} (cobalamin)	Liver, beef, pork, lamb, poultry, fish, low-fat milk, oysters, yeast.	Helps produce red and white blooc cells. Essential for a healthy nervou system.
Folic acid (folacin)	Liver, green leafy vegetables, mushrooms, lima beans, kidney beans, whole-wheat bread, nuts, peas, beans.	Helps produce red and white blooc cells and other cells of the body.
C (ascorbic acid)	Tomatoes, citrus fruits, strawberries, cantaloupes, bell peppers, broccoli, cabbage, cauliflower, potatoes.	Many and varied roles in growth a health of body cells, including thos gums, bones, and teeth. Helps wi response to infection and stress. Assists the body in using iron. He maintain strong capillaries.
D (cholecalciferol)	Fortified low-fat milk, fortified low-fat dairy products, fortified cereals and breads, cod liver oil. (Your skin also manufactures vitamin D with the help of sunlight.)	Essential for good bone structure normal teeth. Helps in absorption calcium and phosphorus. Helps ir maintenance of nervous system a muscles, and in blood clotting.
E (tocopherol)	Vegetable oils, soft margarine, eggs, fish, green leafy vegetables, whole-grain products, dried beans.	Assists in formation of red blood and protects red blood cells from damage and degeneration.
K	Green leafy vegetables, cauliflower, grain products, potatoes, fruits, low-fat milk, low-fat cheese, eggs, cabbage.	Essential for efficient clotting of

SYMPTOMS OR EFFECTS OF A DEFICIENCY
Rough, dry skin, poor night vision, lowered resistance to infection, weak bones, absence of tooth enamel in children.
Cardiomyopathy (p.430), numbness of hands and feet (in the severe form, called beriberi), mental confusion, depression, fatigue, loss of muscle coordination, fluid accumulation, calf tenderness.
Cracked lips, sore tongue, skin eruptions.
Muscular weakness, indigestion, skin eruptions, sore tongue, pellagra (characterized by dermatitis, diarrhea, and dementia).
Skin eruptions, nervousness, irritability, anemia (p.450), insomnia.
Anemia (p.450), sore tongue, spinal cord abnormalities.
Anemia (p.450), lowered resistance to infection.
Bruising of the skin and other tissues, bleeding gums (in the severe form, called scurvy), poor healing of wounds, loosening of teeth, tender joints, susceptibility to infection.
In children, short stature, bowed legs (rickets). In adults, softening and deformity of long bones (osteomalacia). With aging, a tendency to bone fracture.
Uncommon unless there are problems with absorbing fat. Anemia (p.728) in premature or low-birth-weight infants.
Abnormal bleeding tendencies in newborns and adults.

best balance of nutrients. Moreover, excessive amounts of certain nutrients such as vitamins A and D can be toxic (poisonous) if taken over a prolonged period. An adequate intake of vitamins and minerals is assured if you eat a well-balanced diet (see p.26).

Although serious vitamin and mineral deficiencies are uncommon in the US, some people, especially the elderly and the poor, may not get enough nutrients to fully meet their needs. The tables on pp.533–535 summarize the facts and theories about the most significant known vitamins and minerals, their sources, and their functions.

Who lacks vitamins and minerals?

In the US and other developed countries, unmistakable vitamin deficiency diseases such as scurvy (caused by lack of vitamin C) or pellagra (caused by lack of niacin) are rare. It is difficult to determine if mineral deficiencies are common because clear-cut deficiency diseases have not been identified for most minerals. However, iron-deficiency anemia (see p.450; for children, see p.728) is very common worldwide.

Vitamin and mineral deficiencies are not likely to be severe, since they are usually caused by not getting enough of these nutrients rather than a complete lack in diet.

Mild deficiencies are most common among children, teenage girls, pregnant women, and older people. People of any age who eat too many processed foods or who go on crash diets to lose weight may also develop deficiencies. People with marginal diets may not have obvious symptoms of deficiencies, but they have few reserve stores of vitamins and minerals to help them withstand the stress of an illness or injury.

Children are most likely to be deficient in iron and vitamin A, which are needed for growth. Low intakes of vitamin C are also common. Concern about weight often prevents teenage girls from eating enough to get proper amounts of many nutrients, including calcium, iron, zinc, and folic acid.

Most women of childbearing age obtain enough iron from food. Greater-than-average blood loss during menstruation increases the need for iron. Pregnancy further increases this need. Many women may need iron supplements at some point during their lives if they have anemia. Folic acid deficiency (see p.451) may also occur during pregnancy. The requirements for iron and folic acid as well as for other nutrients are higher if you are pregnant or breast-feeding, so your physician may recommend that you take a vitamin-mineral supplement.

Many older people live alone on fixed incomes, which may decrease their desire or ability to eat properly.

Homeless people or other poor people may have the classical symptoms of malnutrition, including a swollen abdomen, skin changes, and cracked lips. Poor or not, people with alcoholism find that it exaggerates the effects of low vitamin and mineral intakes. Alcoholics often have deficiencies of vitamin B_6 (pyridoxine), vitamin B_1 (thiamine), folic acid, and magnesium.

In extremely rare cases, people who are not poor or alcoholic and who eat a reasonably well-balanced diet may have a vitamin deficiency because they have a metabolic abnormality. For instance, some people have anemia because their bodies cannot absorb vitamin B_{12} (see p.451). In addition, some women who use oral contraceptives may show signs of a vitamin B_6 deficiency and may need to take a supplement.

You may acquire a vitamin or mineral deficiency after surgery on the intestinal tract. If you develop a severe intestinal disorder such as Crohn's disease (see p.508), you may eventually have deficiencies because your body cannot absorb vitamins and minerals.

Should you eat differently?

Your chance of having a deficiency of a vitamin or mineral depends on how available that vitamin or mineral is in your diet and how effectively your body can store it. If you eat a well-balanced diet, you should have an adequate intake of vitamins and minerals.

Keep in mind that a healthful diet should be low in fat, cholesterol and sodium (salt), while supplying you with adequate amounts of essential vitamins and minerals. Your diet should also include plenty of fiber.

To ensure that your diet is well-balanced, always choose a wide variety of naturally occurring foods, and use the US Department of Agriculture's Food Guide Pyramid (see p.28) as a general guide. Make your daily food choices from each of these food groups: Bread, cereal, rice, and pasta group 6–11 servings per day); Vegetable group (3–5 servings per day); Fruit group (2–4 servings per day); Meat, poultry, fish, dry beans, and nuts group (2–3 servings per day); Milk, yogurt, and cheese group (2–3 servings per day); and Fats, oils, and sweets (use sparingly). The number of servings you need every day from each food group depends on several factors, including your age, sex, build, and how active you are (see p.29).

Vitamin C is important in the healing of wounds and enhancing iron absorption. However, no evidence conclusively proves that vitamin C helps fight the common cold.

Citrus fruits, including oranges, lemons, limes, and grapefruit, are the main sources of vitamin C. Vitamin C is present in many other foods too, including strawberries, cantaloupe, bell peppers, and potatoes.

Vegetables supply vitamin C as well as other vitamins and minerals. To preserve as much of their nutrients as possible, cook them with little water at low temperatures for a short time; or, better yet, eat them raw.

Are supplements necessary?

Many people believe they can improve their health by supplementing their diet with vitamin and mineral pills. Many physicians, however, continue to discourage the use of such supplements for several reasons. So long as you have no special difficulties with your metabolism, you will probably obtain all the vitamins and minerals you need if you eat a varied diet of fresh food and expose your skin to enough sunlight to increase vitamin D reserves (but see also Sunburn, p.274).

Taking vitamin and mineral supplements may not harm you, but you are unlikely to need the extra-large doses of vitamins and minerals found in some mega-vitamins, and in some cases an especially high dose can be harmful. This is particularly true of vitamins that the body can store efficiently, such as vitamins A and D. Too much vitamin A causes skin changes, hair loss, enlarged fat-infiltrated liver, and various symptoms in muscles and joints. Too much vitamin D leads to excess calcium in the blood, which can cause gastrointestinal, nerve, and muscular disorders. An excess of vitamin B_6 can cause nerve damage. Large doses of minerals may also be harmful. An excess of calcium, for example, may increase the need for magnesium, zinc, and iron. Too much iron can lead to gastrointestinal disorders and liver damage. Too much vitamin C can interfere with copper absorption, and copper intakes are already marginal in the US.

It is important for you to realize that taking vitamin and mineral supplements is a poor substitute for eating a well-balanced diet of naturally occurring foods. A healthy diet is one that gives you most of your energy requirements from foods containing natural fiber and mostly unsaturated rather than saturated fats (see p.32). Such a diet reduces the risks of heart disorders, many gastrointestinal disorders, and some forms of cancer. If your diet mainly consists of high-fat, high-calorie foods, your risk of some day developing heart disease and various other disorders is increased, regardless of how many vitamin supplements you take.

Vitamin and mineral supplements may possibly benefit anyone attempting to lose a substantial amount of weight over a relatively long period of time by dieting. In these circumstances, you should talk to your physician for advice on a safe weight-loss program and on the possible need for vitamin and mineral supplements. The best supplement is probably a multivitamin and mineral preparation with no more than 100 percent of the recommended daily allowances (RDAs) for healthy people.

Children in good health do not need extra vitamins and minerals. Parents should encourage their children to eat a varied diet that includes as much fresh fruit and vegetables as possible. A child who has a piece of fruit as a snack rather than a candy bar develops good eating habits and may not need vitamin or mineral supplements.

Gout

Uric acid, one of the body's waste products, normally passes out through the kidneys in your urine. If there is more of it than the kidneys can process, gout is a likely outcome.

Gout is a common form of joint disease in which uric acid accumulates and forms crystals that may become lodged in certain areas of the body. When uric acid crystals are caught in the spaces between one of your joints, the tissue surrounding the joint becomes inflamed and irritates the nerve endings, which causes extreme pain. Crystals also accumulate in the kidneys, which may cause kidney failure (see p.550).

What are the symptoms?

The main symptom of gout is severe pain, sometimes in your elbow or knee but more often in your hand or foot, frequently at the base of your big toe. The pain usually occurs without warning, although once you have experienced several bouts of gout, you may learn to recognize early twinges. Within a few hours your joint is swollen and tender, and you cannot endure even the weight of a sheet. There is often a fever of up to 101°F (about 38.5°C). The inflamed skin over the joint is often reddish-purple, shiny, and dry.

Gout can affect males after puberty. The first attack usually involves only one joint and lasts only a few days. Sometimes no more attacks occur, but there is usually a second, which may not come on for months or years. After the second attack, the gout may occur at shorter intervals, last longer, or involve more joints.

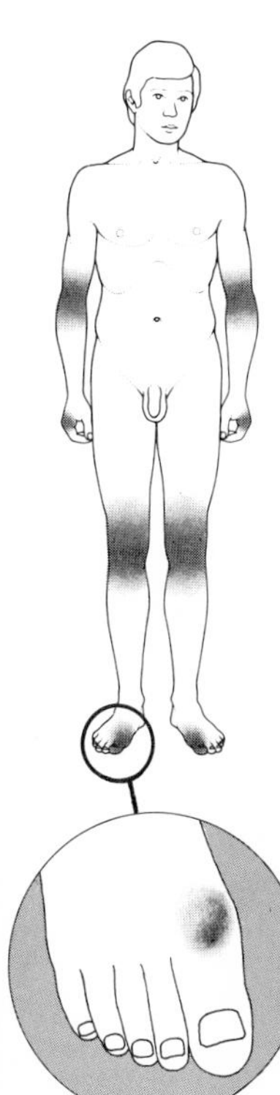

Sites of gout

What are the risks?

Gout is one of the most controllable of the metabolic disorders. Untreated, it can lead to joint deformity, death from kidney disease, or high blood pressure (see p.411).

What should be done?

Even though your first attack will subside on its own in a few days and there will be no immediate recurrence, see your physician. Do not try to ease the pain with aspirin, which can slow down the excretion of uric acid. Your physician may prescribe another nonsteroidal anti-inflammatory drug, such as ibuprofen or indomethacin. Because you may have only one attack, no further treatment is usually recommended. But inform your physician of any subsequent attacks.

Your physician may advise you to make changes in your eating and drinking habits. A high daily water intake is important in controlling uric acid levels, particularly in the urine where uric acid crystals accumulate to form stones. You may need to stop drinking alcohol, because it, like aspirin, inhibits your body's ability to excrete uric acid. Avoid organ meats (liver, kidney, sweetbreads, brain) and other protein-rich foods to cut down on your uric acid levels.

What is the treatment?

There are three lines of treatment. The first is control of pain. The second is control of joint inflammation caused by uric acid crystals. For these objectives your physician may prescribe a nonsteroidal anti-inflammatory drug, a corticosteroid drug, or colchicine, a drug used to reduce joint pain.

Since the symptoms may disappear after the first attack, or the disease may be dormant for months or years, your physician may not prescribe any additional drugs at first. If the symptoms recur, however, you may need the third line of treatment, which involves two drugs to control your metabolic problem.

One drug increases the excretion of uric acid, but you won't receive this drug if tests show you are already excreting large amounts of uric acid. Your physician may recommend that you help this process by increasing your intake of nonalcoholic fluids. The second and most widely used kind of drug reduces the amount of uric acid produced by your body. If you take the drugs exactly as prescribed, the disorder should not recur.

Hyperlipoproteinemia

(including hypercholesterolemia)

As explained in the article on cholesterol (see Your healthy body, p.12), many Americans have higher levels of cholesterol and fats (triglycerides) in their blood than is healthy. Because fats and cholesterol do not mix with water, these substances are transported around the body in the blood in chemical envelopes called lipoproteins, which have an oily core and a coat made in part of protein. A person whose blood contains high levels of cholesterol, triglycerides, or both has high levels of lipoproteins, and the term for that condition is hyperlipoproteinemia.

The most common cause of hyperlipoproteinemia is eating a diet containing too much saturated fat for years and exercising too little. In many cases, however, hyperlipoproteinemia is also caused by an inherited fault in the person's body chemistry. Less commonly, it is caused by a hormonal disorder that has upset the chemical balance. Pinpointing the cause of hyperlipoproteinemia is important so that you can receive treatment before the excess lipids lead to disease of the blood vessels. Atherosclerosis (see p.398), heart attacks (see p.406), and strokes (see p.285) in people under 50 to 55 are often the result of unrecognized and untreated hyperlipoproteinemias.

What are the risks?

A cholesterol test is especially important for anyone with a blood relative who has had a heart attack or stroke before age 50. Inherited hyperlipoproteinemia disorders are somewhat common, affecting about 1 person in 500. All kinds involve hypercholesterolemia or high levels of cholesterol in the blood, and one form involves elevated triglycerides. The dozen or so disorders called hyperlipoproteinemia account for the majority of heart disease in early middle age.

What should be done?

If your cholesterol level is below 200 mg per dL, you need not be concerned. Between 200 and 240 your cholesterol level needs watching. If your cholesterol is over 240, the level should be checked by a second test.

If it is still too high, or if you have a family history of heart disease, then further blood tests are taken after you have fasted to determine the blood levels of triglycerides and also the levels of high-density lipoprotein (HDL) cholesterol, which are protective, and low-density lipoprotein (LDL) cholesterol, which are dangerous. These tests should predict whether you have a low, medium, or high risk of heart disease.

Changes in your diet are the first essential step; you must restrict your intake of animal fats and other saturated fats, reduce your total fat intake to no more than 30 percent of your total calories, and reduce your total calorie intake. If the levels remain abnormally high, especially the LDL levels, cholesterol-lowering drugs may also be recommended, regardless of the cause of your hyperlipoproteinemia. If the tests suggest that you have an inherited hyperlipoproteinemia, other members of your family should be tested, including children.

The whole family may be advised to follow a low-calorie, low total fat, low saturated fat, high-fiber diet; often this is combined with treatment with cholesterol-lowering drugs.

Your physician may also arrange to check whether your hyperlipoproteinemia is associated with a hormonal or metabolic disorder such as hypothyroidism (see p.565) or diabetes mellitus (see p.558). If it is, treatment of the underlying disorder will help lower the lipoprotein levels, but additional changes in your diet may be needed.

Porphyria

Porphyria is an inherited disease caused by an abnormality in the red blood cell protein called hemoglobin. This abnormality causes chemicals called porphyrins to accumulate in and injure the liver and digestive system, the brain and nervous system, or the skin.

What are the symptoms?

Symptoms of the disease may appear first in early adulthood. Even then they may not become apparent unless they are triggered by taking certain drugs such as barbiturates or birth control pills, drinking alcohol, becoming pregnant, or even exposing your body to sunlight. The symptoms of porphyria vary, because it occurs in several forms. There may be vomiting, abdominal pain, muscle cramps and weakness, psychological disorders such as manic-depressive disorder (see p.323) or depression (see p.321), or skin conditions such as itching and blistering.

All forms of porphyria are rare. Tests on your urine, stools, and blood can generally determine whether you have porphyria and which type. Treatment is based on avoiding trigger factors and easing symptoms. You may have to avoid certain drugs, foods, or even climates. Women with porphyria need advice on contraception and special care during and immediately after pregnancy.

Disorders of the urinary tract

Introduction

Your body is like a factory that contains a number of machines, all of which need energy in order to work together smoothly. The energy comes from the food you eat. The food is broken down, during digestion, into energy-containing substances that pass into your bloodstream. Once there, these substances circulate throughout your body and are picked up by body cells. In the cells they undergo reactions that release their energy.

As the nutrients and energy are used up, chemical waste products are produced in the cells in the liver and throughout the body. These wastes must be removed, because they would poison the cells if they were allowed to accumulate. The waste products are carried in your bloodstream to the two kidneys. In the kidneys they are filtered out of the blood and in combination with water they are excreted as urine. Thus, production and excretion of urine are essential to life.

Your kidneys are situated behind your intestines and just above your waist, on either side of your spine outside of your abdominal cavity. Each kidney contains more than 1 million tiny filtering units called nephrons, which hold back most protein and allow amino acids, glucose, mineral salts, and other by-products to pass into a tubule. The tubule reabsorbs essential nutrients (amino acids, glucose, salt, and water) and secretes some waste products, which are excreted in the urine. The urine outflow tract is composed of a narrow muscular tube, the ureter, which carries a slow trickle of urine from each kidney down to the bladder, a temporary storage place in the lower abdomen. From time to time the urine, expelled by the bladder, passes out of your body through another tube, the urethra. This system, from kidneys to urethra, is known as the urinary tract. It is subject to a number of disorders. Infection or inflammation of your kidneys or atherosclerosis involving the small arteries inside the kidney can cause scarring of the filtering tissue. Such scarring may ultimately lead to kidney failure. Hard deposits called kidney stones can form and move into the outflow tracts. These stones can cause extreme pain as they pass down the ureters and can obstruct the flow of urine. Stones may also form in the bladder, especially when there is poor bladder muscle contraction. Also, tumors can form in your urinary tract.

The structure of the urinary tract is slightly different in men and women, mainly because of differing anatomy. Problems specific to either men or women are covered in separate sections (see Men's health, p.611, and Women's health, p.623).

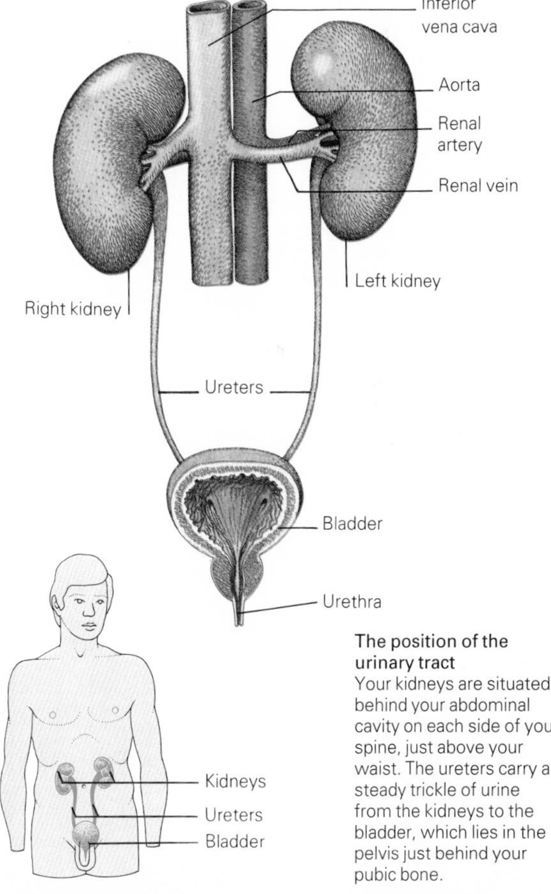

The position of the urinary tract
Your kidneys are situated behind your abdominal cavity on each side of your spine, just above your waist. The ureters carry a steady trickle of urine from the kidneys to the bladder, which lies in the pelvis just behind your pubic bone.

How the kidneys function

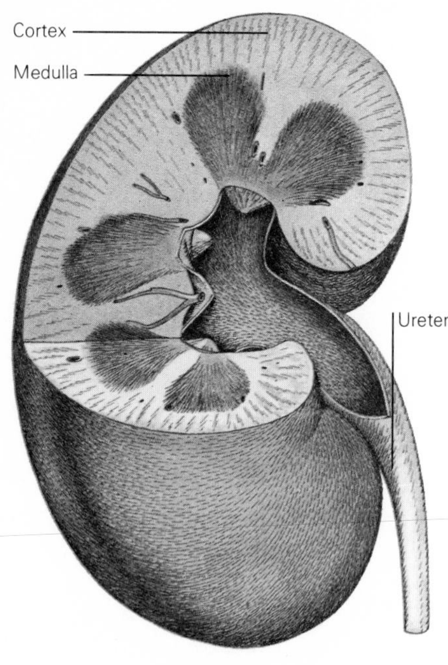

Blood from the renal artery first passes through the glomeruli. These minute, globular structures in the cortex, or outer part, of the kidney filter a liquid containing nutrients and wastes from the blood. The liquid then flows into the medulla, or center, of the kidney via long, thin tubes called tubules. The tubules are surrounded by blood vessels that reabsorb the nutrients from the liquid. The blood leaves the kidneys via the renal vein and returns to circulation. The filtered liquid, which contains waste products from the blood, continues along the tubule, which forms a collecting duct that leads into the ureter, and is collected in the bladder as urine.

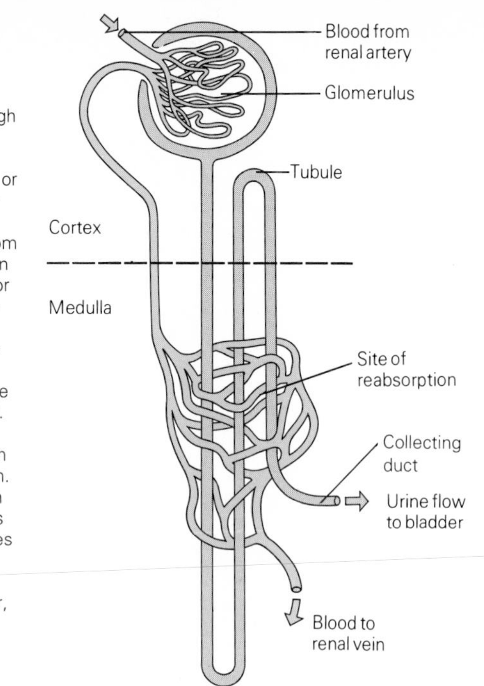

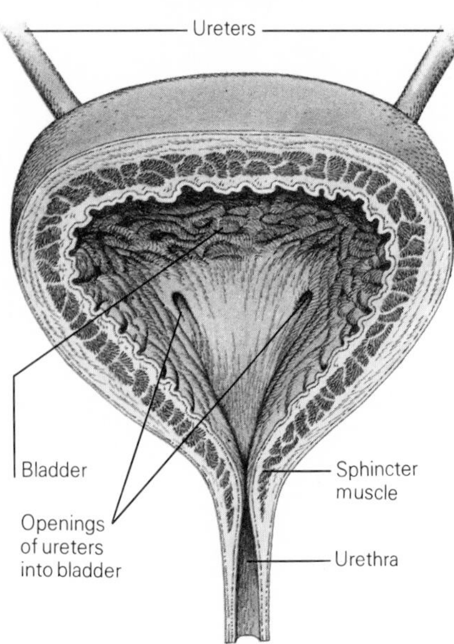

The bladder

Urine trickles down the ureters from the kidneys to the bladder. The bladder has elastic, flexible walls, which allow it to expand as it fills and then contract to expel urine when you urinate. Valves (not shown here) between the ureters and bladder are thought to prevent urine from flowing back up into the ureters.

Male and female urinary tracts

The lower part of the urinary tract is closely related to the reproductive organs and differs in men and women. The male urethra is about 10 in (25 cm) long and provides an outlet for semen as well as urine. A woman's urethra is about 1 in (25 mm) long and lies, with the bladder, just in front of the reproductive organs. Because it is close to the anus and the entrance to the vagina, a woman's urinary tract is more susceptible to infection.

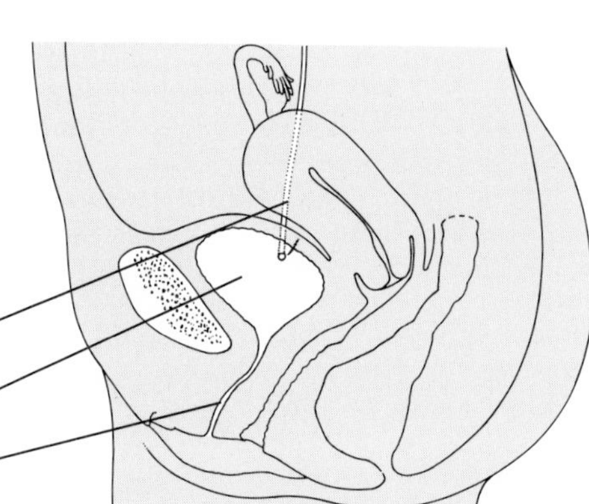

Infections, inflammation, and injury

There are no microorganisms in a healthy urinary tract, and normal urine is sterile. The urinary tract can become infected, however, and infectious agents, especially bacteria, can thrive there. These infectious agents gain access to the urinary tract from outside your body by coming up the urethra and into the bladder. They also may travel to the kidneys from another part of your body through your bloodstream. Either way, once present in the urinary tract they can multiply and spread, thereby disrupting normal functions and causing swelling and inflammation.

Infection of the kidney is known as pyelonephritis. This disorder can be acute, coming on quickly, or it can be chronic, in which case it recurs over many years. Infection of the bladder is called cystitis, and infection of the urethra is called urethritis.

Sometimes swelling and inflammation of the kidney can occur even without an infectious agent. Glomerulonephritis, which affects the glomeruli (the minute filtering units of the kidney) is an example of this type of inflammation. (For forms of glomerulonephritis that typically affect children, see Nephrotic syndrome, p.738, and Glomerulonephritis in children, p.737.)

Injury to the kidneys from a blow or wound is not common, because these organs are tucked away just behind your abdominal cavity and are protected by your rib cage and the fat and muscles of your back. Similarly the bladder lies well protected within the pelvic, or hip, bones. So if your urinary tract is damaged, it often involves a major injury that is associated with other serious injuries and requires hospitalization.

Acute pyelonephritis

Acute pyelonephritis is a kidney infection that develops suddenly. The infection and the inflammation that it causes mainly affect the tissue in which the kidney's tiny filtering units, the glomeruli, are imbedded. This occasionally occurs when infectious agents from another part of your body are carried to your kidneys in the bloodstream. In most cases, however, the infecting bacteria come from the skin around the urethral opening. Poor hygiene in this area, especially when you wipe the area after a bowel movement, can allow bacteria to enter the urethra (the tube between the bladder and the outside) and spread up through the bladder and ureter to your kidneys. This is especially likely if the normal flow of urine is partially blocked for some reason. A stagnant pool results in which bacteria flourish; they are not washed out of the tract as easily as they are when the urine is flowing freely. Although this explains some cases of acute pyelonephritis, the disorder sometimes occurs for no apparent reason in an otherwise healthy person.

What are the symptoms?

In most cases the first symptom is sudden intense pain in your back just above your waist. Although both kidneys may be affected, the pain is usually worse on one side of your body, and it spreads around that side and down into your groin. Your temperature rises rapidly, often reaching 104°F (40°C). This may produce chills or trembling and may be accompanied by nausea and by vomiting. You may also experience difficult or painful urination and you are likely to feel that you need to urinate constantly, even when your bladder is empty. The urine is usually cloudy and may be light red if blood has leaked into it.

What are the risks?

Acute pyelonephritis is a common condition, particularly in women. This is because the urethra, the tube through which urine flows from the bladder, is shorter in women and permits easy access to bacteria. Various conditions that reduce the flow of urine make you more susceptible. These include pregnancy (because of pressure on the ureters from the enlarging uterus), kidney stones (see p.548), a tumor of the bladder (see p.547), or an enlarged prostate gland (see p.615).

With prompt treatment complications are unlikely. In an infant, child, or frail person the infection may spread into the blood and lead to blood poisoning (see p.452). If you have repeated attacks of acute pyelonephritis, you may have a problem in your urinary tract that needs to be corrected.

What should be done?

Consult your physician if you have any of the symptoms described above. In many cases only antibiotics and bed rest are needed, and the attack may subside in a day or so. After you recover, your physician may want you to have blood and urine tests, an X ray of your kidneys, called an intravenous pyelogram (IVP), and cystoscopy for your bladder.

If you are a healthy adult, such diagnostic tests are seldom required after a single episode of acute pyelonephritis. However, for children or for persons who have had previous bouts, tests are usually recommended in order to identify any underlying problems and prevent long-term damage to the kidneys (see Urinary infections in children, p.736).

What is the treatment?

The treatment is bed rest and a light, bland diet that includes extra fluids, particularly large quantities of water. In addition, your physician will probably prescribe antibiotics or sulfa drugs, which you usually take by mouth. The very young or very frail, however, may have to be hospitalized for intravenous medication that requires monitoring or for another serious condition that requires hospital care. Antibiotics generally bring the infection under control in 24 to 48 hours, although treatment may continue for 14 days or longer in some cases.

Chronic pyelonephritis

Chronic pyelonephritis is a condition in which your kidneys become increasingly damaged over the course of several years by repeated, often unnoticed, infections of the urine. In most cases the condition probably starts in childhood and persists unsuspected into adulthood. Years later, symptoms of kidney trouble, including renal failure, appear (see Urinary infections in children, p.736).

The bacteria probably gain access to the urinary tract through the open end of the urethra, the tube that leads from the bladder to the outside. Usually such invasions are confined to the lower parts of the urinary tract (see Cystitis, p.544), since the outflow of urine keeps the infection from spreading upward. When you urinate, your bladder contracts and squeezes urine out the urethra.

At the same time, the bladder muscle acts as a valve and closes off the two ureters where they enter the bladder. This prevents urine from being forced back into the kidneys. Sometimes, however, this valvelike action does not work properly, and urine flows back into the kidney as well as downward. This two-way flow is known as reflux. If this happens with infected urine, the infection may reach the kidneys. A combination of recurring infections and reflux is probably the cause of most cases of chronic pyelonephritis.

Kidney stones (see p.548) may also cause the disorder. Chronic pyelonephritis may be preceded by repeated attacks of other urinary tract infections such as acute pyelonephritis or cystitis, but this is rare.

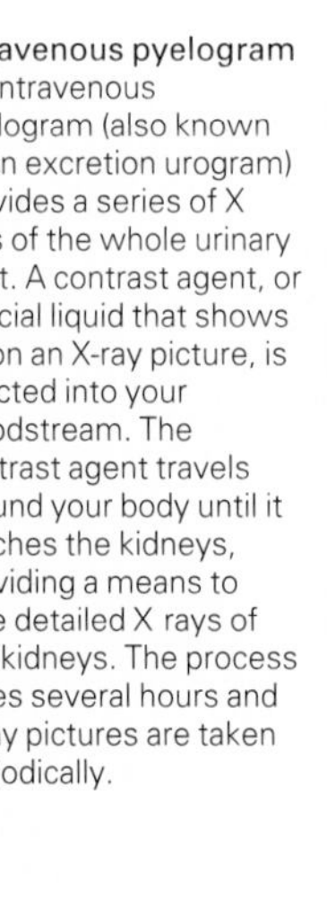

Intravenous pyelogram
An intravenous pyelogram (also known as an excretion urogram) provides a series of X rays of the whole urinary tract. A contrast agent, or special liquid that shows up on an X-ray picture, is injected into your bloodstream. The contrast agent travels around your body until it reaches the kidneys, providing a means to take detailed X rays of the kidneys. The process takes several hours and X-ray pictures are taken periodically.

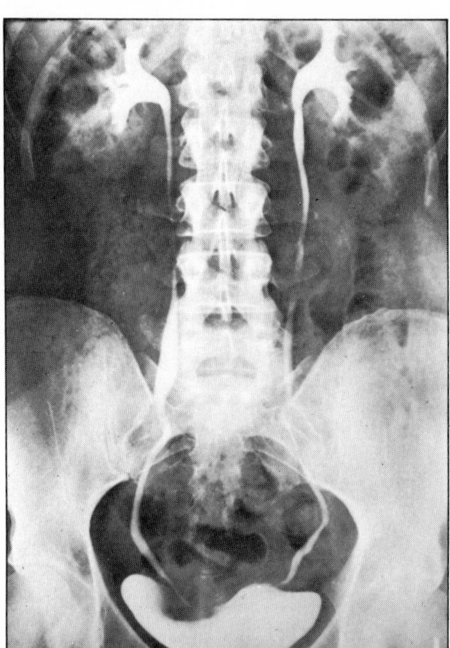

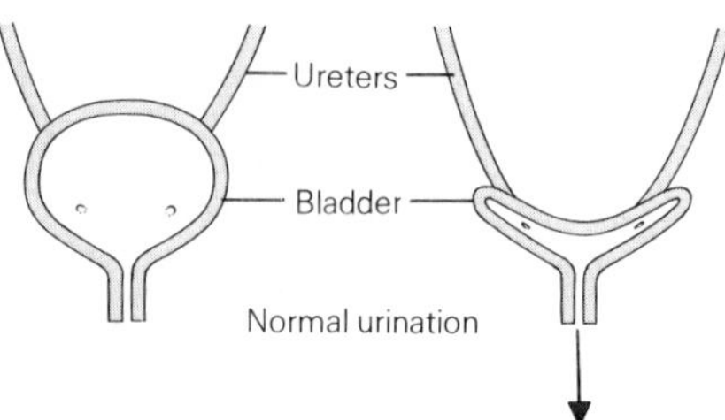

Infected urine in the kidneys
A possible cause of kidney infection is inefficiency of the valves that connect the ureters and the bladder. If these valves do not close properly when you urinate, urine may be squeezed back up the ureters. Any infection in the urine can then travel up to the kidneys.

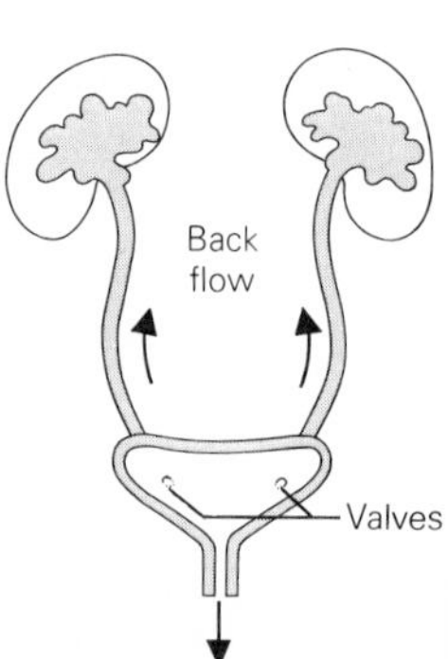

What are the symptoms?

Chronic pyelonephritis seldom produces symptoms until the condition is well established. Eventually, though, early signs of chronic kidney failure (see p.551) may appear; these warning signs include fatigue, nausea, or itching skin.

In many cases the condition is discovered at a much earlier stage of its development through a blood or urine test that is given for some other reason.

What are the risks?

The main risk of chronic pyelonephritis is that the condition may develop undetected until it produces chronic kidney failure. This does not often happen today, however, since there is now more preventive treatment available for urinary infections in young children (see p.736).

What should be done?

If you have repeated mild urinary infections or any symptom of chronic kidney failure, consult your physician. The diagnostic tests are generally the same as those for acute pyelonephritis. They may include blood and urine tests, an intravenous pyelogram (IVP), and cystoscopy.

What is the treatment?

Self-help: If you discover that you have chronic pyelonephritis, but you have no symptoms, your physician may advise you to drink plenty of fluids and restrict your intake of foods high in protein and sodium. Your physician may also suggest that you have blood tests every 6 to 12 months to check on the disorder.

Professional help: Treatment depends on how advanced the disease is when it is diagnosed. Although surgery to repair the faulty valve mechanism in the bladder is sometimes necessary in a child, it is not generally helpful for an adult. Any other cause of repeated infections, such as kidney stones, may respond to appropriate treatment for that condition. Otherwise, you will probably be given a prescription for an antibiotic. Antibiotics are usually used for a short period whenever you have a urinary tract infection. Sometimes with chronic pyelonephritis, however, your physician will prescribe a low dose of an antibiotic for 6 months to 2 years, in an attempt to keep your urine free of bacteria. The disease progresses very slowly, so your physician may advise you to be alert for subsequent kidney trouble and have regular checkups.

Glomerulonephritis

Glomerulonephritis is the term used for several related diseases that damage the glomeruli, the tiny filtering units in your kidneys. Glomerulonephritis is associated with disorders in which your immune system attacks the glomeruli.

In a healthy kidney, your blood passes through the glomeruli, which filter out certain chemicals including waste products. Most of the water and certain chemicals such as glucose that are useful to the body are then reabsorbed into your bloodstream. The remaining waste materials are collected as urine and pass down the ureter to your bladder for storage until you urinate.

This process is adversely affected by the damaged glomeruli. The most obvious disturbance is that red blood cells leak through the glomeruli into your urine. Some proteins also pass from your blood into your urine. If this loss is excessive, which occurs most often in children, it causes an illness called nephrotic syndrome (see p.738). As more of the glomeruli are damaged, the affected kidneys become less efficient as a filter and regulator of the chemical content of your blood. Waste products accumulate and cause kidney failure (see p.550).

Glomerulonephritis can occur in mild or severe forms. It may be acute, flaring up over a few days, or it may be chronic, taking months or years to develop.

What are the symptoms?

Mild, chronic glomerulonephritis produces no symptoms at all. Your physician may notice the condition only when a sample of your urine is tested for some other reason. In some cases, your urine may have a smoky appearance, which results from the presence of small amounts of blood, or it may be bright red, which indicates larger amounts of blood.

In severe, acute glomerulonephritis, you may feel generally ill, with drowsiness, nausea, and vomiting—all symptoms of impending kidney failure. You will probably be producing very small amounts of urine. Fluid may accumulate in your body tissues, causing a condition called edema, which makes your skin, particularly around your ankles, look puffy. If fluid accumulates in your chest, you may become short of breath.

What are the risks?

Glomerulonephritis is not common in adults, but approximately 60 percent of people who have end-stage kidney failure (see p.552) first had signs and symptoms of chronic glomerulonephritis. Acute glomerulonephritis is most common in children (see p.737).

The greatest risk of all forms of glomerulonephritis is that it may lead to chronic kidney failure. The disorder can also eventually lead to high blood pressure (see p.411) because your kidneys play a central part in regulating blood pressure.

What should be done?
Consult your physician, who will arrange for a urine test. If the test results suggest that you may have glomerulonephritis, you may need further tests, including an intravenous pyelogram (IVP) and possibly a biopsy, a procedure in which a small piece of one of your kidneys is removed and examined.

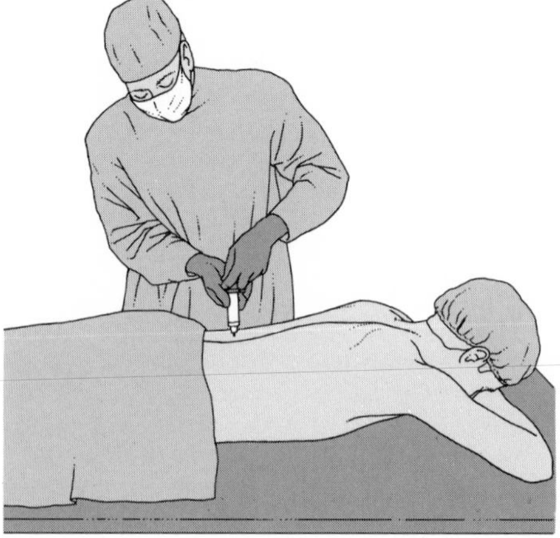

Kidney biopsy
In a kidney biopsy, a small area of skin and muscle over the kidney is first numbed with a local anesthetic. Your physician then passes a hollow needle through the numbed area into the kidney and withdraws a tiny sample of kidney tissue for laboratory analysis.

What is the treatment?
Many forms of glomerulonephritis are so mild that they require no specific treatment other than rest. Other forms of the disease can be treated with corticosteroids and/or immunosuppressant drugs.

If you have edema, diuretics may be prescribed to increase the amount of urine you eliminate and increase the frequency of urination. If you have high blood pressure, it must also be treated, and you may need iron and vitamin supplements if you have become anemic as a result of this disorder. If glomerulonephritis leads to end-stage kidney failure, treatment is as described for that disorder (see p.552).

Urethritis

Urethritis is inflammation of the urethra, the tube that leads from the bladder to the outside. Your urine passes to the outside of your body through the urethra. Typical symptoms of urethritis include pain in the urethral area—particularly when urinating—frequent urination, and a discharge from the opening. In women, urethritis is sometimes the result of bruising during sexual intercourse (see Chronic urethritis, p.644). Urethritis in males is generally caused by sexually transmitted disease (see Urethritis in men, p.619). Two sexually transmitted diseases that can often bring on urethritis are nongonococcal urethritis (see p.655) and gonorrhea (see p.654).

Cystitis

Cystitis is an inflammation of the bladder caused by a urinary infection. The bladder is the temporary storage area for urine. The urine is released regularly from the bladder to the urethra, the tube through which the urine flows to the outside of your body. Cystitis is far more common in women than in men, because a woman's urethra is shorter, providing easier access to the bladder for infectious agents that enter from the outside. Cystitis rarely occurs in men unless an inflamed or enlarged prostate gland or other lower urinary tract abnormality is present.

What are the symptoms?
The major symptom in both sexes is a frequent urge to urinate, which produces only a small amount of a sometimes strong-smelling and bloody urine. With cystitis the urine is likely to burn or sting as you pass it, because the urethra is often inflamed when bladder infection and inflammation are present. You may have a feeling of discomfort just below your navel, where your bladder is located. You may also have a fever.

What is the treatment?
Drinking large quantities of water will help relieve the symptoms, but you should also consult your physician, who will probably prescribe antibiotics. The medication should quickly clear up your symptoms, but you should take the drugs until your physician tells you to stop. For further information, read the articles on cystitis in women (see p.643) and urinary infections in children (see p.736).

Injury to kidneys or ureters

The most likely cause of injury to kidneys or ureters, the tubes that carry urine from your kidneys to your bladder, is either a direct blow to the side of the body just under the ribs (such as that sustained in a football tackle or block), or a crushing force (from being trapped in a vehicle after a collision, for example). Another possible cause of injury is penetration by a knife or bullet. In any injury, a kidney may be bruised or its membranous outer envelope and/or a ureter may be torn. Sometimes a large blood clot forms under the envelope and produces a lump over the kidney that can be felt through your skin. It is also possible for blood or urine to leak into your abdomen through a tear, which may cause peritonitis (see p.503).

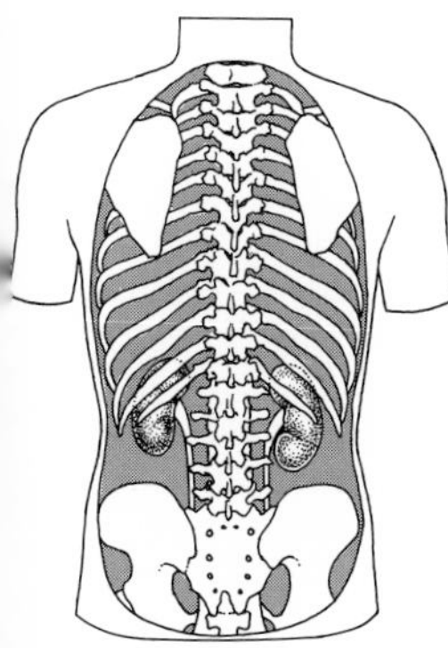

Your kidneys are protected by your rib cage and back muscles.

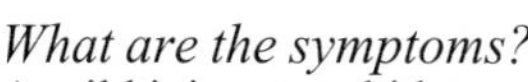

What are the symptoms?

A mild injury to a kidney or ureter may cause pain and tenderness in the lower part of your back. You may also have a fever and occasional traces of blood in your urine. You may not notice the blood until a day or two after the injury has occurred. If you have severe pain and large amounts of blood in your urine, one or both of your kidneys, and possibly the ureters, may have been seriously injured. Bloody urine is a symptom of several potentially serious conditions and should never be ignored. You will probably need to undergo diagnostic tests of the kidneys, including ultrasound, intravenous pyelogram (imaging in which contrast medium is injected into your arm and filtered by the kidney so that it shows up clearly on X-ray films), and/or a CT scan, so that your physician can assess the damage.

What is the treatment?

The ability of kidneys and ureters to heal themselves is remarkable. Even major tears and injuries seldom require treatment other than 7 to 10 days of rest. Unless the injury is very slight, it is usually advisable for you to spend several days in the hospital, where your pulse, blood pressure, and urine can be checked frequently to see if you have serious internal bleeding.

In the unlikely event that your kidney or ureter does not heal after a week or so of bed rest, it may be necessary to repair the torn ureter surgically or to remove the kidney. Removal of a kidney is not usually a complicated operation, and you can lead a healthy, active life with only one kidney.

Injury to bladder or urethra

Because the bladder, in which urine is temporarily stored, lies low inside the abdomen, it is usually protected against injury. When damage does occur, it generally results from a direct blow to your pelvis that fractures a pelvic bone and causes a sharp fragment of the bone to pierce the bladder wall or from a direct forceful blow to a full bladder. Any such rupture usually has serious consequences because it allows urine to leak into the abdominal cavity. In men, rupture of the urethra, the tube that carries urine from the bladder to the outside, is more common but less dangerous. It can be caused by a fall or any kind of impact in the groin. Because the female urethra is very short, urethral damage is rare in women.

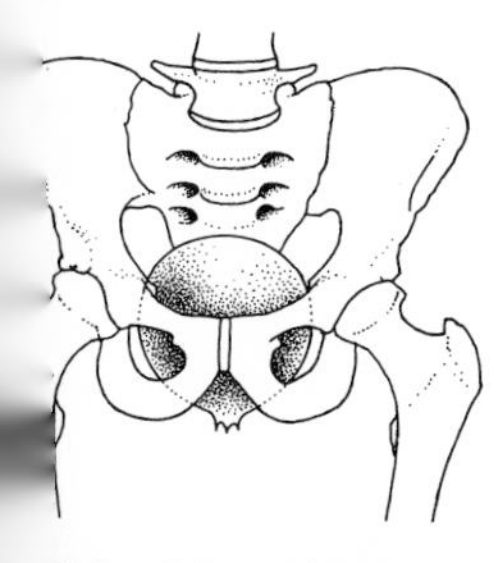

When full, your bladder is less well protected by the circle of bones that form your pelvis.

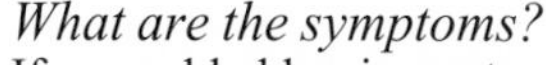

What are the symptoms?

If your bladder is ruptured you will have severe pain in your abdomen, and you may also show signs of shock (see p.414). A urethral injury is also extremely painful and is generally followed by an inability to urinate. Sometimes there is bloody discharge.

What are the risks?

Rupture of the bladder is dangerous because urine leaks into the abdominal cavity and causes peritonitis (see p.503). This condition requires prompt treatment in a hospital. Damage to the urethra, on the other hand, usually does not lead to peritonitis. For a man, the chief risk is that the healed urethra will be scarred, causing a narrowing of the urethra (see p.619).

If you have been injured and you have lower abdominal or urinary symptoms, you should see your physician immediately. You may need special X rays of the abdomen and bladder, a CT scan of the abdomen and pelvis, and cystoscopy.

What is the treatment?

If you injure your bladder or urethra, you will be hospitalized. You will probably be given antibiotics to prevent infection. If your bladder is ruptured and urine escapes, you will need an operation to repair the leak and, if necessary, clean out your abdominal cavity. However, if the tear in the bladder is small and if urine loss is minimal, draining the cavity with a catheter may permit healing. If your urethra is damaged, you will probably have a catheter inserted into your bladder for several days so that urine can drain out. Meanwhile, the urethra usually heals on its own. Occasionally, surgery is necessary.

Cysts, tumors, and stones

A growth or swelling anywhere in your body should be investigated by a physician, and the urinary tract is no exception. The tract can be affected by two kinds of growths—cysts and tumors. Cysts are usually soft, fluid-filled sacs, and are most often, but not always, benign (unlikely to spread). Solid tumors are usually malignant (likely to spread). Cysts and tumors are relatively uncommon in the urinary tract. Another type of growth, the pebblelike kidney and bladder stones (calculi), occurs more frequently. Stones do not represent growth of tissue as do the cysts and tumors; instead, they form in the urine from particles of excreted substances dissolved in it. Although frequently stones may cause great discomfort, they are not often a serious threat to life.

Kidney cysts

There are three main categories of kidney cysts: solitary cysts, acquired cysts associated with kidney failure, and inherited cystic kidney diseases. Solitary cysts, also called simple cysts, are the most common. They are fluid-filled pouches lined with cells called renal epithelial cells. These cysts are single and can occur in both kidneys. They usually cause no symptoms and may be discovered in the course of other investigations. An estimated one fourth of people over 50 have simple kidney cysts.

The second type of cyst occurs only with kidney failure (see p.550). These cysts develop in kidney tubules and progress in number and size as kidney failure progresses. Over 75 percent of people receiving dialysis (see Box, p.551) have acquired cysts after 5 years of dialysis. It is vital to treat acquired cysts because of the increased risk that these cysts may give rise to adenomas, which are benign (unlikely to spread) tumors, or adenocarcinomas, which are malignant (likely to spread) tumors of the kidney.

The third type of cyst is actually a broader category of several different inherited kidney diseases including autosomal dominant polycystic kidney disease, which usually does not affect people until middle age; autosomal recessive polycystic kidney disease, which usually causes death in infancy; and nephronophthisis-medullary cystic disease complex, which usually becomes apparent in people between ages 3 and 17.

What are the symptoms?

A simple cyst may cause pain in the back; it can be large enough to cause pain in the abdomen; if so, it can usually be felt by your physician. Hematuria (bloody urine) is also a symptom. With acquired cysts, chronic kidney failure (see p.551) begins with urinary frequency, tremendous thirst, and anemia. In children, this results in failure to grow. Symptoms of the third type relate to kidney failure and, depending on the type, may be fatal any time from infancy to adulthood.

The presence of cysts in your kidneys is often discovered only when your kidneys are examined for some other reason. Many people have such cysts without knowing it. Severe polycystic kidney disease is rare. In the US it causes about 2 percent of all cases of chronic kidney failure.

What are the risks?

The only risk of a solitary cyst is that a malignancy may develop, and this rarely happens. Polycystic disease may lead to high blood pressure (see p.411) and chronic kidney failure. Cysts develop on the kidneys of people on dialysis and are often malignant.

What should be done?

If you have a single kidney cyst, it will probably be discovered only when tests are done for another reason. Because of the slight possibility of cancerous cells in the cyst or if you are having persistent back pain, your physician may want you to have further tests, such as an ultrasound scan, or even a cyst aspiration, which involves piercing the cyst with a needle that is placed in the cyst with the guidance of ultrasound imaging and withdrawing some fluid and cells for examination. Aspiration of a kidney cyst can usually be done painlessly with a local anesthetic. If the testing of the cells in the fluid shows that they are normal, nothing further needs to be done, unless the cyst enlarges enough to cause either kidney damage or extreme discomfort.

Your physician may discover that you or your children have polycystic disease when testing for a different disorder. But if you know the disease runs in your family, you should talk to your physician about it. A cyst is usually diagnosed with the help of ultrasound or CT scans. To prevent possible problems in the future, you should have regular checkups.

What is the treatment?

No treatment is required for a painless, benign kidney cyst. If it becomes large enough to be painful, fluid can be aspirated (removed with a needle) periodically, or if it is found to be malignant, surgery will be performed to remove the cyst or the entire affected kidney. Removal of one of your kidneys is a simple operation; you can lead an active life with the remaining kidney because one healthy kidney increases in size and level of function and can perform most of the work that was formerly done by two.

There is no specific treatment for polycystic disease. If cysts are discovered, your physician may recommend a low-protein diet and frequent checkups to help you slow the progressive damage to your kidneys that leads to chronic kidney failure (see p.551) or end-stage kidney failure (see p.552). You may need dialysis (see p.551) or a kidney transplant (see p.432).

Tumors of the kidney

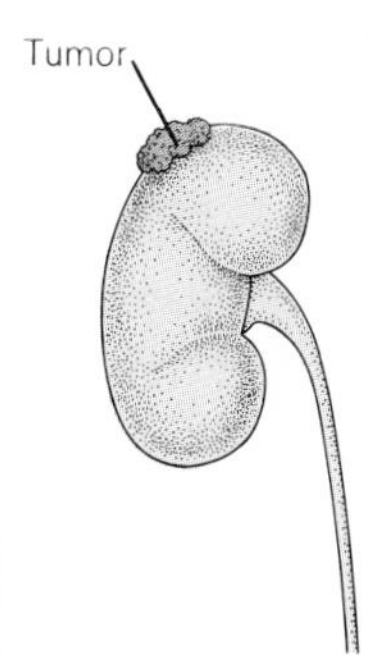

Growths or tumors on the kidney tend to be situated near the top, where they are hidden within the rib cage. Routine examinations may not detect such a tumor.

There are two major types of tumors of the kidney, both of which are malignant (likely to spread and threaten life). One type, which occurs in adults only, is known as hypernephroma, and forms on the edge of your kidney. As the tumor grows, it pushes into healthy kidney tissue, but because the efficiency of the kidney as a filter is affected only at a very late stage in the tumor, eventual kidney failure (see p.550) is rare. The tumor more often makes itself known by causing symptoms such as persistent fever, loss of appetite, and weight loss, or symptoms coming from organs to which it has spread (for example, bone pain or a cough). Your urine may be red or smoky because of bleeding from the tumor.

Hypernephromas are rare; they occur most often in men over 40 and represent a small portion of all cancer deaths. The type of kidney tumor that affects children only is called Wilm's tumor (see p.738).

What are the risks?

The main risk of a hypernephroma is that some of the cells may enter the bloodstream and spread to other parts of your body, particularly the lungs or bones. However, hypernephromas spread less rapidly than many other cancers, and a long-term cure is often achieved if the tumor is discovered and removed at an early stage.

What should be done?

If your urine looks reddish or abnormally cloudy, consult your physician, who will take samples of your urine for laboratory analysis. If a tumor is suspected, you may have diagnostic tests, including an intravenous pyelogram (IVP), an ultrasound scan, and a CT or MRI scan of the kidney.

What is the treatment?

If tests reveal a hypernephroma, the affected kidney will be removed. However, one healthy kidney can generally compensate for the loss of the other. You should have regular checkups to make sure that the cancer does not recur. Interferon and interleukin, drugs made in a genetics laboratory, are being tested on people with kidney tumors, but the outlook is guarded.

Tumors of the bladder

Tumors of the urinary bladder, like those in many other parts of your body, can be either benign (unlikely to spread) or malignant (likely to spread and threaten life). Both types originate from cells that line the bladder, and they tend to produce a growth (or, rarely, more than one) that projects inward, into the space that contains the urine. Cigarette smoking increases the risk of bladder cancer. Any tumor near where the ureter (the tube that carries urine from the kidney) enters the bladder can block the flow of urine and cause the kidney to be stretched from the buildup of urine. This is called hydronephrosis. It makes the kidney susceptible to infection (see Acute pyelonephritis, p.541).

What are the symptoms?

The main symptom of a bladder tumor is hematuria, or blood in the urine. Urinating is not usually painful, but you may have pain after you have finished. You may have a burning feeling and a tendency to urinate small amounts at frequent intervals. These are the symptoms of cystitis (see p.544), which often occurs when a tumor is present. If hydronephrosis has developed, you may also have pain in your back.

What are the risks?

Tumors of the bladder are not common; the disorder is most common in men over 50. A benign tumor is easily treated. A malignant one, however, may damage a large portion of bladder tissue. If the cancerous cells spread to other parts of the body, the prospects for successful treatment are not good.

What should be done?

Always consult your physician if you see blood in your urine. He or she will take urine and blood samples for analysis, and you may also need other diagnostic tests. These may include cystoscopy (in which a long thin tube is passed into your bladder through the urethra), an intravenous pyelogram (IVP), a cystogram, or a CT or MRI scan. If a growth is discovered, you will probably need a biopsy in which a sample of the growth is removed and examined under a microscope to determine whether it is malignant.

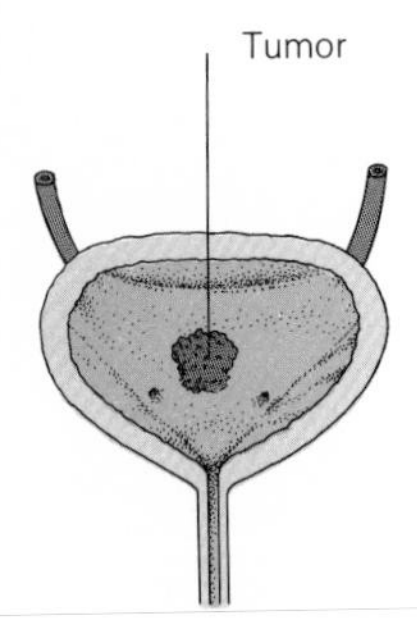

Most tumors in the bladder are warty growths that project from the bladder's inside wall.

What is the treatment?

A common treatment for bladder tumors is to destroy them by burning them with an electric probe passed through a cystoscope. This process is known as fulguration. In another type of treatment, an anti-cancer drug is injected into a vein and then accumulates in the tumor. A laser beam is then transmitted through a cystoscope and causes the drug to destroy the tumor. Chemotherapy drugs or tuberculosis vaccine may be instilled into the bladder periodically for certain stages of bladder tumor. This may clear up the problem, but you will need checkups to make sure that the tumor does not recur.

If a tumor has affected a large area of your bladder, the whole bladder may have to be removed. The ureters are then connected to an opening in the abdominal wall. Thereafter, the urine flows into a bag (an "external bladder"), which must be emptied from time to time. In other cases, the ureters can be attached to a loop of the small intestine, so that urine flows into this reservoir. A valvelike opening on the skin allows you to empty the pouch with a catheter at your own convenience. After surgery, you may need radiation therapy and anticancer drugs to destroy any remaining abnormal cells.

Kidney stones

(renal calculi)

The kidneys are among several organs in your body where stones may form. A kidney stone usually begins as a tiny speck of solid material deposited in the middle of your kidney, where urine collects before flowing into the ureter (the tube connecting the kidney and bladder). As more material clings to the first speck, it gradually builds in size. This process can occur in one or both kidneys. Over a period of years, a stone 1 in (25 mm) or more in diameter can develop. Some kidney stones contain calcium. Other materials, amino acids, or excretory products (such as uric acid) may crystallize in the urine and form a stone.

Tiny stones seldom cause problems, because they are easily carried into the ureter and passed in the urine. Any stone with a diameter of about ⅕ in (5 mm) or more causes severe pain if and when it enters the ureter with urine bound for the bladder.

What are the symptoms?

If stones are too big to pass from the kidney into the ureter, you may have no symptoms or, at most, occasional pain as small pieces break off and are carried down the ureter. The most common symptom of kidney stones is called colic, which is a stabbing pain that tends to come in waves, often a few minutes apart. Colic can be caused by disorders in various parts of the body, including gallstones (see p.526) and intestinal obstruction (see p.503). Typically, it makes you double over with pain. Kidney pain of this type, called renal colic, can occur when a stone passes from a kidney down one of the ureters. It will subside if and when the stone moves into the bladder. The pain almost always occurs on one side of your body at a time, but if you have stones in both kidneys a subsequent attack may occur on the other side.

You usually feel renal colic first in the back, just below the ribs on either side of the spinal column. Over a period of hours or days, the pain follows the course of the stone as it travels along the ureter, around to the front of the body, and down toward the groin. It may make you feel nauseated, and there may be traces of blood in your urine. After the stone reaches your bladder, it will probably pass through the remainder of the urinary tract with little or no pain (see also Bladder stones, next article).

What are the risks?

Because passage of a kidney stone often produces severe pain, the disorder is a frequent cause of brief hospital admissions. It is known that the problem runs in families and that it is more common in hot climates. In very warm weather, people lose a great deal of body water in their breath and in sweat, and unless their fluid intake is substantial, they produce a smaller volume of concentrated urine. This urine contains a higher concentration of stone-forming material.

Men seem more susceptible than women to the disorder, and people over 30 are more susceptible than younger people. In rare cases, children develop a form of kidney stone that is caused by a chemical abnormality in the blood.

Most kidney stones remain harmlessly in the kidneys or are eventually passed in the urine. An occasional stone may get stuck in a ureter and block the flow of urine on one side. Surgery may be required to remove the stone because of the possibility of severe kidney infection and of the destruction of kidney tissue if it were to remain obstructed.

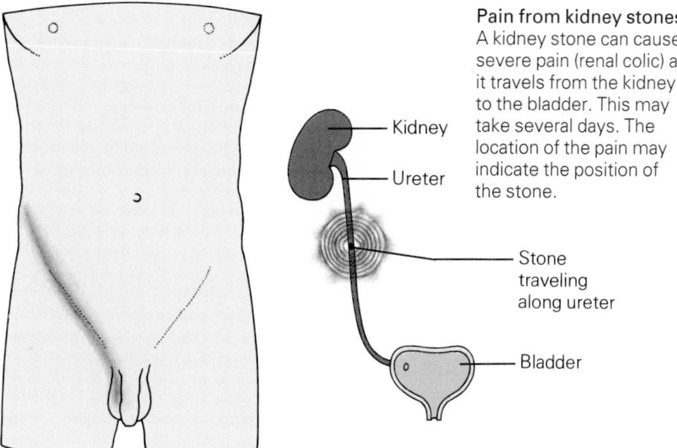

Site of the pain

Pain from kidney stones
A kidney stone can cause severe pain (renal colic) as it travels from the kidney to the bladder. This may take several days. The location of the pain may indicate the position of the stone.

What should be done?

If you know you have kidney stones, see your physician at 6-month intervals to monitor the stones and your kidneys. If you have renal colic, your physician will probably refer you for blood and urine tests and an intravenous pyelogram (IVP) or ultrasound. The tests will help locate stones and will indicate whether further treatment is necessary.

What is the treatment?

Self-help: Consult your physician if you have an attack of renal colic. You should also drink large quantities of water—at least 8 to 10 8-ounce glasses a day. Anyone with kidney stones should develop this habit. Drinking the water helps flush any stones through your urinary tract and helps prevent other stones from forming by keeping the urine diluted. To relieve pain, use the medication prescribed by your physician.

Professional help: There is no satisfactory medical treatment for kidney stones that have already formed. However, if your body forms stones made of uric acid, your physician may prescribe drugs that can prevent stones from forming or sometimes dissolve stones. Thiazide diuretics are prescribed for people whose stones are caused by excessive excretion of calcium in the urine. If a stone causes a blockage in the lower third of your ureter, it can sometimes be removed by manipulation during cystoscopy, using very small instruments that fit through the cystoscope. The physician inserts the instrument through the cystoscope, into the bladder, and up into the ureter where the stone is trapped. When the instrument is withdrawn, the stone often comes out with it. Stones in the ureter may be pulverized by a technique called extracorporeal lithotripsy, in which hydraulically generated shock waves fragment the stones into powder that can then be passed out of the body in the urine. Lithotripsy has made surgery unnecessary in most cases.

In the unlikely event that stones have done irreparable damage to one of your kidneys, the entire kidney may have to be removed. Your remaining kidney will then do most of the work previously done by the two kidneys.

Bladder stones

(vesical calculi)

A kidney stone (see previous article) that has completed the trip, however painfully, through the ureter (the tube that connects kidney and bladder) into your bladder will be relatively small. For this reason the stone can pass out of your body in the urine with comparative ease. Stones that form inside the bladder itself, however, tend to be bigger than kidney stones and may remain in your bladder. This may cause symptoms such as an overly frequent urge to urinate, pain when you pass urine, and blood in your urine. Often the blood seems to be "squeezed out" in the last few drops. Today, however, bladder stones are not a common problem.

If you have bladder stones that are too large to pass naturally through the urethra, the tube that connects your bladder to the outside, they must be removed. This is sometimes done by passing a cystoscope (viewing tube) up the urethra into the bladder; the stones are then either crushed and removed or they are removed in one piece through the cystoscope. In exceptional circumstances, a very large stone or stones may require surgery in which the bladder is opened to remove the stone.

Kidney failure

Kidney failure, also called renal failure, occurs in one of three forms. Acute renal failure is an illness in which your kidneys suddenly stop functioning, sometimes within a few days or even hours. Chronic renal failure, which is also called chronic renal insufficiency, develops over many years and insidiously interferes with your health. In end-stage renal failure your kidneys function so poorly that they can no longer sustain life without the assistance of an artificial kidney machine or a kidney transplant.

Acute kidney failure

Your kidneys may suddenly stop working for various reasons, but usually for one of three main causes. Toxic agents, immune reactions to drugs, and certain infections or diseases such as acute glomerulonephritis (see p.543) can abruptly damage the kidneys enough to cause their failure. A sudden drop in blood pressure, as a result of serious burns, severe bleeding, or a major heart attack, can deprive the kidneys of an adequate supply of oxygen-carrying blood, damaging them. Finally, the flow of urine may be suddenly and completely obstructed by a blockage in the urinary tract or by a crushing injury where myoglobin (the oxygen-carrying pigment of the muscle) filters through the glomeruli and blocks the tubules. The obstruction may be located lower in the urinary tract, such as a blockage of the urethra from an enlarged prostate (see p.615).

As a result, your kidneys cannot produce urine. Waste products build up in your blood and water begins to accumulate in your body. Lastly, there develops a dangerous imbalance of essential chemicals that are normally regulated by the kidneys.

What are the symptoms?

In this severe crisis, symptoms of the condition that has caused the acute kidney failure are more apparent than those caused by the kidney failure itself. You pass drastically less urine than usual, possibly less than a cup a day. Almost immediately you lose your appetite, feel increasingly nauseated, and begin to vomit. Delayed treatment may lead to drowsiness, confusion, seizures, and eventually coma.

Much of the risk depends on the severity of the underlying problem, but this is a potentially fatal condition. Even treatment with dialysis does not always lead to recovery.

What should be done?

If you have acute kidney failure, you urgently need hospital treatment, preferably in a special unit to treat kidney diseases. If the cause is not obvious, you will probably have to undergo an intensive series of diagnostic tests, possibly including a needle biopsy of the kidney, in which a small piece of kidney is removed for examination.

What is the treatment?

When the cause of acute kidney failure is heavy bleeding or a heart attack, treatment of the accompanying shock is required. If the cause of failure is a urinary tract obstruction, you will probably need an operation to relieve the blockage. If the underlying cause is kidney disease, or if the kidneys remain severely affected even though the cause of failure is successfully treated, treatment procedures vary.

If shock or severe fluid loss (from hemorrhaging, vomiting, or diarrhea) has led to acute kidney failure, an intravenous solution of saline, plasma, or blood, sometimes with an adrenalinelike substance, helps restore your blood pressure to more normal levels.

Diuretics occasionally are useful in re-establishing urine flow, but only after your fluid loss is restored to the bloodstream by intravenous solutions. Kidneys will usually recover most or all the lost function within days to several weeks. In some instances, such as cases of acute glomerulonephritis, treatment with specific drugs may be effective. But when little or no urine is being formed and the kidney damage appears massive, your physician may have to use an artificial device that performs the functions of your kidneys until they recover. This type of treatment is called dialysis (see Box, Dialysis: the artificial kidney, next page).

While you are under treatment, you may need a special diet that is high in calories but low in protein, and may include no more than a pint (480 mL) of fluid a day. This provides you with the energy you need but does not overtax your kidneys with waste products from the metabolism of protein.

Dialysis: the artificial kidney

If your kidneys are temporarily unable to function, or if they have become badly damaged by long-standing inflammation, you will probably receive a treatment called dialysis. In dialysis the functions of the kidneys, which include removing waste products from your body and regulating the chemical and water balance, are taken over by a machine.

There are two forms of dialysis. The first is peritoneal dialysis. Your physician makes a small incision in your abdominal wall and threads a thin plastic tube into your abdomen. A special fluid flows slowly through the tube and fills the peritoneal space (the space between the inner and outer layers of the sac lining the abdominal walls). Waste products seep from the blood vessels that line the abdomen into the fluid, which is then drained out along with excess water. The process takes several hours.

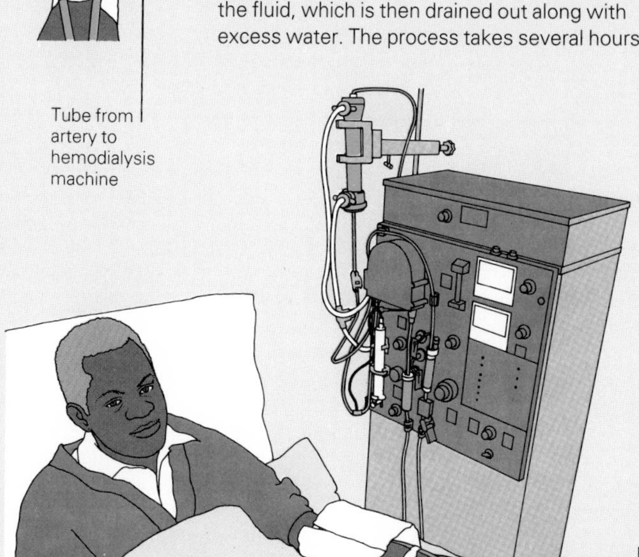

Peritoneal dialysis is a painless procedure. If you have acute kidney failure, you will gradually be weaned off the treatment as your kidneys recover. If the damage to your kidneys is permanent, you may be taught to perform peritoneal dialysis yourself. This procedure (called continuous ambulatory peritoneal dialysis, or CAPD) is performed at home, overnight, enabling you to carry out your normal daily activities.

The alternative form of dialysis, hemodialysis, filters waste products from your blood. To do this, blood from an arm or leg artery is passed along a thin tube to the machine, through its filter (called an artificial kidney), and back along another tube into an adjacent vein. A standard treatment, which lasts 4 hours and is repeated two or three times every week, is enough to control levels of waste products and excess water in your body.

Everyone who begins hemodialysis treatment must first have a minor operation to increase the blood flow in a vein; or if your veins are too small a synthetic vessel is placed under the skin to connect a large artery and vein. Thereafter, you can insert the two needles at the start of each treatment to provide access to the high-volume blood flow required for efficient hemodialysis. Dialysis patients learn how to insert their own needles and run the machine themselves. Some machines are now small enough to be portable so home hemodialysis patients may travel and take their machines with them. People who receive a kidney transplant (see p.432) are able to discontinue dialysis.

Chronic kidney failure

Chronic kidney failure is the phase of gradually deteriorating kidney function that ultimately leads to end-stage kidney failure (see p.552), when dialysis, either peritoneal dialysis or hemodialysis (see Box, above) becomes necessary to sustain life. Chronic kidney failure may result from generalized diseases that affect blood vessels such as glomerulonephritis (see p.543) or from causes of kidney inflammation such as chronic pyelonephritis (see p.542). Diabetes mellitus (see p.558) is a frequent cause of renal failure. Overuse of drugs containing phenacetin and poisoning from heavy metals (such as lead or mercury) may also lead to chronic kidney failure.

If you have chronic kidney failure, chemicals gradually build up in your blood, and your kidneys become increasingly unable to excrete waste products and water. One function of the kidneys is to control blood pressure. Hypertension can thus be a cause as well as a result of chronic kidney failure.

What are the symptoms?

Symptoms appear gradually and you may not have any for years. In fact, your kidney function can decrease 25 percent with no

Painkillers can cause kidney failure
A word of warning: Excessive consumption of certain analgesics, or painkillers, can lead to a disease called analgesic nephropathy, which may result in chronic kidney failure. To develop analgesic nephropathy, you have to take several analgesic pills every day for several years. The preparations most likely to cause the disease are those in which several drugs are combined in a single tablet that you can buy without a prescription. To help avoid problems, tell your physician about painkilling medications you are using, especially combination drugs.

outward signs or symptoms of failure. Then you may notice that you are urinating more often than you used to. This is because your kidneys can no longer concentrate the urine as efficiently, so you pass urine at night and more frequently during the day. You may also feel progressively more tired and lethargic. If your chronic kidney failure continues to get worse, you will have the symptoms of end-stage kidney failure (see next article).

The main risk of chronic kidney failure is that the scarring of the kidneys will become progressively worse and eventually lead to end-stage kidney failure. There are also the risks associated with high blood pressure (see p.411), anemia (see p.450), and hyperparathyroidism (see p.569) causing osteodystrophy (bone damage associated with kidney failure). These three diseases sometimes occur as a result of the failing kidneys' inability to control the levels of blood chemicals and hormones.

What is the treatment?

Self-help: Follow your physician's advice about diet. If you have kidney failure, he or she will probably advise you to eat a low-protein diet (see Acute kidney failure, previous article). Do not take medication without asking your physician about any possible danger resulting from overaccumulation of the drug, which will be excreted more slowly by the less efficient functioning of the damaged kidney.

Professional help: There is no treatment available that can reverse the course of chronic kidney failure, but close medical supervision can sometimes help to slow down the disease and counteract your symptoms. Your physician may prescribe medications to control your blood pressure and to prevent the development of osteodystrophy. With regular checkups, a diet carefully planned with your physician's advice, and appropriate medication, you should be able to lead an active life despite your kidney problem.

End-stage kidney failure

End-stage kidney failure is the most advanced form of kidney failure. It usually occurs when, despite treatment, chronic kidney failure (see previous article) progresses to the point where your kidneys can no longer sustain life. An event such as pneumonia that places added stress on the already limited filtering capacity of the kidneys often tips the balance between chronic failure and end-stage failure.

What are the symptoms?

The importance of the kidneys to your health is demonstrated by the number and variety of the symptoms that occur with end-stage kidney failure. These symptoms may include lethargy, weakness, headache, confusion, delirium, seizures, a furred tongue and unpleasant breath, oral thrush (see p.484), nausea, vomiting, diarrhea, an accumulation of water (edema) in the lungs (producing shortness of breath) and just under the skin (producing generalized swelling), pain in the chest or bones, and/or intensely itchy skin. Profound anemia is a feature of kidney failure, since the kidneys cease production of a hormone, erythropoietin, that stimulates the bone marrow to manufacture blood cells. A woman with end-stage kidney failure may stop menstruating.

What is the treatment?

If you develop end-stage kidney failure, you will probably already be under treatment for chronic kidney failure. Your physician will probably have told you to report any illness or any change in your condition.

Treatment for end-stage kidney failure is a complex team effort. The various aspects of the treatment program will be tailor-made to your individual case.

The anemia of people with end-stage kidney failure is relieved with regular injections of erythropoietin. But because the kidney damage is irreversible, the only satisfactory form of treatment is one that takes over the kidneys' functions. This means either dialysis (see Box, Dialysis: the artificial kidney, previous page) or an operation to transplant a healthy, donated kidney, in which the main risks are rejection and infection (see Transplants, p.432).

Unfortunately, some patients with end-stage kidney failure are too ill for treatment by either dialysis or transplantation.

What are the long-term prospects?

End-stage kidney failure is no longer a swiftly fatal disease because of dialysis, kidney transplantation, erythropoietin to control anemia, and other drugs that are effective for symptom control. Well over half of those who have had the disease are able to live comparatively normal lives 10 years after it begins; dialysis has greatly improved the prospects for survival. A good percentage of transplant recipients are still well many years after receiving a new kidney.

Hormonal disorders

Introduction

Hormones are messenger chemicals made in organs called endocrine glands. These glands are essentially hormone-producing cells clustered around blood vessels. The hormones are released directly into the bloodstream, rather than through a duct, as in some other glands. Together with the nervous system (see p.283), hormones coordinate and control the functioning of various organs and tissues so that all parts of the body work together smoothly, efficiently, and correctly.

When a hormone is released into your bloodstream it circulates to all parts of your body, but it affects only a certain part or parts of the body. The part affected is called the target organ for that hormone. The amount of each hormone that is released into the bloodstream depends on your body's needs at that particular moment. The hormone levels in your blood change in response to events such as infections, stressful situations, and shifts in the chemical composition of your blood. In some cases the level of one hormone in your blood regulates the level of another. For example, several hormones produced by your pituitary gland specifically regulate the amount of other hormones released by certain other endocrine glands. The pituitary gland, a peanut-sized yet centrally important endocrine gland located at the base of the brain, is largely under the control of the hypothalamus, a center of the brain that exerts wide-ranging control of your hormonal system.

Only the more common hormonal problems are discussed in this book. This section addresses those that occur in endocrine glands found in both men and women. They include disorders of the pituitary gland, the pancreas, the adrenal glands, and the thyroid and parathyroid glands. There are several other endocrine glands that occur exclusively in one sex. They are the ovaries and placenta in women and the testes in men. Disorders of these glands are discussed in other sections of the book (see Men's health, p.611; Women's health, p.623; and Pregnancy and childbirth, p.661). Many hormonal disorders require the expert diagnosis and treatment of an endocrinologist, a physician who specializes in such problems.

Hormone-producing glands

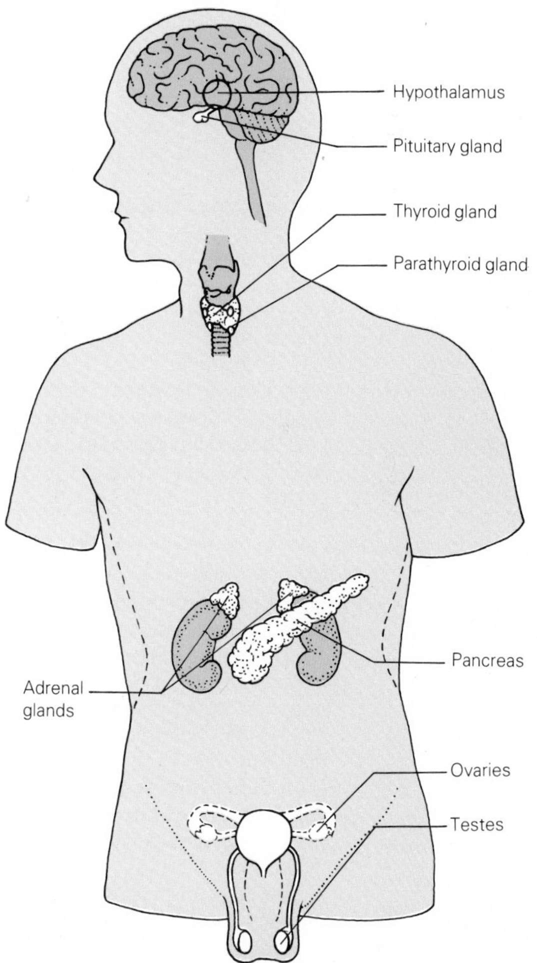

Pituitary gland

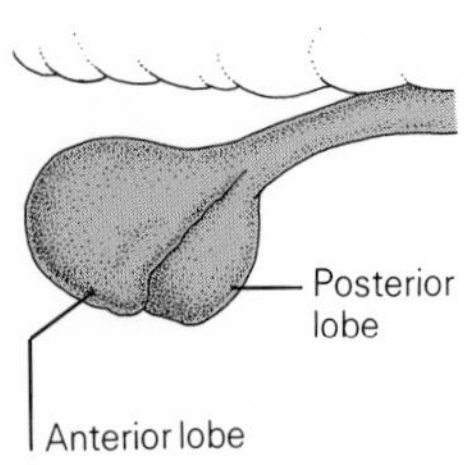

The pituitary gland has two parts, the anterior and posterior lobes.

The pituitary gland, a peanut-sized organ situated just beneath the hypothalamus in the brain, is a very important endocrine, or hormone-producing, gland. It is like a central control switch that regulates many aspects of your body's growth, development, and everyday functioning. The gland has two distinct parts, the anterior, or front, lobe and the posterior, or rear, lobe.

The anterior lobe produces six hormones. Growth hormone, as its name implies, regulates the physical growth of most parts of your body. Prolactin stimulates the breasts to produce milk (see Galactorrhea, p.558). The four other hormones made by the anterior lobe (thyroid-stimulating hormone, corticotropin, follicle-stimulating hormone, and luteinizing hormone) stimulate four other hormone-producing glands; the thyroid and the adrenals, and the ovaries in women and testes in men. These glands, in turn, produce hormones of their own.

The posterior lobe of the pituitary gland produces two hormones. One is antidiuretic hormone, which acts on the kidneys and plays a large part in regulating the concentration and quantity of your urine. It also raises blood pressure. The other hormone produced by the posterior lobe, oxytocin, stimulates contractions of the uterus during childbirth.

The release of hormones from the anterior lobe of the pituitary gland is controlled by the hypothalamus (the region of the brain that lies immediately above the gland). A network of portal veins directly links the anterior pituitary gland to the hypothalamus. The anterior lobe of the pituitary gland is indirectly connected to the other parts of the brain by means of the hypothalamus. This acts as a strong link between the nervous system and endocrine system.

Because of these links, mental processes (including emotions) and events that take place outside of the body (including seasonal changes) may influence the secretion of hormones and therefore the chemistry of the body. For example, intense stress causes secretion of corticotropin, which stimulates the adrenal gland to secrete steroids that help the body cope with stress.

Acromegaly

In this rare condition, the pituitary gland produces too much growth hormone, which causes excessive growth. However, an adult cannot grow taller, since the bones mature and vertical growth stops at the end of adolescence. Instead, the excess growth hormone produces acromegaly, in which your bones thicken and all other structures and organs grow larger. Overproduction of growth hormone is usually caused by a pituitary tumor (see p.557).

What are the symptoms?

Acromegaly generally can occur at any time after adolescence. Usually, the first symptom is enlargement of the hands and feet, typically revealed by the tightening of a ring on the finger, or an increase in glove or shoe size.

After the hands and feet increase in size, the head and neck grow broader, and the lower jaw, brows, nose, and ears become prominent. The skin and tongue thicken, and features become generally coarser. The voice may become deeper.

Many people with this disorder experience tingling in the hands, fatigue, headaches, increased sweating, stiffness, and generalized aches. In a woman, the amount of hair on the body and limbs may increase.

In some cases of acromegaly, diabetes mellitus (see p.558) develops and causes the symptoms of that disorder. If a large pituitary tumor is present, it may cause a number of other symptoms.

What are the risks?

The longer acromegaly is left untreated, the greater the risks become. The heart continues to enlarge; high blood pressure (see p.411) and possibly heart failure (see p.408) develop in time. In addition, a large pituitary tumor can cause serious problems with the eyesight. Also, certain cancers are more common in people who have acromegaly.

What should be done?

If your physician suspects acromegaly, you or your family member will probably be referred to a few specialists. A blood sample will be taken to find out how much growth hormone is circulating in the body. CT or MRI scans will definitely show the extent of the tumor. Tests of your visual field—your side vision—will probably also be required.

What is the treatment?
If the blood test shows that the growth hormone level is high and cannot be reduced, and if the presence of a tumor is confirmed by CT or MRI scans, you should be treated as soon as possible. Your physician will probably recommend either radiation therapy or surgery. Drugs such as bromocriptine can sometimes control a pituitary tumor.

The best form of treatment depends on a number of factors. The drug somatostatin is often used to treat acromegaly; it inhibits growth hormone, which in turn checks the growth of the pituitary tumor.

What are the long-term prospects?
Surgical removal of the pituitary tumor may be effective in improving problems with the eyesight. Also, tumors can now be selectively removed, leaving behind only healthy tissue. Complete cosmetic recovery may not be possible, however, since the changes in your bones and your appearance are largely irreversible. However, treatment halts the progress of the disease.

If all or almost all of your pituitary gland is removed or destroyed, you will need lifelong treatment with hormone replacements, such as sex hormones or thyroid hormone.

Gigantism

Gigantism is the same disorder as acromegaly (see previous article), except that it begins in children and adolescents instead of in adults. The pituitary gland overproduces growth hormone, usually because of a pituitary tumor (see p.557). Overproduction of this hormone causes excessive growth of all parts of the body. The main difference between the two forms of the disease is that acromegaly occurs when the arm and leg bones have stopped growing, and gigantism occurs when they are still growing so that the young person grows to giant proportions.

What should be done?
If a young person seems to be growing excessively, consult your physician as soon as possible. The treatment for gigantism is similar to treatment for acromegaly, and in most cases it is possible to stop the disorder.

Short stature

The causes of slow growth in childhood include inherited short stature, celiac disease (see p.731), hypothyroidism (see p.567), asthma (see p.381), and congenital heart disease (see p.702). Correcting or controlling these underlying conditions permits growth to resume. In rare cases, children fail to grow to normal heights because from birth the pituitary gland has not produced enough growth hormone. Treatment with growth hormone (available since the mid-1980s in synthetic form) is used for children with little or no pituitary growth hormone. It is being investigated in the treatment of Turner's syndrome, a condition in which girls fail to grow and to develop ovaries. Hormonal treatment should be considered only after careful investigation and determination of the cause of the slow growth.

Deficiency of growth hormone may be present from birth or may develop at any age. Except when the deficiency is caused by a pituitary tumor (see p.557), its cause is unknown. When a deficiency of growth hormone develops after birth it is usually accompanied by underproduction of other hormones, which leads to retarded sexual development (see Adolescent health, p.755, and Hypopituitarism, p.557).

What should be done?
All infants and children should be weighed and measured regularly. Failure to grow at a normal rate is usually detected during routine checkups. If you are worried that your child seems small for his or her age, consult the growth charts on p.691. If there seems to be a problem, take your child to your family physician or pediatrician. An examination and blood test will be performed to determine the cause of your child's slow growth. If a

In gigantism or dwarfism, the body is not only of abnormal size, but also is proportioned differently.

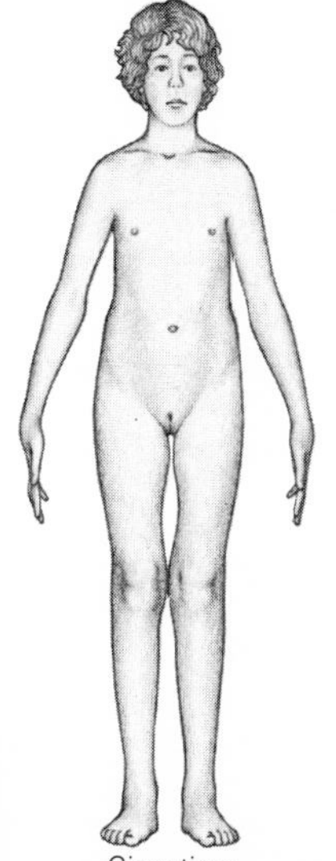
Gigantism

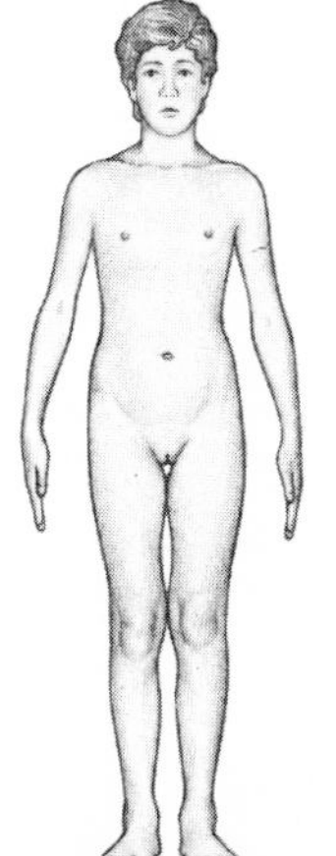
Normal

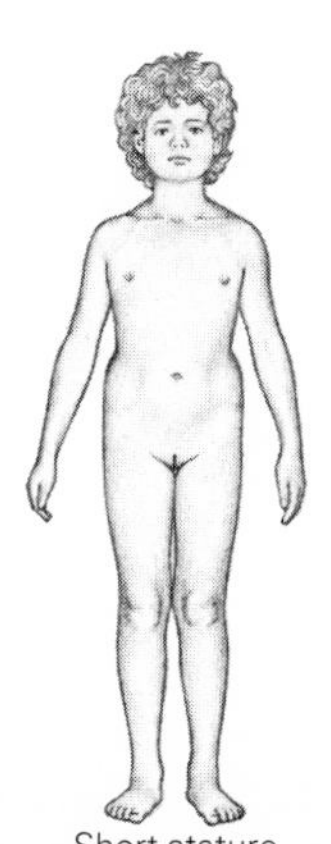
Short stature

growth problem results from some other disorder, it is important to identify and treat the underlying cause. Deficiency of growth hormone is detected by measuring the amount of the hormone in blood samples taken before and after stimulation of the pituitary gland by drugs such as arginine or insulin, or by exercise.

If your child's short stature is caused by deficiency of growth hormone, he or she will need injections of the hormone until the end of adolescence. The synthetic form of the hormone, a product of genetic engineering that is completely safe, was introduced after doubts about the safety of using the natural hormone extracted from pituitary glands after death. In most cases, the child's response to treatment is excellent; provided that the condition is recognized in infancy, the child may grow to normal adult height.

Diabetes insipidus

In the normal production of urine, your kidneys first filter water and other substances from your blood. The kidneys then reabsorb almost all of the filtered water, leaving urine ready to be excreted from your body. The absorbed water is returned to the bloodstream to maintain the correct concentrations of minerals, proteins, and other nutrients in blood and body fluids. If you lose a lot of body water because of fever, perspiration, vomiting, or diarrhea, for example, the kidneys reabsorb almost all of the filtered water and a small amount of concentrated urine is excreted. On the other hand, if you drink large amounts of water, the kidneys reabsorb less filtered water, and a large amount of dilute urine is produced. The process of water reabsorption is regulated by antidiuretic hormone (ADH), a hormone that is produced by the posterior lobe (back part) of the pituitary gland. Diabetes insipidus is a disorder in which there is a deficiency of ADH, causing your body to pass large quantities of urine that contain a high percentage of water.

The most common cause of the disorder is damage to the pituitary gland from a severe head injury. The condition may also result from scarring or damage caused by an operation on the pituitary gland, or may be due to the effects of radiation therapy on the gland or on the surrounding area. Rarely, diabetes insipidus is caused by pressure on the posterior lobe of the gland from a pituitary tumor (see next page). In a form of the disorder called nephrogenic diabetes insipidus, the condition results from an insensitivity of the kidney tubules to ADH. In this condition the level of pituitary secretion of ADH is normal.

Diabetes insipidus should not be confused with diabetes mellitus, which is sometimes known as "sugar diabetes" (see p.558).

What are the symptoms?

The main symptom is that you pass large quantities of colorless urine, as much as 21 qt (20 liters) every 24 hours. This great fluid loss results in an unquenchable thirst. You will constantly be interrupted during the day and awakened at night by the strong need to urinate and drink. Potentially fatal dehydration can occur rapidly.

What should be done?

As soon as symptoms appear, see your physician, who may arrange for you to have a water deprivation test. You will not be allowed to drink any fluid for 8 hours, during which time the volume and concentration in your urine will be measured several times. In a healthy person deprived of fluid for so long, ADH would be secreted and act to conserve water. If the volume of water in your urine remains high and the concentration of the urine is dilute, this shows that you have a deficiency of ADH. Deficiencies can be partial or complete. The effect of an injection of synthetic ADH on your urine output can confirm an insufficient ADH level.

What is the treatment?

Self-help: Continue to drink as much water as you need.

Professional help: In the common form of diabetes insipidus, the most effective treatment is the use of a synthetic form of ADH, taken either as nose drops or by injection. The length of time you must take the drops or receive the injections is determined mainly by what has caused the disorder. If it was caused by a head injury, surgery, or radiation therapy, the defective gland may return to normal within a year, which means that you will be completely cured. If this fails to happen, you will probably have to take medication for the rest of your life. If the disorder is caused by a pituitary tumor (see next page), the tumor will probably have to be removed.

In the nephrogenic form of the disorder, you may only need to restrict your salt intake and take certain diuretics or other medication to help your kidneys conserve water.

Hypopituitarism

The pituitary gland regulates body growth, general metabolism, and sexual development, chiefly through the six hormones that are produced in its anterior, or front, lobe (see Pituitary gland, p.554). In hypopituitarism, the anterior lobe of the gland is underactive and fails to produce adequate amounts of these six hormones. This results, ultimately, in insufficient levels of these substances in the body. The effects of this deficiency are wide-ranging. They include sexual underdevelopment or infertility, prematurely aged, pallid appearance, generalized weakness, and often generally poor health.

The most common causes of hypopituitarism are serious head injuries, complications of childbirth, a pituitary tumor (see next article), or the side effects of treatment for such a tumor. Occasionally the disease develops for no known reason.

What are the symptoms?

Because the pituitary gland stimulates several other hormone-producing glands, the symptoms of hypopituitarism are a combination of the symptoms of several other disorders, each related to another affected gland. These include hypothyroidism (see p.567), adrenal underactivity (see Addison's disease, p.564), infertility (see p.649), absence of menstrual periods (see p.624), and short stature (see p.555) in children.

What are the risks?

If hypopituitarism is not treated promptly, it can sometimes be fatal. This is mainly because your body cannot respond to stress or a major infection.

What should be done?

See your physician if you suspect that you have hypopituitarism. If your physician shares your suspicion, you will probably need blood and urine tests. These tests will measure the function of your anterior pituitary gland. If the tests confirm that you have hypopituitarism, you may also have CT or MRI scans to determine whether a pituitary tumor has caused the disorder.

What is the treatment?

If you have hypopituitarism, you will need lifelong treatment with oral medication and injections that replace the hormones of the pituitary gland and the other glands that are affected. Hormone-replacement therapy may be required to make up for underproduction of hormones by the sex glands (the ovaries in women and the testes in men), the thyroid gland, and the adrenal glands.

Pituitary tumors

Your pituitary gland is divided into two parts, the anterior, or front, lobe and the posterior, or rear, lobe. Pituitary gland tumors almost always occur in the anterior lobe. Why they occur is not known.

More than 10 percent of all tumors inside the skull develop in the pituitary gland. There are two main types. Pituitary adenomas are overgrowths of one or more of the cell types in the gland. These tumors are almost always benign (unlikely to spread). Most are less than ½ in (12 mm) in size. But because they grow in a confined space they may run out of room and may damage the nerves leading from the eyes, cause headaches, and eventually cause serious brain disorders if they begin to increase further in size.

About 50 percent of all pituitary adenomas secrete abnormal amounts of the hormone prolactin. This may cause no symptoms. Or it may result in impotence, absence of menstrual periods, or galactorrhea (see Box, next page). Pituitary adenomas may also secrete other hormones, and this can lead to acromegaly (see p.554), gigantism (see p.555), or Cushing's disease (see p.563). The tumor may also enlarge and press upon surrounding areas, causing other disorders.

The other type of tumor is called a craniopharyngioma. This type of tumor does not cause overproduction of any hormones, but it does progressively enlarge and can exert pressure either on the anterior lobe, which causes hypopituitarism (see previous article), or on the posterior lobe, which

Hormone-producing tumors

Several kinds of cancerous tumors may secrete hormones or chemicals that behave like hormones, causing symptoms similar to those of overactivity of an endocrine gland. For example, lung cancers may secrete hormones that are similar to corticotrophin (the pituitary hormone that stimulates the adrenal glands), parathyroid hormone, or antidiuretic hormone. These same hormones may also be secreted by carcinoid tumors of the intestine (see p.505). Tumors of the islet cells in the pancreas also often secrete abnormal hormones. Because similar hormones may be secreted by a wide range of tumors, the identification of the tumor that is causing the problem may prove difficult. Removing the tumor or destroying it by radiation therapy may ease the symptoms.

causes diabetes insipidus (see p.556). It can also press on the nerves to your eyes and, as a result, eventually cause headaches, double vision, and deteriorating sight (see Brain tumors, p.301).

What is the treatment?

Pituitary tumors that secrete prolactin (prolactinomas) often can be treated successfully with drugs such as bromocriptine that shrink the tumor. But with some prolactinomas and all other types of pituitary tumor, the most effective treatments are surgery or radiation therapy, or sometimes both.

Surgery to remove the tumor is a delicate procedure that is performed as the surgeon looks through a powerful microscope. He or she reaches the tumor through either a nostril or a hole made in the bridge of your nose. If the tumor is large and pressing on the nerves to the eyes, you may need to have open-brain surgery. You will probably recover quickly from the operation, but there is a risk that the rest of the pituitary gland will be damaged during surgery. If this occurs, hypopituitarism, diabetes insipidus, or both may develop. This is usually considered an acceptable risk, since either disorder can be treated by lifelong hormone-replacement therapy.

Instead of removing the tumor, the surgeon may destroy it by using extreme cold or by placing a tiny radioactive implant in it.

If the tumor is large or if it is difficult to pinpoint, radiation therapy of the whole gland may be necessary. Like surgery, radiation therapy may cause damage to the rest of the gland. The long-term outlook depends largely on the size of the tumor, but with treatment a complete cure is possible.

Galactorrhea

Galactorrhea is production of breast milk when it is not supposed to be produced. Milk production normally occurs in a woman a few days before, and in the months following, the birth of a baby. Production at any other time in a woman, and at any time in a man, is called galactorrhea. The problem is not a serious threat to health, although it may be annoying. However, the underlying cause of galactorrhea may be a pituitary tumor, which is more serious and may lead to other symptoms. Because the disorder most often affects women, it is discussed fully in Women's health (see Galactorrhea, p.632).

Pancreas

The pancreas is a long, thin gland that lies crosswise just behind your stomach. It has two major functions. The first is to produce enzymes that help to digest food (see Liver, gallbladder, and pancreas, p.522, for digestive disorders of the pancreas). The second is to produce the hormones insulin and glucagon. These two hormones play a very important part in regulating the level of glucose in your blood.

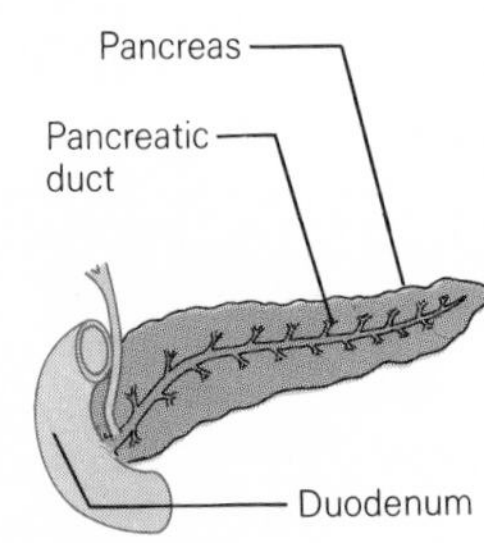

The pancreas is a gland about 6 in (15 cm) long. It lies close to the duodenum and is linked to it by the pancreatic duct.

Glucose is a form of sugar. It is found in many foods, including some that do not taste sweet. Glucose is the main source of energy for all the cells in your body. Insulin stimulates cells to absorb enough glucose from the blood for the energy they need, and stimulates the liver to absorb and store the rest. Insulin thus lowers the glucose level in your blood. Glucagon has the opposite effect; it helps raise the glucose level in the blood by stimulating your liver to release glucose. Therefore, glucagon is used to correct severe hypoglycemia (low blood sugar) sometimes accidentally induced by insulin use among people who have diabetes.

Diabetes mellitus

Diabetes mellitus is a common disorder that occurs when your pancreas either totally stops producing insulin or does not produce enough of the hormone for your body's needs. This lack of insulin results in a low absorption of glucose, both by the body's cells, which need it for energy, and by the liver, which stores it. This results in an abnormally high level of glucose in your blood, along with a spillover of some of the excess glucose into the urine. Do not confuse this disorder with the disorder known as diabetes insipidus (see p.556).

There are two main forms of diabetes mellitus. They are type I (also called juvenile onset or insulin-dependent) diabetes and type

II (also known as maturity onset or insulin-independent) diabetes.

Type I (insulin-dependent) diabetes: In this form of the disorder, which occurs mainly in young people, the pancreas produces very little or no insulin. The defect is caused by damage to the insulin-producing cells. Your body, unable to use glucose because of the lack of insulin, is forced to obtain energy from fat. As the fat is burned, ketones (a dangerous chemical substance) are produced. This can lead to a life-threatening condition called ketoacidosis, in which you become dehydrated and have very high levels of blood sugar.

Type II (insulin-independent) diabetes: In this form of diabetes mellitus, which usually affects people over 40, the insulin-producing cells in your pancreas function, but the output of insulin is not adequate for your body's needs. People who have this form of the disorder usually overeat and are overweight (see Obesity, p.530).

Heredity is also an important factor. In most cases, there is a family history of the disorder. Age is also a factor, because the efficiency of your pancreas decreases as you become older.

Either form of diabetes may be brought on by other diseases. Acromegaly (see p.554), hyperthyroidism (see p.565), Cushing's syndrome (see p.563), and pancreatitis (see p.529) are some examples of diseases that can bring on diabetes. Such cases are known as secondary diabetes, and in some instances the condition continues even after the main disease has been treated successfully.

What are the symptoms?

All forms of diabetes cause the same main symptoms. You urinate much more than usual, sometimes as often as every hour or so, throughout the day and night.

The excessive loss of fluid can make you unusually thirsty, and drinking sweetened beverages increases the amount of urination and makes your thirst worse.

Your cells do not get enough glucose, so you feel extremely tired, weak, and apathetic—so much so that you may be unable to get up in the morning. Some people with diabetes, especially children and young adults, lose a lot of weight, since their fat and muscle are burned up to provide energy and because the glucose lost in the urine is a major source of calories. Other symptoms that you may experience with diabetes include tingling in the hands and feet, reduced resistance to infections (boils, urinary tract infections, and fungus vaginal infections are sometimes the first signs of diabetes mellitus), blurred vision caused by excess glucose in the fluid of the eye, and impotence in men (see p.621) or the absence of menstrual periods in women (see p.624). Certain microorganisms are attracted to the sugary urine, and these agents can cause various complications, such as bladder infections (see p.541) and other urinary tract problems.

Symptoms of type I (insulin-dependent) diabetes usually develop rapidly, within weeks or months. Symptoms of type II (insulin-independent) diabetes often do not appear until many years after the actual onset of the disease. Sometimes the disorder is detected during a routine medical examination, before any symptoms appear.

What are the risks?

Diabetes mellitus becomes increasingly common with age. The type II form occurs most often among those who are overweight, especially middle-aged and older women.

Most people with type II diabetes have a relative with the disease. However, even if both your parents have diabetes, there is only a 1 in 20 risk that you will have it.

The effectiveness of today's treatment has changed this disease that once was often fatal into one from which deaths are extremely rare. However, there are still risks. People with type I diabetes risk ketoacidosis and unconsciousness. You may have such a crisis before your diabetes is discovered, during an infection such as influenza (see p.597), or if you neglect your treatment. You may have to be hospitalized to treat ketoacidosis but you will probably recover completely.

Other complications, which can affect those with both types of diabetes, usually occur 15 to 20 years after the onset of the disease. Such risks include diabetic retinopathy, an eye disorder (see p.349) that often causes blindness; peripheral neuropathy, a nerve disease (see p.302); and chronic kidney failure (see p.551).

People with diabetes also run a higher than average risk of developing atherosclerosis (see p.398), with its risks of stroke, heart attack, and high blood pressure. The blood vessels to your legs become narrowed, which can cause cramps, cold feet, pain when you walk or climb stairs, and even skin ulcers or gangrene (see p.447). Do not cut your toenails too short; try to have them cut by someone who is trained. Always wear shoes that fit properly and be sure to get treatment for such foot problems as corns or ingrown toenails. If any cut fails to heal within 10 days, see your physician as soon as possible.

Medical myth

Children who eat a lot of sugar will get diabetes.

Wrong. The exact cause of diabetes mellitus is unknown, but it does not seem to be directly related to sugar. Children who eat a lot of sugar are, however, more prone to tooth decay.

What should be done?

If you suspect you have diabetes mellitus, see your physician, who will ask you for a urine sample to be tested for glucose and ketones. The presence of both will show that you probably have the disease. If only glucose is present, your physician will ask for a blood sample to measure the amount of glucose in your bloodstream. This is necessary because it is possible to have some glucose in your urine without having diabetes. If there is still no clear result, you will need to have a glucose tolerance test. A series of blood samples are taken before and after you swallow a glucose liquid. If the level of glucose in the later samples is not normal, this shows that you are not producing enough insulin and that you have diabetes mellitus.

Peripheral neuropathy, chronic kidney failure, and, in particular, diabetic retinopathy are possible complications that are treatable and preventable with good glucose control. The best results come from early recognition and assessment of how far the disorder has advanced. It is important that you assume some of the responsibility for your care, which includes diet and weight control, checking your urine for sugar, exercising appropriately, and regular comprehensive medical checkups.

Your physician can give you a card to carry at all times that lists your name, address, the fact that you have diabetes, and instructions on how to help you if you are ill. Or you can buy a bracelet or necklace to wear each day, indicating in a code that you have diabetes, so that emergency medical personnel can treat you promptly and correctly if you are found unconscious. Such aids can help you to feel reassured that someone will be able to help you readily in an emergency.

What is the treatment?

No cure has yet been found for diabetes mellitus, and you will need treatment for the disorder all your life, once it has been diagnosed. Since you administer most of that treatment yourself, its effectiveness will depend mainly on you.

Evidence is growing that shows that the serious complications of diabetes, especially retinopathy and kidney failure, seem to be less common in people who keep their diabetes under control—that is, people who keep the amount of sugar in their blood close to the levels in the blood of people without diabetes. Some people with diabetes have learned to measure their blood sugar values at home; others use urine testing. Whichever method you choose you should maintain a close watch on how your diabetes responds to diet and other treatments (see next page).

Type I diabetes: This form of the disorder is treated with a combination of a measured diet and daily injections of insulin (usually once or twice, sometimes three times, a day) to replace the missing hormone. The insulin used to treat diabetes is extracted from the pancreas of pigs or cattle, or is synthesized by bacteria that have been modified by gene splicing so that their DNA produces the human form of the hormone insulin. This insulin has become widely used in the past few years. However, many people with diabetes who established control of their diabetes using cow or pig insulin have continued to use it.

Insulin can be taken only by injection. If you take insulin by mouth, it is destroyed by digestive juices before it can be absorbed into your bloodstream. Your physician will show you how to use a syringe to inject the insulin just under the skin of your thigh, arm, or abdomen. Most people learn how to do this within a few days. Parents of children with diabetes need to administer the injections until the child is about 10, when the child usually is able to learn to do it independently.

You must follow rigorously the timetable of meals and snacks recommended by your physician. This keeps the supply of glucose to the blood steady, so that regular doses of insulin always act on approximately the same amount of glucose. Insulin is available in various types and strengths, and the type of insulin and the schedule that your physician prescribes will depend on many factors, including your age and the severity of your diabetes. Always make sure that you obtain the same type and strength of insulin each time you renew your prescription.

Even when insulin is given by injection once, twice, or three times a day it is not possible to maintain a steady concentration of insulin in the blood. Research teams have developed several devices that are designed to continuously deliver insulin via a pump and a needle inserted under the skin and so administer insulin at a steadier rate. Some of the devices have an attachment to measure the blood glucose level and modify the dose of insulin released into the bloodstream accordingly. All of these devices are still being developed and evaluated, but they have so far proved somewhat disappointing.

For use in the longer term, research teams are evaluating various ways to transplant the insulin-secreting cells in the pancreas from a healthy person to one with diabetes. This procedure is sometimes performed during a kidney transplantation (see Transplants, p.432) on a person with diabetes. Currently, however, the considerable drawbacks and risks associated with any transplant operation (such as an increased susceptibility to infection and rejection) are too great for the treatment to be offered to people with diabetes who are otherwise in good health.

Self-discipline is essential if you are to control your diabetes successfully. Ask your physician if you can engage in strenuous activities such as fast-paced sports or even heavy digging in the garden, since exercise burns up glucose and may bring on hypoglycemia. Your physician may suggest that you eat extra food beforehand or adjust your dose of insulin.

Any illness, from a cold to a heart attack, places stress on your body and thus increases the amount of insulin you need. If you are not able to eat according to your usual schedule, take glucose drinks, but do not reduce your dose of insulin; consult your physician immediately.

Diabetes can cause problems during pregnancy (see Diabetes and pregnancy, p.672) and in children. Young children may not understand why they must stick to a diet and not have candy and soft drinks, but you must be firm in enforcing the diet. Many teenagers go through periods of rebellion, and teenagers with diabetes may react against the restrictions the disease imposes on them.

If you have diabetes, always tell physicians or dentists before any treatment, so that they can take any necessary precautions.

Type II diabetes: Diet alone can control this form of the disease in many cases. A diet to control diabetes restricts the amount of carbohydrates you eat at one meal. If you are overweight, staying on this diet will reduce your weight significantly. The number of calories you are allowed each day will vary between 800 and 1,500, depending on your motivation, your height and weight, and other factors. Try to eat small portions of carbohydrates at regular intervals, so that there are no extreme variations in the glucose

Monitoring your diabetes

If you have diabetes you should test your urine or blood for sugar (glucose) levels at least once a day, or as often as your physician recommends (for example, just before meals and at bedtime). Urine tests, which can be easily done at home, involve the use of chemically impregnated strips (a different chemical is used in each of two strips). When urine comes into contact with the strip, a chemical reaction occurs and the strip changes color according to the concentration of sugar in the urine. The result of each test can be determined by comparing the strip with a special color chart or by using an instrument known as a reflectance meter. The color chart shows possible shades of color that the strip may turn and the level of sugar that they represent. A reflectance meter does the comparison automatically and gives a digital readout of your approximate sugar level.

You can test your blood sugar level by using a machine that provides a digital readout (see right). A pricking device that comes with the machine enables you to take your own blood sample quickly and easily. The results obtained by the machine provide valuable information on how well your diabetes is being controlled. They will enable you and your physician to improve the control of your diabetes by adjusting your diet, insulin intake, or treatment with drugs when your sugar level fluctuates.

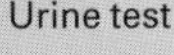

Urine test

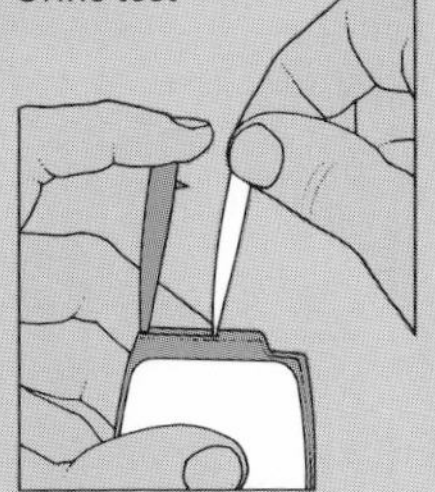

1 Tear a strip of tape about 1½ in (35 mm) long, from the container provided in the kit. Be sure the strip is dry.

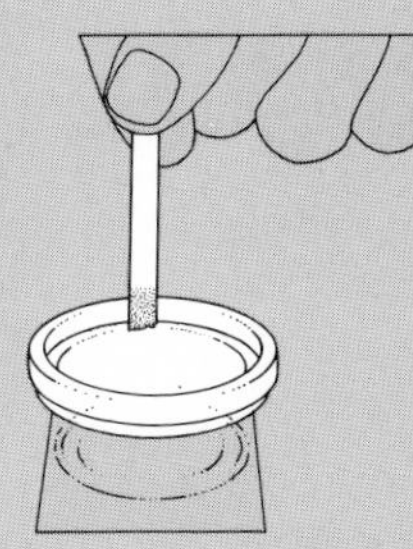

2 Dip one end of the strip very briefly into a sample of urine. Then wait for one minute, until the end has changed color.

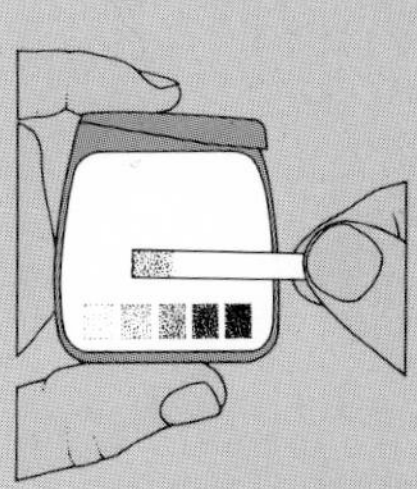

3 Find the color on the chart that most closely matches the color on the strip. The figure below the color on the chart shows the level of glucose in your urine.

Home blood test

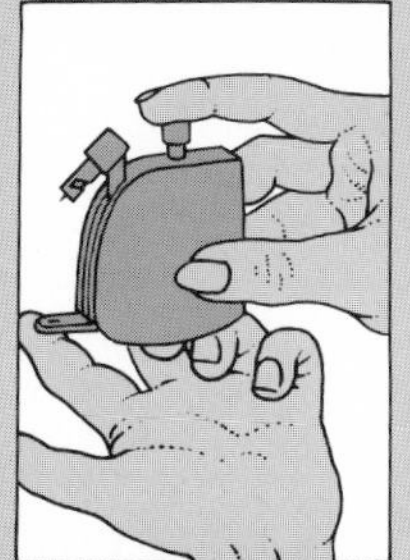

1 By using a pricking device, you draw a few drops of blood, which are then spread on a special chemically coated strip.

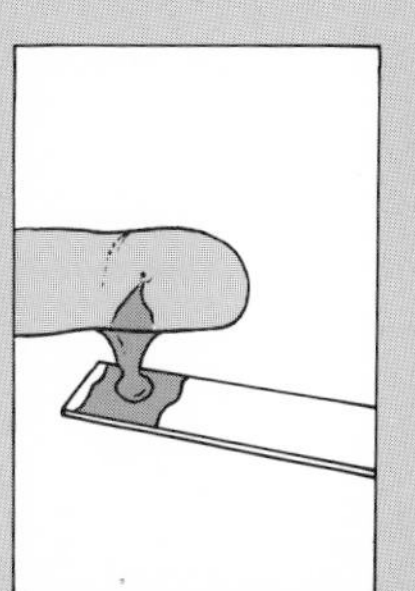

2 After inserting the strip into a blood glucose monitor, you get a reading

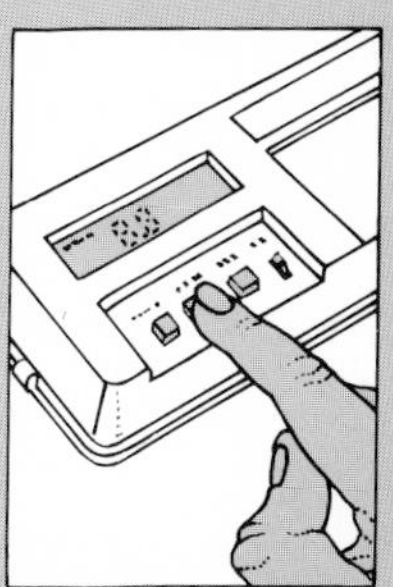

to help you determine the appropriate dose of insulin.

content of your blood. Do not eat sugar or foods that contain sugar. Make sure your diet contains enough fiber by eating whole-grain bread and plenty of salads, fruit, and vegetables. Avoid smoking, which can increase your risk of getting atherosclerosis.

In mild cases, merely avoiding the concentrated sugars of candy, cake, cookies, and sugar-sweetened drinks can be enough to bring your blood glucose level down to normal. This is particularly true if you can reduce your weight and keep it within the recommended range for your height and build (see p.35), because then the insulin that your pancreas produces may be enough to cope with the needs of your reduced body size.

Your progress in keeping your blood glucose near normal will need to be checked, and your physician will want to see you at regular intervals. To keep appointments to a minimum, however, you will probably be encouraged to check your progress with a urine testing kit. You should test your urine as often as your physician recommends and keep a record of the results. This record will assist your physician in evaluating the dosage of your medications. You may notice that any increases in urine sugar loss may be correlated with infections or emotional stress.

Even if you stay strictly on your diet, you may find that your tests show your blood sugar level is still too high. Then your physician may prescribe oral hypoglycemic medication to lower your blood glucose. There are several different kinds of medication available, and if you have side effects from one type, your physician may prescribe another. If you take too high a dosage, hypoglycemia, or low blood sugar (see next article), may result. If you have the symptoms of a hypoglycemia attack, eat something sweet immediately to avoid losing consciousness, and contact your physician about a possible adjustment of the dosage. If your blood sugar levels remain high and resist control, your physician may recommend that you use insulin, as described earlier in the section on Type I diabetes (p.560), instead of oral hypoglycemic medication.

What are the long-term prospects?

As long as you treat your diabetes sensibly, you can expect to lead a full and healthy life. However, if you are taking insulin, you should avoid shift work that interferes with the regular timing of your diet and injections. Also avoid heights, and do not drive buses or other public service vehicles without the advice of your physician, because of the risk of an attack of hypoglycemia.

If you develop complications, they can be minimized by regular medical checkups and strict control of your diabetes. Your best assurance for maximum health and an active life comes from your own responsible attitude and from following the advice you get from your physician.

Hypoglycemia

Hypoglycemia is a low level of glucose in the blood. When this occurs, the muscles and cells in your body are deprived of energy-providing glucose. The condition occurs almost exclusively in people with diabetes mellitus, especially those who are taking insulin injections or oral hypoglycemic medication. Taking too much insulin, not keeping to the prescribed meal schedule, or unusually strenuous or prolonged exercise can all bring on an attack, which if severe is called diabetic coma. Other causes include stomach surgery, some types of cancer, reaction to various drugs, alcohol, liver disease, pregnancy, and high fevers.

What are the symptoms?

The symptoms of hypoglycemia vary considerably from person to person, but they often start with a feeling of being hot and uncomfortable, which is followed by profuse sweating. Other symptoms that you experience may include dizziness, weakness, trembling, unsteadiness, hunger, blurred vision, slurred speech, tingling in the lips or hands, or headache. Also, you may become aggressive or uncooperative without being aware of it, a condition that is sometimes mistaken for drunkenness. Seizures (see p.713) may occur, particularly in children. If symptoms occur during the night, they usually awaken you. In extreme cases you may become unconscious.

What are the risks?

Episodes of hypoglycemia are almost always treated and halted before they can become serious. The chief danger for most people is that you might have an attack when you are swimming, operating machinery, or driving a car. If you have frequent attacks, you should not participate in these activities. However, nighttime attacks, especially in older people, may go undetected for prolonged periods, resulting in severe, sometimes permanent brain damage.

What should be done?
In the process of establishing an insulin program for you, if you have an attack of hypoglycemia your physician will use it to teach you to recognize oncoming bouts.

If you have an unexpected attack, think about what caused it, and try to prevent another one. If you have attacks with any frequency or recurrence, see your physician. He or she may reduce your dose of insulin or oral hypoglycemic medication.

What is the treatment?
Self-help: If you are prone to hypoglycemia attacks, you should always carry glucose tablets, sugar cubes, or candy. At the first sign of an attack, chew or suck some until you feel normal again, which should be within a few minutes. Make sure your family and friends know about the symptoms, so that if you become disoriented or uncooperative, they can give you something sweet. Tell them that if they give you a small drink of fruit juice, you will probably recover enough to eat properly. However, they should never try to feed you if you become unconscious (diabetic coma), because this could choke you. If your hypoglycemia could be caused by drugs you are taking for another disorder, discuss this with your physician, who may either discontinue them or suggest an alternative.

An alternative to glucose tablets that is being used more and more is an injection of glucagon, a hormone that helps raise your blood glucose level. This is especially helpful if an attack makes you unconscious. Many people who have hypoglycemia attacks teach their family and friends how to inject the hormone into an arm or leg muscle.

Instruct your friends and family that if the measures described do not work, or are not available, they should get you to a hospital emergency department right away.

Professional help: The physician will give you an injection of glucose in a vein in your arm. This works so quickly that you may even regain consciousness while the injection is being given.

Adrenal glands

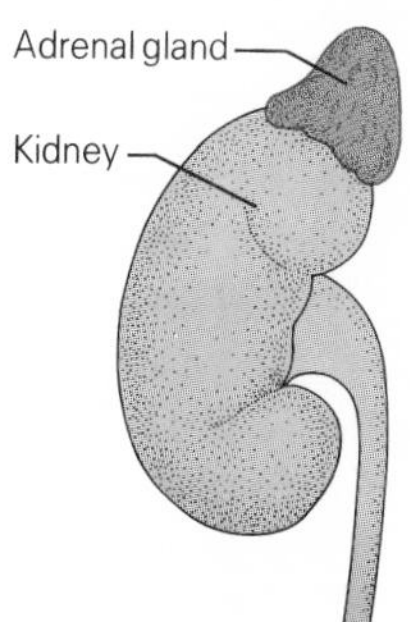

The adrenal glands, situated on top of each kidney, produce hormones that help you cope with physical and mental stress.

You have two adrenal glands, one on top of each kidney. Each adrenal gland has two parts. One part of the gland is the medulla, or central core, and the other part is the cortex, or outer layer.

The medulla produces two hormones, epinephrine and norepinephrine. These hormones play an important part in controlling your heart rate and blood pressure and your body's response to stress. Signals from your brain stimulate the adrenal glands to begin producing these hormones.

The adrenal cortex produces three groups of corticosteroid hormones. The hormones in one group control the concentration and balance of various chemicals in your body. For example, they prevent the loss into the urine of too much sodium and water. The most important hormone in this group is aldosterone. The hormones in the second group have a number of functions. One is helping to convert carbohydrates, or starches, into energy-providing glycogen in your liver. Hydrocortisone is the main hormone in this group. The third group consists of male hormones called androgens and female hormones called estrogen and progesterone; these hormones influence sexual development. The sex hormones are mainly produced by the testes and the ovaries. Both sexes produce both male and female hormones, but androgens predominate in a man, and estrogen and progesterone in a woman. Production of all corticosteroid hormones except aldosterone is controlled by the pituitary gland (see p.554). Aldosterone production is stimulated by another hormone, renin, which is produced by the kidneys.

Cushing's syndrome

(including Cushing's disease)

In Cushing's syndrome there is an excess of corticosteroid hormones in your blood. In the majority of cases it is caused by large doses of corticosteroid drugs that are being taken for prolonged periods for another illness, such as rheumatoid arthritis (see p.589) or asthma (see p.381). Rarely, the condition appears because the cortex, or outer layer, of one or both adrenal glands is producing excess corticosteroid hormones. This can be caused by a tumor in the adrenal gland or elsewhere in your body that is overstimulating your adrenal glands. If the tumor is in your pituitary gland (see Pituitary tumors,

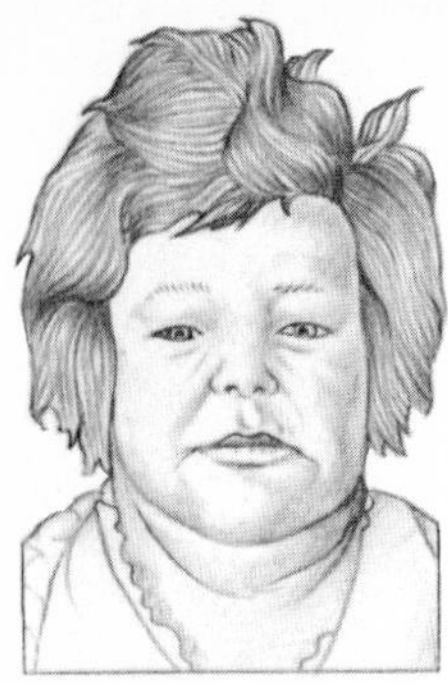
A person with Cushing's syndrome or Cushing's disease gradually grows fatter. Also, the face can become red and moon-shaped.

p.557), the condition is called Cushing's disease rather than Cushing's syndrome.

What are the symptoms?
The symptoms of this disorder usually appear over several months. First, your face becomes fatter than usual, round, and red. Your body also becomes fatter, and often a pad of fat develops between your shoulder blades, making you look round-shouldered. At the same time you lose muscle from your arms and legs. You will feel weak and tired, your skin may become thinner, and bruises sometimes appear spontaneously on your arms and legs. Your bones become thin (see Osteoporosis, p.581) and fracture easily.

Cushing's syndrome is uncommon. It sometimes occurs in people on long-term corticosteroid treatment. Cushing's disease also is extremely rare. It mainly affects young to middle-aged women.

What should be done?
If your physician suspects that you have Cushing's disease, you will be tested for a pituitary tumor. If you are on long-term corticosteroid treatment, signs of Cushing's syndrome should be apparent.

What is the treatment?
If corticosteroid drugs taken for another disorder are the cause, your physician will gradually reduce your dosage and provide other treatment. Unfortunately, the dangers of recurrent disease sometimes prevent such a change in medication. Never abruptly stop taking corticosteroid drugs yourself. You could develop acute adrenal failure (see Addison's disease, next article).

When a tumor of the pituitary gland is the cause, it can be treated by surgery or radiation therapy. An alternative treatment may be to remove your adrenal glands. If this treatment is chosen, you will have to take medication daily for the rest of your life, to replace the missing hormones. If you have a tumor on one adrenal gland, you need surgery to remove the gland. You should, however, be able to function normally with the remaining adrenal gland. If the treatment is successful, you can expect to return to normal or near normal health.

Addison's disease

(including acute adrenal failure)

In Addison's disease, the production of corticosteroid hormones by the cortex, or outer layer, of your adrenal glands gradually decreases. The most common cause of the disease today is destruction of the cortex, probably caused by an autoimmune problem, in which your body's immune system attacks one of your tissues or organs. Tuberculosis (see p.602) may also cause Addison's disease, but this is very rare today.

What are the symptoms?
The symptoms, which usually develop very gradually, include loss of appetite, weight loss, a feeling of increasing tiredness and weakness, and anemia (see p.450). You may also have bouts of diarrhea, constipation, or mild indigestion with nausea or vomiting. In addition, your skin may become noticeably darker and stay that way.

If the disease is not treated, you risk acute adrenal failure. This may be triggered by the stress of even a mild infection. Acute adrenal failure causes vomiting and diarrhea, dehydration, and shock. To prevent death, immediate emergency treatment is essential.

What should be done?
Consult your physician, who will request blood and urine samples for corticosteroid hormones. If Addison's disease is diagnosed, you will need to take corticosteroid medication daily for the rest of your life. The treatment will clear up all of your symptoms. You will be given a card that describes the treatment you need if you have acute adrenal failure. Always carry it with you. If you have any illness or infection, however minor, promptly consult your physician, who may increase your dose of corticosteroids to prevent acute adrenal failure. If you are having surgery, be sure the surgeon is aware that you have the disorder. As long as you take your medication and follow the above precautions, you should be able to lead a normal, healthy life.

Aldosteronism

(Conn's syndrome)

Aldosteronism is a rare illness in which an overproduction of the hormone aldosterone, a product of the cortex of the adrenal glands, leads to high blood pressure. Aldosteronism is caused by either a tumor in one adrenal gland or by an enlargement of both adrenal glands. When a tumor is present, the disorder is known as Conn's syndrome.

The main symptoms are those of high blood pressure (see p.411). Other symptoms include tingling and weakness in your limbs, muscle spasms in your hands and feet, and increased thirst coupled with excessive urination. Your physician will probably first arrange for you to have both blood and urine tests. If the results indicate that you have aldosteronism, you may need a CT scan to find out if a tumor is causing the disorder. If an adrenal tumor is found, it can be removed surgically, and this often cures the disorder. When the condition is caused by another disease, it is controlled by drugs.

Pheochromocytoma

The hormones epinephrine (adrenalin) and norepinephrine (noradrenalin), which are produced by the medulla, or core, of each adrenal gland, work together with your autonomic nervous system (see p.283) to control your heart rate and blood pressure. Very rarely, in a condition called pheochromocytoma, a tumor, usually benign (unlikely to spread), develops in the medulla of an adrenal gland and causes it to produce excess hormones. As a result, slight exercise, exposure to cold, standing up, or a minor emotional upset produces the racing heart, paleness, and sweating normally associated only with intense fear or overexcitement. In addition, you may feel faint and have a severe headache. During an attack your blood pressure is very high, which can lead to several problems (see p.411).

What should be done?

Blood and urine tests may show an excess of the adrenal medullary hormones. If so, further tests, such as a CT scan, may be necessary to locate the tumor. While these tests are being performed, your physician will prescribe medication that will prevent further attacks of hypertension.

If a tumor is discovered, it will be removed surgically; this usually cures the disorder.

Thyroid and parathyroid glands

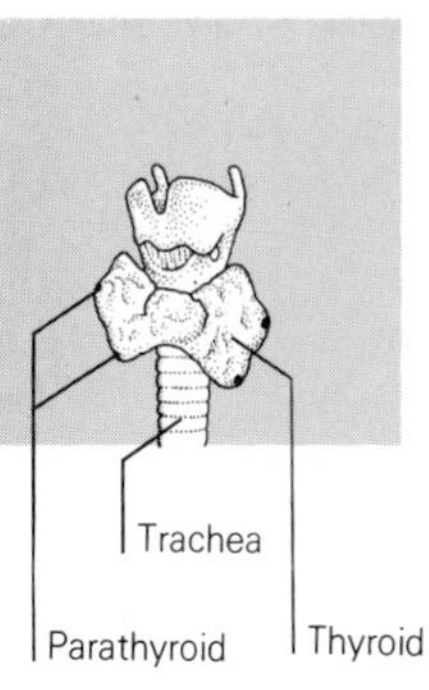

The thyroid gland is a butterfly-shaped structure that consists of two lobes in the lower part of your neck, one on either side of the trachea, or windpipe. The lobes are joined by a thin strand of thyroid tissue. The gland makes a hormone called thyroxine, or T_4, under the control of thyroid-stimulating hormone (TSH), which is produced by the pituitary gland. TSH in turn is regulated by thyroid-releasing hormone. Thyroxine controls the rates at which metabolism takes place in your body; generally, the more thyroxine secreted, the faster your metabolism works. Thyroxine contains iodine. Most people get sufficient iodine in their diets from fish, fish products, and drinking water. Iodine is often added to table salt and bread.

On the four corners of your thyroid gland, but unrelated to the thyroid gland itself, are four parathyroid glands, each one about the size of a pearl. They produce parathyroid hormone. This hormone works with another hormone called calcitonin, which is made by the thyroid gland, and with vitamin D, to control the level of calcium in your blood. Your body requires certain amounts of calcium to develop bones and teeth. Calcium also has a role in the functioning of your nerves and muscles. Parathyroid hormone and vitamin D raise the calcium level in several ways—by causing your intestine to absorb more calcium from food, by making you excrete less calcium in your urine, and by causing calcium to be released from bone.

Hyperthyroidism

(thyrotoxicosis, toxic goiter, Graves' disease)

This relatively common disorder is caused by overactivity of the thyroid gland (see also Hypothyroidism, next article). Activity of the thyroid gland is normally controlled by thyroid-stimulating hormone, which is made in your pituitary gland. In hyperthyroidism, the control mechanism begins to malfunction. Despite the decreased levels of thyroid-stimulating hormone, which is caused by the increased amounts of thyroxine (thyroid hormone) in the blood, the thyroid gland itself continuously produces very large quantities of thyroxine. Increased amounts of thyroid hormones coursing through your system causes a general speeding up of all the chemical reactions in your body. This reaction affects your mental as well as physical processes.

What are the symptoms?

There are many different symptoms typical of hyperthyroidism, but it is highly unlikely that you will have them all at once.

As your mental processes speed up, you become fidgety and anxious. You may be constantly active and thinking of more things to do. You may be tired but unable to relax or sleep. You may feel shaky and your hands may tremble; this is especially noticeable when you are trying to write or perform other tasks that require delicate movement.

You may become insensitive to cold and feel comfortable in lighter clothes even on cold days. You may perspire often.

Your heartbeat may become irregular and much faster, even when you are trying to relax. This causes palpitations, or a fluttering or racing feeling in your chest, which is disturbing, particularly when you are sitting or lying still. You may become breathless after mild exertion. You may have diarrhea.

Because more rapid body processes require more energy, you may develop a gigantic appetite and eat more, yet still lose weight. Your muscles may waste away and you may become so weak that you find it difficult to climb a flight of stairs, or even to lift and keep your arms above your head for a couple of minutes (when combing your hair, for example). Women may have light menstrual periods or their periods may stop. You may notice a swelling in the front of your neck, resulting from the enlarged thyroid gland, which is called a goiter.

The final group of symptoms concern your eyes. These symptoms are less common and become serious in only a few cases. Your eyes may feel gritty and uncomfortable and look wide open and protruding (see Exophthalmos, p.352). This can cause double or blurred vision, but usually causes only red, puffy eyelids. In some cases, these symptoms may not subside as the disorder is brought under control and need further treatment.

What are the risks?

Hyperthyroidism can occur at any age, but it very rarely affects children. It is eight times more common in women than in men. Like its symptoms, the risks of hyperthyroidism are variable. Most people recover completely, although some have recurrent bouts.

If you are older and already have high blood pressure (see p.411) or hardening of the arteries (see p.435), you are at the greatest risk. Additional strain on your heart and circulation can cause angina (see p.403), abnormal heart rhythms (see p.416), or heart failure (see p.408).

What should be done?

Hyperthyroidism may be confused with psychological disturbances such as anxiety states (see p.324) or agitated depression (see p.321). Consult your physician, who will examine you and arrange for you to have a sensitive thyroid-stimulating hormone level test that shows either high or low activity by the glands. You may also have a free T_4 (thyroxine level) test, which measures the thyroid hormone concentration in the blood. Once the diagnosis is made, your physician may arrange for a thyroid scan to see if all of your gland is affected, or only a part of it (see Thyroid nodules, p.568).

What is the treatment?

Hyperthyroidism can be treated in one of three ways. Any complications that arise will also be treated.

The first possible treatment for hyperthyroidism is to prescribe medication that contains antithyroid drugs. In most people the disorder is brought under control in about 8 weeks by this method, although you will have to continue to take the medication for a prolonged period, sometimes for at least a year. The drugs eventually cure some people, but most of those who receive this treatment have the symptoms again, and require some additional treatment.

The second treatment is surgery. An operation may be performed to remove either a lump in the thyroid gland or most of the gland if it is generally overactive. Surgery cures the disorder in about 90 percent of these cases. In a few cases, however, either the disease recurs or the thyroid or parathyroid may become underactive as a result of the surgery (see Hypothyroidism, next article, and Hypoparathyroidism, p.569).

The third form of treatment consists of taking a dose of radioactive iodine in the form of a clear, slightly salty drink. Iodine is an essential component of thyroid hormone, so the radioactive material becomes concentrated in the thyroid gland. There it acts on the glandular tissue to control the cellular overactivity slowly without exposing the rest of the body to radiation. If enough radiation is administered, the thyroid gland may become underactive, and you may have to take medication to compensate (see Hypothyroidism, next article).

Each form of treatment has its advantages and disadvantages, and your physician will help you determine which is most appropriate for you. Despite the wide-ranging effects of hyperthyroidism, it is likely that you will be restored to normal health.

Symptoms and signs of hyperthyroidism

Your thyroid gland produces three hormones that are essential to body metabolism (cell activity that regulates body energy). Overproduction of thyroid hormones may contribute to weight loss, increased appetite, increased sensitivity to heat, diarrhea (in some cases), and sweating. You may also have tremors and a rapid heart beat (palpitations), and you find that you easily become out of breath. In severe cases, your thyroid gland becomes enlarged, forming a goiter.

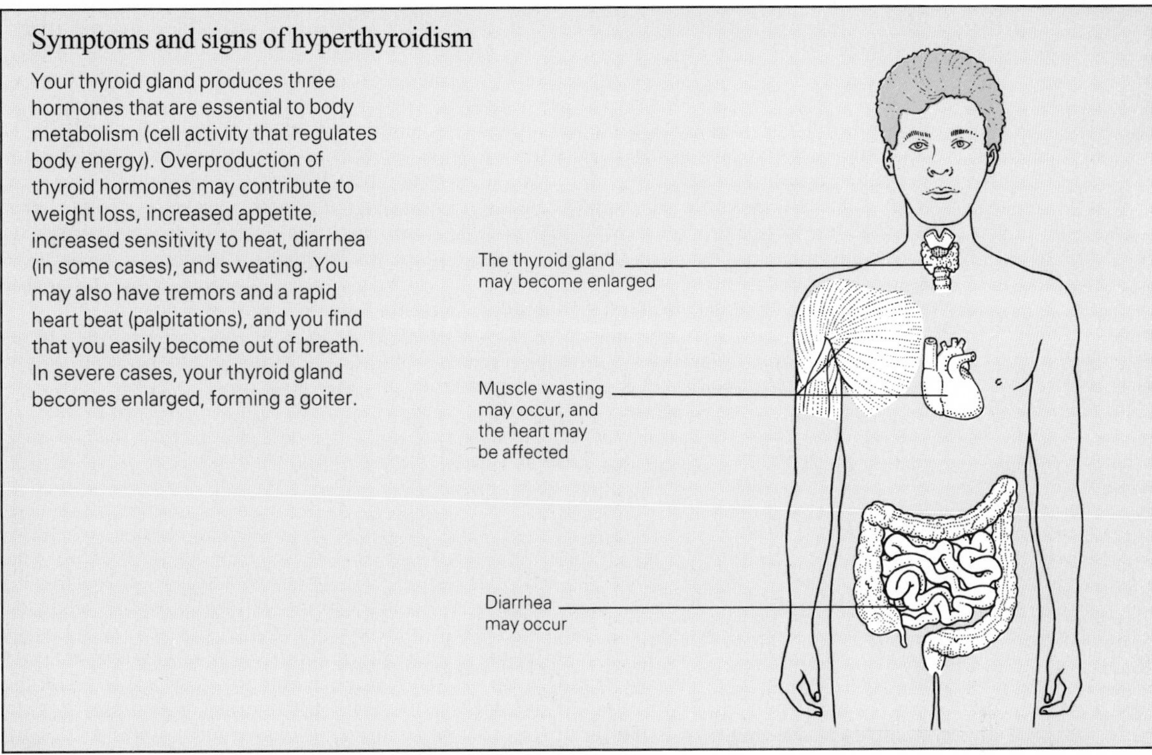
The thyroid gland may become enlarged
Muscle wasting may occur, and the heart may be affected
Diarrhea may occur

Hypothyroidism

(including Hashimoto's disease)

Hypothyroidism, sometimes called myxedema, is caused by underactivity of the thyroid gland. When it occurs, your thyroid gland produces only small amounts of thyroid hormone, and all chemical processes in your body slow down as a result.

Underactivity of the thyroid gland can be due to one of several causes, or it can occur for no apparent reason. One occasional cause is treatment for hyperthyroidism (see previous article), which carries a significant risk that the overactive thyroid gland may later become underactive. Another possible, but much rarer, cause of underactivity is a lack of thyroid-stimulating hormone resulting from a disorder of the pituitary gland or hypothalamus (see p.554). Hypothyroidism may also occur in the course of Hashimoto's disease, a disorder in which an inflammatory thyroid condition (thought to be caused by an autoimmune reaction) destroys your thyroid gland. In such a reaction, antibodies, or biochemical substances in your blood that normally protect you from infection, attack a part of your body.

Very rarely, an infant is born with a defective thyroid gland, or with no gland at all. The result is little or no thyroid hormone. If it is not detected and treated, this condition can lead to irreversible mental deficiency.

What are the symptoms?

The symptoms of hypothyroidism develop slowly, taking months or even years. A person who has not seen you for a few months may be struck by the deterioration in your appearance and mental health.

If you have hypothyroidism, your whole body slows down. You feel continually tired and worn out. Even simple mental tasks, such as adding up a bill, seem to take longer. You may have general aches and pains and move more slowly than usual. Your heart may slow to 50 beats per minute or less (the normal range is usually anywhere from 60 to 100 beats per minute) and your digestive system may become constipated.

Because slowed body processes need less energy, you eat less but gain weight. You feel cold more often, so you wear far more clothing. Your hair becomes dry and lifeless. Your skin becomes dry and thickens because of a mucuslike substance that collects in it. Why this happens is not known, but it makes your face look puffy.

Puffy tissue also collects on your vocal cords, which makes your voice deeper than usual and hoarse; in your ears, which causes hearing loss; and in your wrists, where it presses on the nerves going to your hands and causes numbness and tingling in them. These last few symptoms are more prevalent in myxedema, which is a more severe form of hypothyroidism.

Women may have heavy, prolonged menstrual periods, and both women and men may lose interest in sex. Contrary to popular opinion, hypothyroidism causes less than 1 percent of cases of obesity.

In very severe cases of hypothyroidism you become very cold and drowsy, and may eventually become unconscious. This rare condition is called myxedema coma. It may be brought on by cold weather or by taking certain drugs, especially sedatives.

A baby born with hypothyroidism is lethargic and difficult to feed, has a large tongue and an umbilical hernia (see Hernias, p.505). The child often develops Neonatal jaundice (see p.693) soon after birth.

What are the risks?

Hypothyroidism is common and it affects primarily women at all ages. However, the disorder is very rare at birth, occurring in only about 1 in 5,000 births.

An infant with hypothyroidism, left untreated, will not grow and develop properly. Instead, the child will have short stature (see p.555) and mental retardation. In adults the condition is unlikely to be fatal unless myxedema coma develops.

What should be done?

Many people feel tired and generally "down" at some time or other. However, most of them do not have hypothyroidism. Depression (see p.321) mimics many of the symptoms of hypothyroidism. If you notice several of the symptoms described in this article occurring together, visit your physician promptly.

After examining you, your physician will probably take blood samples for analysis. If the samples contain a high level of thyroid-stimulating hormone, hypothyroidism is the diagnosis. If the samples also contain antibodies that are active against the thyroid gland, the diagnosis is Hashimoto's disease.

Hypothyroidism in infants is sometimes detected during the physical examination performed immediately after birth. More often, however, children who have congenital (from birth) hypothyroidism are detected before signs and symptoms develop, through screening of blood samples taken from newborns for thyroid-stimulating hormone.

What is the treatment?

Whatever its cause, the treatment of hypothyroidism is straightforward. You will take medication containing artificially made thyroid hormones every day for the rest of your life. After a few days of treatment, you will feel much better, and after a few months you should be returned to normal health. Myxedema is also treated with artificially made thyroid hormones.

An infant with the disorder is started on the medication as soon as possible. If treatment is started before the baby is about 3 months old, he or she is likely to grow and develop normally. The child must take the medication exactly as prescribed by the physician.

Thyroid nodules

A thyroid nodule is a lump growing in the thyroid gland. There are four types of nodules: a fluid-filled cyst; an area of bleeding called a hematoma; a benign (unlikely to spread) growth called an adenoma; and a malignant (likely to spread) growth called a carcinoma. Why thyroid nodules develop, or why some people have more than one, is not known.

What are the symptoms?

Thyroid nodules are usually hidden swellings in the front of your neck that your physician discovers when examining you. They can be painful, but are rarely big enough to make breathing or swallowing difficult.

What should be done?

All nodules except carcinomas are fairly common, and usually harmless. About 1 in 200 may become cancerous. However, if you have had radiation treatments to the head or neck as a child, your chance of having a cancerous nodule increases to one in five. If a benign nodule is small, your physician may advise you to leave it alone. A large, unsightly cyst can be aspirated (reduced in size by suction with a needle). If a thyroid scan shows that a nodule may be a carcinoma, the gland will be removed surgically; if it is an adenoma, the gland will be removed surgically or destroyed with radioactive iodine. Once the gland is removed, you must then take thyroxine tablets for the rest of your life, because you will no longer have a natural source of this important hormone.

The outlook for those who get thyroid cancer is generally good. Young people are often completely cured, either through surgery to remove the gland or through a combination of surgery and radioactive-iodine treatments.

Hyperparathyroidism

Hyperparathyroidism is a condition in which your parathyroid glands, which help control bone growth, produce too much hormone. In most cases this occurs because of a small growth in one of the four parathyroid glands. The growth is usually benign (unlikely to spread). Occasionally the disorder occurs because of a generalized enlargement of all four glands. It is not known what causes the growth or the enlargement. The excess parathyroid hormone creates a higher than normal level of calcium in your blood, most of which comes from your bones. Your kidneys pass more calcium into your urine, trying to lower the blood calcium level, but the effects of this activity are limited. Over the years the calcium level gradually builds up.

What are the symptoms?

Loss of calcium from the bones may make them more easily fractured. Excessive amounts of calcium passing through the kidneys can cause kidney stones (see p.548). Symptoms of fatigue, muscle aches, indigestion, constipation, and the need to get up during the night to urinate are common.

What should be done?

If you have the symptoms mentioned above, consult your physician. He or she will take a blood test. Sometimes hyperparathyroidism is diagnosed as part of a checkup. If your blood calcium level is elevated, or if there is a possibility that you have hyperparathyroidism, your physician will arrange for a parathormone (parathyroid hormone) blood level test, to confirm the diagnosis. If the diagnosis is questionable, an ultrasound scan or isotope scan and possibly an angiogram may be performed to attempt to determine which of the four glands is responsible.

What is the treatment?

Surgery to remove a growth or to remove three of the enlarged parathyroid glands cures the disorder in most cases. If, however, the blood calcium is only slightly raised in a person over age 50 and in otherwise good health, the physician may recommend that he or she wait and monitor progress for a year or two, evaluating the health of the kidneys and bones from time to time. There is a risk that after the operation the amount of parathyroid hormone produced will not be enough to maintain a normal level of calcium in your blood (see Hypoparathyroidism, next article).

If your hyperparathyroidism causes kidney stones (see p.548), you may need treatment with extracorporeal sound wave lithotripsy (see p.549), conventional surgery, or drugs.

Hypoparathyroidism

In hypoparathyroidism, your parathyroid glands, the glands involved in controlling bone metabolism, fail to produce enough hormones. This causes the level of calcium in your blood to fall below normal. The disorder can occur either alone or in conjunction with the failure of other endocrine gland functions (for example, those of the thyroid or adrenal glands). In either case, the cause of the defect is not yet known. Hypoparathyroidism is very rare, and affects children more commonly than adults.

Hypoparathyroidism can also be caused by surgery on the thyroid gland to control overactivity in that gland (see Hyperthyroidism, p.565) or to remove a cancerous tumor. An operation on the parathyroid glands to control overactivity (see Hyperparathyroidism, previous article) may also trigger hypoparathyroidism by removing too much functioning parathyroid tissue.

What are the symptoms?

The main symptoms are painful cramplike spasms in your hands, feet, and throat. These spasms are known as tetany (not to be confused with tetanus, see p.603). Other symptoms include tingling and numbness in your face and hands, dry skin, thin hair, and often oral thrush (see p.484) or vaginal yeast infection (see p.645). If the disease is not detected in a child, he or she may have vomiting, headaches, seizures (see p.713), and poor tooth development. The child may also become mentally retarded.

What should be done?

See your physician, who will arrange for you to have blood tests. The results of these tests will show whether you have the disease.

What is the treatment?

Once the illness has been diagnosed, you require lifelong treatment with calcium and vitamin D supplements, which will restore your blood calcium to normal levels. If you have an attack of tetany, your physician will give you an injection of calcium. This usually provides almost immediate relief. The correct dose of vitamin D and calcium will return you to near-normal health. However, to help check your condition and the necessary treatment, you will need tests periodically on the level of calcium in your blood.

Disorders of the muscles, bones, and joints

Introduction

Muscles, bones, and joints provide your body with a supportive framework that allows flexibility of movement. All movement, including the movement of both the body itself and the organs inside the body, is carried out by muscles, which can do their jobs because they are composed of tissues that can contract.

Voluntary muscles, such as those in your arms and legs, are under conscious control, and contract only when your brain tells them to contract. For example, if you want to bend your elbow, your brain instructs your biceps muscle to contract; if you want to straighten your arm, your brain signals your biceps muscle to relax and instructs your triceps muscle to contract. These brain signals are sent via your nervous system.

Involuntary muscles, such as those that are in your heart and digestive tract, normally function without your conscious control or awareness. The articles in this section address only voluntary muscles, mainly those of the arms and legs, neck, and trunk. Disorders that affect involuntary muscles are discussed in sections dealing with the organs controlled by involuntary muscles; for example, irritable colon is discussed in Disorders of digestion and nutrition.

The 206 bones of your skeleton serve mainly as a support system for the various parts of your body. In addition, some bones also cover and protect certain organs. For example, the skull protects the brain, and the rib cage and vertebrae shield the heart, lungs, and, to some extent, upper-abdominal organs such as the stomach, liver, spleen, and kidneys.

Bones are not lifeless structures. They are composed of living cells embedded in a dense framework of protein (collagen), saturated with the minerals calcium and phosphorus. This framework acts partially as a storage and supply area for these minerals. Inside some bones is a soft core, the marrow, that manufactures blood cells (see Bone marrow, p.460).

Some bones, such as those of the skull, are joined closely together by almost immovable connective fibers called sutures. But when most people speak of a "joint," they generally mean the special hingelike structure between certain neighboring bones that permits them to move in relation to each other.

There are several different types of joints in your body. Each of your vertebrae can move only slightly in relation to its neighbors, but this provides enough flexibility over your entire spinal column to allow you to bend your back considerably. The finger joints are called hinge joints, because they permit movement primarily in one plane (backward and forward). The shoulder is a ball-and-socket joint, which is more versatile. It allows your arm to bend, twist, and turn, and, therefore, move in almost any direction.

Each joint is a complicated structure. It is bound together on the outside by fibrous bands called ligaments. Inside each ligament is a capsule made of fibrous tissue surrounding the joint. The capsule is lined on the inside by the synovium, a thin membrane that continuously produces tiny amounts of fluid to lubricate the joint. Where the bone ends meet, the surfaces are covered by smooth, flexible cartilage.

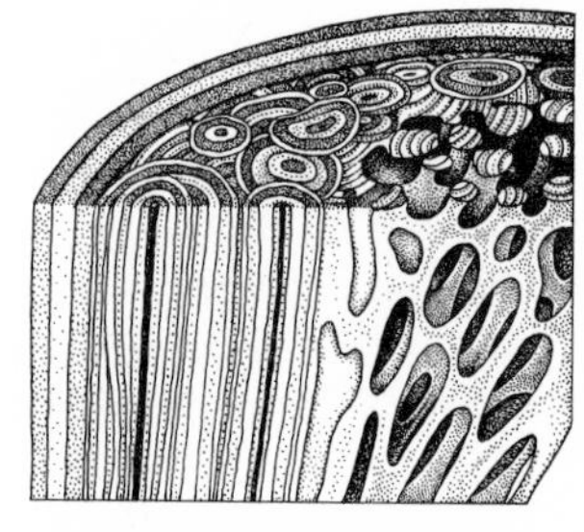

Bone tissue
Magnified bone tissue reveals many tiny cylinders made of organic material containing deposits of minerals, mainly calcium and phosphorus. These cylinders provide much of bone's strength.

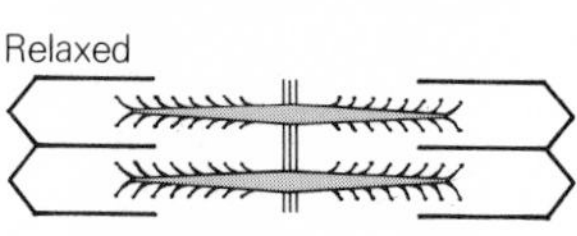

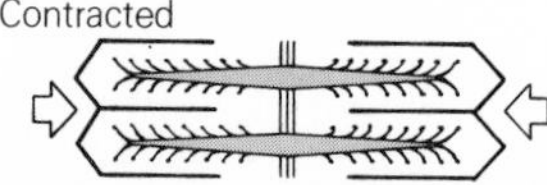

Muscle tissue
A muscle is composed of tiny filaments that move in relation to each other when stimulated by a nerve impulse. This movement results in the contraction and relaxation through which a muscle does its work.

Musculoskeletal system

How the skeleton and muscles work together

Skeletal muscles are attached to two or more bones. When a muscle contracts, the bones to which it is attached move. Muscles usually work in coordinated groups; contraction of one muscle is accompanied by relaxation of another, while other muscles stabilize nearby joints.

Head and neck muscles
Contraction of these muscles produces facial expressions and head movements. They are also responsible for speech and swallowing.

Abdominal muscles
This large group of muscles assists in the regular movements of breathing, balances the muscles of the spine during lifting, and keeps the abdominal organs firmly in place.

Arm muscles
The bulk of arm muscles is at the shoulder and below the elbow. Long tendons connect the muscles in the forearm to the wrist and fingers.

Leg muscles
Leg muscles are among the most powerful in the body and have strong, broad anchorage points, especially at the pelvis.

Involuntary muscles

Involuntary muscles are not under conscious control. That is, they do not contract or relax in response to your decision to make a movement. Instead, they work automatically under the influence of the autonomic nervous system. Involuntary muscles include those that propel food through the intestines and muscles that control sweating and blood pressure.

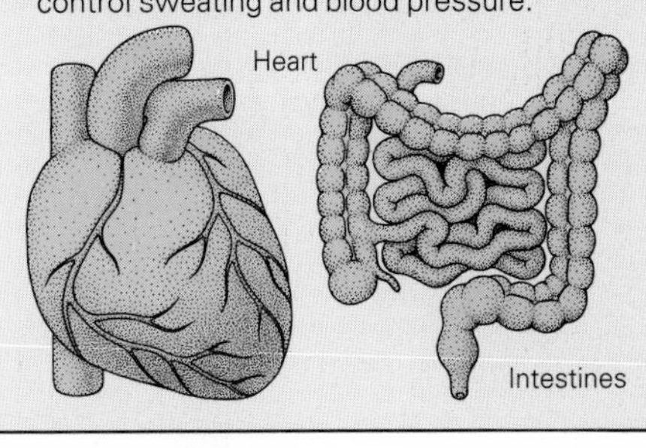

Male and female pelvis

Most bones in the female skeleton are the same shape as the bones in the male skeleton, but usually a little smaller. One exception is the pelvis. A woman's pelvis is usually broader than a man's and has a larger space in the middle. The space accommodates the head of a baby as it passes from the uterus through the pelvis during childbirth.

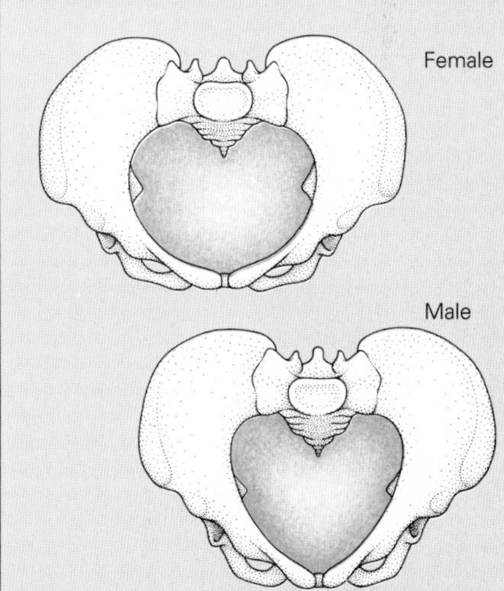

Protection of internal organs
Besides providing a rigid internal framework, the skeleton also provides some protection for certain vulnerable internal organs. The brain is encased in the bony container, the skull. The rib cage shields the lungs and heart and forms a protective umbrella over upper abdominal organs such as the liver and kidneys. The pelvis is a solid ring of bone at the base of the abdomen; it shields the bladder and portions of the genital tract.

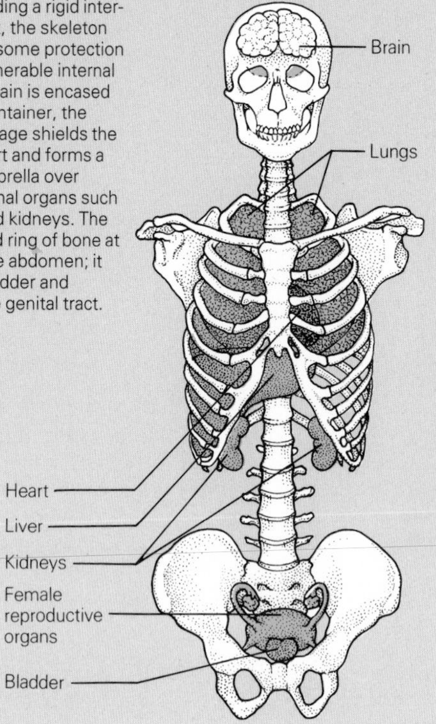

Brain
Lungs
Heart
Liver
Kidneys
Female reproductive organs
Bladder

Different types of joints
Some joints, like the fibrous sutures that join the bones of the skull, allow little or no movement and effectively weld the bones into one rigid structure. Others permit limited movement. Each vertebra can move only slightly, although this adds up to considerable flexibility over the whole spinal column. Other joints—such as the shoulder joint—have a wide range of movement.

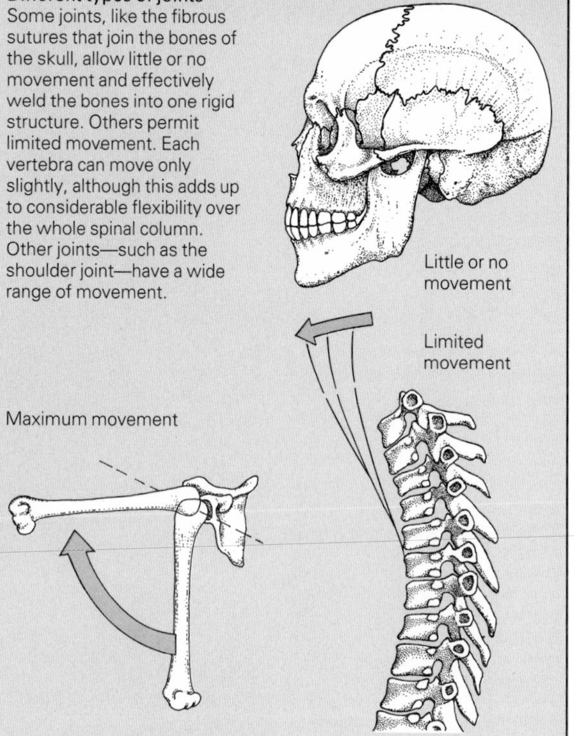

Little or no movement
Limited movement
Maximum movement

Types of joint movement
The finger joints (right) are typical "hinge" joints. They move primarily in one plane, that is, backward and forward. Elbow joints move in the same way. A ball-and-socket joint such as the shoulder joint (below) or a hip joint allows movement on two planes: backward and forward (1) and sideways (2). It also allows the limb to rotate (3). Most actions of the arm involve a combination of these types of movements.

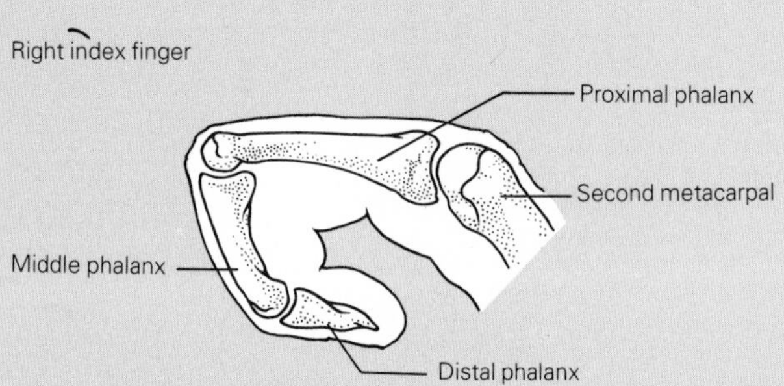

Planes of movement of shoulder joint

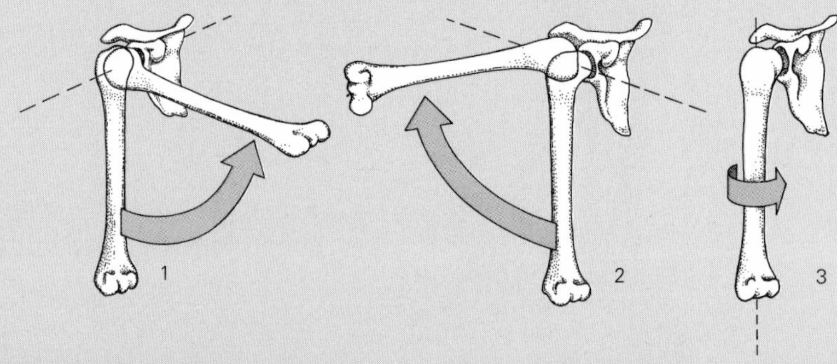

Injuries

Muscles, bones, and joints are all more susceptible to damage from injury than most other parts of the body. Because every muscle has a limited pulling strength, it will be torn or otherwise damaged if it is required to overcome a force too powerful for it, such as when you try to lift something that is too heavy for you. Similarly, bones cannot change shape quickly in response to extreme force (although they can change shape over time in response to prolonged stress), so they will break if they are subjected to too much stress. Each joint in the body allows a particular range of movement. If a joint is overflexed or forced to move in an unnatural direction, the ligaments or other tissues that bind adjoining bones together will be damaged or the bones will break.

Pulled muscle

(strain or tear)

If a muscle is overstretched, some muscle fibers may tear. If this happens, the muscle contracts and may also swell because of internal bleeding. Occasionally, the muscle may be ruptured, or torn completely.

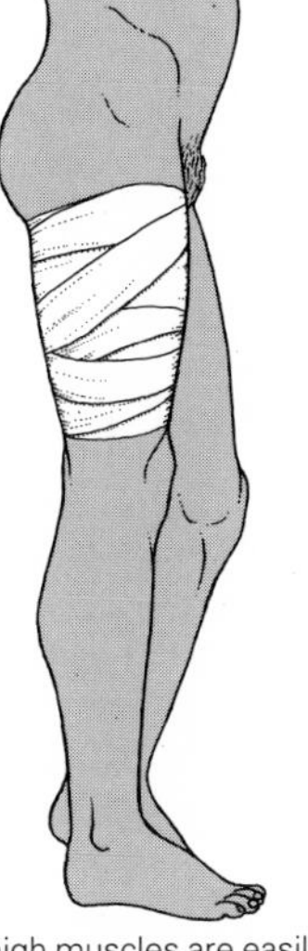

Thigh muscles are easily strained, especially during sports. An elastic bandage around the vulnerable area provides support.

What are the symptoms?

The main symptom is pain when the injury occurs. The pulled muscle feels tender, may become swollen, and will not function efficiently until the torn fibers have healed. If the muscle is ruptured, it will not function at all. A muscle that gradually becomes stiff, painful, and tender (often overnight) has probably been strained. In addition, a few of its fibers may have been torn.

What are the risks?

Almost everybody pulls, or strains, a muscle at some time. People who are active in sports are particularly susceptible to such injuries. Ruptured muscles are much less common.

In most cases recovery from a pulled muscle is quick and complete, and there is no danger of permanent loss of mobility. The older you are, the greater the damage you can do and the more slowly you recover. A strain that tears muscle, however, may permanently impair the working of the muscle unless it is successfully treated.

What should be done?

If you pull a muscle and it does not seem to be severely damaged, try the self-help measures suggested below. If you are in great pain or the affected area becomes badly swollen, consult your physician, who may be able to evaluate the extent of injury by carefully examining the affected area.

What is the treatment?

Self-help: Apply ice wrapped in a cloth or an ice pack to the area to help prevent further swelling and to decrease the pain. Try not to use the pulled muscle for several days, or while pain persists. Bandaging or wrapping the affected area will help decrease swelling, but be careful not to bind it too tightly. This could cause further swelling, which might then interfere with blood circulation.

Professional help: Treatment depends on the severity of the injury. Your physician may prescribe a painkiller. You may be advised to use crutches for a leg injury or a sling for an arm injury. In severe cases your physician may also recommend physical therapy. As pain and swelling subside, a graduated program of exercises may help restore motion and strength to the injured muscle.

If the muscle is torn, the best treatment is often surgery to repair it.

Sprain

If excessive demands are made on a joint, the ligaments that hold the neighboring bones together and keep the joint in position may be stretched or torn. This injury is a sprain, and the severity of a sprain depends on how badly the ligaments are torn.

Any ligament can be sprained, but the ligaments at the knees, ankles, and fingers are especially susceptible because greater force is more often applied to these joints.

What are the symptoms?

The amount of pain and tenderness in the injured area varies depending on the extent of damage to the soft tissue and cartilage that support the joint. A sprained ligament often still functions, but is painful to use. There may also be swelling and, later, skin discoloration. In a sprain so severe that all supporting ligaments are torn, the joint may be misshapen as well as swollen.

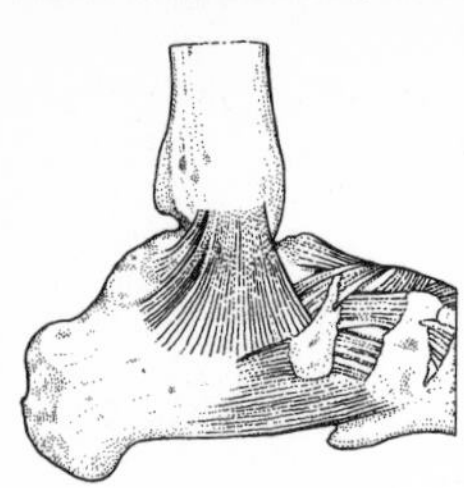

Sprained ankle
The tough, fibrous ligaments of the ankle hold the ankle bones firmly in place. If you put your weight on your ankle in an abnormal position, you may stretch or tear the ligaments. This is a sprained ankle.

What are the risks?

There is no danger in a minor sprain. Any joint will weaken eventually if its ligaments are repeatedly stretched and torn. This is particularly true of the ankle joint. If it is sprained often, the ankle may begin to give way occasionally for no apparent reason.

What should be done?

For a mild sprain try the self-help measures recommended in this article. If the pain is severe or if it lasts for more than two or three days, see your physician. He or she will examine the joint and may take X rays because a severe sprain is often difficult to distinguish from a fracture.

What is the treatment?

Self-help: If you have a mild sprain, support the joint with an elastic bandage and rest it. An ice pack helps reduce the swelling for the first 24 to 48 hours. After a day or so, start to exercise the joint as much as possible, but without forcing it to bear weight. When you are not exercising your damaged arm or leg, keep it in an elevated position to help drain away fluids that cause swelling.

Professional help: If you have a severe sprain, your physician may put a cast or splint on the affected portion of the injured arm, leg, or finger. Occasionally, you may need surgery on the ligaments. Usually after ligament surgery the joint is immobilized in a protective brace, and you are told to use the recovering joint right away. Ultrasound therapy may be used for some sprains to improve circulation to the injured area and promote healing. Physical therapy can usually help restrengthen the joint and get you back to normal more quickly.

Severed tendon

If you cut or otherwise injure your forearm, hand, calf, or foot, one or more tendons may be partly or completely cut. Tendons are long, fibrous cords that connect muscles and bones, such as those that move your fingers, thumbs, and toes. The muscles that move your fingers are located in your forearms, and those that move your toes are in your calves and feet. If you sever a tendon you may be unable to move one or more of your fingers or toes properly.

Muscle tendons sometimes rupture (tear) during physical effort. The main tendon of the ankle (Achilles tendon) is the one most commonly torn.

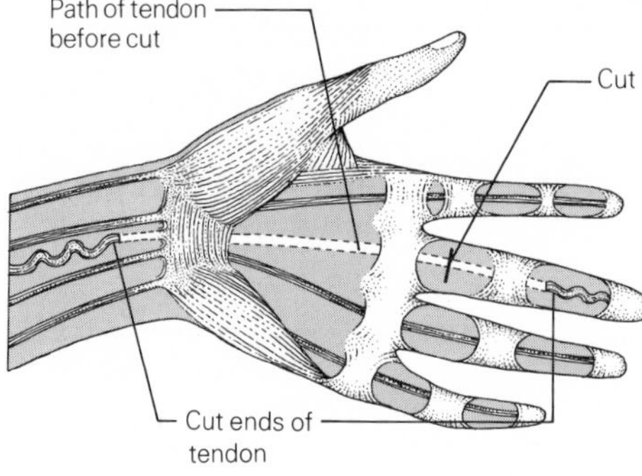

Locating the severed tendon ends
When a tendon is severed, the muscle to which it is attached contracts, causing the tendon to spring back from the site of injury. In such cases, surgery is required to locate the severed ends so they can be rejoined.

What should be done?

Get to your physician or a hospital as soon as possible if you think you have severed a tendon. Depending on the injury, a surgeon may attempt to sew together the two ends immediately. Tendons are under considerable tension, so when one is severed, the cut ends snap back from the cut and may be difficult to retrieve. A large incision may be required to find the two free ends of the tendon for repair.

The results of tendon repairs are usually satisfactory, although in some cases an affected digit may be stiff and less maneuverable than it was before the injury.

The RICE routine for first aid

RICE, which stands for **rest, ice, compression,** and **elevation**, is usually the best way to treat minor soft-tissue injuries such as bruises, strains, sprains, and bursitis.

Rest
Rest the injured part of your body to reduce further bleeding and swelling. Avoid moving the injured part.

Ice
Apply an ice pack to the injured area for 20 to 30 minutes every 2 or 3 hours for the first 48 hours after an injury. This will help relieve pain and minimize bruising and swelling.

Compression
Wear a compression bandage for at least 2 days to help reduce bleeding and swelling. Extend the bandage well above and below the injured area. Do not wrap the bandage so tight that it cuts off circulation. (Increased pain or numbness and tingling are signs that the bandage is too tight.)

Elevation
Raise the injured part of your body (above your heart when possible) to help reduce swelling. Elevation also helps drain any fluid that has accumulated in the injured area.

Dislocation

A joint is dislocated if the bones that should be in contact are pulled apart so that the joint no longer functions. The cause is usually a severe injury that exerts a force great enough to tear the joint ligaments. In addition to displaced bones, there also may be serious damage to the joint capsule (the membrane that encases the joint), and occasionally to surrounding muscles, blood vessels, and nerves. Occasionally, the injury that causes the dislocation also produces a fracture (see next article) in one or both of the bones. Dislocations that are not caused by an injury may be congenital (present from birth; see p.710) or may infrequently occur as a complication of rheumatoid arthritis (see p.589). A dislocation may happen repeatedly, without apparent cause, to a person with a joint weakened by an earlier injury. The jaw and shoulder joints are especially susceptible to this spontaneous type of dislocation.

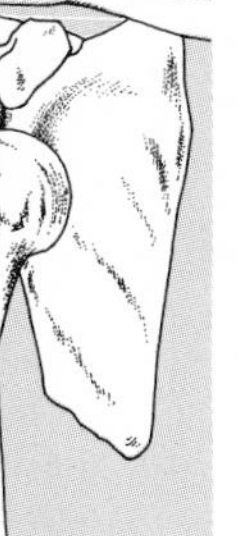

Dislocation of the shoulder
The shoulder joint is a ball-and-socket joint. The ball of the upper-arm bone fits into a cup-shaped socket in the shoulder blade. The shoulder is a very maneuverable joint, and so tends to become dislocated more easily than most other joints.

What are the symptoms?
A dislocated joint may look misshapen, is usually painful, and often is swollen, discolored, and immovable. Other symptoms of a dislocation are related to and depend on the extent of damage to surrounding tissues, nerves, and blood vessels.

What are the risks?
Dislocation of spinal vertebrae can damage the entire spinal cord, sometimes causing paralysis of the body below the level of the injury (see Spinal cord injury, p.296.) Similarly, dislocation of a shoulder or hip can damage the main nerves to the affected arm or leg and cause paralysis of part of the limb. Some joints that have been dislocated may be susceptible to osteoarthritis (see p.588).

What should be done?
Do not let anyone try to manipulate your dislocated joint unless you are sure they know exactly what to do. There may be a fracture or other damage that can be made worse if the injury is handled incorrectly. Protect the injured area as well as you can (see Injuries and emergencies, p.842) and get to a physician or hospital as quickly as possible. Do not eat or drink; this is a problem if you need to have a general anesthetic to have the dislocation repositioned. The physician will X-ray the joint and surrounding area to determine the extent of damage.

What is the treatment?
Self-help: No treatment is feasible in most situations. If you have recurrent spontaneous dislocations, you may be able to learn how to reposition the joint by yourself. Even so, you should see your physician promptly to make sure the repositioning is correct.
Professional help: After 15 to 30 minutes a dislocated joint usually becomes so swollen and painful that repositioning may have to be done under a general anesthetic. Afterward, if the blood vessels, nerves, and bones are in place and undamaged, the joint will probably be protected in a brace for 2 to 3 weeks so that other damaged tissues can heal. Follow your physician's instructions about when and how to use the joint again. Failure to do so can result in reinjury. Physical therapy is often used during the rehabilitation period.

Sometimes surgery is necessary to achieve satisfactory repositioning. Also, if one of your joints has become very weak because of repeated dislocations, your physician may recommend an operation to tighten the ligaments that bind the adjoining bones.

Fractures

A fractured bone is a broken bone. The break occurs as a result of the bone being stressed by a force greater than it can withstand. For purposes of diagnosis and treatment, fractures are classified as closed or open.

A closed fracture is one in which the bone is broken but does not protrude through the skin. In a closed fracture, surrounding muscles and other tissues remain generally undamaged. In an open fracture there is significant damage to surrounding muscles and other tissues, and the broken bone protrudes through the skin.

A fracture is usually caused by severe stresses on the bone from an accident or injury, but this is not always the case. Any bone weakened by bone cancer (see p.583) or a bone disease such as osteoporosis (see p.581) may break with little or no apparent cause. This is called a pathologic fracture. Such fractures are common in the hips of older people, whose bones may be weakened by a combination of lack of use, changes associated with aging, and sometimes disease. Another type of fracture, called a stress fracture, may occur in healthy bone that has been subjected to prolonged or repeated periods of excessive stress.

What are the symptoms?
A fracture makes the area around the injury look swollen, bruised, and sometimes deformed. If you fracture a bone, you will probably be in severe pain, which is increased

by any pressure on the area or any attempt to move that part of the body. A minor fracture may cause only minor symptoms, and can be mistaken for a sprain (see p.573).

What are the risks?

Few people go through life without breaking a bone. The bones most likely to break are those in the wrists, hands, and feet, which are often broken during a fall. Fractures of other bones, such as arm and leg bones and those of the spine and hip, are usually the result of much more powerful forces, such as those that can occur in a traffic accident.

The older you get the more likely you are to break a bone. This is because children, although they are very active and susceptible to injury, have springy, resilient bones that tend to bend rather than snap. The bones of older people fracture more easily as calcium is lost and the bones become weak and brittle. Also, age-related problems with balance and coordination can make falls more likely.

There are two main risks if you fracture a bone. The first is related to the bone itself. If a fracture is not treated, or if treatment is delayed, the broken pieces of bone may begin to rejoin out of alignment. In such cases, the bone may have to be separated and realigned surgically. In a severe open fracture, the bones may sometimes become infected. This complicates the healing process (see Osteomyelitis, p.742). It is possible for a fragment of broken bone, cut off from its blood supply, to die gradually.

Types of fractures

Closed

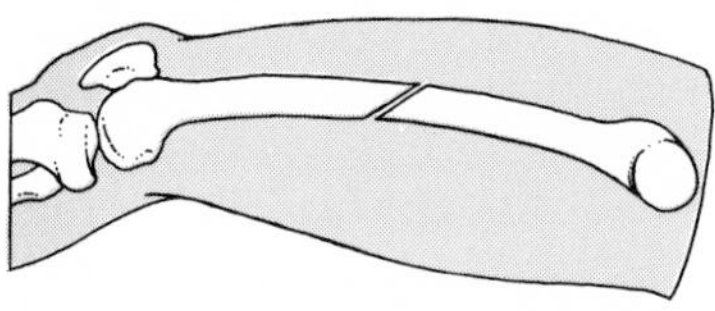

Open

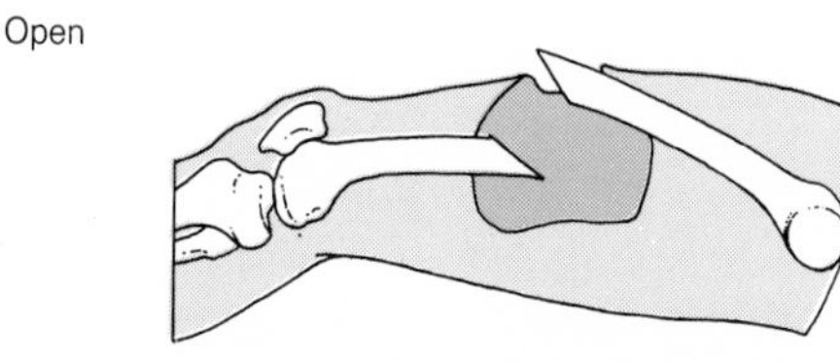

The second risk that is associated with fractures is damage to neighboring tissues. Sharp bone fragments may compress or sever nearby blood vessels or nerves. Fractures of the skull or spine can damage the brain or spinal cord (see Brain injury, p.294, and Spinal cord injury, p.296). Occasionally, other internal organs are damaged by a fractured bone. For example, a broken rib can puncture a lung (see Pneumothorax, p.388). Damage to soft tissues may have to be repaired surgically. This is often done at the same time that the fracture is treated.

What should be done?

If you or someone you know suffers a possible fracture, apply first aid (see Injuries and emergencies, p.842), and seek medical help immediately. Do not give an injured person anything to eat or drink. This may delay treatment because a general anesthetic is usually used and is safer 6 to 8 hours after a person has last eaten or had anything to drink.

Any sprain that has not improved after 2 or 3 days may be a fracture. See your physician, who will confirm the diagnosis of a fracture by an X ray of the injured area.

What is the treatment?

The first task in the treatment of a fracture is to realign the broken pieces of bone if they are in the wrong position. The medical term for this process is reduction. It is often performed under a general anesthetic, and may involve cutting open the tissues around the fracture to reposition the bones correctly.

The second part of treatment is immobilization, which is holding the bone fragments together in the correct alignment while they heal. Plaster casts or lightweight plastic or resin casts and splints are not the only ways to immobilize a fracture during the healing process. In fact, some bones are held together naturally, and need no cast or splint. A broken rib, for example, is held by many chest muscles to nearby unbroken ribs. In a similar way, a fractured finger or toe can be bandaged to a finger or toe next to it, to stabilize it while the bone heals.

In many cases, a fracture is held in position internally. An operation is performed to insert one or more metal screws, rods, or plates that will hold the broken ends in place. Internal immobilization offers a great advantage, because use of the injured limb can be resumed after a few days rather than in weeks or months. This is important because it contributes to the third part of treatment, rehabilitation of any joints or muscles that have not been used during immobilization.

Thighbone (femur) fractures in children are often treated with a body cast, or with traction followed by a cast.

Whatever the type of fracture, follow your physician's advice about when and how to move and to exercise your injured limb.

Particular attention is given to keeping nearby joints as active as possible, within limits of not disturbing the healing of the broken bones. This helps prevent swelling in the immobilized area, and stimulates blood flow to aid bone healing.

The time needed for healing a fracture depends on many factors, including the age of the injured person and whether the fracture is open or closed. A child's broken finger may heal completely in 2 weeks; an adult's shin bone may take 3 months or longer.

Occasionally, even with proper treatment, a fracture does not heal. If your physician suspects that your broken bone is not fusing properly, you may need to have additional X rays taken. Steps may have to be taken to promote healing of the fracture. The most common procedure to accomplish this is a bone graft, in which small pieces of bone are taken from a bone bank (a collection of bone donated for transplantation) or from some other site in your body (often the hipbone) and packed around the break.

Sports injuries

Athletes and others who exercise vigorously run a high risk of injuring muscles, ligaments, bones, or joints (see Pulled muscle, p.573, and Sprain, p.573). Sports injuries are most common at the beginning of an athletic season. Sports injuries frequently occur in people who begin to exercise after long periods of relative inactivity, people who are new to a particular sport, or those who exercise vigorously without first performing a proper warm-up that includes stretching exercises.

If you are injured during a game, you may be eager to return to the game as quickly as possible, but treatment that allows you to do this may have long-term risks. If the injury is a cut or bruise that does not involve serious damage to muscles or ligaments, it is reasonable for your coach or trainer to relieve pain with an icepack or an anesthetic spray, but if there is a possibility of muscle or ligament damage, painkillers may make it possible for you to damage the tissue even more without realizing it. When the extent of your injury is uncertain, or when you become dizzy, disoriented, or unconscious, even for only a few seconds, you should stop playing and see your physician as soon as possible.

Many injuries require no treatment other than rest and sometimes physical therapy to increase the circulation of blood to damaged tissues and strengthen the affected muscles. Some injuries require surgery. If you have a recurring injury, you may have to consider giving up your sport or exercise. If an injury to a ligament or bone recurs, there is a strong possibility of permanent damage, and a price of not stopping the activity may be early development of osteoarthritis (p.588) or some other joint problem. Before you reach a decision, get an accurate diagnosis of the extent of the damage. This may involve X rays, CT and MRI scans, or arthroscopy.

Common injuries requiring medical attention

Stress fracture This fracture is common in the tibia (shinbone) and the metatarsals (foot bones) but can occur in any bone as a result of prolonged or repeated periods of excessive stress. It most commonly occurs in walkers, runners, and those who do aerobics and produces pain in the ball of the foot that worsens on exertion. There are many ways to treat stress fractures, including the use of bandages and braces.

Shin splints This term refers to pain at the front of the lower part of the leg that may have a number of causes. Shin splints may result from a minor muscle tear, inflammation of the fibrous covering (periosteum) of the tibia (shinbone), a stress fracture, or anterior compartment syndrome (the muscles swell and press on nearby blood vessels). In most cases, the symptoms disappear after a week or two of rest. But if pain is severe and recurrent, surgery may be necessary.

Knee injuries Strain on the knee may stretch or rupture the ligaments around the joint, or may damage the internal ligaments or the 2 semicircular pads of cartilage that act as padding beween the surfaces of the joint. If you damage your knee, surgery is performed through an arthroscope (viewing tube).

Hand injuries Injury to the bones or tendons of the hands commonly occurs in boxing, rock climbing, handball, and basketball. If you injure your hand, seek medical attention as soon as possible. If you need to have damaged tendons repaired surgically, treatment may be more successful if surgery is performed soon after the injury.

Head injuries If you lose consciousness even briefly after a head injury see a physician as soon as possible and refrain from vigorous activity for at least 24 hours.

Muscle and tendon disorders

Tendons are tough, fibrous bands or cords of tissue that join some muscles to bone.

Muscles are composed of special elongated cells that contract to produce movement. At each end of most muscles there is a band of fibrous tissue that connects the muscle to a bone. In some parts of the body these bands of tissue are very short or their fibers are inextricably mixed with the muscle tissue to which they are joined. But in other areas, especially in the hands and feet, the tissue forms long, tough cords known as tendons.

Both muscles and tendons can be damaged by injury or disease. Damage from injury is discussed on p.577. The following articles deal with damage from other causes.

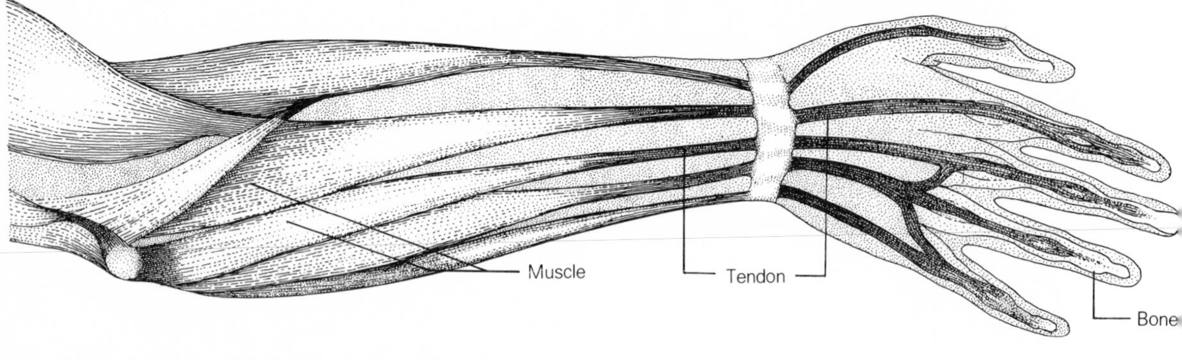

Cramp

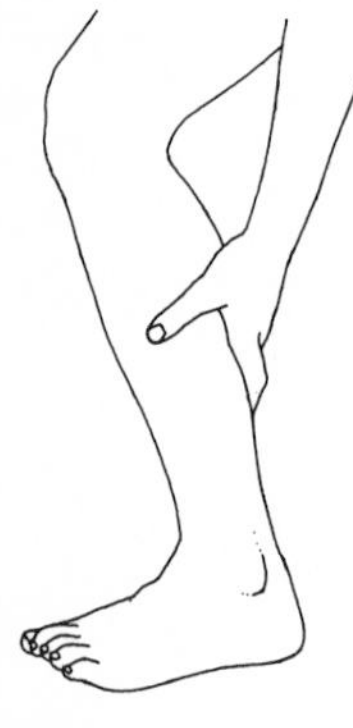

Massage the affected muscle

A cramp is a painful spasm in a muscle. It happens occasionally to almost everybody, and there is usually no underlying cause other than unaccustomed exercise or a prolonged period of sitting, standing, or lying in an uncomfortable position. Some people are roused from sleep regularly by sudden, severe cramps, usually in the legs or feet. In most cases there is no reason for concern. If you think your cramps may be related to an underlying disease, consult the self-diagnosis chart on cramps (see p.179).

What are the symptoms?

When you try to move the cramped muscle, it contracts violently. There is usually a visible distortion of the affected area along with the sudden pain. If you touch the muscle, it feels hard and tense, and you cannot control it. However, when you stand and take a few steps on a cramping leg or foot muscle, the pain is temporarily relieved.

What should be done?

An ordinary cramp lasts no longer than a few minutes and will quickly clear up on its own. You can speed and ease the process by massaging and gradually stretching the cramping muscle. If you continue to have cramps, first be sure you are warming up before exercise by stretching. Adequate fluid intake may help prevent cramping. While there are many electrolyte solutions that help prevent cramping, drinking enough water during exercise may be the most effective prevention. Or consult your physician, who may be able to determine the cause and prescribe a drug such as quinine.

Tendinitis

If a tendon, the tissue that connects muscles to bones, becomes torn and inflamed, the affected area becomes swollen, tender, and painful. Also, the tendon is usually slow to heal because the muscle is constantly in use and there is very little blood supply to the tendon. When it does heal, the inflamed fibers may leave a painful scar in the tendon. The pain generally disappears after a few weeks or months, but it can persist and even become worse, especially in older people. Tendinitis can occur in any place where a tendon joins muscle to bone, but it is most common at the shoulders or heels, on the outside of the elbows (called tennis elbow), or on the inside of the elbows (called golfer's elbow). This condition may result from overexertion in sports or other activities.

What is the treatment?

Rest the painful arm or leg for a few days by putting your arm in a sling if necessary. Take aspirin, ibuprofen, or other nonsteroidal anti-inflammatory drugs to help relieve the pain. After a few days, start to exercise the joint gradually, to prevent it from getting stiff. If the pain persists or becomes much worse, your physician may want you to have an X ray. He or she may also inject a corticosteroid drug and a local anesthetic into the affected area. This procedure may need to be repeated. Physical therapy consisting of anti-inflammatory treatments (application of ice and use of ultrasound) followed by gentle, controlled exercises designed to stretch and strengthen the muscles are also used to treat the pain and inflammation.

Tenosynovitis

(including repetitive strain disorder)

Some tendons, particularly those that work fingers and thumbs, are covered by a membrane, called the synovium, that helps move the tendon. The synovium may become inflamed and swollen, especially if you constantly use your fingers in repetitive fashion, as in typing or assembly-line work; this kind of tenosynovitis is called repetitive strain disorder. In time, the synovium heals, but it may become too tight or narrow. A tight or narrow synovium restricts movement of the tendon it covers, gradually resulting in tenosynovitis. One example of what may happen is the minor disability called "trigger finger," in which a tight synovium makes it hard for you to straighten your finger once you have bent it. The straightening mechanism becomes jammed for a few moments before the tendon suddenly overcomes the obstruction and the finger completes its movement with a sudden jerk. As a result, the area over the tendon may become painful and tender, and the affected finger may hurt and make a soft, crackling sound whenever you bend or straighten it.

Tenosynovitis is sometimes caused by an infection rather than by mechanical factors. In such a condition your sore finger or thumb becomes painful and difficult to use, and you may have other symptoms of infection. This kind of tenosynovitis is a serious infection requiring prompt treatment.

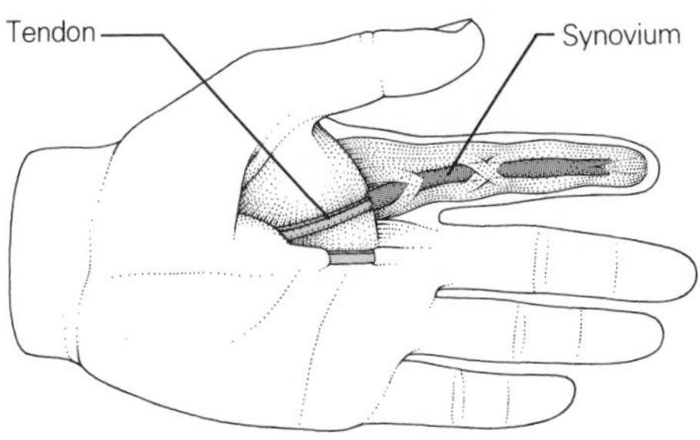

The synovium
The synovium is a membrane that lines the interior of a joint. It makes and contains synovial fluid, which lubricates joints and tendon sheaths.

What should be done?

If your symptoms suggest the possibility of infection, see your physician immediately. You may require treatment with antibiotics, and you may also need surgery to release pus that is produced by the invading bacteria that have caused the infection. Noninfectious tenosynovitis can sometimes be cured by injections of corticosteroid drugs. Repetitive strain disorder may be treated with a combination of injections of corticosteroid drugs and rest; splinting of the hand may be required in some cases. If tenosynovitis persists, a simple operation to open the constricting synovium will allow the tendon within it to move freely again.

Fibromyalgia

(fibrositis, myofascial pain)

Fibromyalgia is stiffness and pain felt in fibrous tissues, usually deep within the muscles. Its cause is unknown, but it seems to be accompanied by emotional tension reflected in the knotting up of muscles. If you have an attack of fibromyalgia, there is nothing basically wrong with the muscles themselves. Yet you are likely to have localized pain, and you may even feel slight swelling within the affected muscles. Fibromyalgia often casues a backache (see p.584). It is common, especially in people past middle age, and usually clears up on its own. Hot baths and aspirin or other nonsteroidal anti-inflammatory drugs should help relieve pain. If it persists, see your physician, who may prescribe antidepressants, other painkillers, or muscle-relaxant drugs. In some cases, physicians prescribe injections of local anesthetics, with or without corticosteroid drugs. However, the effectiveness of this treatment is unproven.

Ganglion

A ganglion is a cystic swelling under the skin, generally in the wrist or the upper surface of the foot. A ganglion develops when a jelly-like substance accumulates in one of two places, a joint capsule or a tendon sheath, and causes it to balloon out. The size of ganglia varies. They may be soft to the touch or quite hard, and they are usually either painless or only mildly painful. As a rule, a ganglion on the wrist does not interfere with movements of the wrist. However, when a ganglion is on the foot, it can make it difficult to wear some types of shoes.

Although a ganglion is harmless, you should not ignore it. It is reasonable to consult a physician about any swelling. Removing fluid with a syringe (aspiration) is effective about half the time. Aspiration is sometimes accompanied by corticosteroid drug injection. Ganglia that are especially painful can be cut away.

The wrist is one of the most common sites for a ganglion.

Dupuytren's contracture

(palmar fasciitis)

In Dupuytren's contracture a layer of tough, fibrous, connective tissue that lies directly under the skin on the palm of your hand progressively thickens and shrinks. This shrinkage eventually causes your ring finger and little finger (most commonly) to be permanently bent (pulled in toward the palm) at the knuckles. Although it is not usually painful, the condition weakens your grasp. One or both hands may be affected, and you may also have thickened skin pads over your other knuckles and on the balls of your feet. This is not an uncommon condition but the causes are not known.

You cannot fully straighten out your ring finger and your little finger at the base of your fingers and in the middle of your fingers when you have Dupuytren's contracture.

What should be done?

Because Dupuytren's contracture can make your fingers permanently useless, see your physician if it begins to develop. If the condition is treated early enough, stiff fingers can be unbent by an operation that either removes or cuts through thickened tissue. With the help of physical therapy, you can then regain the use of your hand. In some cases the condition recurs.

Muscle tumors

Tumors are very rare in muscles. When they do occur, they are usually benign (unlikely to spread). It is not yet known why muscle tissue seems to resist tumors. A malignant growth in a muscle is a rare but serious matter, since malignant muscle tumors grow and spread and are difficult to treat.

The first sign of a growth in a muscle is pain or a detectable lump in the affected area; usually there are no further developments. In some cases, the tumor may grow at a moderate pace over a prolonged period of time. If the growth is malignant, however, it enlarges rapidly and may become more painful. Also, a large muscle tumor can interfere with muscle contraction.

What should be done?

See your physician without delay if you develop an unexplained lump anywhere on your body. Your physician will examine you and, if necessary, may recommend X rays, a CT or MRI scan, and possibly a biopsy to make a diagnosis. In a biopsy, a sample of the growth is removed for examination. The treatment for a benign tumor can range from having you look for any symptoms to having your physician look at the tumor periodically for signs of malignancy. In the unlikely event of malignancy, possible treatments include surgery, chemotherapy, radiation therapy, or a combination of these, depending on the type, location, and extent of the tumor.

Bone diseases

The bones that make up your skeleton are active, living structures. They consist of several different types of cells embedded in a framework of protein (collagen) saturated with calcium phosphate. The cells constantly break down old bone and replace it with new bone, so that your skeleton is gradually but continuously renewed. If this maintenance system goes wrong, one or more of the bone diseases described here may result.

Inside some bones are spaces occupied by marrow, a tissue composed largely of fat, but which contains the primitive cells that form many of the blood cells found in the body. Diseases of the bone marrow therefore mostly affect the blood and are discussed elsewhere (see Bone marrow, p.460). An injury to a bone may lead to a fracture, or a break in that bone whether the bone is diseased or not (see Fractures, p.575).

Osteoporosis

Osteoporosis is a loss in protein structure and mineral content of the bone. In healthy bone, there is a balance between the breakdown of old bone tissue and the manufacture of new, replacement bone tissue. In osteoporosis breakdown occurs faster than replacement and the bones become soft and weak.

Osteoporosis may occur in one or more bones after prolonged immobilization of part of the body. Some hormonal disorders (see Cushing's syndrome, p.563) may cause some osteoporosis. Osteoporosis may also result from a diet low in protein or calcium, which are needed to maintain healthy bones. Osteoporosis sometimes occurs along with osteomalacia (see next article). However, the most common cause is aging. Women are especially susceptible after going through menopause because they lack estrogen, which plays a vital part in the process of depositing calcium on the bones. There is a serious risk of fractures.

What are the symptoms?

Osteoporosis does not usually produce any symptoms unless a spinal fracture occurs. If this happens you will have a severe backache, and you may also notice that you are becoming shorter and more round-shouldered as a result of the gradual compression of your weakened vertebrae. In rare cases of osteoporosis, one vertebra or a few vertebrae may collapse and you will have sudden and extremely severe back pain.

A bone weakened by osteoporosis is much more likely to break if you fall. The wrists, hips, and vertebrae are the most likely to break under these conditions.

If your physician suspects that you have osteoporosis, you will probably need to have X rays to confirm the diagnosis and to determine the proper treatment.

What is the treatment?

Self-help: Research has shown that regular exercise maintains the strength of bones and prevents osteoporosis. If you are a woman and are approaching or are in menopause, you can take steps to keep your bones healthy. Participate in daily physical activity such as cycling, swimming, jogging, or walking. Eat a balanced diet rich in calcium and vitamin D, good sources of which are skim milk and green leafy vegetables.

Aspirin or another nonsteroidal anti-inflammatory drug recommended by your physician should help relieve the pain. Take precautions to avoid falls: use a cane if you are unsteady on your feet; remove hazards such as loose rugs or electrical wires that may trip you; hold the railing when using stairs; and keep your house well lit during the evening and use night-lights too (see also Older people's health, p.765).

Professional help: Once osteoporosis has been established, it is difficult to reverse, so the best strategy is based on prevention. Many physicians recommend hormone replacement therapy (see Menopause, p.627) for women who have reached menopause, as protection against development of osteoporosis, but it remains controversial because some studies have linked it with breast cancer. Women who have severe menopausal symptoms, an early menopause, or female relatives who have suffered from osteoporosis may be offered hormone replacement therapy, since osteoporosis is, in some cases, hereditary. You may also be treated with hormone replacement therapy as a means of protection against the onset of osteoporosis if you have had an artificial menopause—that is, menopause that has occurred early after treatment such as radiation therapy, hysterectomy, or removal of the ovaries.

If you have osteoporosis your physician will want to try to increase the density of your bones. Treatment may include calcium supplements or drugs of the diphosphonate category. Although treatment for women also depends on whether or not you have reached menopause, treatment will always include recommendations for exercise. For more information on prevention of osteoporosis, see Your healthy body, p.24.

Osteomalacia

(adult rickets)

Osteomalacia is softening and weakening of the bones due to the body's inability to absorb calcium or to deposit mineral salts on the protein structure of the bone, usually because of vitamin D deficiency. If you lack vitamin D, you cannot absorb calcium and phosphorus from your food; both of these valuable dietary minerals are required for the growth, hardening, and maintenance of healthy bones. A healthy person gets vitamin D from two sources: food and the action of sunlight on your skin.

Vitamin D deficiency is sometimes caused by a specific disease such as chronic kidney failure (see p.551) or celiac disease (see p.509). Other rare causes are prolonged drug treatment for epilepsy (see p.306) and some forms of digestive tract surgery (see also Vitamin and mineral deficiency, p.532).

What are the symptoms?

Your bones become tender and painful, causing symptoms that can be mistaken for rheumatoid arthritis (see p.589). In addition, you will probably feel generally tired and stiff; you may also have frequent cramps and find if difficult to stand. Depending on how severe they are, these symptoms can cause varying degrees of debilitation.

What are the risks?

Osteomalacia is rare in the US. The main risk of the disease is that weakened bones tend to break under slight stress.

What should be done?

A balanced diet provides ample vitamin D, even if you are pregnant. However, if you seem to have osteomalacia, see your physician, who may arrange for blood and urine tests, X rays, and sometimes a biopsy. Osteomalacia is much less common than osteoporosis, but they look identical on an X ray. A biopsy is the only certain way to make the diagnosis.

What is the treatment?

Self-help: To prevent and treat the disorder, make sure your diet contains plenty of vitamin D and calcium.

Professional help: If you have the disorder, your physician will probably prescribe regular amounts of vitamin D and treat any underlying disease.

Paget's disease

(osteitis deformans)

In Paget's disease, new bone is produced faster than old bone is broken down. There is another disorder called Paget's disease of the nipple that is a form of cancer. The disease occurs in two stages. In the first stage, called the vascular stage, bone tissue is broken down but the spaces are filled with blood vessels and fibrous tissue instead of new bone. In the second, or sclerotic, stage, the blood-filled fibrous tissue becomes hardened and appears to be bonelike, but is actually weak and fragile.

Paget's disease can occur in part or all of one or many of your bones. The hipbone (pelvis) and shinbone (tibia) are the most common sites of the disorder. The thighbone (femur), skull, spine, and collarbone (clavicle) are also frequently affected.

What are the symptoms?

Paget's disease does not always produce symptoms, but when it does, bone pain is the most common symptom. The pain is virtually continuous, and often grows worse at night. The affected bones become enlarged and misshapen, and they feel warm and tender. Depending on which bones are diseased, your head or feet may enlarge, or you may appear shorter, bent, or bowlegged. Headaches also are a common symptom.

What are the risks?

Men seem to be more commonly affected than women. Paget's disease is more common in Europe than in the US, and is rare in certain places. The significance of this uneven distribution is unknown.

Bones weakened by Paget's disease are more likely to break (see Fractures, p.575). Rarely, Paget's disease of the skull can compress the auditory nerve that carries signals from the ear to the brain, at the point where the nerve passes through the skull. This can cause deafness. Another possible risk is heart failure (see p.408), because your heart is strained from trying to maintain the greatly increased blood flow through the diseased bones. In rare cases, a malignant (likely to spread) bone tumor develops (see next article).

What should be done?

If you think that you may have Paget's disease, consult your physician. He or she will perform a physical examination and may request X rays, a CT scan, and blood and urine tests to confirm the diagnosis.

What is the treatment?

The most common symptom of Paget's disease is pain, which can be controlled by aspirin, ibuprofen, and other nonsteroidal anti-inflammatory drugs. If the pain is severe, your physician may recommend that you have injections of a hormone called calcitonin. Or he or she may advise treatment with an anticancer drug such as mithramycin, or a diphosphonate drug such as etidronate disodium. These three treatments all slow or stop the development of new bone. However, each drug may produce side effects.

Bone tumors

Most bone tumors are secondary tumors; they develop from cancer cells that have metastasized, or spread, from a primary malignant (likely to spread) tumor in an organ such as the breast or prostate gland.

Primary bone tumors, which originate in the bone, are very rare. Most are benign (unlikely to spread), but some are malignant. Benign tumors include osteochondromas (consisting of bone and cartilage), which tend to develop close to joints such as the knee or elbow; osteomas (hard knobs of bone), which may form on the skull; and cysts, which may develop in long bones, making them more susceptible to fractures. Malignant bone tumors, such as osteogenic sarcomas and Ewing's sarcomas, are rare.

What should be done?

If you develop any lump on a bone (or anywhere else on your body), see your physician, who will examine you and order X rays, blood tests, and other tests such as a CT or MRI scan. If the lump is benign, your physician may recommend surgery to avoid fracture. Treatment of both primary and secondary tumors involves a combination of surgery, radiation therapy, and cytotoxic (anticancer) drugs. If the bone of an arm or leg is affected and the tumor does not respond to treatment with drugs and/or radiation therapy, amputation of the affected arm or leg may be necessary. An arm or leg may be saved by removing the portion of bone that contains a tumor and replacing it with a bone graft. Bone for the graft may be obtained from a bone bank. Depending on the type of tumor, the chances of complete cure are good with early detection and treatment. If a secondary tumor has become large enough to fracture the bone, the break may be treated by inserting metal plates and rods.

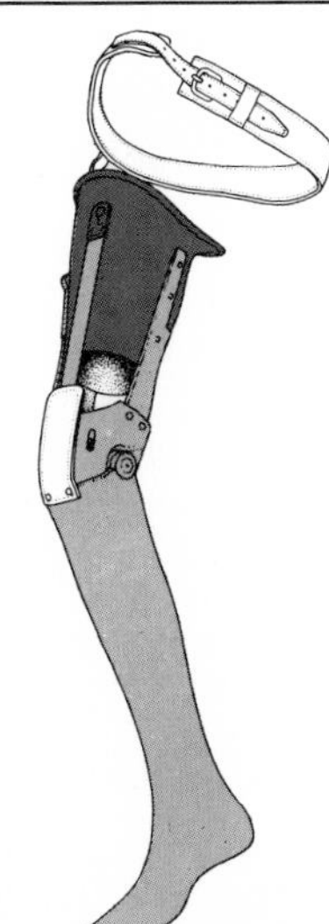

Artificial arms and legs (prostheses)

An artificial arm or leg is used when part or all of an arm or leg is lost. In recent years there have been great advances made in the materials used for prostheses that make them lighter, better fitting, more functional, and more natural looking.

Ideally, an artificial arm or leg should provide mobility and flexibility, and it should look natural. It is important that you discuss your needs and preferences with your physician and the technician who designs your prosthesis so that it will meet as many of your needs as possible.

Once you have your prosthesis, your physical therapist will teach you how to use it. Many people, even those with more than one artificial arm or leg, learn to use these devices quickly. Your age, health status, and attitude are all factors in how quickly you can return to an active life. The extent of your perseverance is particularly important.

Some artificial arms and legs are operated by electric motors or other devices that are stimulated by nerve impulses from the user's arm or leg. These so-called "bionic" arms and legs are very versatile. Prostheses of a more traditional design often incorporate simple hinge joints, sometimes with pendulum counter-weights, that usually give many years of trouble-free service.

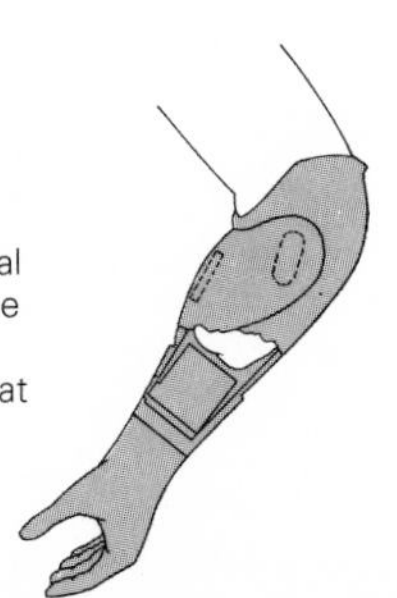

Backaches

The spinal column, or backbone, stretches from the base of the skull to the bottom of the buttocks. It consists of more than 30 separate bones called vertebrae. The vertebrae are linked by strong ligaments, and flexible, flattened discs lie between them. Each disc is constructed of a tough, fibrous outer covering wrapped around a jellylike inner substance; this construction provides enough elasticity to permit some movement over the entire spinal column. It is partly the restrictions imposed by this limited flexibility that are responsible for most back troubles. If you twist the wrong way or overstrain any part of the spinal column, it can have a painful effect on the vertebrae and on the muscles and ligaments that connect the vertebrae.

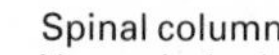

Spinal column
Your spinal column is made up of more than 30 separate bones (vertebrae) that form a protective casing for your spinal cord.

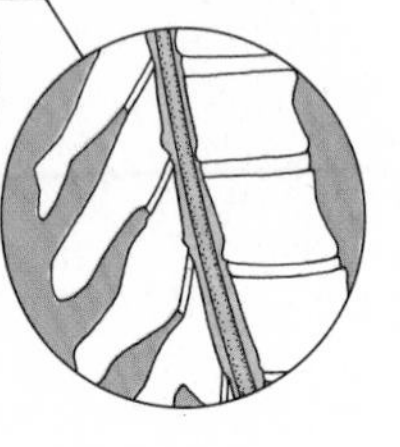

Spinal cord
Your spinal cord runs through a canal inside your vertebrae. It transmits nerve signals between your brain and your body.

Standing correctly
To avoid back problems, do not slouch when you stand. Keep your head up, your shoulders straight, and your chest forward. Try to balance your weight evenly on both feet.

Susceptibility to pain is increased because the spinal cord, which is a major part of the central nervous system, is located in a channel that runs the length of the spinal column. The spinal column also has narrow side channels through which peripheral nerves pass on their way to and from the rest of the body. Thus, any problem with a vertebra, supportive ligament, or disc may lead to pain and weakness in an extremity.

Nonspecific backache

The vast majority of backaches are often called nonspecific because they have no obvious cause. There are also no obvious, easy cures. Many different factors, including psychological factors, are involved in this type of backache, and the cause or causes may vary somewhat from person to person. Most nonspecific backaches may be caused by muscle strain and injury to the surrounding ligaments or joints (called facet joints). In other cases, pain is caused by fibrositis (see p.579) in the back muscles. In addition, some people may develop back pain when they are under stress, just as other people develop tension headaches.

Backaches are a major health problem and common cause of absence from work.

Although a nonspecific backache is often very painful and may interfere with your daily routine, there is virtually no risk of complications. These backaches generally heal without treatment but may recur.

Symptoms of backache

Pain, usually with stiffness, may develop slowly or suddenly. It may begin after you lift a heavy object, fall, stay in an awkward or cramped position for some time, do some unusual exercise, or for no apparent reason. Pain may be continuous or it may occur only when you are in a certain position or at certain times of the day or night. Coughing, sneezing, or bending and twisting the back may aggravate the pain. Sometimes pain seems to occur only in one location or it may travel from one location to another. Three common sites for localized back pain are shown on the next page.

What should be done?

Always protect your back (see Box, next page). If you have what seems to be a nonspecific backache, first try a self-help treatment (see Treating a backache, p.586). If pain persists for more than 3 or 4 days, consult your physician.

Nonspecific backache is difficult to diagnose. After examining your back, your physician may arrange for X rays to be taken of your spine to make sure that you do not have osteoarthritis (see p.588). But in most cases where a physician suspects nonspecific backache, you will be advised to continue with self-help measures for a few days. Your physician may prescribe painkillers or a muscle-relaxant drug.

Gentle massage performed by a well-trained, experienced person may provide temporary relief of symptoms.

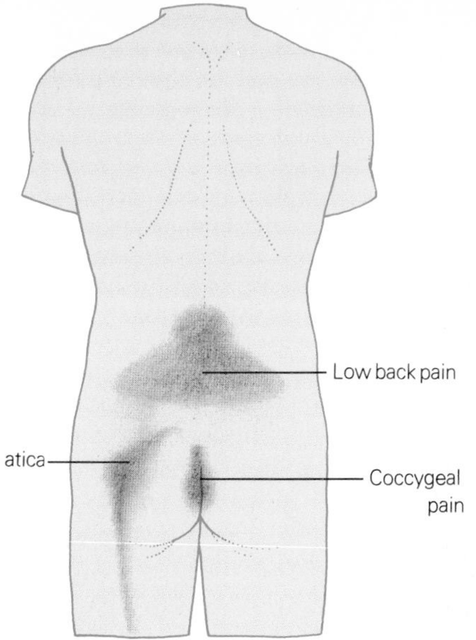

Types of back pain

Low back pain: Low back pain is centered in the small of the back and spreads from there. It is often caused by unusual exertion such as moving furniture or heavy digging in the garden. It may develop either abruptly or overnight. Low back pain may be severe, and sometimes you may be completely unable to move. Physicians disagree about the exact cause of this condition. It is probably a mixture of pulled or strained muscles, muscle spasm, or sprained ligaments.
Coccygeal pain: This term describes nonspecific backache (see previous page) that is located in the area of the coccyx, at the base of the spinal column. It can be continuous pain that is worse when you sit. It may be caused by falling on your buttocks or an injury from being hit. Women occasionally experience temporary pain in this area after childbirth. Some relief from the pain can be obtained by sitting on a soft cushion specifically designed for this purpose.
Sciatica: Sciatica is pain caused by pressure on the sciatic nerve (the largest of all the nerves, with branches throughout the lower body and legs) as it leaves the spinal cord. The pressure is generally caused by either a prolapsed disc or osteoarthritis (see next two articles). You may feel burning pain shooting into your buttocks and down along the back of your thigh, along with numbness and tingling. If you cough, sneeze, or try to bend your back, the pain may get worse.

Whatever type of back pain you have, you should consult your physician if it persists for more than 3 to 4 days.

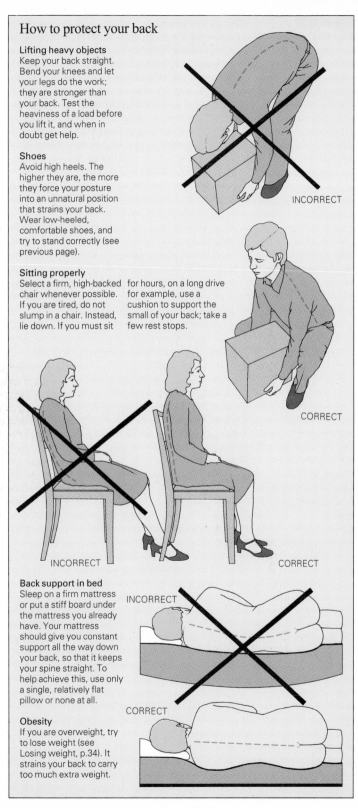

How to protect your back

Lifting heavy objects
Keep your back straight. Bend your knees and let your legs do the work; they are stronger than your back. Test the heaviness of a load before you lift it, and when in doubt get help.

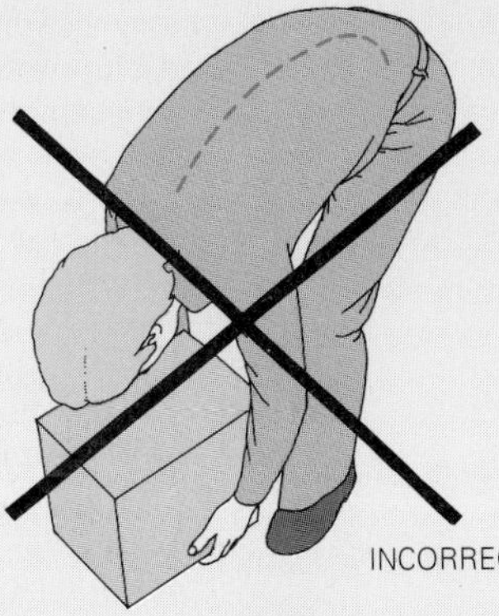

INCORRECT

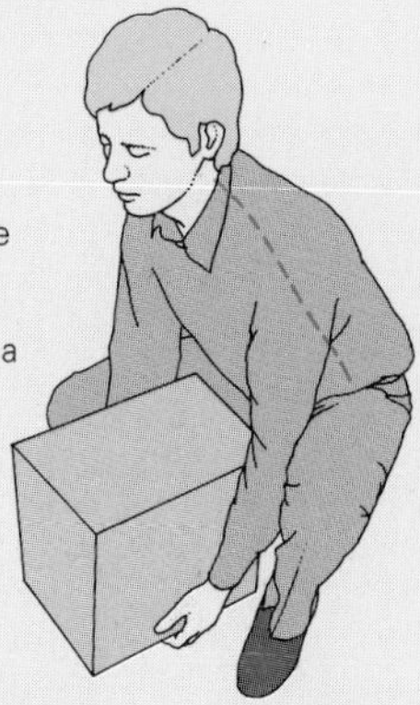

CORRECT

Shoes
Avoid high heels. The higher they are, the more they force your posture into an unnatural position that strains your back. Wear low-heeled, comfortable shoes, and try to stand correctly (see previous page).

Sitting properly
Select a firm, high-backed chair whenever possible. If you are tired, do not slump in a chair. Instead, lie down. If you must sit for hours, on a long drive for example, use a cushion to support the small of your back; take a few rest stops.

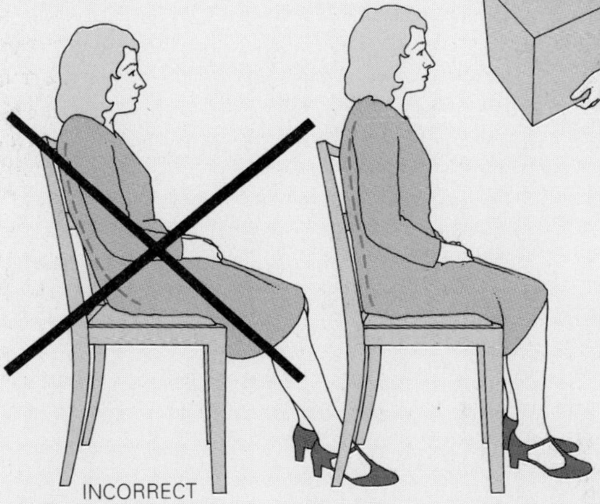

INCORRECT

CORRECT

Back support in bed
Sleep on a firm mattress or put a stiff board under the mattress you already have. Your mattress should give you constant support all the way down your back, so that it keeps your spine straight. To help achieve this, use only a single, relatively flat pillow or none at all.

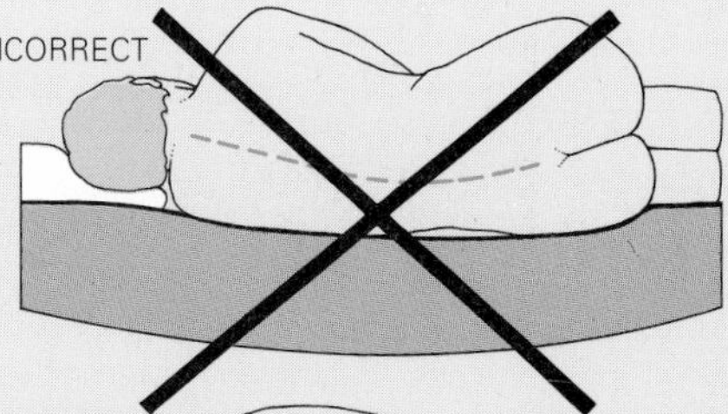

INCORRECT

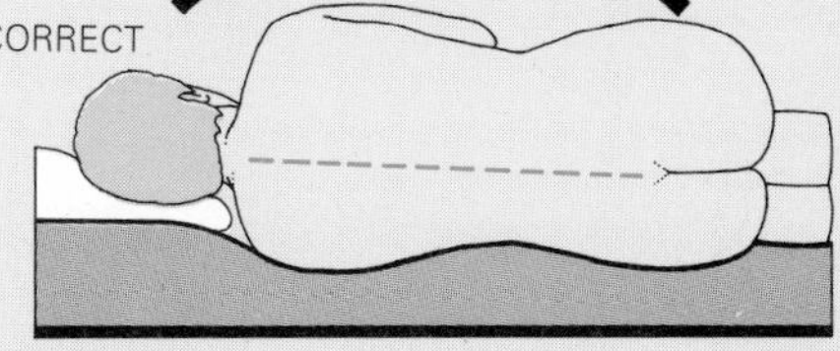

CORRECT

Obesity
If you are overweight, try to lose weight (see Losing weight, p.34). It strains your back to carry too much extra weight.

Prolapsed disc

(herniated disc)

The term "slipped disc" is often used very loosely. If you have a backache, you probably have a nonspecific backache (see previous article), not a slipped disc. A slipped disc, more correctly called a prolapsed or herniated disc, is a specific disorder. Between each vertebra and its neighbors there is a disc made up of a fibrous outer layer surrounding a jellylike inner substance. If a disc begins to degenerate and become less supple, because you are growing older or because you have been overstraining your back, the disc may prolapse. The pressure squeezes some of the softer central material out through a weak point in the harder outer layer. The result is a loss of the cushioning effect of the disc, and painful pressure on a nerve at the squeezed-out portion of the disc. Any disc may prolapse, but those in the lower back are especially susceptible. This can also occur in the neck, where pressure on a nerve root may cause pain and tingling down the arm.

What are the symptoms?

If you have a prolapsed disc in the neck portion of your spinal column, you may wake up with a sore neck. On the other hand, you may gradually become aware of numbness, tingling, or weakness in your arm.

Symptoms of a prolapsed disc may start abruptly or develop gradually. When bending over or lifting something, for example, you may suddenly feel intense pain in your back, often along with a burning pain down one or

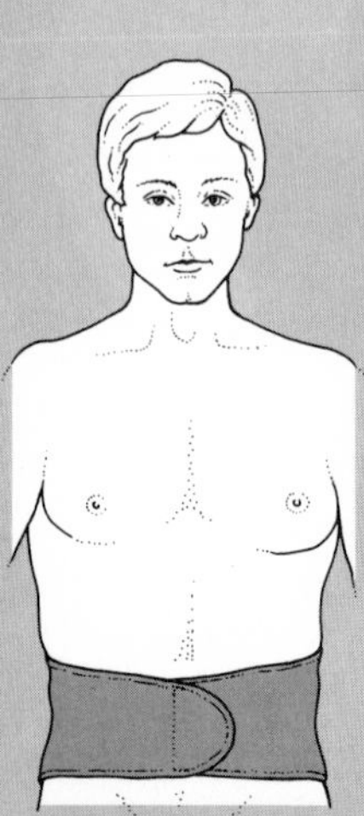

For some types of back pain, your physician may recommend that you wear a special corset (above) that supports your back. Other types of backaches respond better to complete bed rest on a firm mattress that gives overall support.

Treating a backache

The exact causes of back pain are often difficult to pinpoint. Consequently, if you develop a backache, it may be difficult for your physician to make an accurate diagnosis and prescribe immediate, precise treatment. Physicians know that a person with a backache will probably recover in a few days with the help of the simple self-help measures described below. But if your backache is severe, persistent, or recurrent, your physician may order X rays and other diagnostic tests to discover the underlying cause of the problem. Once the cause is known, you will receive more specialized treatment for your particular type of backache.

Self-help for backache

Whatever the cause of your backache, there are measures you can take to ease pain and speed healing. Take simple painkillers such as aspirin as instructed on the package. Apply heat to the painful area to ease pain. You can use an electric heating pad or a hot water bottle wrapped in a towel. Lie flat on your back for as long as you can on a bed with a firm mattress, or on an ordinary mattress with a stiff board under it. It may help to put a pillow under your ankles and calves. If your backache persists for more than 3 or 4 days despite these measures, consult your physician.

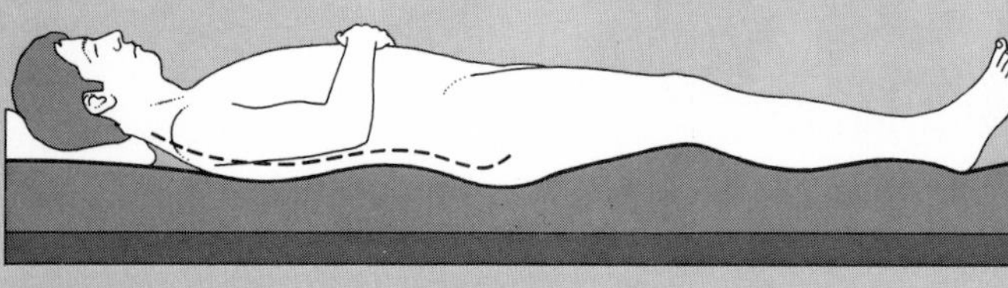

Professional help for backache

Much depends on your history of back trouble and your physician's assessment of your condition. Your physician may prescribe stronger painkillers or a muscle-relaxant drug. If you have a definable sensitive spot in the back muscles, one or more corticosteroid injections may relieve the backache rapidly but usually only temporarily. If your back pain has come on suddenly or does not respond promptly to treatment with medication and rest, your physician may recommend physical therapy. If your symptoms and signs indicate that you have a prolapsed disc, however, your physician may advise you to lie flat on your back on a firm mattress for 2 weeks. This may mean having meals in bed, using a bedpan, and having bed baths. If you get up, this can ruin the treatment. It must be complete bed rest if the treatment is to be effective.

Occasionally, backache is not relieved by these treatments. If this happens, your physician may refer you to an orthopedic surgeon or neurosurgeon for further examination and treatment. Treatment with the enzyme chymopapain is sometimes successful. In other cases, surgery may be necessary to remove the damaged portion of the disc.

As you gradually recover from your backache and cautiously resume your normal routine, your physician may advise you to do exercises to strengthen your back muscles and joints. While the condition is most likely to recur in the first few months after the first episode, you must be aware that throughout your life you will continue to be at risk for backache. Therefore remember to protect your back (see previous page) and follow any recommended exercise routine to avoid back trouble in the future.

How a prolapsed disc causes pain

The flexible discs between your vertebrae act as shock absorbers to cushion the bones from each other as you move your spine. Each disc has a hard outer layer and a soft, jellylike core. When your back is strained, pressure may push some of the soft substance through a weak point in the hard outer layer. It presses against a nerve where it leaves the spinal cord, causing pain.

A common site of pain

Spinal cord

Vertebra

Disc

Inner-disc material pressing on nerve

Ruptured disc

Nerves

both legs. The sudden strain has caused the prolapsed part of the disc to press on a nerve. Or you may have back and leg pains that come and go and build up over several weeks. If the prolapsed disc is in the lower part of your back, you may develop symptoms of sciatica (see p.585).

What are the risks?

Episodes of pain from a prolapsed disc may recur, sometimes resulting in a chronic backache or neck ache. The most serious risk is damage to the nerve roots of the spinal cord (see Spinal cord injury, p.296).

What should be done?

If you have symptoms of a prolapsed disc, see your physician. He or she will carefully examine your back and legs and may arrange for an X ray and other tests of the nerves of your spine. To locate a prolapsed or herniated disc, your physician may want you to have a CT scan or MRI scan.

Treatments for a prolapsed disc vary. If the prolapsed disc is in your neck, you may simply need to wear a supportive collar for several weeks and possibly have some graduated cervical traction (with pulleys attached to a neck collar), diathermy (heat treatment), and massage. Much will depend on your own situation and attitude and on your physician. Read the self-help and professional treatment procedures for backache that are summarized on the previous page.

Osteoarthritis of the spine

(spondylosis)

Degenerative joint disease, or osteoarthritis of the spine, is a hardening and stiffening of the spinal column that results in loss of flexibility. This happens if some of the spaces between vertebrae are narrowed because the discs between the vertebrae have degenerated and lost their elasticity through aging, overuse, or injury. In some people, bony outgrowths (spurs) develop on the vertebrae or along the edges of degenerating discs, and these may press painfully on various nerves where they join the spinal cord. Narrowing and stiffening of intervertebral joints (called facet joints) put additional strain on the backbone and its supporting structures: muscles, ligaments, and other discs. In some cases, osteoarthritis affects only one section of the spine.

What are the symptoms?

Mild cases of osteoarthritis usually do not cause symptoms. You may have the disease for many years, even your entire life, without knowing it. Often, however, you have intermittent pain in the part of your back that is most severely affected (see also Cervical osteoarthritis, p.299). Your back may become increasingly tender and difficult to bend or twist. If the lower part of your back is affected, you may have shooting pains in your buttocks and thighs; these pains are characteristic of sciatica (see p.585).

What are the risks?

If you have had frequent difficulty with a prolapsed disc in your spine (see previous article), you may be especially susceptible to osteoarthritis of the spine.

What should be done?

If you have some symptoms that suggest osteoarthritis, try the recommended self-help measures (see Box, previous page). If the symptoms persist, consult your physician, who, after examining you, may arrange for X rays, a CT scan, or an MRI scan.

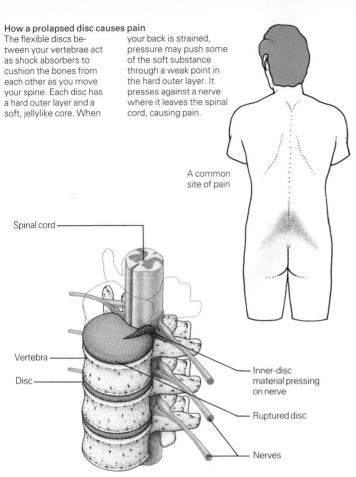

Joint disorders

Because you use one or more joints every time you move, you quickly notice any problems with them. A highly maneuverable joint, such as the hip, is a complicated structure. The entire joint is bound together by fibrous bands called ligaments. Inside the ligaments is a fibrous joint capsule lined on the inside by the synovium, a thin membrane that continuously produces tiny amounts of fluid to lubricate the joint. Where the bone ends are in contact, the surfaces are covered by cartilage.

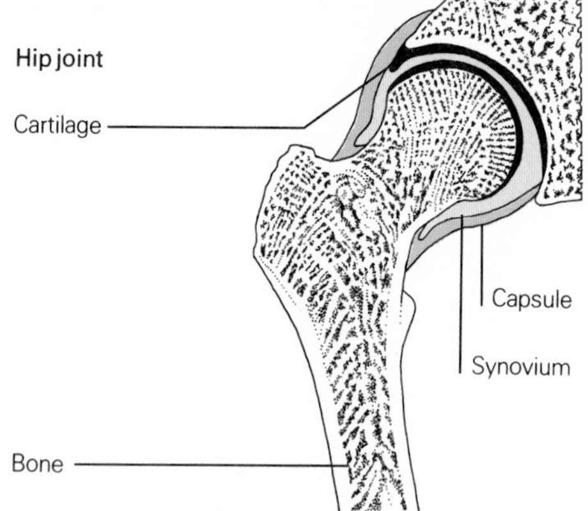

Most joint disorders are discussed in the following pages, but there are three main exceptions. Certain problems of the spinal column, which has a somewhat different construction than most other joints, are covered under backaches (see p.584). Sprains and dislocated joints are discussed under injuries (see p.573). Gout, a joint disease that is affected by diet and metabolism, is discussed in the section on disorders of digestion and nutrition (see p.467).

Osteoarthritis

(degenerative joint disease)

Osteoarthritis is a condition of unknown cause accompanied by wear and tear on the joints. It usually becomes apparent in older people, in the larger, weight-bearing joints including the hips, knees, and spine. Many people also develop changes in their finger joints, which give their hands a gnarled appearance. The smooth lining of a joint, known as the articular cartilage, begins to flake and crack. As the cartilage deteriorates, the underlying bone is affected, and may become thickened and distorted. Moving the joint becomes painful and restricted, causing you to use associated muscles less often. The unused muscles may gradually waste away, which is a natural reaction of any muscles that are unused.

What are the symptoms?

Episodes of pain, swelling, and stiffness in the affected joint occur at intervals of months or years. Although osteoarthritis often affects several joints, it is rarely severe enough to cause symptoms in more than one or two joints at a time. Pain that begins as a minor discomfort may, in some cases, eventually become severe enough to disturb sleep and interfere with everyday life.

The amount of swelling in an affected joint varies. You may hardly notice it, or your affected joint may become extremely knobby and enlarged. The pain is frequently deceptive. You may feel it directly in the area of your affected joint, or it may be transmitted to other parts of your body. This type of pain is known as referred pain. For example, osteoarthritis of the hip is sometimes felt most painfully in the front of the thigh and knee.

What are the risks?

Osteoarthritis is the most common joint disorder. If you live long enough, you are very likely to have the condition in some joints. You may or may not have symptoms from it. X rays show some degree of osteoarthritis in one or more of the joints of most people who are over 40. It seldom becomes a serious problem, however, and the disease involves no life-threatening risks. Thus, if you have osteoarthritis with no severe symptoms, there is no reason to worry about it or treat it.

Certain occupations and sports are more often associated with eventual development of osteoarthritis. Many ballet dancers get it in their feet after years of standing on their toes. Football players have also been particularly susceptible to problems with their joints as a result of repeated trauma and injuries to the joints that occur during games.

What should be done?

If you occasionally experience mild pain and stiffness in a joint, there is no cause for concern. If symptoms persist, try the self-help

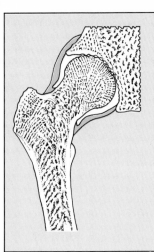

Replacing damaged joints

The replacement of natural joints with artificial ones made of metal or a combination of metal and plastic or porcelain is a constantly developing and improving form of treatment for joints that are causing chronic pain and have become almost completely immobile from an arthritic condition. If the replacement is successful, it improves movement and relieves pain. The most common and generally satisfactory replacements are of hip and knee joints, but replacement ankles, shoulders, elbows, and finger joints are also available. Improvements in design and in ways of securing the joints in place have gradually improved the long-term results, and surgeons are now more willing to operate on younger patients and at an earlier stage in the disease. Nevertheless, there is a small risk of failure; joint replacement is considered only after your physician has tried other treatments and they have not worked for you. Also, your physician evaluates the risk in terms of your general health.

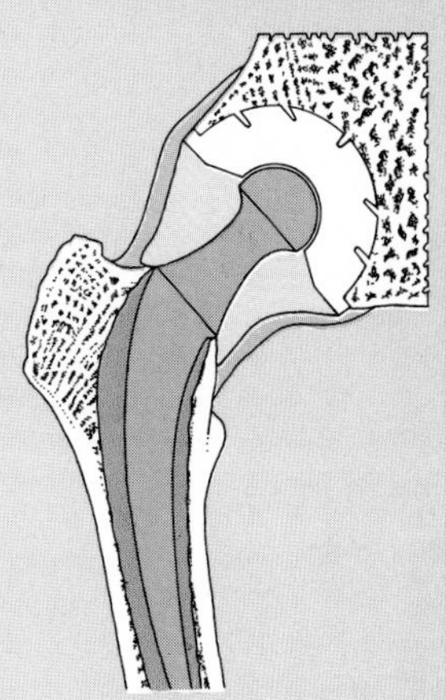

measures recommended below. Then, if necessary, consult your physician, who will examine you and may want you to have blood tests along with X rays of the affected joint or joints. If these tests do not indicate anything out of the ordinary, it is likely that your problem is osteoarthritis.

What is the treatment?

Self-help: Wear and tear on weight-bearing joints is greatest in people who are severely overweight. If this applies to you, take off some of the strain by losing weight. Use a cane (in the hand opposite the hip or knee that is affected), rest frequently, and sleep on a firm mattress. Stay warm, since heat often helps to ease joint pain.

It is important that you do not allow the muscles around the affected joints to become weak through decreased use. Regular exercise will strengthen your muscles and, in the long run, minimize your symptoms. Do not use nonprescription products that boast miracle cures. Take aspirin or other nonsteroidal anti-inflammatory drugs, such as ibuprofen, but do not use other painkillers unless they are prescribed by your physician.

Professional help: Your physician may prescribe a stronger painkiller than aspirin. Some anti-inflammatory drugs seem to ease the symptoms of osteoarthritis. If pain becomes severe, an injection of a corticosteroid drug into the painful joint may help, but this type of treatment can do more damage to the joint cartilage if it is used too often. Your physician may also arrange for you to have physical therapy, usually including exercise, massage, and heat treatments.

Surgery is sometimes recommended. A common operation is joint replacement (see Box above). Replacement of hip and knee joints is highly successful in most cases. Other joints are replaced less frequently as a result of osteoarthritis.

If you wonder whether a change in your diet might have a beneficial effect on your arthritic symptoms, the answer is simple: the only kind of diet that helps is a weight-loss diet (see p.34), since excess weight can further damage the joints and surrounding tissues. Other possible treatments, none of which can be guaranteed to help, include wearing special kinds of warm clothing (so-called thermal wear), applying heat to the affected area, and swimming regularly in a heated pool. There are no magic cures.

Do not forget that there are many devices available to assist people who are disabled by diseases such as osteoarthritis. Ask your physician for information and assistance.

Rheumatoid arthritis

Rheumatoid arthritis is a chronic disease of the joints characterized by alternating periods of active inflammation and absence of symptoms, both of variable duration. Its exact cause is unknown, but for some reason your immune system begins to form antibodies that help create a chronic inflammation of the joints. In rheumatoid arthritis the synovium, a thin membrane surrounding a joint, gradually becomes inflamed and swollen, which leads to inflammation of other parts of the affected joint.

After a series of episodes, the bones linked by the joint are slowly weakened. In severe cases, bone tissue may eventually be destroyed. The joints that are usually affected are the small ones in your hands and feet, mainly the knuckles and toe joints, but rheumatoid arthritis can occur in any joint, including your wrists, knees, ankles, or neck. It occurs less often in the spine or hips, which are much more susceptible to osteoarthritis (see previous article). The disease can also cause inflammation of the eyes, heart, lungs, and blood vessels, and changes in the tissues that are just beneath the skin.

What are the symptoms?

Rheumatoid arthritis may begin without obvious symptoms in the joints. Over several weeks or even months you may feel generally ill, listless, and without appetite. You are likely to lose weight and to have vague muscular pains and possibly a low-grade fever. Only later do you develop the joint symptoms that are typically characteristic of rheumatoid arthritis. In other cases, the inflammation flares up suddenly, without previous symptoms of any kind.

When your joints are affected, they become red, warm, swollen, tender to the touch, painful to move, and stiff. The stiffness is usually most noticeable first thing in the morning. As you move and exercise the joints, the pain and stiffness gradually become less severe.

In some people, these joint symptoms are accompanied by bursitis (see p.592). Other people become anemic (see p.450). Only one or two joints may be affected, or the disease may rapidly become widespread. Some people have only one mild episode, while others have episodes that may or may not leave them increasingly disabled. In a few cases, and it is important to emphasize that these cases are quite uncommon, continuous deterioration of joint and bone tissues produces deformities in the joints and surrounding area and makes it difficult to live an active life.

What are the risks?

Most cases of rheumatoid arthritis occur in the 20 to 40 age group, but the disease may develop in people of any age. In severe cases, swollen, deformed joints may collapse and become partly or completely dislocated. This can cause great discomfort and problems with walking if knee, ankle, or foot joints are affected. Tendons may also become so weak that they snap, making it impossible to control certain movements.

What should be done?

If you develop the symptoms described, consult your physician, who will examine your joints, and may want you to have X rays and some special blood tests. Rheumatoid arthritis can usually be diagnosed with these tests, but it may be necessary to perform a biopsy or observe the progress of the disease for several weeks or months.

What is the treatment?

Self-help: The best thing you can do is to come to terms with what may be a permanent but almost always manageable condition. Follow the advice of your physician, get plenty of rest, and exercise regularly and moderately. Swimming in a heated pool is good for stiff joints. A firm mattress and warm but lightweight covers will help you to sleep comfortably.

Professional help: If you are having an episode of rheumatoid arthritis, your physician will probably prescribe nonsteroidal anti-inflammatory drugs. He or she may recommend heat applied to the affected joints. You may be referred to a physical therapist who can teach you some helpful exercises and who may also provide you with removable splints that can be strapped onto painful joints when they need rest.

If your rheumatoid arthritis remains active, your physician will probably add a medication such as chloroquine, penicillamine, gold compounds, sulfasalazine, or methotrexate, which sometimes interrupt the process that produces arthritis.

Rheumatoid arthritis is a disorder of the immune system and, in some cases, treatment

Rheumatism and arthritis

Rheumatism and arthritis are virtually interchangeable words. They are loosely used to describe disorders characterized by red, stiff, and sometimes swollen joints and muscles. Strictly speaking, however, there is no medical condition called simply rheumatism or arthritis.

Many people believe that rheumatism is a milder condition than arthritis. According to this theory, rheumatism comes and goes, is often brought on by wet weather or strenuous activity, and is easily treated by a hot bath and a couple of aspirin. On the other hand, many people believe that arthritis is a more severe, perhaps crippling, condition—a chronic disorder that can be made bearable only with routine use of painkillers and other drugs.

In fact, no such simplified distinction between rheumatism and arthritis can be made. Do not assume that you have rheumatism because you were told that your grandparents had it. If your physician tells you that you have arthritis or rheumatism, ask for a more detailed description; then read the articles on Osteoarthritis, Rheumatoid arthritis, and other conditions in this chapter.

consists of reducing the levels of antibodies in the blood by giving the person chemotherapy (anticancer) drugs.

Surgery is playing a stronger role in the management of rheumatoid arthritis. In the early stages, a synovectomy (removal of the inflamed synovium) may be recommended if only one joint is badly affected. In later stages, replacing damaged joints may be considered (see Box p.589).

What are the long-term prospects?

Rheumatoid arthritis is as variable in its outlook as it is in its severity. Statistics indicate that in a little less than half of all cases, the person recovers completely after one or more episodes of painful joint inflammation. About the same number of people remain somewhat arthritic. Only about one in ten people who have the disease are severely disabled by it.

Infectious arthritis

(septic arthritis, bacterial arthritis)

Infectious arthritis is a rare disease caused by bacterial invasion of a joint. Bacteria may enter a joint through a wound, spread directly from a nearby infection, or be carried to a joint through the bloodstream from a distant infection. Once in a joint, the bacteria multiply and cause redness, warmth, pain, and swelling due to inflammation and accumulation of pus. More than one joint is rarely affected. The infection also causes a fever, sometimes as high as 104°F (40°C). Although many nonbacterial diseases, such as rheumatic fever, rubella, mumps, and chickenpox, can cause joints to become swollen and painful, these symptoms are not the same as infectious bacterial arthritis.

What should be done?

If you have symptoms of infectious arthritis, see your physician as soon as possible. If it is not treated, your joint may become stiff and almost useless because the cartilage can be destroyed. Your physician will examine your swollen joint, and may use a needle and syringe to draw out some of the accumulated fluid. Examination of the fluid should confirm the diagnosis. Antibiotic drugs are used to treat the disease. In addition, a surgeon may need to open the affected joint so that the pus can be drained. Once the infection is eradicated, you will be taught how to exercise your joint carefully but thoroughly to prevent it from becoming permanently stiff.

Ankylosing spondylitis

Spondylitis is inflammation of the joints that link the vertebrae; it usually occurs in young men. In ankylosing spondylitis, the inflammation subsides but leaves behind damaged joints and thickened long spinal ligaments that, in effect, fuse together the individual bones of the spine. The cause of this debilitating disease is not known.

The first joints to be affected are the sacroiliac joints, which link the base of the spine to the pelvis, or hip bone. Bony growths fuse the normally separate bones together, and the resultant stiffness may move slowly up your spine until it affects many, if not all, of the joints between your vertebrae.

What are the symptoms?

Ankylosing spondylitis often starts with pain in the lower portion of the back, which may spread to the buttocks. The pain and stiffness are generally most severe in the morning. You may also have stiff, painful hips and a general feeling of stiffness in your spine. Other possible symptoms are vague chest pains. You may also have loss of energy, weight loss, a poor appetite, and a slight fever. For reasons that are not clear, your eyes may become red and painful.

What are the risks?

Ankylosing spondylitis is much more prevalent in men than in women and occurs mainly in the 20 to 40 age group. It also seems to run in families.

The disease may be confined to the lower part of the spine, or it may be more generalized, resulting in a stiff spinal column that may cause your head to be permanently bent down onto your chest. The ribs can also become involved at the point where they join your spine, and this reduces your ability to breathe. Chest infection then becomes a risk. Also, your jaw may be stiff, which causes difficulty in both eating and speaking.

What should be done?

If you have symptoms of ankylosing spondylitis, consult your physician, who will examine you with special attention to the range of your back movements and chest expansion. You may need to have blood tests and X rays of your back and pelvic area before a diagnosis can be made.

What is the treatment?

Self-help: A regular daily exercise routine is essential. Swimming is especially beneficial.

Breathe deeply, sleep on a firm mattress, and do not use a pillow. Try to teach yourself to sleep on your stomach rather than on your back or side. All of these self-help measures help keep your back muscles strong and provide more mobility.

Professional help: Your physician may refer you to a physical therapist, who will teach you appropriate exercises. Your physician may prescribe painkilling and nonsteroidal anti-inflammatory drugs.

If your spine is very badly bent, it may be improved by osteotomy, a surgical procedure that is sometimes used to straighten bent, fused bones. However, osteotomy is performed only in extreme cases.

Bunions

(hallux valgus)

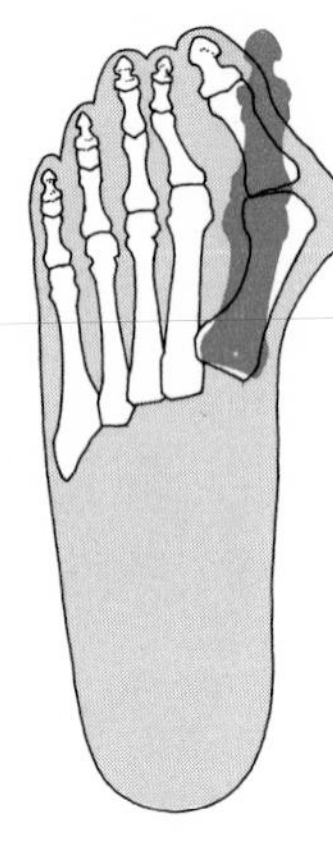

Normal position of big toe shown in color

A bunion is a bony protrusion from the inside edge of the joint at the base of the big toe. Bunions are part of "hallux valgus," which refers to a big toe that points toward your little toe. Occasionally, the toes may overlap. Hallux valgus tends to run in families. Poorly fitted shoes, especially those with very high heels and pointed toes, make it worse. One result of the deformity is that the bony base of the twisted big toe is pushed out beyond the normal outline of the foot and forms a bump known as a bunion. As this rubs on the inside of your shoes, the overlying skin toughens and thickens into a callus (see p.269).

What are the risks?

Although bunions are common, they are not usually troublesome. Three times as many women as men have bunions.

Sometimes the persistent pressure of a shoe on a bunion causes painful bursitis (see next article). The affected joint is likely to develop degenerative joint disease (see p.588) sooner than it normally would.

What should be done?

Without treatment, a bunion will get worse. If you have a bunion that causes pain and makes it difficult to walk, consult your physician, who will examine your feet and may refer you to an orthopedic surgeon.

What is the treatment?

Self-help: Always make sure your shoes fit comfortably and leave plenty of room for your toes. If you have bursitis, you can relieve pressure on the bunion and give it a chance to heal by wearing a shoe with extra room for the toes (for example, by cutting a hole in the top of an old, comfortable shoe and wearing it until the inflammation subsides). Occasionally, the symptoms can be helped by a bunion splint.

Professional help: If you have a severe hallux valgus, you may be advised to have surgery. After an operation, the foot is usually protected in a special shoe or a cast for 6 to 12 weeks, depending on the type of surgery that was performed.

Bursitis

A bursa is a soft sac that contains a lubricating liquid that minimizes friction between body tissues that must constantly move by each other. Bursae are usually found near joints, either between the skin and underlying bones or between tendons and bones. If a bursa is irritated by pressure over it or by injury to the nearby joint, the sac may become inflamed and distended with fluid. This is called bursitis. It is a fairly common condition that causes pain and swelling in the area around the bursa.

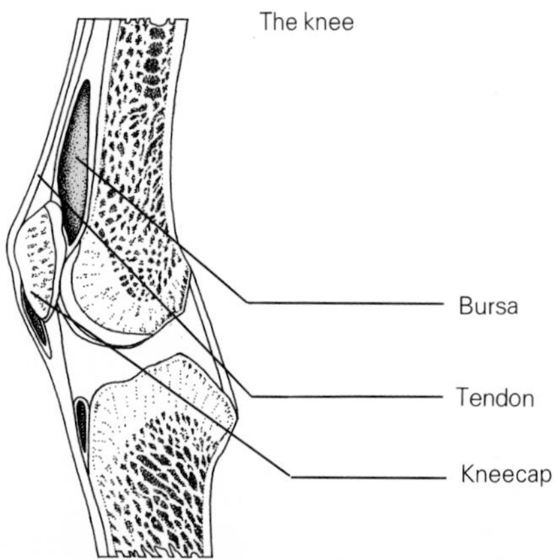

Olecranon bursitis is a familiar type of bursitis that occurs around the elbow. Other joints that are particularly susceptible to bursitis include the kneecap, the hips, the heel, the base of the big toe (see Bunions, previous article), and the shoulders.

What should be done?

Bursitis often is not a serious disorder. It may clear up on its own in a week or so, especially if you keep pressure off the tender spot while it remains swollen. If bursitis persists, consult your physician, who will examine your joint to make the diagnosis. To bring down any swelling and relieve pain and stiffness, nonsteroidal anti-inflammatory drugs may be prescribed. Your physician may draw off the fluid with a needle and give injections of a corticosteroid medication along with a local anesthetic, to relieve pain and inflammation.

Bursitis often recurs in the same place. Ask your physician to tell you about exercises to help prevent formation of scar tissue, and do them faithfully. It is important to learn to avoid putting pressure over the area that is inflamed. Occasionally, a bursa can become infected and surgery becomes necessary. If conservative treatment fails, surgical removal of the bursa is needed.

Frozen shoulder

(adhesive capsulitis)

In a frozen shoulder, the shoulder becomes stiff and painful, so that normal movement is impossible. It usually starts as a slight injury or a minor problem such as tendinitis (see p.578), or bursitis (see previous article), which prevents you from using the joint. This lack of use leads to more stiffness and pain, followed by more disuse, weakening of the tissues, and loss of function of the shoulder. Eventually, you can hardly move your arm, and the pain is often severe enough to disturb your sleep. The pain may be localized either in your shoulder or (more frequently) it may spread to the upper part of your arm, your neck, or both.

If it is not treated, the condition runs a slow course. Symptoms gradually become worse over several months, resulting in a stiffened, immobile shoulder. Symptoms may remain the same for a few months, sometimes followed by a slow period of partial improvement. Thereafter, you usually feel no more pain, but your shoulder mobility often remains permanently impaired and may interfere with your activities. It is important to seek professional help quickly if you think a frozen shoulder may be developing.

What is the treatment?

A frozen shoulder should be kept in motion as much as possible. Use a nonsteroidal anti-inflammatory drug such as aspirin. Your physician may teach you, or may refer you to a physical therapist who will teach you, how to improve your mobility with exercises, including those to preserve or increase the range of motion of your shoulder. Injection of corticosteroid drugs into the shoulder increases the pain for about 24 hours, but sometimes proves helpful in the long run. If your problem is severe and persistent, your physician may recommend that you have your shoulder manipulated as far as possible under a general anesthetic. With treatment and regular exercising, your chances for recovery of pain-free mobility are good.

Connective tissue diseases

Connective tissue is an essential part of every structure in the body. Its major component is a protein known as collagen. Through inflammatory changes in blood vessels and other connective tissue, diseases of the connective tissue can affect virtually all body systems. Although each condition is separate and distinctive, the symptoms are often similar. While joint areas are frequently affected, very little destruction of bone and cartilage occurs.

The causes of this group of diseases are unknown. Physicians do know that the body's natural defense system, called the immune system, starts to work abnormally, and antibodies formed in the body begin to attack a person's own body cells and their components (normally the immune system attacks only those things that are foreign to the body, such as bacteria or viruses). The resulting inflammation damages the body's own connective tissue; this effect has led to connective tissue diseases being described as "autoimmune disorders."

These disorders are unpredictable; some people have a fluctuating pattern of improvement and relapse while other people never regain full health. Sometimes a person's disease will "burn out," never to recur. Although there is no specific cure for these disorders, treatment with drugs relieves their symptoms and slows their progression. Many people with autoimmune disorders continue to lead active lives.

One of these disorders, systemic lupus erythematosus, is described in detail below, but all autoimmune disorders share some common characteristics.

Systemic lupus erythematosus

(SLE)

In systemic lupus erythematosus, often called SLE, connective tissue in any part of the body may become inflamed, damaging the skin, joints, and internal organs. The underlying reason why the immune system forms antibodies against cell nuclei, DNA and RNA, cell proteins, phospholipids, red and white blood cells, and other structures is unknown. These antibodies become joined to their targets as immune complexes that provoke the inflammation. Typically, the disease flares up for a few weeks and then goes into a period of inactivity.

What are the symptoms?

Because the disorder affects so many body systems, general symptoms are common, including fatigue, a sense of ill health, loss of appetite, loss of weight, and fever.

The skin is affected in 80 percent of cases, usually with a butterfly-shaped rash over the cheeks and the bridge of the nose. A more general rash often affects those areas of the skin exposed to sunlight. You may lose some or all of your hair. Skin ulcers and skin nodules may form.

Around 95 percent of people with lupus have some problems with their joints and muscles, with pain more common than deformity. About 85 percent have anemia or another blood disorder, including either ineffective blood clotting or unwanted clotting in the veins or arteries causing an embolism, stroke, or other problems.

About half the people with lupus have kidney damage, revealed by protein in the urine. In a minority of people, progressive damage to the kidneys causes symptoms of kidney failure (see p.550).

About 60 percent of people with lupus have symptoms related to damage to the brain and nervous system, such as mild mental dysfunction, seizures, a partial paralysis, impaired coordination, or damage to nerves in the arms and legs. Chest pain may result from inflammation of the pericardium (the membrane that encloses the heart), pleurisy, or inflammation of the lungs.

Virtually every body system may be affected—from the eyes to the intestines. SLE affects mostly women. Because of the blood-clotting abnormalities, miscarriages are common in pregnant women with SLE. The disease often flares up in the early months of pregnancy. Nevertheless, many women with the disease have successful pregnancies and give birth to healthy infants.

What are the risks?

SLE affects about one person in 20,000 in the US; most of these are young women. The disease usually becomes chronic and requires some form of continuing treatment. More than three fourths of people with the disorder remain in reasonably good health 10 years after the first symptoms, but in a minority of cases kidney failure or repeated infections may be life-threatening or even fatal.

What should be done?

Your physician will arrange for a thorough medical evaluation, including blood tests for the presence of antibodies. SLE sometimes develops as a side effect of treatment with drugs, especially if you take hydralazine for high blood pressure, and your physician will want details of all medications you have taken recently. Further tests of specific organs, such as kidney biopsy, are sometimes needed. Occasionally, it is not possible to make a certain diagnosis, and a period of observation is recommended.

In about one third of patients, the disease remains mild and the only treatment required is with nonsteroidal anti-inflammatory drugs. In more severe cases the usual mainstays of treatment are corticosteroid drugs and immunosuppressive drugs. To avoid the rash associated with exposure to sunlight, wear a sunblock lotion and protective clothing (including a hat) when necessary.

Several experimental treatments aimed at the immune system are under evaluation, including plasmapheresis, in which part of the fluid portion of blood is removed repeatedly, taking with it the damaging antibodies and immune complexes. People in whom end-stage kidney failure develops require treatment with dialysis or kidney transplantation.

Polyarteritis nodosa

(periarteritis nodosa)

In polyarteritis nodosa your small and medium arteries become inflamed, causing damage to one or more of the organs of your body in which the arteries are located. The effects of the condition may be localized or generalized, depending on which of your arteries are inflamed.

What are the symptoms?

Most commonly your skin, joints, peripheral nerves, intestines, and/or heart are involved. Lung damage produces shortness of breath. Liver, gallbladder, and intestinal damage may cause abdominal pain. Weakness and numbness of your arms and legs can occur.

Kidney involvement may produce blood in the urine or swelling of your face, arms, and legs, or both. Such symptoms often are accompanied by fatigue, pain, persistent fever, weight loss, and rapid heartbeat.

What are the risks?
Polyarteritis nodosa is a rare condition. Three times as many men as women get it. Without treatment, the disease can be rapidly fatal.

What should be done?
With treatment, some damage may be prevented. If you survive 1 year of the disease with treatment, you have a good chance of living for many more years. Many tests, including arteriography, may be needed before the diagnosis of polyarteritis nodosa can be made. Treatment depends on which organs are damaged. Corticosteroids or anticancer agents, or both, may be prescribed.

Scleroderma

(systemic sclerosis)

In scleroderma the connective tissue becomes inflamed in and around tiny blood vessels called capillaries. Scarring occurs that makes the tissues shrink and become stiff.

What are the symptoms?
Your skin and underlying tissues and your esophagus are almost always affected. Your lungs, kidneys, and other organs are also occasionally involved. If you have Raynaud's phenomenon (see p.440), your blood vessels may be involved. Patches of skin become shiny and uncomfortably tight. Your esophagus may stiffen so that swallowing difficulties may occur. Also, there may be a persistent slight fever, loss of weight, and a feeling of general ill health.

What are the risks?
Kidney failure (see p.550), heart failure (see p.408), scarring of the lungs with progressive shortness of breath, and joint impairment similar to that caused by rheumatoid arthritis (see p.589) may be present with scleroderma.

What should be done?
Scleroderma is rare, but if you suspect you have it, see your physician, who will arrange for blood tests and other investigations. If the diagnosis is confirmed, many of the symptoms can be prevented with drugs. Physical therapy can help maintain independent function. However, the tight skin and stiffness usually remain.

Polymyositis and dermatomyositis

Polymyositis is inflammation of multiple muscles, most commonly those around your shoulders and pelvis. The inflamed muscles gradually become weak. If the disease is accompanied by skin inflammation, it is called dermatomyositis. In such cases, a rash often spreads over your face, shoulders, arms, and bony prominences such as your knuckles. In all cases of polymyositis and dermatomyositis, you feel generally ill.

Two thirds of those who get polymyositis and dermatomyositis are women. A diagnosis is made based on blood tests, electromyography (tests of the electrical properties of the painful muscles), and by muscle biopsy. In a biopsy, a small sample of tissue is removed for examination.

What is the treatment?
Treatment is aimed at suppressing inflammation and minimizing symptoms. High doses of corticosteroid drugs are often prescribed. In some cases, immunosuppressive drugs are also prescribed. A physical therapist can teach you exercises to minimize weakness and shrinkage of muscles. Occasionally, the disease disappears by itself after a few years.

Polymyalgia rheumatica

This is a fairly common disease after age 50, and it occurs twice as often in women as in men. It affects many muscle areas, particularly those of your neck, shoulders, and buttocks. The involved muscles and adjacent joints become weak and stiff, especially in the morning. You may also have a slight fever and feel ill. In some cases temporal arteritis (see p.439) also develops and visual disturbances may occur, including blindness.

When you consult your physician, in addition to blood tests, a biopsy of one of the temporal arteries at the side of your head may be performed. Often, ordinary painkillers and nonsteroidal anti-inflammatory drugs such as aspirin or iboprofen may control your symptoms. In severe cases, corticosteroid drugs are prescribed, and improvement may be dramatic. Usually, the condition disappears on its own after a few years.

General infections and infestations

Introduction

The articles in this section deal with diseases caused by identifiable organisms that live in or on the human body. Infections are caused by minute organisms invisible to the naked eye that invade and multiply within the body. Some bacteria, viruses, *Chlamydia*, protozoa, and fungi cause infections in healthy people, while others cause infections only in people whose natural defenses have been weakend. The body's natural defenses are known as the immune system. In general, the body is capable of mounting a counterattack, through the immune system, against such invading organisms. An infection occurs when the counterattack fails to control the organisms.

The infections discussed in the following pages have general effects on the body. Infections that attack specific parts of the body, such as pneumonia, bronchitis, and dysentery, are discussed in the relevant sections; for example, hepatitis, which is an infection of the liver, is discussed in Liver, gallbladder, and pancreas, see p.522. Infections that are primarily children's diseases, such as mumps or chickenpox, are discussed in Childhood infectious diseases (see p.744).

The parasites that cause infestations are larger organisms than those that cause general infections. The problems caused by bites from some common insects, including ticks, are also included in this section.

Many of the organisms that are responsible for general infections and infestations are contagious; that is, they spread from person to person.

Some diseases that could be classified as general infections are not included because they are very rare in the US. One is leprosy, a bacterial disease that causes permanent damage to skin and nerves but is very minimally contagious. Leprosy can be treated effectively with modern medications.

Viruses and bacteria

The two major infectious agents are viruses and bacteria. Viruses cause damage by taking over cells, including their reproductive mechanisms, and manufacturing thousands of new viruses in your body. In the process, your cells are usually destroyed and others are invaded. Only a few viral infections can be treated with antiviral drugs; most cannot (including the common cold).

Bacteria live virtually everywhere, including in and on your body. Problems arise, however, when the harmless bacteria in your body multiply in great numbers and cause infections or when harmful bacteria enter your body—for example, through a cut on the skin or in the food you eat. Bacteria cause disease by producing toxins (poisons) that damage cells. Most bacteria can be controlled by use of antibiotic drugs, and diseases caused by bacteria are less common than they once were and less threatening when they do occur.

Three types of bacteria

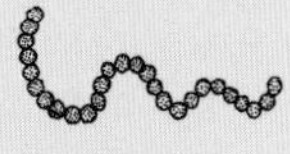

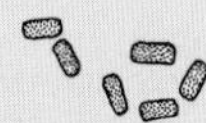

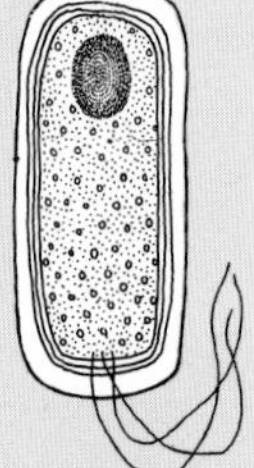

Infections

The organisms that enter your body and cause infections are spread in various ways. People spread infectious organisms by coughing or sneezing them into the air or by direct contact such as a handshake. Some infectious agents spread to humans from animals or animal products (meat or eggs). If the spread of an organism that causes an infection can be halted, the disease may possibly be eradicated, as for example smallpox has been.

If you have an infectious disease, you should take precautions against passing it on to relatives, friends, and coworkers. There are several ways in which you can prevent the spread of infection. Infectious organisms enter the air when you cough or sneeze and can be transmitted to your hands when you blow your nose. When you have a cold avoid shaking hands and handling food that someone else might eat (such as during cooking). Blow your nose into tissues rather than handkerchiefs so that you can discard them or flush them down the toilet.

Gastrointestinal infections are commonly transmitted by poor hygiene, especially among those who prepare food in restaurants. People who have diarrhea and/or bouts of vomiting should wash their hands thoroughly after using the toilet. Do not let anyone use your towel or washcloth.

If you suspect that you have a sexually transmitted disease (see p.654), it is important that you use a condom or abstain from sexual contact until your physician tells you that you do not have such a disease, that the disease is in a stage when it cannot be transmitted, or that you have been cured.

Once infectious agents enter your body, it takes time for them to multiply and cause symptoms. This period before symptoms appear is called the incubation period. It generally varies from a few days to several months, depending on the disease. Physicians know the incubation periods for certain infectious diseases, so if you get one of those diseases, it is often possible to figure out when, where, and how you caught it.

The symptoms of an infection are caused by the body's reaction to fighting infection. Your white blood cells attack invading organisms either by trying to engulf them or by producing antibodies to inactivate them. This process causes symptoms.

Immunization (see p.748) along with antibacterial, antibiotic, and antifungal drugs are often used to assist your natural defenses. However, antibiotics do not work against most viruses. That is why viral diseases such as colds and infectious mononucleosis are not treated with antibiotics.

Influenza

(flu)

Influenza, usually called flu, is caused by a virus that spreads from one person to another in the spray from coughs and sneezes and more commonly from hand-to-hand contact such as hand shaking. The virus enters the upper part of the respiratory tract through the nose or mouth and may also invade the rest of the tract, including the lungs. Symptoms appear after an incubation period (the time between the infection and the beginning of symptoms) of 1 to 4 days. Influenza epidemics, affecting many people within a community, occur in winter or early spring.

What are the symptoms?

Among the early symptoms are chills, a temperature that may be as high as 104°F (about 40°C), sneezing, headache, muscle pain, and a sore throat. These are usually followed by a dry, hacking cough and, often, chest pains. The fever generally lasts for 3 to 5 days and leaves you feeling weak for another few days. If there are no complications, you should be fully recovered within 1 or 2 weeks. The weakness may persist for several weeks after recovery.

What are the risks?

Epidemics of influenza occur at unpredictable intervals. A winter may pass without an epidemic, or may bring 2 or 3 epidemics. In a severe outbreak, most people in an affected area have at least a mild form of the disease.

Epidemics die out when everyone who has been infected by a particular strain, or type, of flu virus becomes immune (resistant) to further attack by that strain. There are several strains of influenza virus; the most common are A and B types. Public health officials name new strains according to their assumed place of origin, such as Bangkok flu or Leningrad flu. Immunity from one strain is only temporary and may not protect you from other flu viruses.

The danger of flu
Sometimes flu symptoms are confined mainly to the upper respiratory tract. But if you have a bacterial infection complicating the flu, infectious organisms may spread through the trachea down to the lungs, causing pneumonia.

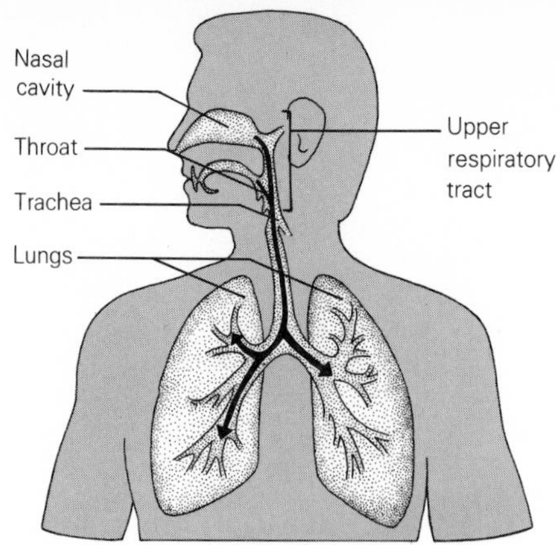

The main risk of influenza is that a complicating bacterial infection may spread from the upper respiratory tract down into the lungs and cause bronchitis (see p.379) or even pneumonia (see p.384). Such complications usually occur in very young children, older people, heavy smokers, people with diabetes, or people with chronic chest disorders and chronic heart disease.

What should be done?
Influenza must run its course, but you can ease the symptoms by using the self-help measures recommended here. You probably do not need to see your physician unless you are among the groups most susceptible to complications, as discussed above. If you seem to be the only person in your area with the flu, you may have a different viral disease (for some examples, see Infectious mononucleosis, p.601, and Fungal diseases of the lungs, next article).

What is the treatment?
Self-help: Go to bed as soon as symptoms begin and stay there until your temperature returns to normal. Take aspirin or an aspirin substitute if you are an adult. A child or a teenager should take an aspirin substitute rather than aspirin, because of association between aspirin and Reye's syndrome (see p.713). Drink as much water or fruit juice as you comfortably can. If your fever lasts for more than 3 or 4 days or if you become short of breath while resting, call your physician. You may feel weak, and possibly depressed, for a week or more after your temperature drops, and you should rest as much as possible until you have completely recovered.
Professional help: There is no specific treatment for influenza, since antibiotics are not effective against viruses. However, amantadine (an antiviral drug) sometimes prevents or relieves symptoms caused by an influenza A virus if the drug is started just as symptoms develop. Or your physician may recommend amantadine before symptoms start, especially if there are many cases of flu in your area and you are older or have a chronic disease. If a complication such as bacterial pneumonia develops, however, antibiotics will be prescribed.

Physicians advise people who are most at risk from complications (including infants, older people, and those with chronic lung diseases) to have annual injections of an anti-influenza vaccine. Because the virus changes almost every year, the vaccine must be updated each year and cannot guarantee protection. The vaccine protects you for only one winter or less, even against the strain for which it is effective.

Fungal diseases of the lungs

Several diseases are caused by different types of fungus (mold) that primarily infect the lungs. Fungal diseases of the lungs include blastomycosis, cryptococcosis, histoplasmosis, and coccidioidomycosis; they begin when you breathe in fungus spores.

Different types of fungus occur in different environments. The fungus that causes cryptococcosis is carried in chicken and pigeon droppings; while the coccidioidomycosis fungus lives in semiarid desert soil, most commonly in parts of Arizona and the San Joaquin valley. The histoplasmosis fungus is mostly found east of the Mississippi River. It flourishes in soil enriched with bird and/or bat droppings.

Fungal diseases may clear up without treatment. However, they can also spread throughout the body via the bloodstream and cause dangerous complications.

What are the symptoms?
Most of these diseases begin with flulike symptoms (see Influenza, previous article) that may include fever, a cough, chest pain, and muscle aches; severity of the symptoms varies. In cryptococcosis, you may have no symptoms, or you may have weight loss, night sweats, and shortness of breath in addition to the flulike symptoms mentioned above. With coccidioidomycosis, some people also have a red rash on the skin that looks like measles.

Blastomycosis sometimes causes painless skin lesions and can lead to prostatitis (see p.617) in men.

What are the risks?

Although most people who get fungal diseases of the lung recover in a few weeks without treatment, in some cases the disease spreads through the bloodstream to other parts of the body. People who have diabetes, chronic lung, blood, or kidney diseases, or cancer are particularly susceptible to complications. Pregnant women are especially at risk for coccidioidomycosis. Older people and young children are also more likely to have severe symptoms and complications. Also, fungal lung infections can lead to chronic lung disease.

If a fungal lung disease spreads, one of the possible complications is meningitis (see p.290), an inflammation of one of the membranes that surround the brain. The symptoms of this serious condition include fever, headache, confusion, and stiff neck.

What should be done?

If you have the symptoms listed above and they do not improve within about 2 weeks, see your physician. He or she will perform an examination and may order some blood tests and take samples of phlegm from a cough; spinal fluid; urine; or some other body fluid to test for signs of a fungal infection or some other cause of your prolonged symptoms.

What is the treatment?

If your physician diagnoses a fungal lung infection and if the symptoms are severe or you are particularly susceptible to the spread of the disease, your physician will probably prescribe an antifungal medication. The medication may be given intravenously. This treatment can sometimes clear up the infection, but several weeks of treatment may be required.

Sporotrichosis

Sporotrichosis is a skin disease caused by a fungus (mold). This fungus lives in soil and decaying vegetation, and the infectious spores are often picked up from rose thorns and splinters from rotting wood. Gardeners, farmers, and children are often infected.

The disease occurs when a contaminated thorn or sharp object punctures the skin and introduces the spores into a wound. A warty, crusting sore appears within 2 weeks. The ulcer is painless, but it does not heal, and the infection spreads to the lymph nodes directly above it. The infected area has a large sore with a series of small ulcers or inflamed lymph nodes in a line above it.

If you have been exposed to spores and think that you have an infected area that looks like this, see your physician, who will probably take a sample of pus from the sores for laboratory tests. If sporotrichosis is diagnosed, your physician will prescribe an antifungal medication to heal the sore.

Staphylococcal infections

Staphylococcus aureus bacteria normally live in the nose, mouth, rectum, or genital area without causing any kind of infection. However, when an injury such as a puncture wound introduces the organism into some other part of the body, the *Staphylococcus* bacteria can secrete toxic substances that tunnel into tissues, destroying and dissolving matter along the way. The bacteria can produce pus-containing abscesses anywhere on or in the body. If you have an illness such as chronic liver or kidney disease, diabetes, or cancer, you are particularly susceptible to infection by *Staphylococcus* bacteria.

Staphylococcal skin infections

Several fairly common skin infections can be caused by *Staphylococcus* bacteria. Boils (see p.267), impetigo (see p.273), cellulitis (see p.273), and paronychia (see p.281), which affects the nails, are some examples. *Staphylococcus* bacteria can infect any open cut or wound on the skin.

Folliculitis This staphylococcal infection is a smaller version of a boil. Small, white-headed pimples erupt around hair follicles anywhere on the body. Friction, blockage of the follicle, or injury (such as a cut from shaving) can cause a rashlike eruption.

Staphylococcal scalded skin syndrome This infection occurs only in infants and young children. A form of the *Staphylococcus* bacteria produces a toxin (poison) that forms fluid-filled blisters that dislodge the top layer of skin.

Toxic shock syndrome In this disease a staphylococcal infection somewhere in the body releases a toxin into the bloodstream that causes fever, diarrhea, and a sunburnlike rash that leads eventually to skin peeling. Toxic shock syndrome was widely publicized in the early 1980s because of an epidemic associated with staphylococcal infections caused by using super-absorbent tampons. Toxic shock syndrome may also occur less commonly along with infected wounds, surgery, or other staphylococcal infections. The full-blown syndrome may lead to profound lowering of blood pressure and damage to the liver, kidneys, and other organs; it can be fatal if not treated promptly.

Wound complications Any skin wounds, whether they are caused by an injury or made during surgery, can be complicated by infections caused by *Staphylococcus* bacteria ordinarily found on the skin. Symptoms and signs are the oozing of pus, pain, redness, heat, and fever and chills.

Other staphylococcal infections

Staphylococcus bacteria can infect any part of your body. In the eye, they can cause styes (see p.340), some types of conjunctivitis (see p.343), and orbital cellulitis (see p.353). In the breast they can cause a breast abscess (see p.632), particularly in nursing mothers.

Staphylococcal infections may develop in bones and joints from bacteria that spread through the bloodstream. As the organism circulates in the bloodstream, it tends to lodge in the long bones of the arms and legs, or somewhere within the vertebrae. In the lungs, staphylococcal pneumonia can develop (see Pneumonia, p.384). This type of pneumonia may occur if the bacteria circulates in the bloodstream, if an abscess lodges on one of the valves on the right side of the heart, or along with influenza (see p.597).

If *Staphylococcus* infects the inner lining of the heart, endocarditis will develop (see p.422). This disorder can cause irreversible heart damage and is fatal in some cases. Staphylococcal food poisoning with cramps, vomiting, and diarrhea can occur if you eat food that contains toxins produced by the bacteria (see Box, p.495).

Staphylococcus infrequently causes a colon infection if you take an antibiotic medication that kills many kinds of bacteria, including those that normally live in the digestive tract. This may upset the balance of microorganisms in the intestines, so that staphylococci then overmultiply and cause abdominal pain, a swollen abdomen, and bloody diarrhea.

What is the treatment?

In mild cases of staphylococcal infection such as folliculitis or boils, cleaning the infected area with soap and water and eliminating the cause of the infection often clears up the problem. If the infection persists despite self-help treatment, or if you have severe symptoms, see your physician. He or she will probably prescribe an antibiotic to combat the infection.

Streptococcal infections

Like *Staphylococcus aureus*, streptococci are bacteria commonly found on the skin, in the nose and throat, and elsewhere in the body where they seem to cause no harm. However, *Streptococcus* bacteria are also responsible for a substantial number of sore throats and wound infections.

Streptococcal sore throat

It is impossible to distinguish between sore throat caused by infection with *Streptococcus pyogenes* ("strep throat") from that caused by a virus infection without seeing your physician. Both the bacterial and virus infections are common in childhood between ages 5 and 15. If the tonsils are substantially enlarged and fiery red, strep throat is likely. To determine if you have strep throat, your physician will take a sample of secretions from your throat (a throat culture) for laboratory analysis. An "instant" strep test, taken in your physician's office, can produce results in as few as 10 to 30 minutes. If you do not have strep throat, you may have a virus infection. Initial symptoms of virus infections mimic those of a cold, such as runny nose and watery eyes.

Streptococcal skin infections

Streptococcus bacteria are responsible for many types of skin infections, including those associated with burns and simple cuts and bruises, and with infected surgical incisions. Streptococci also cause cellulitis (see p.273) and impetigo (see p.273).

Other streptococcal infections

Streptococcus viridans bacteria live harmlessly in the mouth, but if the heart is damaged (from a congenital defect or rheumatic fever) the bacteria may infect the heart valves, causing a life-threatening illness, subacute infective endocarditis (see p.422). Other streptococci may cause urinary infections and infections of the female genital tract.

What is the treatment?

Because of the risk of serious complications, all streptococcal infections should be treated by a physician. Your physician may use swabs to take samples from your throat or other areas of the body or use other diagnostic tests, including blood tests, to determine the cause of the infection. Treatment with antibiotics is usually rapidly effective.

Infectious mononucleosis
("mono")

Infectious mononucleosis is a virus infection sometimes known as "mono." It is also called "the kissing disease" because it is passed from one person to another through oral contact. It is more common in teenagers and young adults, often those who are away from home at school, and seems to strike them during stressful periods such as final examination times. Infectious mononucleosis is caused by either the Epstein-Barr or cytomegalic virus. If you get mononucleosis, the virus may spread to almost any organ.

What are the symptoms?
You may think at first that you have influenza, since the early symptoms of infectious mononucleosis are similar to those of flu. These include fever, chills, headache, sore throat, and a profound feeling of illness and weakness. After a day or so, you may also notice that you have painful, swollen glands in your neck, armpits, and/or groin. In addition, you may develop jaundice (see p.522) or a skin rash similar to that of rubella (see p.746). The skin rash is sometimes aggravated if your physician prescribes ampicillin for your sore throat before mononucleosis is diagnosed. All these major symptoms usually disappear within 2 to 3 weeks, but you will probably feel weak and lack energy for a couple of weeks to several months. You may also be depressed.

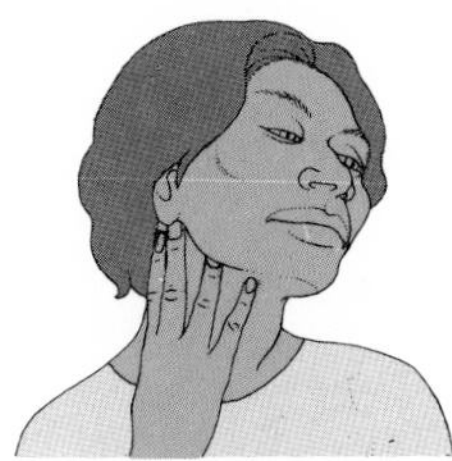

Swollen glands that you can feel in the neck are a common symptom of infectious mononucleosis.

What are the risks?
When you have mononucleosis, your spleen enlarges along with the lymph glands. If you are struck in the upper left abdomen, your spleen could rupture, causing hemorrhage and peritonitis (see p.503). You will then need emergency surgery.

What should be done?
If you have symptoms of influenza that persist for more than a few days, see your physician, especially if you have swollen glands and a sore throat. A blood test is usually necessary to determine whether you have infectious mononucleosis.

Self-help: Even if it is painful to swallow, drink plenty of water and fruit juice, especially while you have a fever, and stay at home. To relieve discomfort or pain, take aspirin or an aspirin substitute recommended by your physician. (Do not give aspirin to adolescents because of the risk of Reye's syndrome, see p.713.) Rest is essential.

Professional help: Infectious mononucleosis is a virus disease, so antibiotics are not effective in treating it. The disease must simply run its course.

Chronic fatigue syndrome

The term chronic fatigue syndrome refers to a set of symptoms that vary from person to person and last for prolonged and variable periods of time. A person who has chronic fatigue syndrome feels weak and exhausted and finds that his or her ability to function is severely reduced. An affected person may have great difficulty performing even nondemanding, routine activities.

Whether the cause of chronic fatigue syndrome is physical, psychological, or some combination of both is still being investigated. Some symptoms indicate that the immune system (the body's natural defense mechanism) is affected. The syndrome may be associated with stress or depression. Currently it is not known whether the syndrome is caused by an underlying disease or infection, or whether it is simply a collection of symptoms that have no specific cause.

What are the symptoms?
Some people with chronic fatigue syndrome have symptoms similar to those caused by a virus infection. Common symptoms are mild fever (99.5°F to 100.5°F), sore throat, tender lymph glands under the arms and/or in the neck, muscle aches, muscle weakness, joint pain, and headache. An affected person may eventually develop emotional symptoms, such as anxiety or depression. He or she usually feels extremely tired and weak after any physical exertion. The person may also be forgetful, have difficulty sleeping, and find it hard to concentrate. Your physician will not consider a diagnosis of chronic fatigue syndrome unless you have had these symptoms for at least 12 weeks and your physician has not found any other cause. The symptoms may last for months or years.

What is the treatment?
Your physician will examine you and perform tests to try to determine the cause of your symptoms. Severe fatigue can be caused by any chronic infection or disease, including depression (p.321), tuberculosis (p.602), Lyme disease (p.605), hepatitis B and C (p.523), rheumatoid arthritis (p.589), congestive heart failure (p.408), and infection with HIV (human immunodeficiency virus, the virus that causes AIDS, p.465).

The cause of chronic fatigue syndrome is not known and thus has not been treated effectively. But it is possible to treat many of the symptoms. Your physician may prescribe acetaminophen or aspirin, or another non-steroidal anti-inflammatory drug to help relieve headache, muscles, and joint pain. (Do not give aspirin to a child or adolescent who is ill with a fever because aspirin has been linked with Reye's syndrome, p.713, a potentially fatal condition.)

Most people who have chronic fatigue syndrome recover; their symptoms disappear and they eventually return to their usual level of activity. In some cases, however, the disorder persists indefinitely.

Shingles

(herpes zoster)

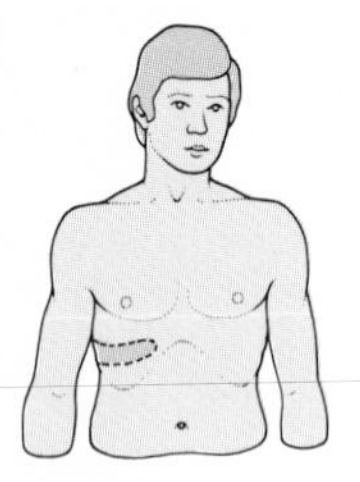

A common site of shingles

Shingles is the result of infection by the varicella zoster virus, the virus that causes chickenpox (see p.747). During an attack of chickenpox the virus may invade the root of a nerve in the brain stem or spinal cord. It lies dormant for years, until it is reactivated. Then the virus multiplies and produces intense, knifelike pain. It also causes a rash in the form of groups of blisters on the skin that lies above the nerve. It is not known what re-activates the dormant varicella zoster virus.

What are the symptoms?

Severe burning pain in the affected area often precedes the blisters by several days. Almost any part of the body may be involved, but the disease is especially common on one side of the trunk, and it is most dangerous if it affects the face and the eyes. The pain often lasts for weeks after the blisters disappear.

Blisters caused by shingles are itchy; they gradually become encrusted and less con-tagious. The blisters usually disappear after about 7 days, but they leave scars like those that are caused by chickenpox.

What should be done?

If the infection is in its early stages and you are older or have a chronic illness or infection near the eye, your physician may prescribe acyclovir, an antiviral medication, to speed recovery. If your face is affected, your physician will advise you on how to protect your eyes. Always keep the rash clean.

Tuberculosis

(TB)

Tuberculosis, often called TB, is a disease that develops slowly and can lead to chronic poor health and death if it is not treated. In people who are healthy, tuberculosis is caused by a specific bacterium that is usually transmitted from one person to another through the air. The bacteria usually attack the lungs, but can also spread to other parts of the body, especially the brain, kidneys, or bones. As the bacteria multiply, they create an area of inflammation in which your tissue is destroyed. They may then spread to the nearest lymph nodes.

During the primary, or first, phase of the infection, which may last for several months, the body's natural defenses resist the disease by destroying or walling off most of the bacteria in a fibrous capsule. Often the dis-ease never develops beyond this phase. Some of the walled-in bacteria remain alive, how-ever, and may reactivate the infection if you become weak, ill, or undernourished—all of which may undermine your immunity. You may also become reinfected if you are in close, prolonged contact with someone who has active tuberculosis.

The secondary phase of tuberculosis most commonly affects the lungs, and the resulting lung damage reduces your ability to breathe. Similarly, little pockets of trapped bacteria elsewhere in the body may become active again. Such secondary outbreaks of tuber-culosis can usually be stopped if they are adequately treated with antibiotics.

What are the symptoms?

The primary stage of tuberculosis often causes no symptoms or very mild symptoms that mimic a cold. You may never even know that you have had tuberculosis until years later when you have a chest X ray or positive skin test for TB. If the infection progresses to the secondary stage, you are likely to de-velop a slight fever, night sweats, weight loss, and tiredness without obvious cause. Tu-berculosis of the lungs, the most common type, causes a cough that is dry at first but eventually produces pus-containing phlegm, or sputum that is sometimes blood-streaked or bloody. Shortness of breath and chest pain may also develop. If any other organ is affected, the symptoms of an infection of that organ appear gradually.

What are the risks?

Tuberculosis was becoming a less common disease in the US until the mid-1980s, when it began to increase in frequency partly as a result of the AIDS epidemic. People who are infected with the human immunodeficiency virus (HIV) are more susceptible to tuberculosis because their immune systems are compromised. Anyone with apparently inactive tuberculosis who becomes infected with HIV is more likely to develop an active TB infection. Also at risk are those who come into contact with people born in other countries where there is a high rate of tuberculosis. Another group with a high risk of tuberculosis is people who live in long-term care facilities; tuberculosis spreads rapidly in older people.

Nevertheless, tuberculosis remains an infrequent risk for most people. All cattle in the US are routinely checked for tuberculosis, and most milk is pasteurized, so milk is no longer a source of infection from the bovine form of tuberculosis.

What should be done?

Consult your physician if you lose weight without trying to do so, become generally ill, or develop a fever with sweats and a persistent cough. Your physician will examine you, will probably take samples of sputum for tests, and arrange for a chest X ray.

What is the treatment?

Self-help: Follow your physician's instructions carefully. Take the prescribed drugs regularly and eat a well-balanced diet of naturally occurring foods. If you neglect your treatment, antibiotic-resistant bacteria will develop, making a cure more difficult. You must also be sure you get enough rest, which is also essential for a complete recovery from tuberculosis.

Professional help: Antibacterial drugs and antibiotics are used to treat tuberculosis, and combinations of these drugs must be taken continuously for several months. If an infected organ is damaged severely, you may need surgery to have it removed. After successful treatment, have periodic checkups as often as your physician recommends, to ensure the disease does not flare up again.

Tetanus

(lockjaw)

Tetanus is a serious and often fatal disease. It is caused by clostridia bacteria that live in the soil. These bacteria can invade the human body through contamination of any wound that comes in contact with soil containing the bacterium. Infection can also occur from a puncture wound from a contaminated object, such as a nail or a thorn. A toxin, or poison, produced by the bacteria attacks the nerve cells in the spinal cord that control muscle activity. After an incubation period that may be as short as 2 days or as long as 2 weeks or more, your muscles become rigid and subject to painful spasms.

Because immunization against tetanus is now routine (see p.748), it is rare in the US. Only 100 or fewer cases are treated each year. Infants are immunized against the disease during their first year, and booster injections are usually given at 10-year intervals.

Despite treatment with anticonvulsant drugs and muscle-relaxant drugs, about 40 percent of all tetanus cases end in death, often because of suffocation.

What should be done?

Make sure that each family member is immunized against tetanus and has a booster shot every 10 years. Keep a record of the dates when family members received antitetanus injections so that you can be sure they are protected. Always clean out small cuts with soap and water and apply an antiseptic. This is especially important with cuts that occur outdoors, where contamination is more common, and with puncture wounds that break the skin, such as that from a rusty nail, because they are hard to clean and they provide an environment particularly favorable to the growth of the bacteria.

If you have never had a tetanus injection and if you suffer a puncture wound, it is vital that you call your physician's office or go to a hospital emergency department without delay, so that you can receive an antitetanus injection as soon as possible and have the wound cleaned.

If tetanus develops, you will need to be hospitalized as soon as possible. Treatment includes antibiotics, along with injections of an antitoxin. You may be given muscle-relaxant drugs, and your breathing may need to be aided or taken over by a mechanical ventilator. The goal of treatment is to keep the body functioning for several weeks while the disease runs its course.

Rabies

(hydrophobia)

Rabies is a virus disease of animals and humans that can be spread through a bite or scratch. Once you are bitten or scratched by an infected animal, the rabies virus travels to the nerve nearest to the bite and then continues on through the nerve pathways to the brain. Rabies is virtually always fatal. The earliest symptom of this dangerous disorder is a fever and a general sense of illness, as you might feel with any virus infection. After 2 or 3 days of feeling ill, however, you become irrational and have violent mouth and throat spasms. Although you are very thirsty, these spasms are made worse by trying to drink water (hydrophobia means "fear of water"). At this point, death is likely to occur within a few days.

The incubation period—the time it takes from infection until the appearance of symptoms—varies from 10 days to 2 years, but is usually 1 to 3 months. In the US, the animals that most often carry rabies are skunk, fox, bobcat, badger, bat, coyote, dog, raccoon, and cat.

What should be done?

A safe, reliable rabies vaccination is now available, and veterinarians or anyone who comes into regular contact with wild animals should be vaccinated regularly. If you have been bitten or scratched by an animal that may have rabies, see a physician without delay. Any time lost may place you in increasing danger of fatal infection. The animal should be captured if possible, but not destroyed. Tests can be performed to determine if the animal has rabies. Meanwhile, you will probably be given a series of injections of antirabies vaccine to help prevent the disease from developing. (The vaccine has changed, and the shots are no longer given through the abdomen.) Have your pets immunized.

Rocky Mountain spotted fever

Rocky Mountain spotted fever is a disease caused by rickettsia bacteria. Rickettsia can live inside ticks, and people are infected with them through tick bites (see p.610). However, an infected person may not notice the tick bite that caused the disease.

What are the symptoms?

About 2 days after the tick bite, you have three major symptoms of the disease: severe headache; a high temperature (up to 103° to 105°F, or 39° to 40°C); and severe muscle aches and weakness.

Most people also develop a characteristic rash. It usually begins as flat red spots or splotches on the palms of the hands and the soles of the feet, then spreads to the wrists, ankles, legs, arms, and finally the trunk.

Rocky Mountain spotted fever also causes other symptoms, including chills, abdominal pain, nausea, spasms in your back, mental confusion, and finally unconsciousness. The kidneys, liver, and lungs can be damaged in the later stages of the disease.

What are the risks?

Although ticks that carry Rocky Mountain spotted fever rickettsia are found all over the US, the disease most frequently occurs in the southeast, from Maryland to Georgia. It usually occurs in the spring and summer in children who spend a lot of time outdoors.

There is a greater risk of becoming infected if a tick has remained attached to your body for several hours or if you crush the tick while removing it.

Left untreated, the infection can become severe. Seven percent of all cases are fatal.

What should be done?

The best preventive measures are to avoid tick-infested areas and wear protective clothing (especially long pants and socks). If you are traveling through a tick-infested area, inspect your body thoroughly several times a day and at bedtime to remove any ticks (see illustration, p.610). See your physician at once if you know that you have had a tick bite and you develop the symptoms described.

Your physician will confirm the diagnosis with two consecutive blood tests. The second test, to measure the number of antibodies (proteins produced by the body to fight infection), is done 10 to 14 days after the illness begins. Your physician must treat the infection as soon as it is suspected, however, because there is a greater risk of heart damage and death if treatment is delayed.

Antibiotics usually provide a cure. If the disease is not treated right away, you may have to be hospitalized to be treated for the damage to your kidneys, liver, and lungs.

Yellow fever

This virus disease, which usually attacks the liver, is carried by mosquitoes. It usually occurs in Central and South America and in parts of Africa. Immunization is very effective and is required for anyone visiting countries in which yellow fever is a known risk (and recommended for other countries).

Attacks of yellow fever range from mild to fatal. A mild attack may produce symptoms similar to those of influenza (see p.597).

However, symptoms of more severe cases include nausea, vomiting, gastrointestinal bleeding (visible in the stool or in vomit), abdominal pain, and yellowing of the skin (see Jaundice, p.522). You may feel very depressed and confused and may even go into a coma. As with many virus diseases, there is no effective treatment for yellow fever, but a person who has recovered from the disease is immune (protected) for life.

Smallpox

Smallpox disease has been eliminated as the result of a successful worldwide vaccination campaign. Vaccination is no longer necessary and in 1980 the World Health Organization declared the disease officially extinct. The disease was severe, highly infectious, and often fatal. People who survived it were left with varying degrees of scarring on their skin caused by the smallpox rash.

Smallpox viruses are now maintained in medical laboratories under safe, secure conditions for research purposes.

Candida infections

Candida albicans is a fungus that often exists in small, harmless quantities in the mouth, intestinal tract, vagina, and on the skin. The fungus grows rapidly and causes an obvious illness, sometimes called thrush, if your normal immune defenses are impaired. *Candida* infections often occur in people who are being treated with immunosuppressive anti-cancer drugs or who have AIDS. *Candida* infections also occur when antibiotics destroy bacteria normally present in the mouth, intestines, or vagina. *Candida* often infects the surface between folds of skin in people who are overweight.

What are the symptoms?

Oral thrush (*Candida* of the mouth) causes white patches on the lining of the mouth and throat and cracks at the corners of the mouth. These sores may be painful but often are not. Thrush can also affect the moister, warmer skin in folds under the breasts, between the buttocks, and in the genital region. Men may develop balanitis (see p.620) and women, vaginal thrush (see p.645).

Infection of the intestinal tract with *Candida* may cause ulceration and lead to other symptoms such as bloody diarrhea, abdominal cramps, shaking chills, and high fever. In people whose immune system is seriously impaired, *Candida* may spread via the bloodstream to all parts of the body, including the brain, eyes, and bones. This form of candidiasis is life-threatening.

What should be done?

Anyone with an impaired immune system should watch for signs of *Candida* infection; if any occur, see your physician promptly so that you can be treated with antifungal drugs.

Lyme disease

Lyme disease (named for the village where it was first identified) is an infection caused by a bacterium, the spirochete *Borrelia burgdorferi*, which is transmitted to humans by the bite of an infected tick. These ticks are parasites on animals such as deer and mice that live in bushes, tall grasses, or woods. Lyme disease occurs in people who live in or visit tick-infested areas.

What are the symptoms?

A person bitten by an infected tick usually develops a red spot on the skin that gradually increases in size. The center of the spot returns to its normal color after a day or two, so the skin has the appearance of a bull's-eye on an archery target. This spot on your skin is very noticeable but may not be painful.

In some cases the skin clears up and there are no other symptoms. However, in other cases within a day or two more red spots appear and you have a headache, fever, swollen lymph glands, and pain in the joints and muscles. You feel ill and weak.

If your Lyme disease is not recognized or treated, you go on to the second stage of the illness in which the disease affects the heart and nervous system. Meningitis (inflammation of the meninges, or coverings of the brain and spinal cord) and partial paralysis of the muscles served by the facial and other nerves often occur; the meningitis causes severe headache, muscular weakness, and numbness or tingling. Irregular heartbeat and inflammation of the heart and pericardium (the heart's covering) are common.

Those who remain untreated move to the third stage of Lyme disease, in which chronic arthritis often develops, usually affecting the larger joints such as the knees.

What are the risks?

Lyme disease became well known only in the 1980s, but the first case in the US may have occurred in 1962. Probably around 8,000 people are infected each year in the US. If Lyme disease is recognized in its early stages and treated with tetracycline or another effective antibiotic drug, the outlook is good. Once chronic arthritis has developed, however, treatment is less successful.

What should be done?

Anyone who goes into wooded areas should consider using tick-repellent that contains DEET or permethrin. Be aware of the risks of tick bites and wear clothing that protects you against ticks (including long pants and socks). If you find a tick embedded in your skin, see the article Ticks, p.610, for the correct way to remove it. If a tick bites you and a rash develops, treatment with tetracycline is recommended for at least 10 days for adults (children are treated with penicillin). Additional treatment may be necessary if symptoms recur. If symptoms of late-phase Lyme disease occur, treatment is usually given with penicillin or a cephalosporin antibiotic. Prolonged use of antibiotic drugs may be needed for those with arthritis from Lyme disease.

Chlamydial infections

Chlamydiae are a type of microscopic organism that are not bacteria, viruses, or fungi. However, they can be eliminated with certain antibiotics. Chlamydiae are responsible for several diseases, including some diseases that are sexually transmitted.

Going out of the country

If you are planning a trip out of the country, make sure that you are adequately protected against any diseases that may occur in your country of destination. Many developing countries do not have the most up-to-date water or sewage systems. As a result, diseases associated with contaminated water supplies, such as dysentery (see p.494), typhoid (see p.494), and polio (see p.292), are common in developing countries.

About 6 weeks before you leave, find out from either your travel agent, the country's embassy or consulate, your local public health department, or your physician which vaccinations are compulsory for entry into the country and which are recommended. The US Centers for Disease Control and Prevention, located in Atlanta, Georgia, is a good source of information too. At least 1 month before you travel, consult your physician or local public health department about when and where to get the immunizations you need; many vaccinations are not immediately available or must be taken well in advance of your trip. For example, if you plan to visit, even if only for a few hours, any of the countries in which malaria is endemic (always present) you should begin antimalarial drug treatment 2 weeks before your trip and continue it for 6 weeks after you leave the malaria-infested country. You can be protected against typhoid and polio by vaccination.

Tropical countries have many insects, such as mosquitoes and flies, that transmit diseases such as malaria (see p.608) or yellow fever (see p.604).

If you swim or bathe in developing countries, or walk barefoot, you risk becoming infested with parasitic worms such as schistosomes and hookworm. Schistosomes, or blood flukes, can be found in freshwater and can enter your body through your skin. In some cases these parasites only cause dermatitis (see p.269), a skin condition. In other cases, however, infestation with schistosomes results in a disease known as schistosomiasis, or bilharziasis. In this disease the parasites travel from the skin to the bladder and the intestines, from where they may spread to other parts of the body. The severity of the disease depends on the number of parasites that enter your body.

Hookworms are parasitic roundworms that are found in developing countries, particularly in areas of poor sanitation. Larvae of the parasite live in the soil, and you risk infestation if your skin comes in contact with infested soil or if you eat or drink contaminated food or water. The roundworms enter the bloodstream and travel to the small intestine, where they attach or "hook" themselves to the lining and suck blood. In severe cases, the presence of roundworms can result in anemia.

While you are out of the US, take some precautions. Boil water or milk unless you are certain that it is safe to drink. Alternatively, there are purifying tablets that you can use to treat water and other liquids by the glassful. However these pills may have a slightly unpleasant taste, so some people add a fruit-flavored powder to purified water to make it more palatable. Carbonated beverages such as colas in sealed cans and bottles are generally safe since the chemical composition of the liquids helps retard growth of bacteria. Avoid salads and reheated foods, and do not eat unpeeled fruit. Always wash your hands before handling or eating food, and do not use tapwater for brushing teeth.

If you plan to visit rural areas or remote areas, make sure that you take adequate clothing for protection against insect bites, especially if you plan to sleep outside or travel at night, when insects can be the most annoying.

Finally, remember that the health problems most commonly encountered by tourists are sunburn and food poisoning, which are preventable.

Trachoma This is a chlamydial infection of the conjunctiva, the moist tissue that lines the eyelids and the white portion of the eyeball. Although this infection is rare in the US, it is the major cause of blindness in North Africa and the Middle East.

Nongonococcal urethritis Chlamydiae also cause one of the most common STDs, nongonococcal urethritis (NGU), a urinary-tract inflammation (see p.655). Symptoms of this type of urethritis include pain when urinating and a watery, mucous discharge. In men, the bacteria that produce gonorrhea (see p.654) also cause a type of urethritis, but the chlamydial infection is milder than the gonorrheal infection and the discharge from the penis is less copious.

Nongonococcal urethritis is passed on through sexual intercourse. In a woman, the infection can result in pelvic inflammatory disease (see p.639) and cause infertility.

Lymphogranuloma venereum Some strains of chlamydiae produce lymphogranuloma venereum, another STD. The organism is rarely found in the US, but is more common in tropical climates. People who have multiple sexual partners are especially likely to get this disease.

The initial sign of infection is a painless pimple or blister that develops on the penis or the outer lips of the vagina, 5 to 20 days after exposure. About 2 to 12 weeks later, the lymph nodes in the groin enlarge painfully, mat together, redden, and ooze pus.

The infection sometimes seems to improve without treatment, but sores appear on the genitals. Complications include scarring, which causes strictures (small bridges of tissue that narrow the opening) in the urethra, vagina, or rectum.

Psittacosis Also called ornithosis, this is a chlamydial disease that infects the lungs of people who inhale organisms from the feathers and droppings of infected birds, particularly parrots and parakeets. Psittacosis is most common in pet store workers and those who keep birds as pets.

The infection spreads rapidly from the lungs to the bloodstream. Symptoms vary from a mild flu to a severe pneumonia (see p.384), with temperatures ranging from 103° to 105°F (39.4° to 40.6°C).

What should be done?

If you have the symptoms of any of these diseases, see your physician. Chlamydial disorders are usually identified by a laboratory test of secretions from the penis and vagina to measure the levels of certain antibodies, the substances that the body produces to combat infection. Your physician will probably prescribe an antibiotic, which usually clears up the infection.

In cases of nongonococcal urethritis and lymphogranuloma venereum, which are transmitted sexually, all sexual partners should be treated so that they do not transmit the infection to others.

Infestations

Infestations occur when parasites invade your body and live either on it (such as lice) or in it (such as tapeworms). Parasites that live only on the skin usually cause no symptoms other than discomfort. Some of these, ticks for example, can cause infections because they may carry disease. Those that infest the inside of the body sometimes cause vague, ill-defined symptoms that you hardly notice, so they may remain undetected. If, however, parasites lodge in a vital place or multiply rapidly, they can cause severe problems.

Many people believe, incorrectly, that parasitic infestations only occur in people who bathe infrequently, or who rarely wash their clothes. In fact, anyone, regardless of personal hygiene, may become infested with lice, scabies, or any other parasite.

It is almost impossible to get rid of parasites without treatment because your body does not have natural defenses against them. Most types of dangerous infestations are rare in the US and today's parasite-killing drugs are highly effective.

Trichinosis

Trichinosis is a serious, occasionally fatal, infection caused by the parasitic roundworm *Trichinella spiralis*. Infection results from eating raw, undercooked, or inadequately processed meat containing trichinae (the larvae of the parasite). Pork is the most common source of infection, but bear meat has also caused trichinosis in rare cases. The more larvae you have unknowingly eaten, the more severe are your symptoms. Generally, however, diarrhea, abdominal pain, and fever develop within a few days of eating infected meat. Also, your muscles may become painful and your eyes swollen and bloodshot. Later, the lungs, nervous system, or heart may be affected, which may lead to coughing up bloodstained phlegm, heart failure, paralysis, or even coma.

What should be done?

Make sure all meat is thoroughly cooked or has been properly processed before eating it. Never eat rare pork or uncooked bacon or sausages. If you develop symptoms, consult your physician immediately. If you suspect that you may have eaten infected meat, see your physician within 24 hours. He or she will probably prescribe thiabendazole, a drug that is effective against trichinosis when it is taken promptly. If your trichinosis is not diagnosed early, your physician may prescribe corticosteroids or other anti-inflammatory drugs to relieve symptoms.

However, despite treatment, trichinosis usually runs its full natural course. Most people recover completely 6 to 8 weeks after infection, but in a few very severe cases the disease is fatal.

Malaria

Malaria is a disease caused by minute single-celled parasites called plasmodia, which are transferred from one person to another by the *Anopheles* mosquito. There is no other carrier; plasmodia enter your bloodstream only if you are bitten by an *Anopheles* mosquito that has bitten someone who has malaria.

Once in your bloodstream, the plasmodia travel to the liver, where they multiply very rapidly. After several days, thousands of them flow back into your bloodstream, where they destroy red blood cells. However, many plasmodia also remain and continue to multiply in the liver cells, and some of these plasmodia are released to invade the red blood cells in your bloodstream. When the parasites mature, they rupture the red blood cells and enter the bloodstream. This is why a person with malaria usually has repeated attacks unless the disease is treated. Each attack signals the release of plasmodia.

A particularly dangerous type of malaria is caused by *Plasmodium falciparum*, one of the four species of plasmodia that infect humans. If you have falciparum malaria, all the organisms are released from your liver into your bloodstream at the same time. Thus there is only one bout of the disease, but that bout is extremely severe.

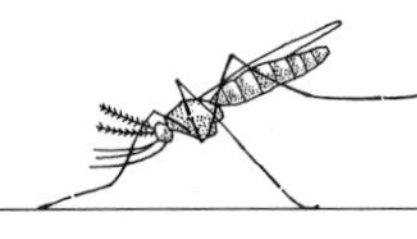

The female *Anopheles* mosquito carries the tiny organisms that cause malaria. The mosquito gets the organisms by biting someone who has malaria and sucking in some blood. The organisms then multiply in the mosquito and enter the bloodstream of the next person whom the mosquito bites.

What are the symptoms?

Malaria causes no symptoms at first. About 8 to 30 days after the mosquito bite, depending on the type of plasmodium, a full day of headache, fatigue, and nausea is followed by 12 to 24 hours of chills alternating with fever. A sudden chill is followed by a feverish stage with rapid breathing but no sweating. A final sweating stage is accompanied by a drop in temperature. Similar bouts occur whenever more plasmodia are released into your bloodstream, generally every 2 or 3 days.

If malaria is not treated, attacks can continue to occur for years, but your immune system slowly builds up a defense against the disease, and the attacks come less often. In falciparum malaria, the bout of chills alternating with fever is likely to last for 2 or 3 days and to be so severe that it can be fatal. If you recover, it does not recur.

Children with malaria are likely to have prolonged high fever without chills. The fever sometimes affects the brain, causing unconsciousness or seizures (see p.713).

What are the risks?

The *Anopheles* mosquito lives in the southeastern and western US and is widespread in tropical and semitropical countries. Mosquito abatement programs have eradicated malaria in the US. With the exception of a handful of cases each year, the only malaria in the US is brought back by travelers.

Since plasmodia destroy red blood cells, anemia (see p.450) may develop. Also, the damaged blood cells are apt to form small clumps, which may block blood vessels and lead to brain or kidney damage. This is particularly true if you have falciparum malaria, which carries a risk of massive blood-vessel blockage and possibly death.

What should be done?

If you develop symptoms of malaria, consult your physician without delay. Your physician will probably arrange for you to have blood tests. Because it is not always easy to detect the presence of plasmodia, you may need to have the blood tests taken periodically.

What is the treatment?

Self-help: To guard against malaria, if you are going to visit an area in which the disease is a problem (see Going out of the country, p.606), be sure to wear protective clothing, and ask your physician to prescribe anti-malarial drugs to protect you. You must start taking them before you travel and continue to take them after you return. In many parts of the world, malaria parasites have become resistant to some of the common drugs such as chloroquine, but new and effective drugs are constantly being developed.

Professional help: Your physician will prescribe drugs to prevent malaria if you expect to be at risk. If blood tests show that you have malaria, your physician will prescribe other drugs.

Tapeworm

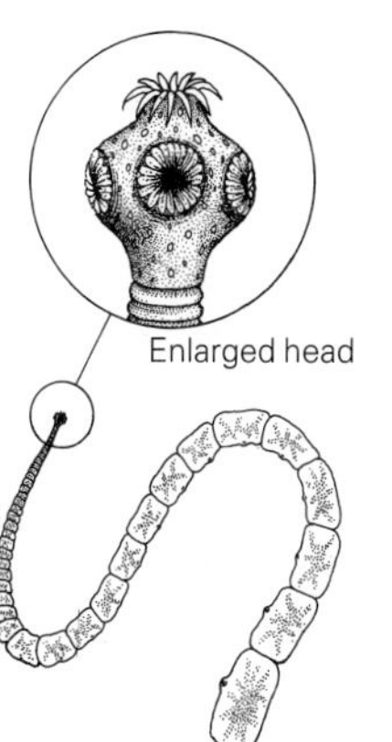

Tapeworms are parasites that sometimes infest pigs, cattle, and fish. They can be passed on to a human who eats infested pork, beef, or fish that has not been adequately cooked. Once in the intestines, a tapeworm can anchor itself by embedding its head end into the intestinal wall. The tapeworm then absorbs food and may grow to more than 30 feet (about 10 meters) long. Segments of the worm break off and are excreted in stools. These segments look like short pieces of narrow white ribbon. If the worm remains in the intestines, it often causes symptoms such as weight loss, occasional abdominal pain, loss of appetite, and irritation around the anus. A pork tapeworm can cause brain and liver damage; a beef or fish tapeworm can cause anemia. Despite strict regulations for control of meat-packing procedures, meat that contains tapeworms occasionally gets on the market. However, thorough cooking kills any worms in your meat.

What should be done?

If you think you may have a tapeworm, consult your physician, who will probably want to examine a specimen of your stools. There are a number of medications that kill parasitic worms, and, if necessary, your physician will prescribe medication for you.

You will need to return to your physician's office with stool samples until you excrete the tapeworm's head, indicating an end to the infestation. This may take several days.

Scabies

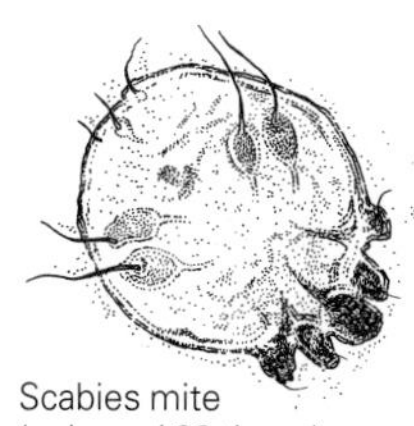
Scabies mite (enlarged 88 times)

See p.256, **Visual aids to diagnosis, 67.**

Scabies is caused by a mite that burrows into the skin and lays eggs from which additional mites emerge. The result is intense but relatively harmless itching, especially at night. Scabies rarely occurs on the head or face. It most often affects the hands, wrists, armpits, buttocks, or genital area. Scabies is highly contagious. The mites are spread through casual physical contact such as shaking hands, but are more likely to be spread through close physical contact, such as sexual intercourse. Mites are also spread through contact with infested clothes or bedding, so if one family member has scabies, often everyone in the household has scabies.

What are the symptoms?

The main symptom of scabies is intense itching. Continual scratching causes sores and scabs to form.

What should be done?

Although scabies occurs most commonly in unhygienic conditions, anyone can get it. If your physician diagnoses scabies, you will need to scrub all infected areas and apply a prescribed medication to your entire body below the neck. It is important to follow the directions on the label carefully.

The mites that cause scabies do not live long once they are removed from human skin.

Lice

(pediculosis)

Human head louse (enlarged 45 times)

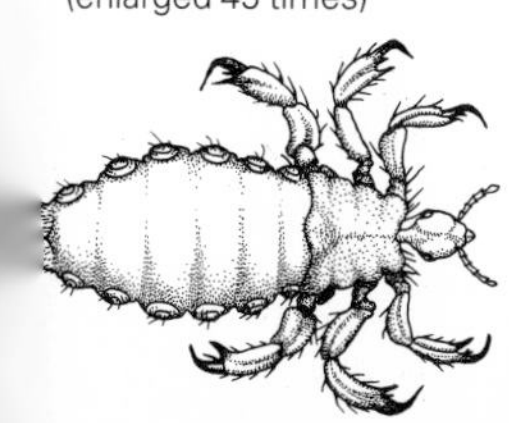

Lice are tiny but visible insects that live in the hair and suck blood from the skin. Often lice are spread among children at school. Crab lice (see p.657) live in pubic hair and are usually spread by sexual intercourse.

The eggs of lice are known as nits, and they, too, are visible. They look like tiny white grains clinging to the hair. The bites of lice cause itching in affected areas, and there is a slight possibility of infection. For the most part, however, these parasites simply irritate the person who has become a host.

What should be done?

If your child has lice, report it to his or her school. Lice infestations are considered a public health problem, and it is necessary to trace them to their source and prevent them from spreading further. For treatment, whether for a child or an adult, consult your physician, who will recommend a special shampoo, lotion, or both. Hairbrushes, hats, and any other clothing should be washed in hot water and dried in a hot dryer. If these items are not washable, discard them.

Fleas

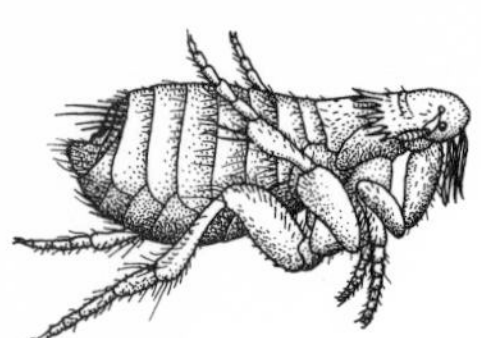

Flea
(enlarged 9 times)

There are many species of fleas, and each one is a parasite of a different animal. Animal fleas do not stay long on human skin. Fleas can leap great distances, and isolated flea bites on human skin can be caused by animal (usually cat or dog) fleas that have left their hosts temporarily. Flea eggs hatch in bedding about 7 days after they have been laid. The fleas may then live in the bedding and feed off their animal hosts and, occasionally, humans. Their bites cause intense irritation for up to 2 days. Flea infestation of humans occurs in all parts of the world, but is most common in developing countries and other places where there are crowded living conditions, close contact between people and domestic animals, or poor hygienic conditions.

What should be done?

To avoid infestation, use antiflea spray, powder, or shampoo on your pets' skin, and spray their bedding regularly as well. Flea collars for pets may also be helpful. If you suspect infestation in your bedding, furniture, or rugs, apply a flea repellent to your skin and spray the suspected items. In severe cases, you may not be able to eliminate the fleas, and you may need to call a professional exterminator to do so.

Ticks

Ticks are parasites that feed on blood. Tick bites are potentially dangerous because of the viruses and bacteria that ticks carry and transmit as they feed. Infections transmitted through tick bites include Rocky Mountain spotted fever (see p.604), Lyme disease (see p.605), and encephalitis (see p.291). Some ticks also harbor a toxin, or poison, that paralyzes the nerves in the legs, then moves toward the trunk. The paralysis is relieved by removing the tick.

The tick embeds its head into your skin, then swells as it feeds, sometimes to several times its original size. The skin around the bite hardens into a lump surrounded by a red halo. Usually, the lump subsides after the tick is removed, but it can persist, especially if the tick's head remains embedded in your skin after its body has been removed.

Tick
(enlarged 9 times)

Ticks are usually found in wooded areas or tall grass. Wear a long-sleeved shirt and long pants tucked into your socks when walking through these areas. Use an insect repellent that works against ticks. If you have been in the woods or fields, it is a good idea to check your body for ticks. They often lodge in your hair, around the ankles, and in the genital area, so you may have to search for them. If you find a tick right away, remove it as shown in the illustration below, before it becomes embedded in the skin.

Removal of the entire tick including the head is necessary, because any part of a tick can continue to release toxic substances, bacteria, or viruses.

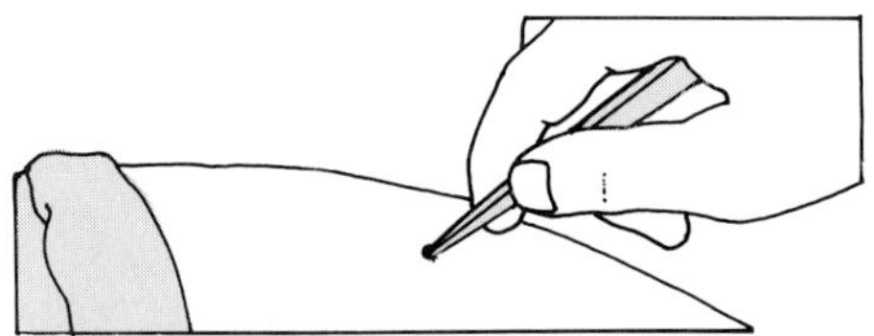

Removing an embedded tick
Using tweezers or small curved forceps, grasp the tick's head (not just the body) as close to the skin as possible. Pull steadily. After you remove the tick, preserve it for your physician without touching it and disinfect the bite with alcohol. If necessary, your physician can remove the head with a small incision. Do not use a lighted match or cigarette on the tick.

Chiggers

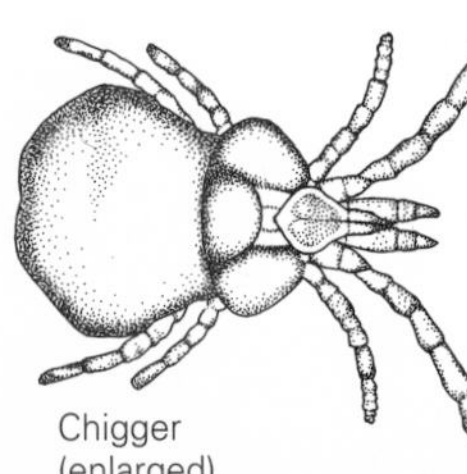

Chigger
(enlarged)

Chiggers are a type of mite, sometimes called a red bug or a harvest mite. They live in grasses, shrubs, and vines in the southern US and sometimes as far north as Canada. Farmers, hikers, hunters, and others who spend a lot of time outdoors are most likely to get chigger bites.

The larva, or immature mite, is only about one hundredth of an inch (0.3mm) long. It attaches to the ankles, groin, belt line, or wherever clothing is tight, and attaches to a hair follicle or an area of hairless skin. The mite releases enzymes that dissolve the skin, then inserts a feeding tube to reach a supply of blood. It remains in one spot for 1 to 4 days, then drops off, engorged with blood.

The skin's response to the mite varies from an allergic skin reaction with hives (see p.272) to an itching, red, pimplelike lump. Sometimes blisters, swelling, or large red patches develop. Usually, the bites itch severely, making it very difficult to keep from scratching. Medications for chigger bites include antihistamines to relieve itching, corticosteroid creams to reduce irritation and allergic reaction, and antibiotics to take by mouth or to apply directly to the affected area if an infection occurs.

Men's health

Introduction

The male reproductive system, which includes two testicles (testes) suspended in a sac (scrotum) and a penis, is closely connected with the organs of the male urinary tract. A disorder in one system may cause symptoms in the other. Each of your testicles is a gland that produces sperm and the male sex hormone testosterone. A long, tightly coiled tube called the epididymis lies behind each testicle. Sperm are continually produced in each testicle. Sperm pass into the epididymis, where they mature over a period of 2 or 3 weeks before they pass into a duct called the vas deferens, which acts as a storage system.

When you have a sexual climax (orgasm), sperm pass from the seminal vesicles into the urethra, and are ejaculated in the seminal fluid. The urethra, which runs from your bladder along the length of your penis, carries both semen and urine. The muscular action of urination automatically closes the passageway for semen, while the muscular action of ejaculation automatically closes the passageway for urine.

Sperm makes up only a small portion of semen, which is composed mainly of secretions from various glands. The secretions may act to mobilize and nourish the sperm and provide them with additional nutrients for their passage through the male and female reproductive tracts. The largest of these glands is the prostate, which surrounds the top section of the urethra at the point where the urethra leaves the bladder. Prostate problems, therefore, can seriously affect both the genital and urinary systems. The urethra is much longer in a man than it is in a woman. It is surrounded in the penis by spongy, heavily veined tissue that makes erections possible when blood fills the tissue and is temporarily held there. The length of the male urethra provides an effective barrier against infection of the reproductive and urinary tracts. Infections of the reproductive and urinary tracts are rare in men, while they are fairly common in women.

The disorders discussed in the following articles are grouped according to the part of the urinary tract or reproductive system in which problems can occur. These parts are the testicles and scrotum, the prostate gland, and the bladder, urethra, penis, and rectum.

Male reproductive organs

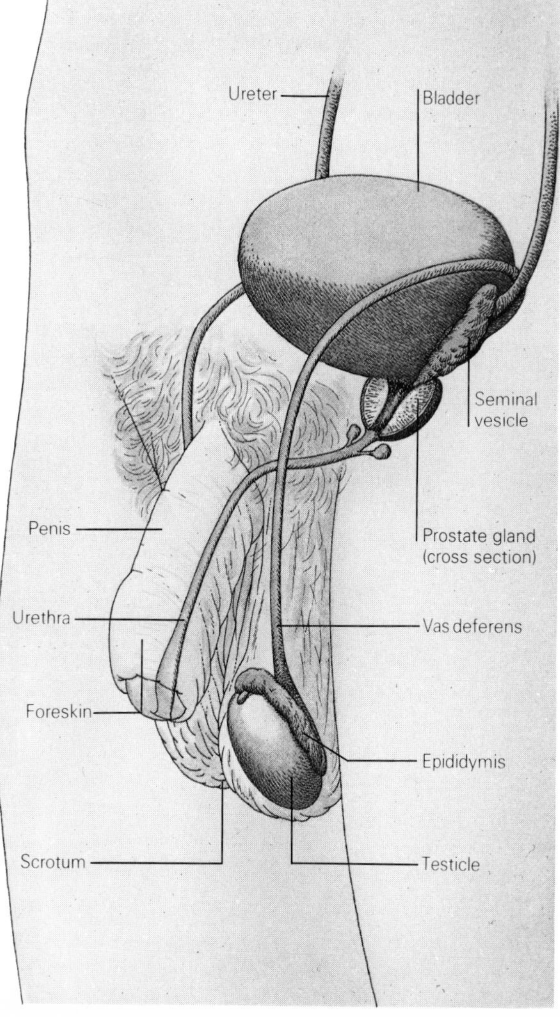

Testicles and scrotum

The two male sex glands, called testes or testicles, develop inside the abdomen of a male fetus. Usually by the time of birth they have descended through the abdominal wall of the fetus to the familiar external position, where they hang suspended in a pouch of skin called the scrotum (see also Undescended testicles, p.739). Each testicle is connected to the body by a single spermatic cord, which is composed of the vas deferens, or sperm duct, and a number of nerves and blood vessels.

Sperm that each testicle produces remain in the epididymis, a coiled tube that lies behind the testis, for about 3 weeks, until they mature. The fully developed sperm then pass into the vas deferens, where they are stored. If sperm are not eventually ejaculated, they gradually disintegrate. The following articles describe disorders of the testicles, scrotum, and epididymis. The spermatic cord, which helps move sperm to outside the body, is not usually susceptible to disease.

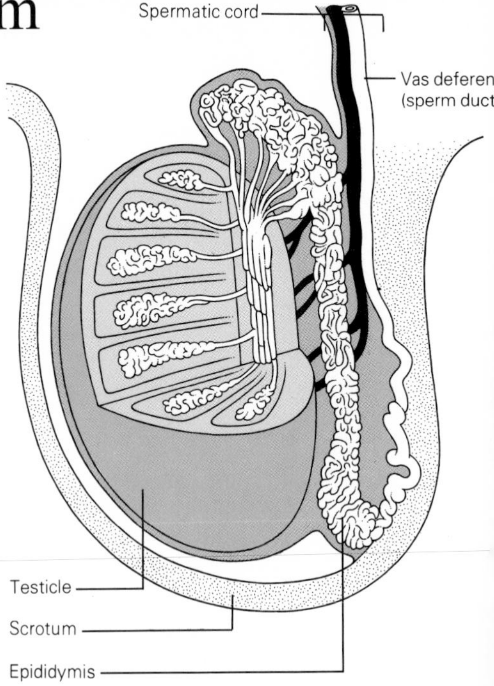

Cancer of the testicle

(cancer of the testis)

Cancer of the testicle is a rare type of cancer that occurs most commonly in young to middle-aged men. It is also an easily cured type of cancer. However, if it is not treated early, it can metastasize (spread) through the lymphatic system (see p.463) to lymph nodes in the abdomen, chest, and neck, and may eventually spread to the lungs. Because there is no direct lymphatic connection between the two testicles, the disease is unlikely to spread from one testicle to the other.

What are the symptoms?

The main symptom of cancer of the testicle is a lump in the testicle. The lump grows slowly, and you may not be aware of it for some time unless you examine your testicles regularly (see Self-examination of the testicles, below).

What are the risks?

Cancer of the testicle is rare, although it is a common type of cancer in men between ages

Self-examination of the testicles

Cancer of the testicle is a common cancer in men under age 40, but it is curable if detected and treated at an early stage.

All men should routinely examine their testicles once a week. Perform the examination after a bath or shower when the scrotum is relaxed. Hold each testicle with both hands, gently rolling it between your fingers and thumb. Gently feel the surface of each testicle to search for any lump or swelling. Spend about 30 seconds to 1 minute examining each testicle. If you find a lump or swelling, whether it is painful or not, consult your physician immediately.

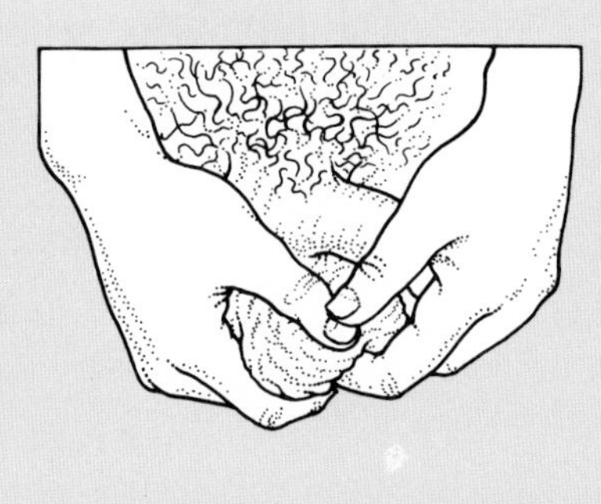

18 and 40. However, with early detection and treatment, the chances of a complete recovery are excellent.

What should be done?
Not every swelling in the scrotum is dangerous; there are often small, insignificant swellings in the epididymis (see Cysts of the epididymis, p.614). A lump in the testicle, however, is usually a serious matter that requires a biopsy. In a biopsy, a small sample of tissue is removed for examination to find out if the lump is cancerous.

What is the treatment?
If you have cancer of the testicle, treatment is surgical removal of the diseased testicle. The operation usually leaves one testicle intact, so there is usually no significant effect on your potency or fertility. Radiation therapy, chemotherapy, and a lymphadenectomy, in which nearby lymph nodes are surgically removed, may be performed to further treat the cancer. In 10 to 15 percent of men treated for cancer of the testicle, the disease recurs. In such cases, high-dose chemotherapy and bone marrow transplant are very effective.

Torsion of the testicle

In this disorder, one testicle is twisted out of its normal position. Each testicle is enclosed by a fibrous two-layered covering. A small amount of lubricating fluid lies between the two layers, which allows the testicles to move around. (These coverings should not be confused with the scrotum, a loose pouch of skin in which the testicles rest.) The covered testicle is attached to the spermatic cord in a way that usually prevents it from twisting out of its natural position. However, when an extreme twist, or torsion, occurs, it can cause the blood vessels to become kinked, preventing blood flow to and from the testicle. This can happen at any time, is extremely painful, and is a medical emergency.

What are the symptoms?
The main symptom is sudden pain in one testicle. Your scrotum then becomes swollen, red, and tender. Intensity of pain varies from case to case, but it can be so severe that you may feel nauseated and may vomit.

In many cases of testicular torsion, the testicle somehow untwists by itself. If this happens, you will feel immediate relief of both pain and swelling.

What are the risks?
Torsion of the testicle is uncommon. The problem usually occurs in adolescence, but it can happen at any age, even in infancy.

If your testicle does not return to its usual position naturally and you do not see your physician immediately, the entire testicle may be destroyed or the sperm-producing parts of the testicle may be permanently damaged. This may reduce your fertility, although sperm can still be produced by your other testicle.

What should be done?
Even if the problem seems to have cleared up by itself, it is vital to see your physician immediately. Pain from injuries, inflammation, and even cancer of the testicle can sometimes resemble torsion of the testicle, so a review of your medical history and examination by your physician are especially important. If the diagnosis is torsion of the testicle, your physician may try to untwist your testicle by careful, gentle manipulation. Even if manipulation relieves the pain, the torsion may recur. If your physician cannot untwist your testicle, or if your testicle does not stay untwisted, the situation is a surgical emergency. Surgery is usually performed as soon as possible. The surgeon untwists the testicle, then attaches it in a position that will help prevent the problem from recurring. Removal of the affected testicle may be necessary if it has been severely and irreversibly damaged because of a prolonged lack of blood flow.

Injury to the testicles

An injury to the testicles usually causes severe pain, but you can assume that there is no serious damage if the pain subsides within an hour or so and your scrotum is not bruised or swollen. Continued pain, bruising, or swelling may indicate internal injury. If you have these symptoms, see your physician or go to the nearest hospital emergency department immediately. If the problem is not treated, accumulated blood may cause the testicle to swell and press against its membranous covering, which may damage healthy tissue. Surgery may be necessary to stop any bleeding and remove any blood clot.

Epididymitis

Inflammation of the epididymis (a coiled tube behind each testicle) is called epididymitis. It is caused by an infection that spreads from the urinary tract into the vas deferens (sperm duct). The first symptom is often swelling on the back of one of your testicles. The swollen area is hot, tender, and very painful. Swelling develops over the course of a few hours and is followed by a painful swelling and stiffening of the scrotum. The testicle may also be affected and may be sore.

What should be done?

If you think you have epididymitis, consult your physician immediately. Laboratory tests of your urine and prostate secretions can help to identify the cause of infection. In younger men, the disorder usually results from nongonococcal urethritis, caused by microorganisms called *Chlamydia* (see Chlamydial infections, p.606). Treatment with antibiotics usually cures epididymitis.

It may also be necessary to treat your sexual partner. This will help prevent chronic sexually transmitted infection in both partners. If swelling of the scrotum is especially painful, bed rest and ice packs may help reduce the swelling. Rarely, in severe or chronic cases, your physician may recommend surgery to drain the infection.

Cysts of the epididymis

(spermatoceles)

Sometimes the tubes through which sperm pass from a testicle to its epididymis develop cysts, or sacs of fluid. Although the cysts may increase in size because sperm accumulates in them, causing them to expand, they are harmless. Cysts of the epididymis are common. If you have a cyst, you will notice a painless swelling in the upper, rear portion of one or both of your testicles.

Although these cysts sometimes resemble tumors of the epididymis, the cysts are not life-threatening. If a physical examination or ultrasound scan does not show that you have a serious problem, you may require no further treatment, but you should watch carefully for increased swelling. Sometimes cysts of the epididymis grow large and cause varying degrees of discomfort. In such cases the cysts generally need to be removed.

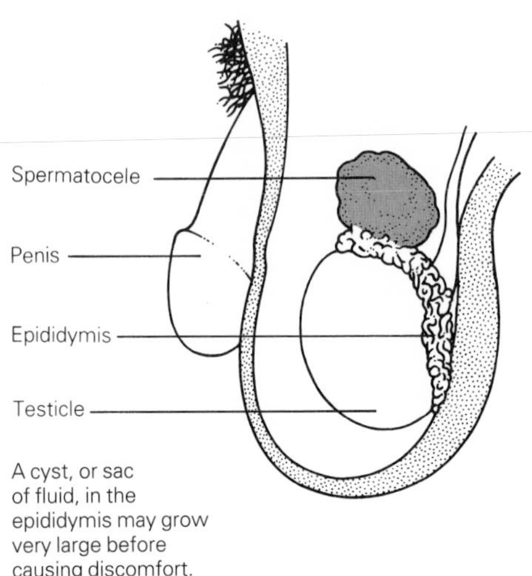

A cyst, or sac of fluid, in the epididymis may grow very large before causing discomfort.

Hydrocele

The membranes that form a covering around each testicle (see Torsion of the testicle, previous page) contain just enough fluid for good lubrication. Sometimes, however, an excessive amount of fluid may be produced and a hydrocele, a soft, usually painless swelling around the testicle, forms and fills the scrotum. Hydroceles are sometimes caused by inflammation or injury of the area, but there is usually no obvious cause. Hydroceles are harmless and common, especially in older men.

Treatment of a small hydrocele is rarely necessary. If the hydrocele becomes very large or painful, however, the fluid can be drained with a needle and syringe. This is a simple procedure that is usually performed under a local anesthetic. The fluid may reaccumulate in the same area. If you have a recurring hydrocele that is causing you some discomfort, your physician may recommend that you have surgery to tighten or remove the covering to prevent the lubricating fluid from accumulating.

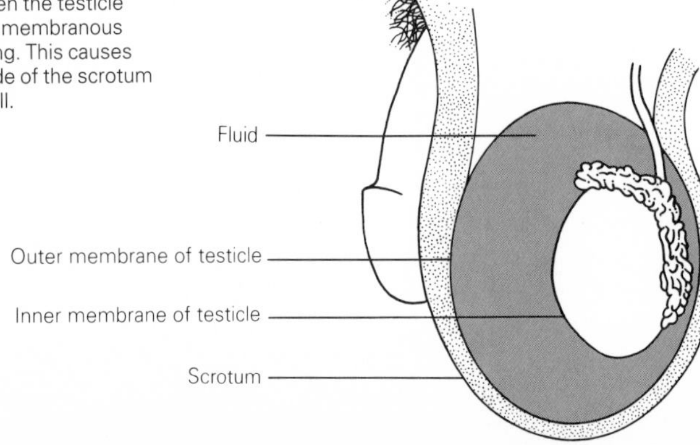

Fluid accumulates between the testicle and its membranous covering. This causes that side of the scrotum to swell.

Varicocele

If the veins that drain one of your testicles become abnormally expanded (see Varicose veins, p.441), you have a mild disorder called varicocele. There is usually no obvious cause for this condition, which produces swelling around the testicle. The swelling may disappear when you lie down, but it is sometimes accompanied by a heavy, dragging feeling in the scrotum, especially during hot weather or after exercising.

To relieve the discomfort, wear tight-fitting underpants or an athletic supporter. No other treatment is usually necessary unless you plan to have children; a varicocele may reduce fertility but it does not affect your ability to get and maintain an erection. If you are worried about fertility or if the varicocele continues to cause discomfort, see your physician. He or she may recommend surgery to remove the affected veins.

Prostate gland

The prostate gland is not one single gland, but a cluster of small glands that surrounds the urethra at the point where it leaves the bladder. The glands are tubular and have muscles that squeeze their secretions into the urethra. The exact function of the prostate gland is not clear. It is thought that the addition of prostatic secretion to the semen somehow stimulates active movement of sperm. Common disorders affecting the prostate are infections and growths. In older men, cancer of the prostate is relatively common. Because the prostate gland encircles the urethra, any prostate disorder may interfere with the free flow of urine, an uncomfortable and sometimes risky problem.

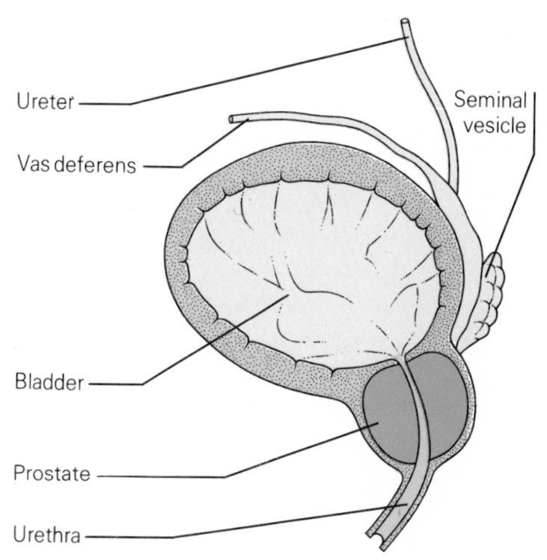

Enlarged prostate

(benign prostatic hypertrophy)

Nearly every man over 45 has some degree of enlargement of the prostate gland, which slowly progresses throughout the aging process. Harmless overgrowths of normal prostate tissue are a natural result of aging. As you age, nodules gradually develop inside the prostate, and as they accumulate the size of the gland changes. The change may cause no problems even if the prostate becomes quite enlarged. The size of a harmless enlargement is less important than whether the portion of the urethra, which connects the bladder with the penis and passes through the prostate, is narrowed by the enlarging gland. However, as the gland grows larger and constricts the urethra, the muscles of the bladder may compensate by becoming stronger. This extra strength is often enough to keep the urethra open indefinitely. Serious problems with urination occur only when the bladder muscles are unable to overcome resistance caused by the enlarging prostate, and the flow of urine is blocked.

What are the symptoms?

Symptoms of severe prostate enlargement vary widely, but one very common symptom is a weak stream of urine. You are likely to have a frequent urge to urinate (an urge so strong that it may wake you several times a night), yet you can pass only a dribble whenever you try to urinate. You may also find that it is difficult to start urinating no matter how strong the urge. This may be most obvious first thing in the morning. There is usually no pain, surface swelling, or lump, because the prostate gland lies deep inside the lower abdomen. Occasionally, however, there may be hematuria, or blood in the urine.

What are the risks?

Prostate enlargement, although very common in men over 45, rarely causes problems before age 60. Urinary problems caused by this disorder are common in older men.

Prostate enlargement is not risky in itself, but the condition may lead to major problems. First, if your bladder is never entirely emptied, pools of stagnant urine inside it can become infected (see Cystitis in men, p.618). Second, when the flow of urine is hampered or blocked, pressure inside the bladder increases and the kidneys and ureters (tubes that carry urine to the bladder from the kidneys) may be affected. This can lead to kidney infection (see Acute pyelonephritis, p.541). Third, if severe enlargement of the prostate is not treated, your bladder may not be able to expel urine. This may happen suddenly or gradually.

Sudden failure of your bladder to expel its contents is called acute urinary retention. It is rare, but very painful, and requires emergency treatment. Passing a catheter through the urethra and into the bladder provides immediate but temporary relief.

Gradual failure, which is more common, occurs when the amount of urine emptied from the bladder is gradually reduced. If the condition is allowed to persist, the amount of urine left in the bladder may become so great that the abdomen swells. In this condition, some of the accumulated urine dribbles out whenever you cough, sneeze, or strain. Urination becomes a prolonged process, and urine may continue to dribble out after you think you have finished urinating. The disorder seldom reaches this stage, but if it does, and is not treated, it will eventually lead to either acute urinary retention or kidney failure (see p.550).

What should be done?

If you have symptoms of an enlarged prostate, consult your physician, who may examine your prostate by inserting a gloved finger into your rectum. You may be referred to a urologist, a physician who specializes in urinary and genital diseases. The urologist will observe your urinary stream and perform various tests to evaluate the health of your bladder and kidneys. He or she may insert a cystoscope (viewing tube) into your bladder and possibly measure the fluid pressure as you urinate. He or she may also arrange for blood tests and for ultrasound and X-ray examination of your kidneys. The results of these tests will show whether your symptoms result from an enlarged prostate.

If you have symptoms of acute urinary retention, see your physician or go to a hospital emergency department immediately. Your bladder must be emptied with a catheter before treatment can begin.

What is the treatment?

If your symptoms are mild and tests indicate that immediate surgery is not necessary, your physician may take no action. In at least 1 in 3 mild cases of an enlarged prostate, the symptoms clear up without treatment or with drug treatment, so it often makes sense to wait for a while. But if the problem does not go away, if it gets worse, or if tests show that urine flow is seriously blocked, the affected tissue must be removed.

The operation is called a prostatectomy. It may be performed by surgery through an abdominal incision or by a method known as transurethral resection of the prostate. Either method requires that you have anesthesia. To remove the excess tissue, your surgeon makes an incision in the lower part of the abdomen. In transurethral resection, no incision is made. Instead, a thin tube is passed up the penis to the prostate. In the tip of the tube is an electric cutting loop that removes the enlarged tissue. The electric cutting loop is guided with the help of a miniature telescope that is also in the tube. This procedure requires a hospital stay of about 4 days as compared with about 7 days for surgery to remove the prostate. In some cases, however, a transurethral resection is not possible.

What are the long-term prospects?

Regardless of the technique that is used, most prostatectomies are successful. They relieve urinary difficulties, and prostate problems seldom recur. Occasionally, a man becomes impotent after the operation. Almost all men who have had prostate surgery become sterile because their semen is expelled backward into the bladder instead of being ejaculated, but they are still able to have an orgasm. Semen in the bladder causes no harm. It is simply eliminated in the urine.

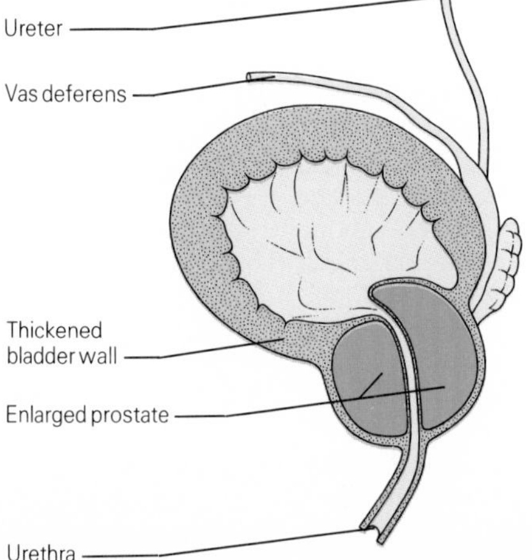

An enlarged prostate can obstruct the urethra, reducing the flow of urine and causing the muscular wall of the bladder to thicken as it works harder to force urine out.

Cancer of the prostate

Cancer of the prostate is the most common cancer in men in the US. The disease occurs more frequently after age 45, and by age 80 many men are found to have a small prostate cancer if tested. In most such cases, however, the cancer causes no symptoms and requires no treatment.

Early prostate cancer may be discovered by rectal examination during a physical checkup or the cancer may cause the prostate to enlarge, producing the same symptoms as an enlarged prostate. About half the men found to have cancer of the prostate have an early form of the disease that has not spread outside the prostate gland. If the cancer is not discovered at an early stage, however, it may metastasize (spread) to another part of the body, usually the bones. If cancer of the prostate spreads to the bones, the symptoms are those of bone cancer. Symptoms of bone cancer often indicate the presence of underlying cancer of the prostate.

What are the risks?

Cancer of the prostate rarely causes any symptoms before age 50, but it is a major cause of cancer death in older men. However, the symptoms and possible disability from cancer of the prostate can often be controlled for several years by hormone treatment.

What should be done?

A blood test along with a rectal examination may indicate the possible presence of prostate cancer. If cancer of the prostate is suspected either during a routine physical examination or because of the presence of urinary symptoms, your physician may refer you to a urologist, a specialist in urinary and genital diseases, or an oncologist, a cancer specialist. The urologist or oncologist may recommend a biopsy of the gland, in which a small sample is removed for examination. He or she may also recommend an ultrasound examination and X-ray tests of the kidneys and bladder. Your physician may examine the inside of the bladder using a cystoscope (viewing tube) to check for metastasis.

If the biopsy shows that a cancer is present, further tests such as a CT scan or radioisotope scan may be performed to look for cancer that has spread to the bones.

What is the treatment?

Treatment of prostate cancer usually requires a choice between treatment aimed at cure and less radical treatment aimed simply at relieving the symptoms. The man's age, his general health, how much importance he places on preserving sexual function, and whether the disease has spread are factors in determining the choice of treatment.

When the disease has not spread further than the prostate gland, there is a high chance of cure with surgical removal of the entire gland or by radiation therapy. Complete removal of the prostate gland offers the highest cure rate, but surgical removal can cause sexual impotence. In many men, the nerves controlling the ability to have and maintain erections can be saved, thereby preserving sexual function.

If the cancer has spread to the bones, surgical cure is not possible, but the cancer and its metastases in the bones can usually be controlled by hormone treatment. One effective method of halting the spread of the cancer is surgical removal of the testicles, but this treatment is used less often today, since the development of hormone treatment. In most cases, symptoms can be controlled for long periods without any serious side effects.

Prostatitis

Prostatitis, or inflammation of the prostate gland, is usually the result of a urinary tract infection that has spread to the prostate. Prostatitis may improve on its own, may become abscessed and form pus, or may persist and become chronic.

What are the symptoms?

An acute episode of prostatitis usually begins suddenly, with a high fever, chills, and pain in and around the base of your penis and behind your scrotum. Your rectum feels full, which produces an urge to move your bowels. Later, as the prostate gland becomes more swollen and tender, you may find it difficult and painful to urinate. This is because the prostate surrounds the urethra, and swelling of the gland narrows the urethra and blocks the flow of urine. Chronic prostatitis, however, often comes on gradually with some minor but persistent pain.

What are the risks?

Chronic prostatitis is common, especially in older men with enlarged prostates (see p.615). The disease may recur once you have had an initial acute attack.

If prostatitis is not treated, or if treatment with drugs is unsuccessful, the prostate may become abscessed and form pus, burst, and release blood and pus into the urethra. Such an abscess requires surgical treatment.

What should be done?

If you suspect you have prostatitis, consult your physician, who may perform an examination of your rectum to feel your prostate gland and determine whether it is swollen and tender. Your physician also may request a urine sample in order to identify the infectious agents that may be causing the inflammation.

What is the treatment?

If your symptoms are the result of a bacterial infection, your physician may prescribe antibiotics or antibacterial drugs. Occasionally, however, drugs do not completely cure prostatitis. Your physician may also recommend that you take hot tub baths 1 or 2 times a day to relieve discomfort, aid circulation, and promote healing.

Bladder, urethra, penis, and rectum

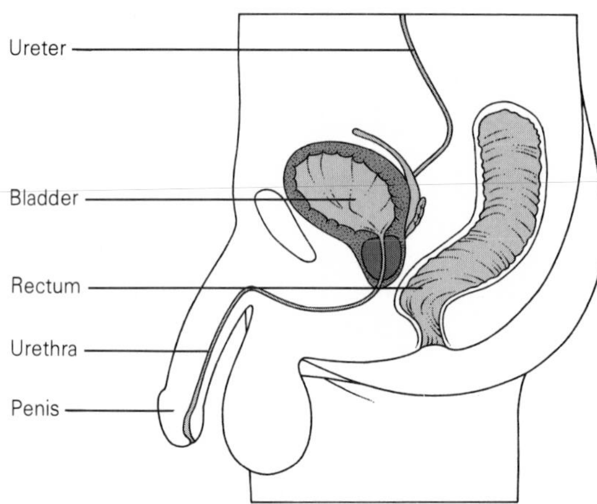

In men, several ducts join the urethra near the point where it leaves the bladder. The ducts lead from the testes, the seminal vesicles, the Cowper's glands, and the prostate gland. These ducts carry semen or seminal fluid to the outside during ejaculation. The prostate gland (see p.615) surrounds the passageway. For a full discussion of the structure of the bladder and urethra and their relationships to the rest of the urinary tract, see p.539. In a man, most of the urethra lies inside the penis. The penis is composed of spongy tissue filled with tiny blood vessels that are capable of holding large amounts of blood. In an erect penis this spongy tissue is engorged with blood. In a relaxed penis the spongy tissue is empty and the penis appears smaller. The slightly bulbous end (glans) of the penis is covered by a loose flap of skin, the foreskin or prepuce. In the US foreskins are frequently removed at birth in a procedure called circumcision (see p.698).

The rectum is the last segment of the large intestine, and it is connected to the outside of the body by the anus. The function of the rectum is described in the section of the book that describes the digestive system (see Large intestine, p.512).

With good personal hygiene, the male bladder, urethra, penis, and rectum are not particularly susceptible to disease. For additional information on disorders that can affect these parts of the body but that originate elsewhere in the body, consult the sections on disorders of the urinary tract (see p.539) and sexuality (see p.648).

Cystitis in men

Cystitis, or inflammation of the bladder, is a common, often uncomfortable, but relatively harmless condition in women (see p.643). Cystitis is rare in men, but potentially more serious because it is usually caused by either an underlying urinary tract problem such as an obstruction or a tumor, or by an infection that has spread from elsewhere in the urinary tract, such as the urethra or the prostate gland. The symptoms of cystitis include pressure or pain in the lower abdomen, itching, burning, blood in the urine, a sense of an urgent need to urinate, and/or increased frequency of urination. The symptoms may be secondary; that is, indicate that you also have some other disorder, so you should see your physician immediately. Your physician may prescribe antibiotics or antibacterial drugs and may also recommend tests to discover the underlying disorder. Such tests may include cystoscopy, ultrasound, and an intravenous pyelogram (special X rays of the kidneys, bladder, and ureters taken after injecting a solution into a vein). Once the underlying disorder has been identified, your physician will discuss appropriate treatment with you.

Penile warts

Warts on the penis are similar to warts elsewhere on the body and are caused by similar viruses that are members of the human papillomavirus family (see Warts, p.268), but they are usually transmitted by sexual contact. Do not assume, however, that any wartlike growths on your penis or just inside the urethral opening are harmless. Rarely, but occasionally, a growth that resembles a wart may be an early sign of either cancer of the penis (see p.620) or syphilis (see p.655). So always consult your physician if you develop what looks like penile warts. If your physician confirms the diagnosis of penile warts and recommends or prescribes a lotion for removing them, be sure to use it exactly as directed. Never try to treat warts on your penis with an over-the-counter preparation designed to treat warts elsewhere on the skin. Penile skin is much more sensitive than, for example, the skin on your hands or feet. Skin on the penis can be damaged by the powerful chemicals used in over-the-counter wart removal lotion.

Like all warts, those on the penis are caused by local virus infection and are therefore contagious. Warts on the genital area can be transmitted to your sexual partner during intercourse. So if you have (or have had) penile warts, it is a good idea for your sexual partner to consult a physician, who may check for genital warts. Unless both partners are successfully treated, the virus can be passed back and forth indefinitely. Viruses from the human papillomavirus family have been implicated as a possible cause of cancers of the penis, vulva, vagina, cervix, and anus.

Urethritis in men

Urethritis, or inflammation of the urethra, in men usually results from an infection transmitted through sexual intercourse with an infected partner. The major symptoms of urethritis are a plentiful thick, yellow, pus-filled discharge from the tip of the penis and dysuria, burning pain when you urinate. The urine may be bloodstained. The most common forms of urethritis in men are non-gonococcal urethritis (see p.655) and gonorrhea (see p.654). Because these diseases can be passed back and forth between sexual partners, they are discussed in the section on sexuality (see p.648).

Urethral stricture

Urethral stricture is a rare condition in which the urethra gradually narrows as a result of shrinking scar tissue inside the urethral walls. The scarring is often caused by an injury in the genital area. A common cause of urethral scar tissue once was persistent urethritis (see previous article) due to infection, but early antibiotic treatment of diseases such as gonorrhea (see p.654) has all but eliminated them as causes of scarring by shortening the duration of the infection. However, the risk still exists for those men in whom recurring or chronic urethritis develops.

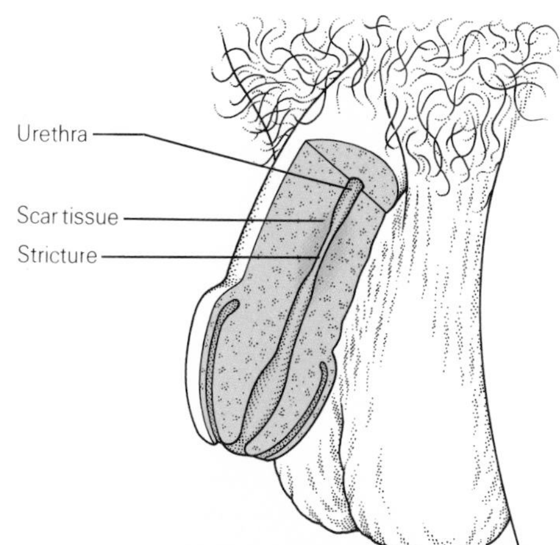

Scar tissue in a urethra previously damaged by disease or injury can narrow the channel and may completely block the flow of urine.

What are the symptoms?

The narrowed urethra of a man who has urethral stricture may make it increasingly difficult for him to urinate. This problem can be painful and can lead to urinary infections.

What should be done?

If your urethral stricture continues to become more narrow, your physician may refer you to a urologist, a specialist in urinary and genital diseases. The urologist may try to stretch the urethra using a long, flexible instrument. The instrument is inserted through the opening in the penis with the help of a local anesthetic. You will need several of these treatments, called dilatations, over several weeks, and you may need follow-up treatments.

If this does not widen the stricture, the urologist may recommend surgery to remove the scar tissue or to remove and replace the scar tissue with tissue taken from another part of your body and grafted on the area. No treatment has been completely satisfactory.

Balanitis

Balanitis describes several types of inflammation of the foreskin and glans at the tip of the penis. The cause of this common problem may be infection (see Genital herpes, p.656), accumulation of a thick, cheesy skin gland secretion called smegma, friction with damp clothing, or irritation from certain chemical substances in your clothing, condoms, or spermicides. Uncircumcised men are more susceptible to this condition. Balanitis can cause an increase in soreness and swelling at the end of the penis and in the foreskin, making it difficult for uncircumcised men to pull the foreskin back to wash the area.

Most types of balanitis clear up if you determine and treat the underlying cause. If necessary, particularly if it is painful or difficult to pull back your foreskin, consult your physician, who may prescribe an antibiotic lotion or oral medication to help relieve the inflammation. In persistent cases, your physician may recommend surgical loosening of the foreskin or circumcision, in which the foreskin is removed.

Priapism

An erection that persists in the absence of sexual arousal and will not subside is known as priapism. This rare and painful condition is usually caused by sudden, unexplained obstruction of the outflow of engorging blood from the erect penis. Occasionally, however, priapism is caused by disease or injury of the nerves in the spinal cord that control erection. If the priapism lasts for several hours, the spongy tissues of the penis may be permanently damaged, which can make future erections impossible.

What should be done?

If you have an erection that persists for no apparent reason, call your physician or go immediately to a hospital emergency department. Priapism is an emergency. It may be treated with surgery to bypass the blockage, spinal anesthesia, or drugs that will relieve the muscle spasm in the blood vessels that prevents blood from leaving the penis. If priapism is treated quickly, the erection will probably subside, and you should eventually be able to have normal erections again.

Cancer of the penis

The cause of cancer of the penis is not known, but there appears to be a strong relationship between development of the disease and many years of poor hygiene under the foreskin. Circumcised males are less susceptible than uncircumcised males.

What are the symptoms?

The major symptom of cancer of the penis is a sore spot, skin ulcer, or warty lump that slowly spreads across the skin of the penis and deep into the tissues of the penis. If the disease is not treated, it will metastasize, or spread to other parts of the body, most often via the lymphatic system (see p.463) or the bloodstream. Cancer of the penis may spread first to the lymph glands in the groin and may cause them to swell.

What should be done?

If you have a draining sore or any type of growth on your penis, consult your physician, who may recommend a biopsy. In this procedure, a small sample of tissue from the penis is removed for examination. The biopsy is necessary to distinguish cancer of the penis from syphilis (see p.655) and penile warts (see p.619), both of which may look similar to a cancerous growth. If cancer of the penis is diagnosed, your physician may recommend surgery. However, radiation therapy is another possible form of treatment.

Hemospermia

Hemospermia means blood in the semen. Blood usually appears as pinkish, reddish, or brownish streaks in your semen. Hemospermia results from rupture of a small vein or veins in the upper part of the urethra. This can happen at any time during an erection. It is common and usually goes unnoticed. If you notice a small amount of blood in your semen, do not be concerned. The ruptured vein or veins usually close up within a few minutes without treatment. If your semen remains discolored for more than several days, consult your physician.

If you are not sure that the blood was actually in your semen, and if you think it may signify bleeding from your urethra after ejaculation, you should see your physician. He or she may want to rule out the possibility of bladder problems as a cause of the bleeding. Hematuria, or blood in the urine, may be a symptom of serious illness (see, for example, Tumors of the bladder, p.547).

Anorectal abscesses

Abscesses, or enclosed pockets of pus, can develop around the anus and rectum. These infections, called anorectal abscesses, are more common in men and in people with digestive diseases (see Ulcerative colitis, p.516), leukemia (see p.457), and diabetes mellitus (see p.558).

Anorectal abscesses can occur either in the tissue surrounding the anus, deeper in the rectum between the sphincter muscles, or in the tissues higher up in the rectum. Symptoms include intense rectal pain, swelling, and warmth, sometimes resulting in fever and chills. If the abscess is inside the space surrounding the rectum, it may be difficult for your physician to locate it until it ruptures. However, an examination of the rectum performed with a gloved finger often helps the physician find the abscess. An ultrasound examination may also be performed.

What is the treatment?

If you have intense pain in the rectal area, see your physician. He or she may treat an anorectal abscess by surgically opening the abscess and allowing the pus to drain. Abscesses near the skin's surface are easily operated on, but deeper ones may require more exploration and probing. In such cases, you may need general anesthesia.

Proctitis

Proctitis is inflammation of the rectum. It may be related to ulcerative colitis (see p.516), and is the mildest form of that disease. However, if the rectum is the only area of inflamed bowel, proctitis usually results from a sexually transmitted disease.

Proctitis caused by the bacterium that causes gonorrhea produces a discharge that ranges from cloudy mucus to a puslike material. This discharge may be accompanied by burning, itching, bleeding, and painful bowel movements. Proctitis from syphilis causes a chancre, or open sore, either in the rectum or around the anus. The herpes virus can cause blistering ulcers inside the rectum or near the anus. Often these causes of proctitis may lead to itching and pain around the rectum and anus. The herpes virus can also infect the nerves that extend from the spinal cord into the lower back and cause recurrent pain in the back, thighs, or buttocks, difficulty in urinating, or problems with erections (see Impotence, next article). Penile warts (see p.619) can also affect the rectal area but do not cause proctitis.

When proctitis results from these sexually transmitted diseases, it can be spread further through anal or vaginal intercourse. If you have any of these symptoms, see your physician right away. He or she may want to analyze a sample of any discharge from sores to find out what is causing the problem. Your physician may prescribe antibiotics if the infection is caused by bacteria. Warts can be treated with a special solution. No effective treatment is currently available for the herpes virus, so the infection must be allowed to run its course, and it may recur in a milder form.

Impotence

Impotence is the loss of a man's ability to have and maintain an erection. Impotence may result from either physical or psychological factors, or a combination of both. These psychological factors may be complicated and difficult for the man to admit. Men who cannot have or maintain an erection may still have a strong sexual drive and can feel very vulnerable and frustrated about the impotence.

Often temporary situations such as marital difficulties, job or money loss, stress, fatigue, or anxiety lead to loss of sexual interest or desire and may result in impotence. Impotence may also be a symptom of severe depression (see p.321).

Even when a man cannot maintain an erection for psychological reasons, he usually continues to have erections during the night. He may have erection problems with one sexual partner but not with others. (See also Loss of sexual desire in men, p.658.) In such cases, the man would also be able to sustain an erection with masturbation.

During an erection, the penis becomes engorged with blood as the spongy tissues expand and allow blood to flow into the tissues, and then temporarily keep it from flowing back out again. Because this action is controlled by muscles in the blood vessels, which, in turn, are controlled by nerves that are controlled by the brain, some drugs prescribed to treat other conditions may affect the brain and interfere with an erection. Some commonly prescribed medications can have this effect, such as various drugs used to treat hypertension, including diuretics. Tranquilizers and medications used to treat depression (antidepressants) can also inhibit sexual function.

Alcohol often affects a man's ability to have and maintain an erection, even when he does not drink excessively. Chronic alcohol abuse (see p.329) and the liver disease it may lead to (see Cirrhosis of the liver, p.524) lowers the amount of testosterone circulating in the bloodstream. Testosterone, the major male sex hormone, is produced in the testicles. Testosterone affects male physical characteristics such as body hair and stimulates the sex drive and sperm production. Therefore, decreased testosterone production may interfere with a man's sexual function.

Diseased blood vessels can prevent the inflow or interfere with the retention of blood necessary to produce an erection. Severe arteriosclerosis (see Hardening of the arteries, p.435) in the blood vessels of the lower half of the body causes narrowing of the vessels that restricts the inflow of blood needed to produce an erection. Men who have severe, chronic diabetes (see Diabetes mellitus, p.558) also are at risk for impotence because the nerves and blood vessels may be damaged by the disease. Hypertension, or high blood pressure (see p.411), and chronic illnesses such as kidney failure (see p.550) may also be associated with impotence.

Diseases that inhibit the production or action of the male hormone testosterone can also reduce sexual interest and performance. Sometimes, rare conditions such as tumors of the pituitary (see p.557) or hypothalamus affect these vital centers in the brain that regulate and produce hormones.

What should be done?

If you are consistently unable to have an erection, consult your physician. He or she will want to find out whether the problem is caused by physical or psychological factors, or a combination of both. If you are able to have erections on waking or with masturbation, your impotence may have psychological origins. Your physician will also want to know about your drug or alcohol intake or if you are taking any medication that may have an effect on your ability to have and maintain an erection.

Your physician may recommend using a sensitive gauge to take measurements of changes in the size and firmness of your penis as you sleep. He or she may also recommend X rays of spongy erectile tissues to see whether blood drains from them too rapidly. In a very few cases, blood pressures in these tissues may be measured.

What is the treatment?

If your impotence appears to be caused by psychological problems, your physician may refer you to a psychiatrist, a psychologist, or a sex therapist. Psychological treatment is usually given to couples, not individuals.

If impotence results from an underlying physical condition, treatment is usually straightforward. If the cause is arterial or nerve disease, or if psychological treatment is unsuccessful, erections may be induced by injections of drugs into the penis. Thousands of men have learned how to inject themselves in this way. Often a few erections induced by injection are enough to break the psychological cycle of failure. Also available are external vacuum erection devices that draw blood into the penis; a rubber band helps keep the erection for no more than 20 minutes.

Surgery to slow blood flow from the penis or to reestablish blood flow in narrowed arteries has also been used in some instances. Persistent impotence may also be treated by surgical insertion of a prosthesis into the penis. Several different designs are in common use. However, surgical insertion of a prosthesis should not be considered a guaranteed solution to sexual problems, and such treatment should be attempted only after consulting an experienced sex counselor.

Hygiene for men

Daily soap and water washing of the penile shaft and scrotum are important. If you are not circumcised, be sure to wash the glans (the head of the penis) under the foreskin by pulling back the foreskin.

Thorough washing will not prevent gonorrhea (see p.654) or syphilis (see p.655), since the bacteria that produce these diseases are inside the body. However, organisms that produce minor infections such as nongonococcal urethritis (see p.655) and nonspecific vaginitis in women may be removed by washing the genital area thoroughly with soap and water.

As you wash, always look for sores or ulcers that could result from a sexually transmitted disease, and see your physician as soon as possible if you find any.

Women's health

Introduction

The topics discussed in this section are those that primarily affect women. Aspects of women's health that are not discussed here, such as pregnancy and childbirth, problems of adolescent girls, problems of older people, problems of couples (including sexually transmitted diseases), and all the conditions that affect women in much the same way as they affect men, are discussed in other sections of this book.

The topics described in the following pages are divided into several categories. First, there are disorders of the menstrual cycle: the monthly cycle of egg ripening, egg release, and shedding of the lining of the uterus. The menstrual cycle is controlled by a complex system of hormones that are produced and released by the hypothalamus, pituitary gland, and the ovaries. The cycle can be disturbed if the hormonal balance is upset by any of a number of factors, both physical and emotional.

Several of the other groups of articles are concerned with a variety of structural abnormalities, infections, inflammations, and growths that can occur in female organs. These are disorders of the breast, ovaries, uterus and cervix, and of the vagina and vulva.

Of particular importance are the boxes related to breast cancer, a major concern of women today because breast cancer affects 1 out of 9 women in the US. One box describes and illustrates the proper way to examine your breasts for signs of cancer. Another box tells you what you should know about having a mammogram.

There is also a group of articles that describe disorders of the bladder and urethra. These articles appear in this section because disorders of the bladder and urethra are more common in women and often cause different problems in women than they do in men.

If you suspect that you have one of the disorders described in this section, consult your physician. This section also contains several informative boxes that discuss some health aspects not necessarily directly related to a specific disease. These include menstrual care and vaginal douching. A box on hysteroscopy explains how physicians have developed improved technology for diagnosing problems of the uterus.

The female reproductive organs

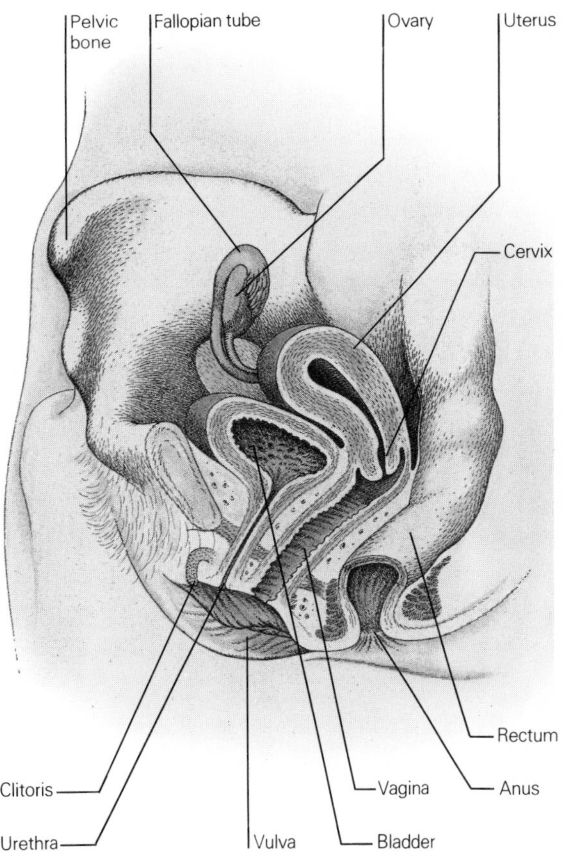

Menstruation and menopause

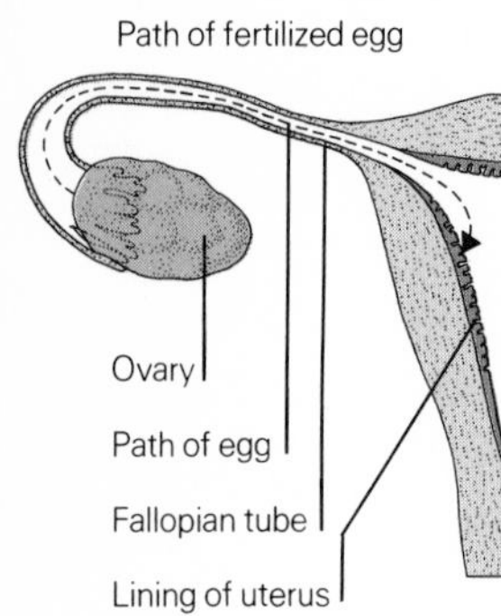

Each month, if you are fertile, you experience ovulation, or egg release. One of your 2 ovaries releases an ovum, or egg. The egg is a tiny single cell, barely visible. It travels down your fallopian tube to your uterus. This takes about 5 days. You can become pregnant if you have sexual intercourse within a day or 2 before or after the egg is released. After intercourse, sperm usually make their way up into the fallopian tubes. Sperm can live for as long as 6 days, so if you have sexual intercourse between 5 days before release of the egg and 24 hours after, a sperm will be able to fertilize the egg.

A few days before ovulation, the lining of your uterus becomes thickened and engorged with blood. This prepares your body for the possibility of fertilization. By the time a fertilized egg reaches the uterus, the lining is prepared for the egg to attach itself to the uterus. Once attached, the egg will start developing into an embryo. If this happens, you are pregnant.

If the egg is not fertilized, the thickened, blood-filled lining of the uterus is shed along with the unfertilized egg, about 14 days after ovulation. The menstrual fluid passes out of the cervix (the neck of the uterus), into the vagina, and out of your body. This discharge, called menstruation or a menstrual period, lasts an average of 5 days. During the next 9 days a new lining grows in the uterus, and then the process of ovulation starts again.

The entire cycle lasts an average of 28 days. But in most women the cycle fluctuates by a day or two or sometimes longer. Each stage in the menstrual cycle is controlled by interrelated hormones produced in the hypothalamus, pituitary gland, and ovaries.

Menstrual periods usually start between ages 11 and 14. The first period is called menarche. Periods are irregular for the first year or 2 because ovulation does not initially occur regularly. Periods also become irregular after about 45 because of irregular ovulation, and finally stop permanently. This is called menopause.

Problems related to the length, frequency, and effect of menstrual periods are discussed in this section.

The menstrual cycle (28 days)

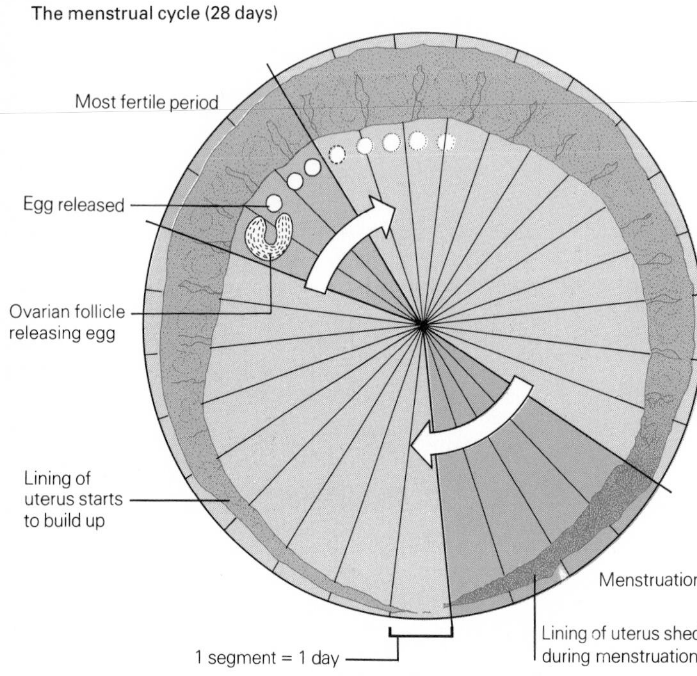

Absence of periods

(amenorrhea)

The temporary or permanent absence of menstrual periods is known medically as amenorrhea. In some girls, periods fail to start at the normal age, usually between 11 and 14. This is called primary amenorrhea, which is usually the result of a naturally late onset of puberty, but it can be caused by an abnormality in the reproductive or hormonal system. The search for such abnormalities does not usually begin until a girl has reached age 16 or 17 without having a period.

In a woman who has had regular periods, a delay or absence of periods is called secondary amenorrhea; it is caused by a change in the balance of hormones that control the release of an egg from the ovary. One cause of secondary amenorrhea is pregnancy. Hormones may also be disrupted by emotional factors (such as heightened emotions or a new job), a rapid weight loss (see Anorexia nervosa, p.758), illness, or taking certain drugs. Women who have just stopped taking oral contraceptives may experience secondary amenorrhea for a few months. Sometimes absence of periods is a result of a disorder affecting egg release (see Abnormalities of the hypothalamus, pituitary, and ovaries, p.628).

Periods stop permanently at menopause (see p.627) or when the ovaries are removed as treatment for another disorder.

What are the risks?

Absence of periods is common; secondary amenorrhea occurs much more often than primary amenorrhea. In rare cases, it may indicate a more serious disorder. In addition, a woman with amenorrhea may not be able to get pregnant without special treatment. Also, there are risks to prolonged anovulation (absence of egg release).

Normally, there is a balance between estrogen and progesterone (the two main female sex hormones) in a woman's body. When periods are absent, no progesterone hormones are produced, leaving only estrogen. Estrogen, without progesterone, can lead to endometrial cancer or may lead to breast cancer. This risk is probably greater in obese women or in women with other medical problems, such as hypertension (high blood pressure) or diabetes.

What should be done?

If you are 14 and have not had a period, not had an increase in growth, and not begun to develop breasts or pubic hair, talk to your physician. If you are over 16 and you have never had a period but are fully physically developed, you should also consult your physician, who will examine you. In most cases, there is no reason for you to be concerned. Usually no treatment is necessary, and you can simply wait for your periods to start on their own. Young women who are very thin or who are in intense athletic training programs sometimes have a delayed onset of menstruation.

If your periods have already started and become fairly regular, and your period is delayed for 2 weeks or more, consult your physician. If there is a possibility that you are pregnant, your physician may recommend that you have a pregnancy test. If you are not pregnant and are otherwise well, your physician will probably advise you to wait for a few months to see if your periods will start again on their own.

If you have amenorrhea, it is important to remember that an egg may be released at any time. If you want to avoid getting pregnant, and you expect to have sexual intercourse, you must use some form of contraception.

If you do not have a period for 6 months, your physician may arrange for you to have some diagnostic tests to look for any underlying problem. If none is found, no treatment may be given for the absence of periods unless you want to become pregnant. In that case, your physician may prescribe a fertility drug to restart ovulation (see Infertility, p.649).

Irregular periods

(oligomenorrhea)

A woman's periods are irregular when there are wide variations in the number of days between them, their length in days, or the amount of blood lost.

Variations in your pattern of menstruation may result from stress, travel, or a change in contraceptive method. Since menstruation depends on a balance of estrogen and progesterone hormones (the two main female sex hormones), irregular periods may result from a disturbance of your usual hormone cycle (see Abnormalities of the hypothalamus, pituitary, and ovaries, p.628). After menstrual periods begin and for several years before menopause (see p.627), your periods may be irregular and ovulation (release of an egg) may or may not occur.

Vaginal bleeding between periods may also result from an unrecognized pregnancy or an early miscarriage. Sometimes underlying disorders of the uterus, ovaries, or pelvic cavity (see Endometriosis, p.638) can result in irregular periods or painful periods (see next article). Irregular periods may not affect your general health and usually do not require treatment.

Painful periods

(dysmenorrhea)

Painful periods, especially menstrual cramps, are also called dysmenorrhea. If the pain starts within about 3 years of menarche, it is known as primary dysmenorrhea, which is thought to be a result of normal hormonal changes during menstruation and can persist for years until menopause.

If periods become painful in a woman who has been menstruating longer than 3 years, the condition is known as secondary dysmenorrhea. Secondary dysmenorrhea may be caused by disorders such as endometriosis (see p.638), pelvic inflammatory disease (see p.639), or fibroids (see p.636).

What are the symptoms?

Menstrual pain varies considerably. Some women have dull pain in the abdomen or

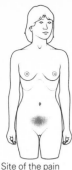

back, others have severe cramping abdominal pain. The pain is usually worse at the beginning of a period. Sometimes there is also nausea and vomiting.

Painful periods are very common but most cases are mild and do not require treatment. Painful periods do not affect your general health. However, they may be a symptom of a more serious underlying disorder.

What is the treatment?

If the pain is not severe, you may only need to take a nonsteroidal anti-inflammatory drug such as aspirin or another pain-relief medication sold over the counter. Your physician may prescribe nonsteroidal anti-inflammatory drugs. Oral contraceptives may provide both pain relief and contraception. Exercise may also help relieve the pain. Bed rest is usually not necessary.

Consult your physician if you develop severe menstrual pain following 3 or more years of relatively pain-free periods, or if the pain is worse than usual. He or she will examine you to determine what is causing the pain, and treat any underlying disorder.

Site of the pain

Heavy periods

(menorrhagia)

Unusually heavy and prolonged periods are known medically as menorrhagia. You have them if your periods last longer than 7 days, if especially large clots of blood are passed, or if the flow is very heavy. The condition is often brought on by a spontaneous disturbance of the hormones that control the menstrual cycle. It can also be caused by fibroids (see p.636), pelvic inflammatory disease (see p.639), or, rarely, endometriosis (see p.638). An intrauterine device (IUD) may also cause the condition.

What are the risks?

Heavy periods are common. Some women regularly have heavy periods; others have them only occasionally. The condition frequently occurs in young women who have not yet established regular ovulation cycles, and it is especially common in women approaching menopause.

Apart from being very inconvenient, menorrhagia can be distressing. However, the condition rarely indicates a serious underlying disorder. One risk is that if you regularly have heavy periods and you do not consume enough iron-containing foods, you may develop iron-deficiency anemia (see p.450).

What should be done?

If you have been having heavy periods for some time, consult your physician. If you have a single unusually heavy period, follow the self-help measures suggested later in this article. If your period was late as well as heavy and there was a chance of pregnancy, you may be having an early miscarriage. In this case, see your physician immediately. Your physician will question and examine you to determine the extent of bleeding and to see if there is any abnormality of your uterus. A Pap test may be done to check for cervical cancer, and an endometrial biopsy (taking a sample of the uterine lining) may also be performed. A blood test may be done to find out if menorrhagia has made you anemic and to check for other blood and hormone problems that can cause the condition.

What is the treatment?

Self-help: If you have an unusually heavy period and do not think you are pregnant, reduce your activity. If the bleeding does not lessen within 24 hours, call your physician.

Professional help: If your physician does not find a reason for your heavy periods, he or she may prescribe a hormone medication that contains estrogen, a progesterone replacement, or both, to reduce the bleeding. These are the same ingredients as those used in oral contraceptives. If you are already taking oral contraceptives, or if you cannot take them for some reason, your physician can prescribe another drug to reduce the bleeding. If you are using an IUD, your

Hysteroscopy

A hysteroscope is a flexible, lighted viewing instrument that is inserted through the vagina, through the cervical canal, and into the uterus. Hysteroscopy is the name of the procedure using this instrument; it can be performed in a hospital outpatient clinic or your physician's office using a local anesthetic.

A hysteroscopy allows your physician to view your uterus directly and to evaluate and diagnose certain uterine disorders. It may, for example, confirm the presence of uterine fibroids, endometrial polyps, hyperplasia (thickening of the lining of the uterus), and tumors that may be benign (unlikely to spread) or malignant (likely to spread). A hysteroscope may be used as a viewing aid during a D&C (see Box, p.637) and can also be used to look for lost IUDs.

Another technique to evaluate the status of your uterus is a hysterogram, an X ray during which dye is injected into the uterus through a small tube. If the dye outlines not just your uterus but also your fallopian tubes, the procedure is called a hysterosalpingogram.

physician may recommend that you consider using another method of contraception. If blood tests indicate that you are anemic, you may have to take an iron supplement.

If this treatment is not effective after a few months, your physician may take a sample of the lining of your uterus (an endometrial biopsy); this may be done with or without hysteroscopy (see p.626). Another alternative is dilatation and curettage (D&C) (see Box, p.637), which can help determine the cause; even if no abnormality is found, the D&C may temporarily reduce bleeding. Endometrial ablation is a new procedure in which the surgeon destroys all or most of the lining of the uterus; it sometimes offers benefits for women who do not want a hysterectomy or to become pregnant. In some circumstances, however, a hysterectomy (see Box, p.638) is the best solution.

Premenstrual syndrome

(PMS)

Each month various glands in your body release hormones into the bloodstream. The two main sex hormones in women are estrogen and progesterone, both of which are made in the ovaries. They control various changes in your body, including changes in the uterus during the menstrual cycle (see Menstruation and menopause, p.624), and associated physical changes such as increased breast tenderness. In addition, the monthly cycle of hormonal changes may affect your mood and produce mental or emotional changes. The combination of physical and emotional changes that may occur in the 7 days or so before you have your period may cause premenstrual syndrome (PMS).

What are the symptoms?

Mood changes usually take the form of increased irritability, aggressiveness, and/or depression. Physical changes may include an increase in weight because of fluid retention, slightly enlarged and tender breasts, food craving, and bloated stomach. The degree of severity of these symptoms may vary considerably. In many cases, the symptoms are moderate. But occasionally the symptoms are so pronounced that they affect personal relationships or performance at work.

What should be done?

Consult your physician if your symptoms are severe. Although there is no clear evidence that the symptoms result from an excess of either progesterone or estrogen in the body, some women find that their symptoms are relieved by treatments that alter the activity of these hormones, such as the combined oral contraceptive pill. Other women obtain relief with monthly injections of progesterone or brief periodic use of diuretics or vitamin E supplements. You and your physician may need to experiment with different treatments to find the one that suits you best. Aerobic exercise, good nutrition, and adequate rest all help diminish PMS symptoms.

If your symptoms are not relieved by such treatment, your physician may prescribe analgesics or tranquilizers to take on days when symptoms are most severe. If you have severe depression, your physician may refer you to a psychologist or psychiatrist.

Menopause

Menopause is the term used to describe the normal, permanent ending of menstrual cycles, including both ovulation and menstrual periods. The term is often used in a broader sense to mean the months or even years before and after this natural event occurs. This time is sometimes called the climacteric or the change of life. The last period usually occurs between ages 40 and 54, but can happen as late as 60. In the years leading up to menopause, your menstrual cycle changes and periods may become irregular.

What are the symptoms?

About 25 percent of women do not notice any changes at menopause, except the cessation of periods. Another 50 percent notice slight physical and/or mental changes. The remaining 25 percent have inconvenient or distressing symptoms that may include sweating, hot flashes, dryness of the vagina (sometimes causing soreness during sexual intercourse), palpitations, joint pain, and headaches. More seriously, after several years about one woman in five develops osteoporosis (see p.581), which, in severe cases, may lead to increased susceptibility to fractures of the wrists, hips, and spine. Other symptoms may include depression, anxiety, irritability, difficulty concentrating, lack of confidence, and sleeping difficulties. These symptoms may last from a few weeks to several years.

What should be done?

Some symptoms are more likely to occur during menopause—such as irregular menstrual bleeding and hot flashes—but will eventually stop. Diseases occur during any period of your life, however, and you should not automatically attribute all symptoms to menopause. Instead, discuss them with your physician. He or she will examine you to find out the cause of your symptoms.

You should see your physician immediately if you have bleeding between periods, prolonged or excessive menstrual bleeding, or another period 6 months or longer after what appeared to be the last. Any of these symptoms could indicate a malignant growth such as cancer of the uterus (see p.637).

What is the treatment?

Self-help: Regular exercise and a diet rich in calcium (good sources of calcium include skim milk and green vegetables) give the best protection against osteoporosis. Exercise can also help combat depression, another common symptom of menopause.

Remember that you may still be fertile as you start menopause. If you are under 50 and are sexually active, you should continue to use contraceptives for 24 months after the date of your last period. If you are over 50, you should protect yourself for 12 months after the last period.

If you are having hot flashes and sweating, keep in mind that you are usually the only person who is aware of them. If sweating is a nuisance at night, wear absorbent cotton night clothes. If you find that intercourse makes your vagina sore, use a lubricant such as a water-soluble jelly; your physician can also prescribe a vaginal cream that contains estrogen, which can help relieve the dryness of your vagina.

Professional help: Symptoms of menopause are mostly due to lack of estrogen, so the logical treatment is to replace it. Hormone replacement therapy has been prescribed for millions of women, and its advantages and drawbacks are still being researched.

Hormone replacement therapy not only relieves menopausal symptoms and helps prevent osteoporosis, but there is also growing evidence that estrogen reduces the risk of coronary heart disease. Many physicians now recommend that treatment be continued indefinitely after menopause.

Most women take medication that contains estrogen and a progestin (a synthetic form of progesterone). This hormone combination is used because estrogen given alone may slightly increase the chance that cancer of the uterus will develop. If you have had your uterus removed, however, there is no need to take progesterone. Still being debated is the possibility of a slightly increased risk of breast cancer.

The combined hormone preparation is usually taken in a cyclical fashion (like an oral contraceptive), and menstrual bleeding may occur every 1 or 2 months after you stop using the drug. In some circumstances, estrogen is taken via a patch applied to the skin, as a long-acting injection, or as a vaginal cream.

There are medications other than hormones that can help alleviate menopausal symptoms. These may be prescribed for women who for some reason should not take hormone therapy. You may benefit from discussing your concerns with other women who are going through menopause; ask your local hospital if it has a menopause support group.

If you have mainly emotional or psychological symptoms, your physician may prescribe antidepressants. However, unless you have severe anxiety, it is unlikely that your physician will prescribe tranquilizers because of the risk of addiction.

Abnormalities of the hypothalamus, pituitary, and ovaries

A number of problems can be caused by a disturbance of the interrelated system of sex hormones in a woman's body. The menstrual cycle is regulated by several hormones. Each month the hypothalamus, which is part of the brain, produces chemicals known as releasing hormones. Releasing hormones pass into the pituitary gland and stimulate the production of pituitary hormones, which in turn affect the ovaries and cause ovulation, the release of an egg. These hormones also stimulate the production of the female sex hormones estrogen and progesterone in the ovary.

This cycle can be disturbed by a number of factors. The hypothalamus may be affected by emotional factors, drug abuse, extreme changes of weight (see Anorexia nervosa, p.758), or another severe illness. Occasionally, the hypothalamus is disturbed if you stop taking oral contraceptives. Some brain disorders such as meningitis (see p.290) or a brain tumor (see p.301) can also affect the hypothalamus.

The pituitary gland is less susceptible to disturbances. Tumors of the pituitary gland (see p.557), although they are very rare, almost always cause abnormalities in sex hormone production. Certain rare disorders of the ovary may also affect hormone production. These include some ovarian cysts (see p.635), and polycystic ovary disease. For other disorders of the ovaries, see the articles beginning on p.635.

What are the symptoms?
The main symptom of abnormal sex hormone production is disruption of periods (see Absence of periods, p.624). If the pituitary gland is the cause, there may also be other symptoms (see Pituitary gland, p.554).

In some disorders of the ovaries or adrenal glands, production of the male sex hormone testosterone (also produced in women) may increase. This may cause hairiness (hirsutism) on the face and body, deepening of the voice, acne, and weight gain.

Each month the hypothalamus produces releasing hormones that, in turn, stimulate production of pituitary hormones. Pituitary hormones then affect the ovaries, triggering ovulation.

What should be done?
If your periods become irregular or stop completely, consult your physician, who after examining you to see if either pregnancy or an underlying disorder is causing the problem, may advise you to take no further action unless you have no periods for at least 6 months. If your physician suspects an underlying disorder, you may need to have blood and urine tests to determine hormone levels in your body, along with a CT or MRI scan of your pituitary gland.

If an underlying disorder is causing your symptoms, your physician will treat it. Treatment consists of oral contraceptives or progesterone medication, unless you want to become pregnant (see Infertility, p.649).

Breasts

Each of a woman's breasts consists of 15 to 20 groups of milk-producing glands surrounded by fatty tissue. From each group a milk duct runs to the nipple. Around the nipple is a dark area, the areola, that contains small sebaceous, or lubricating, glands that keep the nipple supple.

During pregnancy, the release of hormones from the placenta and the pituitary gland causes the breasts to enlarge and, after delivery, to produce milk (see Pregnancy and childbirth, p.661). The breasts may also become a little larger, and sometimes tender, before a menstrual period.

The following group of articles discusses some of the problems that can develop in the breast. Such problems may be caused by abnormal growths such as cysts or tumors or they can also result from a breast infection.

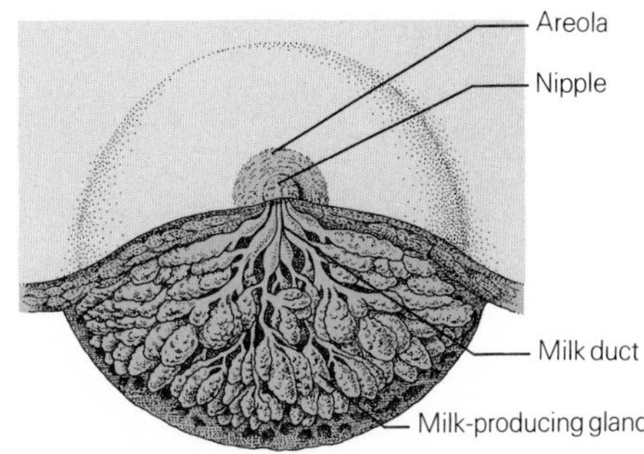

Breast cancer is the most common cancer in women. Every woman should examine her breasts regularly, have regular physical examinations, and have her first mammogram between age 35 and 40 (see Box, p.631) to detect any signs of possible breast cancer.

Lumps in the breast

Some women's breasts are irregularly shaped, uneven in texture, or have lumps in them. This is usually not a cause for concern. Lumps in the breast may cause no discomfort at all. Sometimes a lump is slightly tender or even painful. The appearance of a new lump is more important. There are five possible causes of a lump in the breast. The first is a cyst, which is a fluid-filled sac of tissue. The second is an infection, which usually involves additional symptoms (see Breast abscess, p.632). The third cause of a breast lump is fibrocystic changes, which are a thickening of the milk-producing glandular tissue. The fourth cause is a benign growth. None of these lumps is harmful. But the fifth possible cause of a lump in the breast is a malignant (likely to spread) tumor.

How to examine your breasts

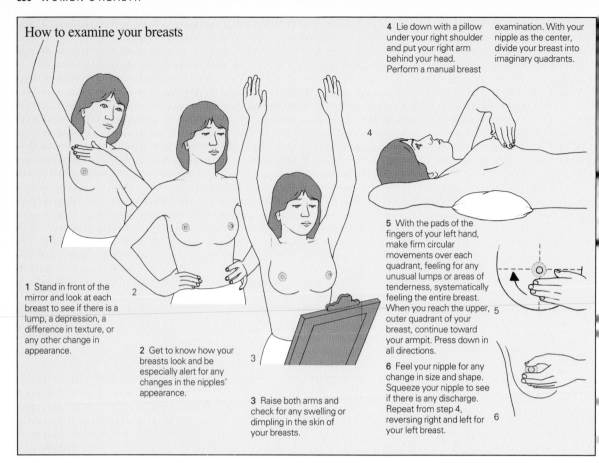

1 Stand in front of the mirror and look at each breast to see if there is a lump, a depression, a difference in texture, or any other change in appearance.

2 Get to know how your breasts look and be especially alert for any changes in the nipples' appearance.

3 Raise both arms and check for any swelling or dimpling in the skin of your breasts.

4 Lie down with a pillow under your right shoulder and put your right arm behind your head. Perform a manual breast examination. With your nipple as the center, divide your breast into imaginary quadrants.

5 With the pads of the fingers of your left hand, make firm circular movements over each quadrant, feeling for any unusual lumps or areas of tenderness, systematically feeling the entire breast. When you reach the upper, outer quadrant of your breast, continue toward your armpit. Press down in all directions.

6 Feel your nipple for any change in size and shape. Squeeze your nipple to see if there is any discharge. Repeat from step 4, reversing right and left for your left breast.

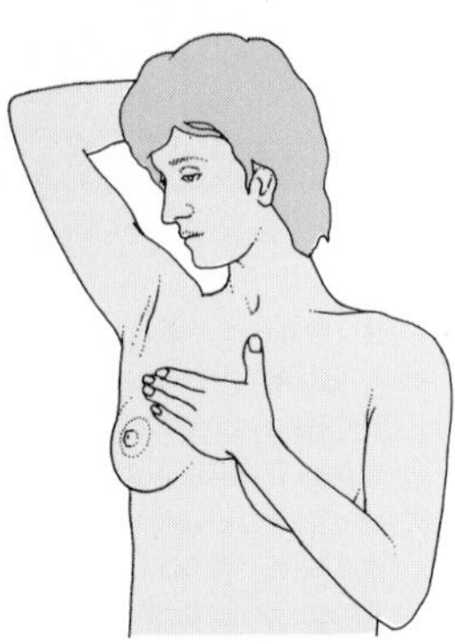

Self-examination is vital because lumps in the breast usually cannot be seen and rarely cause symptoms.

What should be done?

Read the box Having a mammogram, on p.631. In addition, examine your breasts each month (see illustration above), so that you can detect a lump early. Many women decide on a specific time to examine their breasts every month, such as at the end of their period, or on a specific date.

If you feel a lump that you did not find the last time you examined your breasts, whether it is painful or not, see your physician as soon as possible. Also, if you have always had a lump but it feels different in some way—becomes painful, harder, or bigger—see your physician immediately. He or she will examine you and may recommend that you have a mammogram. He or she may also refer you to a surgeon. The surgeon will also examine you and may arrange for one or more diagnostic tests to find out the nature of the lump and to determine the cause. Tests usually include mammography, CT scan, and a biopsy of the lump. In a biopsy, a small piece of tissue is removed for examination under a microscope.

What is the treatment?

Treatment depends on the nature of the lump. If it is a cyst, it may be drained through a needle into a syringe. This simple procedure may not even require a local anesthetic and usually clears up the problem.

When the cause of the lump (or lumps) is thickening of the glandular tissue in the breasts (fibrocystic changes), treatment is not essential. However, if such a lump feels tender or painful, your physician may recommend that you limit your caffeine intake or may prescribe sex hormones or drugs that affect your hormone balance. In addition, your physician may advise you to wear a bra that gives firm support.

If diagnostic tests show that the lump is a tumor, you will need to have it removed. The type of surgery depends on the type of tumor. If it is benign, it is usually necessary to remove only the tumor. This procedure is usually performed in a hospital outpatient surgery unit and may not require an overnight stay. For treatment of a malignant tumor, read the next article.

Breast cancer

A malignant (likely to spread) tumor may develop in the breast and not spread at first. But by the time it has grown to about ¾ in (about 20 mm) or more across, it may have shed cancerous cells that metastasize, or spread, through the bloodstream and the lymphatic system to other parts of the body, where new tumors develop. In about 10 percent of cases, tumors develop in both breasts.

What are the symptoms?

A lump, which may or may not be painful, develops in the breast, usually in the upper, outer part. The lump is usually not easily noticed and is most often detected by mammography or breast self-examination. Sometimes when the tumor has spread at least locally (in the region of the tumor), the skin over the lump becomes dimpled or creased. There may also be a dark-colored discharge from the nipple, or the nipple may turn inward and invert.

What are the risks?

Cancer of the breast is the most common cancer in women; in the US the disease develops in about 1 of every 9 women, most often in women in their 40s and 50s. Several factors contribute to the risk of breast cancer. It is slightly more common in women who have never had a baby, in women who have a family history of the disease, and in women who have had a late menopause (see p.627). If it is not treated, or treated too late, the disease is usually fatal. Most lumps are not cancerous, but you should report any new breast lump to your physician. The outlook is good if the cancer is diagnosed and treated early (see Box, p.633).

Having a mammogram

The earlier breast cancer can be detected—preferably before you feel a lump—the greater the chance of cure.

Studies have shown that regular mammograms reduce the death rate from breast cancer. Around the age of 40, all women should have their first mammogram (a special X ray of the breast). Between age 40 to 50, all women should have a mammogram every 1 to 2 years. After age 50, all women should have a mammogram each year.

Women at high risk for breast cancer (anyone with a close relative who has had cancer) should have a mammogram every 1 to 2 years, beginning at age 35. During a mammogram, each breast is compressed between 2 plates and X rays are passed through the breast to form an image on an X-ray film. The doses of radiation used in this technique are so low that there is very little risk involved. Having a mammogram is painless for most women.

What should be done?

Examining your breasts every month will help you detect a lump early. Read the box How to examine your breasts on p.630 to learn how to perform a breast self-examination. Then read the box Having a mammogram on this page. From the age of 40 onward, all women should have their breasts examined by mammography. If you detect a lump during self-examination, or if an abnormality is found during mammography, your physician will examine you to determine whether it is breast cancer or another disorder. Further tests may include another mammogram and CT (computed tomography) scanning. Your physician may perform a biopsy (taking a sample of the lump for examination), or remove fluid from the lump with a syringe (aspiration). If any of these procedures indicate that the lump is a malignant tumor, there are several methods of treatment available.

What is the treatment?

The treatment of breast cancer is complex and depends on many variables, including the microscopic appearance of the tumor (which can indicate whether it will grow rapidly), whether there are any metastases (tumors that spread from a primary cancer to another organ), whether the cancer has spread to the lymph glands, the sensitivity of tumor cells to hormones such as estrogen or a progestin, and the general health of the woman. In a very few cases when the entire tumor can be removed during a biopsy, radiation treatment alone can effectively eliminate breast cancer. In most cases, however, surgery (see Box, p.633) is necessary to remove the tumor (which may involve removing part or all of the breast), followed by radiation therapy and/or chemotherapy. Hormonal treatment may be prescribed instead of surgery.

Depending on the size of the tumor, with minimal surgery there is a risk in about 20 percent of cases that the cancer will recur in the breast. When radiation therapy is used in conjunction with surgery, the recurrence rate is only about 5 percent. Recent studies, however, make it clear that if breast cancer is discovered early, a woman who has minimal surgery followed by radiation therapy has as good a chance of survival as a woman who has a mastectomy, surgery to remove part or all of a breast. However, there is the possibility with minimal surgery that the entire breast may have to be removed later. A woman with breast cancer should decide carefully whether she prefers to have minimal surgery initially. Ask if a lumpectomy, or simple removal of the tumor, is appropriate for your situation.

After the operation, you may be given radiation therapy, especially if you have had a lumpectomy. If you are under 50, you may also have chemotherapy with a combination of anticancer drugs. Under these circumstances, when chemotherapy is not the main treatment, it is called adjuvant chemotherapy. Or, if you have passed menopause, treatment with hormones will inhibit the cancer's growth. The effectiveness of anticancer drugs given just before or during surgery rather than afterward is being researched.

Today's chemotherapy and hormonal therapy have greatly increased the survival rate from breast cancer, and chemotherapy drugs are much less unpleasant than they once were. Tamoxifen, an antiestrogen drug used to treat breast cancer, has almost no side effects. The length of time you must stay in the hospital depends on the extent of the surgery and other treatment.

Losing a breast is highly distressing. However, many women who have had a mastectomy also have breast reconstruction surgery (see Box, Plastic surgery, p.279). This involves inserting an artificial breast implant or reconstructing a breast with muscle and fat from elsewhere in the body. The procedure may be performed during a mastectomy operation or after you recover from surgery. Another option is a prosthesis worn in the bra. It can be matched to the other breast and is almost undetectable. Make sure you take adequate time to choose the prosthesis that suits you best, and that it is fitted as soon after surgery as possible. Some large department stores offer private prosthesis consultation.

What are the long-term prospects?

If the tumor is removed at an early stage, you can expect either a complete cure or many years of good health. After treatment, your physician may recommend semiannual or annual checkups. If the cancer recurs, it can be limited for many years by drugs, radiation therapy, and sometimes more surgery.

Even after widespread metastasis of the cancer, experimental treatments may help. Very-high-dose chemotherapy may be used alone or combined with radiation therapy and bone marrow transplants.

Breast abscess

An abscess is a pus-filled infected area of tissue. A breast abscess begins to form when infectious agents enter the breast tissue through the nipple and infect the milk ducts and glands. The infection usually comes from the skin surrounding the nipple, and as the infectious agents multiply they cause a red, tender, painful swelling or lump in your breast. The glands in the armpit next to the affected breast may also be tender, and you may have a fever. Breast abscesses are not common. In many cases, the disorder occurs in a woman who is breast-feeding a newborn child. This is because cracks in the nipples, which may occur during the first week of breast-feeding, make it easier for infectious agents to enter the breast tissue.

What should be done?

If you are breast-feeding, you can reduce your risk of developing an abscess by keeping your nipples clean and dry between feedings, preventing irritation from clothing, and not allowing your infant to "chew" instead of suck.

Whether you are breast-feeding or not, see your physician if an abscess develops. The treatment is the same, whatever the cause. You may be given antibiotics to fight the infection, and perhaps aspirin to reduce any pain and fever. You may be asked to apply a warm, moist washcloth at the inflamed site.

You may be advised to stop breast-feeding from the affected breast until the infection clears up. Your physician may also recommend that you express the milk from your breast to prevent it from becoming engorged.

Occasionally, antibiotics do not clear up the problem and you may need to have the abscess drained. A small cut is made at the edge of the areola (the darker skin surrounding the nipple) to allow the pus to drain. Draining the pus, together with taking antibiotics, quickly clears up the infection.

Galactorrhea

(milk production)

The breasts normally produce milk only after childbirth, and sometimes for a few days before childbirth. If milk production occurs at any other time in a woman, or at any time in a man, it is called galactorrhea. The milk is usually produced by both breasts and is whitish or gray-green in color.

Galactorrhea is uncommon in women and rare in men. It is usually caused by excessive amounts of the female sex hormone estrogen,

OPERATIONS: Surgery for breast cancer

(lumpectomy and mastectomy)

If a lump in your breast is malignant (likely to spread), you need not lose your entire breast. Although mastectomy (removal of the entire breast) has been the usual treatment, removing the lump, sampling the lymph glands in the armpit to see if you will need further treatment, and radiation therapy may produce similar results if the cancer is detected early. The type of surgery performed and the amount of tissue removed depend on the size and location of the tumor and whether the cancer may have spread.

In lumpectomy, the tumor and a small amount of surrounding tissue are removed. Some lymph glands in the armpit are also sampled. Lumpectomy is followed by radiation therapy to reduce the risk of recurrence.

In partial mastectomy, one form of which is quadrantectomy, a segment of the breast that contains the tumor is removed. Some lymph glands in the armpit are also sampled. Partial mastectomy is usually followed by radiation therapy to help prevent recurrence of the cancer. In subcutaneous mastectomy, the tissue inside the breast is removed, but the skin and nipple are left intact. Lymph glands in the armpit are examined, and biopsies (removal of tissue for laboratory examination) are performed. An implant is inserted to replace the breast tissue that was removed.

In simple mastectomy, the entire breast is removed. This operation is performed for precancerous growths in the breast or for a tumor that has not spread beyond a limited area of the breast. Lymph glands and muscles on the chest wall are not removed (but a few lymph glands are removed for examination).

In modified radical mastectomy, the entire breast and all of the lymph glands in the armpit are removed. The chest muscles are not removed in this procedure.

In radical mastectomy, the entire breast, all of the lymph glands in the armpit, and the chest muscles are removed. This operation is no more effective than simple or modified radical mastectomy. Radical mastectomy is deforming and is almost never performed today.

Implants to restore the appearance of your breast may be inserted either during the mastectomy operation or after you recover. Your breast can also be reconstructed using your own tissues including skin, fat, and muscle from the side of your abdomen or your back. This procedure is usually performed about 6 months after the original surgery.

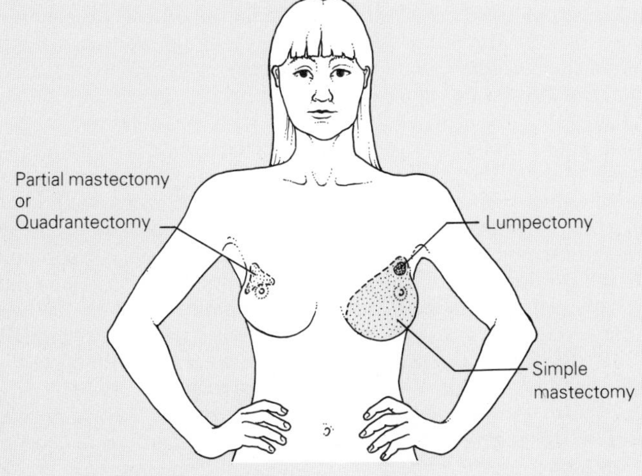

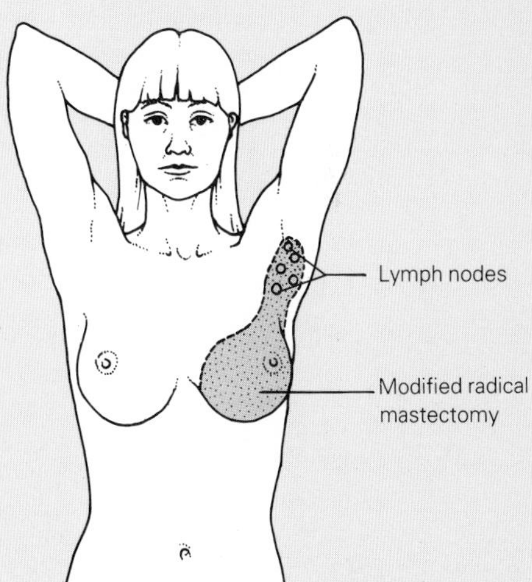

which can occur during pregnancy or from taking oral contraceptives or some other medications. Another possible cause is excessive production of the hormone prolactin. Prolactin is made by the pituitary gland and stimulates milk production. Galactorrhea can also be caused by a disorder of the pituitary gland such as a tumor (see p.557) or may occur for no apparent reason. In women, galactorrhea is often coupled with an absence of periods (see p.624).

What should be done?

If you think you have galactorrhea, consult your physician. If a pituitary tumor or another underlying disorder is suspected, your physician will probably refer you to a specialist for diagnostic tests, which may include a CT scan or an MRI scan of the brain and blood and urine tests.

If tests fail to reveal any cause for the condition, you will probably not need any treatment. If the problem is caused by drugs, discontinuing the drugs will clear it up. If galactorrhea is caused by a pituitary gland disorder or some other disease, your physician may prescribe hormone treatment or the drug bromocriptine to prevent milk production. Your physician will also treat the underlying disorder.

Nipple problems

Most nipple problems do not affect your general health. But in rare cases, a nipple disorder may be an early sign of a serious underlying disease. In such cases, early diagnosis means early treatment and an increased chance of a cure.

Nipple discharge

A whitish or gray-green discharge is likely to be breast milk, especially if it comes from both nipples. If it occurs at any time other than just before or after childbirth, it is called galactorrhea (see previous article), which can be a sign of an underlying disorder.

Any dark-colored discharge (usually dark red or black), especially if it comes from only one breast, should be reported to your physician. Note which nipple the discharge comes from and whether it comes from one nipple duct (the tiny holes in the tips of the nipple) or many. The coloring is usually due to blood discharge, often from a tiny benign growth called a duct papilloma. But the cause could be breast cancer (see p.631).

Your physician will examine your breasts and, if possible, analyze a sample of the discharge. You may also need other tests, including a mammogram and a biopsy of any unusual tissue found on the mammogram. In a biopsy, a small sample of tissue is removed for examination under a microscope. If a papilloma is found, it can be removed by simple surgery.

Nipple retraction

Nipple inversion, or retraction, that first appears at puberty, usually affects both of your nipples. Such retraction is not actually a health problem, but it may make breast-feeding a little difficult later in life.

Retraction at other times or a pulling back of the nipple or any part of the breast, especially if it affects only one breast, may be a sign of breast cancer. You should report it to your physician immediately.

Cracked nipples

Mothers who are breast-feeding often find that the skin of their nipples becomes cracked and painful. See Breast conditions, p.688, for advice on coping with the problem.

Cysts or boils in the areola

The areola is the darker area around the nipple. It contains sebaceous glands that produce a waxy substance to lubricate the nipple. If the duct of one of these glands becomes blocked, a cyst (fluid-filled sac) forms in the duct. If the gland then becomes infected, a boil results.

Consult your physician if you have a cyst or boil in the areola. In general, treatment is the same as for a cyst or boil elsewhere on the body (see Sebaceous cysts, p.276, and Boils and carbuncles, p.267).

Paget's disease of the nipple

Paget's disease of the nipple is an uncommon form of breast cancer that starts in the milk ducts of the nipple. The disease resembles eczema and usually affects only one nipple. The nipple will itch and burn, and there may be a sore on the nipple that will not heal. Without treatment, the cancer may gradually spread deeper into the tissues of the breast.

If you think that you have symptoms of Paget's disease of the nipple, your physician may perform a biopsy (removal of a small piece of tissue for examination) of the affected breast. Early detection and treatment are your best chances for recovery. Treatment is much like that for breast cancer (see p.631), depending mostly on the extent of the cancer when it is diagnosed.

Ovaries, uterus, and cervix

The two ovaries and the uterus are the primary female reproductive organs. The ovaries sit on either side of the uterus, just above your pubic bone. They move freely within a small area. Each ovary contains thousands of eggs, which you are born with. During your fertile years, one egg (or sometimes more) ripens each month and is released into the fallopian tube connected to the ovary from which the egg came. As the egg travels slowly down the tube toward the uterus it can be fertilized by a sperm cell. The uterus lies at the front of your lower abdomen, behind the urinary bladder. Its walls are composed of powerful muscles, which are mainly used to push out the baby during childbirth. In the lower front end of the uterus is a narrow, thick-walled structure, the cervix, which leads into the top of the vagina.

The following disorders are for the most part structural problems and various kinds of growths or infections in the ovaries, uterus, or cervix. Disorders of the menstrual cycle, which are usually caused by hormonal disturbances, are discussed in the articles on menstruation and menopause (see p.624).

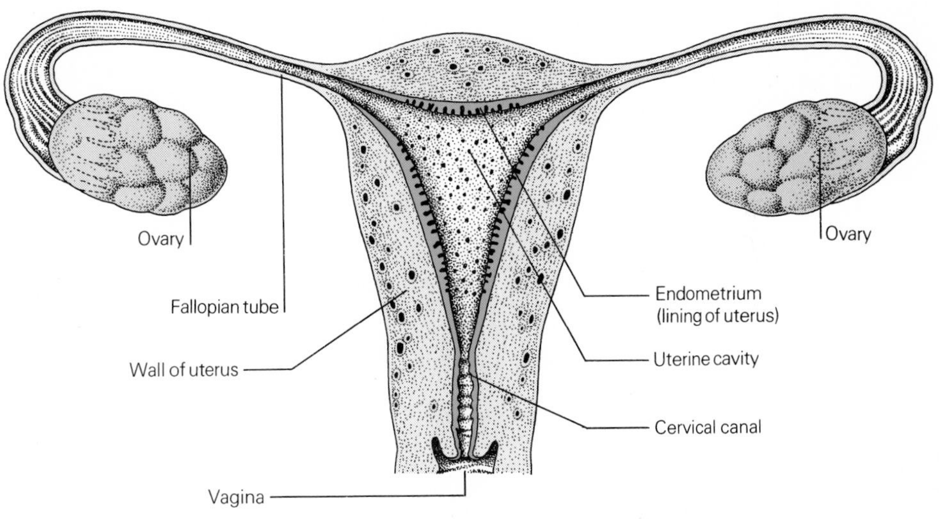

Ovarian cysts

An ovarian cyst is a sac full of fluid that forms on an ovary. The cyst can grow to a considerable size and in a very few cases interferes with production of sex hormones in the ovary.

In some cases, an egg develops abnormally inside the ovary and forms a small cyst. This type of cyst usually causes few if any symptoms and disappears within a month.

What are the symptoms?

Ovarian cysts most often produce no symptoms, but you may notice pain during sexual intercourse and, with a large cyst, firm, painless swelling in your lower abdomen. Sometimes a large cyst can press on the area near the bladder, causing urine retention. When a cyst affects hormone production, there may be symptoms such as irregular vaginal bleeding or an increase in body hair (see Abnormalities of the hypothalamus, pituitary, and ovaries, p.628).

A cyst may become twisted. This causes severe abdominal pain, nausea, and fever and requires immediate attention.

What are the risks?

Ovarian cysts are common, but seldom require any treatment. Cysts that have caused no problems are often discovered during a routine checkup. The most immediate risk is that a cyst may become badly twisted, or burst to cause peritonitis (see p.503). It is also possible that, instead of being an ovarian cyst, it may be a malignant (likely to spread) tumor (see next article).

What should be done?
Consult your physician if you have any of the symptoms described. If your physician's examination reveals a lump on your ovary, you may need to have an ultrasound and a laparoscopy (examination of the inside of the abdomen with a laparoscope) or laparotomy (abdominal exploration, see Box, Laparotomy and acute abdomen, p.513).

What is the treatment?
An ovarian cyst that is not malignant can be removed from the ovary with a device called a laparoscope (a tube equipped with a light, lenses, and a clawlike attachment that can be passed through the tube for cutting). Often this can be done without affecting the ovary, but occasionally the only way to ensure complete removal of the cyst is to take out the entire ovary and possibly the fallopian tube as well. Since you have two ovaries and two fallopian tubes, you can still get pregnant if one set is removed.

If you do not want children in the future or are past menopause, your gynecologist may recommend surgery to remove both ovaries and possibly your uterus (see Box, p.638). This is because certain types of cysts are more likely to recur, and there is a slight risk that they will be cancerous.

Cancer of the ovary

Cancer of the ovary is one of the leading causes of death from cancer in women. Although it can occur at any age, the disease is most common after age 50. It can occur as a primary growth originating in the ovary, or as a secondary growth that has metastasized (spread) from elsewhere in the body. The cause is unknown.

What are the symptoms?
Cancer of the ovary is very difficult to detect in its early stages because the ovaries lie deep inside the lower abdomen; swelling often is not noticed until the disease is advanced. At this stage there may also be lower-abdominal pain, weight loss, and general ill health. Sometimes the tumor produces fluid that causes the abdomen to swell.

What are the risks?
Cancer of the ovary is uncommon. If it is not discovered and treated promptly, it can be fatal within a few years. If it is discovered and removed early, there is a chance of complete cure. Tell your physician if your mother or sister had cancer of the ovary.

What should be done?
If you think that you have any of the symptoms of cancer of the ovary, see your physician or gynecologist immediately.

If your physician suspects cancer, he or she will arrange for you to enter the hospital as soon as possible for further examination, which may include a laparoscopy.

What is the treatment?
If cancer is present, an operation is necessary to remove not only the affected ovary but also the other ovary, the fallopian tubes, the uterus, any tumor inside the abdomen that may have spread from the ovary, and affected lymph glands to make sure that no cancer is left to grow and spread to other parts of your body. Radiation therapy or cytotoxic (anti-cancer) drugs are usually given to prevent the disease from recurring or to slow down the progress of the disease if it has already begun to spread. Periodic blood tests may be performed to monitor the effects of the chemotherapy treatment. Any fluid from the tumor that collects in the abdomen can be drained periodically.

Fibroids

(leiomyomas)

A fibroid is a benign tumor in the uterus. Such tumors may grow larger, but they are unlikely to spread. The tumor develops either within the muscular wall of the uterus or attached to the uterus wall by a stalk of tissue. Some fibroids take many years to grow to the size of a pea, while others may reach the size of grapefruit within a few years. Also, if you have one fibroid, you are likely to develop others. However, after menopause fibroids often shrink.

Most women with fibroids have no symptoms, especially if the fibroids are small.

What are the risks?
Roughly 30 percent of women over 30 have fibroids. They are seldom found before age 20, and are most common between 35 and 45. Only a small proportion require treatment.

If your fibroids are located just under the lining of the uterus, they can cause heavy menstrual periods, which may produce iron-deficiency anemia (see p.450) because of the extra blood lost. Sometimes, a fibroid attached to the outer surface of the uterus becomes twisted and loses its blood supply, or starts to wither away. Sudden sharp pain

OPERATION: D&C

(dilatation and curettage)

In this operation, the uterine lining is scraped to determine the cause of frequent or heavy periods (see Heavy periods, p.626), to terminate a pregnancy (see Termination of pregnancy, p.671), or to treat an incomplete abortion or miscarriage.

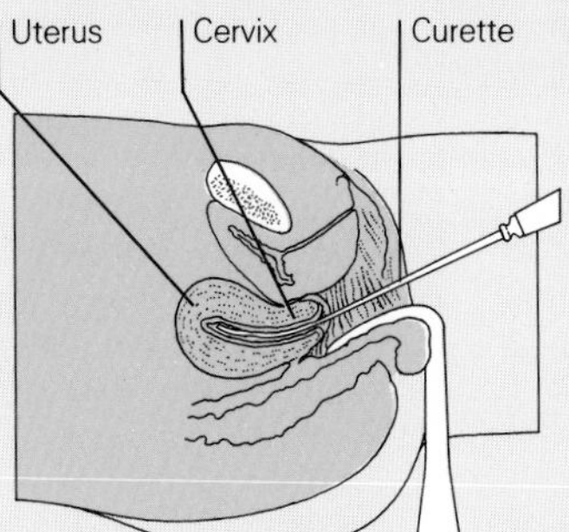

During the operation You will probably be under general anesthetic. Your cervical opening is widened with rods of increasing size, the lining of the uterus is scraped with a curette, and the scrapings are examined under a microscope. The operation usually takes about 30 minutes.

After the operation You will bleed from the uterus for a few days and may have some pelvic and back pain. You will probably be able to go home the same day or the next morning.

Convalescence Sexual intercourse and use of tampons should be avoided for several weeks, but most other activities can be resumed after a few days have passed.

low in the abdomen may follow, and an emergency operation may be required to remove the fibroid. Occasionally, a fibroid enlarges rapidly during pregnancy and may cause pain, a miscarriage, or obstruction during delivery.

What is the treatment?

Self-help: If your periods are heavy, you can help prevent iron-deficiency anemia by including plenty of iron-containing foods in your diet. The growth of fibroids is stimulated by excess estrogen, but the estrogen used in hormone replacement therapy (after menopause) usually does not affect fibroid growth.

Professional help: Small, symptomless fibroids do not require any treatment. After menopause, when levels of the sex hormone estrogen usually decline, fibroids tend to get smaller or even disappear. If your fibroids are causing problems, such as heavy menstrual bleeding, your physician may recommend endometrial ablation (a surgical procedure that destroys the uterine lining). Or in cases of severe bleeding or when fibroids grow large enough to cause swelling of your abdomen, you may need a hysterectomy (see Box, next page). Your choice depends on your age, whether you want to have children in the future, and your general health.

Cancer of the uterus

Cancer of the uterus starts in the endometrium, or lining of the uterus. After growing in the lining, the cancer invades the wall of the uterus and, if it is not treated, spreads to the fallopian tubes, ovaries, lymph glands in the area, and other organs. Why cancer of the uterus occurs is not known, but there are some factors that can make it more likely to occur. These risk factors include high blood pressure (see p.411), obesity (see p.530), diabetes mellitus (see p.558), and estrogen replacement therapy. However, the risk caused by estrogen replacement therapy is eliminated when the hormone progesterone is added to the treatment program.

What are the symptoms?

Women who are past menopause may have slight bleeding from the vagina, and women who are still menstruating may have very heavy periods, or some bleeding between periods. There may also be a discharge that ranges from a watery, pink fluid to a thick, brown, foul-smelling one. It may cause intermittent pain similar to menstrual pain. The most suspicious symptom is vaginal bleeding in a woman who has had menopause and who has had no spotting for some time.

What are the risks?

Cancer of the uterus is the most common form of cancer of the reproductive organs in women. It occurs mainly between 50 and 70, and is more common in women who have not had children than in women who have.

This type of cancer grows and spreads very slowly, so the risk that the tumor will be fatal is much lower than in some other cancers.

OPERATION: Removal of the uterus

(hysterectomy)

The uterus, and sometimes the ovaries and fallopian tubes, may be removed to cure several different gynecological disorders, especially if you are at or near menopause. You may want to get a second medical opinion before deciding to have a hysterectomy.

During the operation In the most commonly used method the surgeon removes the uterus through an incision in the lower abdomen. Or, the incision is made at the top of the vagina. Either operation takes about 1 to 2 hours under a general anesthetic.

After the operation You may have some vaginal bleeding and discharge for a few days. You will be encouraged to get out of bed and walk around a little the day after the operation and you usually can go home in several days.

Convalescence Convalescence may vary, but full activity is usually possible in 6 to 8 weeks. In a woman who has not reached menopause (see p.627), removal of the ovaries brings about an early menopause with the accompanying symptoms. Your physician may recommend estrogen replacement therapy.

What should be done?

If you have any irregular vaginal bleeding or an abnormal discharge, it is essential that you consult your physician as soon as possible. If cancer is suspected, diagnostic tests will be done, including possibly a Pap smear (see p.641), a hysteroscopic examination (see Box, Hysteroscopy, p.626), a biopsy, and a dilatation and curettage (D&C; see Box, previous page) to confirm the diagnosis.

What is the treatment?

If cancer of the uterus is confirmed, the uterus is usually removed (see Box, left), along with the ovaries and fallopian tubes. Radiation therapy and sometimes chemotherapy are used instead of, or in addition to, surgery. Or you may receive hormone therapy in the form of oral medication. If the cancer is detected at a fairly early stage, your prospects for complete recovery are excellent; about 80 percent of women operated on in the early stages of cancer of the uterus are completely cured.

Endometriosis

The tissue that lines your uterus is called the endometrium. Each month part of the endometrium thickens, becomes engorged with blood, and then, if conception does not occur, is shed as a menstrual period. In endometriosis, endometriumlike tissue develops in other places—within the muscular wall of your uterus, in or on your ovaries, or (less commonly) in or on the fallopian tubes, in the vagina, on the intestine, or even in scars that have formed in the abdominal wall after surgery. Each month these fragments of endometriumlike tissue bleed like the lining of the uterus. But because the fragments are embedded in tissue the blood cannot escape. Instead, blood blisters form or bleeding occurs that irritates and scars the surrounding tissue, which in turn forms a fibrous covering around each bleeding area, which may result in adhesions.

What are the symptoms?

In most cases endometriosis causes no symptoms, or symptoms so mild that they pass unnoticed and require no treatment. If you have symptoms, they may include abdominal and/or back pain during menstrual periods, which often becomes worse just after the period is over. Sometimes periods are heavy (see Heavy periods, p.626), and sexual intercourse may be painful.

Because endometriosis is linked to menstruation, it occurs only during the fertile years. With menopause, development of endometriumlike tissue subsides. Therefore, the condition appears most often between ages 25 and 50. It occurs most frequently in women who have not had children. Endometriosis in its mild form is common. Only a few cases are severe enough to require treatment. In very rare cases, the condition causes a major problem, such as an intestinal obstruction (see p.503).

What should be done?

If you start to have painful periods as described, see your physician. You may need to have a laparoscopy (see Glossary) to confirm the diagnosis.

What is the treatment?

Often mild endometriosis can be treated during laparoscopy with diathermy (heat treatment using sound waves, for example), cauterization (destruction of tissue by chemical or physical means), or laser surgery. Your physician may prescribe daily treatment with hormones or hormonelike drugs for several months. This allows your body gradually to destroy the abnormal tissues.

If endometriosis affects the ovaries, the treatment resembles that for an ovarian cyst (see p.635). In severe cases that do not respond to treatment, your physician may recommend a hysterectomy with removal of the fallopian tubes and the ovaries.

Trophoblastic tumors

(including hydatidiform moles)

A trophoblastic tumor is a rare type of growth that may occur during pregnancy. It grows in the placenta and may prevent the fertilized egg from developing into a fetus. A tumor can also develop in placental tissue left in the uterus after childbirth or miscarriage, up to 5 years after pregnancy. Trophoblastic tumors are often called hydatidiform moles and are either benign (unlikely to spread) or malignant (likely to spread). Both types are rare and grow large; a physician may suspect the presence of a trophoblastic tumor from the rapid expansion of the uterus. A benign growth usually remains confined to the uterus. A malignant growth, if not treated, rapidly invades the wall of the uterus and spreads to other parts of the body.

The main symptoms of a trophoblastic tumor are irregular vaginal bleeding, nausea, and vomiting.

What should be done?

If you have a combination of the symptoms described, consult your physician without delay. An ultrasound scan and a blood test may be performed. A trophoblastic tumor causes excessive production of the hormone HCG, which is normally made by the placenta. This hormone passes into the blood and can be easily detected (see Pregnancy testing, p.666). If a trophoblastic tumor is present in the uterus, the growth is removed surgically in a procedure similar to a dilatation and curettage (D&C; see Box, p.637). No further treatment is necessary for a benign tumor besides regular checkups and blood tests over the following year to make sure the tumor has not occurred again. Pregnancy is not advisable during this time, and your physician may prescribe oral contraceptives for birth control.

If the tumor is malignant, it may be necessary to remove the uterus (see Box, previous page). Cytotoxic (anticancer) drugs are given for several months to prevent spread of the disease. After this treatment, regular checkups are necessary. The prospects for a complete cure are good.

Pelvic inflammatory disease

(salpingitis)

Pelvic inflammatory disease or pelvic infection occurs when infectious agents invade the uterus and then spread to the fallopian tubes, ovaries, and surrounding tissues. The infection may not have any obvious cause but is often introduced through the vagina during sexual intercourse. Sometimes it occurs after an intrauterine device (IUD) is inserted or if an infection develops after a miscarriage or abortion. Pelvic infections can be acute (sudden) or chronic.

What are the symptoms?

An acute pelvic infection causes severe pain and tenderness in your lower abdomen and may also cause a high fever. A chronic pelvic infection causes recurrent mild pain in the lower abdomen and sometimes backache and a low-grade fever. In both acute and chronic forms of pelvic inflammatory disease, you may have pain during intercourse, your periods may be early or heavy, and you are likely to have an abnormally heavy and foul-smelling vaginal discharge.

What are the risks?

Pelvic infection, while not common in general, is most common in young, sexually active women, and least common in women who have reached menopause. If the infection is not treated, an abscess may form in a fallopian tube or ovary, which can cause scarring, and may result in damage to the fallopian tubes and prevent conception. Rarely the infection spreads quickly and causes peritonitis (see p.503) or blood poisoning (see p.452).

What should be done?

See your physician as soon as symptoms occur. Your physician will take a swab of tissue from inside your vagina. Analysis of this material helps identify the infectious agents that are causing the condition.

What is the treatment?

Your physician may perform an internal examination and a laparoscopy (examination of the inside of the abdomen with a laparoscope) to make a diagnosis. He or she will usually prescribe antibiotics to clear up the infection or recommend aspirin or acetaminophen to help relieve abdominal pain. Your physician may also recommend bed rest until the symptoms have disappeared and may advise you to avoid sexual intercourse for 3 or 4 weeks. This treatment usually leads to a complete recovery. If there is no improvement after about 5 days, you may need to be admitted to a hospital for a short time for treatment with another antibiotic or a combination of drugs. If the examination reveals blocked fallopian tubes or an abscess as a result of the infection, your physician may recommend surgery to unblock the tubes or to drain the abscess.

Prolapse of the uterus or vagina

Your uterus, vagina, and other lower abdominal organs are held in place by strong muscles and ligaments at the base of your abdomen. Weakness of these pelvic-floor muscles can lead to stress incontinence (see p.644), or slight urine leakage. Prolapse of the uterus or vagina occurs when the muscles and ligaments become extremely stretched, slackened, or torn. Slackening of the muscles may occur as a result of childbirth, and as you get older as a result of decreased estrogen, which may weaken the supporting tissues. In some cases, the muscles and ligaments no longer hold the uterus firmly in place, so it falls and causes the vagina to sag downward. This causes the prolapse, a bulge of the front or back wall of the vagina. Sometimes the uterus may descend so far that it bulges out of the vagina, a complete prolapse.

What are the symptoms?

A lump or bulge appears in the vagina and may project outside the vagina. This may cause a feeling of heaviness and discomfort, and occasionally backache, especially after lifting or otherwise straining your muscles. In some cases, stress incontinence appears, but in others the prolapse may make urination more difficult. If the back wall of the vagina has descended, you may find bowel movements difficult. Pushing too hard while having a bowel movement makes the problem worse by causing further prolapse.

What are the risks?

Minor degrees of prolapse are common, especially for a few months after childbirth and in later life. Prolapse can be uncomfortable and inconvenient, but there are few risks to general health.

What should be done?

Exercises to tone the pelvic muscles after childbirth may prevent prolapse (see What is the treatment? below). If you think you have a prolapse, consult your physician.

What is the treatment?

There is a lot you can do to relieve symptoms of a prolapsed uterus. Lose weight if you are overweight. Eat plenty of high-fiber foods, so that you will be able to move your bowels without straining. You can also strengthen the muscles of your pelvic floor by doing exercises. Exercise your pelvic muscles for several minutes each day by alternately contracting and relaxing them as though you were trying to interrupt a flow of urine.

If there is no improvement, your physician may recommend hormone replacement therapy to help strengthen the pelvic-floor muscles, or he or she may recommend that you be fitted with a pessary, a device inserted into the vagina to support the uterus. Or your physician may recommend a hysterectomy, which will enable him or her to tighten the pelvic-floor muscles and ligaments.

Retroversion of the uterus

(tipped uterus)

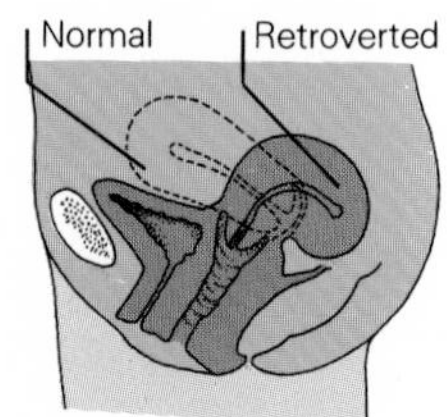

The uterus is normally tilted upward and forward and lies immediately behind the bladder. In about 20 percent of women, however, it inclines downward and backward and lies close to the anal canal. It is then said to be retroverted or tipped (see illustration); this condition is usually congenital (present from birth), but occasionally occurs after childbirth. Retroversion of the uterus is diagnosed by physical examination of the pelvis. This is not a disease and is usually considered to be a variation of the normal position of the uterus. In nearly all cases, the condition is completely symptomless and requires no treatment. Occasionally, it causes backache, especially during menstruation.

In very rare cases, you might feel some pain during sexual intercourse when your partner's penis penetrates deeply and presses on tissue next to an ovary. Talk to your physician if this happens to you.

Sometimes retroversion of the uterus may result from an underlying disease, such as a tumor, endometriosis, or pelvic inflammatory disease. In such cases, the underlying disease may require treatment. In rare cases with symptoms, surgery may be performed to move the uterus into a forward position.

Cervical dysplasia

Cervical dysplasia occurs when there are changes in the cells of the lining of the cervix. Normal cells are replaced by abnormal cells. There are no symptoms with cervical dysplasia, and it usually does not affect your health. However, certain types of dysplasia, if not treated, can change into cancer of the cervix. It is vital to have regular Pap smears to detect these changes early.

What should be done?

You should have a regular Pap smear (see p.641). If the Pap test reveals any abnormal cells, your physician may examine you with a colposcope, an instrument with a magnifying lens that allows a closer examination of the cervix to identify abnormal areas that might need to be removed and examined in a biopsy. Whether or not treatment is necessary depends on the results of the biopsy.

What is the treatment?

If colposcopy reveals that the cells lining the cervix show precancerous changes, the tissue must be removed or destroyed. This can usually be done with a laser. In most cases, laser treatment allows faster healing and has fewer side effects than cone biopsy, a procedure in which a cone-shaped section of tissue is surgically removed. Cauterization by heat, electricity, or chemicals may also be used to destroy the tissue. All these procedures can be performed during a visit to the hospital as an outpatient.

If the area of abnormal tissue extends up the cervical canal, a cone biopsy may be required. This is usually performed with a local anesthetic during an outpatient visit, and afterward you may need to rest for a day. In very rare cases, a cone biopsy can lead to the tendency to miscarry. If you have had a cone biopsy and become pregnant, you should inform your physician, especially if you have had a prior miscarriage. Your physician will monitor your pregnancy.

If you have cervical dysplasia and you do not want children, and especially if you also have heavy or painful periods, your physician may recommend a hysterectomy (see Box, p.638) to avoid the risk of cancer.

After treatment, you should have a Pap smear twice a year for the next 2 years, and once a year thereafter, so that any recurrence can be detected and treated early.

Pelvic examination and Pap smear

A pelvic examination is often performed as part of a physical checkup. The examination is usually painless if you do not tense up your pelvic muscles. For the examination, you will lie on your back on an examining table, with your knees bent. An instrument called a speculum is inserted into your vagina to hold it open while your physician uses a light to look for any abnormalities of the cervix and vaginal walls.

A few cells are scraped from the cervix and sent to a laboratory, where they are examined for conditions that might lead to cancer and for signs of cancer of the cervix (see next article). This procedure is called a Pap smear (after its developer, G.N. Papanicolaou) or a cervical smear test. It should be done at least every 3 years after two consecutive annual Pap smears have been normal, or as often as your physician recommends.

After taking the cells, the physician removes the speculum, inserts two gloved fingers of one hand into your vagina, and carefully feels for any abnormalities of the uterus, ovaries, and fallopian tubes. Your physician may examine your rectum as well.

The results of your Pap test usually are known in a few days. The test is negative if the cells are normal, and positive if they are precancerous or cancerous. If the results are inconclusive, the test may be repeated every 3 months until something definite can be determined or a colposcopy (examination of the cervix with a special viewing instrument) is done. If the results indicate cancerous or precancerous cells, your physician will arrange for further tests and treatment.

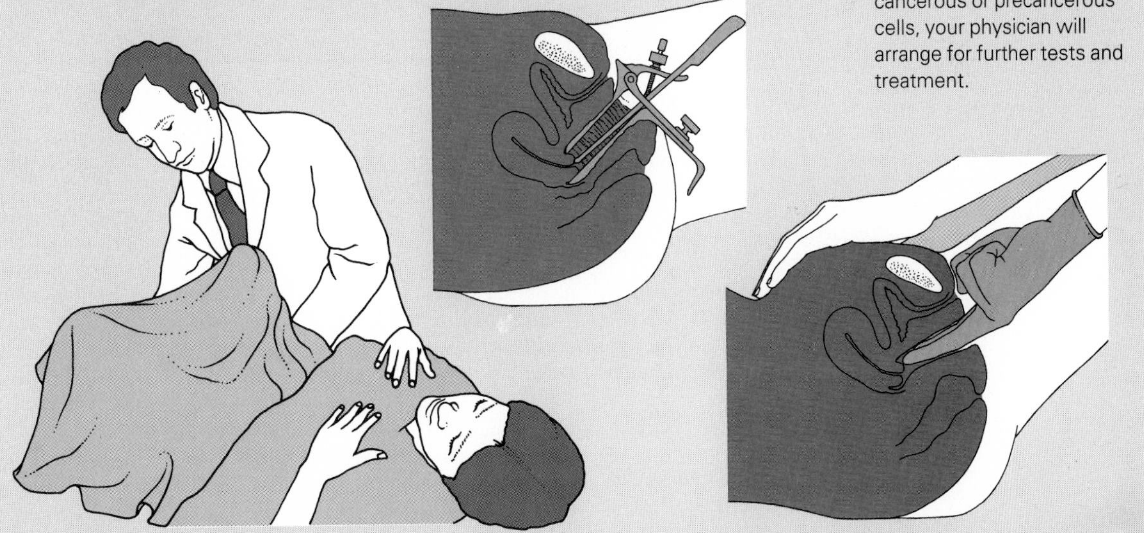

Cancer of the cervix

Cancer of the cervix frequently develops in women who have either untreated cervical dysplasia (see previous article) or its more advanced form, called carcinoma in situ. Cells have turned malignant (likely to spread) in carcinoma in situ but have not yet invaded nearby cells. The cancer, if it is not treated, spreads deep into the tissues of the cervix, to nearby lymph glands, and up into the uterus.

What are the symptoms?

Two main symptoms are a watery, bloody discharge, which may be heavy and foul-smelling, and vaginal bleeding between periods, after intercourse, or after menopause.

What are the risks?

Cancer of the cervix is a common form of cancer in women. It occurs mostly in women over age 40. Early detection and treatment of cancer of the cervix may help prevent metastasis (spreading) and can often lead to a complete cure.

What should be done?

To help prevent cervical cancer, see your physician regularly—every 1 to 3 years, as your physician recommends—for a Pap smear (see previous page), a procedure that makes early detection of cervical dysplasia possible. Pap smears are important on an annual basis in either of the following cases: if you become sexually active at a very early age, or if you or your partner have had multiple sexual partners. The earlier you become sexually active and the greater the number of your sexual partners, the higher your risk of cancer of the cervix. The importance of the Pap smear is not that it detects cancer, but that it can help to prevent it by detecting precancerous changes in the cervical cells, which can then be destroyed.

If you have any of the symptoms described here, see your physician. If cancer is suspected, you may have a Pap smear, a colposcopy (examination of the cervix with a special viewing instrument), and a biopsy of the cervix. In a biopsy, a small sample of tissue is removed for examination under a microscope.

What is the treatment?

Cancer of the cervix is usually treated by surgery to remove the cervix, the rest of the uterus, the ovaries, the fallopian tubes, and samples of lymph nodes in the pelvis or near the uterus (see Box, p.638), and/or by radiation therapy. Discuss the risks and benefits of each form of treatment with your physician before choosing the best course. The samples of lymph nodes are examined in a laboratory to help determine any further treatment you may need.

What are the long-term prospects?

The chances of treatment providing a complete cure when cancer has not spread beyond the uterus are extremely good; in fact, much better than with most other cancers. However, treatment prevents you from becoming pregnant.

Even if your reproductive organs are not removed, the radiation therapy will probably disrupt your menstrual cycle. A woman who is still having menstrual periods may experience some symptoms of menopause.

For a few months after radiation therapy, you may have diarrhea and difficulty retaining urine. After treatment, have regular checkups as your physician recommends.

Cervical polyps

A cervical polyp is a grapelike growth on the mucus-producing lining of the cervix or hanging outside of the cervix. Polyps usually are single, but may be multiple, and can grow up to almost 1 in (20 mm) in width. They usually produce an excessively heavy, watery, bloody discharge from the vagina, and sometimes bleeding between periods, after sexual intercourse, or after menopause (see p.627). Cervical polyps are fairly common, particularly in women who have not had children.

What should be done?

If you have the symptoms described, report them to your physician. Cervical polyps are harmless, but they produce symptoms similar to those that are produced by cancer of the cervix (see previous article) and uterus. Do not take unnecessary risks; see your physician immediately.

Your physician may examine you and perform a Pap smear (see previous page). If a polyp is found, it may be removed by a quick, painless procedure. When a polyp has been causing irregular bleeding as well as a discharge, you may need to have an endometrial biopsy (removal of a small piece of tissue from the lining of the uterus for examination), hysteroscopy (see Box, p.626), or a dilatation and curettage (D&C; see Box, p.637). This ensures that a more serious disorder is not causing the bleeding. Once a polyp is removed, it does not recur.

Bladder and urethra

The bladder is a muscular-walled reservoir that is located in the lower portion of the abdomen. It touches the lower surface of the uterus, just above the pubic bone. Urine trickles slowly from the two kidneys down two thin tubes, called the ureters, into the bladder, where it is stored. Eventually, you eliminate the urine by squeezing it out of the bladder along a short passage, the urethra.

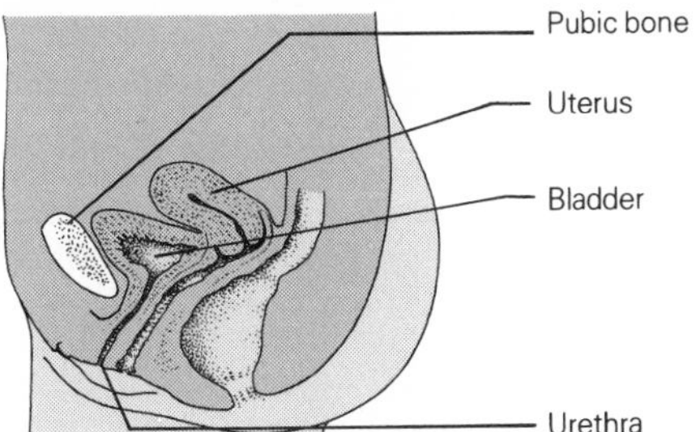

Disorders of the bladder and urethra that affect both sexes are discussed in the section on disorders of the urinary tract (see p.539). Disorders included here either affect women only, or, like cystitis, affect women and men in very different ways (see also Cystitis in men, p.618, and Urethritis in men, p.619).

Cystitis in women

Cystitis is inflammation of the bladder. It is usually caused by bacteria that travel up the urethra and infect both the urethra and the bladder. There are several other urinary tract problems, such as urethritis (see next page) and irritable bladder (see next page), that may produce similar symptoms.

What are the symptoms?

If you have cystitis, you may feel a frequent urge to urinate, but when you try, only a small amount of urine comes out. This urine may have a strong smell, may have blood in it (hematuria), and can burn or sting as you pass it (dysuria). The urge to urinate is sometimes so strong that you cannot control it. This is called urge incontinence. You may also have a fever and a dull pain in your lower abdomen and lower back.

What are the risks?

Most women have cystitis at some time in their lives. It is particularly common during the first few months of pregnancy.

Cystitis is annoying and inconvenient, and sometimes, if it is untreated, this infection of the bladder may spread to the kidneys (see Acute pyelonephritis, p.541).

What should be done?

If you increase your intake of fluids by 2 quarts for a day, it may relieve the symptoms. See your physician if the symptoms persist or are severe. Your physician may give you a small container for a midstream urine specimen. Your physician or nurse will probably give you paper towels to wipe yourself with first before you urinate. While sitting on the toilet, spread your labia (genital lips) with the fingers of one hand. Start to urinate; in the middle of urinating, catch a small amount of urine in the container. The sample is examined in the office for pus cells that indicate infection and then sent to a laboratory to identify the agents responsible for the infection.

What is the treatment?

Self-help: Drink plenty of fluids. Try to empty your bladder completely each time you urinate, and follow the self-help measures described for chronic urethritis (see next page). To prevent infections, always wipe yourself from front to back after a bowel movement, and empty your bladder immediately after you have had sexual intercourse.

Professional help: Your physician may prescribe antibiotics, antibacterials, or other drugs to treat the condition.

If you have more than two or three episodes of cystitis, your physician may refer you to a urologist, a physician who specializes in urinary tract disorders, to see if you have any urinary tract abnormality that is making you particularly susceptible to bladder infection. The urologist will examine you and may ask for additional midstream specimens of urine. Sometimes an ultrasound scan is performed. Also, you may need an intravenous pyelogram (IVP, a special X ray of the kidneys and bladder), and a visual examination of the bladder (cystoscopy).

If these examinations and tests reveal an abnormality of the urinary tract, your physician will treat it. If not, the urologist may prescribe antibiotics or antibacterial drugs for a month or more. This may solve the problem. However, cystitis often recurs.

Stress incontinence

At the base of your abdomen you have a sheet of muscles called the pelvic-floor muscles. These muscles support the base of the bladder and close off the top of the urethra, the short channel through which you pass urine. In stress incontinence, the pelvic-floor muscles are weak. When you exert pressure on them by coughing, laughing, or lifting something, you lose a little bit of urine. This happens only when the muscles are under stress, not when you are resting or sleeping.

What are the risks?
Some stress incontinence is very common. The pelvic-floor muscles are weakened by childbirth or by obesity. Also, when your ovaries stop making estrogen at menopause, the lack of estrogen results in weakening of the muscles, which can lead to prolapse of the uterus or vagina (see p.640).

What should be done?
If you have stress incontinence, see your physician, who will examine you and ask questions about the history of your condition.

You may be asked to provide a midstream urine specimen (see previous article), which will show whether a urinary tract infection is a factor. You may also need to have a voiding cystogram (special X ray of your bladder taken while you are urinating), a cystoscopy (examination of the inside of your bladder), and urodynamic testing (filling the bladder with water and inserting a device that measures pressure).

What is the treatment?
Treatment for stress incontinence usually consists of exercises to strengthen your pelvic-floor muscles (see Prolapse of the uterus or vagina, p.640). If you are overweight, you will probably need to lose weight (see Obesity, p.530). In women past menopause, hormone replacement therapy may be prescribed to strengthen the pelvic-floor muscles. If these measures do not cure the condition you may be advised to have surgery to tighten your pelvic-floor muscles.

Irritable bladder

With irritable bladder, your bladder contracts uncontrollably. You have a sudden urge to urinate (urgency) and often pass a small amount before you can reach a bathroom. You may also have to get up at night to urinate. This is called urge incontinence.

Why certain people have an irritable bladder is not known, but it sometimes occurs in conjunction with stress incontinence (see previous article), prolapse of the uterus or vagina (see p.640), or, more often, an infection of the urinary tract (see next article). It is a fairly common, inconvenient, and distressing disorder, but it is not risky.

What should be done?
See your physician, who will examine you and arrange for you to provide a midstream urine specimen (see previous page). It will be analyzed for indications of any urinary tract infection. Your physician may also arrange for urodynamic testing (see previous article), a voiding cystogram (a special X ray of your bladder taken while you are urinating), and a cystoscopy (examination of the inside of your bladder with a viewing tube).

What is the treatment?
If you have an irritable bladder, your physician may recommend that you try to hold back your urine for as long as possible in order to strengthen your bladder muscles. He or she may also prescribe a drug to relax your bladder muscles or reduce the activity of the nerves that control muscle contraction. You may also be advised to avoid stress.

Chronic urethritis

Chronic urethritis, a common disorder, is recurrent inflammation of the urethra. The symptoms are similar to those of cystitis (see p.643), except that they last for only 1 or 2 days. Chronic urethritis may be caused by bruising during sexual intercourse. It may also result from exposure to soapy bath oils, some spermicides, or other chemical irritants. However, it is more often caused by an infection, often by *Chlamydia* (see p.606), although the microorganism that is responsible cannot always be identified.

What should be done?
See your physician, who may ask you for a sample of urine for analysis. If the underlying cause is an infection, it can usually be treated successfully with antibiotics or antibacterial drugs. However, in some cases of chronic urethritis, no infecting microorganism can be found. If this is the case, you may want to try some self-help measures each time you have sexual intercourse; if you use a lubricant, make sure it is water-soluble; also, empty your bladder completely after intercourse.

Vagina and vulva

The vulva is the area around the opening to the female urinary and reproductive systems. It consists of two folds of tissue (the labia) on each side of the openings from the urethra and the vagina. The clitoris and several lubricating glands are also located inside the vulva. The vagina is the passage between the vulva and the uterus. The tissues of the vulva are susceptible to skin problems such as warts or severe itching. The lining of the vagina and glands in the vulva produce fluid that cleanses the vagina, facilitates intercourse, and makes sperm passage easier. Benign tumors or cysts may occur on the vulva, but they can be treated effectively with surgery. Cancer of the vulva is rare and is also treated surgically or by radiation therapy.

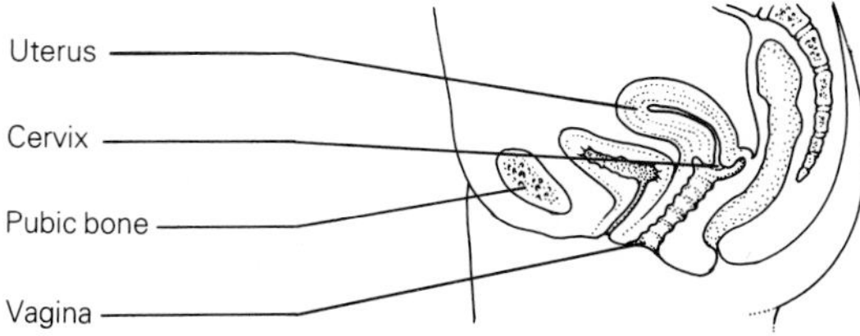

Vaginal yeast infection

(candidiasis, moniliasis)

A yeast infection occurs when the fungus *Candida albicans* overgrows in the vagina. Many women have small amounts of the fungus that may not cause symptoms. If vaginal conditions change and become more favorable for the fungus, it grows and displaces the harmless bacteria that normally control the fungus.

Anything that kills these helpful bacteria allows the fungus to increase. Helpful bacteria may be killed by feminine hygiene sprays, douches, and, occasionally, antibiotics. Similarly, hormonal changes that occur if you are pregnant or if you take oral contraceptives can change conditions in the vagina and allow the infection to develop. Also, women with diabetes are especially susceptible to candidiasis. Yeast infections are a nuisance but not risky.

What are the symptoms?

Vaginal yeast infection causes itching and irritation of the vagina and swelling and redness of the vulva. You may notice an unusual thick, white discharge, and you may have pain or soreness during sexual intercourse. You may urinate more frequently than usual, and the urine may sting or burn.

What should be done?

Avoid wearing nylon underpants. Unlike cotton, nylon cannot "breathe" and therefore offers a warm, moist breeding area for the infection. Do not use feminine hygiene sprays or powders, and do not douche.

If you develop symptoms of a yeast infection, consult your physician, who will examine you and take a sample from the inside of your vagina to verify that a fungal infection is present.

What is the treatment?

Treatment for yeast infection is an antifungal drug in the form of a nonprescription vaginal suppository or cream. Using the medication for about a week usually clears up the problem. However, if you have repeated episodes, your physician may want to check your blood sugar for diabetes and may prescribe an oral antifungal medication.

Trichomonal vaginitis

(Trichomonas)

Trichomonal vaginitis is infection of the vagina caused by *Trichomonas*, a tiny, one-celled organism. Symptoms of the infection are similar to those that result from a yeast infection (see previous article). However, the discharge for trichomonal vaginitis is usually heavy, unpleasant smelling, and greenish-yellow.

Trichomonal vaginitis is common and is not thought to be risky, but it can be irritating and painful. And because the disease is usually transmitted through sexual intercourse, it is likely that your sexual partner also has it. The infection often does not cause symptoms in a man, but a male partner who has it can reinfect you.

If you have the symptoms, consult your physician, who may take a sample from the inside of your vagina for microscopic analysis. Treatment is usually an oral antibiotic medication that your physician will prescribe for both you and your partner.

Pruritus vulvae

Itching of the vulva with no identifiable disorder such as infection, allergy, or a generalized skin condition is called pruritus vulvae. It often occurs in girls before they begin to have menstrual periods and in women after menopause (see p.627). It may be related to production of sex hormones, particularly the low level of estrogen that commonly occurs after menopause. It also occurs in women with diabetes mellitus.

What are the symptoms?
Your genital area is very sensitive, easily irritated, and intensely itchy. A sore and dry vagina, especially during intercourse, often accompanies pruritus vulvae. You may have a thin, white discharge.

What are the risks?
Pruritus vulvae is common, particularly in women over age 45. There are no risks directly associated with the condition, but if white patches of abnormal skin called leukoplakia form in the irritated area, there is an increased risk of developing cancer of the vulva (see below).

What should be done?
Do not scratch the itchy area; scratching will only make the soreness and irritation worse. Wash with water and unscented soap once a day (no more) and apply a soothing cream recommended by your physician. Do not douche or use talcum powder or feminine hygiene sprays, because they are likely to increase the irritation. A water-soluble lubricant jelly is helpful during intercourse. Wear cotton underpants and avoid panty hose. If the condition does not improve within 2 weeks, see your physician.

What is the treatment?
If there are patches of abnormal skin, your physician will take samples for a biopsy. He or she may then prescribe corticosteroid cream or oral or topical hormonal treatment.

Vulvar warts

Warts are small, occasionally itchy areas of viral infection on the skin. Warts on the vulva are fairly common and are much the same as those on other parts of the body (see Warts, p.268). Because they are believed to be caused by a contagious virus, warts on your vulva may have spread from warts on your fingers, or from warts on your sexual partner's penis. They spread more easily in moist and unhygienic conditions, and often appear in conjunction with a disorder that produces an increased vaginal discharge, such as vaginal yeast infection (see previous page). Warts may also develop during pregnancy when there is a natural increase in the moistness of the vagina.

Warts present for many years may, in rare cases, become malignant (likely to spread). If you think you have vulvar warts, see your physician, who will examine you. A blood sample may be taken to test for syphilis (see p.655), since some vulvar warts may be caused by the bacterium that causes syphilis. There may be an association between the virus that causes genital warts and cancer of the cervix, vagina, or vulva.

What is the treatment?
The virus that causes the warts lives inside human cells; to kill the virus the cells must be destroyed. Therefore, your physician may treat small warts by applying a paint that kills the virus. The treatment may have to be repeated a few weeks later. If it fails, or if the warts are large or inaccessible, they can be removed in your physician's office or in the outpatient surgical department of the hospital. The warts can be removed by other means such as freezing, laser, or electrical cauterization. If you got the warts from your partner, your partner must be treated to prevent you from becoming reinfected.

Cancer of the vulva

Cancer of the vulva starts as a small, hard lump in the skin, which gradually breaks down to form an ulcer. The ulcer has thickened, raised edges, and may ooze or bleed. The ulcer gradually enlarges and, if it is not treated, will eventually metastasize, or spread to other parts of the body. Cancer of the vulva tends to grow very slowly, and early detection and treatment usually lead to a complete cure.

If you have any lump or ulcer on your vulva, your physician may perform a biopsy, in which a small sample of tissue is removed for examination. If the growth is malignant (likely to spread), the usual treatment is a vulvectomy, in which the growth and surrounding skin, or the growth, the lymph glands in the groin, and the skin between the two areas, are removed. Radiation therapy may be used.

Menstrual care

PMS

Premenstrual syndrome (PMS; see p.627) is a group of symptoms that can occur during the week before your period. Severity of these symptoms varies from person to person. Although moderate in many women, symptoms may be nearly intolerable in others. See your physician if your symptoms are severe.

Odor

To minimize odor during your period, change pads or tampons frequently and bathe or shower with soap and water daily. Perfumed or deodorized tampons and pads provide no additional benefit over soap and water washing, and the chemicals they contain can cause skin allergies, with symptoms such as itching and a rash.

Tampons vs. pads

Although almost half of American women use tampons, some misconceptions about their use still exist. For example, girls and women who are virgins can use tampons comfortably and safely. However, after childbirth or surgery involving the vagina, uterus, or cervix (for example, episiotomy, dilatation and curretage, or even a biopsy of these areas), use pads rather than tampons until healing is complete.

Toxic shock syndrome

In the early 1980s, there was an epidemic of a disorder called toxic shock syndrome (see Staphylococcal infections, p.599) associated with prolonged use of tampons that were advertised as superabsorbent. This type of tampon was taken off the market, and toxic shock syndrome is now very rare. Nevertheless, if you are menstruating and using tampons, you should change them several times a day. Be careful not to forget to remove a tampon toward the end of your period. You should be alert for any flulike symptoms that quickly get worse, especially if they are accompanied by a rash. If symptoms appear, call your physician immediately or go directly to the nearest hospital emergency department.

Menstrual cramps

The medical term for menstrual cramping is dysmenorrhea. Intrauterine contraceptive devices (IUDs) and specific disorders such as endometriosis, fibroid tumors, and pelvic inflammatory disease sometimes cause constant discomfort with occasional cramps. See painful periods (p.625).

If you have premenstrual syndrome or severe cramps, consult your physician, who can examine you for any underlying problem. No treatment works for everyone, but nonsteroidal anti-inflammatory drugs such as ibuprofen often help. Studies have shown that diuretics (see Drug glossary in this volume) are not effective during the premenstrual cycle. Discuss with your physician whether one of the nonprescription medications might work for you, or if you should take a prescription drug.

Vaginal hygiene

Most physicians believe that washing the area around the vaginal opening (including the minor and major labia, urethra, and clitoris) daily with unscented soap and water provides the best hygiene available. Do not use deodorant sprays, which are unnecessary and which contain chemicals that can irritate the vaginal lining, the labia, and other areas of the skin.

The vagina cleanses itself by secreting a mucous discharge that flows downward, removing bacteria, old cells, and menstrual blood when present. Normal vaginal discharge is minimal in amount, is either clear or white and sticky, and has a mild odor. The discharge dries as a yellowish stain on underclothes. The consistency and volume of the discharge may change when you ovulate, which happens about midway between menstrual periods. Infections of the vagina and cervix can produce more plentiful, creamier vaginal secretions that may be foul smelling and cause redness, dryness, flaking, itching, and irritation.

Douching is not recommended. It is important to realize that douching is not a method of birth control. Douching may also wash away the protective mucous plug that covers the cervix to prevent organisms from entering the uterus. In addition, it can spread a vaginal infection into the uterus and fallopian tubes by forcing contaminated water upward from an infected vagina. Some douching preparations can irritate the mucous membrane that lines the walls of the vagina. In some women, these preparations have caused an allergic reaction.

If you have a foul-smelling or unusual discharge and think you have a vaginal infection, see your physician. He or she will examine you and take a sample from inside your vagina for testing. Do not decide to treat yourself by douching (especially for 3 days before your appointment). Douching will wash away secretions that can help your physician diagnose the infection, and the lack of these secretions, which serve as the vagina's natural cleansing method, may actually prolong the infection.

Sexuality

Introduction

In recent years many aspects of sexuality have been changing. Attitudes toward sex have been changing, and in the US there is a renewed awareness of the value of monogamy (having only one partner who has only you for a partner). As sexually transmitted diseases (STDs) have become more widespread, physicians strongly recommend using condoms for sexual intercourse to prevent such diseases. With technical advances, many sexual problems such as infertility can now be treated medically or surgically.

Topics in this section are divided into three groups. The first group deals with infertility and contraception. When a couple is not able to have a child, a variety of factors may be involved. Many of the causes can be treated, resulting in successful pregnancies.

If, on the other hand, you want to avoid pregnancy, there are several reliable contraceptive techniques available, and each one has advantages and disadvantages. Some contraceptives require a prescription, while others are available over the counter. Be sure to discuss with your physician the possibilities and the risks and benefits associated with each one before choosing a method of contraception. Consider the factors of reliability, side effects, and protection against sexually transmitted diseases.

The second group of articles in this section addresses sexually transmitted diseases. The term venereal diseases was once applied to such infections. The three main venereal diseases were syphilis, gonorrhea, and non-gonococcal urethritis (see Chlamydial infections, p.606). During recent years, however, it has been discovered that other disorders, among them human immunodeficiency virus (HIV) infection (AIDS) (see p.465) and hepatitis B (see p.523), can also be transmitted either by sexual intercourse or by other forms of intimate sexual contact. The diseases covered in this section of the book are those that are usually spread by sexual contact.

The third group of articles deals with sexual problems. It is usually most helpful to look at these problems as difficulties for both partners to tackle. Also included in this section is a box on homosexuality and bisexuality, which are discussed more openly today.

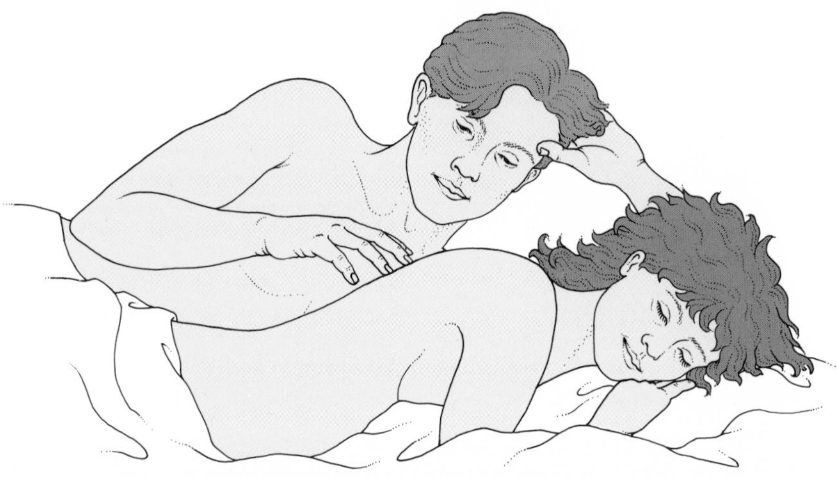

Infertility and contraception

Some couples invest a lot of energy in trying to avoid having children, while others do everything they can to try to conceive. Medical science can be helpful in both cases. New diagnostic techniques and drugs as well as sophisticated surgical procedures offer most infertile couples an eventual pregnancy. Similarly, a number of contraceptive techniques are also available for your use. Health considerations, religious views, reliability (see Table at right), and convenience may all influence a couple's choice of contraceptive method. Your physician should be able to help you make your decision.

Method	Number of pregnancies per 100 women*
Combined pill	less than 1
Condom plus contraceptive foam	less than 1
Contraceptive foams, creams, suppositories, and sponges	5 to 15
Diaphragm plus contraceptive cream or jelly	2
IUD	less than 1
Natural (see p.652)	2 to 20
Sterilization	less than 2 out of 1,000
No contraception	90

*Using method for 1 year

Infertility

If you are planning to have a baby, make sure you know as much as possible about the best conditions for conception (for more information, see p.662).

If you have not conceived after 12 months of trying, both partners should visit a physician. Initially, your physician will ask you how often you have sexual intercourse and about the timing of intercourse. He or she will probably refer you to a physician who specializes in treating fertility problems.

The fertility specialist will perform a number of tests, the first of which is usually a microscopic examination of the man's semen to count the number of healthy sperm. Many factors can contribute to a low sperm count. Among them are certain drugs, emotional stress, overwork and fatigue, excessive use of tobacco and alcohol, and a raised temperature inside the scrotum (sometimes caused by tight underwear).

If sperm production and ejaculation are found to be normal, the next step is to make sure the woman's reproductive system is functioning properly. A woman must ovulate to become pregnant. Ovulation is the process in which an egg ripens in the ovary, is released, and migrates into a fallopian tube. This occurs about 14 days before the beginning of each menstrual period. After ovulation, the ovary produces the hormone progesterone, which alters the endometrium, or lining of the uterus, and the consistency of the mucus in the cervix. Your physician may test samples of your cervical mucus.

He or she may also measure the levels in your blood of progesterone and other hormones at various times during your menstrual cycle and may also recommend ultrasound scans of your ovaries. The process of ripening and release of the egg is detectable by scanning.

If the reason for your infertility is that you are not ovulating, treatment may be given to stimulate ovulation. The first step is to check your general health and, in particular, to look for treatable causes such as stress, which may alter your hormonal balance. If you are healthy, you may start by taking a fertility drug such as clomiphene, which may stimulate the ovaries into producing eggs. If this does not work, a series of gonadotrophin hormones may be started, consisting of oral medication and injections. This treatment may continue for several months, may be repeated, and needs careful monitoring, since overstimulation of the ovaries might result in a multiple pregnancy or adverse effects such as hot flashes, headache, nausea, and fatigue.

Since fertilization occurs in the fallopian tubes, they must be unobstructed for the fertilized egg to travel into the uterus and implant in the uterine wall. Previous pelvic infections can scar and block the fallopian tubes, and this can prevent pregnancy. Your physician may use a special test called hysterosalpingography (special X rays of the uterus and fallopian tubes) to check for any obstruction in these organs.

Much publicity has been given in recent years to new techniques of treatment, originally known as "test tube baby" methods. These techniques are designed to help couples with infertility caused by damaged fallopian tubes, but extend to other types of infertility. During in vitro fertilization the ovaries are stimulated to produce eggs, which are then removed from the ovaries, usually through the wall of the vagina with ultrasound guidance. These eggs are then fertilized in the laboratory by semen from the male partner or from a donor if the partner is infertile. The fertilized egg is observed while cell division begins and several embryos at early stages of cell division are then introduced into the uterus. In GIFT (gamete intrafallopian transfer), the egg and some sperm are placed into the fallopian tube—a method that is suitable only for women with healthy tubes. In ZIFT (zygote intrafallopian transfer), the fertilized egg is put into the tube.

Sometimes endometriosis (see p.638) or adhesions (fibrous tissue from old infections or previous surgery) interfere with fertilization. This can be diagnosed by using laparoscopy (examination of the inside of the abdomen with a viewing instrument). The problem can usually be corrected surgically if adhesions are found.

Artificial insemination is another possibility. In this procedure, semen is introduced into the woman's cervical canal or directly into the uterus.

If the partner's semen is fertile, but conception is prevented because of erection difficulties or premature ejaculation (see p.657), your physician can obtain semen from the partner if he can have a partial erection. The woman may then place the semen into her cervical canal herself by using a syringe, or it can be done by the physician. In the case of a low sperm count, sperm can be concentrated and also put in this way.

Sometimes a man's fertility is affected because his sperm are sensitive to the secretions of a woman's vagina or cervical canal. The sperm will then need to be released directly into the uterus with a syringe.

These methods offer the possibility of pregnancy to couples with infertility that is resistant to ordinary treatment, but they are expensive and success rates (as measured by the number of healthy babies born to couples undergoing treatment) for fertility centers are low. Before you begin treatment, ask about the success rate for each center.

Contraception

Oral contraceptives (The pill)

The contraceptive pill is currently the most effective method of temporary birth control. Physicians know more about the pill's side effects than about most other medication. Some good and bad side effects of birth control pills are described here, but ask your physician for the latest information about this form of birth control.

The most effective and commonly used birth control pills are called "combined" pills. This is because they contain synthetic versions of estrogen and a progesteronelike hormone, the hormones that control the female reproductive cycle. The mini-pill contains a progestin only, and while it is less effective as a means of birth control, it is believed to be safer because it causes fewer side effects.

Birth control pills work primarily by signaling the pituitary to stop causing the ovaries to release eggs. Also, the pills make it difficult for sperm to enter the uterus by stimulating production of mucus to plug the opening of the uterus.

The natural female sex hormones determine the amount and time of menstrual bleeding. Because small amounts of these hormones are made by the ovaries when they are prevented from releasing an egg, most women notice changes in their menstrual cycles when they take birth control pills. Periods occur after every 28 days and are usually shorter and lighter.

A change that fewer women experience is bleeding between menstrual periods. Called breakthrough bleeding, this is not uncommon during the first few months of using birth control pills and requires no treatment. If it keeps occurring, your physician may increase the estrogen content of your pills for several months.

Side effects Serious possible side effects of taking birth control pills include heart attack (see p.406), stroke (see p.285), and the formation of blood clots in veins (see Deep-vein thrombosis, p.445). However, physicians in the US have studied thousands of women who used birth control pills for up to 10 years and have discovered that serious side effects are not likely to occur in women under age 30. Today's low-dose pills contain less than half the amount of estrogen used in and are safer than their predecessors. More recent research has shown that there is still a significant risk for women over age 35 who are on the pill and smoke cigarettes. Other women who may be advised not to use oral contraceptives include those with a history of blood clots, high blood pressure, diabetes, uterine fibroids (see p.636), or breast or uterine cancer.

In addition to preventing pregnancy, birth control pills have other beneficial effects. A woman who takes birth control pills is much less likely to have an ovarian cyst (see p.635) than a woman who does not, and is also less likely to have breast lumps (see p.629), anemia (see p.450), rheumatoid arthritis (see p.589), and pelvic inflammatory disease (see p.639). The combined pill also helps prevent ectopic pregnancies (see p.675).

(continued on next page)

Cancer and the pill

Some research studies have suggested links between birth control pills and both breast and cervical cancer. However, since manufacturers reduced the levels of estrogen in the combined pill, the link with breast cancer has weakened, and recent studies suggest that the risk of developing cancer, if any, is extremely small.

Every woman who takes the pill should have regular Pap smears (see p.641) for early detection of cervical cancer. More positively, birth control pills are known to protect a woman against both cancer of the ovary and of the uterus.

Taking the pill

Birth control pills are easy to use. Your physician will probably recommend that you begin taking the pills on the fifth day after your menstrual bleeding has started. Then you take a pill every day at the same time for 3 weeks. Some pill packages include seven inactive pills to take during the last week of the cycle. After you take the last of the hormone-containing pills, the hormone levels in your blood fall quickly, and menstrual bleeding occurs. If you miss a pill, you should take it as soon as you notice the mistake. If you miss two or more pills from one package, continue to take the pills from the package, but use an additional method of birth control until you begin a new package of pills. If you miss taking a pill, the sudden withdrawal of the hormones may cause menstrual bleeding.

Birth control pills should not have any effect on your ability to become pregnant after you stop taking them. Your physician may recommend that you wait about 3 months, or until you have had two periods after stopping the pill, before you try to become pregnant.

The mini-pill

If you have been advised not to take the combined pill, you may be able to take the mini-pill. This pill contains only a progesterone hormone and may be safer if you have high blood pressure, diabetes, a history of blood clots, or other diseases that estrogen might make worse. Because they do not contain estrogen, which helps prevent the lining of the uterus from shedding during the pill cycle, a small amount of bleeding may occur at any time. In addition, some women may go for a long time without having regular menstrual periods. The mini-pills are less effective than combined birth control pills. On average about 2 out of every 100 women who use the mini-pill for a year will become pregnant. Your physician will probably advise you to begin taking the mini-pill on the first day of a period, and to take one each day for as long as you want contraception to continue. It is especially important that you take the mini-pill at the same time each day; because the mini-pill has its greatest contraceptive effect about 4 hours after it is taken, early evening is usually the best time to take it if you normally have sex at bedtime.

The IUD (intrauterine device)

An IUD (intrauterine device) is a T-shaped device made of copper or plastic that your physician inserts into your uterus, where it prevents pregnancy. It is not clear how an IUD prevents pregnancy; it may stop the fertilization of the egg by the sperm, or it may prevent implantation of a fertilized egg in the lining of the uterus. One device currently approved for use in the US releases a progesteronelike hormone to help prevent menstrual problems caused by IUDs. An IUD is often inserted during a menstrual period when your cervix—the opening to the uterus—is more open, but it can be inserted any time during your menstrual cycle once your physician determines that you are not pregnant.

The most common problems with wearing an IUD are the risk of increased menstrual bleeding and increased menstrual pain. Therefore, the IUD is usually not the best contraceptive method if you already have long, painful periods. Sometimes spotting occurs between periods during the first 2 or 3 months after an IUD is inserted, but this usually goes away. Menstrual bleeding usually becomes less heavy after a year or 2 of wearing an IUD.

The IUD must be inserted by a trained health professional using special equipment. The insertion takes only a few minutes, but it sometimes causes cramping pain for a short time. In some cases, this pain can be relieved by the administration of a local anesthetic at the time of insertion. The progestin and copper-containing IUDs must be replaced every 1 and 6 years, respectively.

Once inserted, the IUD protects you from pregnancy as long as it remains in the uterine cavity. Since any accidental expulsion of the IUD generally occurs in the first several months of use, you should check frequently to make sure the IUD is in place. You can check this by putting a finger inside your vagina and feeling for the string up against the cervix. If you can feel the string, you can be confident that the IUD is still in place. If you feel the hard plastic of the IUD, the device must be removed and replaced with a new one by a nurse or physician.

Although cramping pain and increased menstrual bleeding are the most common problems with wearing an IUD, the most dangerous problems are pelvic inflammatory disease (see p.639) and ectopic pregnancy (see p.675). Women who wear IUDs are more likely to have pelvic infections than women who do not. Since a very severe pelvic infection can cause sterility, your physician may recommend that you not use an IUD if you want to have children in the future. Infections are also more common in IUD users who are 20 or younger and in women who have not had children.

Because pelvic infection and ectopic pregnancy are serious side effects, you should see your physician immediately if you have pelvic pain, have an unexplained fever, have a foul-smelling vaginal discharge, or believe you may have become pregnant while wearing an IUD.

(continued on next page)

Implanted hormones

Another form of contraception is a hormonal implant (a progestin) placed under the skin of the arm. The chief advantages are that you do not have to remember to take a pill or use a device; also, you only need to replace the implant about every 5 years. Some women have experienced spotting as a side effect.

Condoms

A condom is a tube-shaped piece of thin latex rubber, closed at one end, which is rolled onto the erect penis before intercourse. Condoms are not only contraceptives, but also a method for preventing sexually transmitted diseases. When your partner ejaculates, the sperm are trapped in the closed end of the condom. During withdrawal of the penis after intercourse, the condom should be held at the base to prevent it from slipping off and spilling the contents. For maximum reliability you should use condoms in conjunction with some form of spermicide, a sperm-killing substance (see Table, p.649). Some condoms are already lubricated with spermicide.

Condoms come in a variety of designs and are easy to obtain. Many couples incorporate the use of the condom into their foreplay. It is important to avoid tearing the condom, however.

A variation of the condom is the female condom. This thin rubber tube fits inside the vagina and has an outer rim that remains outside. The female condom acts both as a contraceptive and as protection against sexually transmitted diseases.

Diaphragm and cervical cap

The diaphragm is one of the most effective barrier methods of contraception, in which the sperm is blocked from entering the uterus. The diaphragm is a rubber cup stretched over a flexible wire frame. Diaphragms are fitted to each user's vagina to cover the cervix.

Using the diaphragm correctly is very important: The diaphragm must be inserted every time before intercourse, but not more than 6 hours before. A spermicidal cream or jelly (see Spermicides, next column) must be put on the diaphragm every time it is inserted. A ring of spermicide is put around the edge of the diaphragm, and about ½ tsp. is placed in the center before the diaphragm is put into the vagina. Diaphragms bend into a partial circle when they are squeezed together to be inserted. Check immediately after insertion to make sure that the rubber of the diaphragm covers the cervix (the opening to the uterus) and that the edge of the diaphragm is behind your pubic bone. If the edge rests on top of the cervix, sperm are not blocked from entering the uterus and pregnancy can occur.

After sex, the diaphragm must be left in place for at least 6 hours to allow the spermicide to kill any sperm. If you have sex again within 6 hours, put more spermicidal cream or jelly in your vagina using the plastic applicator that is supplied with the spermicide. If more than 6 hours have passed, remove the diaphragm, wash it, put spermicidal cream or jelly on it as before, and replace it in your vagina. The diaphragm can be an effective method of birth control if these directions are followed (see Table, p.649).

The cervical cap, like the diaphragm, is a barrier method of birth control. It is much smaller than the diaphragm and fits tightly over the cervix rather than filling the vagina. There are several types of cervical caps, but the one most commonly used attaches to the cervix by suction. A cap must be fitted carefully. Most women use a cervical cap in the same way as a diaphragm, with spermicidal cream or jelly and following the same precautions. Used in this way, a cap is about as effective as a diaphragm.

Spermicides

Spermicides are chemicals that kill sperm. They are available in cream, jelly, or foam, and are inserted into the vagina shortly before intercourse. Once there, they tend to lose strength, so you should use more spermicide for each session of intercourse. Always use a spermicide with a condom, a diaphragm, or a cervical cap (see Table, p.649). Very rarely, a spermicide may cause an allergic reaction, with itching and redness in the genital area of either partner.

Vaginal sponge

The vaginal sponge is made of absorbent polyurethane foam saturated with spermicide. To use it correctly, you moisten the sponge and insert it high into your vagina. The sponge can be inserted at any time from 24 hours to immediately before intercourse, but you must leave it in place for at least 6 hours after intercourse. The sponge is effective as a carrier of spermicide, but ineffective as a barrier. It can be easily displaced and should be used along with a condom. The sponge is available without a prescription but has a relatively high failure rate.

Natural method

The natural method of contraception is based on predicting the day in the menstrual cycle when you will ovulate, or release an egg. Intercourse for that day, the following day, or for about a week before carries a high risk of conception. This is because sperm can live in the woman's body for as long as 6 days after intercourse (an average of 4 days), and an egg can be fertilized by a sperm for about the first 24 hours after ovulation.

Natural birth control methods are the least reliable of the methods of contraception discussed here (see Table, p.649), because each woman's cycle may vary, so the methods depend on an estimate of the time of ovulation. Also, the effectiveness of natural methods depends on abstaining from intercourse on unsafe days. You will need to keep records over several months in order to determine the pattern of your cycle. There are four ways to calculate the time of ovulation. Ovulation occurs in most women about 14 days before the first day of a period.

(continued on next page)

The temperature method: In most women, morning temperature (called basal temperature) rises slightly just after ovulation and does not fall again until the next period begins. Take your temperature each day as soon as you wake up—before you get out of bed or eat or drink anything—using a basal body thermometer designed to record small changes in temperature. Keep a chart of each temperature recording to determine your pattern of ovulation. To prevent pregnancy, avoid intercourse from the first day of a period until 3 full days after the temperature rise. The disadvantages of this method are that you have no warning when ovulation will occur, and that false readings may be obtained—illness, alcohol, and some drugs can cause a rise in body temperature.
The mucus inspection method: About 4 days before ovulation the mucus in the cervix becomes thinner, clearer, wetter, and more plentiful than when you are not ovulating. You can learn to examine this mucus and determine your pattern of ovulation. You should avoid intercourse from the time the wet mucus appears until 4 days after the mucus becomes noticeably thicker and drier.
The mucothermal method: This method is a combination of the temperature and mucus inspection methods. It is the most reliable natural method, especially when performed with the guidance of your physician. But you must avoid intercourse 3 days after your temperature rises and 4 days after your mucus thins (as described above).
The calendar method: This is the least reliable natural method. To detect ovulation you keep an accurate record of the lengths of your cycles for at least 12 months. Subtract 18 from the number of days in the shortest cycle (14 from ovulation to your period, plus 4 for average sperm life span) to find the first unsafe day in your cycle, counting the first day of your period as day 1. Subtract 10 days from the longest cycle (14 from ovulation to your period, less 1 for egg life span and 3 for good measure) to find the last unsafe day in your cycle. The calendar method is impractical if the woman has an irregular cycle; you would need to abstain from intercourse most days each month.

Sterilization

If you are certain that you do not want children in the future, sterilization offers an almost completely safe and reliable form of birth control. Most physicians recommend male rather than female sterilization to couples because it is safer and simpler. Because sterilization is simply a sealing off of the tubes that carry sperm or eggs, it has no effect on the production of sex hormones. If you are a man, you will produce a sperm-free seminal fluid. If you are a woman, you will produce eggs but they will not reach the uterus. Menstrual periods are not affected. Sterilization does not physically affect masculinity or femininity, but some people may develop emotional problems.
Male sterilization (vasectomy): A vasectomy is a simple operation that usually involves no hospitalization. It requires a local anesthetic and takes about 20 minutes. Your physician cuts the two vas deferens, the tubes that carry sperm from the testicles. The man still ejaculates after the surgery, but the seminal fluid contains no sperm.

Some sperm may already have been stored in the seminal vesicles before the operation is done, so you will probably be advised to use some other method of contraception for the first 6 to 8 weeks after the operation. During that same time, you will have to bring in a specimen of semen at least twice over a 6- to 8-week period. When two consecutive specimens are found to be sperm-free, you are considered sterile. How soon you have sexual intercourse is up to you. Vasectomy does not affect the man's ability to have an erection or an orgasm.
Female sterilization (tubal ligation): Female sterilization can be done with either a general or a local anesthetic. The operation takes less than an hour to perform, and can be performed with a laparoscope (a viewing tube equipped with blades for cutting) as outpatient surgery.

In the most commonly performed operation, two tiny cuts that leave virtually no scars are made just below the navel. Through this a laparoscope is inserted, and an attachment to this instrument is used to seal off the fallopian tubes by electrocautery (sealing with heat), tiny metal or plastic rings and clips, or cutting and tying off the ends of the fallopian tubes.

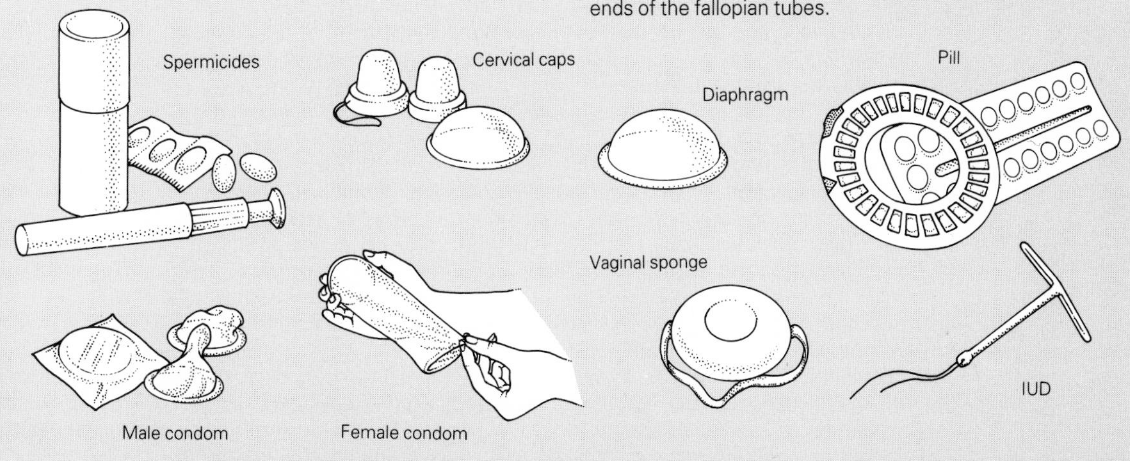

Sexually transmitted diseases (STDs)

A sexually transmitted disease (STD), once called a venereal disease, is an infection transferred from person to person during sexual contact. Most of the organisms responsible for STDs thrive and infect only in moist, warm conditions, and are unable to survive outside a person's body for more than several minutes. You are most likely to become infected with an STD through having sexual intercourse (vaginal or anal) with a person who is already infected. Other forms of sexual contact, including oral sex, can also spread an STD.

People who are most at risk for STDs are those who have multiple sexual partners. The risks are minimized if a condom is always used during sexual intercourse. There is evidence that if you contract one STD, such as gonorrhea or syphilis, you may also be at risk of contracting others, including human immunodeficiency virus (HIV). The risk of acquiring HIV, the virus that causes AIDS, from an infected partner is especially increased with anal sex, possibly through abrasions made in the wall of the rectum.

An increasing number of people are becoming infected with HIV through heterosexual vaginal intercourse.

Hepatitis B (see p.523) and possibly hepatitis C may be transmitted through sexual contact. Some STDs—trichomonal vaginitis (see p.645) and nongonococcal urethritis (see p.655), for example—may develop within a relationship in which neither partner admits to having had any outside sexual contact.

If you suspect you have acquired an STD, you should consult your physician immediately. Gonorrhea and syphilis can be cured, but delaying treatment can have serious long-term consequences. Also, infected people can infect their sexual partners. You should therefore use a condom or abstain from sexual relationships until you are cured and also make sure that anyone with whom you have had sexual contact seeks treatment without delay.

You can go to your physician for treatment, or to a clinic that specializes in diagnosis and treatment of STDs. In either case, your visit will be treated confidentially.

While some sexually transmitted diseases, including syphilis (see p.655), have been less common, their incidence is once again increasing, along with that of other STDs such as genital herpes (see p.656) and non-gonococcal urethritis.

A number of STDs are fully described elsewhere in this book, including scabies (see p.609), penile warts (see p.619), *Chlamydia* (see p.606), and AIDS (see p.465).

Gonorrhea

Gonorrhea is an infectious disease caused by *Gonococcus* bacteria and transmitted through sexual contact. These bacteria usually infect the man's urethra (the tube that carries urine and semen through the penis) and the woman's cervix (the opening to the uterus). Gonorrhea is one of the most common sexually transmitted diseases.

What are the symptoms?

Men with gonorrhea commonly find it extremely painful to urinate and have a cloudy discharge from the penis that looks like pus. Women may have a cloudy discharge from the vagina, some discomfort in the lower abdomen, or abnormal bleeding from the vagina. Sometimes women with the disease also find urinating painful. But frequently, women have no symptoms at all. When they do occur, symptoms usually appear about 2 to 8 days after infection or at the beginning of the next menstrual period.

Gonorrhea can also infect the rectum or mouth through anal or oral sexual contact. These infections often cause few symptoms. A person with rectal gonorrhea may feel some rectal pain, especially during a bowel movement, or have a cloudy discharge. With a gonorrhea throat infection, a person may have a sore throat.

What are the risks?

Untreated gonorrhea in men can spread from the urethra to the prostate gland and the epididymis, two internal structures that play roles in semen production. Often the urethra becomes narrowed from scar formation, which may make urinating difficult.

Untreated gonorrhea in a woman can infect the lining of the uterus or the fallopian tubes and cause damage and scarring that may make her infertile. Bacteria can also infect the uterus and the surrounding abdominal cavity, causing peritonitis (see p.503).

In both sexes, untreated gonorrhea can spread via the bloodstream and infect the joints, skin, bone, tendons, and other parts of the body. As the bacteria multiply in the bloodstream, blood poisoning (see p.452) can develop. This is a medical emergency.

What should be done?
If you suspect you have gonorrhea, consult your physician or go to a clinic that specializes in treating sexually transmitted diseases. It is important to use a condom or abstain from sexual relations until your condition has been diagnosed and treated and your symptoms have subsided. Gonorrhea usually is diagnosed by analyzing a sample of the cloudy discharge from the man's urethra or the woman's cervix.

What is the treatment?
Gonorrhea can be cured with antibiotics. This treatment can be given orally or by injection. Both you and your partner or partners should be treated.

Nongonococcal urethritis *(NGU)*

Nongonococcal urethritis (NGU), sometimes called nonspecific urethritis, is the most common sexually transmitted disease. It is an infection of the urethra, the tube through which urine passes from the bladder to outside the body.

The organisms that cause NGU are transmitted through sexual activity and may also contribute to long-term problems such as infertility. About half of the cases of NGU are caused by an organism called *Chlamydia* (see Chlamydial infections, p.606).

What are the symptoms?
Many men and women who have NGU have no symptoms but can still pass the infection to their sexual partners. In men the symptoms (when they occur) often resemble those of gonorrhea, with a painful, burning sensation when urinating and a cloudy, mucous discharge from the penis. Only a laboratory analysis of this discharge determines whether you have NGU or gonorrhea.

In women, symptoms (when they occur) may resemble those of a urinary tract infection (see Cystitis in women, p.643), including a painful, burning sensation when urinating, and the need to urinate frequently without expelling much urine. A test of the urine, however, will show that no bacterial infection is present. Other symptoms include pelvic pain, a heavy vaginal discharge, or abnormal uterine bleeding (either between your periods or heavy period bleeding).

What should be done?
Any man who has a cloudy discharge from his penis should consult his physician or a sexually transmitted disease (STD) clinic to find out if the problem is caused by gonorrhea. If the gonorrhea test results are normal, the problem may be NGU. Women whose urine shows no bacterial infection although they still have the symptoms may have NGU. There are laboratory tests available to diagnose many causes of NGU.

Antibiotics, taken 4 times daily for about a week, usually clear up the infection. Despite treatment, however, NGU may recur.

If you have NGU, do not have sexual intercourse until you have completed the entire course of antibiotic medication. This will help prevent reinfection and will also help prevent your partner from getting your infection. Your sexual partner or partners should also have medical treatment.

Syphilis

Syphilis is transmitted through sexual activity when a bacterium called *Treponema pallidum* penetrates the moist mucous membranes of the mouth, the vagina, and the penis's urethra, through which urine passes from the bladder to the outside.

If it is not treated, syphilis has three stages that can appear throughout a lifetime. Usually the painless skin ulcers that occur during the first stage and the rash that occurs in the second stage are highly infectious and contaminate others through contact with the infected mucous membranes and, rarely, through open sores. The third stage of syphilis is usually not contagious unless the blood from an infected person is somehow transfused to someone else. All donated blood is tested for syphilis.

What are the symptoms?
First stage Any time between 1 and 8 weeks after infection, a small painless sore called a chancre (pronounced "shanker") appears. Usually a chancre is red and solid and protrudes above the skin. The initial chancre usually occurs in the genital area. Chancres on the penis are usually visible, but when they occur in a woman's vagina or cervix

they may not be noticed. They can occur elsewhere on the body, frequently on the mouth or rectum. The chancre heals in 1 to 5 weeks, leaving a thin scar. During this period, the syphilis-causing bacteria circulate in the blood throughout the body.

Second stage This stage is called secondary syphilis. About 6 weeks after the chancre has healed you may feel ill, have a sore throat, fever, and a headache. Glands in your neck, armpits, and groin may swell. You may also develop a skin rash of small, red, scaling bumps that do not itch. Spots may appear on the palms of the hands and the soles of the feet. Gray patches of skin, which are different from chancres, can occur in the mucous membranes of the mouth, vulva, and penis. A rash around the rectum may also develop. All of these skin conditions are highly infectious and heal in 2 to 6 weeks.

Third stage This is also called latent syphilis or late syphilis. The symptoms of the first two stages disappear for several years, and unless you have a special blood test, you have no way of knowing that you have syphilis. This final stage can last anywhere from 2 years to a lifetime.

During this stage, the disease flares up without warning. It can affect the brain, causing paralysis, dementia, loss of equilibrium, loss of sensation in the legs, and, rarely, blindness. The disease can also infect the aorta (the large blood vessel that leads from the heart), weaken its walls, and cause an aneurysm (see p.436), which may rupture. Sometimes third-stage syphilis affects the functioning of the aortic valve of the heart, leading to inflammation of the aorta or insufficiency of the aorta.

Rarely, syphilis can also infect the liver, stomach, eyes, meninges (the membranes that cover the brain), and other organs.

What should be done?

Anyone with a suspicious sore in his or her mouth or on the genitals should see a physician. Syphilis is highly contagious during the first and second stages, so you should notify your sexual partner or partners since they may be infected.

Syphilis can be diagnosed by a blood test and is easily cured in the first stage with antibiotic injections. Some cases may be cured in the second stage. If you are allergic to penicillin, another antibiotic can be prescribed. In the third stage, syphilis cannot be reversed once the blood vessels and brain are damaged.

Genital herpes

(herpes genitalis)

The herpes simplex virus can produce a painful infection of the genitals called genital herpes (herpes genitalis). Groups of blisters develop and eventually rupture and become shallow ulcers or sores. Genital herpes is transmitted through sexual activity.

A similar virus that causes cold sores in the mouth (see p.484) also causes about 15 percent of cases of genital herpes usually as a result of oral-genital contact.

What are the symptoms?

About 6 days after contact with an infected person, you may feel pain, tenderness, or an itchy sensation near the penis or vulva. These symptoms may be accompanied by fever, headache, or a generally ill feeling.

Single and multiple blisters soon appear along a man's penis or on a woman's vulva. They sometimes also occur on the thighs or buttocks. The blisters also form in a woman's vagina or on the cervix, where they cannot be seen, so it is possible to unknowingly infect a sexual partner. When the blisters break, they form extremely painful open sores, which last from 1 to 3 weeks.

Since the virus may remain in the body after the blisters subside, about half of the people who get genital herpes will have recurrences in the following months or years. Usually these recurrences are less severe, and the problem disappears altogether with time.

What are the risks?

The major risk is infecting another person, which can occur only when you have an active infection, so do not have sexual contact until the infection clears up. The herpes virus can spread into the bloodstream and infect other organs in people who have difficulty fighting infection, such as people who have cancer or kidney, lung, or blood diseases.

If you are pregnant and have herpes near the time of delivery, your physician will perform the delivery by a cesarean section (see p.686) to avoid infecting your infant.

What should be done?

There is no cure for genital herpes, but your physician may prescribe an analgesic such as aspirin or the antiviral drug acyclovir, which may speed healing. Frequent warm baths may help reduce inflammation. The herpes virus may be implicated in some cases of cancer of the cervix, so women with herpes should have an annual Pap smear.

Pubic lice

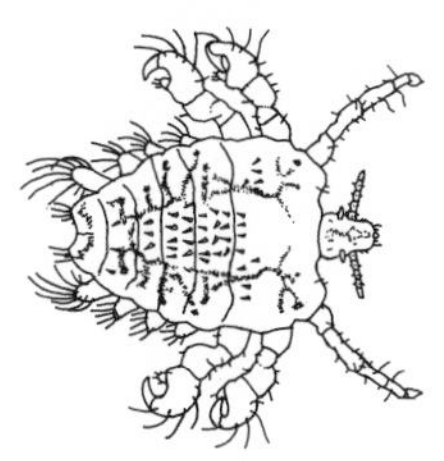
Pubic louse about 20 times actual size.

Pubic lice, also known as crab lice (or "crabs"), are blood-sucking lice that usually appear only in the pubic hair and the hair around the anus. Occasionally, however, they occur on other body hair and sometimes on the eyebrows and eyelashes. The louse, which can be clearly seen if you look closely, is 1 to 2 mm across and resembles a small, flat crab. It clings tightly to hair with its clawlike legs. The female's pale, white eggs, called nits, can just barely be seen with the naked eye. They are attached so firmly to hairs that normal washing does not remove them.

Pubic lice are acquired from sexual contact with someone who is infested with them.

What are the symptoms?
Many people have no symptoms, but others have itching in the pubic region, particularly at night, when the lice are active.

What should be done?
If you have pubic lice, go to your physician, who will recommend a nonprescription lotion or shampoo to kill the lice and their eggs. At the same time, your physician may want to perform a checkup to make sure that you do not have any other sexually transmitted diseases. You should also notify your sexual partner or partners that they may have lice and need treatment.

Sexual problems

Sometimes a couple cannot fully enjoy sexual intercourse, or cannot have intercourse at all, because of physical or psychological problems. Although these problems are discussed separately in the following articles, many couples suffer from a combination of physical and psychological problems that interfere with sex. For example, premature ejaculation by a man may result in lack of orgasm for his partner. Treatment of sexual problems is usually far more successful if it is applied to the couple rather than only one partner. Talk to your physician, who may refer you to a sex therapist.

Impotence

An impotent man is one who fails to achieve or maintain an erection. This problem can prevent a couple from having any sexual relationship, but often it can be successfully treated. If you are impotent, consult your physician. There are a number of courses of treatment he or she may recommend.

Physicians once thought that most cases of impotence had psychological causes, but more physical causes of the problem have been discovered. Among the physical factors that can cause impotence are conditions in which the level of the male sex hormone testosterone in the blood is drastically lowered. Extreme stress, fatigue, chronic illness, use of illegal narcotics, and the heavy use of alcohol can also be contributing factors in impotence, as can certain prescription medications.

Most men experience impotence for a day or 2 or longer at some time in their lives. The experience can be embarrassing and can cause concern and stress about poor sexual performance so that the impotence lasts longer than it otherwise would. Impotence may also develop as a result of concern over other sexual problems, such as premature ejaculation (see next article). For a discussion of the causes of impotence, read the article in Men's health (see p.611).

Premature ejaculation

Premature ejaculation is rapid orgasm immediately after, or before, the penis penetrates the woman's vagina for sexual intercourse. It is one of the most common sexual problems of men. Most men have probably ejaculated prematurely at least once when very excited or anxious. Some sex researchers consider it to be premature ejaculation when a man reaches orgasm before his sexual partner in more than half of his sexual experiences with her. This is a controversial definition, since some women take 20 minutes to achieve climax.

There seems to be little if any relationship between premature ejaculation and psychological problems. However, it is thought that some men may develop premature ejaculation through social conditioning in their youth. For example, if a young man's first sexual experiences were with prostitutes, they may have coaxed him to ejaculate rapidly. Premature ejaculation may also result from a young man's anxiety about his parents' reactions to masturbation or premarital sex. Some men develop impotence (see previous article) as a result of anxiety about sexual performance and premature ejaculation.

A couple in which the man has premature ejaculation should consult a sex therapist. Premature ejaculation often leads to conflict, hostility, and distrust between partners if it is not treated. Treatment usually requires the participation of both partners in order to be effective. Relaxation, body massage, and open and honest communication are crucial for a successful recovery.

What is the treatment?

Although several modes of therapy are available, the "squeeze" technique is an effective method used to delay ejaculation. The partners massage each other first. The man then lies down on his back, while the woman stimulates his penis until ejaculation is imminent. At his signal, she firmly squeezes the glans (the head of the penis) where it is joined to the shaft for about 15 seconds. The male partner should then lose his urge to ejaculate and his erection will diminish by 10 to 30 percent. After about 30 seconds, the couple can resume sex play, including stimulation of the penis. Should the man feel the urge to ejaculate again, the squeeze technique can be repeated.

Lack of orgasm

Lack of orgasm may be due to lack of sex education and early inhibitions. It may be caused by underlying psychological problems, but it may also be the result of a lack of sexual interest that began with a physical problem such as damage to the vagina after childbirth or thyroid disease, or a side effect from a drug.

Lack of orgasm is rare among men. However, only about one in three women regularly reaches orgasm through intercourse alone, without additional stimulation of the clitoris. Up to 10 percent of women cannot reach orgasm, even by stimulation.

If you are dissatisfied with the frequency or ease with which you or your partner reaches orgasms, discuss it openly and honestly. You may find that you need to change your sexual techniques. For example, it may help to spend more time with massage or foreplay by stimulating each other's whole body and then the genitals before intercourse.

Sometimes a new position during intercourse helps. If both partners are willing, experiment with some new positions. One position that women report to be very stimulating is with the woman on top, astride her partner. In this position, the woman can

Loss of sexual desire in men

The male sex hormone testosterone stimulates the male sexual drive. If your testosterone level is lowered your sexual interest and capacity for arousal are likely to decrease. The conditions underlying a drop in testosterone level may be a physical problem such as liver, kidney, or pituitary disease, or it may be a side effect of a drug you are taking. The loss of sexual desire also may be due to fatigue, stress, or pain. However, the root of the problem may be psychological or a combination of psychological and physical factors. Severe depression (see p.321), for example, may cause you to lose interest in sex.

Loss of sexual interest in a familiar partner or the stress of a divorce are common problems that may result in a loss of sexual desire in men. This can also happen when there are other problems, either sexual or nonsexual, in a relationship. Other conditions such as impotence (see previous page) or premature ejaculation (see previous page) can interfere with the enjoyment of sexual intercourse and cause a man to avoid sex.

If self-help measures such as reading sexually explicit materials or using fantasy do not help you to regain your sexual desire, consult your physician, who may examine you to look for a physical cause for your loss of sexual desire. If no obvious cause is found, you may be referred to a sex therapist for treatment.

What can you do?

It may help to discuss the issue openly with your partner. This may clear up misunderstandings or uncover other problems in the relationship that may be affecting you both. If you are bored with a long-standing relationship, try new ways of having intercourse that are mutually agreeable to both partners.

What treatment is available?

Treatment depends on the underlying condition. Psychotherapy can be helpful if your physician is unable to identify any underlying physical condition. Self-help measures, fantasy, and relaxation techniques may also be helpful. Ask your physician to recommend a book on sexual technique that is suitable for you.

control the intensity and exact location of her clitoral and vaginal stimulation.

If lack of orgasm persists, see your physician, who may refer you to a sex therapist. Drugs are seldom prescribed unless they are needed for related problems. Sex therapy usually involves therapy sessions and exercises to be done at home.

Painful intercourse

Painful sexual intercourse, or dyspareunia, has a number of causes and can affect both men and women. There are often physical reasons that your physician can identify by asking questions and examining you.

Painful intercourse in women

Many medical conditions can make sexual activity painful for women. Infections or irritations of the vulva such as genital herpes (see p.656) or candidiasis (see p.605), cysts

Loss of sexual desire in women

If you are a woman who is frustrated and unhappy during sexual activity, effective treatment is available.

Many factors shape the sexual desire and response of women, including cultural conditioning and learned sexual attitudes. Research is now being done on how women's bodies (such as the blood vessels, nerves, and muscles) change during sexual arousal and intercourse. A major difficulty in analyzing diminished sexual desire involves defining what is normal sexual behavior. The meaning of "normal" changes with the cultural and social climate.

Generally, very few women lose interest in sex as a result of disease, drugs, or hormonal imbalance. However, anger, conflict, stress, alcohol, fatigue, and some drugs can temporarily affect sexual desire. Drugs that can decrease sexual desire include narcotics and tranquilizers.

Female sexual arousal

Before a woman can feel sexually responsive, there are usually some essential preliminaries. One condition that is necessary for most women's enjoyment is a relaxed and secure environment, both physically and emotionally. Fears of rejection, desertion, or pregnancy may prevent optimal sexual pleasure. One requirement during sexual intercourse is that a woman must receive adequate physical stimulation to the erogenous (sensitive) areas of her body, including the clitoris, if she is to respond with vaginal lubrication and finally orgasm. Lubrication is provided by a moist substance secreted by the walls of the vagina. This substance allows the penis to enter comfortably and glide easily in and out.

Research has shown that the amount of time for arousal varies with the individual, as does the type of foreplay each woman prefers. In some cases, poor or no communication between sexual partners about what is pleasurable causes a loss of sexual interest. Some women find it difficult to express or even to identify specific preferences. This is often because they have been culturally conditioned to be sexually passive and unassertive, thinking that their partner should take responsibility for the pleasure of both of them during sexual intercourse. Some women tell their partners about a desire for foreplay but the partner forgets or ignores the request. An orgasm includes intensely pleasurable reflex contractions of all body muscles, including muscles in the vagina. Occasionally the uterus contracts briefly during peak arousal.

Disorders of female sexual response

The quality of a woman's relationship with her partner greatly influences her ability to respond. Most women need to feel love and/or affection for and from their partners. Power struggles, hidden hostilities, ambivalence, passivity, fear of losing control, fear of rejection and abandonment, a poor marital relationship, low self-esteem, memories of previous sexual trauma (rape or molestation), or psychological disturbances can inhibit a woman's sexual response. When a woman receives adequate sexual stimulation in a relaxed and undemanding environment and is still unable to enjoy sexual activity, there may be an underlying problem in one of two general categories. One is general sexual dysfunction, which refers to women who are not aroused by erotic foreplay and so do not lubricate. The other is orgasmic dysfunction, which refers to women who are sexually stimulated and lubricate, but do not experience orgasm.

In both conditions, unconscious feelings and attitudes about sex such as shame, fear, or guilt can block all or part of the natural response to sexual stimulation. A woman may have some unconsious conflict about her sexuality, or she may feel guilty about freely expressing her sexuality.

Women with general sexual dysfunction may need to learn more about their bodies, since they may unconsciously block their erotic feelings and physical responses. They can be treated with a combination of psychotherapy (see p.323) and sex therapy. Qualified sex therapists use special exercises to teach the woman how to get in touch with her body's erotic sensations and encourage using sexual fantasy to attain arousal. A secure and undemanding atmosphere, whether she is alone or with her partner, is important for successful treatment.

Women with orgasmic dysfunction may unconsciously overcontrol the orgasm reflex, usually because of some of the feelings discussed above. Counseling and psychotherapy, combined with performing sexual exercises at home, are usually helpful. If you decide to seek treatment, consult your physician, who can refer you to reputable professionals for sex therapy.

or boils, and rashes or allergic reactions all can cause sexual discomfort. Vaginal infections irritate the vaginal walls and can cause painful intercourse. Episiotomy scars (see Box, Special procedures in childbirth, p.685) may also cause pain during intercourse.

Diseases that affect the uterus can cause pain when the man thrusts his penis deeply into the vagina. These include pelvic inflammatory disease (see p.639), ectopic pregnancy (see p.675), endometriosis (see p.638), and ovarian cysts (see p.635) and tumors.

Bladder disorders such as cystitis (see p.643), urethritis (see p.655), and cystocele (when the bladder loses its pelvic support and collapses into the urethral canal) all make both foreplay and intercourse uncomfortable. Arthritis or chronic pain in the lower back also can cause pain during intercourse. Painful intercourse from these causes can sometimes be relieved by taking aspirin or an aspirin substitute about an hour before engaging in intercourse, and by adopting a new position for intercourse.

Painful intercourse in men

Men, too, can experience painful intercourse. The causes are usually physical. A tight foreskin in an uncircumcised man may need to be released. Infection or irritation of the skin of the penis, such as genital herpes (see p.656) or allergic rashes, can cause pain during intercourse. Some spermicides used as contraceptives (see p.652) may cause a burning sensation on the surface of the penis.

Infections of the prostate gland, urethra, or testicles can also make sexual intercourse painful. Cancer of the penis or testicles and arthritis of the lower back also make thrusting uncomfortable.

If intercourse is painful for you, you should consult your physician.

Vaginismus

In vaginismus, the lower vaginal muscles tighten into spasm. This prevents sexual intercourse. Vaginismus is a natural vaginal protection mechanism. When no infection or other disorder exists, anticipation of pain or fear of becoming pregnant are other possible causes. The problem may occur when a woman's natural sexual arousal is somehow inhibited for psychological reasons (see Box, Loss of sexual desire in women, p.659).

Vaginismus can be relieved by working with a physician or therapist trained in treating sexual disorders. The physician or therapist may prescribe a series of dilators or tubes of varying size. You insert the smallest one into the vagina, then the next size and so on, until you are comfortable with inserting a dilator that is the size of an erect penis. This treatment may be supplemented with exercises that are designed to teach you how to contract and relax the vaginal muscles at will, as when you wish to stop the flow of urine. Another treatment is for the woman to lie down, relax, use sexual fantasy, breathe out slowly, and insert one finger in her vagina for 5 minutes twice a day for 2 days. Then she inserts two of her fingers in the same way twice a day for 2 days.

Homosexuality and bisexuality

Homosexuals do not choose homosexuality any more than heterosexuals choose heterosexuality. Both "just know" or are "aware" of their sexual orientation from an early age. Reversing either orientation is equally difficult. Trying a same-sex encounter does not necessarily indicate that you are homosexual.

Psychiatrists differ in their approach to homosexuality, but most consider it a normal variation of sexual behavior. Homosexuality is neither congenital (present from birth) nor inherited. Theories on homosexuality are abundant and confusing, and so far none has received universal acceptance. Infants have no sexual orientation, and many variables influence their sexuality. In all cultures, in every socioeconomic group, 90 to 95 percent of men and women are heterosexual, and 5 to 10 percent are homosexual. Homosexuals differ widely in their emotional and social adjustment, as do heterosexuals.

The word bisexual describes people who can regularly enjoy and engage in sexual activity with either men or women. It refers to more-than-occasional teen experimentation. Bisexuality is poorly understood, and no one knows how many people are bisexual.

The well-adjusted homosexual person does not need psychotherapy. All homosexuals experience the same physical, emotional, and behavioral ups and downs as heterosexuals. A homosexual who is alienated or troubled about his or her identity may want to seek psychotherapy, group therapy, family therapy, or joint therapy with a spouse or homosexual partner to reduce physical and emotional distress. If you have recently learned that a friend or relative is homosexual or bisexual, you can seek further information or emotional support from an organization such as Parents and Friends of Lesbians and Gays (PFLAG).

Pregnancy and childbirth

Introduction

If you are planning to get pregnant or are pregnant, you may want to read through the entire section on pregnancy and childbirth. Many changes take place in your body during pregnancy—most of them predictable. In fact, a majority of pregnancies and deliveries do not involve major problems for the woman or the child.

Conception, or fertilization of one of your eggs, can occur shortly after a mature egg has been released from one of your two ovaries, which happens approximately halfway through your menstrual cycle (for more information on ovulation, see p.624). The egg travels along the fallopian tube toward the uterus. If you have sexual intercourse during this time, the millions of sperm that your partner has ejaculated travel from your vagina, through the uterus, and up to the fallopian tube. If one sperm penetrates the cell wall of one of your eggs, fertilization occurs. The fertilized egg reaches the uterus 2 to 7 days later and embeds itself in the uterine lining. This happens at about the time your next period is due. By the time you think you might be pregnant, the egg has already become an embryo and is developing in your uterus. A full-term pregnancy lasts about 38 weeks from the time of fertilization, also called conception, to delivery. Although conception usually occurs halfway through a woman's menstrual cycle, the delivery date is calculated from the first day of your last period because the precise day the egg is fertilized is usually not known. This means that if you conceive halfway through a regular 28-day cycle you will be 4 weeks pregnant 2 weeks after conception, and the entire pregnancy will have lasted 40 weeks, not 38.

Some articles in this section cover general concerns of pregnancy, which range from the common problem of heartburn to the comparatively rare disorder of Rhesus factor blood incompatibility. Other articles discuss disorders that can occur in early, middle, or late pregnancy. The most common problems of childbirth are described, as well as the techniques available to assist you during pregnancy and childbirth. In the final part of this section, problems that may affect women shortly after childbirth, such as postpartum depression, are discussed.

Problems that can affect newborns, such as respiratory distress syndrome, neonatal jaundice, gastroenteritis, and feeding problems, are described in the section called Children's health (see p.690).

Rubella (German measles) and pregnancy

If you contract rubella (German measles, see p.746), during pregnancy, there is a risk that your child will be born with a heart defect. The risk is highest if you have had the illness in the first 3 months (first trimester) of pregnancy. If rubella occurs during the first 4 weeks of pregnancy, more than 50 percent of babies are born with a major defect, such as a complicated heart disorder (see p.702) that will often require surgery soon after birth. By the 13th week (early in the second trimester), that figure has dropped to 8 percent, and the risk steadily decreases after that.

If you have already had rubella, you are not likely to get it again. However, do not rely on your own or a relative's memory that you have had the illness. Make sure before you try to get pregnant, by asking your physician to give you a blood test that will show whether your immune system (your body's natural defenses) has developed antibodies (substances in the blood that fight infections) to the rubella virus. If the test shows you have not had rubella, your physician may immunize you against it by injecting you with a vaccine that gives you a mild form of the disease. You should avoid conception for 3 months after the vaccination because the virus may still be present in your body during this period and can infect the developing embryo.

The biology of pregnancy

Egg production and ovulation

A woman has two ovaries, one on each side of the uterus, which contain thousands of immature eggs. After puberty, a single egg normally ripens each month in one of the ovaries. The maturing egg and about 100 cells that cluster around it and nourish it form what is called a follicle. The follicle is filled with liquid. About halfway through the menstrual cycle, the follicle bursts and the ripe egg is released (ovulation) and drawn into the fallopian tube nearby.

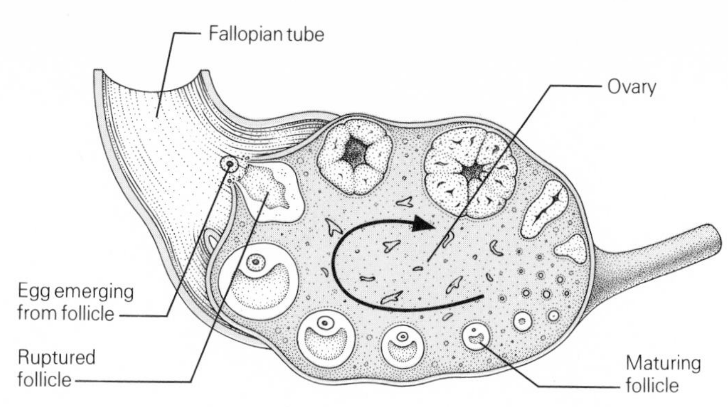

Sperm production

Sperm are minute cells produced in the many coiled tubes, called seminiferous tubules, inside the two testicles. The sperm pass from the testicles into the epididymis, and then to the seminal vesicles, where they are stored until ejaculation.

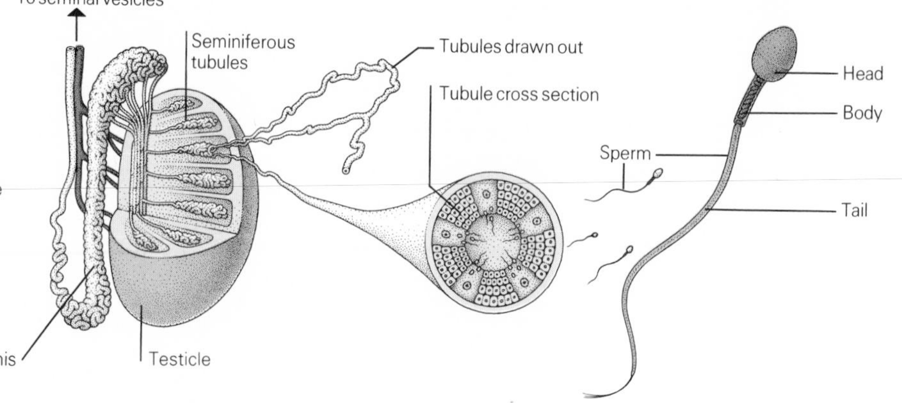

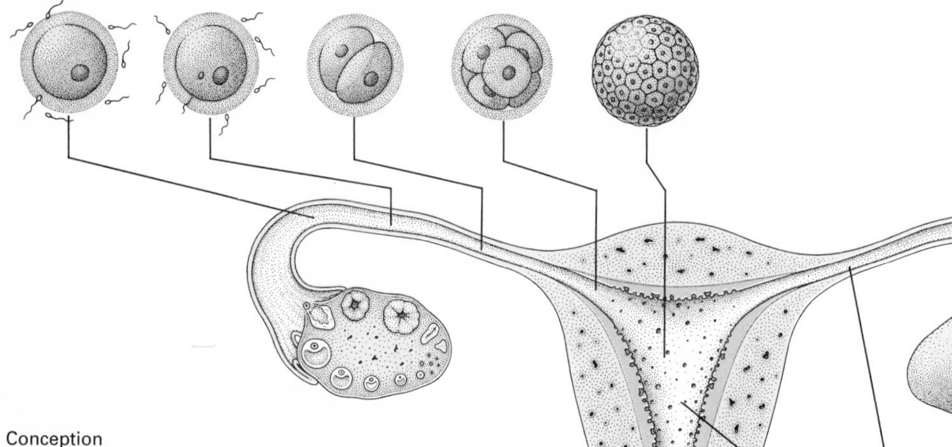

Conception

Conception, or fertilization of an egg by a single sperm out of the millions ejaculated, takes place in the fallopian tube shortly after ovulation. The sperm's nucleus joins with the egg's nucleus, combining their genetic material, and the cell divides into two cells. Each of these cells then divides into two, which divide again and so on. The group of dividing cells travels along the fallopian tube toward the uterus, where it embeds itself in the lining 2 to 7 days after fertilization. In a few weeks, it develops into an embryo and placenta.

A growing embryo

Until about the 12th week of pregnancy, the fertilized egg is known as an embryo. (From 12 weeks until delivery, it is called a fetus.) The embryo develops extremely rapidly. At 5 weeks, it is about the size of a grain of rice, but by 12 weeks it is about 2½ inches (6 cm) long. At 28 days, the most developed organ is the heart. The arms and legs first develop as buds. The nervous system, eyes, and ears are all obvious by 6 weeks. The proportions of a developing embryo are very different from those of an adult human being. The illustrations below show the embryo (enlarged) at different stages of development and (in outline at top) at actual size.

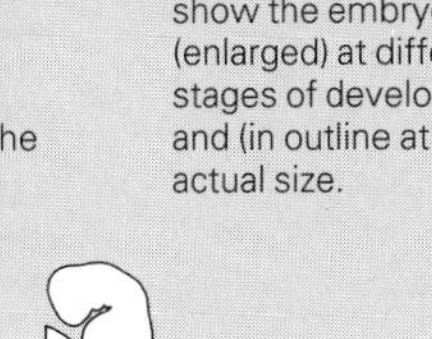

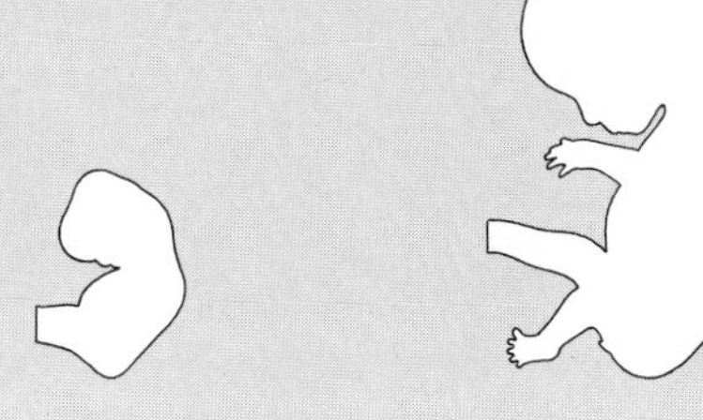

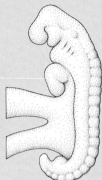

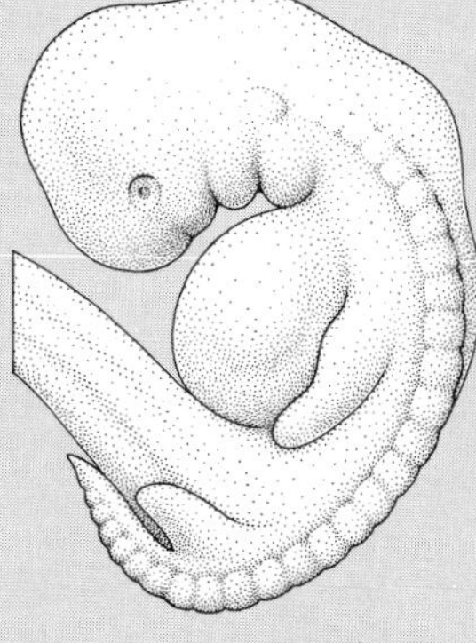

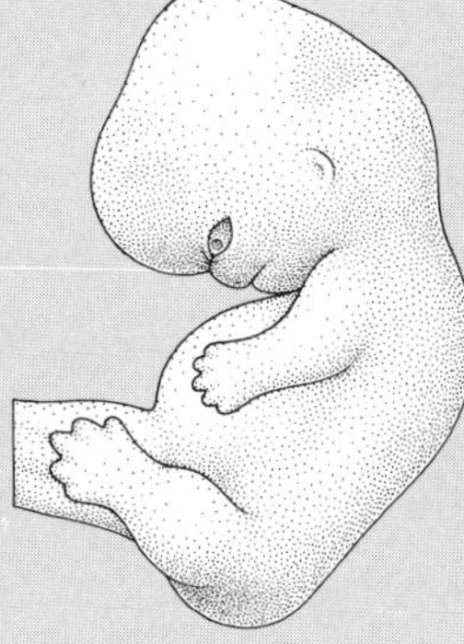

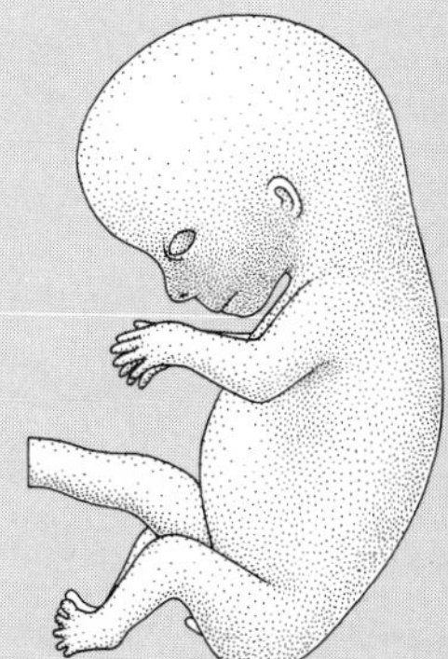

Time since last period — 6 weeks (enlarged) — 7 weeks (enlarged) — 9 weeks (enlarged) — 10 weeks (enlarged)

Your changing profile

During the first weeks of pregnancy, there is little obvious change in your body, although your breasts may seem a little larger and feel tender and heavy. By about the 12th week, your enlarging uterus causes a bulge in the abdominal wall. By the time you are 20 weeks pregnant, your abdomen may be swollen and, instead of being indented, your navel may protrude. Toward the end of pregnancy the fetus's head may move down slightly to settle in the pelvic cavity. This may make breathing easier, but you may need to urinate more often than is usual, because of pressure on your bladder.

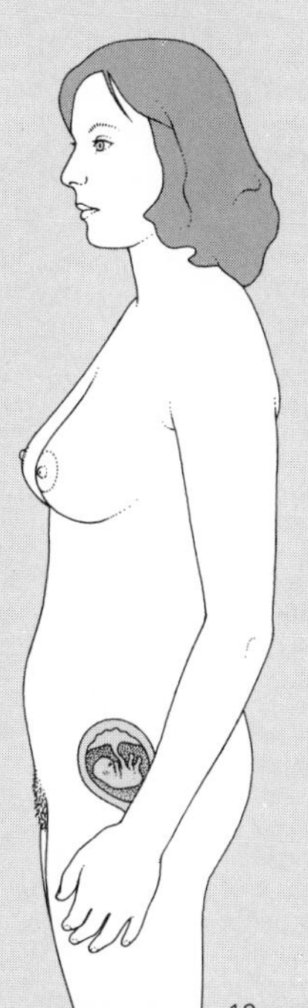

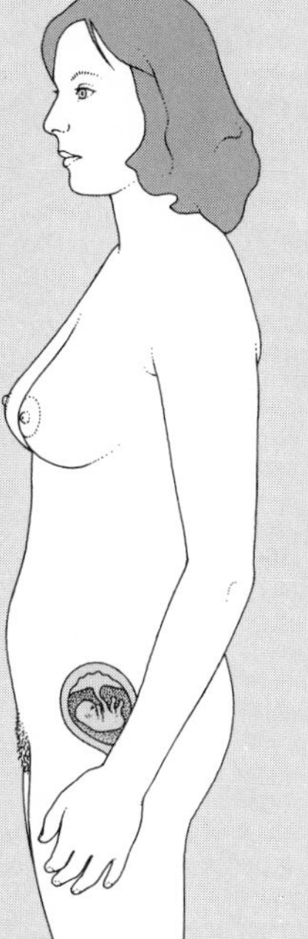

12 weeks

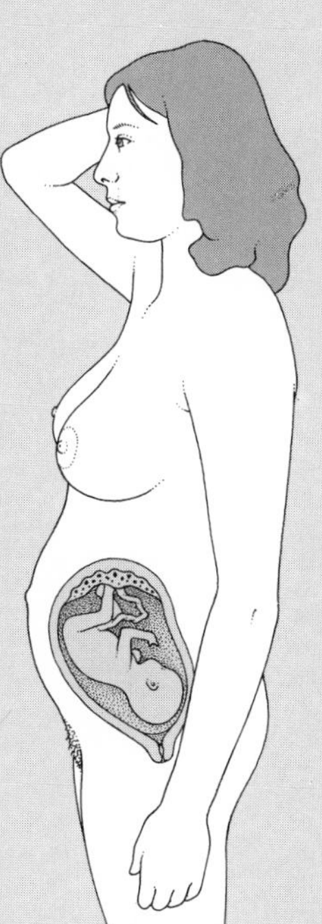

28 weeks

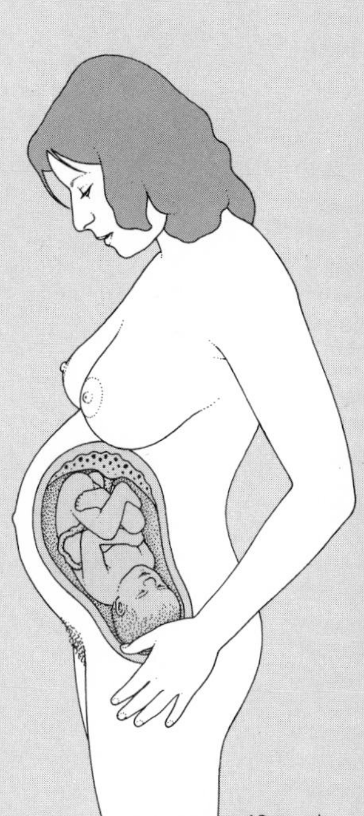

40 weeks

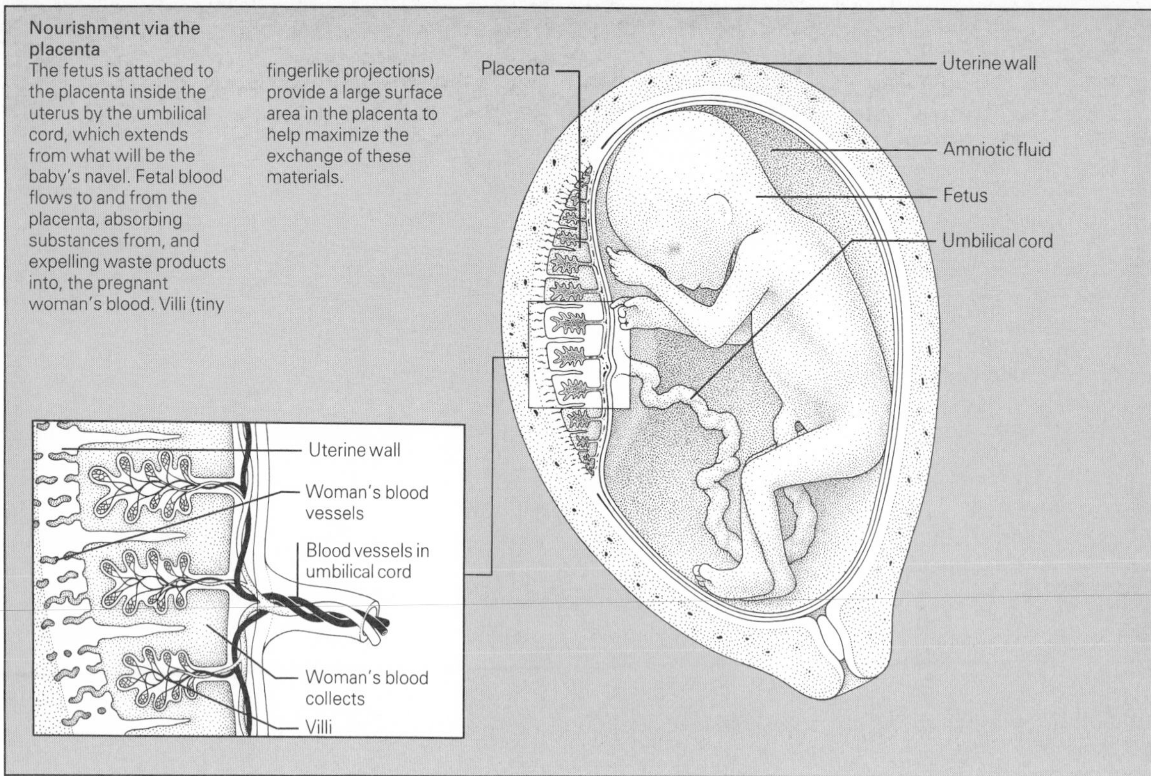

Nourishment via the placenta
The fetus is attached to the placenta inside the uterus by the umbilical cord, which extends from what will be the baby's navel. Fetal blood flows to and from the placenta, absorbing substances from, and expelling waste products into, the pregnant woman's blood. Villi (tiny fingerlike projections) provide a large surface area in the placenta to help maximize the exchange of these materials.

Genetic counseling

As medical understanding of inherited disorders has improved, genetic counseling services have become available, often at major medical centers. The purpose of genetic counseling is to help people who are concerned about the possibility of having a child with a birth defect or passing along an inherited disorder to a child. Knowledge of genetic disorders is advancing very rapidly, and anyone who suspects he or she may carry an inherited disorder, perhaps because a particular illness appears to run in the family, should seek genetic counseling.

A child may be born with a physical or mental disorder or defect for one of four reasons: 1) The child may have inherited one or more abnormal genes from one or both parents who are carriers of the disorder, such as cystic fibrosis and some cases of hemophilia. 2) The child may have one or more abnormal genes because of a mutation that occurred in the egg or sperm of one of the parents. This explains how parents who are completely healthy can have children with genetic disorders such as muscular dystrophy or hemophilia. 3) Faulty cell division that occurred just before or just after fertilization may have led to a chromosomal disorder such as Down syndrome or Turner's syndrome. 4) The child's chromosomes and genes may be normal but the development of the embryo in the uterus may have been faulty, which may result in a disorder such as spina bifida.

Of every hundred children born, two or three have a serious mental or physical handicap that is genetic in origin or results from damage to, or faulty development of, the fetus during pregnancy. The harmful agent during pregnancy may be excessive intake of alcohol or an infection such as rubella (See Rubella (German measles) and pregnancy, p.661). Genetic disorders include disorders of the blood, such as hemophilia (see p.455), thalassemia (see p.454), and sickle cell anemia (see p.453); muscular dystrophy (see p.741); cystic fibrosis (see p.732); and disorders of the brain, such as Huntington's chorea (see p.313) and Tay-Sachs disease.

It is now possible, with many genetic disorders, to have tests to determine whether or not you are a carrier. Most people who suspect that they may carry a genetic disorder wait until they are planning to have children before they are tested. However, if one child in a family has, for example, thalassemia, his or her relatives can be tested to find out if they carry the thalassemia gene in their cells.

If one or both parents are found to be carriers of a genetic disorder, genetic counselors can calculate the chances of their children inheriting it depending on whether the abnormal gene that carries the disorder is dominant or recessive. For some genetic disorders, an exact calculation can be made. For example, a child may have a 25 percent chance of inheriting the disorder. In other cases, however, it is more difficult to make an exact calculation.

As part of genetic counseling, you will be asked for detailed information about the health of parents, brothers, sisters, cousins, and other relatives. It will help if you have this information in writing when you go for counseling. You will need to give details of the exact causes of deaths in the family, and the age at which relatives died. This is particularly relevant if any relatives died during infancy. Ethnic and racial background is also considered. Increasing age of parents is also a risk factor for some disorders such as Down syndrome.

If a woman has a stillborn child, she should ask her physician whether the child may have had a genetic disorder. If there is a possibility of a genetic disorder, a genetic counselor should be informed.

Most genetic disorders are inherited as recessive disorders (see Genetics, p.752). If only one of the two parents has the defective gene (and thus is a carrier), all of their children will be healthy. Each child, however, will have a 50 percent chance of also being a carrier of the disorder (see illustration, below). If two carriers marry, each child has a 25 percent chance of inheriting the disorder. The exceptions to this genetic pattern are sex-linked disorders, such as Duchenne muscular dystrophy and hemophilia, and the dominant disorders, such as Huntington's chorea. In sex-linked disorders, the defective gene occurs in the pair of chromosomes (the threadlike structures that the genes form) that determines whether the fetus will be a boy or a girl; a boy will be affected if only one of the two chromosomes is abnormal. Such disorders are almost entirely limited to boys. In dominant disorders, only one of the paired chromosomes needs to be abnormal for the disease to appear.

Recent advances in genetics have made it possible, in some cases, to determine whether the developing fetus has a genetic disorder. Chorionic villus sampling (see p.684), for example, may be performed early in pregnancy, during the 6th to 8th weeks. In this procedure, a sample of the placenta is removed and examined. If results of chorionic villus sampling are inconclusive, another test may be performed later in pregnancy (see Amniocentesis, p.684, and Fetoscopy, p.685). As individual genes involved in disease are isolated, protein and DNA analysis are used to provide more information about the parents' genes and those of the developing fetus (see Genetics, p.752). This is already possible for many of the disorders mentioned earlier, such as cystic fibrosis. Some tests may be carried out on the pregnant woman's blood. Such tests include an examination of the level of a chemical known as alpha-fetoprotein in the blood. This chemical is normally present in the blood, and a higher than average level of alpha-fetoprotein indicates that the fetus may have a brain or spinal cord defect, such as spina bifida (see p.700); a lower than average level may indicate Down syndrome.

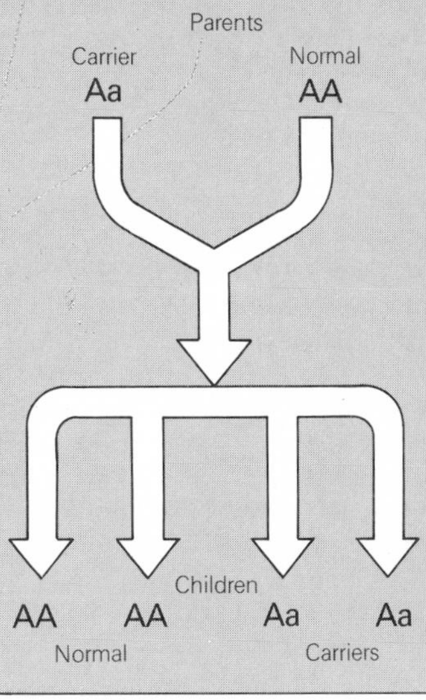

Certain invasive tests performed during pregnancy, such as amniocentesis and chorionic villus sampling (see Box, Special procedures in pregnancy, p.684), however, carry a slight risk to the developing fetus. There is also a small chance, with some tests, that an infection of the uterus or even a miscarriage may result. The parents need to discuss with their physician the risks that both the tests and the disorder carry. This will enable them to decide whether they are prepared to risk losing or harming the fetus, which may otherwise be healthy, and whether they would want the pregnancy terminated if the fetus has a genetic disorder.

The severity of genetic disorders varies according to the disorder involved. For example, Duchenne muscular dystrophy is always fatal during adolescence or early adulthood. Hemophilia, however, can be treated so that the affected child can lead a relatively full life. In sickle cell anemia, the severity of the disorder is unpredictable. During genetic counseling, prospective parents are advised on the potential severity of the disorder their children may inherit, and the treatment currently available for it. Treatment for many genetic disorders continues to improve. For example, the treatment for hemophilia has advanced greatly in recent years. Many parents prefer not to have the tests, accepting the possibility that the child may be handicapped.

Disorders that are congenital (present from birth) but do not result from a child's genetic makeup are more likely to occur when the pregnant woman has a disease such as diabetes mellitus (see p.558). Environmental factors such as maternal alcohol consumption or other drug use may also contribute to birth defects. Often, however, disorders occur for no apparent reason. For example, the cause of many congenital heart defects is not known. Even so, genetic counselors are often able to estimate the risks of the condition occurring in any subsequent children. It is rare for the risk to be more than 1 in 20 for each child. In some cases, a couple may choose to terminate a pregnancy if the fetus has a serious physical or mental handicap. As with genetic disorders, tests may be performed during pregnancy to determine whether the fetus is healthy. In many cases, congenital disorders can be corrected, including most congenital heart disorders (see p.702).

This illustration shows the possibilities that can occur when only one parent carries a gene for a recessive disorder. The carrier may give either a normal (A) or a defective (a) gene to each offspring. The partner will give one of two normal genes. Each child therefore has a 50 percent chance of becoming a carrier (Aa), but none will have the disorder (aa). Carriers may pass a defective gene through several generations without the disorder occurring.

General concerns of pregnancy

The concerns discussed in this section are those that may occur at any time during pregnancy. Many women say that they are aware, at a very early stage, that they are pregnant. Other women can tell only when they experience some of the early symptoms of pregnancy. These symptoms may include missing a period when you were previously having regular periods; having a short, scanty period and tender, swollen breasts with darkened nipples; feeling nauseated, especially in the morning; needing to urinate more frequently; having an increased vaginal discharge; feeling tired; or suddenly losing your taste for some foods.

Diagnosis of pregnancy

If you miss two menstrual periods and you know that your periods are usually regular, then you are probably pregnant and should see your physician to confirm it. At this time, your physician can usually diagnose pregnancy by a pelvic examination. However, you may want to know if you are pregnant before being examined by your physician, especially if you have had trouble with previous pregnancies or you do not want to be pregnant. In such cases, as soon as you suspect you are pregnant you should have a pregnancy test. Testing can be arranged through your physician, a family planning clinic, or a reputable commercial pregnancy-testing service. You can also use a simple home pregnancy test to determine if you are pregnant (see Box, below).

Once your pregnancy has been confirmed, your physician may recommend that you have prenatal care. Appointments for prenatal care are usually scheduled monthly, and more frequently in the last 2 months before delivery. Ideally, prenatal care should begin before conception. During the first 3 months of pregnancy, the fetus is very sensitive to environmental factors such as smoking, alcohol, any medication or drug use, poor nutrition, and maternal illness. Your physician may refer you to an obstetrician if he or she does not handle deliveries. Prenatal care consists of checkups and any necessary medical care before birth and also provides information about labor and delivery. Studies have shown that prenatal care helps prevent complications of pregnancy and childbirth, so keeping your prenatal care appointments and following your physician's recommendations are important.

Diet during pregnancy

When you are pregnant, what you eat also provides food for the fetus, so it is important that you eat regular, well-balanced meals. Pregnant women need more protein, calcium, iron, and zinc. Meat, fish, cheese, beans, lentils, and eggs are excellent sources of protein. Low-fat dairy products are rich in calcium. Eggs, liver, kidneys, whole-grain or enriched bread and cereal, dried fruit, and green leafy vegetables will supply you with the iron you need to avoid anemia (see p.450). Lean red meat, whole-grain cereals, nuts, and peas and beans are good sources of zinc. Your physician may recommend that you take multiple vitamins especially formulated for pregnant women.

Do-it-yourself pregnancy testing

Kits for do-it-yourself pregnancy testing are available at many drugstores. They work by detecting the hormone HCG, which is present in the urine of a pregnant woman about 2 weeks after the first missed period. The negative result (that you are not pregnant) is less reliable than the positive result (that you are pregnant), especially if you are taking antidepressant drugs, nearing menopause, or having irregular or infrequent periods.

Be sure that you follow the testing kit manufacturer's instructions carefully. Also, to get the most accurate results, it is best to test your urine first thing in the morning, before you drink anything.

Pregnancy testing that is more reliable and not necessarily more expensive than do-it-yourself testing can be obtained at family planning clinics, your physician's office, or your local or county health department.

Your physician may suggest a range of weight that you should gain, usually about 20 to 30 lb (10 to 15 kg). Either too much or too little weight gain may harm the fetus. Alcohol harms the fetus, and alcohol and other drugs have been shown to cause many birth defects and complications. Consult your physician before taking any medications or drugs. Smoking during pregnancy can cause your child to be underweight at birth. Smoking during pregnancy also increases the risk of premature delivery.

Physical activity during pregnancy

(including sex)

Exercise: Continue your usual physical activity while you are pregnant, unless your physician recommends some changes. Exercising regularly may help you feel well and keep you in good physical condition. Walking and swimming are frequently recommended. Avoid strenuous sports and sports that carry a risk of injury. But as a general rule, after discussion with your physician, you can continue the forms of exercise you enjoy as long as you do not overtire or overstrain yourself. It is probably also a good idea to avoid saunas, steam baths, hot tubs, and hot baths at home.

Travel: Traveling may tire you more than usual, and you should allow for this possibility when planning any kind of trip. If travelling by car, be sure to pull over at frequent intervals so that you can get out and stretch. Most airlines will not carry women who are in the last weeks of pregnancy, because of the risk of delivery in flight. If you are planning to fly, check with your physician and the airline before you make reservations.

If your physician has given you any records concerning your pregnancy, carry these with you so that in an emergency the information will be easily available. Avoid traveling far from home if you have recently had spotting (see Miscarriage, p.674), if you are within about 2 weeks of the expected time of delivery, or if your pregnancy has some complication that would require special care at the time of delivery.

Work: Many pregnant women continue to work until the labor and delivery. If your physician thinks your activities at your job are too strenuous, he or she may recommend that you arrange to take a maternity leave. However, if you are physically well and your pregnancy has been uneventful, there may be no medical reason not to continue working until much nearer the time of birth, even up to the day of delivery. Whether you are at work or at home, do not lift heavy objects. Also, it is important to get plenty of rest, whether you are working or at home.

Sex: If your pregnancy is uneventful, you can safely have sexual intercourse. Some women feel increased desire for intercourse during pregnancy, while others lose desire.

If you have had repeated miscarriages during the early weeks of past pregnancies, or if you have recently had spotting, talk to your physician about whether you should have intercourse during pregnancy.

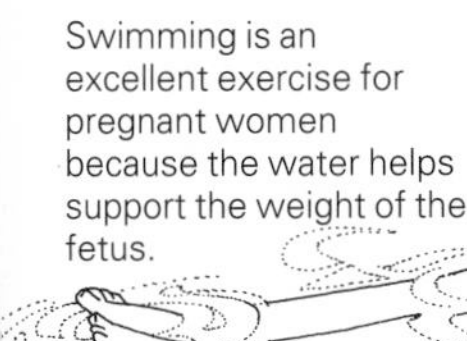
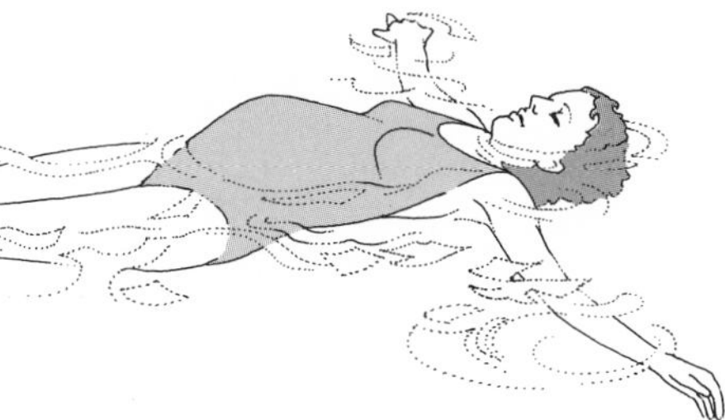

Swimming is an excellent exercise for pregnant women because the water helps support the weight of the fetus.

Nausea and vomiting during pregnancy

(morning sickness)

Many women have nausea and vomiting during early pregnancy, and in some cases it occurs throughout pregnancy. This usually happens in the morning, often immediately after waking, but it can occur at any time of the day or night. The problem usually begins during the first month of pregnancy and continues until the 14th to 16th week. Although the cause of morning sickness is unknown, some research indicates that increased hormone production during pregnancy may trigger nausea and vomiting. The vomiting is usually harmless, though unpleasant. In a small percentage of cases, it develops into severe vomiting, known as hyperemesis, which drains your body of fluids and minerals and harms your health.

Nausea, and sometimes vomiting, occur in about half of all pregnant women in the first 3 months of pregnancy.

What should be done?

If you have been vomiting during your pregnancy, do not overfill your stomach. It is a good idea to eat small frequent meals during the day instead of three large meals. Also, drink plenty of fluids, including milk and fruit juice. If you wake up feeling nauseated, eating dry toast or a cracker before you get up may help. Do not take any drugs for your vomiting without first consulting your physician.

If your vomiting continues, see your physician. He or she will evaluate whether the vomiting has caused a harmful loss of body fluids and minerals and check for the unlikely possibility that some disorder is causing the vomiting.

Hyperemesis requires immediate hospital treatment. The severe vomiting is controlled with antiemetic drugs (see Antiemetics in Drug index in this volume), and the lost body fluids and minerals are replaced with intravenous fluids.

Heartburn during pregnancy

Heartburn is a burning pain in the center of the upper abdomen that rises into the chest. Despite its name, heartburn has nothing to do with the heart. (See Reflex esophagitis, heartburn, and hiatal hernia, p.488.)

Heartburn is common during pregnancy; it affects almost half of all pregnant women. This is because during pregnancy the muscle that helps close off the esophagus from the stomach relaxes and allows stomach acid to reenter the esophagus and irritate its lining. In late pregnancy the enlarging uterus presses on the stomach and aggravates the condition.

Heartburn is a symptom that usually disappears after childbirth unless it is not related to the pregnancy.

What should be done?

You can minimize heartburn by eating small, frequent meals, which ensures that there is always food in your stomach to soak up much of the stomach acid. If this does not solve the problem, you should consult your physician, who may prescribe an antacid and recommend changes in your diet that may help you reduce heartburn.

Preparing for birth

During pregnancy, the growing fetus and the hormones that nurture its growth produce dramatic changes inside a woman's body. If you are a pregnant woman, it is important to learn not only about pregnancy but also about labor and delivery.

Many organizations sponsor prenatal education classes; your physician may be able to recommend a suitable one. These classes may include teaching you techniques that use breathing patterns to help deal with uterine contractions and labor pains. To prepare for delivery, both you and your partner or a close friend with whom you would like to share your childbirth experience (called a coach) may attend several classes starting at about the 7th month of pregnancy. Most women who attend these classes have a more positive childbirth experience since they are calmer and more relaxed during delivery and they know what to expect.

What are the options?

Trends in the care of women during labor and delivery are changing. Most women deliver in hospitals, but some hospitals offer alternatives to the labor and delivery room. One alternative is called a birthing center. This is a private room with windows, curtains, and a large bed where a woman spends both labor and delivery. Her coach can share the time spent in labor as well as provide help and support. If any problems arise during labor, the woman can be easily moved into the labor and delivery suite, where the medical and nursing staff can manage complications.

To qualify for this type of childbirth, a woman must have no medical problems complicating her pregnancy, and she must have adequate prenatal care. She and her coach must also attend prenatal classes.

Hospitals vary in their policies about caring for women and their infants. Some offer a family centered approach in which the infant can stay in the mother's hospital room and both your partner and other children in the family can feel free to visit frequently.

Some women prefer home childbirth. If any difficulty should arise that requires emergency treatment in a hospital, however, home childbirth can be risky. Nurse-midwives can provide a valuable service, especially in areas where a physician may not be readily available. To minimize any risk, however, it is important that the pregnant woman be healthy, the pregnancy uncomplicated, and that a physician is on call if any complications occur during labor or delivery. Medical research studies are being conducted to evaluate the safety of this method in healthy, low-risk pregnant women, but results are not yet available.

If you are pregnant, many options are available to you, and you can decide how and where you want to deliver your baby. Discuss the possibilities thoroughly with your physician. Also discuss your physician's policy about the use of midwives and nurse practitioners, episiotomy, pain medications during delivery, and the circumstances that may require a cesarean section (see Box, Special procedures in childbirth, p.685). You may also want to discuss breast-feeding (see p.688).

Anemia during pregnancy

One of the most important components of blood is hemoglobin, a protein that carries oxygen to the body's tissues. If the hemoglobin in your body falls below an adequate level, you are anemic. The most common cause of this problem is a deficiency of iron in the body (see Iron-deficiency anemia, p.450). Another possible cause of anemia is an inadequate amount of folic acid in the body (see B_{12} deficiency anemia and folic acid deficiency, p.451).

You may not notice mild anemia, but if the condition is more pronounced, you might have any of the following symptoms: paleness, weakness, tiredness, breathlessness, fainting, and palpitations, or an abnormal awareness of your heartbeat.

Even if you have an adequate amount of iron and folic acid in your diet, you may become anemic when you are pregnant. In addition, in about the fifth month of your pregnancy the developing fetus will use more iron and folic acid.

What are the risks?

Anemia in pregnancy makes a woman less able to cope with physical or emotional stress. Anemia also may make you more likely to have a premature baby and more vulnerable to infection.

What should be done?

You can help prevent anemia during your pregnancy by eating foods that are rich in iron, such as liver, beef, whole-grain bread, eggs, and dried fruits. Eat citrus fruits and fresh vegetables, because the vitamin C in them helps your body absorb iron more efficiently. Make sure you eat plenty of green leafy vegetables, since these are one of the best sources of folic acid.

Early in your pregnancy, your physician may perform a blood test to find out if you are anemic. If you are anemic, your physician will probably prescribe iron and folic acid supplements. He or she may also recommend that you take a multiple vitamin.

Other types of anemia such as sickle-cell anemia (see p.453) can cause complications during pregnancy. Discuss any family history of sickle cell disease with your physician before you plan to become pregnant. You and your partner may want to be tested for sickle-cell trait (see Box, Genetic counseling, p.664).

Constipation during pregnancy

Constipation is common in pregnancy. In about the fourth month of pregnancy it is aggravated by the pressure of the enlarged uterus on the intestines. Constipation is not a risky condition, but it often aggravates hemorrhoids by causing you to strain harder to have a bowel movement.

You can help avoid constipation by eating plenty of fruit and vegetables and other foods high in fiber (see The components of a healthy diet, p.26), by drinking 8 to 10 glasses of liquids each day, and by moving your bowels when you get the urge. Never strain to move your bowels. Safe, nonprescription glycerin suppositories often help.

Do not take laxatives without consulting your physician, who may prescribe a medicine to soften your stools.

Varicose veins during pregnancy

Many women have varicose veins (see p.441) during pregnancy. The problem is especially common in the last 3 months. This is because when a woman is pregnant, her blood vessels have to accommodate an increased volume of blood in order to supply the needs of the developing fetus. As the uterus enlarges and presses on some of the major veins, the flow of blood from the leg veins up to the pelvis slows down. This combination of factors sometimes produces pressure that causes the veins in the calves and thighs to become swollen and painful. The veins around the entrance to the vagina and rectum may also be affected as a result of the same kinds of pressure. Varicose veins are more likely to develop if there is a history of varicose veins in your family.

What should be done?

Do not wear clothing that fits tightly around your waist or legs. Avoid standing for long periods of time; rest with your feet up as often as possible. If you are working and you spend a lot of time on your feet, sit down and rest as much as possible. Also, avoid gaining too much weight during your pregnancy.

Elastic stockings relieve the discomfort of varicose veins significantly. You can ask your physician to prescribe specially fitted stockings or buy them over the counter. Put them on first thing in the morning, before you get out of bed.

Varicose veins that develop during your pregnancy usually will become considerably less swollen or will disappear within 6 to 12 weeks after childbirth.

Sleeping problems during pregnancy

Many women find it difficult to get to sleep or stay asleep when they are pregnant. This may result from changes in hormone levels, a need to urinate more often, worry about your health and the health of the fetus, and other concerns. In the last 3 months of pregnancy, you may also have difficulty finding a comfortable position. Anxiety about losing sleep may make it even harder to fall asleep.

What should be done?

Try the self-help measures described on p.40. It may also help if, before you go to bed, you do some relaxation exercises. Your physician may recommend that you take a warm bath each night before bedtime, drink a glass of warm milk at bedtime, avoid daytime sleeping, exercise during the day (but not right before bedtime), or read when you get in bed. If you can't sleep, don't stay in bed. Get up and read or otherwise occupy your mind until you get sleepy, then go back to bed.

If you are losing a lot of sleep, do not take any drugs, but consult your physician. He or she may prescribe a sedative, but most physicians prefer not to because of the possibility of affecting the fetus. This is especially true in the first 14 weeks of pregnancy, when there is the risk that the drug could harm the fetus, or close to your due date, when the drug could make the baby very sleepy or affect its breathing after birth.

Backache during pregnancy

When you are pregnant, the ligaments and fibrous tissue that normally support your joints become slightly more elastic. This allows your pelvis to expand during delivery. However, this loosening of the joints also has a potentially harmful effect: it makes them more susceptible to strain. In particular, the joints of your spine are placed under additional strain during pregnancy. The growth of your uterus shifts your center of balance and your posture changes in response, so standing can give you what is called a nonspecific backache (see p.584).

Many women also have abdominal pain during pregnancy, probably because of stretching of the ligaments that attach the uterus to the abdominal wall. This is called round ligament pain, and it is usually most severe in the middle 3 months of pregnancy, when the uterus expands most rapidly.

What should be done?

You can keep the strain on your back during pregnancy to a minimum by sleeping on a firm mattress. Also, wear low-heeled shoes, avoid lifting heavy objects, and do not gain too much weight (see Diet during pregnancy, p.666). You may learn exercises that can help strengthen your muscles and relieve back pain in prenatal classes. For the treatment of backaches in general, see p.586.

Round ligament pain can often be relieved by lying on the aching side. Like many other problems of pregnancy, these types of pain usually disappear after childbirth.

Relieving backache
A gentle exercise for relieving backache is to get on your hands and knees and arch your lower back a few times. When you relax, do not allow your back to sag; this can cause more backache.

High blood pressure and pregnancy

At routine checkups in early pregnancy, some women are found to have high blood pressure (see p.411). This condition may have been present for some time before pregnancy, or it may be related to the pregnancy. Anxiety alone can raise blood pressure for short periods of time. If anxiety is the cause, the blood pressure will return to normal. It is common for blood pressure to fall slightly during the middle weeks of pregnancy and to rise slightly at the end. There are generally no symptoms, but extremely high blood pressure is associated with pregnancy complications and can harm the fetus.

High blood pressure in the last 3 months of pregnancy can be a symptom of preeclampsia (see p.676). It can also lead to hemorrhage (see Antepartum hemorrhage, p.677), intrauterine death (see p.678), and intrauterine growth retardation (see p.678).

What should be done?

The earlier preexisting high blood pressure is discovered, the greater your chances of having a safe pregnancy. If you have high blood pressure, you should have frequent examinations. Not only will your blood pressure be monitored, but blood and urine tests will also be done to check on the function of your kidneys and the condition of the fetus. Ultrasound (see p.684) is used to see if the fetus is developing at the usual rate.

Your physician may advise you to rest, and if your blood pressure is above a certain level, one or more drugs may be prescribed to lower it. Most women with the condition have a normal delivery.

Heart disorders and pregnancy

Pregnancy involves extra work for your heart, and if your heart already has a serious underlying defect such as those caused by congenital (present from birth) heart disorders (see p.702) or heart valve diseases caused by rheumatic fever (see p.421), there is a risk of heart failure (see p.408).

What should be done?

If you know you have a heart disorder, talk to your physician before you decide to get pregnant. He or she can tell you what, if any, special risks pregnancy involves for you. If you become pregnant, you may be referred to a cardiologist for additional care. In all such cases, it is vital that your health be monitored for any signs and symptoms of possible complications.

Although your physician usually can tell if you have a heart disorder, sometimes such a disorder shows up for the first time under the extra demands that pregnancy places on your body. Such disorders may produce a heart murmur, which your physician can detect during a routine examination. You can have a murmur without having a disorder, however, and most heart murmurs discovered in the first 3 months of pregnancy are insignificant. If, however, your physician suspects that you have a heart disorder, an echocardiogram, an electrocardiogram (ECG), and other tests may be performed.

What is the treatment?

The main treatment is rest, so that extra strain is not placed on a heart that is already working harder than usual. If you develop heart failure, it will be treated as described on p.408. If you smoke, your physician will strongly recommend that you stop.

Delivery in a hospital is necessary. If there are no complications, a pregnant woman with a heart disorder should go into labor normally at term. When you go into labor, your physician's main goal will be to help you have as easy a delivery as possible—one with a minimum of pushing, since this puts a strain on the heart and deprives it of oxygen.

Termination of pregnancy

Learning that you are pregnant may require some serious decision making. If you believe that you cannot raise a child now, you can continue the pregnancy until delivery and arrange to have the baby adopted through an adoption agency or foster home, or you can terminate the pregnancy with an abortion.

In 1973, the US Supreme Court struck down restrictive state regulation of a woman's right to choose abortion up to the 24th week of pregnancy. Up to the 12th week of pregnancy, an abortion is a private matter between a woman and her physician. Some states have enacted laws to govern termination of a pregnancy after the 12th week and until the 24th week. There have been attempts to ban abortions in some or all cases. So far, this decision can still be made by a woman and her physician in most cases.

Vacuum suction, the simplest type of abortion, can be performed up to the 16th week of pregnancy. After dilating the cervix with slender rods, a flexible tube connected to a suction machine is inserted into the cervix. The end of the tube, placed in the uterus, removes the pregnancy tissue (the embryo or fetus, the placenta, and the lining of the uterus).

From the 16th to the 24th week, termination of a pregnancy is riskier; labor may be induced (see p.685) with drugs administered as suppositories in the vagina, intravenously, or injected through the uterine wall into the amniotic fluid that surrounds the fetus.

RU-486 (mifepristone), a hormone drug, can induce abortion in women who are up to 6 weeks pregnant, when taken with prostaglandins (drugs that cause the uterus to contract). RU-486 is not yet available in the US.

Diabetes mellitus and pregnancy

Diabetes mellitus (see p.558) can be a risky condition for a pregnant woman. If the diabetes is not carefully controlled, the risks of the child having a congenital (present from birth) disorder or of a stillbirth increase. However, when the diabetes is carefully controlled before and during pregnancy, the risks are greatly reduced or eliminated. If you have diabetes, consult your physician before you become pregnant. To ensure that your blood sugar level remains stable, he or she may recommend a special diet and an insulin regimen, and may arrange for regular tests of your blood sugar level. For every woman who knows that she has diabetes before pregnancy, there are several who find out they have gestational diabetes during pregnancy. In most instances, gestational diabetes disappears after delivery; this should not be confused with diabetes mellitus.

What should be done?

During the early third trimester (26 to 28 weeks), you should have a 1-hour glucose tolerance test to look for gestational diabetes. If the test results show that you have elevated levels of blood sugar, a 3-hour glucose tolerance test will be performed to determine if you have chronic diabetes.

What is the treatment?

If you have diabetes, you may first be given a diet to follow to control the disease. If this diet is not effective, you may need to take insulin. If the disease is severe, which is rare, you may be admitted to the hospital for the last days or weeks of the pregnancy, so that the diabetes can be controlled precisely, the fetus's condition can be monitored, and early induction of labor or cesarean section performed if needed.

Rhesus (Rh) incompatibility

Rhesus (Rh) incompatibility is an incompatibility between the Rhesus blood groups of the pregnant woman and the developing fetus. Blood groups are determined by the presence or absence of certain protein molecules on the surfaces of blood cells. Which proteins and whether these proteins are present depends on genes inherited from the parents.

Rhesus incompatibility occurs only if the mother has Rh-negative blood and the fetus has Rh-positive blood because it has inherited Rh-positive genes from the father. However, there is a chance that a fetus may inherit Rh-negative genes from a father whose blood is Rh-positive. In that case, the fetus would have Rh-negative blood, which does not lead to Rhesus incompatibility

At childbirth, and following miscarriage (see p.674), abortion (see previous page), ectopic pregnancy (see p.675), hemorrhage (see Antepartum hemorrhage, p.677), chorionic villus sampling, or amniocentesis, some of the fetus's blood may enter the

Rh disease in pregnancy

When a Rhesus (Rh)-negative woman gives birth to an Rh-positive child, some of the child's blood can move into the woman's bloodstream during childbirth. If the woman is not given a vaccine within 48 hours of delivery, she will develop antibodies to Rh-positive blood. These antibodies will cause no problem unless the woman becomes pregnant with another Rh-positive fetus, when her antibodies may cross the placenta and destroy the fetus's red blood cells.

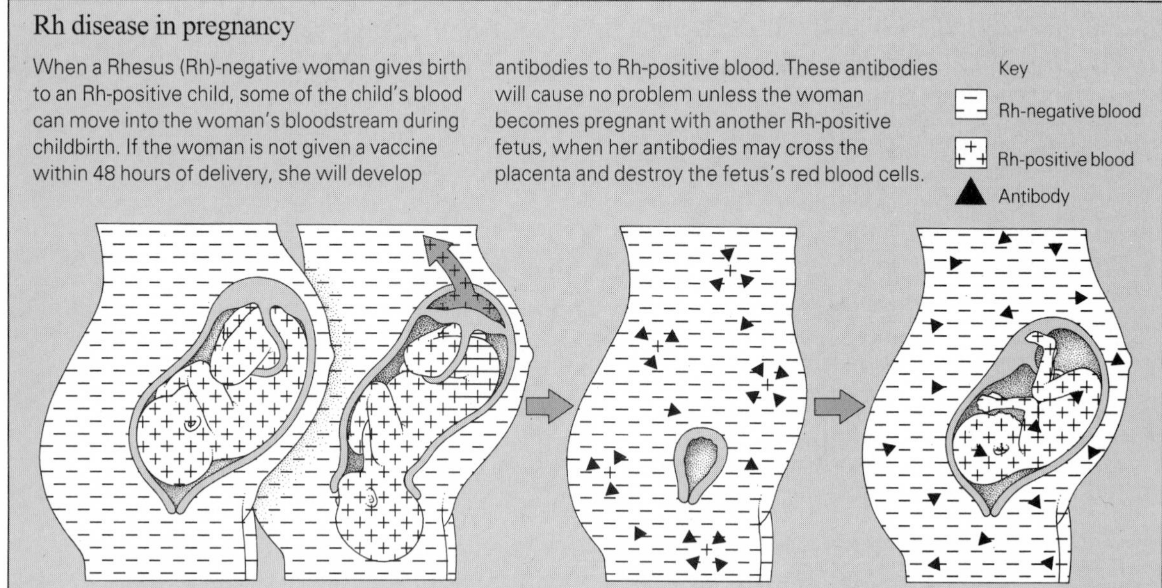

woman's circulation. An Rh-negative woman's body reacts to the fetus's Rh-positive blood as foreign material and produces antibodies to fight it. Because this usually happens as a delayed reaction after childbirth, the first child may not be harmed. However, the woman will continue to produce these antibodies after delivery, and in any subsequent pregnancy these antibodies may pass from the woman's bloodstream into the bloodstream of the developing fetus and will start to destroy the fetus's red blood cells, if the fetus has Rh-positive blood.

What are the risks?

About 15 percent of the white population of the US has Rh-negative blood. The trait is less common in other races. About 10 percent of pregnancies involve an Rh-negative woman and an Rh-positive man. However, with today's diagnosis and treatment Rhesus incompatibility is now uncommon.

Rhesus incompatibility is a silent condition that produces no symptoms in the pregnant woman. When it occurs, the child may develop hemolytic anemia (see p.454) and neonatal jaundice (see p.693) at birth or, in extreme cases, may be stillborn. These risks increase with each subsequent Rhesus-incompatibility pregnancy.

What should be done?

At the beginning of the pregnancy, you will be given a blood test to determine (among other things) whether your blood is Rh-negative or Rh-positive. If your blood is Rh-negative, it will be tested for the presence of antibodies, then the father's blood will also be tested to determine whether his blood is Rh-negative or Rh-positive. If your first pregnancy occurred before the Rh vaccine was available, the tests will show the concentration of antibodies in your blood. When antibodies have formed, any effect they are having on your fetus can be detected in one of two ways: by amniocentesis (see p.684), an examination of the amniotic fluid that surrounds the fetus in the uterus; or by taking samples of the infant's blood from a vein in the umbilical cord.

What is the treatment?

The development of a vaccine has almost eliminated the many risks of Rhesus incompatibility. The vaccination is given by injection to the woman in the early third trimester, soon after every delivery, or after miscarriage, chorionic villus sampling, amniocentesis, hemorrhage, or abortion. The vaccine destroys any red blood cells from the fetus that may have entered the woman's circulation, before her body has had time to develop antibodies. In this way, a subsequent pregnancy has no additional risk.

In cases where antibodies begin to destroy the fetus's red blood cells, labor may be induced, or started artificially (see p.685), in the hospital if the fetus is sufficiently mature. If the fetus is not mature enough to be delivered, it may be given a blood transfusion while still in the uterus. This may give the fetus a chance to mature to the stage where delivery is feasible.

After delivery, the child may have jaundice. If the jaundice is severe, he or she may need an exchange blood transfusion. Neonatal intensive care units have been established in many hospitals to deal with various problems of sick and premature infants. As a result, the health outlook for infants with Rhesus incompatibility has improved significantly.

Complications of early pregnancy

During the first 3 months (the first trimester) after conception, the fetus is especially vulnerable. Because so much is happening to the fetus during early pregnancy, any infection in the pregnant woman (see Box, Rubella (German measles) and pregnancy, p.661) or unfavorable environmental factors may cause damage. In addition, any severe genetic defect of the fetus or disorder of the pregnant woman's reproductive system that affects implantation of the fertilized egg can case serious complications that usually occur in early pregnancy. A common problem is miscarriage, in which the pregnancy ends naturally and too early. Another complication is ectopic pregnancy, in which the fetus starts to develop outside the uterus, usually in a fallopian tube. A box on vaginal bleeding (see next page) during pregnancy gives you practical advice on how to handle this symptom. Complications of the second or third trimester are covered later.

Miscarriage

Miscarriage (known medically as a spontaneous abortion) occurs when a pregnancy ends naturally before the beginning of the 20th week of the pregnancy counted from the 1st day of the last period. After that time, the natural end of a pregnancy is known as a stillbirth if the child is born dead and a premature delivery if the child is born alive. When a pregnancy is ended intentionally, it is an elective abortion.

Miscarriages are common, occurring in 20 percent of women who know they are pregnant. Miscarriage is due to the separation of the developing fetus and the placenta from the inner wall of the uterus. This may occur because of a developmental defect in the fetus or because the placenta is not attached properly. At least 50 percent of miscarriages result from a chromosomal abnormality in the fetus. Often the cause of miscarriage is not known. Miscarriages from falls or other injuries are uncommon, because the fetus is well protected inside the uterus.

Some women have what is called a "threatened" miscarriage in early pregnancy. There is usually spotting from the vagina. However, there is sometimes slight bleeding when the fertilized egg implants in the uterus, and this may be misinterpreted as a threatened miscarriage. About one in five women has some bleeding in the first 3 months, but if care is taken, the pregnancy usually proceeds normally.

An "inevitable" miscarriage occurs when the fetus has died, so nothing can be done to prevent miscarriage. In an "incomplete" miscarriage, parts of the fetus and placenta remain in the uterus. A "missed" miscarriage means that the fetus has died in the uterus, but there are no symptoms. Any miscarriage can be very emotionally distressing.

Vaginal bleeding during pregnancy

Vaginal bleeding at any time during your pregnancy can be a signal of a serious problem, so you should notify your physician promptly. In early pregnancy, about 20 percent of women have some vaginal bleeding (see Miscarriage, this page). Vaginal bleeding in the final 3 months of pregnancy affects less than 2 percent of women. It may indicate the onset of premature labor (see p.680) or bleeding from the placenta (see Placenta previa, p.677). Immediate treatment is usually needed, and you should contact your physician immediately if bleeding occurs in the second half of pregnancy.

What are the symptoms?

The first symptom you are likely to notice when a miscarriage begins is bleeding from your vagina. This can range from a few drops of blood to a heavy flow. The bleeding may start with no warning or may be preceded by a brownish discharge.

A threatened miscarriage is often painless, but an inevitable miscarriage is usually accompanied by cramping pain in the lower abdomen or back. The pain may be either dull and constant or sharp and intermittent. At some stage during an inevitable miscarriage, you may pass some solid tissue through your vagina. Try to save this tissue so that your physician can examine it.

In an incomplete miscarriage, you may have either constant or intermittent bleeding and pain for several days. With a missed miscarriage, you may have no bleeding or pain, but the symptoms of early pregnancy will disappear. Often the only symptom is that your physician discovers that your uterus has not increased in size.

What are the risks?

Although exact figures are not available, about 20 percent of all pregnancies end in miscarriage, most during the first 8 weeks. Miscarriages usually do not threaten health unless the miscarriage is incomplete. If an incomplete miscarriage is not diagnosed, you may continue to bleed and the tissue left in your uterus may become infected.

If you are pregnant and have bleeding from the vagina, with or without pain, contact your physician. If the bleeding stops or is not very heavy, your physician may recommend that you rest at home. However, if bleeding is heavy or pain is severe, you should see your physician immediately.

If the pregnancy seems to be continuing, even though you have had some bleeding, your physician may arrange for you to have another pregnancy test, and perhaps an ultrasound scan, to confirm that the developing embryo is still alive. It is best not to have sexual intercourse for a few weeks after bleeding, to give the pregnancy a chance to become more stable. Talk to your physician about other precautions.

What is the treatment?

In the case of a threatened miscarriage, there is no medical treatment, and you may simply be told to rest in bed as much as possible.

If your miscarriage is inevitable, missed, or incomplete, you may have the remains of the fetus and placenta removed from your uterus by your physician, usually in the hospital but sometimes in your physician's office or in a clinic. Often the uterus can be emptied by a simple suction procedure.

If you were trying to become pregnant, you will probably become deeply depressed after a miscarriage. Consult your physician if you think you need short-term counseling to recover from your loss. However, you can safely start trying to conceive again soon afterward. Most physicians recommend that you give your body at least 6 to 8 weeks to return to normal. You should wait until you have had at least one normal period, which makes it easier to estimate a due date.

Ectopic pregnancy

In ectopic (or tubal) pregnancy an egg is fertilized by a sperm but develops outside the uterus, usually in one of the fallopian tubes. The placenta burrows into the surrounding tissue, which usually tears and causes internal bleeding. The tissue cannot sustain a placenta and fetus, and the pregnancy cannot continue. In this condition, you may have cramping abdominal pain, often with vaginal bleeding. You may not suspect you are pregnant.

About 1 in every 100 pregnancies is ectopic, and most are discovered in the first 2 months. You are more likely to have an ectopic pregnancy if you have had some abnormality of your fallopian tubes from birth, if your fallopian tubes were previously operated on or infected, or if you are using an intrauterine device (IUD; see p.651).

An ectopic pregnancy usually occurs in a fallopian tube when the fertilized egg does not make its way down into the uterus.

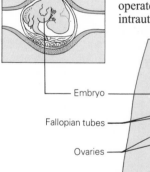

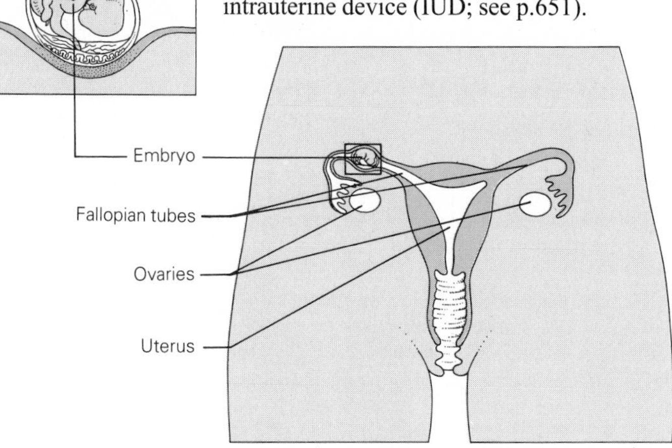

What should be done?

If you experience abdominal pain that lasts for more than a few hours, see your physician as soon as possible. There is a risk of severe internal bleeding that can lead to shock (see p.839) and death.

Your physician will examine you carefully, since abdominal pain of ectopic pregnancy can be similar to that of several other conditions, including miscarriage (see previous article), appendicitis, and infection of the fallopian tubes. An ultrasound scan may allow an accurate diagnosis, but in some cases a laparoscopy (an examination of the inside of the abdomen using a viewing tube) may be required.

Once an ectopic pregnancy is confirmed, you are hospitalized if you have not already been admitted. Any severe loss of blood is treated with intravenous fluids or a blood transfusion and an operation is performed immediately. The developing fetus, placenta, and surrounding tissue are removed and the damaged blood vessels are repaired.

Even if one of your fallopian tubes has been damaged by an ectopic pregnancy, it is possible to have a normal pregnancy, although chances of conception are slightly reduced. You may also need extra checkups and tests should you become pregnant again, since ectopic pregnancies can recur. If you want to become pregnant again, physicians usually recommend a healing interval of one to two periods at least.

Complications of mid-pregnancy

During the middle 3 months of pregnancy (the second trimester), many women feel quite healthy, perhaps because the physical changes associated with the fetus's development proceed more slowly at this time.

It is vital to start prenatal care early. Your physician will evaluate your health, recommend iron and vitamin supplements, and will examine your blood and urine regularly.

Most pregnancies continue smoothly during the middle 3 months. The main complications that may occur during this period are incompetent cervix, hydramnios, intrauterine growth retardation (see p.678), urinary tract infections (see Cystitis in women, p.643), and either excessive or insufficient weight gain by the pregnant woman (see Diet during pregnancy, p.666).

Incompetent cervix

In this condition, the cervix opens up during pregnancy, usually after the 14th week. The fetus and placenta escape from the uterus, which causes a miscarriage (see p.674). Weakness of the cervix may trigger this, but usually the cause is not known.

If it is known or if your physician suspects that you may have an incompetent cervix, a miscarriage may be prevented by surgery during early pregnancy. While you are under a general anesthetic, a piece of strong thread is sewn through the cervix and tightened to hold the cervix firm. After surgery, you may be given a drug to reduce chances that the operation might stimulate premature labor (see p.680). The thread is cut when labor starts or at about the 38th week of pregnancy if labor has not yet started.

Hydramnios

Hydramnios is a usually harmless condition that can occur in the middle or late stages of pregnancy. The condition occurs when an excessive amount of amniotic fluid is produced around the fetus. In most cases, the swelling of the uterus is only slightly greater than normal, and the condition produces either no symptoms or a gradual onset of slightly more breathlessness than is usual, indigestion, and tension in the muscles of the abdomen. In some cases, swelling may be pronounced, symptoms may begin suddenly and may be accompanied by nausea, and there is risk of premature labor. Hydramnios is more common in women with diabetes mellitus, when a fetus has a malformed gastrointestinal system or spine or brain malformations, and in a twin or other multiple pregnancy (see Box, p.678).

What should be done?

For a minor case of hydramnios, your physician may obtain a detailed ultrasound scan to rule out fetal malformations. If hydramnios comes on suddenly, your physician may advise you to rest completely and may prescribe drugs to relax your uterus and reduce the risk of premature labor. Rarely, amniocentesis is performed to reduce the woman's discomfort.

Complications of late pregnancy

Because most infants stand a better chance of survival the nearer to full term they are born, some of the treatment you may receive in the last 3 months (the third trimester) of your pregnancy is designed to prevent you from going into labor too early (see Premature labor, p.680). This is accomplished mainly with rest and sometimes with drugs to relax the uterine muscles so that they do not begin the contractions that lead to childbirth. However, if your physician suspects that the fetus would have a better chance of survival outside the uterus, he or she may induce labor (see p.685), or deliver the fetus by cesarean section (see p.686). A cesarean section may also be necessary if you have recurrent outbreaks of genital herpes and the infection is active at the time of labor. It is important that you continue to keep your prenatal appointments during the last weeks of pregnancy, so that any complications can be diagnosed and treated.

Preeclampsia and eclampsia

(toxemia of pregnancy)

Preeclampsia is a disorder that occurs during late pregnancy. In this disorder, the woman's blood pressure rises and there is excess fluid in her body. In addition, the woman's urine may contain protein. Preeclampsia, the cause of which is not known, may lead to eclampsia (seizures), which are hazardous to both the woman and fetus.

In mild preeclampsia, you may not have any symptoms and feel perfectly well. You should therefore go to all your prenatal checkups, so that the condition can be spotted early. The symptoms of more severe preeclampsia, which can develop during the last 3 months of pregnancy, are headaches, blurred vision, intolerance of bright light, upper abdominal pain, nausea and vomiting, and salt and water retention.

Preeclampsia seems to occur particularly in the first pregnancies of women between ages 18 and 30 and in women who have diabetes mellitus, high blood pressure, or a family history of high blood pressure. Physicians believe that chronic high blood

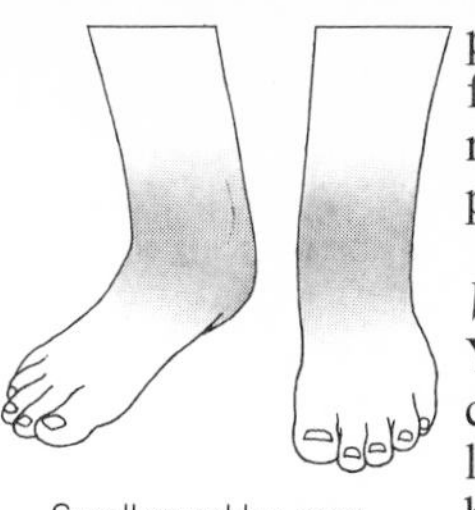
Swollen ankles may indicate preeclampsia

pressure plays a role in retarded growth of fetuses. This is because high blood pressure reduces the efficiency of the placenta, which provides the fetus with oxygen and nutrients.

What is the treatment?

Your physician may prescribe a drug to control your blood pressure. You can help lower it yourself by getting plenty of rest and by reducing your salt intake.

If you develop symptoms of severe preeclampsia or eclampsia, contact your physician immediately. You may be admitted to a hospital, where you may be given drugs to lower your blood pressure, remove excess fluid from your body, and prevent other complications. Delivery of the baby may be advisable, either by inducing labor (see p.685) or by cesarean section (see p.686). These procedures involve some risks, which must be weighed against the possible risks of eclampsia. Your physician can discuss your situation with you and outline the choices of treatment.

Antepartum hemorrhage

Antepartum hemorrhage is any bleeding from the vagina after the end of the 20th week of pregnancy. Earlier bleeding is known as a threatened miscarriage (see Miscarriage, p.674). Antepartum hemorrhage may be the result of placenta previa (see next article), a vaginal varicose vein that has burst, damage to the cervix, or partial or complete separation of the placenta from the wall of the uterus. In most cases, antepartum bleeding is mild and harmless. An antepartum hemorrhage caused by placental separation can cause intrauterine growth retardation (see next page), however, and if the placental bleeding is heavy it can threaten both the pregnant woman and the fetus.

If you have bleeding during pregnancy, call your physician as soon as possible. He or she may arrange for blood tests and an ultrasound scan. If bleeding is severe, you will be hospitalized, and you may receive transfusions. The baby may be delivered as soon as possible, either by inducing labor (see p.685) or cesarean section (see p.686).

Placenta previa

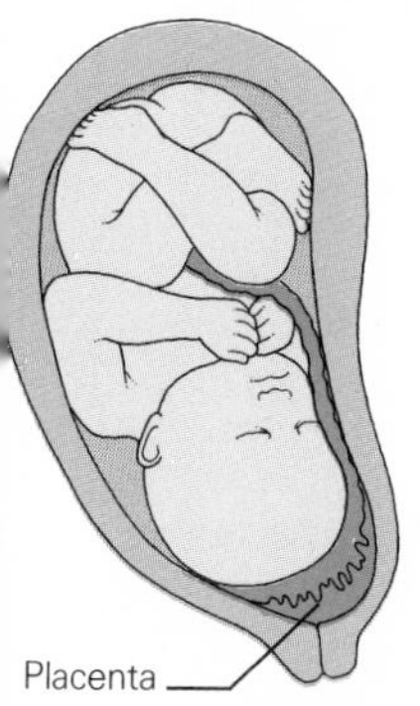

In placenta previa, the placenta develops low in the uterus, either partially or completely over the cervix. Any part of the placenta that is near the cervix is poorly supported and vulnerable to damage. The condition occurs in about 1 pregnancy in 200 that have continued past the 28th week. The cause is unknown, but it occurs more frequently in women who have already given birth to several children or who are pregnant with twins.

In some cases, the placenta starts off low in the uterus, but as the pregnancy develops it moves up the wall of the uterus to a more normal position and causes no problems.

What are the symptoms?

There may be no symptoms, but if the placenta becomes partly detached from the uterus, you will have sporadic, painless bleeding from the vagina, usually late in the pregnancy. If you have bleeding from the vagina during pregnancy, call your physician immediately and go to bed. Do not put anything in your vagina, not even a tampon.

What is the treatment?

When a slight degree of placenta previa exists, your physician may recommend that you have an ultrasound scan to determine if normal labor may eventually be possible. Sometimes placenta previa bleeding is heavy and may require a blood transfusion, and the infant will be delivered as soon as possible by cesarean section (see p.686) to prevent further hemorrhaging of the placenta. Such bleeding can cause damage to the fetus, or even death. It can also cause the woman to lose a dangerous amount of blood.

Premature rupture of membranes

When labor starts, the membranes surrounding the fetus may rupture, releasing amniotic fluid. This is called "breaking the bag of waters." Occasionally, the membranes may rupture before labor has begun. The main risks associated with premature rupture are that it may be followed by premature labor (see p.680) or an infection of your uterus.

What should be done?

If your membranes have ruptured prematurely, contact your physician, who will examine you and may admit you to a hospital. Fluid from your vagina may be collected, or an amniocentesis (see p.684) may be performed to find out if the fetus's lungs are developed enough for it to survive. If your expected delivery date is in 2 or 3 weeks, and tests confirm that the fetus is mature enough, labor may be induced (see p.685), but if your due date is further ahead, you may be hospitalized for bed rest until labor begins or evidence of infection makes delivery necessary. Sometimes a small tear in the membranes surrounding the fetus heals naturally and allows the pregnancy to continue to a full-term delivery, but the risk of infection of the uterus remains, so your condition must be watched carefully.

Intrauterine death

Intrauterine death is the death of a fetus in the uterus after the 20th week of pregnancy. In many cases, it is the result of severe preeclampsia or eclampsia (see p.676), a hemorrhage (see Antepartum hemorrhage, previous page), postmaturity (see next page), or a severe abnormality of the fetus. It may also be related to diabetes mellitus in the pregnant woman (see pp.558, 672). In other cases, the cause is not known.

Usually, the only symptom of intrauterine death is that the pregnant woman no longer feels any movement from the fetus. If the physician cannot hear any heartbeat, a fetal electrocardiogram (ECG) and ultrasound scan are done. If these tests show an absence of fetal life, intrauterine death is confirmed.

If the woman does not go into labor naturally, labor is brought on artificially (see Induction of labor, p.685).

Except when the pregnant woman has diabetes mellitus, the outlook for any future pregnancy after an intrauterine death is usually the same as for any first pregnancy.

Intrauterine growth retardation

(retarded fetal growth)

In some pregnancies, the placenta does not supply enough nourishment to the fetus. The result is that the fetus's development in the uterus is stunted. The deficiencies of the placenta in this disorder include obstruction of blood flow to some areas of the placenta. This leads to destruction of the tissue, which is replaced with scar tissue. If scarring is extensive the fetus is denied nutrients. This may be caused by severe preeclampsia (see p.676), high blood pressure (see pp.411, 670), hemorrhage (see Antepartum hemorrhage, previous page), or placenta previa (see previous page). Retarded growth may also result from heart disease (see Heart disorders and pregnancy, p.671), diabetes mellitus (see pp.558, 672), smoking, alcohol or other drug use, or malnutrition in the pregnant woman.

What are the risks?

At birth, the infant will have less body fat and therefore less resistance to cold than normal

Twins

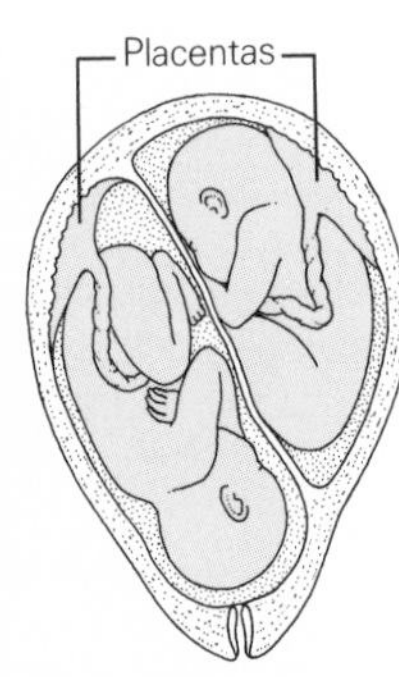

Fraternal twins each have their own placenta.

Twins occur as the result of either the splitting of a single egg or the parallel development of two eggs. They account for 1 in 90 births in the US. Triplets, by comparison, are uncommon. They occur in about only 1 in 8,000 pregnancies. Seven of 10 pairs of twins are binovular, which means that two eggs were fertilized by two sperms. These are fraternal twins. Identical, or mono-ovular, twins develop from one egg that has split shortly after fertilization. Fraternal twins each have a placenta, but identical twins have only one between them.

The outlook for both the pregnant woman and the twins is good, particularly if the mother has adequate nutrition, rest, and prenatal care. But there are risks associated with every pregnancy, and in a twin pregnancy the risks of anemia (see p.669), preeclampsia (see p.676), placenta previa (see previous page), and postpartum hemorrhage (see p.683) are slightly higher than in a single pregnancy. Also, about one fourth of twin pregnancies end 4 or more weeks early (see Premature labor, p.680).

A multiple pregnancy is usually discovered by your physician during a routine prenatal examination and confirmed by ultrasound (see p.684). As with any pregnancy you should get enough rest and be sure to eat a balanced diet. To avoid the risk of anemia, your physician may recommend that you take additional vitamin and mineral supplements.

If you have contractions in late pregnancy or have a watery discharge from your vagina, contact your physician; you may be going into premature labor. If you are, you may be admitted to a hospital so that your uterine contractions can be closely monitored.

and will be susceptible to hypoglycemia (see p.562). Such infants have more medical and developmental problems and may even die. If the infant is delivered early, he or she may have some of the complications of premature labor (see p.680), including respiratory distress syndrome (see p.692).

What should be done?
Pregnant women should keep all prenatal appointments. If you are beyond the 30th week of your pregnancy and you think your fetus is not moving as much as before, count the movements carefully. Choose 2 days when you are not planning to leave the house, and on each day make a note of each movement you feel between nine in the morning and five in the afternoon. Then discuss your notes with your physician. Your fetus is probably healthy. In fact, there is a complete absence of movement in some normal pregnancies. But it is always wise to check rather than take any chances.

Your physician may recommend that you have an ultrasound scan (see p.684) and fetal heartbeat tests (see p.685) to check on the fetus's condition.

If it is determined that fetal growth is retarded, your physician can discuss with you the best time for the infant to be delivered. If the fetus is not growing well, it may actually develop better in an intensive care nursery where it won't have to depend on a placenta that may be functioning inefficiently. You may need to have the baby in a hospital that has a neonatal intensive care unit, which specializes in treating such problems in newborns. Labor may be started artificially (see Induction of labor, p.685) or you may need to have a cesarean section (see p.686).

Postmaturity

Ideally, labor starts when your fetus is fully mature and able to survive. When labor does not occur until long after this stage, the fetus can be harmed. This condition is known as postmaturity. An aging placenta can fail to provide a large fetus with enough oxygenated blood, and this can result in brain damage or even death. The stillbirth rate in postmature infants is almost double that in infants that are carried to term.

Postmaturity may be more likely to occur if you have a family history of diabetes mellitus, and is extremely likely if you have been carrying a fetus for more than 40 weeks. If postmaturity is suspected, your physician will probably induce labor (see p.685). Your physician will monitor labor and delivery; if the infant is in distress, the delivery may be by the use of forceps (see p.686) or cesarean section (see p.686).

Childbirth

There are several signs of approaching childbirth. The first sign in normal labor is contractions of the muscles of the uterus. At first, these contractions may seem like irregular bursts of indigestion like pain or twinges of backache. As childbirth approaches, however, the contractions come at more regular intervals and there is less time between them.

Contractions are not always a reliable sign that labor has started. Throughout pregnancy, the uterus has been contracting in preparation for labor. These contractions, called Braxton Hicks' contractions, are usually not noticeable until the last weeks of pregnancy. If you have contractions, but they are not accompanied by other signs of labor and they do not increase in frequency, you are probably not in labor.

As labor starts, the mucous plug that has formed a barrier between your uterus and vagina during pregnancy may be expelled as a bloody discharge. This episode, which is called the "show," is no cause for concern.

Another sign of labor is the bursting of the membranes that surround the amniotic fluid in which the fetus floats. When this occurs, you may have a slow trickle from your vagina or you may have a sudden gush. This is called "breaking water" or "breaking the bag of waters."

Notify your physician when you have any of these signs of labor. You may be advised to go to the hospital. If you have planned a home birth, your physician or nurse-midwife should be called when these signs appear.

In the hospital, there is usually an admission procedure. Your physician performs a vaginal examination to see how far your labor has progressed and to find out the fetus's position and heart rate, and the contractions of the uterus are monitored.

Stages of labor

Labor is divided into three stages. The first stage starts with the first contractions, which help open the cervix, through which the fetus leaves the uterus. With each contraction, the cervix is gradually pulled open and up (dilated), so that it becomes effaced—that is, it merges with the walls of the uterus. Full dilation is reached when the opening of the cervix with the baby's head protruding is about 4 inches (10 cm) in diameter.

The average duration of the first stage of labor is 12 hours for a first baby and 4 to 8 hours for a subsequent birth. For some women who are having their first baby, the first stage can last for more than 24 hours. For some women who have had several children, it may last only a few minutes.

When the cervix is fully dilated, there is a transition period between the first and second stages of labor; labor seems to come to a temporary halt. As the second stage begins, contractions may be accompanied by an urge to push the baby out and down the birth canal. As the baby moves through the birth canal, it presses on the rectum and may make you feel that you want to have a bowel movement. You will be advised to push only when you are having a contraction. This is so that the two physical forces (your pushing and the contractions) combine to expel the baby and you can conserve energy by resting as much as possible between contractions. Episiotomy (a surgical incision in the vagina to enlarge the birth canal) may be performed toward the end of the second stage of labor, before the baby emerges. Episiotomy is performed to avoid irregular tearing of the vagina, which may be difficult to repair.

The second stage of labor ends when the baby emerges completely from the birth canal. The second stage can last up to 2 or 3 hours for a first baby, and up to 1 or 2 hours for a subsequent baby.

After the baby is delivered, the umbilical cord that connects the baby to the placenta while it is inside the uterus is tied and cut.

The third stage of labor is delivery of the placenta (afterbirth). Your uterus contracts to expel the placenta. There is some bleeding, and the umbilical cord moves a little farther out of the vagina. The third stage of labor usually lasts about 15 minutes.

After the placenta has been delivered, you may be given a medication to prevent excessive bleeding. Any tears or incisions in the vagina are cleaned and stitched.

Premature labor

Labor is called premature if it occurs between the 24th and 36th weeks of pregnancy and results in the birth of a pre-term baby. This means that the child has had less than 37 weeks of development in the uterus.

Severe preeclampsia and eclampsia (see p.676) cause about a third of all cases of premature labor. High blood pressure during pregnancy, placenta previa (see p.677), hemorrhage (see Antepartum hemorrhage, p.677), cigarette smoking by the pregnant woman, and other factors account for some cases of premature labor. About 5 percent of pregnancies result in premature labor.

The earlier in a pregnancy that a baby is born, the less the baby's chance of survival. Babies who do survive risk having respiratory distress syndrome (see p.692), neonatal jaundice (see p.693), or other medical or developmental problems. The risk of having one of these disorders is greater the more premature the birth.

What should be done?

If you think you are starting labor prematurely, contact your physician at once. If your physician is not immediately available, ask someone to drive you or call an ambulance to take you to the hospital where you plan to deliver your baby. Call the hospital to say that you are on your way. If the hospital is far away, call them for advice. In the hospital, you will be examined to see if labor has started. There are many false alarms. Amniocentesis (see p.684) may be performed to check on the fetus's lung development. Medication may be given to control contractions so that the fetus will stay in the uterus until it is mature.

What is the treatment?

If your physician decides to let the labor proceed, you may have an episiotomy (see p.686) to allow easier passage of the baby's head, which is more fragile than a full-term baby's head. Forceps (see p.686) may also be used to protect the baby's head. After birth, the baby will be placed in a neonatal intensive care unit, where its heartbeat, respiration, and temperature will be carefully monitored and any problems that develop will be treated promptly.

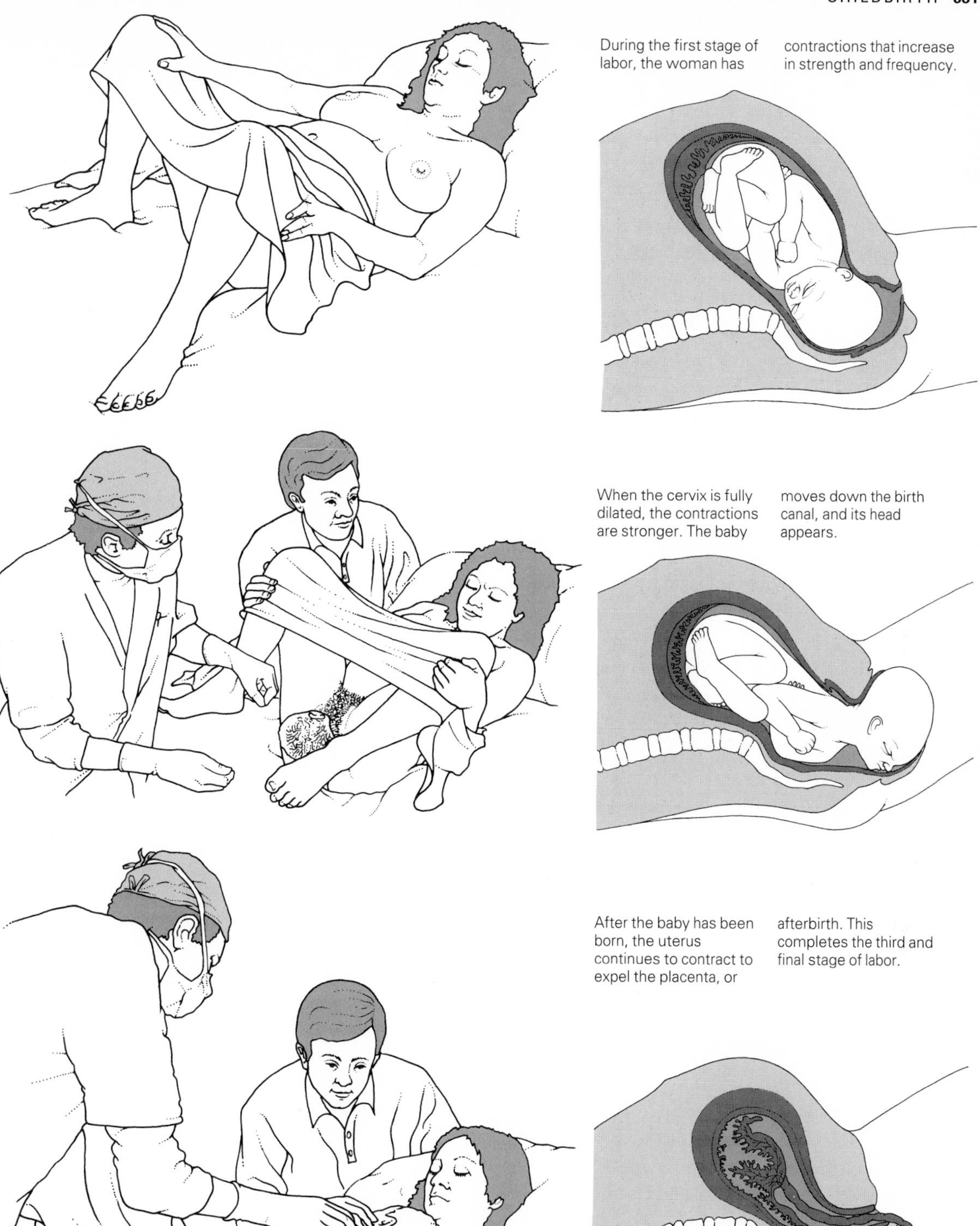

During the first stage of labor, the woman has contractions that increase in strength and frequency.

When the cervix is fully dilated, the contractions are stronger. The baby moves down the birth canal, and its head appears.

After the baby has been born, the uterus continues to contract to expel the placenta, or afterbirth. This completes the third and final stage of labor.

Pain relief in labor

Epidural anesthesia
The injection for epidural anesthesia is given between contractions with the woman lying on her side and curled up as much as possible to allow the anesthetist to insert the needle between the vertebrae.

The intensity of pain in labor varies significantly from woman to woman, and is partly influenced by your expectations. If you are frightened or tense, you may feel pain more acutely. This is one reason why you and your partner, or a close friend, should attend childbirth classes if they are available in your community. Some classes include breathing and relaxation exercises.

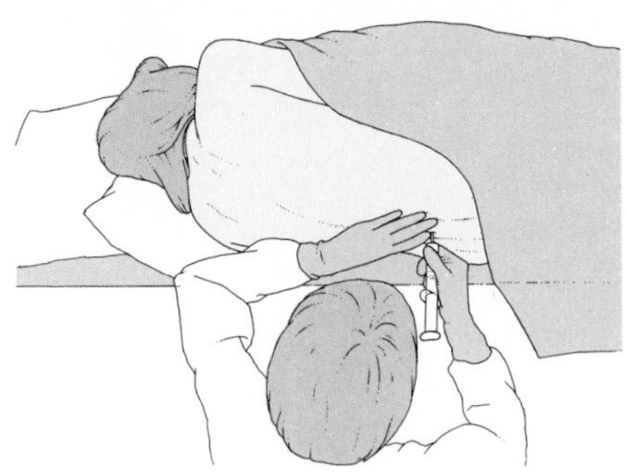

You may not need pain relief during labor, but if you do, there are several options available. If the first stage of labor is very painful, you may be given medication to help reduce tension and pain. This is done only if your physician is fairly sure that delivery is not imminent, because the drug can affect the baby's breathing if given late in labor.

Vaginal pain can be relieved by an anesthetic injected into the tissues of the vagina. This is called pudendal block. It is often used just before a forceps delivery or before an episiotomy, in which an incision is made in the vagina to aid delivery.

A painkilling method called epidural anesthesia involves injecting an anesthetic into the base of your spine to temporarily deaden the nerves running to the lower half of your body. A catheter is then usually placed in the lower part of your back and small doses of anesthetic are given if needed as labor progresses, or during delivery.

Malpresentation

The part of the fetus that has settled at the outlet of the pregnant woman's pelvic cavity immediately before birth is called the presenting part. In most cases the presenting part is the head, with the top of the head settled into the cavity of the pelvis, and the face to the woman's back. This presentation positions the fetus for the easiest passage through the birth canal. The fetus, however, may be in one of several other positions that cause problems and which are called malpresentation.

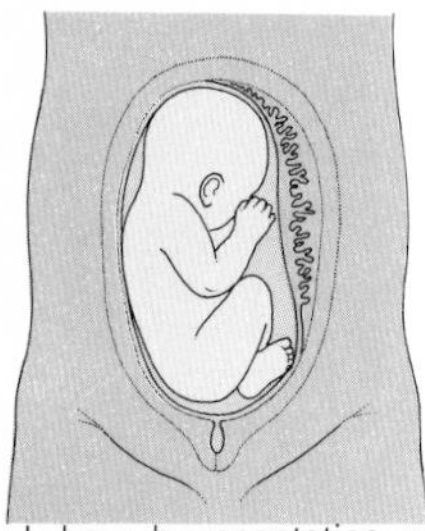

In breech presentation, the fetus passes into and comes down the woman's birth canal buttocks first.

Two common malpresentations are occipital posterior presentation and breech presentation. An occipital posterior presentation is head down, but with the face toward the woman's front. This puts the fetus in a difficult position to travel through the birth canal, but usually the fetus rotates naturally to the proper position. Delivery by forceps and sometimes by cesarean section may be necessary. Breech presentation is common in premature labor (see p.680) because a fetus may not assume a normal position for delivery until late in pregnancy. The fetus is positioned with its buttocks down, and one or both feet may emerge first. In a buttocks-first delivery, the fetus's head is more vulnerable to pressure as it passes along the birth canal, which is not sufficiently enlarged by the buttocks. Such a delivery may have to be by cesarean section or forceps.

In some cases of breech presentation, a physician can manipulate the fetus into the normal presentation position during the last few weeks of pregnancy. If breech presentation persists, but there are no other problems, your physician may suggest that you allow labor to start naturally, while being prepared for a cesarean section if labor is difficult.

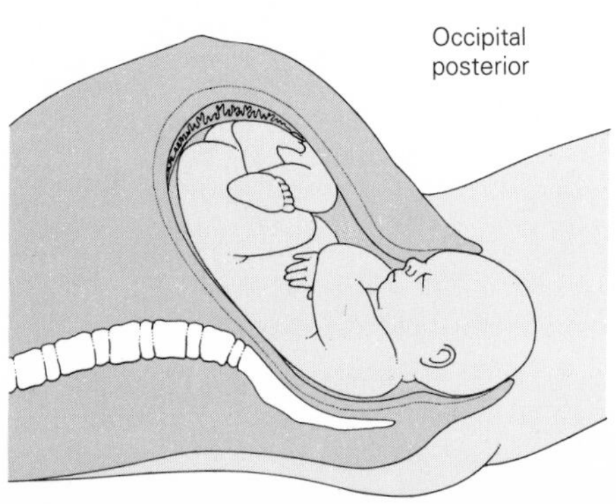

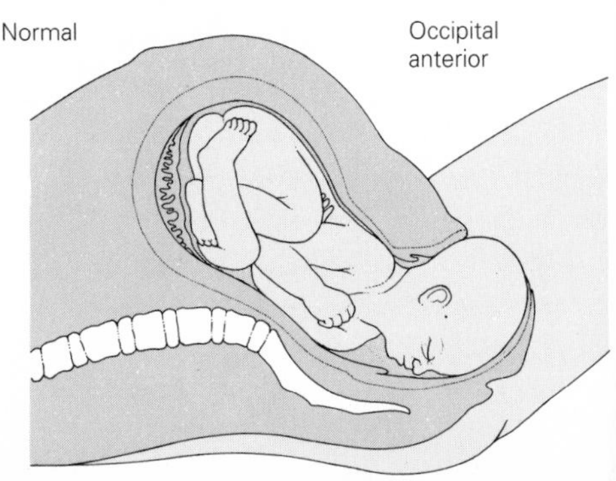

In occipital posterior presentation (right), the fetus's chin is pushed down onto the chest, so that the neck cannot be flexed to get around the curve of the birth canal as in the normal occipital anterior presentation (far right).

Prolonged labor

Prolonged labor is usually caused by one of two things. The muscles of the uterus may not produce sufficiently strong or regular contractions. This can be the result of receiving a spinal anesthetic, which interferes with muscle contraction. Or in some cases, there may be an obstruction to normal delivery. Obstruction occurs in disproportion (see below), when the fetus's head is too large for the bony outlet from the pelvic cavity, or malpresentation (see previous article), when the fetus's position makes delivery difficult.

Your physician may use intravenous medication to stimulate contraction of the uterine muscles (see Induction of labor, p.685). In some cases, delivery may be performed by cesarean section (see p.686) or forceps (see p.686), depending on the stage of labor and the position of the fetus.

Disproportion

(cephalo-pelvic disproportion)

The term disproportion means that the woman's pelvic cavity is too narrow for the passage of the fetus's head. This can happen in small-boned women and in women who are under 5 ft (1.5 m) tall. In some cases, a woman's pelvis is disproportionately small because of an injury received earlier in life. Disproportion may also occur if the fetus's head is abnormally large, as in hydrocephalus (see p.701).

If your physician suspects disproportion, you may be given an ultrasound scan to confirm this. If you appear to have severe disproportion, your physician probably will recommend delivery by cesarean section (see p.686). Pelvimetry, or X rays to outline the bony structure of the fetus and the woman, is usually performed only if labor has already begun. It is not recommended before labor since X rays may harm the fetus. If your physician decides to proceed with a vaginal delivery, labor will be allowed to continue, but the fetus's condition will be closely monitored.

Postpartum hemorrhage

Postpartum hemorrhage is excessive loss of blood from the uterus or vagina after delivery. It often occurs when the uterine muscle does not contract firmly enough to cause the uterus to shrink and compress the blood vessels in the uterus. This causes failure to control the bleeding produced when the placenta separates from the uterus. This problem may occur if you had a very long labor or if the uterine muscles have been stretched excessively by twins or by many births. Another possible cause of postpartum hemorrhage is that parts of the placenta can remain inside the uterus and prevent it from tightening up sufficiently after childbirth. A hemorrhage can also occur if vaginal tissues have been torn during delivery.

Bleeding from the uterus is controlled by medications that encourage the uterus to contract. If fragments of placenta remain in the uterus, they should be removed. If bleeding is from torn vaginal tissues, the tear may be stitched up after the area has been numbed with a local anesthetic.

Retained placenta

Usually, the placenta separates from the wall of the uterus after delivery and, with the help of your physician who presses on your abdomen and pulls gently on the umbilical cord, it is expelled. Occasionally, the placenta becomes trapped in the uterus, in some cases because it has not separated completely from the uterine wall. If it has not been expelled within 30 minutes after delivery, it is called a retained placenta.

If necessary, a retained placenta can be removed manually by your physician. While you receive an anesthetic, your physician places his or her hand inside your uterus and removes the placenta. You will then be given a drug to encourage your uterus to contract in order to prevent excessive bleeding.

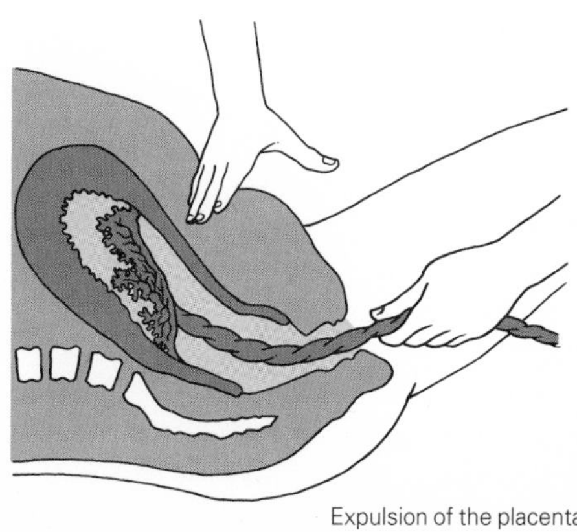

Expulsion of the placenta

Special procedures in pregnancy

Amniocentesis

In amniocentesis, the physician inserts a hollow needle through the abdomen and the uterine wall into the amniotic sac to withdraw a sample of amniotic fluid, which surrounds the fetus. Amniocentesis is performed if there is a possibility that the fetus has Down syndrome (see p.699), spina bifida (see p.700), or some other serious genetic abnormality. If you have already had a child with a severe birth defect, if there is a family history of some abnormality, or if you will be age 35 or older when the baby is due, amniocentesis may be performed between the 16th and 18th weeks of pregnancy.

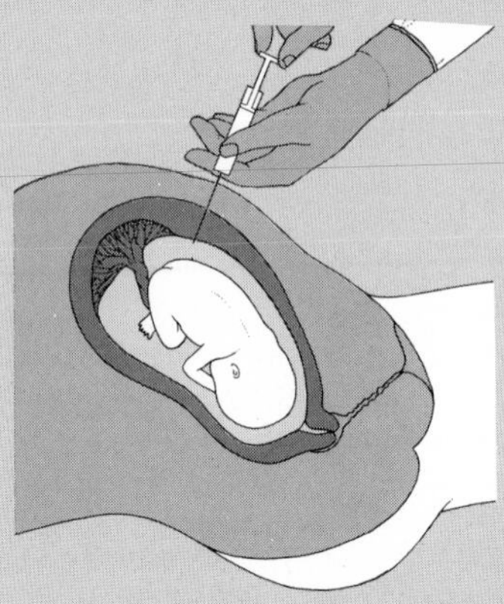

Amniocentesis, in which a sample of amniotic fluid is withdrawn from the uterus, is done if your physician suspects an abnormality that can be diagnosed by examining cells shed by the fetus into the fluid.

Amniocentesis is also used to determine the level of maturity of the developing fetus's lungs if premature labor (see p.680) is expected or if the baby will be delivered by cesarean section. An ultrasound scan (see next column) is performed before amniocentesis to determine the exact position of the fetus and placenta; your abdomen is numbed with a local anesthetic before the needle is inserted.

Tests of amniotic fluid can identify many genetic abnormalities. The procedure involves a slight risk of terminating the pregnancy.

Amniocentesis may also reveal the sex of the developing fetus. So, if you are having this procedure done for some other purpose, you can ask your physician to tell you the sex of the fetus before birth. Given this opportunity, many parents choose not to learn the fetus's sex.

Chorionic villus sampling

Chorionic villus sampling (CVS) is a procedure that enables the accurate diagnosis of certain genetic disorders between the 6th and 10th weeks of pregnancy. Because this procedure can identify various genetic disorders so early in pregnancy, parents have the option of deciding whether or not to terminate the pregnancy if the developing embryo is found to have a genetic disorder.

In CVS, a small piece of the placenta is removed and examined. The sample is removed under ultrasound guidance, either through the cervix by means of a minor suction procedure or through the abdomen. The placenta contains the same genes as the embryo, and an examination of the sample therefore reveals whether the embryo has a genetic disorder. CVS carries a small risk of inducing a miscarriage. For this reason, the test is performed only when there is a clear risk that the embryo may have a serious genetic disorder.

CVS cannot detect all inherited disorders, and, in certain cases, must be postponed until between the 16th and 18th weeks of pregnancy, when amniocentesis (see previous column) and fetoscopy (see p.685) can be performed.

Ultrasound

Ultrasound is a device that transmits sound waves through body tissues, records the echoes as the sounds bounce off tissues inside the body, and transforms the recordings into a photographic image. When used on a pregnant woman, the surface of the abdomen is first covered with a film of oil, and the transmitter is then moved slowly over the surface of her abdomen.

Ultrasound can be used to measure accurately the size and shape of the fetus to help establish the stage of a pregnancy, to detect twins, to show the rate of development if intrauterine growth retardation (see p.678) is suspected, to determine the position of the fetus during late pregnancy (see Malpresentation, p.682), to locate the position of the placenta if placenta previa (see p.677) is suspected, and to detect body malformations that are present in the fetus. Ultrasound is a painless procedure that does not harm either the fetus or the woman.

(continued on next page)

Fetoscopy

Ultrasound techniques (see text, previous page) allow a physician to obtain very clear images of a developing fetus at all stages of pregnancy. In some cases, however, the physician may require a closer examination of the fetus. This is possible after the 22nd week of pregnancy.

In the procedure called fetoscopy, a laparoscope (a viewing instrument) is passed into the uterus. The technique used is similar to amniocentesis (see previous page). Once the laparoscope is inside, the physician can examine the fetus. He or she may also remove a blood sample by using a special attachment on the laparoscope. The physician may even perform an operation during this procedure, such as bypassing an obstruction in the urinary system of the fetus.

Fetal monitoring

Fetal monitoring records the fetus's heart rate and movements and the contractions of the uterus. Fetal monitoring is most commonly used during labor, but it is also sometimes used during the last few weeks of pregnancy.

During pregnancy, fetal monitoring may be performed if the woman has previously had a stillbirth, if she has had symptoms of preeclampsia (see p.676), or if the growth of the fetus has been slower than expected. The purpose of monitoring during pregnancy is to establish how the fetus is likely to react to the stress of labor. For fetal monitoring, recording devices connected to an electronic monitor are strapped to the woman's abdomen. The heart rate and other responses of both the woman and fetus may be recorded, or a stress test may be performed. In the stress test, the woman is given a carefully calculated dose of a drug that stimulates the uterus to contract, and the responses of both the woman and fetus are recorded; alternatively, the woman inhales a specially prepared mixture of oxygen and nitrogen, which reduces the amount of oxygen in her blood. The effect on the fetus is then monitored. Through analyzing such responses, the physician can decide whether, when labor begins, the birth should proceed naturally or whether it may be safer to deliver the baby by cesarean section.

Fetal monitoring during pregnancy is performed routinely when there is some reason to observe the fetus more closely than usual. Many physicians believe that fetal monitoring should be performed at least intermittently during all labors. At the start of labor, once the membranes that surround the fetus have ruptured (see Childbirth, p.679), an electrode may be attached to the fetus's scalp to observe its response to labor. If there are any signs of distress, the physician may decide that it is safer to deliver the baby by cesarean section.

Special procedures in childbirth

Induction of labor

Inducing labor is the deliberate starting of labor by a physician. Labor is usually induced when the risks of allowing the pregnancy to continue appear to outweigh the risks of inducing labor. This is often true in intrauterine growth retardation (see p.678) or postmaturity (see p.679). Your physician first examines you internally to find out if your cervix has begun to dilate, or open. Then your physician locates the membranes around the amniotic fluid, the liquid that surrounds the fetus in the uterus, and may make a small, painless incision in the membranes to drain the fluid.

Sometimes this is enough to start labor. If not, you may receive an intravenous injection of the synthetic hormone oxytocin, which encourages the uterus to contract as it would in natural labor. However, in about 1 in 50 inductions of labor, the uterus fails to respond to the hormone. In such cases, the baby may be delivered by cesarean section (see next page) so that you and the fetus can avoid possible infection.

When labor is induced, the condition of the fetus is monitored throughout delivery by fetal monitoring (see above) and by frequent physical examinations. Usually, labor proceeds safely to a normal delivery, but there are some slight risks involved any time that labor is induced. There is also a chance that you will have a premature baby with the associated risks, because it is sometimes difficult to identify the exact stage that a pregnancy is in before inducing labor.

(continued on next page)

Episiotomy

Episiotomy is an incision sometimes made during labor to widen the opening of the vagina. It is often performed when labor is premature, expecially when a forceps delivery is necessary, because the baby's head is vulnerable to pressure in the birth canal. Episiotomy may be performed to avoid tearing the vagina as the baby's head emerges from the birth canal. The incision usually is made after injecting a local anesthetic. After delivery, the cut is sewn up, usually with stitches that gradually dissolve. The incision heals rapidly, although the scar may cause discomfort for up to 3 months. To relieve any discomfort in the area around the incision, use an ice pack, sit in a shallow tub of warm water, or sit on an inflatable pillow. To help prevent infection, rinse the area with warm water and pat dry every time you go to the toilet.

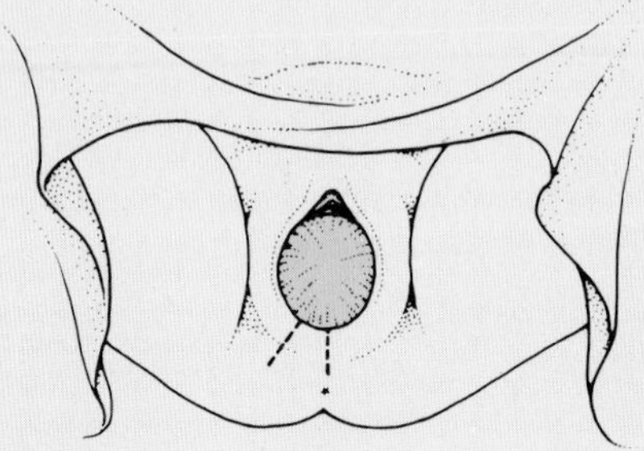

The two most common incisions (dotted lines) for an episiotomy are midline (down toward the anus) and mediolateral (to the side).

Forceps

Obstetrical forceps consist of two wide, curved blades designed to fit around a baby's head. There are several different types of forceps, and they are used to assist delivery when, for example, your uterus is not contracting efficiently, or when a baby appears to be suffocating and needs oxygen as soon as possible. Forceps may be used to protect the baby's head in a breech presentation (see Malpresentation, p.682) or in premature labor (see p.680). When epidural anesthesia (see p.682) has been used toward the end of labor, forceps are often needed to "lift" the baby out. Before forceps are used, an episiotomy is usually performed. The forceps are then inserted into the birth canal, and the baby is gently lifted out. The risks of using forceps range from temporary marks on the baby's cheeks or ears, to damage to the baby's nerves, or damage to the woman's vagina. However, a forceps delivery is usually less risky than a cesarean section, for both the woman and the infant.

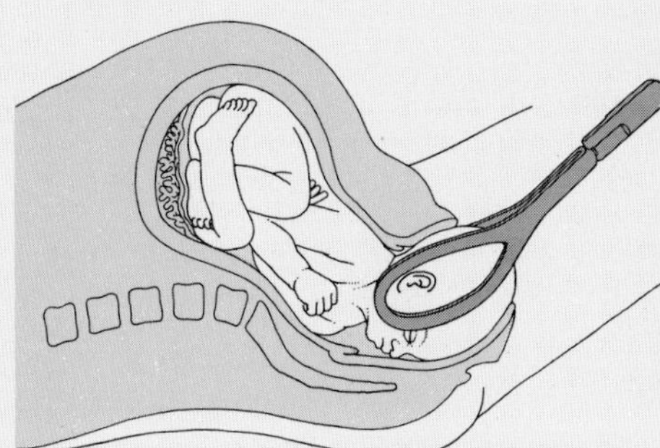

A cross section of the birth canal shows forceps helping delivery.

Cesarean section

Cesarean section is a surgical procedure that enables the safe, quick delivery of a baby. Most cesarean sections are performed under a general anesthetic, but sometimes a spinal, or epidural, anesthetic may be used (see p.682). In cesarean section, an incision is made in the woman's lower abdomen, just above the pubic hair, and through into the uterus, through which the baby is delivered. For the woman, recovery from the surgery takes longer than it would from a vaginal birth, and the procedure has the risks of a major operation. You are usually able to go home in 3 to 4 days.

The number of babies born by cesarean section in the US has been increasing in recent years and in some parts of the country accounts for as many as one fourth of all deliveries. The reasons for this trend include an increase in the number of women having their first child late in life, when the risks of pregnancy and birth are greater to both woman and fetus. Other reasons include the use of monitoring techniques before and during labor (see previous page) that can identify fetuses that might be damaged as a result of a prolonged labor, and the belief among many obstetricians that cesarean section is the safest way of delivering a baby presenting as a breech (see Malpresentation, p.682). Obstetricians fear professional liability lawsuits may follow if difficult childbirth results in complications for the woman or baby. If you have previously delivered a baby by cesarean section and are considering having a vaginal delivery in this pregnancy, talk to your physician. Most women who have delivered a baby by cesarean section may have a successful vaginal delivery on a subsequent pregnancy.

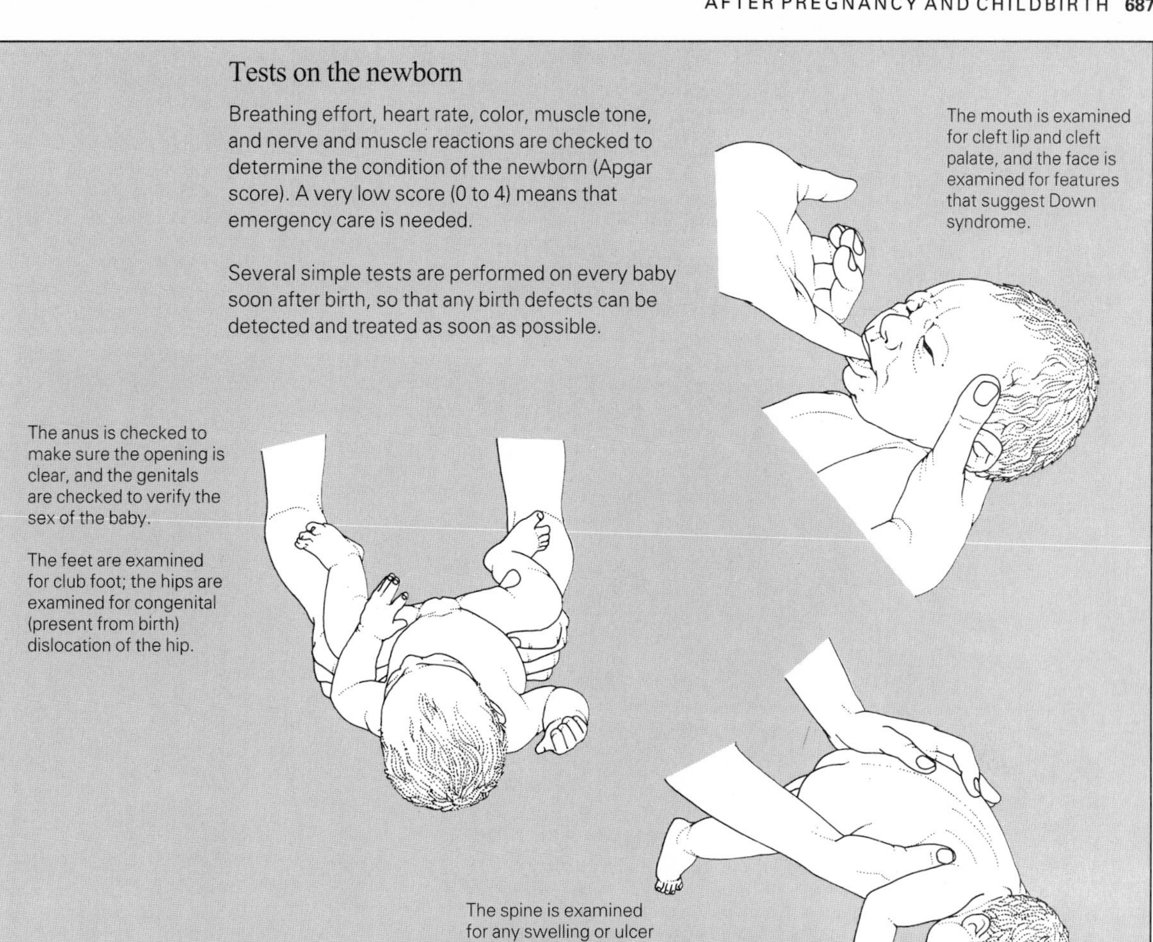

Tests on the newborn
Breathing effort, heart rate, color, muscle tone, and nerve and muscle reactions are checked to determine the condition of the newborn (Apgar score). A very low score (0 to 4) means that emergency care is needed.
Several simple tests are performed on every baby soon after birth, so that any birth defects can be detected and treated as soon as possible.
The mouth is examined for cleft lip and cleft palate, and the face is examined for features that suggest Down syndrome.
The anus is checked to make sure the opening is clear, and the genitals are checked to verify the sex of the baby.
The feet are examined for club foot; the hips are examined for congenital (present from birth) dislocation of the hip.
The spine is examined for any swelling or ulcer that may indicate spina bifida, and the navel is examined for any swelling resulting from umbilical hernia.

After pregnancy and childbirth

It is easy to view the whole experience of pregnancy only as a preparation for childbirth and not look beyond the baby's birth. However, gradual changes that have happened in your body over a period of 9 months are reversed in a much shorter time after you have gone through childbirth. Your body changes quickly while, especially if this is your first baby, you are attempting to meet the needs of your newborn and getting less sleep. These changes may cause you to feel depressed for the first week or two.

During pregnancy, you probably have considered whether to breast-feed or bottle-feed your baby. Breast-feeding has several advantages over bottle-feeding. Breast-feeding has psychological benefits for you and your infant because it helps promote a warm, close relationship between mother and child. Also, breast milk provides the ideal balance of nutrients for your infant. In addition, breast milk can help protect your baby against infections to which you are already immune. The composition of breast milk also seems to vary with your baby's needs, whereas the composition of canned milk or formula stays constant. You can put your baby to your breast as often as he or she seems to want it, and the baby will not gain weight too quickly, but a baby may become overweight with too much bottle-feeding.

There are advantages and disadvantages to each method. In most women, breast milk is always available and requires no preparation. There may be times when you need to be elsewhere at feeding time or you may be tired or sick. You can arrange for someone else to feed your baby either by pumping milk with a breast pump into a sterile bottle or by substituting a bottle of formula.

If you choose artificial feeding, formula provides the necessary nutrients for your infant. Make sure that you prepare the formula according to directions. Some people prefer the convenience of feeding the baby from a bottle.

If you have any problems in the first few days of breast-feeding, do not be discouraged. Talk to your physician for support and advice on breast-feeding, or ask your physician's office for information from or a local telephone number for La Leche League International, a group that offers practical advice and moral support for women who are breast-feeding.

About 6 weeks after childbirth, you should have a postnatal checkup. In this examination, your physician will examine you to make sure that your uterus and bladder are in the correct positions and that any scar tissue from the delivery is healing satisfactorily. The visit also provides an opportunity for you and your physician to discuss any questions that you may have.

Breast conditions

Breast-feeding provides benefits to both mother and child, as discussed above in the introduction to this section. Breast-feeding strengthens the bond between the mother and child and reduces the baby's risk of infection. However, getting started can be difficult. Since most of these problems can be overcome, you should not let them prevent you from breast-feeding. During pregnancy, your physician may have instructed you on care and preparation of your breasts for breast-feeding.

Engorgement

In most women, milk supply arrives quickly and forcefully a few days after delivery. The breasts become tightly swollen and sore, and are said to be "engorged." This can also happen when you decide to stop breast-feeding and milk accumulates in your breasts.

Breast pumps remove milk without nursing. The milk can be used immediately or refrigerated or frozen for use later.

A baby cannot get milk from a swollen nipple, so some excess milk must be removed before you can breast-feed. Excess milk can be removed (expressed) either by hand or with a breast pump. Your breasts should also be softened by bathing them in warm water. If your breasts are engorged because you have stopped breast-feeding, support them with a firm bra and take aspirin or acetaminophen. After a few days, the build-up of milk will prevent additional milk from being produced and your breasts will gradually become less full and less painful.

Cracked nipples

You may feel a sharp pain in your nipple while your baby is nursing, which may mean that there is a thin crack in your nipple. This can happen if you do not dry your nipples thoroughly after each feeding. Tell your physician, who may recommend a soothing cream to apply to your nipple. The crack should take only a few days to heal; meanwhile, feed your baby from the other breast until the nipple heals.

Blocked milk duct and abscess

If you feel a small, hard lump in your breast, you may have a blocked milk duct. Try massaging your breast and bathing it in warm water. If the lump does not disappear in a day or two, see your physician immediately. The lump may be a breast abscess (see p.632). Your physician will examine the breast and may give you antibiotics to treat the infection. You usually can continue feeding your baby from the affected breast. If the abscess is not treated early enough, you may have to have a minor operation to drain it.

Postpartum depression

Many women feel depressed a few days after childbirth. This is a common feeling that is called postpartum depression. Postpartum depression may have several causes. One factor is that the sudden change in your body hormones caused by childbirth can affect your mood. Also, you may have a sense of letdown after an event that you have anticipated for so many months.

Many new mothers are very tired and may feel afraid and underconfident. Postpartum depression usually goes away quickly with the support of friends and family. It may be reassuring even to know that this is a very common experience among new mothers.

It is also common to feel mildly depressed during the first weeks after childbirth. The fatigue that is inevitable when you are taking care of a new baby and the sudden change in your life-style all contribute to this.

A small number of women become much more seriously depressed after childbirth, to the extent that they are unable to take care of themselves or the baby. Such an illness (see Depression, p.321) usually starts within about a month of childbirth.

What should be done?

It is important for you to avoid becoming overtired. Keeping your baby in the same bedroom with you at night is usually not recommended, because it can disturb you not only when the baby is hungry, but also when the baby moves in his or her sleep and makes noises while awake. You need all the sleep you can get, so you should put your baby in another room at night.

Try to schedule a shift system with your partner, so that you do not have to take care of your baby every time he or she needs attention. In addition, family or friends may be willing to do shopping for you or take care of your baby while you get some rest during the day.

Most women who feel depressed after childbirth work through their feelings and do not need treatment. However, if you find that you cannot get rid of your depression, and that it is affecting your life so that you can no longer care for yourself and your baby properly, consult your physician. He or she may prescribe an antidepressant drug or suggest a support group. In rare cases, if your depression does not respond to treatment and is very severe, your physician may refer you to a psychiatrist for possible psychotherapy treatment. Very rarely, your physician may advise that you go into a hospital psychiatric unit for treatment. If this is necessary, you and your partner should discuss who will take care of the baby. It is sometimes possible for you to be admitted to a hospital psychiatric facility that is equipped to care for you and your baby. This may be a good idea even if you feel that your baby is the cause of your illness. A separation at this stage may make it even more difficult for you to develop a close relationship with your baby.

Sex after childbirth

After a normal delivery, discuss with your physician when you can resume sexual intercourse. In some cases, you can start intercourse a few days after childbirth. Most physicians recommend that you wait until your postnatal examination about 6 weeks after childbirth.

Since you can become pregnant again after childbirth, talk to your physician about the steps you can take to avoid pregnancy. Breast-feeding and absent periods do not prevent pregnancy. If you want to become pregnant again soon, ask your physician about the risks and benefits.

Your vagina may be extremely tender for the first 10 days or so after childbirth, or possibly for several weeks if you had an episiotomy (see p.686) or your vagina was torn during labor. If intercourse is painful, see your physician. Such pain may be caused by an area of raw skin in the vagina or a stitch that has not disappeared completely. Both of these problems can be treated.

You may find that your vagina has lost some elasticity. To correct this, you can tone up the muscles around your vagina by repeatedly interrupting and resuming flow in mid-stream each time you urinate.

Taking care of a new baby can be extremely tiring and emotionally exhausting and can leave you no energy for sex. Use the techniques recommended for avoiding over-tiredness suggested in Postpartum depression (see previous article).

Especially with a first baby, your partner may feel left out of the new developing relationship between you and your child and may seek the reassurance of your continuing affection and attention. Just as he must realize that you are going through a period of adjustment, you should make an effort to understand that he, too, may be feeling confused and vulnerable now that the baby needs so much attention. Talk to your partner openly about his role in caring for the baby and how the baby affects your relationship.

Children's health

Introduction

Some of the problems discussed in this section are found only in infants and children, while others can affect people of all ages but require special diagnostic tests or treatment in infants and children. Also, the outlook for some diseases is very different for infants and children.

The first group of articles in this section describes problems of newborns and infants up to about 6 months old. First-time parents in particular tend to worry about the health of a newborn baby. How can you tell if your child is ill? What are the signs of serious illness? Sometimes a symptom such as skin rash, fever, loss of appetite, change in the quality and intensity of your baby's cry, or diarrhea make it clear that your baby is ill. At other times, changes in your baby's behavior will indicate that something is wrong, but the cause of the problem may not be obvious. Consult the self-diagnosis charts in Part II of this book. If your baby has a high fever, cries loudly and persistently, and does not stop crying when picked up, or if he or she is listless or refuses to eat, call your physician. (To check your baby's development, see Milestones, next page.)

Some infants have health problems that are congenital, or present from birth. Congenital disorders may not be discovered immediately. Such problems have a variety of causes. Some congenital disorders can be treated.

Most of the problems in this section are grouped according to the part of the body affected.

Psychological and nervous system disorders, as well as eye and ear problems, can affect a child's learning ability.

Common respiratory infections included in this section represent almost half of all childhood illnesses. While gastroenteritis (see p.695) commonly causes digestive problems in children, the other digestive disorders included here are far less common. Like respiratory tract infections, however, they are usually easy to diagnose.

Unlike respiratory and digestive disorders, blood and urinary tract disorders are not always obvious, because they often cause mild and varied symptoms or no symptoms at all. Muscle, bone, and joint disorders need prompt treatment.

The last group of articles describes the most common infectious diseases in children. If you think your child has one of these disorders, see Symptoms of childhood infectious diseases (p.744) or the appropriate self-diagnosis chart, and see your physician if necessary. Also, see p.745 for suggestions on how to care for a child who has one of these diseases. Today, it is possible to immunize a child against most common infectious diseases. Immunizations are vital to ensuring your child's health, and proof of immunization may be required for school attendance. Check with your local health department or school district, and read the Immunization schedules on p.748. An immunized child is less likely to contract or transmit an infectious disease.

Newborn and early infants

The disorders discussed here are most common in children during the first year of life. Some, such as asphyxia and respiratory distress syndrome, occur mainly in infants who are premature or who go through a difficult delivery. These disorders are treated in the hospital. Other problems covered here, such as diaper rash and excessive crying, are very common and are usually very easily treated at home.

Many common infections that are usually not serious in adults can be very serious in infants. Gastroenteritis (inflammation of the stomach and intestines), for example, usually

Milestones

All children acquire mental and physical skills in the same order. For example, a child will not stand before learning to sit. But the rate for acquiring these skills varies enormously, and the age given below for each milestone in a child's development is only a rough average with a wide range.

Your baby may be able to:

- Smile at 6 weeks
- Roll over from a sideways position onto the back at 9 or 10 weeks
- Raise his or her head and shoulders from a face-down position at 3 to 4 months
- Sit supported at 6 months
- Say simple two-syllable "words," such as "Dada" or "Mama," at 9 to 10 months
- Move to a sitting position at 9 months
- Understand simple commands at 12 months

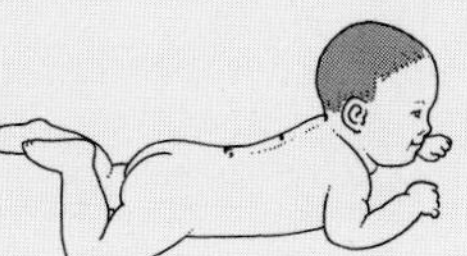

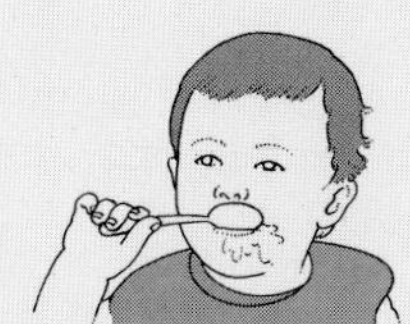

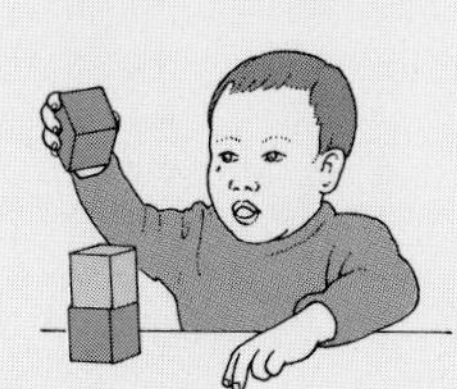

- Stand unsupported for a second or two at 12 months
- Try to feed himself or herself with a spoon at 18 months
- Walk without help at 18 months
- Make a three-block-high tower at 18 months
- Be toilet trained at 2 years
- Stay dry during the day at 2 years
- Talk in simple sentences at 3 years
- Get dressed and undressed (with help) at 3 years
- Hop, skip, and draw a figure with separate head, body, arms, and legs at 5 years

For information about progress in seeing and hearing, see p.722.

Growth charts

These charts show normal height and weight ranges for boys (right) and girls (far right) from ages 1 to 12. Children's growth rates vary, so the charts show a normal range of height and weight for each year of growth. Assume that your child's growth is normal if his or her height and weight fall within the shaded areas in line with his or her age.

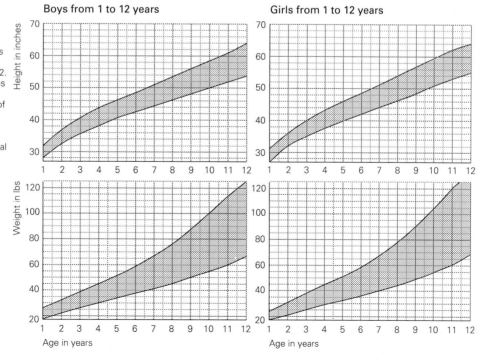

requires treatment with intravenous fluids to prevent dehydration, which is a medical emergency that can lead to shock, coma, and even death. This section also discusses Down syndrome, which is caused by an abnormality in the child's chromosomes. To see if your child is developing normally during the first few years of his or her life, see the box on milestones in a child's mental and physical development, previous page.

Asphyxia in the newborn

Some babies do not breathe at birth. This condition is called asphyxia. Because the brain controls breathing, failure of the baby's brain to function normally can result in asphyxia. Sometimes an infant's brain does not function normally because of an inadequate oxygen supply from the placenta to the baby during labor. An inadequate supply of oxygen may occur when the baby is small for the length of the pregnancy (smoking during pregnancy is one cause of this), significantly overdue, or if the umbilical cord is flattened or twisted during labor.

Brain damage may occur before or after the baby is delivered.

What are the symptoms?
The baby does not breathe or cry at birth. In milder cases, the baby's skin is blue and the arms and legs may feel stiff, although they may move. In severe cases, the baby is gray in color, immobile, and limp.

What are the risks?
Today, fewer newborns need help with their breathing than before because health care for pregnant women and their infants (obstetrics) has continued to improve. However, babies born to women who smoked during pregnancy are more likely to be small and prone to asphyxia and other respiratory problems.

Obstetricians, physicians who specialize in the treatment of pregnant women and their newborn children, are prepared to treat an asphyxiated baby immediately after birth. Because of this, the risks of brain damage (after about 5 minutes without oxygen) or death (after about 10 minutes) are minimal.

The risk of serious complications is higher for a home birth, even when a physician is present, because a hospital has all the equipment and personnel required to handle medical emergencies.

What should be done?
In the unlikely event that you have to revive a newborn baby that is not breathing, or a baby who has stopped breathing, first clear any mucus from the baby's throat with your finger and then perform gentle mouth-to-mouth-and-nose resuscitation (see p.834).

What is the treatment?
It is possible for an obstetrician to identify a baby that is at risk for asphyxia late in the pregnancy, before labor begins. The baby should be delivered in a hospital that has a specialized neonatal intensive care unit. An inadequate supply of oxygen from the placenta is usually detected during the course of labor. In such cases, asphyxia can be prevented or minimized by an emergency delivery of the baby, sometimes by forceps or cesarean section (see p.686).

If the baby is born asphyxiated, secretions of fluid from the uterus, together with mucus at the back of the baby's throat, and often meconium (stool passed by the fetus if it is in distress from lack of oxygen), are quickly sucked out of the baby's mouth and nose through a special tube. In mild cases of asphyxia, the baby will then gasp while inhaling oxygen, which causes the baby's brain to initiate breathing.

To treat severe cases of asphyxia, oxygen is passed into the baby's lungs through a tube inserted into the baby's windpipe and artificial respiration is started. The child usually begins to breathe within a few minutes. Occasionally, if the brain has been damaged during delivery or is underdeveloped, the child may have to be placed on a ventilator for up to several weeks. If the baby's brain has not been deprived of oxygen for more than about 5 minutes, and action is taken immediately, asphyxia of the newborn has no permanent aftereffects.

Respiratory distress syndrome

After a baby's first breath has expanded the lungs, the alveoli (small air sacs in the lungs) are kept open by a chemical in the lungs called surfactant. Keeping the alveoli open is essential, because it is through the capillaries that surround the alveoli that the chief steps in respiration take place: oxygen passes into the bloodstream and carbon dioxide enters the lungs to be exhaled.

However, in some very small, premature babies the lungs do not have enough surfactant, and the alveoli start to close up again

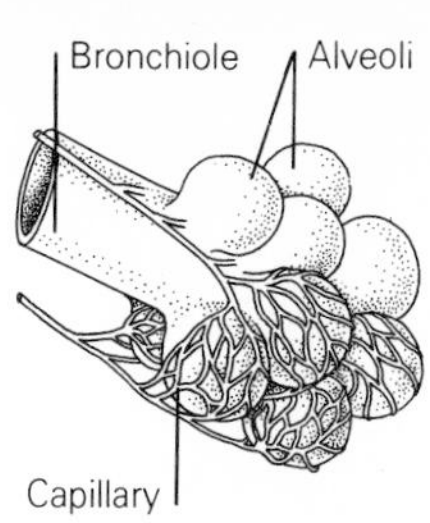

When a baby is born and takes his or her first breath, oxygen moves through the bronchi (large air passages in the lungs) and bronchioles (smallest air passages in the lungs) to the alveoli (air sacs in the lungs). The alveoli fill with air, and oxygen passes into the baby's bloodstream through the capillaries that surround the alveoli.

within a few hours after birth. The baby then develops respiratory distress syndrome, in which the child begins to have increasing difficulty in breathing.

What are the symptoms?

During the first few hours after birth, the baby's breathing gradually becomes more labored and rapid. As the baby breathes in, the chest sinks instead of expanding. When breathing out, the baby grunts.

What are the risks?

The more premature a baby is, the more likely it is that he or she will have respiratory distress syndrome. It is very common in babies that weigh less than 3 lb (1,500 g) at birth. It is also common in infants born to women with diabetes (see Diabetes and pregnancy, p.672).

Current pediatric intensive care technology and treatment have greatly improved the chances of survival for babies with respiratory distress syndrome, but this disorder is still a significant cause of death in infants who have been born prematurely.

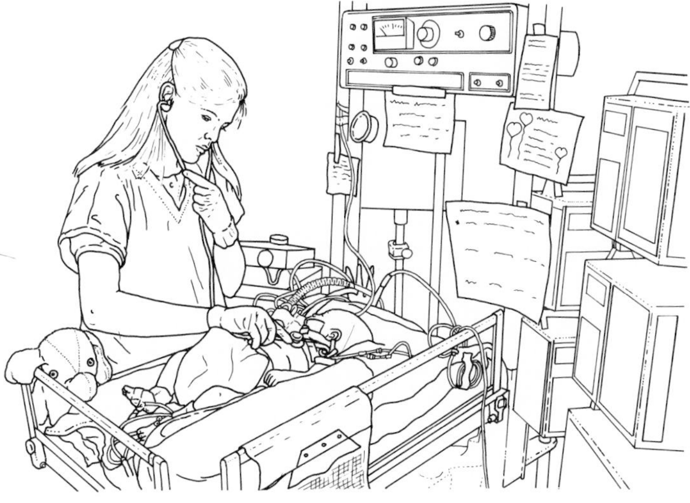

What is the treatment?

When a premature birth is expected, the adequacy of surfactant in the fetus's lungs may be determined by taking a sample of the pregnant woman's amniotic fluid (the fluid that surrounds the fetus in the uterus; see Amniocentesis, p.684). If the supply of surfactant is inadequate, it may be increased by giving the pregnant woman an injection of a corticosteroid medication. This injection is not given if the birth is imminent, because the drug takes about 24 hours to work.

A baby who has respiratory distress syndrome, or who is in danger of developing respiratory distress syndrome, is treated in a hospital intensive care unit. The treatment includes placing an inhaler over the child's face to administer artificial surfactant (to aid the passage of oxygen and carbon dioxide) that helps restore your baby's lungs to normal. Your child may also need artificial respiration, and his or her lungs will need to be continuously monitored with measurements of the levels of oxygen, carbon dioxide, and other chemicals in the blood.

What are the long-term prospects?

Since the introduction of treatment with surfactant the chances of survival for infants with respiratory distress syndrome have improved significantly. However, infants who are very premature (born before the 28th week of pregnancy) or those who are very small (about 3 lb, or 1,500 g) are still at risk because all of their organs are not fully developed. Prolonged lack of oxygen may permanently damage the brain or lungs.

A baby in intensive care A baby who has respiratory distress syndrome may need a mechanical ventilator to breathe properly. Neonatal intensive care units (specialized hospital units for treating newborns) are equipped with these and other machines to treat newborns who are seriously ill.

Neonatal jaundice

Neonatal jaundice causes yellowing of an infant's skin, soon after birth. This condition usually clears up without treatment in a few days. Jaundice is caused by an excess of bilirubin, a waste product of the normal breakdown of red blood cells, in the blood. Normally, bilirubin is removed from the blood by the liver. In newborns, jaundice usually occurs when the liver is not yet functioning completely when the baby is delivered; therefore, the liver does not process the bilirubin fast enough. The result is known as physiological jaundice. This problem often occurs in premature babies.

Another cause of neonatal jaundice is hemolytic disease. In hemolytic disease, antibodies from the mother, which are normally protective substances, enter the fetus's bloodstream and combine with the fetus's red blood cells, causing the cells to break down more quickly than usual (see Rhesus incompatibility, p.672). This early breakdown results in excess release of bilirubin, and the baby is severely jaundiced at birth.

Obstructive jaundice, a more serious form of the condition, is caused by malformed or absent bile ducts. Bile and bilirubin cannot pass out of the liver, and bilirubin builds up in the blood. Other rare causes of neonatal jaundice are neonatal hepatitis, blood disorders, and hypothyroidism (see p.567).

What are the symptoms?

In all types of jaundice, a baby's skin and the white of the eyes turn yellow. The baby's skin may even have an orange-yellow color, as though he or she were sun-tanned. In hemolytic disease the yellow color appears within the first day after birth, in physiological jaundice after about 2 days, and in obstructive jaundice usually after 1 to 2 weeks. In physiological jaundice and mild hemolytic disease, the yellow coloring is slight and usually disappears after a few days, but in severe cases of hemolytic disease and obstructive jaundice the discoloration grows more pronounced, and it must be treated.

What are the risks?

Physiological jaundice occurs in over half of all newborns. However, hemolytic disease is uncommon, and obstructive jaundice is extremely rare.

Jaundice carries the remote risk that a very high level of bilirubin in the blood will cause brain damage. But brain damage almost never occurs, provided that the baby is treated and the level of bilirubin in the blood is checked regularly. In obstructive jaundice, surgery to correct the blockage in the outflow of bile and bilirubin from the liver is needed to prevent fatal liver damage, which can occur within a few months if not treated.

What is the treatment?

In most cases of physiological jaundice, no treatment is necessary. In mild cases of hemolytic disease, jaundice disappears without treatment. Obstructive jaundice usually requires surgery. Otherwise, when the level of bilirubin is high, a physician may expose the baby to blue light (phototherapy), which aids in converting the bilirubin to a form that will pass out of the liver. Severe cases of jaundice, especially those caused by hemolytic disease, are treated by an exchange blood transfusion, in which all the baby's blood is replaced.

Feeding problems

If your baby appears to be getting an adequate amount of breast milk, but still seems to be hungry and irritable, try offering the baby a supplemental bottle of formula after he or she has nursed from both breasts. If the baby takes another 3 or 4 ounces, check with your physician. He or she may recommend that you continue to offer a bottle of formula as a supplement to nursing your baby.

Crying after and between feedings

Many babies cry for a few minutes after eating. Cuddle your baby, and if he or she has had enough to eat, the child will soon go to sleep. If your baby continues to cry, or cries a lot between feedings, it is possible that he or she has not had enough to eat. Try giving your baby more. Do not worry about overfeeding. The baby will stop eating when he or she has had enough.

Some babies cry because they are thirsty, especially in hot weather. Give your baby some boiled and cooled water in a bottle.

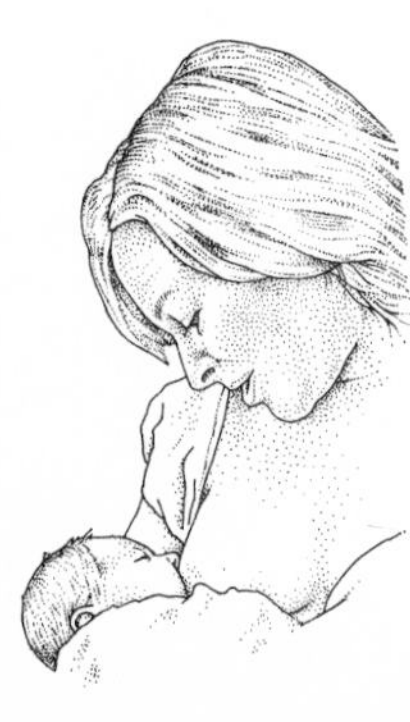

Poor feeding

During their first few weeks, some babies start to eat actively, then fall asleep before they have spent enough minutes at the breast or drunk enough milk. If this happens, gently wake the baby and continue the feeding until you are confident that the baby has taken enough. This phase passes in a healthy baby, but if it continues, he or she may have an infection, and should see a physician. See your physician also if your baby eats slowly for 2 or 3 days after having eaten normally.

Bottle-feeding

Prepared formula is more popular in the US than powders and concentrates that must be mixed with water, although all three types of formula are available. Prepared formula comes in milk-based and soybean-based varieties because some infants are allergic to milk (see Lactose intolerance, p.733).

Always prepare powdered and concentrated formulas exactly as specified in the package directions or as directed by your physician. Formula that is too diluted (too weak) can prevent your baby from getting enough nourishment.

A baby who fusses soon after starting a bottle may be frustrated because the nipple hole is too small or clogged. If you think this might be a problem, substitute another nipple.

Spitting up after feeding

Most babies spit up a little milk, particularly when they burp. This is especially true of bottle-fed babies, because they may swallow air when feeding, and that may overfill the stomach. Some very active babies spit up a lot. This is usually nothing to be concerned about. Spitting up gradually stops after solid food is introduced, when the baby is 4 to 6 months old, and it usually stops completely by the time the baby is 9 months old. Spitting up is also called regurgitation.

Vomiting, rather than regurgitation, may be due to some disorder such as pyloric stenosis (see p.502). Check with your physician, especially if the vomit shoots some distance. This is called projectile vomiting, and it can indicate serious illness.

Beginning solid foods

Infants are usually ready to begin gradually eating solid foods at between 4 to 6 months old. Start by spoon-feeding your child baby cereal twice a day. Then introduce your baby to a variety of pureed vegetables and fruits, one at a time so you can detect any problems that may occur. When your baby is older, you can add finely chopped meat and eggs. Try to start your baby off with good eating habits: do not give him or her foods high in sugar, fat, or salt, or highly refined foods, and only give food at mealtimes. Also, do not use food as a means of pacifying your baby.

Gastroenteritis in infants

If the stomach and small intestine become inflamed from such causes as a bacterial infection or food intolerance, a baby will have diarrhea and will vomit. The disorder may be just a mild stomach upset, or may be a severe episode that leads to dehydration.

Almost all gastrointestinal problems are caused by viruses spread by coughing, sneezing, or poor hand washing. Contrary to popular opinion, most stomach upsets have nothing to do with bottle sterilization.

What are the symptoms?

The baby has frequent loose, green, watery bowel movements. In mild cases, the baby remains happy and eats well. In more severe episodes, the baby is miserable and irritable, eats poorly, has a slight fever, and may vomit. A baby who has as many as 10 bowel movements in a day may become dehydrated. Signs of dehydration are a dry mouth, sunken eyes and soft spot, lethargy, irritability, and in some cases, vomiting up all fluids. In severe dehydration, a dangerous condition, the baby's skin loses its elasticity. That is, when you pinch the child's skin between your thumb and finger, it does not immediately return to its original position. In addition, the baby refuses to eat, and may have either a fever or a below-normal temperature.

What are the risks?

Most cases of gastroenteritis in infants are mild or are treated before severe dehydration can occur, and the child suffers no lasting effects. If dehydration reaches an advanced stage, however, it can cause kidney and brain damage or even death.

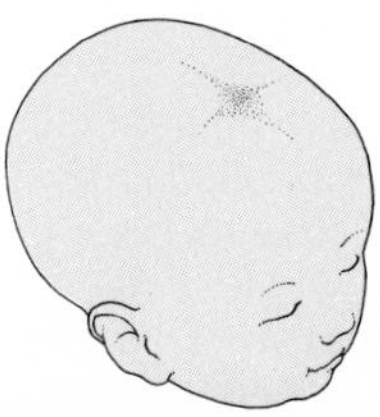

Depressed soft spot
If the soft spot (fontanelle) on top of your baby's head seems to sink, the baby may be dehydrated, possibly because of a stomach upset with diarrhea. Call your physician immediately.

What should be done?

You can treat mild gastroenteritis by following the self-help measures in this article. See your physician immediately or go directly to a hospital emergency department if your baby has symptoms of dehydration, has three large or loose bowel movements and/or vomits all feedings in a 6-hour period.

What is the treatment?

Self-help: Talk to your physician as soon as diarrhea and vomiting develop. If you are bottle-feeding, stop the baby's usual feeding for 24 hours and substitute an electrolyte-sugar solution available at your pharmacy, in order to restore the fluids that your baby has lost. (If the fluids will not stay down, go to a hospital emergency department.) On the second day, replace this liquid with a soybean formula or the usual formula diluted to one half of the normal strength. Use two-thirds–strength formula on the third day, and three-quarter–strength on the fourth day. During this time, give the baby the same volume of food as usual, but feed it in small amounts every hour or so. On the fifth day, return to normal feeding.

If you are breast-feeding your baby, resume feeding after 12 to 24 hours of using the electrolyte-sugar solution.

Professional help: A baby who is having a serious episode of gastroenteritis will usually be hospitalized. In the hospital the baby will be given special liquids to replace the lost water and vital chemicals, first intravenously and then by mouth as the baby recovers.

In most cases, the baby recovers completely, with no aftereffects.

Diaper rash

See p.242, **Visual aids to diagnosis, 4.**

Prolonged moisture and other irritants can inflame the skin on a baby's buttocks, thighs, and genitals and cause diaper rash. The irritants are mainly chemicals in the baby's stools or in soap or detergent left in diapers if they are not thoroughly rinsed. Most babies have diaper rash at some time. The best way to avoid the problem is to change wet or soiled diapers promptly.

What are the symptoms?

The skin in the area covered by the diaper becomes red, spotty, sore, and moist. The rash varies in severity. It may look alarming, especially to new parents.

What should be done?

Diaper rash is generally a problem that parents can deal with themselves. In some cases, however, the inflamed skin becomes infected with the fungus called *Candida*, and treatment with a nonprescription antifungal cream or ointment is necessary. See your physician if the treatment described below does not rapidly improve the rash.

What is the treatment?

The most important first step is to change all diapers promptly when they are soiled. After washing cloth diapers, rinse them several times to remove all traces of soap or detergent. Be aware that fabric softeners may cause skin reactions in the diaper area. Plastic pants usually have nothing to do with whether a baby gets diaper rash. If diapers are not changed frequently enough, however, waterproof pants keep the rash moist, and can aggravate it.

There are several treatments for diaper rash. One is to expose the baby's buttocks to a warm, dry atmosphere. Take the baby's diaper off and lay him or her chest down, with the face turned to one side, on soft towels covering a waterproof sheet. Any stools or urine produced should be cleaned up immediately and the rash bathed with warm water and a mild soap. Change the towels if necessary. Afterward pat the affected area dry with a soft towel, and lightly sprinkle the rash with baby powder.

It may be more practical to obtain a nonprescription cream or ointment from a pharmacy to help relieve the rash. For mild rashes, use a cream that contains zinc oxide and mineral oil. Immediately after cleaning the diaper area, place a thick layer of the zinc oxide cream over the affected area. A cotton ball soaked with mineral oil may be used gently to clean any soiled area. Afterward, reapply the cream.

If the rash is serious or persists, see your physician, who may be able to give you more detailed practical help and a prescription ointment to speed healing.

Cradle cap

(seborrheic eczema)

See p.242, **Visual aids to diagnosis, 5.**

This common skin condition occurs during the first 2 years of life, usually during the first 3 to 6 months. Cradle cap, which occurs on the baby's scalp, is the most common form of seborrheic eczema. The eczema can also appear on the face, the folds of the neck, in the armpits, and in the groin.

In cradle cap, thin, dry scales appear on the scalp. Then yellow, greasy, scaly patches, which sometimes extend over the eyebrows and behind the ears, replace the initial scales. In seborrheic eczema on the face, there are small red blotches and pimples, which become redder when the baby cries, has a bath, or gets hot. Elsewhere, the eczema occurs as red, somewhat scaly patches.

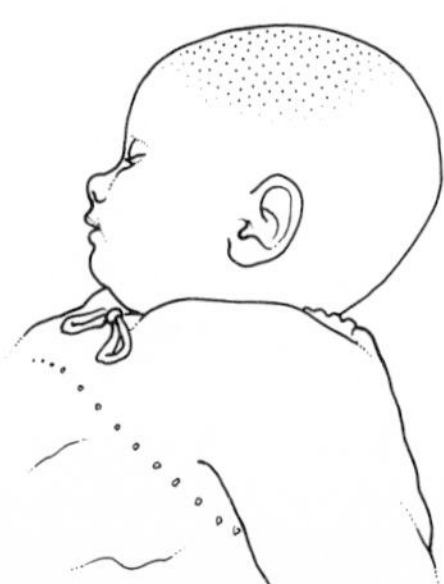

Cradle cap
The thin, dry scales of cradle cap cause no discomfort for the baby (left). They can be rubbed away gently with baby oil or ointment.

The eczema does not bother the baby and has no effect on his or her general health. In rare cases, it becomes infected; to prevent infection, keep the baby's head clean. When infected, the patches become soft, and yellowish pus oozes out.

What is the treatment?

Ask your physician whether you should use baby oil or a prescription ointment. Keep the affected areas clean and dry by bathing them with soap and water and drying them thoroughly. If cradle cap is unsightly, rub the scales gently with unscented baby oil, then comb the hair with a fine-tooth comb. This loosens the scales and they can be washed away during a shampoo. For other affected areas, bathing the baby with a gentle, bland lotion or cream may be helpful.

Be sure to talk to your physician if your baby's rash gets worse or becomes itchy and a nuisance, because an infection may have developed that needs immediate attention.

Excessive crying

During the first few weeks of life, a baby sleeps most of the time but may cry loudly when awake. An infant who has a weak, infrequent cry may be seriously ill. As the baby's awareness of his or her surroundings grows, wakeful periods without crying grow gradually longer until, at about 6 weeks, the baby may be awake and alert without crying for half an hour or so after some feedings. The number of quiet wakeful periods increases as the baby grows.

Babies are very different in their responses and development, so there are no definite rules for how much crying is excessive. Some babies cry more than others because of differences in personality.

Much of a placid baby's contentment may come from the mother, father, and any other loving person who is caring for the baby. In the same way, an anxious parent can transmit anxiety to the baby, who may then sleep badly and cry excessively. A vicious circle can evolve: the more the baby cries, the more anxious the parents become. Parents may become angry with the baby for crying so much, which causes the baby to cry even more. Some common explanations for excessive crying are discussed below.

Colic: The word colic means pain. The term is often used to refer to a baby crying loudly without apparent cause. Babies with colic seem to be miserable and may eat poorly, act as if they have a stomachache by drawing up their legs, and pass gas.

Infantile colic, as it is sometimes called, usually begins at 2 to 4 weeks of age. No one really knows what causes it, but the loud, continual crying of the baby can often be frightening and also exhausting for the parents. In all but a few cases, colic stops by the time the baby is 3 to 4 months old.

There is no specific treatment for colic, but some babies with colic seem to feel better if they sleep in a quiet room, are handled very gently, and get a lot of attention from their parents. If the baby is breast-fed, the mother should talk to her physician about her diet. Chocolate, milk, "gassy" vegetables such as broccoli, cabbage, and beans, spicy foods, citrus fruit, and alcohol are transmitted through breast milk and can cause discomfort in the infant. A bottle-fed baby may do better if you change to a soybean formula. Of course, every baby, especially one with colic, should be burped thoroughly after feeding.

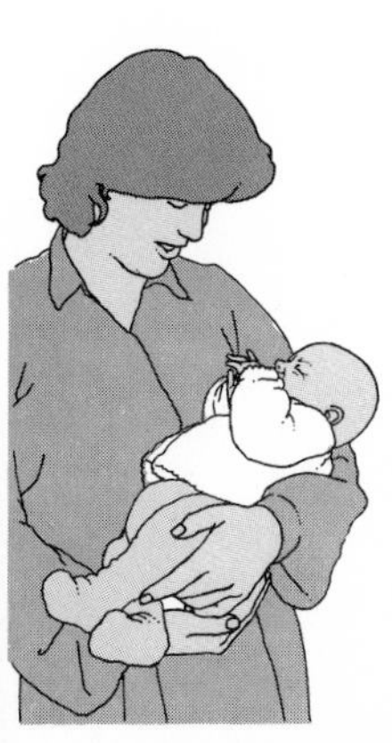

If your baby stops crying when picked up and held in your arms, he or she may simply want more comfort and attention.

Teething: Children generally cut their first teeth between ages 6 months and 2 years. Before the teeth emerge, the gums may be sore, and a baby may drool, rub his or her gums, and cry. Where a tooth emerges, the gum may be slightly swollen and inflamed, and the discomfort will make an infant cry. But the inflammation rapidly subsides, and even if several teeth are coming through, your baby should stop crying after a few days.

Passing urine: Sometimes a baby cries when he or she urinates. This leads some parents to believe that urinating is painful for their baby. In most cases, however, a baby starts crying before he or she urinates.

Some infants cry excessively and inconsolably because they are ill. A runny nose, a cough, vomiting, diarrhea, or poor eating may all be symptoms of an infection. The same symptoms may also indicate a problem such as a hernia in the groin area that is causing pain. If your baby stops crying when you pick him or her up, he or she may just want you to provide affection and attention. It is also possible that your baby may be eating food that upsets his or her stomach or that he or she is not eating enough food (see Feeding problems, p.694).

What should be done?

After you have made certain that your baby is not lonely, hungry, or uncomfortable because of a wet or soiled diaper, ask your physician to examine him or her. You may have success putting a crying baby to sleep by taking the child for a walk in a fabric child carrier, taking the child for a ride in the car, holding the child on your shoulder or across your lap while gently rocking in a chair, or putting a radio in the infant's room tuned to static (white noise).

If you are tired and irritable from getting up to feed your baby at night, try to sleep for a few hours during the day, while your baby sleeps. Talk to your partner about his role in caring for the baby. If possible, arrange a shift system with your partner, so that you are not the only one taking care of your baby. Let housework take second place to the well-being of you and your child.

Accept any offers of help from family or friends. If possible, treat yourself to an afternoon or evening out while someone you trust cares for your baby. If you are breast-feeding, make sure your baby has learned to accept an occasional bottle feeding.

If you still feel stressed, talk with your physician as soon as possible for help in finding practical ways in which you can cope with the situation.

Birthmarks

See p.241, **Visual aids to diagnosis, 1–3.**

A birthmark is any persistent area of discolored skin that is present from birth. A birthmark may be pink, red, or purple; the color results from a concentration of blood vessels in the skin. A birthmark can also be a tan or brown discoloration on the surface of the skin called a pigmented spot.

There are three main types of red marks. A capillary mark is pink or pinkish-brown. Many babies have capillary marks at birth, most of which gradually fade and disappear before the baby is 18 months old.

A strawberry mark or hemangioma is a bright red, raised area up to 4 in (10 cm) across. Such birthmarks occur on any part of the body. At birth this mark may be so small that it is not noticed for a few days. It grows rapidly for a few weeks, then increases in size proportionately with the baby. Occasionally, when there is fatty tissue or deeper blood vessels under the strawberry mark, the red area lies on top of a soft lump, about ⅓ to ¾ in (1 to 2 cm) above the skin. When the baby is about 6 to 10 months old, small, scattered gray-white areas can be seen in the mark. These gray-white spots spread, gradually replacing the red tissue, and at the same time the area becomes flatter. The mark usually disappears by the time the child is 5, but it can persist for a few more years, eventually leaving a slightly pale area of skin.

The third type of red mark, a port wine stain, is usually a purplish-red, often large, and sometimes partly raised area that occurs alone on the face, arm, or leg. Generally a port wine stain persists into adult life, although the mark may fade slightly.

The other type of birthmark, a pigmented spot, is most commonly a flat, irregularly shaped, tan or brown spot. Usually there are only one or two small spots in any area, but in some cases there are many spots, large spots, or both. Pigmented spots are generally permanent. These spots are often referred to as "beauty marks."

Persistent red birthmarks may cause disfigurement and bleed as the child grows older. Large, unsightly birthmarks can be treated by lasers as early as a few weeks of age. If you consider a birthmark to be unsightly, you can also cover it with a special skin-colored cream that can be obtained at a pharmacy. Larger brown pigmented spots may become cancerous later in life. Talk to your physician, who will recommend any necessary treatment.

A large strawberry mark occasionally bleeds, either on its own or if it is bumped or scratched, but pressing on the mark for several minutes usually stops the bleeding. If a strawberry mark near the eye enlarges, see your physician immediately.

Doubtful sex

During the first 3 months of pregnancy, the embryo secretes hormones (see p.553) that regulate the development of sex organs. If this hormone production is abnormal, the baby's sex organs will be malformed at birth.

Minor defects in the sex organs can usually be corrected by surgery. In rare cases, the defect may be so severe that it is impossible to determine the baby's gender by examining the genitals. In such cases, blood is drawn from the infant shortly after birth for chromosome analysis (see Box on Genetics, p.752) to find out the sex of the child.

Once the child's sex is known, treatment can be planned. Plastic surgery can make the appearance of the sex organs match the child's chromosome gender. Surgery is usually performed by age 2, and is sometimes performed as a series of operations over a period of years. In most cases, the surgery, hormone treatment, and psychotherapy will help the child lead a full life.

Should I have my son circumcised?

A 1989 report of the Task Force on Circumcision of the American Academy of Pediatrics concluded that circumcision is a generally safe procedure in infants when performed by an experienced person under sterile conditions. One advantage of circumcision is a decrease in the number of urinary tract infections. Also, with poor hygiene, a foul-smelling, cheesy, white secretion called smegma can accumulate under the foreskin. Research has shown that smegma may be a cancer-causing agent (carcinogen). Therefore, when your son grows up, there may be a decreased risk of cancer of the cervix in his sexual partners if he has been circumcised.

Complications, such as bleeding and infection, are rare. However, only healthy infants should be circumcised shortly after birth, to avoid possible problems with blood clotting.

The report by the American Academy of Pediatrics states that "when considering circumcision of their infant son, parents should be fully informed of the possible benefits and potential risks of circumcising a newborn, both with and without local anesthesia."

Down syndrome

In the normal human body, all cells except egg cells and sperm cells have 46 chromosomes each (see p.752). Sometimes a child is born with 47 chromosomes in each cell. Such a child has Down syndrome.

What are the symptoms?

Infants with Down syndrome are recognizable at birth by their facial appearance. The eyes slope upward at the outer corners, the face and features are small, and the tongue is large and tends to stick out. Other characteristics include a flat-backed head, sometimes a little finger curved toward the third finger, and often double-jointedness.

Children with Down syndrome are mentally impaired (see Learning problems, p.720), but they can still be active, loving participants in family life.

What are the risks?

Down syndrome affects about 1 out of every 600 to 800 babies born. A woman is at greater than average risk of having a baby with Down syndrome if she is over age 35 or if she or her spouse has a rare chromosome abnormality known as "translocation."

Measuring certain chemicals in the blood can identify women at increased risk of having a fetus with Down syndrome. These tests are now performed on pregnant women over age 35. If the test results are abnormal, more tests are needed (see Special procedures in pregnancy, p.684). Chorionic villus sampling or amniocentesis (see Box, p.684) can indicate the presence of Down syndrome.

About a third of children who have Down syndrome also have some form of congenital (present from birth) heart disorder (see p.702). They also have a slightly higher than normal incidence of intestinal atresia (see p.708) and acute leukemia (see p.729). Children with Down syndrome may be more susceptible to respiratory and ear infections.

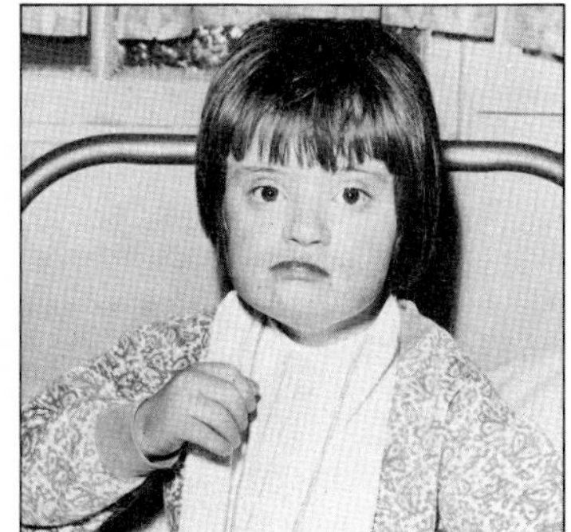

Typical facial features
Most children with Down syndrome have upward-slanting eyes and puffy eyelids. Sometimes the child's tongue sticks out slightly and his or her ears are abnormally shaped and set low.

What is the treatment?

Plans for the care of a child with Down syndrome should be discussed with your physician at the time of birth and frequently thereafter. It is best to raise a child with Down syndrome at home. Support is often available from local social service agencies.

In severe cases of Down syndrome, it may be necessary to send a child to an institution that can provide the care that he or she needs. If this is the case, be sure to visit and inspect any potential facilities, and interview staff members. To ensure that your child can develop physically and mentally to his or her best potential, it is essential that he or she be cared for in a loving, stimulating, challenging environment that is run by skilled staff.

What are the long-term prospects?

Children with Down syndrome usually can make the most of their abilities with education and a supportive environment. They will always, however, need a protective environment, and they will need to be cared for either by their families or in a facility for the mentally disabled. People with Down syndrome do not usually live beyond early middle age. Life expectancy is reduced if the person has severe congenital defects that sometimes accompany Down syndrome, such as congenital heart disorder.

Sudden infant death syndrome

(crib death)

The exact cause of sudden infant death syndrome—in which an apparently healthy baby dies while asleep—is not known. Usually, no cause of death is discovered. The risk of crib death is higher in winter and may be related to immaturity of the part of the brain that controls breathing. The problem does not seem to be hereditary. Crib death is more common in male infants and usually occurs when the baby is 2 to 3 months of age. Sudden infant death syndrome occurs at a rate of 1 per 5,000 live births.

Death of a baby is emotionally devastating, and the parents will need support from relatives and friends. Support groups or group therapy with other parents who have had the same experience can provide great comfort. The reassurance of a counselor that nothing could have been done to prevent the tragedy is extremely helpful. Psychiatric counseling may also be helpful.

If an infant dies suddenly, it is essential that an autopsy be performed to find out the exact cause of death.

Congenital disorders of the central nervous system

The central nervous system (described in detail on p.283) includes the brain and spinal cord. It develops in the fetus within the first 2 months of pregnancy from a strip of cells running along the back of the embryo. The edges of the strip gradually curl inward to form a tube of cells. The front part of this tube expands and forms the brain. The back part of the tube forms the spinal cord. Surrounding and inside the brain and spinal cord is a liquid produced by the brain called cerebrospinal fluid, which cushions the brain and spinal cord. As the bones develop, the skull and spinal column provide further protection.

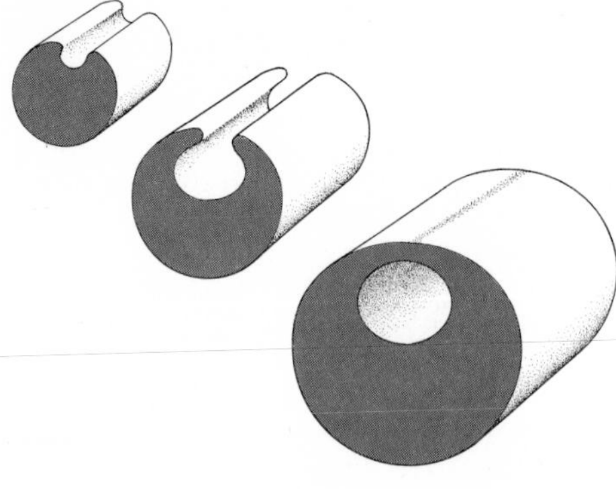

Beginning of the spinal cord
The spinal cord begins to develop when the embryo is about 20 days old. A groove appears in the center of what will be the baby's spine (right). Over a few days, the groove deepens and the edges begin to curve around toward each other (center). Within 3 days, the edges have fused and formed the tube that later develops into the spinal cord (far right).

A congenital disorder of the central nervous system is one that is present at birth, such as spina bifida, in which the spinal column and usually the spinal cord inside it are defective. In hydrocephalus, there is an excess of cerebrospinal fluid (the fluid that surrounds the brain and spinal cord) in and around the brain.

Congenital disorders of the central nervous system usually run in families. If a couple has one affected child, or relatives who have such a child, they should discuss the risks involved in any subsequent pregnancy with a genetic counselor (see p.664).

Spina bifida

In spina bifida, part of the spinal column does not develop fully. The nerves of the spinal cord in that area are exposed and unprotected and may also be defective. The disorder usually affects the lower spine. The spinal nerves in that area control the leg muscles, bladder, and bowels. A child born with spina bifida usually has some weakness or paralysis of the legs and may be unable to control his or her bladder and bowels. The extent of physical disability depends on the severity of the spinal defect.

What are the symptoms?

The defect in the lower spine and the resulting damage to the spinal cord varies from child to child. In some cases, the only visible sign may be a small dimple in the skin over the child's spine. Other children with spina bifida may have a large purplish-red membrane on their backs that covers a gap in the spine. In some children, the spine is also curved abnormally.

What are the risks?

The purplish-red membrane on the child's back is fragile and can be easily damaged. If an infection enters the cerebrospinal fluid through the damaged area, meningitis (see p.715) develops. Infections of the bladder are common in cases of spina bifida, and may result in kidney damage. When the child also has hydrocephalus (see next article), which often happens, there are additional risks.

What is the treatment?

Defects in formation of the spinal cord cannot be corrected. Any paralysis is permanent.

In many cases, surgery to repair the fragile membrane on the child's back is performed shortly after birth. Although it is usually not

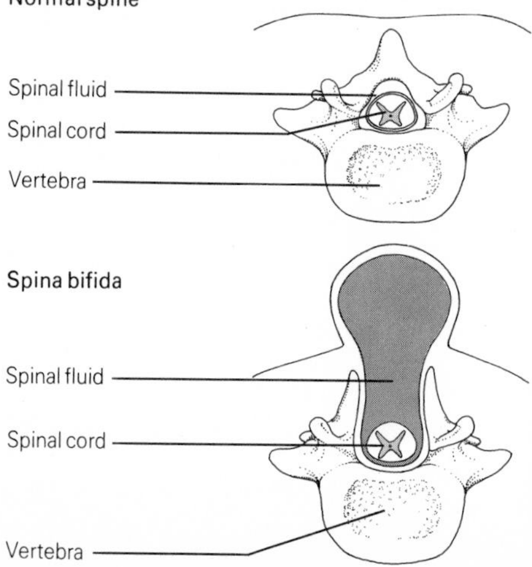

possible to repair the defective spinal nerves, physical therapy can be very helpful. Physical therapy can promote the development of the muscles that are unaffected, and children with spina bifida can learn to move around and become very mobile with the help of wheelchairs, braces, and walkers. For a child with spina bifida to develop his or her full potential, treatment in a children's hospital with physicians specializing in neurology is essential. Treatment with antibiotics may be needed to reduce the risk of urinary and other infections.

What are the long-term prospects?
Prospects for a child with spina bifida vary significantly according to the severity of the disorder and whether or not he or she also has hydrocephalus.

Sometimes surgery to correct deformities of the legs and/or to enable a child to achieve bladder control may be recommended. However, many children with spina bifida manage to achieve delayed bladder control on their own, with toilet training.

Children with spina bifida can often attend regular schools.

Hydrocephalus

Cerebrospinal fluid is found inside and surrounding the brain. This fluid is produced by the brain and passes into the space around the brain, where it is absorbed into a membrane that surrounds the space. If that membrane is defective in a developing fetus, or if the flow of cerebrospinal fluid is blocked, the fluid builds up in the cavities of the brain. The increasing pressure causes the child's brain to swell. To accommodate the swelling, the loosely connected bones of the skull spread apart, and the child's head becomes larger than normal. In particularly severe cases of hydrocephalus, the brain is permanently damaged.

Hydrocephalus may also occur later in infancy as a result of damage to the brain from an infection or a tumor.

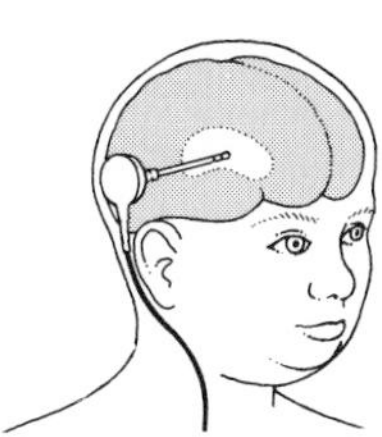

Treatment for hydrocephalus
The surgeon may insert a tube called a shunt in the child's head to drain the fluid from the brain into a vein in the neck or abdomen. The tube usually remains in place for life.

What are the symptoms?
Hydrocephalus may be suspected at birth if the circumference of the baby's head is significantly larger than average, depending on the overall size of the infant. If hydrocephalus is suspected, the head will be measured once a week for a few weeks, and if its rate of growth is greater than normal, depending on the age and size of the baby, an ultrasound scan, an MRI scan, or a CT scan (see Box, p.295) may be performed.

What are the risks?
Hydrocephalus is rare and sometimes occurs with spina bifida (see previous article). If hydrocephalus is well advanced at birth, serious brain damage will usually result. Brain damage severely limits both physical and mental development, and the infant may die of infection.

What is the treatment?
Hydrocephalus is treated surgically. The baby is given a general anesthetic and a small hole is drilled in the skull. A delicate tube with a one-way valve is inserted into the hole and installed between the brain at one end and a major blood vessel leading into the abdominal cavity or the heart at the other. Fluid drains from the brain into the bloodstream through this tube.

After the operation, the size of the baby's head gradually returns to normal. During the first year, the baby will need a checkup about once a month. As the child grows, the tube may become blocked, which allows pressure to build up in the brain. The child will become irritable and vomit frequently. Vomit may spurt out as much as several feet away. This is called projectile vomiting. If this happens, see your physician immediately. The child will be hospitalized to have the blockage removed or the tube replaced.

What are the long-term prospects?
In most cases where surgery is performed early, the chances of normal mental and physical development are good.

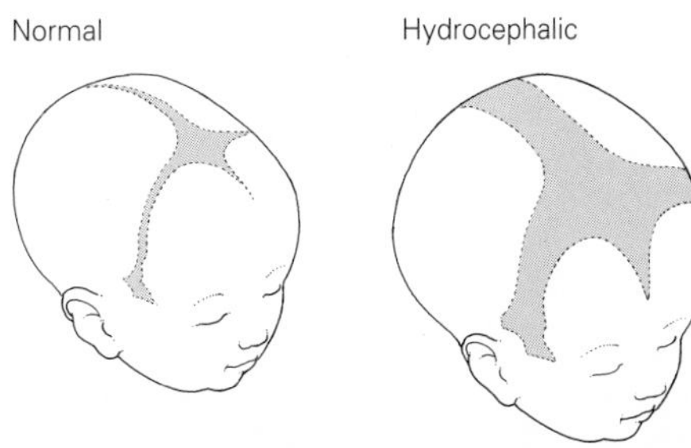

Congenital heart disorders

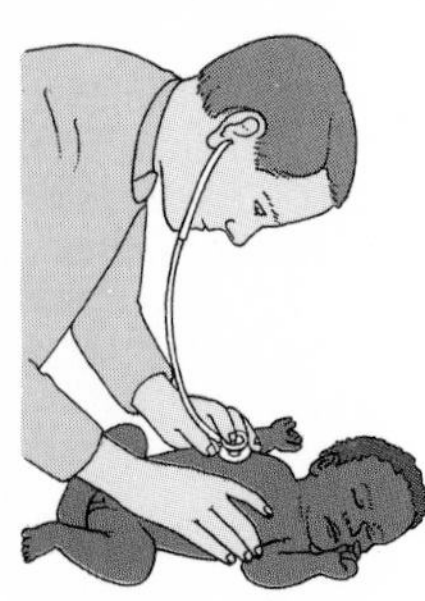

Most heart murmurs heard at birth do not indicate heart disease.

About 8 in every 1,000 babies born will have a heart abnormality of some kind. A congenital (present from birth) abnormality may be so minor that it needs no treatment and has no effect on the child's health. Other congenital heart disorders may be so severe that immediate treatment is necessary.

The development of abnormalities

The heart of a fetus starts to develop early in pregnancy and is fully developed by the third month of pregnancy. Any abnormality of development during this vital period can cause a congenital heart disorder. An abnormality may result if the pregnant woman develops an infection such as rubella (German measles, see p.746) during the early stages of pregnancy. In most cases, however, it is not known what causes the abnormality. An abnormality may result if the child has defective genes. Genetic disorders include Down syndrome (see p.699) and Marfan's syndrome. Marfan's syndrome is a disorder of the fibrous protein tissue called collagen that gives blood vessels and heart valves their strength. Marfan's syndrome causes weakness of the heart valves, especially the aortic and mitral valves, and of the aorta. Children with this disorder grow tall and thin. The lenses in their eyes may also be displaced. Ultrasound (see Box, p.684) examination of the fetus is often part of the assessment during the first few months of pregnancy, and the image obtained gives a clear picture of the internal organs. The heart is usually studied in detail, and any major developmental defect will be visible.

What are the symptoms?

In many cases of congenital heart disease, there are no symptoms, and the abnormality is discovered during a routine examination of the heart. In other cases, symptoms are obvious. Sometimes symptoms appear at birth, and sometimes they do not develop until childhood or much later. Symptoms are not directly related to the need for surgery; many cases without symptoms still require surgery to prevent problems from occurring later in life.

A common characteristic of congenital heart problems is cyanosis, or blueness of the skin. This occurs when the heart problem has allowed an excess of deoxygenated blood to circulate through the system. Mild heart failure (see p.408) in a baby may show up as difficulty in eating. The baby does not have enough energy to suck. The baby becomes underweight and cries less than usual. In severe heart failure, these symptoms are more severe. Breathing is rapid and difficult, and the baby may also have cyanosis.

Children with congenital heart disease may have difficulty breathing when they exert themselves, and if they have heart failure, they will have difficulty breathing even while resting. These children may have cyanosis, and their physical development is slow.

Medical myths

Any child who has a heart murmur must have surgery or lead the life of an invalid.

Wrong. About one fourth of children who have heart murmurs do not have anything wrong with their hearts. Others may have only a slight abnormality and should be encouraged to lead an active life. Restrict your child's activities only if your physician advises you to do so.

What should be done?

Diagnosis of a congenital heart disorder is usually made by examining the heart with a stethoscope (an instrument for listening to internal sounds). The stethoscope helps a physician hear the sounds made by the heart when the ventricles contract and the valves snap shut. Most unusual sounds that the heart makes are called heart murmurs. Presence of a murmur does not always mean that the heart is unhealthy. Some murmurs are a sign of abnormality while other murmurs are not. A particular type of abnormality will usually produce a particular type of murmur. Because of this, a physician can usually determine the type of heart abnormality by making an examination with a stethoscope. Additional tests can be performed to confirm the diagnosis of a disorder. These tests include an echocardiogram (an ultrasound examination of the heart), an electrocardiogram (a recording of the electrical impulses generated by the heart), and a chest X ray.

If your child has an insignificant heart murmur, treat him or her like any other child. Physical activity does not pose any unusual health risks to a child with an insignificant heart murmur.

Once your physician has detected an abnormality, additional tests are performed to determine the extent of the problem. An X ray of the chest indicates abnormalities in the shape and size of the heart chambers. An electrocardiogram (ECG) records the electrical impulses associated with the heartbeat and often reveals any enlargement of the chambers of the heart or abnormalities of rhythm. Also, an echocardiogram is usually performed to measure the thickness of the heart chamber walls and the condition and shape of the valves.

In some cases, a test called cardiac catheterization is required. The child is anesthetized or sedated, and a thin tube called a catheter is passed into a blood vessel, usually through a small incision (cut) in a leg, until it reaches the heart. Your physician watches the tube on an X-ray screen as it moves through the heart and passes through any abnormal openings. The catheter also enables your physician to measure the blood pressure in each chamber of the heart and the amount of oxygen in the blood in each chamber of the heart. Finally, an X-ray moving picture is taken while a liquid that shows up on X rays is passed through the catheter into the heart and lungs. This film shows the shape and size of the chambers, valves, and blood vessels of the heart.

With the information obtained from these procedures, pediatric heart specialists and chest surgeons can usually diagnose the child's problem exactly and can then recommend appropriate treatment.

What is the treatment?

Most cases of congenital heart disease require surgery to correct the abnormality. Surgery is usually delayed until early childhood, unless the disorder is so severe that immediate surgery is necessary. Successful correction is easier to achieve in childhood than in infancy because the child is more able to withstand open-heart surgery. The success rate for most heart surgery on children is high, and children who have had successful operations can usually live a full life.

An infant with heart failure may need to take digitalis to strengthen the heart muscle and diuretics to reduce excess body fluid. Medication is used until surgery is possible.

Now that heart transplantation (see p.432) is an established medical procedure, transplants are being performed on infants who have major heart defects that cannot be corrected with other forms of treatment. There is, however, a severe shortage of appropriate donor organs.

The normal heart before and after birth

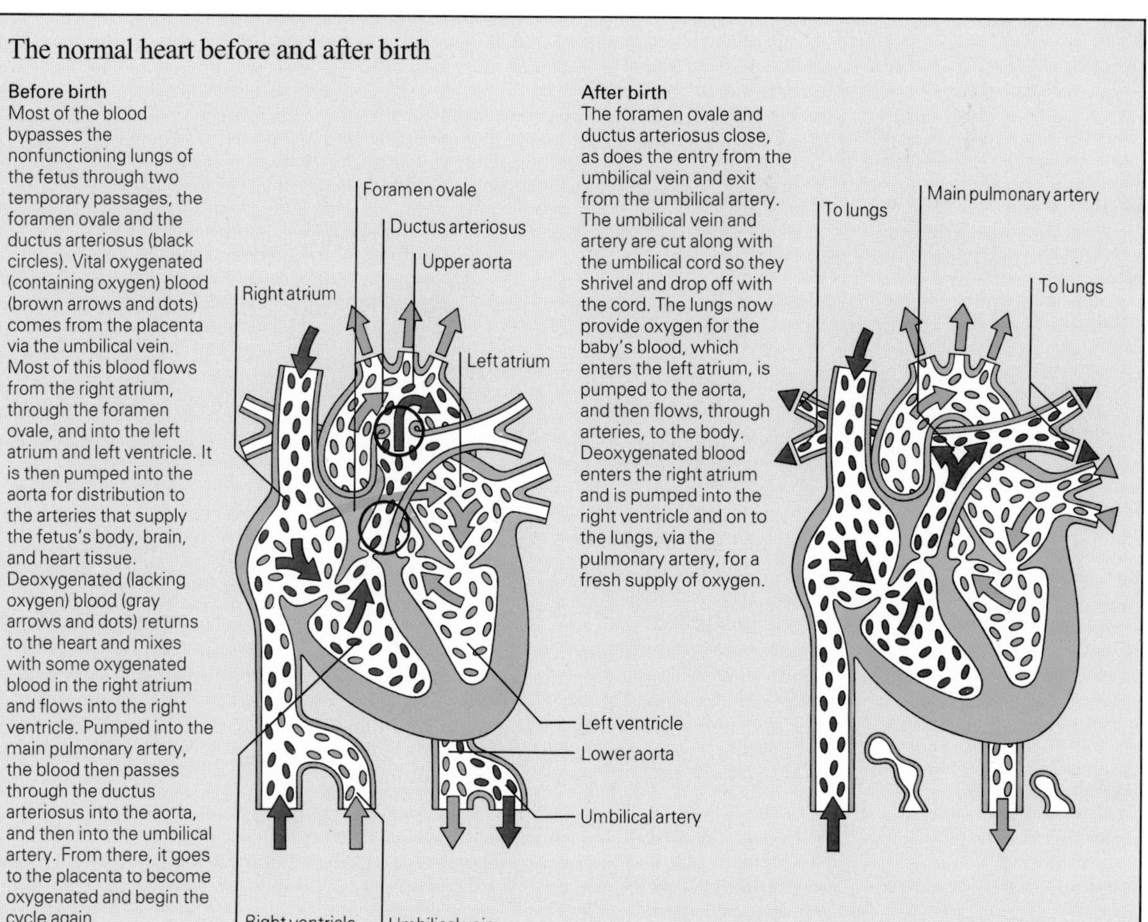

Before birth
Most of the blood bypasses the nonfunctioning lungs of the fetus through two temporary passages, the foramen ovale and the ductus arteriosus (black circles). Vital oxygenated (containing oxygen) blood (brown arrows and dots) comes from the placenta via the umbilical vein. Most of this blood flows from the right atrium, through the foramen ovale, and into the left atrium and left ventricle. It is then pumped into the aorta for distribution to the arteries that supply the fetus's body, brain, and heart tissue. Deoxygenated (lacking oxygen) blood (gray arrows and dots) returns to the heart and mixes with some oxygenated blood in the right atrium and flows into the right ventricle. Pumped into the main pulmonary artery, the blood then passes through the ductus arteriosus into the aorta, and then into the umbilical artery. From there, it goes to the placenta to become oxygenated and begin the cycle again.
Foramen ovale
Ductus arteriosus
Upper aorta
Right atrium
Left atrium
Left ventricle
Lower aorta
Umbilical artery
Right ventricle
Umbilical vein
After birth
The foramen ovale and ductus arteriosus close, as does the entry from the umbilical vein and exit from the umbilical artery. The umbilical vein and artery are cut along with the umbilical cord so they shrivel and drop off with the cord. The lungs now provide oxygen for the baby's blood, which enters the left atrium, is pumped to the aorta, and then flows, through arteries, to the body. Deoxygenated blood enters the right atrium and is pumped into the right ventricle and on to the lungs, via the pulmonary artery, for a fresh supply of oxygen.
To lungs
Main pulmonary artery
To lungs

Congenital aortic stenosis

Aorta

Narrowed aortic valve

Abnormality Narrowing near the beginning of the aorta, and sometimes of the aortic valve as well, that restricts the flow of blood to the body.
Effects Usually none. In rare cases, the child may have severe heart failure and cyanosis (blueness of the skin). The child may have shortness of breath, chest pains, and blackouts. Rarely, a child may die suddenly without symptoms.
Treatment Surgery is generally performed to relieve or remove the constriction (narrowing) when the blood pressure is high in the left ventricle.

Congenital pulmonic stenosis

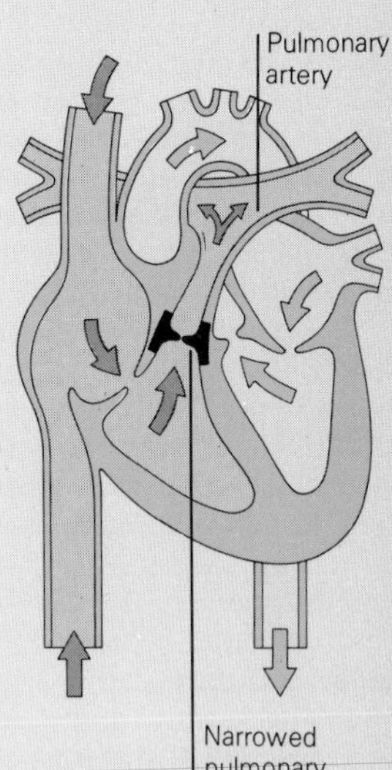

Abnormality Narrowing of the pulmonary valve or, more rarely, of the upper right ventricle. The narrowing reduces the flow of blood to the child's lungs.
Effects Usually none. Some children have shortness of breath when they exert themselves, tire easily, and may have cyanosis (blueness of the skin) if the foramen ovale (see The normal heart before and after birth, p.703) is forced to reopen. Other children may experience severe heart failure.
Treatment If the stenosis is mild, no treatment is necessary. If it is moderate or severe, surgery is performed to relieve or remove the constriction (narrowing).

Ventricular septal defect

(hole in the heart)

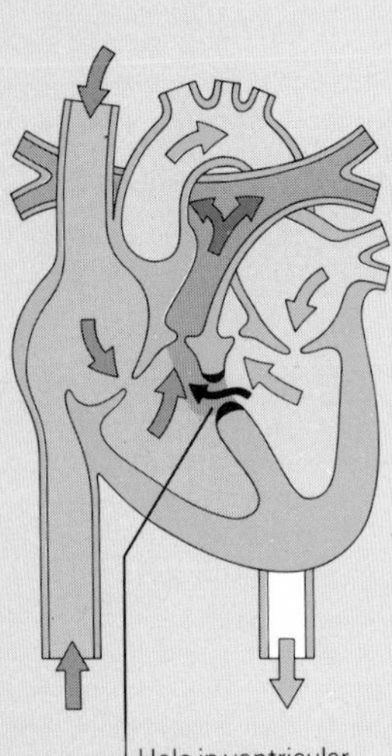

Abnormality A hole in the ventricular septum, or wall. Blood flows abnormally from the left ventricle into the right, sometimes in large quantities, so that excess blood travels to the lungs.
Effects Most children have no symptoms, but if the problem is severe, they may tire easily and have shortness of breath when they exert themselves. Occasionally a child may have severe heart failure or pulmonary hypertension (high blood pressure in the lung vessels).
Treatment Usually a small hole will become smaller or close on its own and does not require treatment. If a hole does not close on its own, or for a larger hole, open-heart surgery is usually needed, although it is often delayed until the child is 2 to 3 years old. If pulmonary hypertension has developed, a preliminary operation to relieve the high blood pressure in the arteries that supply blood to the lungs is performed between 6 and 12 months of age.

Atrial septal defect

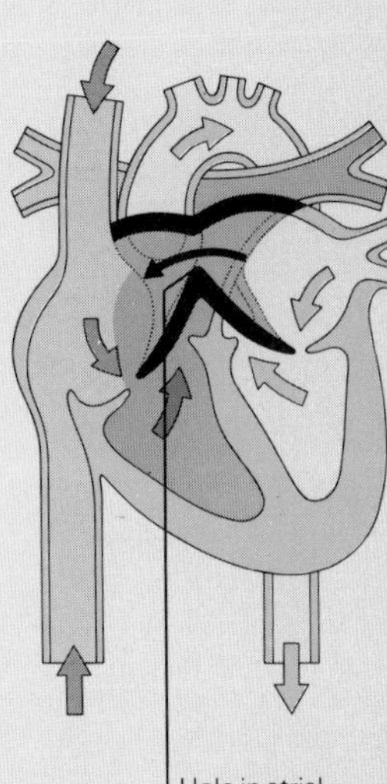

Abnormality A hole in the atrial septum, or wall. Blood passes from the left atrium into the right atrium, sometimes in large amounts, so that excess blood circulates through the lungs. The hole rarely closes without treatment.
Effects Most children have no symptoms, or they may tire easily and have shortness of breath when they exert themselves. If the disorder is not detected and treated in childhood, pulmonary hypertension may develop in late adolescence or in adulthood.
Treatment Surgery is necessary to correct the defect unless the hole is very small so that there is no danger that pulmonary hypertension will develop later. The operation is usually performed when the child is past 2 years of age.

Coarctation of the aorta

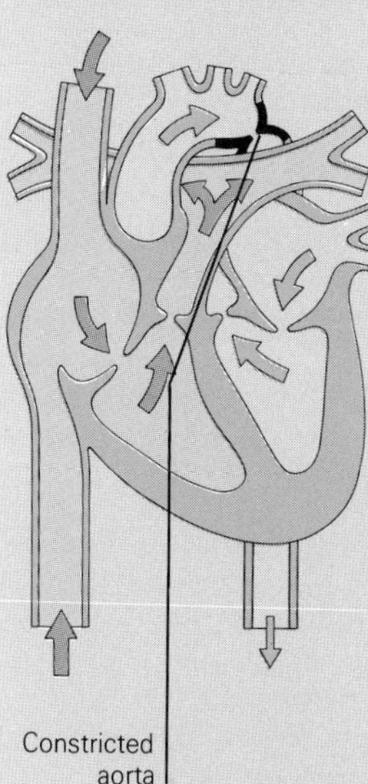

Abnormality Localized (restricted to a limited area) narrowing of the aorta that reduces the supply of blood to the lower part of the body.
Effects Some children have no symptoms. Others develop headaches, weakness after exercise, weak or absent pulses in the groin, and sometimes coldness in the legs. These symptoms are caused by high blood pressure above the narrowed area and low blood pressure below it. If the aorta is too constricted, severe heart failure (see p.408) may occur.
Treatment Surgery is necessary in all cases, even when there are no symptoms. The constriction (narrowing) is removed and the two parts of the aorta are rejoined. The surgery is usually performed around 1 year of age.

Patent ductus arteriosus

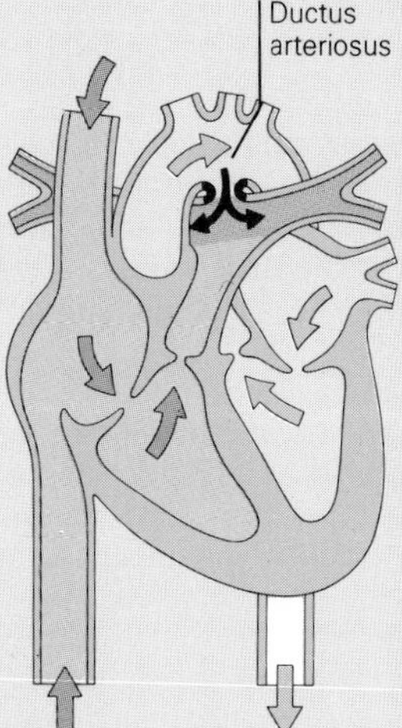

Abnormality The ductus arteriosus, an extra blood vessel in the heart before birth, fails to close after birth. Blood from the aorta continues to flow through it into the pulmonary artery, so that excess blood passes through the lung vessels.
Effects Usually there are no symptoms. In a few cases, the child has shortness of breath during exertion, frequent respiratory infections, and/or cyanosis (blueness of the skin).
Treatment In some cases, if detected early, the ductus arteriosus can be closed by treatment with a nonsteroidal anti-inflammatory medication. In most other cases, a simple operation to close the duct can be performed after the infant is 6 months old, if full term, or after 9 months of age, if he or she was premature.

Fallot's tetralogy

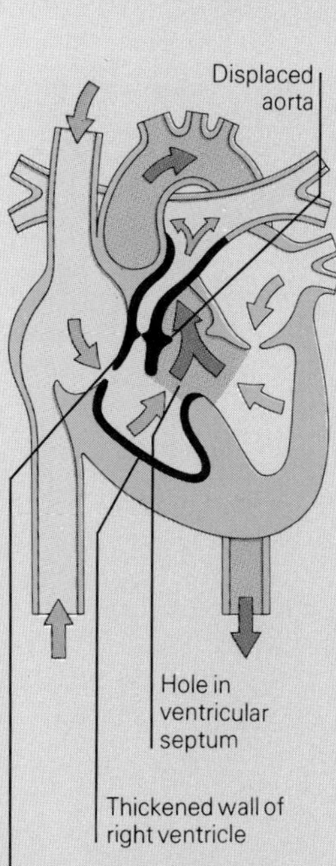

Abnormalities Four abnormalities occur together: a hole in the upper ventricular septum; a displacement of the aorta to the right, so that blood from both ventricles enters it; pulmonary stenosis (see previous page); and a thickening of the right ventricle's wall.
Effects From birth, or shortly afterward, cyanosis (blueness of the skin, particularly the lips), clubbing of the fingers and toes (thickening and broadening of the tips, with increased curving of the nails), and generalized underdevelopment occur. After exertion, the child is short of breath and squats to relieve his or her discomfort.
Treatment Surgery to correct all the abnormalities is usually performed around 1 year of age.

Transposition of the great vessels

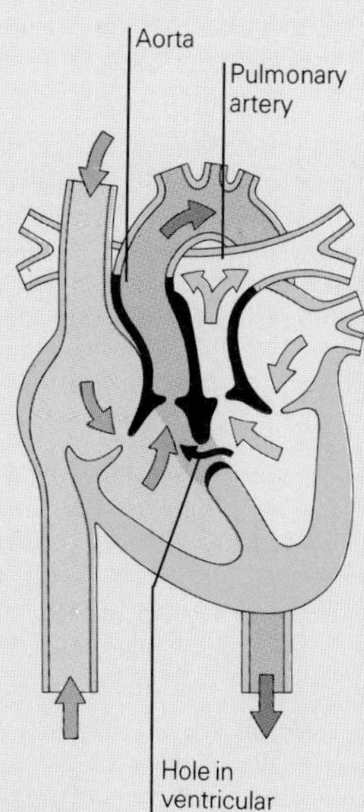

Abnormality The positions of the aorta and pulmonary arteries are reversed, so that oxygenated blood from the lungs passes through the pulmonary artery and back to the lungs, instead of through the aorta and to the tissues. Unless there is a hole in the septum or some other passageway that allows oxygenated blood to pass into the right side of the heart and the aorta, the infant will not survive.
Effects From birth, the child has cyanosis (blueness of the skin), clubbing of the fingers and toes, and underdevelopment.
Treatment Emergency surgery to create a larger hole in the septum is performed before the baby is 2 weeks old. In a second operation, performed before the child is 5 years old, the surgeon creates two artificial blood vessels that restore the circulation to normal.

Congenital disorders of the digestive system

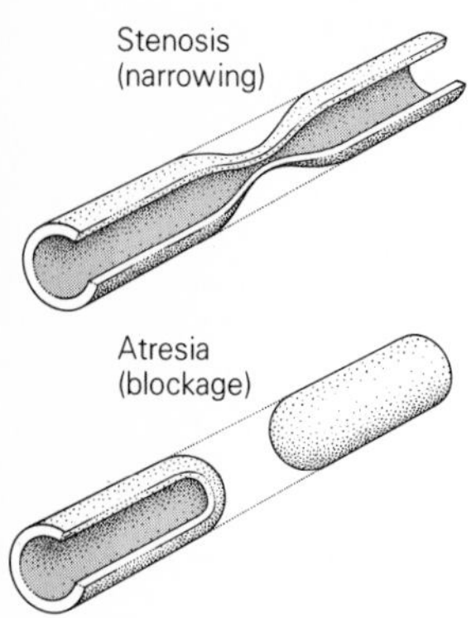

The digestive tract (described on p.468) is a continuous tube that digests food, absorbs nutrients from it, and eliminates what remains as waste matter. Glands connected to the digestive tract include the salivary glands and the pancreas, which produce digestive juices, and the liver, which provides bile to aid in digestion and absorption of food (see Liver, gallbladder, and pancreas, p.522).

While in the uterus, the fetus receives all nutrients from the pregnant woman through the placenta and umbilical vein. It is only after birth, when the baby must eat, that the digestive tract is used. Malformations of the digestive system that may have occurred during development, therefore, affect the baby only after birth. The digestive system is affected mainly by two kinds of malformations. One is stenosis, a narrowing of a tube or duct, sometimes almost to the point of closure. The other is atresia, a blockage in a tube or duct that separates it into two distinct, sealed-off sections. The causes of these defects are not known.

Any serious abnormality in the digestive tract affects an infant's ability to digest and absorb food, but there are also some more immediate risks. For example, in disorders that cause vomiting, a baby may inhale his or her vomit, which can lead to choking or pneumonia. Also, vomiting can lead to severe dehydration. The most common congenital (present from birth) disorders of the digestive system are described in this section. Most of these disorders can be successfully treated by surgery. An infant is prepared for surgery by being fed with intravenous fluid to keep the digestive tract empty and to maintain the correct balance of water and chemicals in the body. An infant usually recovers from successful surgery within 48 hours and can be taken home within a week.

Congenital pyloric stenosis

The pylorus is a short muscular tube that connects the stomach to the duodenum, the first section of the small intestine. In pyloric stenosis, the muscular wall of the tube thickens, and the passageway inside narrows. As a result, little or no milk can pass from the infant's stomach into the intestines and he or she does not receive enough nourishment. Therefore, the infant fails to thrive. The cause of pyloric stenosis is not known.

Duodenum
Stomach
Pylorus

In pyloric stenosis, the walls of the infant's pylorus (the tube connecting the stomach and the small intestine) are thickened, which obstructs the flow of milk from the stomach to the intestine.

What are the symptoms?

Between 2 and 8 weeks after birth, the baby begins to vomit violently after feedings. The infant's stomach makes strong contractions, trying to force food through the narrowed pylorus. Instead, food is forced up the esophagus and out of the mouth, sometimes spurting out as much as several feet away. This is called projectile vomiting. Usually the vomit contains a lot of curdled milk and mucus and has an unpleasant, sour odor. For the first few days, the vomiting does not interfere with the child's health or desire to eat. However, the baby soon begins to lose weight and becomes irritable and restless. At times, the baby will cry inconsolably. Then, the baby eats reluctantly and becomes listless because the constant vomiting dehydrates him or her.

What are the risks?

Pyloric stenosis is most common in first-born males, and usually runs in families.

Risks associated with vomiting include dehydration along with choking and pneumonia from vomit that has been inhaled. If not treated, pyloric stenosis can result in malnutrition and even death.

What should be done?

If your baby is vomiting in the way described, take him or her to see your physician immediately. If your physician suspects pyloric stenosis, he or she will examine the baby and then ask you to feed the baby. During the feeding, your physician will watch the baby's abdomen, looking for the strong contractions that precede vomiting caused by pyloric stenosis. Your physician will feel the abdomen for the swelling caused by an enlarged pylorus. A barium X ray of the upper digestive tract and an ultrasound examination of the pylorus may be necessary to confirm the diagnosis.

What is the treatment?

Self-help: Until your baby has surgery, feed him or her more often than usual, but reduce the amount of each feeding, so that less undigested food is in the stomach.

Professional help: Surgery to treat this disorder should be performed as soon as the diagnosis is confirmed. It is usually necessary to prepare the baby for surgery with intravenous fluids, to keep the digestive tract empty and to maintain the correct balance of fluid and chemicals in the baby's body.

The surgeon makes an incision along the outside of the thickened pylorus, which immediately allows the food to pass through. During the 48 hours after surgery, the amount of the baby's feedings is gradually increased until feeding becomes normal.

What is the long-term outlook?
The success rate of surgery for pyloric stenosis is almost 100 percent. After successful surgery, the infant will have no further feeding problems, and the disorder produces no aftereffects.

Esophageal atresia

In esophageal atresia, part of the esophagus (the tube that carries food from the throat to the stomach) is missing. The top part, which leads from the mouth, is a dead-end, and there is no passageway into the child's stomach. As a result, the infant cannot swallow secretions (saliva and mucus) from its mouth and nose. Instead, these secretions may enter the windpipe and partially block it.

What are the symptoms?
Esophageal atresia interferes with an infant's ability to breathe. Parents can hear continual bubbling noises in the throat, and sometimes the baby's skin turns blue from lack of oxygen. When a physician removes the secretions with a suction tube, the symptoms vanish but return as soon as the secretions build up again. When the baby eats, he or she may cough, gag, or sputter. A baby with this disorder should not be given food or liquids by mouth. Intravenous feeding, which is available in the hospital or through home health care services, is used to provide nourishment until the condition is corrected.

What should be done?
If your child has any of these symptoms, talk to your physician, who may check for esophageal atresia by trying to pass a soft tube down the baby's esophagus.

What is the treatment?
Surgery is performed in one or more stages to open and join the two separate sections of the esophagus. This procedure usually eliminates the problem.

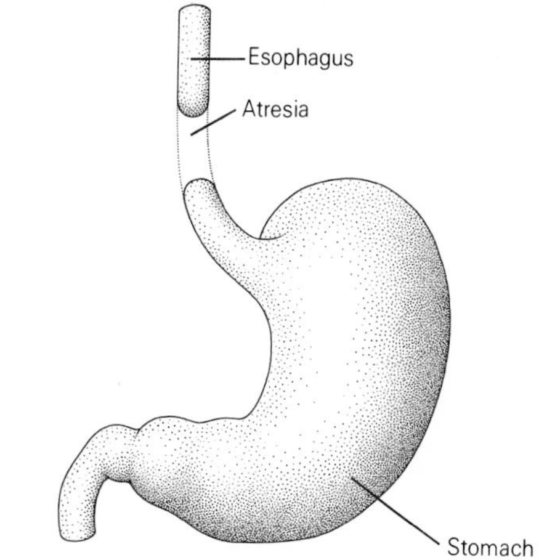

Esophageal atresia is corrected by an operation to join the separated parts.

Bile duct atresia

Bile, a liquid produced by the liver, is involved in many essential processes in the body. One function of bile is to carry a chemical compound called bilirubin (a waste product of the normal breakdown of red blood cells) from the liver into the intestine (see Neonatal jaundice, p.693). Bile travels through a series of tiny ducts in the liver and then through larger ducts outside the liver. The ducts outside the liver join to form the main bile duct that branches off to the gallbladder and then leads to the duodenum (the first section of the small intestine). Very rarely, an infant is born with atresia, in which parts of the bile ducts are missing, either inside the liver or leading away from the liver to the intestine. Bile is trapped in the child's liver and flows back into the bloodstream, causing jaundice. This is bile duct atresia.

What are the symptoms?
Symptoms of bile duct atresia include prolonged jaundice (yellowing of the skin), which usually starts during the second week after birth. The infant may also have pale or white stools and dark urine.

The jaundice is similar to that of neonatal hepatitis (see Neonatal jaundice, p.693), and it may be difficult to tell if the child has hepatitis or bile duct atresia.

What is the treatment?

If atresia is diagnosed, a surgeon will perform an operation, which is usually done when the baby is 2 to 3 months old, or earlier if possible. The inside of the baby's abdomen is examined, and if there is atresia of the ducts directly outside the liver, it is possible in some cases to enable bile to flow from the liver to the intestine by joining the gallbladder to the duodenum. In other cases, a loop of the middle section of the small intestine (jejunum) is attached to the base of the liver and bile drains from the liver into the newly attached loop.

If the bile ducts outside the liver appear normal, a small piece of liver is removed. Examining the fragment under a microscope will show whether the baby has hepatitis (see p.523), which eventually gets better by itself in most cases, or atresia of the small bile ducts in the liver. This form of atresia, and other types that cannot be corrected with surgery, are treated by liver transplantation. Many children have now had a liver transplant and the results have been encouraging (see Transplants, p.433).

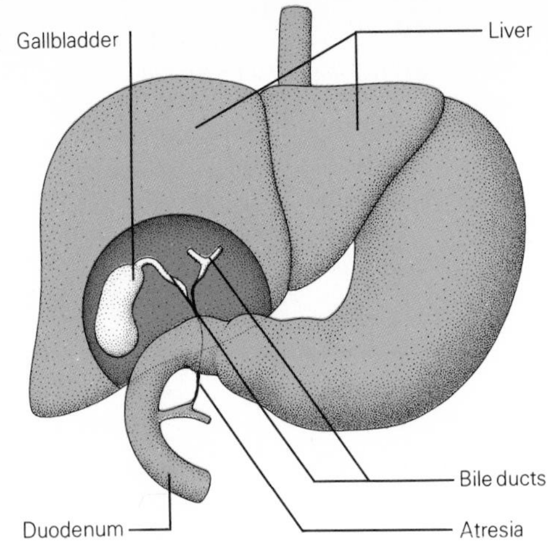

Atresia in the bile duct below the gallbladder can be corrected by joining the gallbladder to the duodenum and bypassing the lower part of the main bile duct. Atresia higher up the bile duct is more difficult to treat.

Intestinal atresia and intestinal stenosis

In intestinal atresia, an infant is born with one or more parts of the small intestine missing or shriveled into a useless cord without a passageway that is attached to two healthy sections of small intestine. In intestinal stenosis, part of the upper intestine is narrowed almost to the point of closure.

What are the symptoms?

An infant with either of these problems begins to vomit bile within a few hours of birth. Bile is a green liquid that is produced by the liver and passed into the intestine, mainly to help in digestion. The vomiting continues on and off, and the baby's abdomen swells as gas builds up in the intestine. Also, the child has no bowel movements. There are other disorders with similar symptoms, such as cystic fibrosis (see p.732) and Hirschsprung's disease (see next article). Diagnosis of any of these disorders may be aided by an X ray.

What is the treatment?

For either problem, surgery must be performed immediately. In atresia, the surgeon joins the separate parts of the intestine. In stenosis, the surgeon widens or removes the narrowed intestine. Surgery performed early is usually successful, and the child normally does not have long-term problems.

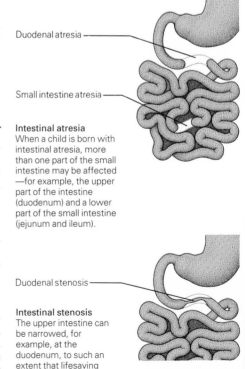

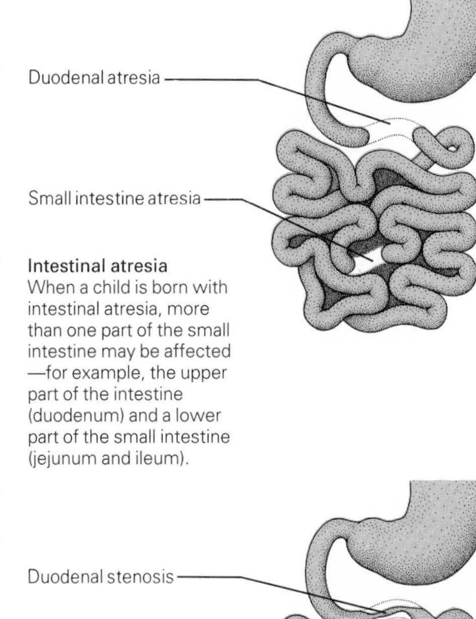

Intestinal atresia
When a child is born with intestinal atresia, more than one part of the small intestine may be affected—for example, the upper part of the intestine (duodenum) and a lower part of the small intestine (jejunum and ileum).

Intestinal stenosis
The upper intestine can be narrowed, for example, at the duodenum, to such an extent that lifesaving surgery to widen the intestine is needed as soon as possible.

Hirschsprung's disease

(congenital megacolon)

The large intestine contracts and pushes its contents toward the rectum to produce bowel movements. In some babies, segments in the lower parts of the large intestine, including the rectum, have no nerve cells to transmit the impulses that stimulate the necessary contractions. Because these segments of the large intestine do not function normally they are abnormally distended. This condition, called Hirschsprung's disease, causes severe constipation.

What are the symptoms?

The baby's bowel movements are infrequent and hard, and his or her abdomen is distended (swollen full of stool) and tight. In some cases, vomiting begins a few hours after birth (see previous article). The child fails to grow or gain weight, has anemia, and cries more easily than most infants.

Diagnosis of the disease is confirmed by a barium enema (see Glossary) and a biopsy of the rectum. In the biopsy, a small section of the rectum is removed and examined.

What is the treatment?

Surgery is performed to remove the affected part of the intestine and join the separate sections. The operation has a high success rate, and the outlook for the child is good.

Imperforate anus

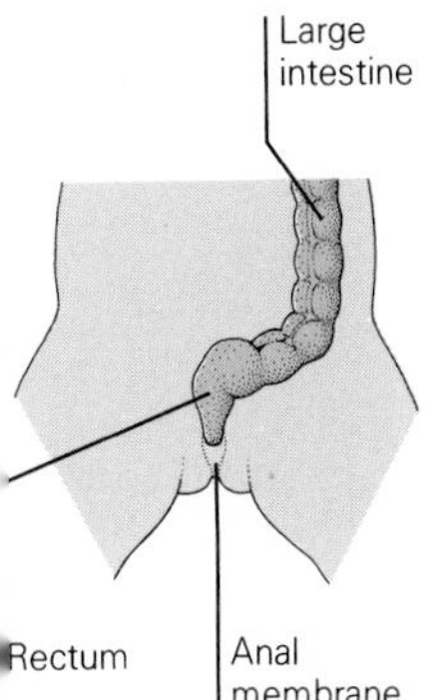

The anal canal is the final section of the digestive tract before the anus, the opening through which stools pass. Some babies are born with the canal imperforate, or closed. There may be a membrane stretching across the canal, or, in rare cases, the canal does not develop and the digestive tract ends at the rectum with no connection between the rectum and the anus.

What are the symptoms?

Examination of the child after birth will reveal the presence of the membrane across the anal canal. However, if the canal did not develop at all, the problem is more difficult to detect. Imperforate anus is suspected if the baby has not passed meconium (a green-black substance that accumulates in the intestines of the fetus) within 12 hours after birth. The diagnosis is confirmed when a finger or catheter inserted into the anus meets a blockage—the end of the rectum.

What is the treatment?

An operation is necessary to remove the membrane or to open the end of the rectum and join it to the anus. Surgery is usually successful, and the child can be trained to develop good bowel control. The training can take several years. The long-term outlook is good unless the muscles of the baby's anus are weak. In such cases, the child will have either severe constipation with hard stools or poor bowel control with soft stools. The child may then need an operation called a colostomy (see p.518), in which the surgeon creates an outlet for stool from the large intestine in the child's abdominal wall.

Diaphragmatic hernia

The diaphragm is a large sheet of muscle that separates the chest from the abdomen and plays a major role in breathing. Some infants are born with an opening in the diaphragm, through which part of the spleen, stomach, and/or part of the large and small intestines may stick up into the chest and press on the lungs, thereby causing breathing difficulties. In such cases, the baby's breathing may be assisted by a ventilator until surgery is performed. However, infants with this condition often die before or after surgery. Diaphragmatic hernia is diagnosed by an X ray.

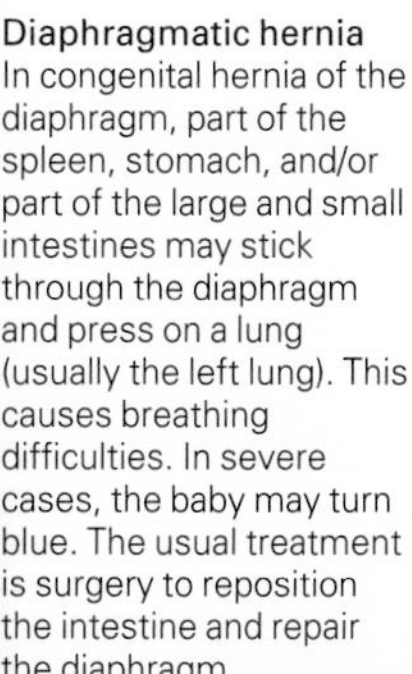

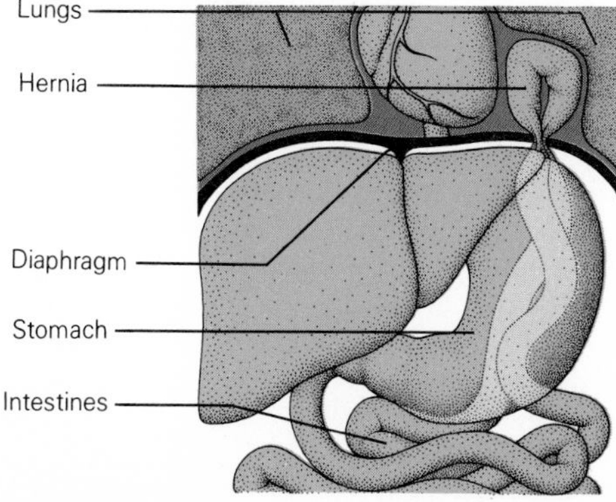

Diaphragmatic hernia
In congenital hernia of the diaphragm, part of the spleen, stomach, and/or part of the large and small intestines may stick through the diaphragm and press on a lung (usually the left lung). This causes breathing difficulties. In severe cases, the baby may turn blue. The usual treatment is surgery to reposition the intestine and repair the diaphragm.

What is the treatment?

Surgery is performed immediately. The chest is opened, the organs are pushed back into the abdomen, and the opening in the diaphragm is sewn up.

In some cases, the infant is placed on a special heart-lung machine, which removes carbon dioxide from the blood and supplies adequate oxygen, thereby enabling the diaphragm to rest and heal. This procedure improves the infant's chances of survival.

Congenital disorders of the skeleton

The four disorders described in this section are dislocation of the hip, club foot, and cleft lip and cleft palate (covered together). These disorders tend to run in families but they can also be the result of an abnormality in the development of the fetus before birth.

A child who has surgery to correct a dislocated hip will have difficulty in learning to walk. A child who has cleft lip and cleft palate will have difficulty in learning to speak and can also have problems eating. For these reasons, and because of the psychological strain on a child who must cope with such a disorder, these conditions should be treated as soon as possible. In the case of a dislocated hip, however, the problem may not be detected until childhood, when treatment is less likely to be successful.

A child who has a congenital (present from birth) disorder may need professional psychological treatment to help him or her cope with the physical and emotional challenges. The same is true if a parent or other family member has difficulty in dealing with a child's disorder. If you are having difficulty coping with a congenital disorder in your child, ask your physician for the names of some self-help organizations.

Congenital dislocation of the hip

Some infants are born with dislocation of the hip. When a hip is dislocated, the head of a thighbone lies outside of its socket in the pelvic bone. Also, the socket is shallow and poorly formed. One or both hips may be affected. The cause of the condition is not known, but about 1 baby in 60 is born with a suspected hip dislocation. The disorder tends to run in families, and it occurs more frequently in girls than in boys.

What are the symptoms?

Symptoms of congenital dislocation of the hip are not obvious. As part of the routine examination of a newborn, the physician manipulates the infant's hip joints, and if one or both are dislocated the physician will hear a click. A more reliable test uses ultrasound imaging to view the hips. The ultrasound image gives a clear picture of the hip joints and allows the physician to assess the severity of the underlying defect in the hip socket or sockets.

What is the treatment?

If the disorder is detected early, the baby is put into a brace to hold his or her hips in place. This treatment lasts for 6 to 8 weeks and is usually successful.

Ask your physician about any special care that your child may need because of the temporary problems the brace may cause.

If dislocation of the hip is not detected until childhood, the child must then have one or more operations on the hip to correct the dislocation. The child is hospitalized and surgery is performed while he or she is under a general anesthetic.

After the operation, plaster casts are put on the child's legs for several months. This may be a difficult time for the child, since casts restrict your child's movements and are uncomfortable.

What are the long-term prospects?

If corrected early with a brace, dislocation of the hip is often completely cured. The child will be able to walk normally. If the dislocation is not detected and corrected surgically until childhood, the child may continue to have problems walking.

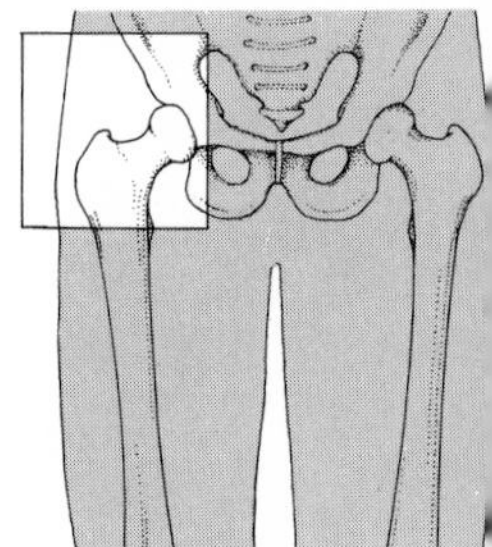

Normal hip joint
In a normal hip joint, the ball at the top of the thighbone fits neatly into the socket in the pelvis.

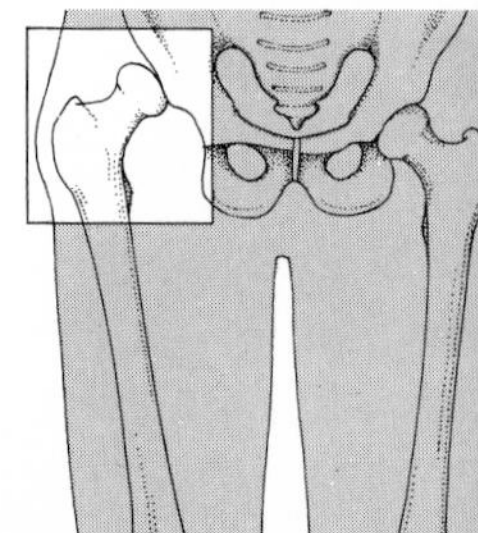

Dislocated hip joint
In a dislocated hip joint, the ball at the top of the thighbone lies outside of the socket in the pelvis.

Club foot

(talipes)

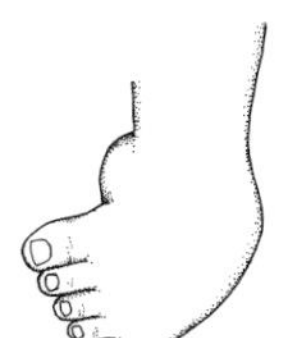

A baby with club foot is born with one or both feet bent either downward and inward or upward and outward. Many babies with normally formed feet persistently turn them inward, but the feet can be pushed back to the proper position. In club foot, it is not possible to push the foot or feet back to the proper position. Club foot may run in families.

Today, nearly all cases of club foot are detected at birth and treated, and the child learns to walk normally.

What is the treatment?

If the club foot is not too severe, the physician will show the infant's parents how to manipulate the foot regularly each day until, as the bones and ligaments continue to develop, it settles into a normal position. In more severe cases, as much correction as possible is done by manipulation, then either splints or a plaster cast are put on the affected foot to keep it from moving back to its former position. Periodically, the splints or cast are removed, the foot is manipulated farther back toward a normal position, and new splints or a new cast are put on to hold it in the new position. This is repeated for 6 to 12 weeks. If splints or a cast are not successful, surgery is needed to correct the deformity. The entire course of treatment may last 4 to 12 months.

Cleft lip and cleft palate

A cleft lip is a vertical split in the upper lip. It may be partial, or it may extend all the way to the base of the nose. In some children with a cleft lip, the nose appears to be flattened. Sometimes there are two splits, affecting both sides of the lip. In some children with cleft lips, the gap continues along the roof of the mouth. This gap, called a cleft palate, runs along the middle of the palate and extends from behind the teeth to the cavity of the nose. Cleft palate makes eating and swallowing difficult. In newborns, cleft palate may cause regurgitated milk to come through the nose instead of through the mouth.

If not treated, a cleft lip usually results in psychological distress for the child because of its appearance. An uncorrected cleft palate will also cause serious speech difficulties (see Learning problems, p.720).

Cleft lip and cleft palate sometimes run in families and may affect more than one child of the same parents. In most cases, the cause of the defect is unknown.

What is the treatment?

Surgery to correct cleft lip is performed when the baby is about 3 months old. From birth until the time of the operation, treatment varies according to the severity of the problem. Infants who do not have problems eating need no interim treatment. However, some bottle-fed babies may need a larger than normal hole in the nipple, or may have to be spoon-fed. The baby will usually stop regurgitating milk through the nose on its own after a few weeks.

In severe cases of cleft palate, a special plate may be placed on the roof of the baby's mouth before each feeding. A special brace may also be placed on the infant's upper gum if the gum is misaligned in the area of the mouth around the clefts.

Plastic surgery (see p.279) can be performed on a cleft lip when the baby weighs about 10 lb (4.5 kg), usually at 8 to 12 weeks old. If the nose appears to be flattened, it can be corrected with plastic surgery when the child is 14 to 16 years old, and his or her facial bones are fully developed. A cleft palate can be repaired by surgery when the baby is about 9 to 12 months old, preferably before the child learns to speak. For each operation, the baby is hospitalized, usually for about 24 hours, and given a general anesthetic for the surgery.

Surgery usually improves the child's appearance and allows the development of normal speech. If a speech defect does develop, speech therapy is recommended. Ask your physician to recommend a qualified speech therapist.

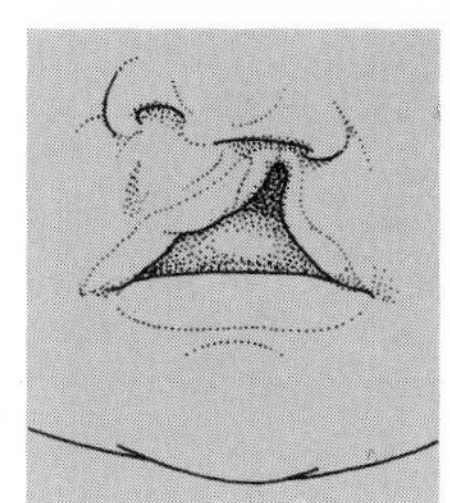

Cleft lip

Cleft lip and cleft palate
A cleft lip (left) can vary in severity from a notch in the upper lip to a split extending to the base of the nose. It may occur on one or both sides of the nose. A cleft palate may be an extension of a cleft lip (below left) or it may occur alone (for comparison, a normal lip and palate are shown below).

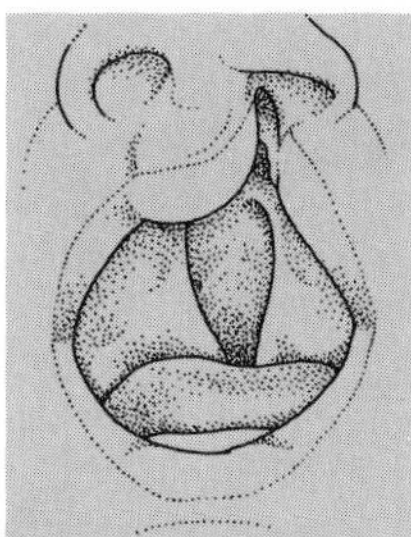

Cleft lip and cleft palate

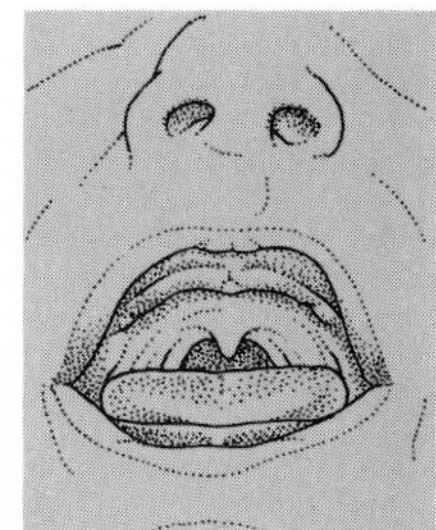

Normal lip and palate

Skin

Many skin problems that affect adults can also affect children (see Skin, hair, and nail disorders, p.266). The two disorders discussed here occur mainly in children. Infantile eczema is an allergic reaction (see Allergies, p.754); while it is not a serious condition, it may indicate that the child will develop other allergies later in life. Infantile eczema results from an inherited sensitivity to certain foods or to other substances, and is not contagious. Ringworm is a fungus infection and is extremely contagious.

Infantile eczema

(infantile atopic dermatitis)

See p.242, **Visual aids to diagnosis, 6.**

Infantile eczema is a red, scaling, sometimes oozing skin condition. It is a form of allergy (see p.754) and is not contagious.

What are the symptoms?

In mild cases of infantile eczema, the skin is somewhat dry, red, and scaly, and a rash appears only in small areas, particularly on the cheeks. In severe cases, the rash is more obvious and covers a larger area. In very severe cases, the rash almost covers the body.

Small red pimples appear, and as the baby scratches them, they begin to ooze and form large oozing areas that become encrusted.

What are the risks?

If the eczema oozes, infection may occur, particularly in the diaper area, where the wet, warm, dark, and contaminated environment is ideal for infection. Also, many infections that affect the skin, such as chickenpox (see p.747), can be unusually severe in children with eczema. If your infant has eczema and is allergic to eggs, extreme caution is urged before he or she receives a measles-mumps-rubella immunization, which is grown on egg. The child should be hyposensitized (given a series of increasing doses of the vaccine that helps the body to becomes less sensitive to the vaccine) or have the vaccine diluted and given in frequent small amounts. Talk to a pediatrician or pediatric allergist (a physician who specializes in treating allergies in infants and children) who is familiar with this procedure.

What should be done?

Mild forms of infantile eczema require no treatment other than applications of a thick moisturizing cream. For more severe cases, you should see your physician.

What is the treatment?

Self-help: If your baby has more than a mild case of infantile eczema, try to prevent him or her from becoming too hot from wearing too many clothes. Make sure that clothes in direct contact with your baby's skin are made of cotton and have been washed and rinsed thoroughly so that they do not irritate your child's skin. Do not use creams or lotions on your child's skin without first checking with your physician.

Professional help: If the baby's skin is very itchy, your physician may prescribe an antihistamine. Severe episodes of infantile eczema are treated with corticosteroid creams or ointments. Cow's milk, wheat, orange juice, eggs, nuts, and chocolate, all of which commonly produce a rash, should be eliminated from your baby's diet.

In some children, infantile eczema goes away on its own after a few months. In others, the condition may come and go for several years. Most children outgrow infantile eczema by the time they reach puberty.

Ringworm

See p.245, **Visual aids to diagnosis, 20.**

Ringworm is not a worm. It is a fungus (*Tinea* in Latin) that infects the skin and causes scaly, round, itchy patches to develop. It may affect the scalp, skin, or nails.

When ringworm affects the scalp, bald patches develop. The skin on these patches flakes and itches. Ringworm on the trunk starts as a small, round, red patch that is scaly and itchy. The patch gradually grows larger until it is about 1 in (2 to 3 cm) across. As it gets larger, the central area of the patch heals and leaves a red ring on the skin. After a week or two, other patches may appear nearby.

Ringworm is infectious and can be caught from a dog or cat that is a carrier or that has mange. Ringworm is not usually a serious condition, but it can be unsightly.

Take your child to your physician as soon as the symptoms appear. Your physician may prescribe an ointment containing a fungicide to be applied at least twice daily to the affected areas. If the ringworm is on the scalp, or if it is on the trunk and is very severe, your physician may prescribe an oral antifungal medication.

Any child with ringworm may go to school once treatment has begun. It takes 1 to 2 months to cure ringworm on the scalp. You should dispose of any combs, hairbrushes, or hats the child has used.

Nervous system and psychological disorders

The first four disorders that are discussed in this section result from an abnormality or disturbance in the nervous system (for a general description of the nervous system, see Disorders of the brain and nervous system, p.283). Three psychological disorders are also included in this section. They range in severity from sleeping problems, which are usually not serious, to autism, which is a serious disorder that may require extensive treatment and special education. Child abuse is also discussed.

If you are concerned about the progress of your child's mental development, consult the Milestones chart (see p.691) and read the article on learning problems (see p.720).

Reye's syndrome

Reye's syndrome is a serious childhood disorder that can be fatal. The disorder has only been widely recognized in recent years, and its cause is still unknown. In most cases, Reye's syndrome begins after a minor respiratory illness, chickenpox (see p.747), or influenza (see p.597). Within 2 or 3 days, the child begins to vomit and becomes drowsy. He or she may then lose consciousness, and seizures may occur. Serious disturbances in the balance of chemicals in the child's blood occur. There is swelling of the liver and damage to the brain and kidneys. In the 1980s, parents were warned that giving aspirin to children who had chickenpox, influenza, or minor respiratory illnesses seemed to increase their child's risk of developing Reye's syndrome, and warning labels were put on aspirin bottles. Since aspirin use has declined in children, Reye's syndrome has become much less common.

What are the symptoms?

Reye's syndrome should be suspected when a child who has chickenpox or another viral infection (such as a cold or a cough) begins to vomit and becomes drowsy.

What are the risks?

Of the cases of Reye's syndrome diagnosed in recent years, about one third were fatal. However, treatment of this disorder is now more successful. And early detection and treatment of Reye's syndrome may save a child's life.

What is the treatment?

Do not give aspirin to your children or teenagers; use acetaminophen instead for minor illnesses with fevers. Children with Reye's syndrome are monitored in the hospital to watch for brain swelling and for disruption of the chemical balance in their bloodstream.

The child is then given intravenous fluids to help restore the chemicals in the blood to normal and reduce swelling of the brain. Your physician may recommend surgery on the skull to reduce the pressure on the brain caused by the swelling.

Seizures in children

A seizure results when abnormal activity of nerve cells in the brain causes abnormal electrical discharges. Seizures occur more often in children than in adults, because a child's developing brain is more sensitive to disturbances such as a fever or changes in the balance of chemicals in the blood than the fully developed brain of an adult.

The causes of seizures in children vary. In most cases, the cause is either unknown (idiopathic epilepsy) or related to a fever caused by a minor infection (febrile seizure). However, seizures may also occur in children with brain damage, cerebral palsy (see p.716), a brain tumor (see p.301), or meningitis (see next article).

Changes in the body's chemical balance can also cause seizures. These changes may be due to congenital (present from birth) enzyme deficiencies, such as phenylketonuria (see p.735), or accidents, such as when a child who has diabetes receives too large a dose of insulin (see Diabetes mellitus, p.558).

What are the symptoms?

Grand mal seizure (also called a major motor seizure): This is the most common type of seizure in children. The child may cry out and suddenly fall to the ground unconscious, with arms and legs held stiff. After 30 seconds or so, the arms and legs, and sometimes the face, start to twitch or jerk rhythmically. The seizure usually lasts for about 2 to 3 minutes, and during this time the child may urinate or, more rarely, have a bowel movement.

During the next few minutes, the child slowly regains consciousness, and may be confused and irritable or have a bad headache. Soon the child falls asleep and sleeps for several hours. The child is usually back to normal when he or she awakens.

One or two grand mal seizures lasting 2 to 3 minutes each are not usually harmful, but prolonged seizures of this kind can lead to brain damage.

Petit mal seizure: This minor type of seizure is caused by epilepsy (see p.306). Seizures can occur as frequently as 20 times in a single day and are often mistaken for daydreaming. The child suddenly becomes motionless, and stares ahead vacantly for a few seconds. Repetitive movements of hands, mouth, or eyelids, or lip smacking may occur. Occasionally he or she may totter or fall. After the seizure, the child is usually unaware that anything unusual has happened. Frequent petit mal seizures may interrupt thinking and interfere with performance in school. Seizures can be controlled and most affected children eventually stop having them. Some children have a mixture of petit mal and grand mal seizures. These children usually do not grow out of their epilepsy and will require anticonvulsant medication to control the seizures as adults.

Psychomotor seizure (also called a temporal lobe attack): This type of seizure may be preceded by dizziness, abdominal discomfort, or intense anxiety. These sensations may be followed by staring, repetitive movements of the hands, lips, or face, and then by behavior such as wandering, undressing, fumbling with objects, or other aimless activity. The child may speak nonsensically. In contrast to a petit mal seizure, children with psychomotor seizures are often drowsy or confused afterward. They usually do not remember the seizures or the events that occurred immediately beforehand.

Psychomotor seizures may continue into adult life, and if they do, an anticonvulsant medication is required to control the seizures.

Infantile spasms: With a sudden jerk, the baby doubles up at the waist for only a second. This type of seizure, which occurs many times each day, first appears at about 3 months to 8 months of age. The seizures may disappear in time, in some cases where no cause is found. Other seizures are associated with abnormal brain development or infections acquired sometime before birth. These children sometimes have other types of seizures as they grow older.

What are the risks?

Seizures may run in families. Mentally retarded children or children who have cerebral palsy may also have seizures. Seizures are often a cause of great concern to parents, but most of them can be controlled with medication. The most serious risk is that a prolonged grand mal seizure may result in brain damage or that a serious injury may occur as a result of the child's falling while having a seizure.

What should be done?

A child who has a seizure for the first time should see a physician as soon as possible. If any seizure lasts for more than 5 minutes, immediate medical care is essential. If a child has a grand mal seizure, lay the child on his or her side. Do not attempt to restrain movements or to force anything between the teeth. For other types of seizures, move any possibly harmful objects out of the child's way. Try to notice and remember the details of any seizure to help your physician make a diagnosis later.

For most cases of first seizure (except for febrile seizures), tests are performed to determine the cause of the seizure. These tests may be performed in the hospital for children with grand mal or very frequent seizures. Tests usually include a thorough physical and neurologic examination, an electroencephalogram (a recording of the electrical impulses of the brain), and a CT or MRI scan of the brain. Sometimes additional tests are also performed to check for conditions that can be associated with seizures, such as meningitis (see p.715), encephalitis (see p.291), or brain tumor (see p.301). If the seizures recur, the child will be placed on an anticonvulsant medication.

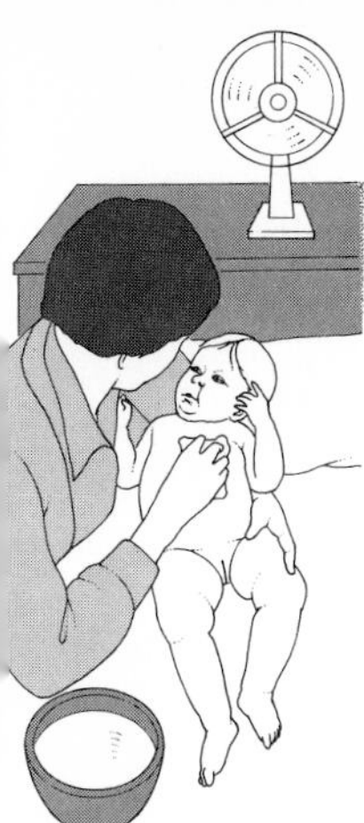

Avoiding febrile seizures
A child who has had previous seizures caused by a high fever may have them again if he or she has another high fever. Keep the child cool, using a sponge soaked in lukewarm water.

What is the treatment?

Self-help: If your child has an infection and has had a previous febrile seizure, take steps to rapidly reduce the child's temperature and avoid a possible recurrence of the seizure. Give your child a fever-reducing medication recommended by your physician, such as acetaminophen. Take the child's temperature every 2 hours. If it is above 100°F (38°C), remove your child's shirt, sponge his or her face and upper body with lukewarm water, and use an electric fan to keep air moving to help the evaporation of perspiration, thereby cooling the child.

Professional help: Some childhood seizures are caused by disturbances in the balance of chemicals in the blood or conditions of the brain such as infections or tumors that can be treated and corrected. When seizures recur and their cause cannot be eliminated, anticonvulsant medications can often effectively control the seizures.

Depending on the frequency and type of seizures, your physician may prescribe one or more medications, starting with a low dose and increasing the dose until the seizures are controlled. If side effects occur, different combinations of medications may be tried. Blood tests may be performed to help adjust the dosage of the drugs. Frequent visits to your physician will be required during this period. It is important that the child take the medications regularly as directed, and that the parents continue to work with their physician to help with their child's treatment.

It is a good idea to inform a child's school about recurrent seizures. If the child must take medication during the school day, most schools require written authorization from the child's parents before allowing the medication to be given at school.

Once the frequency of seizures has been decreased by anticonvulsant medication, the child should be encouraged to participate in his or her usual activities. Supervision should be provided, but the child should not be made to feel self-conscious.

In some cases, if a child being treated with anticonvulsants has been completely free of seizures for at least 2 years, the physician may gradually discontinue the medication in the hope that the condition has been cured.

Meningitis in infants and children

Meningitis is a contagious infection of the three thin layers (meninges) that cover the brain. Meningitis usually occurs alone, but occasionally it occurs as part of a general infection such as mumps (see p.748) or tuberculosis (see p.751). A bacterium called *Haemophilus influenzae* type b (Hib) is the most common cause of meningitis in children under 6. Meningitis can also result from a penetrating head injury.

What are the symptoms?

The infant or child has a fever and a severe headache and will be miserable and irritable. The child will have a stiff neck, will become unusually quiet and withdrawn, and will turn away from bright lights. The child may feel nauseated and may vomit. He or she may also have seizures (see previous article).

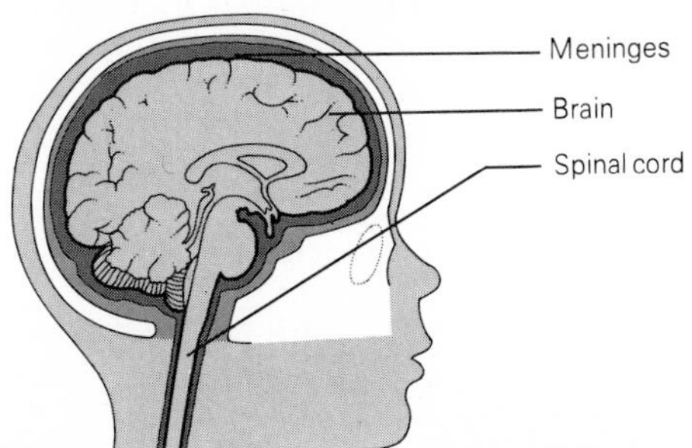

The meninges
The brain and spinal cord are covered by the meninges, which become inflamed in meningitis.

In young babies, the soft spot (fontanelle) may be bulging and taut, instead of slightly sunken as it usually is.

What are the risks?

The risks for babies and young children are greater than those for older children and adults, because very young children may not be able to communicate their symptoms. When meningitis caused by bacteria goes untreated, it may result in brain damage or death. When promptly treated, however, the child usually makes a complete recovery.

What should be done?

Prevention of meningitis by immunization is important. There is a vaccine available for meningitis caused by *Haemophilus influenzae* type b (Hib) bacteria (see Immunization, p.748). Have your physician or local public health department immunize your child against Hib infection. If your child has the symptoms described here, see your physician immediately or take your child to a hospital emergency department. If your physician suspects meningitis, the child will probably be admitted to the hospital, where a lumbar puncture test will confirm the diagnosis. Antibiotics will be prescribed for bacterial infections. If viruses are responsible, the disease will usually clear up by itself.

Cerebral palsy

Cerebral palsy is a condition resulting in weakness of the arms and legs accompanied by either stiffness or floppiness and sometimes twisted postures. Cerebral palsy is caused by a brain abnormality and may become obvious during the first year of life. The severity of the child's handicap varies and some arms and legs may be severely deformed. Even simple movements such as reaching for a cup may be jerky and accomplished only (if at all) after several attempts. The stiffness of the arms and legs associated with cerebral palsy is called spasticity. Some children with cerebral palsy have a degree of mental retardation, although others have normal intelligence. Children with this disorder may also have some degree of hearing loss, visual defects, crossed eyes (see p.721), and seizures (see p.713).

For most children, the cause of cerebral palsy cannot be determined. It is definitely not inherited, and having one affected child does not increase the chances of having another. Cerebral palsy may result from abnormal development of the brain before birth. It is more common in babies born prematurely. Later in life, brain damage can be caused by a head injury (see p.294), meningitis (see previous article), or severe seizures (see p.713).

What are the symptoms?

In many cases, cerebral palsy is not recognized until well into a baby's first year. Floppy muscles may be an early indication of the disorder, but many babies who have cerebral palsy do not have this symptom. The main symptom, stiffening of the arms and legs, does not usually occur until a baby is at least 6 months old. When this happens, normal muscle balance is disrupted, and the arms and legs settle in typical unusual positions. For example, affected arms are usually tucked into the side, with elbows and wrists bent. Legs may be crossed like scissors, and the feet may point downward from the ankle. The baby may move very little, and what little movement there is will be clumsy. The baby may find it difficult to suck and swallow. Normal infant development (see p.691), such as walking and speech, may be delayed, sometimes considerably.

Children who walk very late or who do not learn to walk are not able to explore their environment and learn from their experience at a vital stage of their development. This situation is made worse if the child also has problems with hearing and/or vision.

When speech development is considerably delayed, as is often the case when a child has hearing problems, speech may be distorted and difficult to understand. Children who have cerebral palsy and who also have average or high intelligence can become extremely frustrated by being deprived of normal activity and ability to communicate and may have emotional problems as a result.

Types of paralysis
Cerebral palsy rarely affects the whole body, and the degree of physical and mental disability varies considerably. Three main patterns of muscular weakness and spasticity have been recognized for many years: quadriplegia (affecting all four limbs), hemiplegia (affecting the arm, leg, and trunk muscles on only one side of the body), and paraplegia (paralysis of both legs). In all types of cerebral palsy, the chest muscles are usually unaffected.

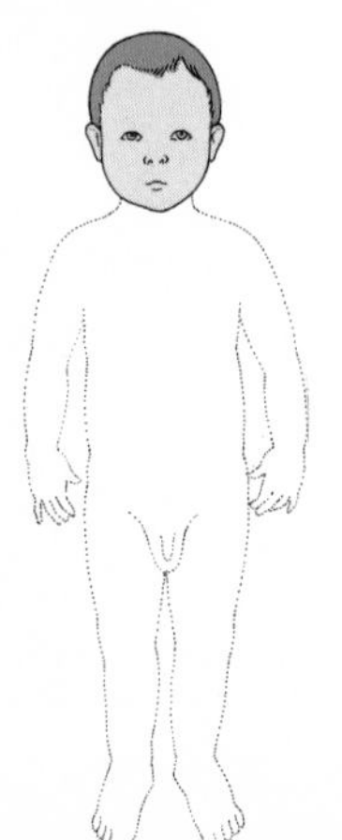

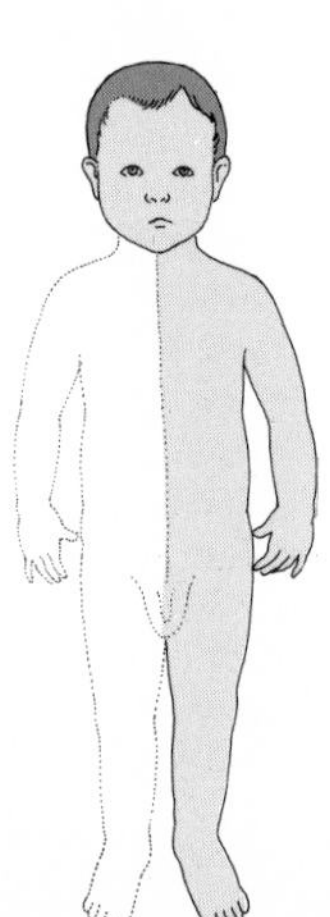

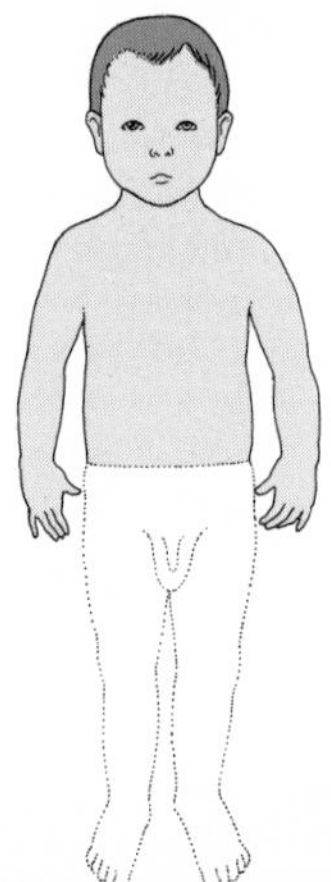

What are the risks?

Cerebral palsy is the most common crippling disorder of childhood. And it is especially common in babies who are premature or under 5½ lb (2½ kg) at birth.

The affected child's stiff muscles can easily become immobile, which further restricts movement. The child may not learn to walk and may have to use a wheelchair.

There is a risk that an intelligent child will not be recognized as such, especially when movement and communication are difficult. An affected child's mental ability and development should be evaluated regularly, and his or her vision and hearing should be tested so that any problems in those areas can be considered when providing for the child's education (see Learning problems, p.720).

What should be done?

If you take your child to see your physician for his or her regular checkups, there is very little chance that any signs or symptoms of cerebral palsy will go undetected.

What is the treatment?

Abnormalities of the brain such as those that cause cerebral palsy do not get worse, but they also do not improve. This does not mean that treatment is unavailable for a child with the disorder. The aim of treatment is to determine the extent of any disabilities, whether physical, mental, visual, or auditory (hearing), and then to minimize the effects of these disabilities.

Caring for a child who has cerebral palsy requires teamwork that involves parents, physicians, physical therapists, occupational therapists, speech therapists, and teachers.

Physical therapy may be provided at hospitals, schools, clinics, or in a child's home. The goals of physical therapy are to prevent additional deformity and to develop posture and muscle function within the limits of a child's condition. Children learn how to prevent development of deformities as much as possible by relaxing stiffened muscles and finding beneficial positions for their affected limbs. Some children learn to walk with such aids as braces, crutches, and walkers. Speech therapy can improve speech and swallowing.

Orthopedic surgery can ease the stiffness in some deformed arms and legs. Surgery enables some children who would otherwise be confined to a wheelchair to walk with braces, crutches, and/or walkers. Hearing problems in many children can be treated with a hearing aid. Crossed eyes can be corrected by an operation, and prescription eyeglasses may also be helpful. A muscle-relaxant medication is sometimes prescribed to make movement easier, and anticonvulsant medications are used to treat seizures.

A child who has cerebral palsy should be examined regularly by a physician to assess his or her general physical and mental progress. Sometimes your physician will refer your child to a physical therapist, an educational psychologist, or a social worker who can help you decide which educational arrangements would be best for your child.

Many children who have mild cerebral palsy have normal or near normal intelligence and can attend a regular school. Children who are moderately to severely disabled by the disorder and have normal intelligence may need to attend a school for the physically disabled, or go to special classes. A child who has limited intelligence may need to attend special classes for the mentally disabled. Different communities have different arrangements for disabled children. Your local school district can tell you about any programs that are available.

What are the long-term prospects?

The prospects for children with cerebral palsy depend on the severity and type of their disability. For children able to attend a regular school, there should be few problems. Most of them do well. For many children who need to attend special schools or classes, there can be moderate to severe problems.

Sleeping problems in children

Normal sleeping patterns

Most babies, in the early weeks of life, wake once or twice during the night, but by the age of 9 months, they sleep through the night. At 1 year, babies sleep an average of about 16 hours in every 24. Two to 3 hours of this sleep will be during the day.

By the time they have reached the toddler stage (18 months), children begin to vary in the amount of sleep they need. Some toddlers require relatively little sleep and wake up very early each morning. Leave plenty of soft toys in the child's crib overnight, to occupy the child and allow you to get your normal amount of sleep in the early morning. Such a child is often very active during the day, may need no daytime nap, and does not become tired until bedtime.

By the age of 3, many children reach the same stage as the very active toddler and give up their daily nap. And by the age of 5, nearly all children stay awake throughout the day.

Combating sleeplessness

Do not make yourself too easily available to your child during the night. Otherwise, he or she may become dependent on your attention and become sleepless and irritable if deprived of it. For example, if your baby cries after being fed at night, do not immediately go and pick up the baby. Listen outside the door of the baby's room. In most cases, the crying will stop after a few minutes, and the baby will go back to sleep. If the crying continues, go in to check on the baby.

Some children have trouble falling asleep, although they may sleep well during the night. In this case, try to make sure that the child is not disturbed by unnecessary noise such as an older brother or sister repeatedly entering the bedroom. Sometimes leaving a radio playing music softly will cover up disturbing noises. You also should not send a child to bed as punishment. If, over a period of time the child associates going to bed with punishment, he or she may fear going to bed, and, once in bed, sleep poorly.

What to do about sleeplessness

Your pediatrician's office may be able to recommend books on helping your baby sleep through the night. In spite of your precautions, your child may still find it very difficult to get to sleep or may wake during the night. Never give a child your own sleeping medication. It is not a good idea to treat sleeping problems with medication. If the sleeplessness becomes a persistent and unbearable problem, talk to your physician, who may refer your child to a specialist such as a neurologist or a psychiatrist.

Nightmares and sleepwalking

Nightmares usually become a problem only after age 3. In most cases, they are caused by a disturbing incident or a frightening story, movie, or television program. Occasionally nightmares are an indication that the child is under stress from unresolved problems at home or school. Some children have night terrors. They may scream, talk or babble, and appear terrified, but are difficult to wake and cannot tell you what has frightened them. Sleepwalking and repetitive jerking movements during sleep are also related to changes in brain activity during sleep.

The immediate remedy for nightmares and night terrors is to comfort your child. Try to get to him or her as soon as possible, and turn the lights on to reassure your child that it was only a dream. Do not question your child about the fear immediately, since this may only make him or her feel worse. Instead, physically comfort your child and take his or her mind off the disturbance by talking soothingly about something pleasant. A child

Child abuse

More than 2 million cases of child abuse and neglect are reported each year in the US. In addition, an estimated 150,000 to 200,000 new cases of sexual abuse occur annually in the US. Sometimes relatives and neighbors of these children suspect abuse, but find it difficult to believe that parents could injure their own child. In such cases, the relative or neighbor should contact his or her local health and/or social services departments and alert them to the possibility that the child is at risk.

Types of injury

Young babies may be abused because parents find their crying annoying. In these cases, the parents may violently shake the baby and damage may be caused to the interior of the baby's eyes or to the brain. In addition, the upper part of the arms or the child are usually marked where the baby has been held too tightly. Older babies may have small burns or bruises on the face, and/or injuries to the lips. Severe assaults may cause fractures of the ribs, skull, and of the arm and leg bones.

Injuries sustained by toddlers and older children can result in bruising and burn marks. In some cases, however, the abuse takes the form of starvation or terrorization. For example, parents may repeatedly lock the child in a dark room at night. In these cases, the child usually appears thin, unhappy, and withdrawn.

Children at risk

Child abuse can occur in families of any intelligence and social class. However, health professionals have identified certain factors that make the incidence of child abuse in a family more likely. Young parents with limited education, living in poor social conditions on a low income are under stress that may contribute to abuse. This seems especially true if the parents have no contact with their own families. There is some evidence to suggest that mothers who do not undergo the usual psychological bonding process with their babies are more likely to abuse their children. The bonding process may be impaired when a mother and newborn are separated immediately after birth, such as when the baby is born prematurely or has to spend several weeks in the hospital in a neonatal intensive care unit. Drug abuse (see p.332), including alcohol abuse (see p.329), by the parents also increases the likelihood of child abuse.

When to suspect abuse

Broken bones, repeated bruising, and burn marks on a child may result from injury inflicted by the parents in one of the following cases: if the parents delay or fail to seek medical help; if the parents offer doubtful or inconsistent explanations for the injuries; or if their reactions to the injuries seem to reflect lack of concern or are otherwise inappropriate under the circumstances. The most reliable indication of continued abuse or neglect is usually failure of the child to grow at a normal pace or to achieve expected levels of physical and mental development. Children who are victims of abuse do not thrive and their weight drops well below the average for their age. Children who are abused often have behavior problems and learning problems in school, in addition to their obvious injuries.

Sexual abuse

Children who are otherwise taken care of adequately may be sexually abused by a parent (usually the father) or another close relative. Often the child feels too guilty, embarrassed, or afraid to tell someone. The adult abuser may also threaten the child into silence. In some cases, the child seeks help from another adult. If you are approached by such a child, respond sympathetically and suppress feelings of shock or disgust, which would only add to the child's unwarranted sense of guilt. Anyone who suspects that a child is being sexually abused should contact his or her local health and/or social services departments.

Attention deficit disorder

Children who have attention deficit disorder have a short attention span, a low tolerance for frustration, and often behave without thinking about the consequences. More than half these children are hyperactive; they are overly energetic and aggressive. Children who are not hyperactive are usually anxious and withdrawn. If your child has attention deficit disorder, try the following:

- Have your child follow a regular daily routine.
- Do not let your child become overtired.
- Do not overstimulate your child, especially near bedtime.
- Set limits for your child and enforce them by withdrawing treats and privileges.
- Encourage and reward your child's good behavior and good performance in school.

Most of the diets and vitamin treatments recommended for hyperactivity have not been proven effective, and some are potentially harmful. Treatment may include counseling; research on medications is continuing.

who has a night terror will probably drift back into a peaceful sleep. Unless the terror persists, it is better not to wake the child. Your child will outgrow his or her night terrors. It is also best not to wake a sleepwalking child. Instead, guide him or her back to bed. Once you have discovered that the child sleepwalks, put a gate across the top of any stairs and close any accessible windows to prevent a serious fall.

If your child is old enough, it is usually a good idea to discuss nightmares with him or her and try to find out what the underlying problem is, so that you can deal with it. If your child has a persistent problem sleeping, see your physician.

Autism

Autism is a child's inability from birth—or a loss of the ability within the first 30 months of life—to develop normal human relationships with anybody, even with parents. In many of its symptoms, autism is similar to schizophrenia in adults (see p.319). While the cause of autism is still unclear, there is some evidence that it is biological because it is sometimes accompanied by several disorders of the central nervous system.

What are the symptoms?

The symptoms of autism vary greatly, but follow a general pattern. As a baby, the autistic child has difficulty with feeding and toilet training. He or she does not give, or stops giving, smiling recognition to either parent's face. It will become increasingly obvious that the child lives in a world of his or her own. Speech, facial expressions, and any other form of communication are absent or unintelligible. In some cases, a few words are spoken, but are repeated endlessly for no apparent reason. An autistic child makes no distinction among people, other living things, and inanimate objects, and treats them all in the same way. He or she cannot evaluate situations and therefore consistently reacts inappropriately to them. For example, the child may become fiercely agitated if the furniture is rearranged in the home or if he or she is taken into new but friendly surroundings, but the same child may also run across a busy street without any sign of fear.

By not communicating, the autistic child remains isolated from other family members. Children with autism behave unpredictably. They may be violent at one moment, and then sit completely still, in some strange position, for many hours. Autistic children may adopt unusual postures and mannerisms that can upset those around them. And although an autistic child may have normal intelligence, he or she may appear to be retarded, or in some cases deaf.

What are the risks?

Autism occurs more frequently in boys than it does in girls.

There is always a risk of injury if a child with autism is left unsupervised, because he or she is unable to recognize danger.

What should be done?

If you feel that your child has always been, or has suddenly become, seriously withdrawn or uncommunicative, take him or her to your physician. Because a deaf child may also be unresponsive, your physician may perform a hearing test. If your child's hearing is normal, and your physician suspects that he or she is autistic, you and your child may be referred to a child psychiatrist. The psychiatrist can determine if the problem is autism.

What is the treatment?

Once autism has been diagnosed, the parents, the physician, and any specialists involved may meet to discuss the alternatives available for helping your child. In many cases, you will be unable to take care of your child at home. You may get support from your child psychiatrist and any other specialists who become involved in the treatment of your child. Support groups for parents of autistic children can be helpful. Ask your physician for the name of a group in your area. Your child may have to attend a special school.

What are the long-term prospects?

Some autistic children improve enough, over a period of several years, to be able to participate in the world around them and lead productive lives. However, most autistic children do not improve, and when they grow older, they almost always need to be taken care of in special institutions.

Learning problems

Every parent wants his or her child to live as well as possible. To do this, a child must learn early in life not only what is taught in school but also what goes on in the environment. Such learning actually begins at birth, but it may only be later, when a child fails to perform measureable tasks as well as friends or siblings do, that parents become aware of possible learning problems.

If your child is having trouble learning to speak, read, or write compared to other children of the same age, it may be that he or she is slower to develop these skills, and will eventually catch up. It is possible that the situation is more serious. Aside from differing rates of development, there are several major causes of learning problems.

Mental retardation

The first possible cause of learning problems is that the child's intelligence, defined as the ability to understand and benefit from experience, is below normal. Many such children can be educated in regular schools. Children who are severely mentally retarded may need to be educated in special classes or in special schools.

If a series of tests and assessments indicate that your child is mentally retarded, talk to your local school district about any programs available in your community and which of them would be most useful for your child. The school staff and your physician may be able to provide you with support and assistance in coping with a retarded child, or they may refer you to another professional or agency.

Speech and hearing problems

The second major cause of learning problems is difficulty in speaking and hearing. To learn to speak, a child must be able to hear other people speaking. The child must be exposed to a variety of words and word combinations in the speech of other people. In time, the child learns to associate a particular sound with a particular person, or an object such as a toy, or a pet. Finally, the child must be able to convert an idea into the organized sounds we call speech. This is accomplished by stimulating the various parts of the mouth and throat to produce the desired sound. If any part of this process does not work, the child will have trouble learning to speak.

Most speech problems are related to hearing problems. If your child is slow to develop speech (see Milestones, p.691), or if you are worried about your child's hearing (see Can my baby see and hear well? p.722), talk to your physician. Once any hearing problem is corrected, you may be referred to a speech therapist. Regular speech therapy sessions enable many children to catch up with their friends or classmates and then progress normally. Become familiar with your child's problem and find out how you can get help for him or her.

Vision problems

Vision problems are another major cause of learning difficulties. A young child learns most about the world by looking at it. But in order to do this, the child must first be able to see clearly. Most vision problems in children result from crossed eyes (see next page), cataracts (see p.345), or nearsightedness (see p.336), all of which can be improved or corrected, or to some degree of blindness. If you are concerned that your baby's vision is not normal, consult your physician as soon as possible. Vision tests can be done at a very early age.

Once you feel confident that your child can see well, he or she must be supplied with sufficient visual stimulation to be able to use his or her eyes to learn about the world. You can help by talking about pictures in illustrated books, magazines, or newspapers, and by encouraging your child to explore the world visually as you talk about what you see when you are doing things together. Sometimes a child's vision problem is not diagnosed until he or she goes to school. If your child needs glasses, have them fitted and encourage the child to wear them.

Reading problems

Finally, your child must be able to understand what he or she sees. Reading problems are often problems of understanding what is read; that is, of translating visual images into ideas. While such problems exist before a child learns to read, they are often identified at school by the child's teacher.

For a child with a true reading disorder, learning to read is difficult and slow. These reading disorders are called dyslexia. One such disorder occurs when the child sees words and letters reversed. Reversing letters such as "b" and "d" occurs as a part of normal development. A diagnosis of dyslexia is made only when this pattern persists. Most reading problems require specific treatments. Discuss your child's reading difficulties with the specialist or teacher, and find out how you can best help your child to overcome them.

Eyes and ears

A child learns about the world by watching, listening, and touching. So even a minor problem with the eyes or ears, if not treated, may interfere with a child's development (see Box, Learning problems, previous page). Therefore, it is vital to check the development of your baby's vision and hearing. Take your baby to your physician or clinic for routine eye and ear tests during his or her first year of life. You can check to make sure that your baby is developing normally by performing some simple tests on your own (see Can my baby see and hear well?, next page).

If your child has crossed eyes, itching eyes, or a discharge from or crusting around the ear, or if he or she seems distracted, take him or her to your physician. Many childhood eye and ear problems, particularly crossed eyes or ear infections, can be completely cured with early diagnosis and treatment.

Crossed eyes in children

In someone who has crossed eyes, the eyes do not look in the same direction. One eye focuses on what the person wants to look at, and the other eye looks in another direction (usually inward, but occasionally outward or upward). This happens because the muscles in the eyes are not properly aligned. Crossed eyes are fairly common.

Crossed eyes usually appear first in infancy or in early childhood, when eyesight is developing. Crossed eyes occur because the muscles that control the movement of the eyes are unbalanced and misaligned. Usually only one eye is affected. The problem may be constant or it may come and go. Most children who have crossed eyes do not see double, because their brains ignore what is seen by the misaligned eye. The misaligned eye will become "lazy." Because it is not being used, the eye will become weak and will eventually be able to see less and less detail. If not treated, amblyopia (impaired vision in the misaligned eye) can occur.

Medical myths

A child with crossed eyes soon grows out of it.

Wrong. You should not expect persistently crossed eyes to correct themselves. It is never too early to bring possible crossed eyes to your physician's attention. The sooner treatment is started, the better the chances of a total cure.

What should be done?

If a baby under 3 months old has eyes that cross occasionally, there is no need to see a physician; the baby's eye coordination is still developing. In cases of occasional crossed eyes past this age, take the child to your physician. The child may not have crossed eyes. Many young children have a fold of skin over the inner corner of each eye that covers part of the iris and often gives the illusion of crossed eyes.

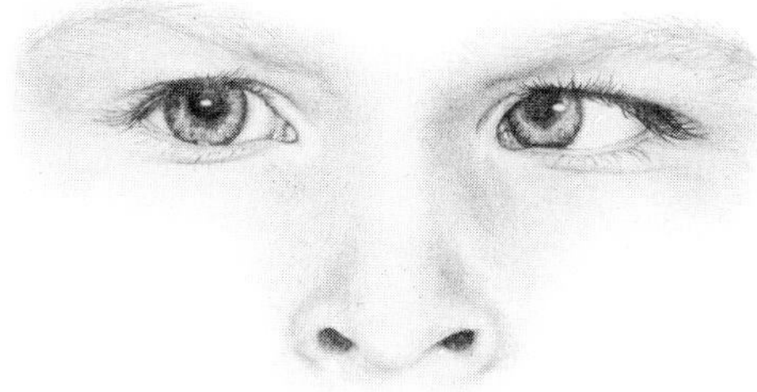

Crossed eyes are rarely obvious in a newborn. They usually become more obvious as the child learns to use his or her eyes.

If your physician suspects crossed eyes, he or she may refer your baby to an ophthalmologist (a physician who specializes in care of the eyes), who can perform tests to discover the cause of your child's crossed eyes and recommend treatment.

What is the treatment?

If a child has crossed eyes, a patch is placed over his or her good eye for several hours each day. This forces the child to use the lazy eye. This treatment is usually effective only before the age of about 24 months. After this, the problem of always avoiding use of the lazy eye becomes a habit, and the condition is very difficult to cure. Eyeglasses may also be prescribed if the child is nearsighted or farsighted. In most children, the combination of a patch and eyeglasses eliminates the problem within a few years.

If a child's eyes are severely misaligned, surgery may be performed before the age of 24 months, both to help the child use the lazy eye and to improve his or her appearance. In the operation, the surgeon shortens the muscles that move the misaligned eyeball. Usually the child stays in the hospital for a few hours after outpatient surgery. Whatever the treatment, it may be accompanied by special eye exercises, to build up the eye muscles. The child learns the exercises under the supervision of an ophthalmologist.

What are the long-term prospects?

The prospect of cure is very good with treatment before age 7. After this age, correcting the problem is still possible, but there is an increased risk of blindness in the affected eye.

Chronic middle ear infection

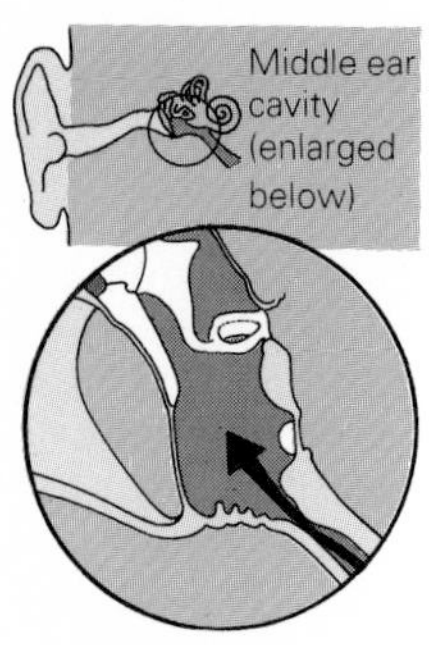

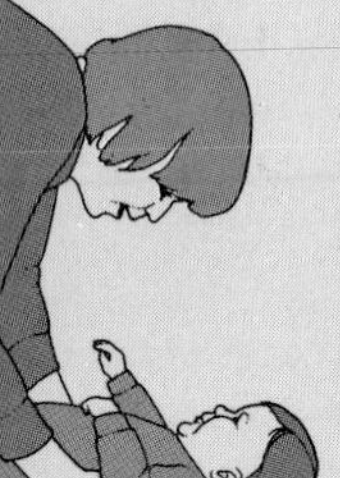

Path of infection through eustachian tube to middle ear

Some children have repeated infections of the middle ear (see p.360), which usually occur because an infection of the nose and throat (such as a cold) passes along the eustachian, or auditory, tube from the back of the nose to the middle ear cavity. Episodes are more frequent in children than they are in adults, because a child's eustachian tubes are relatively short and straight, which makes it easy for infectious agents (microorganisms) to move through them and reach the middle ear. A sticky fluid produced by the infection may gradually accumulate in the middle ear. The fluid cannot drain away through the eustachian tube because the tube has become swollen and blocked.

What are the symptoms?

The main symptom of chronic middle ear infection is partial hearing loss in the affected ear. In most cases, the child can still hear, but sounds are muffled or faint. The hearing loss occurs because the sticky fluid that has accumulated in the middle ear prevents the eardrum and middle ear bones from vibrating freely. These vibrations are essential to hearing. The child may also have a sensation of fullness in his or her head.

If your child does not respond when you speak to him or her, or if he or she is having trouble paying attention at school, it could be because of partial hearing loss from a chronic middle ear infection.

What are the risks?

If chronic middle ear infection is not detected and treated after several months, there is a risk that the bones of the middle ear may become joined. The vibration of these bones is crucial in carrying sound to the inner ear. If the bones of the middle ear become joined, they will not be able to vibrate, which can then result in permanent hearing loss in the affected ear.

A hearing problem in a child may interfere with development of speech, which, in turn, may eventually affect his or her performance in school (see Learning problems and Speech and hearing problems, p.720).

What should be done?

If you suspect hearing loss after your child has had an ear infection, see your physician, who will examine the affected ear and perform a special test to determine whether fluid has accumulated in the middle ear.

What is the treatment?

In mild cases, when there is not much fluid in the ear and hearing loss is minimal, your physician may prescribe a decongestant or an antihistamine. These medications can help reduce swelling of the eustachian tube, which will allow the accumulated fluid to flow down the tube and into the nose and throat. The fluid then can be eliminated when the child swallows, coughs, or blows his or her nose.

In severe cases, the fluid must be removed. This is usually done in the hospital. While the child is under a general anesthetic, a very fine needle is passed through the eardrum into the middle ear, and the fluid is sucked out with a syringe, or a small incision is made in the eardrum (myringotomy).

If your child's adenoids (see p.724) are repeatedly infected and swollen and are blocking the entrance to the eustachian tube, they may be surgically removed, to help prevent middle ear infections from developing in the future.

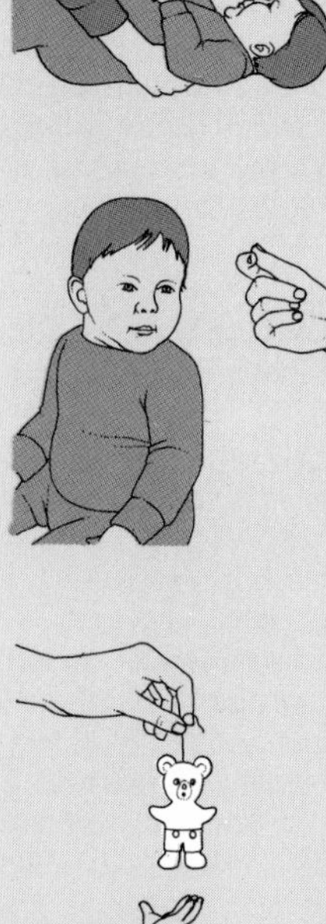

Can my baby see and hear well?

All babies should have a physical examination immediately after birth, so that any obvious defects of vision and hearing can be detected. When a baby is between 4 and 6 weeks old, his or her vision and hearing should be tested again. To check your baby's vision and hearing yourself during the first few months, use the simple tests outlined here.

All infants are nearsighted during the first few weeks of life. At 4 to 6 weeks, your baby may smile if you bring your face to within about 20 in (50 cm) of his or her face. You can test your baby's vision at 3 months by dangling a familiar toy about 8 in (20 cm) away. Your baby should be able to follow the movement of the toy with his or her eyes.

Your newborn is also sensitive to sound. A loud noise will startle a baby, and the sound of somebody talking will be soothing. When your baby is 3 months old, crumple up a piece of newspaper out of sight, about 12 to 18 in (30 to 45 cm) from his or her head. A baby with normal hearing will react to the sound by blinking, or by throwing out his or her arms as if startled. By 4 months old, your baby should turn his or her head to look for the source of a sound.

If you think your baby's vision and hearing may be developing slowly, talk to your physician.

Never hesitate to ask your physician about your child's progress. It is always better to ask questions than to take a chance of overlooking an important problem. Be sure to keep all of your appointments with your physician or health department clinic.

Respiratory system

Children develop much of their immunity from repeated infections (see Box, Immunization, p.748), and infections are the most common cause of respiratory system disorders in children. It is natural for infections of the nose and throat to spread readily to other parts of the respiratory tract, causing various infections, until a child's immunity is fully developed. (For a general discussion of the respiratory system, see p.367).

Before the widespread use of antibiotics, many respiratory tract infections that are now considered minor, such as tonsillitis, often resulted in life-threatening complications. Today, even pneumonia, which at one time was often fatal for children, may usually be treated at home.

The major risk of respiratory infections is that your child will have difficulty breathing (see Croup and stridor, p.725). If your child is short of breath and his or her lips start to turn blue, take the child immediately to a hospital emergency department (see also Injuries and emergencies, p.834).

Tonsillitis and pharyngitis in children

The two tonsils, at the back of the throat, are very small at birth. They gradually increase in size until age 6 or 7. Thereafter they shrink, but they do not disappear as the adenoids do (see next article).

The tonsils have reached maximum size by the time a child reaches age 6 or 7 and the respiratory tract is exposed to a variety of infectious agents (microorganisms). The tonsils drain and help to control infections of the nose and throat.

Both tonsillitis (inflammation of the tonsils) and pharyngitis (inflammation of the pharynx, or throat) are bacterial or virus infections of the back of the throat that cause soreness. Sore throats may also be part of a respiratory infection, such as bronchitis or pneumonia (see p.726). A child's tonsils become enlarged and inflamed when he or she gets tonsillitis and pharyngitis.

What are the symptoms?

Tonsillitis and pharyngitis start suddenly with a sore throat and difficulty swallowing. Within a few hours, the child becomes feverish and may feel very ill. The pain in the throat makes some children vomit and/or cough. In rare instances, the child may have a febrile seizure (see p.713). Children with tonsillitis often have stomach pain. Glands on either side of the neck often swell, especially at the angles of the jaw, and feel tender. The glands can be felt as small, knoblike lumps. Sometimes this swelling persists for weeks after the symptoms have subsided.

Medical myths

Surgical removal of tonsils is a safe, minor operation, which would benefit most children.

Wrong. Like any operation, a tonsillectomy involves risk. Although the risk is small, it increases with age. Except in severe cases of recurrent tonsillitis, or if swollen tonsils interfere with swallowing or breathing, surgery is usually not necessary.

What are the risks?

Almost every child has one or more episodes of tonsillitis, which is contagious and is usually associated with infections of the adenoids (see next article). Children who have frequent episodes of tonsillitis usually begin to have fewer episodes after age 7, as resistance develops to the microorganisms that cause tonsillitis. Tonsillitis is not risky today. Before the use of antibiotics, tonsillitis could easily lead to rheumatic fever (see p.740) or glomerulonephritis (see p.737).

What should be done?

Use a flashlight to look in your child's mouth. You will see the bumpy tonsils on each side of the throat. If there are white spots on the tonsils, or if the tonsils are swollen over the opening of the throat, call your physician. If the tonsils are just red, use the self-help measures recommended below. If your child has not wanted to eat and has had a fever for more than 24 hours, see your physician, who will examine your child's tonsils and recommend treatment.

What is the treatment?

Self-help: Keep your child indoors, but not necessarily in bed, in a warm—but not overheated—room. Symptoms can usually be relieved with medications recommended by your physician, such as the painkiller acetaminophen, as well as plenty of fluids. Older children should be given at least a pint of extra liquids per day. Do not force your child to eat or drink. Offer cold desserts such as ice cream or frozen yogurt to cool the throat. Use of a fan or frequent sponging of the face with lukewarm water will help reduce the child's temperature. In most cases, children with tonsillitis respond quickly to this treatment. Do not give aspirin to children or adolescents who are ill with a fever because aspirin has been linked with Reye's syndrome (see p.713), a potentially fatal condition. Never administer a cold water enema to relieve a child's fever.

Professional help: If the inflammation is caused by a bacterial infection, your physician may prescribe an antibiotic for 10 days, after doing a throat culture that is positive for the type of *Streptococcus* that causes tonsillitis and pharyngitis. If the throat culture is negative, the infection is probably caused by a virus and requires only treatment for relief of symptoms (acetaminophen and rest). Your physician can use a special kit in his or her office to check whether or not strep is present. The results will be available after about 30 minutes. The symptoms of tonsillitis usually subside in a few days. Even if the child seems to be completely well, however, be sure that he or she takes the full course of medication according to instructions.

If episodes of tonsillitis are so severe and frequent that they affect your child's general health, hearing, or breathing, or if the episodes interfere with school attendance, your physician may recommend surgical removal of the tonsils (tonsillectomy, see Box). Most physicians recommend that tonsillectomy be performed only if other treatment methods are not successful.

Most tonsillectomies are performed as outpatient surgery; the child stays at the hospital for only a few hours. Your physician may decide not to perform a tonsillectomy if your child has an active infection of the tonsils, or if there is a history of bleeding problems in your family.

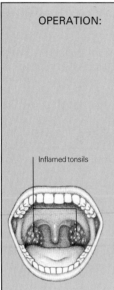

OPERATION: **Tonsils removal**
(tonsillectomy)

The tonsils are removed in cases where recurrent episodes of tonsillitis are interfering with a child's general health or school attendance. The operation is usually performed before the child is 6 or 7. After this age, episodes of tonsillitis usually become less frequent.

During the operation Under general anesthetic, the mouth is held open and the tongue is pulled forward to reveal the tonsils. The tonsils are cut away, and the cut area is left to heal on its own.

After the operation There may be some bleeding of the cut areas, but it is not usually serious. Tonsillectomy is usually performed as outpatient surgery, and the child is at the hospital for only a few hours. He or she should recover completely from the surgery within 2 weeks. Eating ice cream or frozen yogurt will help to soothe the child's sore throat.

Inflamed tonsils

Adenoids

Adenoids are swellings at the back of the nasal cavity, above the tonsils, and they are found in preadolescent children. Adenoids assist the body's defenses against respiratory tract infections and require treatment only if they grow too large. Normally, adenoids begin to grow at about age 3, probably to give extra protection when the child is particularly susceptible to infection. At about 5 years old, the adenoids begin to shrink, and they disappear at puberty. In a few cases, however, the adenoids grow instead, and eventually block the airway from the nose to the throat, the opening of the eustachian tubes from the middle ear to the nose, or both. If either or both blockages develop, various problems usually result.

What are the symptoms?

If the airway from the nose is blocked, a child breathes mainly through his or her mouth, snores, and may speak with a nasal twang. The flow of secretions at the back of the nose is blocked, and the adenoids become infected. Infected secretions drip from the child's nose during the day. Whenever the child lies down, these secretions drip back down into the throat, causing an irritating cough. If the infection is not cleared up, it may spread to the middle ear.

What are the risks?

If infections are not treated and are followed by chronic middle ear infection (see p.360), some hearing loss may result.

What is the treatment?

If your child repeatedly has a stuffy nose, earaches, or an irritating cough at night, your physician may examine your child's adenoids by reflecting a light onto them from a mirror held at the back of the throat.

Infections are treated with antibiotics when necessary. Surgical removal of the adenoids (adenoidectomy) is not often required, because the adenoids shrink on their own as a child reaches puberty. However, when repeated earaches interfere with a child's school attendance or persist after antibiotic treatment, your physician may recommend adenoidectomy. Your physician may decide not to remove your child's adenoids if they are infected, or if there is a history of bleeding problems in your family.

Croup and stridor

Croup is inflammation and narrowing of the air passages in children up to the age of about 4 years. Croup is associated with a condition called stridor, a shrill wheezing or grunting noise that a child makes who is breathing through a narrowed larynx (voice box) or trachea (windpipe). The narrowing usually results from swelling caused by a respiratory infection, often a cold (see Recurrent colds in children, p.727).

What are the symptoms?

In addition to the symptoms of stridor, a child with croup is likely to have a harsh, barking cough and hoarseness. Older children may have discomfort around the larynx or somewhere in the front of the chest. Episodes of croup usually occur at night. The child awakes and breathes with a sudden loud crowing noise, which becomes louder when he or she inhales. The episode of croup usually subsides in a few hours. If a child suddenly develops stridor, sometimes along with a fit of coughing, and does not have a respiratory infection, he or she may have inhaled a foreign object (see Box).

Inhaled foreign object

If a child inhales a foreign object, it can block the air passage. If your child has sudden difficulty breathing and/or if his or her lips appear blue, take him or her to a hospital emergency department immediately (see also Injuries and emergencies, p.835). If an inhaled foreign object causes only a partial blockage of the air passages, the child will make a wheezing or grunting noise and possibly will cough. In this case, see your physician, who will arrange for bronchoscopy (examination of the inside of the lungs with a viewing tube) to look for the inhaled object and, if possible, remove it.

Occasionally an inhaled object passes farther down into the lungs, and causes inflammation and infection (see Pneumonia in children, next page). The inhaled object must be removed with a bronchoscope (a viewing tube), and antibiotics may be prescribed to treat or prevent an infection.

What should be done?

Any young child, especially one under 5 years, with noisy, rapid breathing should be taken to a physician immediately. In most cases, the cause of the breathing problem is croup. In some rare cases, however, noisy, rapid breathing may be a symptom of epiglottiditis, which is a medical emergency that requires immediate hospital treatment. In epiglottiditis, the valve at the top of the windpipe becomes swollen because of an infection and obstructs breathing. If not treated, this condition can cause suffocation.

What is the treatment?

Self-help: During an episode of croup, be calm and reassuring. Panic will only make the situation worse. Your physician may recommend using a vaporizer or steam from a hot shower to help relieve the congestion. Always be careful not to injure your child when you are using steaming water.

Professional help: Your physician may prescribe antibiotics if your child has an underlying respiratory infection that may be caused by bacteria.

A child who is having difficulty breathing may need to be admitted to a hospital. X rays of the larynx may be taken to determine the amount of obstruction of the air passages. Your physician may prescribe antibiotics, and your child may be given oxygen and put in a room with a vaporizer. If the air passages are seriously obstructed because of severe croup or epiglottiditis, it will be necessary either to pass a tube through the mouth into the throat to open the air passage or, in the most severe cases, to make an incision in the throat and insert a tube to enable the child to breathe. The tube is usually removed within 24 to 72 hours. Rarely, breathing must be maintained artificially with a mechanical ventilator. Most children admitted to a hospital for this treatment recover completely within a few days.

Bronchiolitis

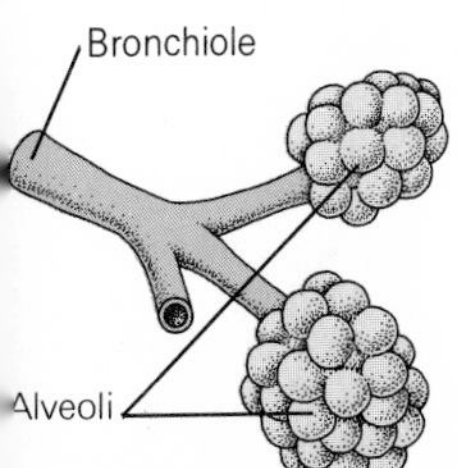

A large part of the lungs is made up of millions of tiny tubes called bronchioles. The bronchioles move air between the larger airways, called bronchi, and the tiny air sacs known as alveoli. In bronchiolitis, the lining of the bronchioles is infected, usually by a virus. The infection may first cause a cold and then begin to spread to other parts of the respiratory tract. The infected lining swells and almost completely blocks the passage of air into and out of the alveoli. The disorder can be rapidly fatal.

What are the symptoms?

The child has a cold and cough that suddenly become worse after a day or two. He or she then starts to breathe very quickly and with difficulty. In some cases, the chest does not expand when the child inhales. The child goes limp, is unable to eat, and his or her skin may turn blue from lack of oxygen.

Bronchiolitis is not common, but is easily diagnosed and should be treated immediately. Rarely, pneumonia (see next article) and heart failure (see p.408) can result.

What should be done?
If your child shows any of the symptoms described, see your physician immediately. You should be especially concerned if your child has a cold that suddenly gets worse after 2 to 3 days and if he or she is breathing quickly and with difficulty.

What is the treatment?
Go to a hospital emergency department immediately. If blueness of the skin has developed, your child needs to be placed in a humid oxygen tent immediately. In most cases, intravenous fluids are given for a few days; then if the child is not eating, a tube is passed through the nose into the stomach to feed him or her with liquids. In severe cases, liquids are given to the child intravenously. Antibiotics are often prescribed to prevent any bacterial infection that may result from the bronchiolitis.

In very severe cases, a child's breathing may have to be maintained with the help of a ventilator. With prompt treatment, most previously healthy children recover completely from bronchiolitis in 2 to 3 days.

Pneumonia in children

Pneumonia (see also p.384) is an inflammation of the lungs that is usually caused by an infection that has started in the upper respiratory tract. The infection produces a patchy inflammation, which is sometimes called bronchopneumonia, usually in the lower parts of both lungs.

Bronchopneumonia can also develop as a complication of measles (see p.745), whooping cough (see p.749), and chickenpox (see p.747) and is common in children with cystic fibrosis (see p.732).

Rarely, the inflammation may involve an entire section (lobe) of a lung. This is sometimes called lobar pneumonia, and it is usually caused by the *Pneumococcus* bacterium. Pneumonia can also be caused by an inhaled foreign object (see previous page).

What are the symptoms?
A child who has bronchopneumonia may start by having a cold for 2 or 3 days. His or her temperature then rises to about 101°F (38.5°C), and he or she develops a dry cough, starts breathing more rapidly than normal, and, in some cases, may wheeze. In very serious cases, a child may have cyanosis, which is blueness of the skin. Cyanosis is usually visible around the lips.

A child who has lobar pneumonia may have a higher temperature (104°F or 40°C). Occasionally, pleurisy (see p.387) develops and causes pain in the child's chest.

What are the risks?
Bronchopneumonia is more common than lobar pneumonia, but both of these infections are uncommon. Bronchopneumonia develops in only a small percentage of upper respiratory tract infections.

The high temperature can cause a febrile seizure (see Seizures in children, p.713). Rarely, the tissue in the inflamed areas of the lungs is replaced by fibrous scar tissue. Bronchiectasis (see p.389) may develop when small pouches form in the lungs during healing, and then become infected. Pneumonia is rarely fatal in children.

What should be done?
If your child has a fever and starts breathing with difficulty, call your physician. These symptoms can signal pneumonia if the child is younger than 6 months.

Most cases of pneumonia in children can be easily treated at home. Hospitalization is necessary only in very severe cases.

What is the treatment?
Self-help: If your child can be treated at home, there are several things you can do to relieve the symptoms and speed recovery. Your child's high temperature can be lowered and his or her pain can be relieved by taking a fever- and pain-reducing medication recommended by your physician, such as acetaminophen, removing the child's pajamas, and sponging his or her body with lukewarm water. Give plenty of liquids; at least a pint more than usual each day. And have your child rest quietly as much as possible.

Lowering a fever
To lower a feverish child's temperature, sponge his or her body with lukewarm water. A high temperature can lead to seizures.

Do not give aspirin to a child or adolescent with a fever because aspirin has been linked with Reye's syndrome (p.713), a potentially fatal condition.

Professional help: For the most part, a child's resistance to the infection leads to recovery. Your physician may prescribe antibiotics to treat the bacterial infection. Antibiotics are usually given by mouth, but the medication may be given intravenously if the infection is very severe.

An otherwise healthy child will usually recover completely from pneumonia after about 1 week.

Recurrent colds in children

It is common for a child to have a number of coughs and colds, especially in winter, and it is not something you need to worry about. Most children catch many colds at day care or during the first few years of school, because they are exposed to all kinds of new viruses. Gradually, however, the child acquires increasing immunity to the viruses.

A child's cold is often accompanied by a cough because, instead of blowing his or her nose, a child usually sniffs mucus down into the throat. The mucus irritates the throat, so the child coughs in an attempt to get rid of the mucus. Abdominal pain is also common in a child with a cold.

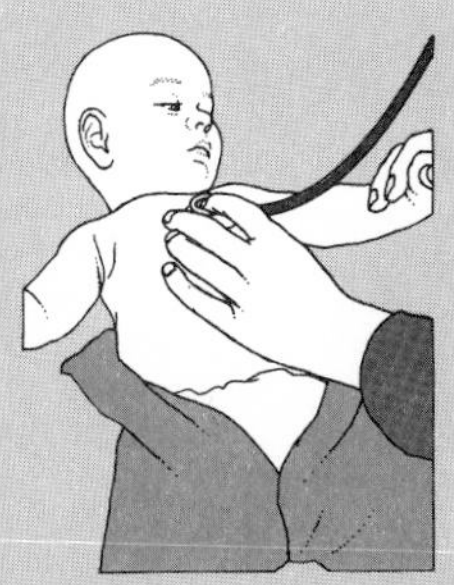

Chest examination
Your physician will examine your child's chest to see if the cold is developing into a more serious disorder such as bronchopneumonia (see p.384) or bronchiolitis (see p.725).

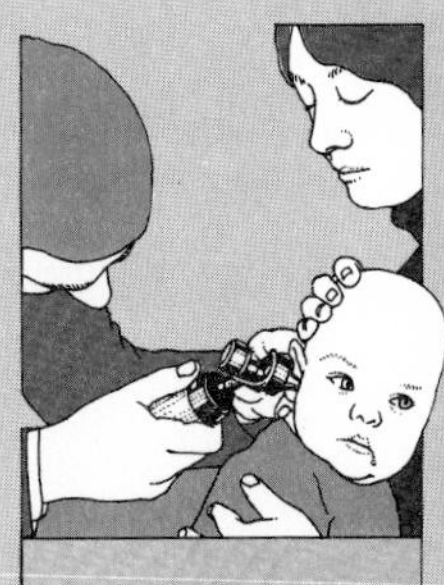

Ear infections
Respiratory infections often travel along the eustachian tube, which connects the back of the nose to the middle ear cavity causing middle ear infections. Ear infections should be treated immediately; they can lead to persistent ear problems.

When to see your physician

In rare cases, recurrent coughs and colds are a symptom of a serious underlying disorder. If that is the case, a child will seem ill most of the time, even without having a cold. If your child seems generally ill, with or without a cough or cold, take him or her to your physician.

In some children, cold symptoms are caused by an allergy. If your child sneezes and has a runny nose and watery eyes during the warm months, he or she probably has hay fever, an allergy to tree or other plant pollen. If the symptoms occur throughout the year, your child may be allergic to dust. Allergies may start when a child is between ages 1 to 3 (see Allergic rhinitis, p.370). If your child has such coldlike symptoms all year long, see your physician.

If a recurrent cough is not accompanied by a cold, or if a cough is accompanied by wheezing, it may indicate asthma (see p.381), or in rare cases cystic fibrosis (see p.732), and you should see your physician.

If a baby with a cold cries continually, refuses to eat, is restless and has skin that feels hot to the touch, develops an earache or pain in the face or forehead, has a high fever (about 102°F or 39°C), or is persistently hoarse and has a dry, painful cough, see your physician. These symptoms may indicate an infection.

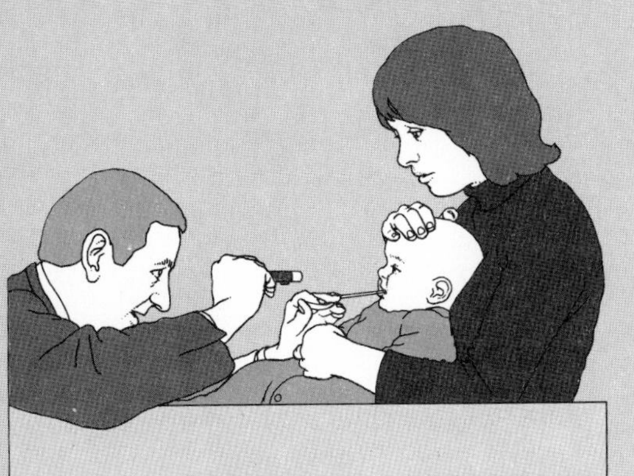

Physician's examination
Your physician will examine your child's throat to see if the tonsils or adenoids are inflamed. Although neither tonsillitis nor enlarged adenoids are usually risky, they can lead to breathing difficulties. If your child has been wheezing or grunting, your physician may suspect stridor (see p.725) and want to see how far the inflammation has spread before making a diagnosis.

What you can do

In some cases, a child with recurrent colds will cough a lot at night. This may be because the child's room is too cold and the air is irritating his or her throat, or because the room is too warm and the air is making the child's throat dry. Adjusting the room's temperature or humidity may solve the problem.

Infants with colds may have trouble eating. This is no cause for concern if the problem lasts no more than a day or so. You can help by keeping your baby's nose clear of obstructing mucus by using a small bulb syringe available in many drugstores and nonprescription saline nose drops.

Try to give an older child liquids before bed, to help clear the back of the nasal passage. Your physician may recommend a mild cough syrup.

Blood disorders

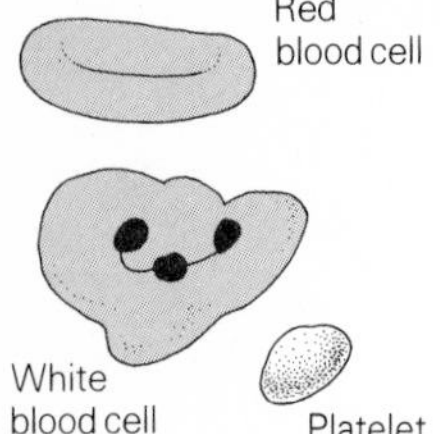

The blood disorders discussed in this section vary greatly in their effects on a child. These disorders, because their symptoms are varied and usually mild, may go undetected. For a child with iron-deficiency anemia or allergic purpura, a delayed diagnosis is not likely to cause any permanent effects. But a child who has leukemia, a cancer that affects white blood cells, has the best chances of recovery if the disease is diagnosed early. Progress in the treatment of leukemia has improved the prospects for children with the disease. Even so, leukemia requires intensive treatment, often in a hospital. This serious disease places great stress on both the affected child and his or her family (see Cancer in children, p.744).

Allergic purpura

(anaphylactoid purpura, Henoch-Schönlein purpura)

In allergic purpura, a rash appears just beneath the surface of the skin. The rash is thought to be due to an abnormal reaction between antibodies (substances in the blood that protect against infection) and blood vessels. The blood vessels become inflamed or burst and produce the rash. In some cases, it is thought that the antibodies are produced to fight an infection caused by *Streptococcus* bacteria. The antibodies can also be produced by the body's reaction to a certain food, a medication, or a virus. Allergic purpura most commonly affects children. Allergic purpura is very rare, and it occurs more frequently in boys than in girls.

What are the symptoms?

Usually a child will have a sore throat 2 weeks before the rash appears. The rash, which causes no discomfort, consists of purplish-red, irregularly shaped spots that vary in size and appear on the ankles, shins, buttocks, and elbows. When the spots appear, some children feel ill and have a slight fever. The rash tends to come and go.

Some children may also have swollen joints, or a stomachache that is often severe and persistent. Occasionally a child who has the disorder may have bloody stools, which indicate bleeding in the bowel, or bloody urine, which signifies kidney damage (see Glomerulonephritis in children, p.737).

The main risk faced by a child who has allergic purpura is permanent kidney damage. Two other, although extremely rare, risks are intussusception (see p.730) and massive bleeding into the intestinal tract and other internal organs.

What should be done?

If your child has any of the symptoms described, see your physician. Treatment is not required in most cases, because the disorder clears up on its own after a month or two. In severe cases, however, corticosteroid medications (hydrocortisone or prednisone) or intravenous gamma-globulin may be used. In some children, the problem may occasionally recur for up to 2 years before it finally disappears for good.

Iron-deficiency anemia in children

Anemia results from an insufficient supply of hemoglobin, a protein in the blood that carries oxygen to the tissues of the body. Iron-deficiency anemia (see p.450) is the most common type of anemia in children. The most likely cause of this disorder is inadequate iron in the diet. In most babies, it does not matter that the milk or formula that they are fed contains little iron, because they can draw on a supply of iron built up before birth. Premature babies, however, may have a low supply of iron and may therefore have iron-deficiency anemia. Other susceptible children are babies who are taken off breast milk or formula and put on a diet of solid foods deficient in iron, and older children who do not eat enough iron-rich foods. But iron-deficiency anemia may reduce a child's appetite, making the problem worse.

Less common causes of iron-deficiency anemia in children are inability of a child's body to absorb iron in the diet, as in celiac disease (see p.731), and undetected internal bleeding, such as the bleeding caused by hookworm infestation (see Box, Going out of the country, p.606).

What are the symptoms?

Mild anemia may produce no obvious symptoms. Symptoms and signs of more pronounced anemia (of any type) include several or all of the following: paleness, especially in the hands and inside the lower eyelids; tiredness; weakness; and, less commonly, fainting; breathlessness; and palpitations (awareness of one's heart beat). These symptoms, when present, are all more obvious after physical exertion.

What should be done?

If your child is less active than his or her playmates and if breathlessness follows minimal activity, see your physician. Do not assume that the child has anemia and try to treat it yourself with iron supplements.

Your physician may take blood samples for analysis and perform further tests, such as checking stools for blood (fecal analysis) and taking X rays of the digestive tract.

What is the treatment?

If, as is most common, the diagnosis is iron-deficiency anemia caused by lack of iron in the diet, your physician may prescribe an iron supplement for 3 months or longer, usually in liquid form. Your physician will also make recommendations about diet. Any underlying disorder will also be treated.

Leukemia in children

Leukemia is a cancer that affects white blood cells, the ones that protect the body against infection. Acute lymphocytic leukemia is the type that appears most often in children. (For a full definition of leukemia and a description of the disease in adults, see p.457.)

Acute lymphocytic leukemia affects the lymphocytes, white blood cells that are produced in the lymph glands (see p.463) and bone marrow. The cancer cells overflow from the lymph glands and bone marrow and circulate in the bloodstream. They can invade and affect any or all organs of the body, including the liver, spleen, and surface of the brain and spinal cord. In the bone marrow, the leukemic cells seriously interfere with the marrow's production of red blood cells, platelets, and the remaining noncancerous white blood cells.

What are the symptoms?

The main symptoms of acute lymphocytic leukemia are increasing paleness, tiredness, and general illness caused, in part, by anemia; a purplish-red rash caused by thrombocytopenic purpura (see Thrombocytopenia, p.456); pain in the limbs; severe headaches; swollen glands in the neck behind the angles of the jaw; an enlarged spleen, which your physician may feel just below the ribs in the upper left portion of the child's abdomen; susceptibility to infections, especially pneumonia (see p.726); and the development of sores and ulcers in the mouth and throat.

What are the risks?

Any form of leukemia in children is uncommon, but leukemia accounts for about half of all childhood cancers. Most children affected by leukemia are under 10 years old. There are about 2,000 cases of leukemia per year in this age group in the US. With recent advances in treatment, leukemia in children is now curable in most cases.

What should be done?

If you are concerned that your child might have leukemia, your physician will examine him or her and take a blood sample for analysis. If the possibility of leukemia cannot be ruled out, your physician will arrange for a bone marrow biopsy, in which a small amount of bone marrow is removed and examined under a microscope. These tests will show whether your child has leukemia.

What is the treatment?

Treatment is performed in a hospital. Basic treatment is with cytotoxic (anticancer) and corticosteroid medications. Some of these medications are given orally, others intravenously. Because the child's immune system is impaired, any infection that develops is treated with antibiotics.

To protect your child against the risk of serious infection, he or she may be isolated from other patients, and when you visit, you may have to wear a mask and gown to avoid spreading any germs that you might bring into your child's room. A sick child may be confused and upset, and will need your love and support. Talk to your child about his or her illness (see Cancer in children, p.744).

In nearly all cases, treatment reduces the symptoms after several weeks. Then the child is allowed to go home. Over the next year or so, the child is given frequent regular checkups and also takes doses of anticancer medications. If symptoms recur, the most effective treatment is bone marrow transplantation. The affected white blood cells and healthy blood and marrow cells are destroyed by radiation and medication; they are then replaced with healthy marrow from a donor (see Transplants, p.433). After the transplant, your child is kept in isolation temporarily to protect him or her against infection. In most cases, treatment of leukemia in children results in a cure.

Digestive system and nutrition

Several of the disorders described in this section occur because the digestive system is unable to handle certain foods (see p.468 for a full description of the digestive system).

Most of these disorders are usually tested for and detected soon after birth, since the symptoms they cause require immediate attention. If your child has such a disorder, your physician will prescribe a strict diet and recommend any specially prepared foods.

A healthy digestive system and a balanced diet are essential for a growing child. If you are concerned about your child's growth, see Growth disorders (p.734).

Intussusception

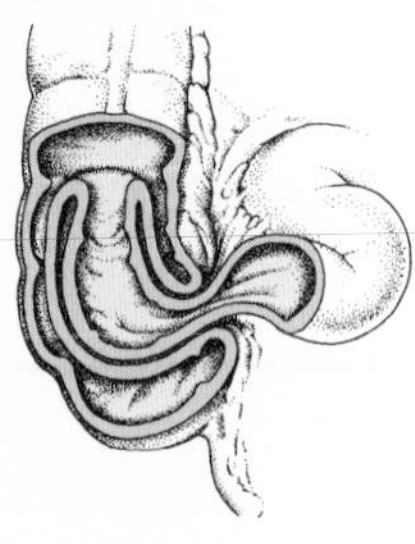

In intussusception, part of the baby's intestine telescopes in on itself.

In this rare disorder, a part of the baby's intestinal tract, usually the small intestine, telescopes into the adjoining part of the intestine. What causes the telescoping is not known. It happens most often in babies 4 to 6 months old, and is more common in boys.

What are the symptoms?

A baby suddenly screams as a strong wave of muscular contraction passes along the telescoped portion of intestine. The screaming may continue for several minutes. The baby then becomes pale and limp. He or she may vomit and may pass a bowel movement of bloody mucus, like red jelly. Screaming episodes recur every few minutes, as each additional wave of muscular contraction occurs.

What should be done?

Call your physician as soon as these symptoms occur. By examining the child's abdomen, your physician may be able to make a tentative diagnosis of intussusception.

The baby will be sent to a hospital for a barium enema X ray (see Glossary, p.822). This will confirm the tentative diagnosis of intussusception, and may also, as the barium is forced back along the intestine, push the telescoped intestine back into its normal position. If the barium enema does not accomplish this, the baby may need to have an operation in which the abdomen is opened and the intestine is pushed back into its normal position. The results of the operation are usually excellent.

Encopresis

In encopresis, children who are old enough to be toilet trained still regularly soil their underpants, even though they have no underlying disease. In most cases, this occurs because large amounts of hard stools accumulate in the rectum and the lower bowel (where your physician can sometimes feel the stools as a lump in the abdomen or by performing a rectal examination), and a liquid that may contain mucus flows past the blockage. Because the stool that comes out of the child is liquid, the condition may be mistaken for diarrhea when the problem is actually constipation (see Constipation in children, p.734). The child cannot control the passing of this liquid.

In a few cases, another type of encopresis develops in which a child soils his or her underpants with solid stools. This uncontrolled or involuntary bowel movement usually results from a stressful situation at home or at school. Parents who mistakenly think that the child is purposely soiling his or her clothing in this way may react with anger, thereby making the problem worse.

What is the treatment?

A child with encopresis should be taken to a physician to make sure the problem is not caused by an underlying disorder, and to get treatment. One treatment is enemas or suppositories used to clear the rectum and the lower bowel. Your physician may recommend that you try this at home.

The child must be encouraged to move his or her bowels at least once a day, at a regular time. In some cases, your physician may prescribe glycerin suppositories or daily laxatives for a few days or longer. The problem is far more distressing to your child than it is to you. For this reason, you should try to continually show the child that you understand the problem and are eager to help him or her overcome it.

You may be able to cure a child who cannot control bowel movements with fluids and a high-fiber diet, and by having the child move his or her bowels at the same time every day. If the problem persists, see your physician, who may refer you to a child psychiatrist or other specialist.

Celiac disease

(gluten enteropathy, nontropical sprue)

Celiac disease is an allergy that affects the small intestine. In this disorder, when gluten (a protein found in most grains) comes in contact with the small intestine, the membrane that lines the intestine loses its usual texture and becomes smooth. As a result, the intestine is less able to absorb nutrients (see Malabsorption, p.511). The disease is usually diagnosed in infancy or early childhood.

What are the symptoms?

Symptoms usually start within a few weeks after cereals are introduced into the baby's diet at 3 to 4 months old or later. The baby gains weight more slowly or may even lose weight. He or she may also have a poor appetite, which will aggravate the problem. The baby will have loose, pale, bulky, foul-smelling bowel movements, together with a lot of gas, several times a day. The gas is produced in such a large quantity that it may make the baby's abdomen swell. The swollen abdomen will contrast with his or her general appearance of being undernourished. In some cases, ulcers develop in the baby's mouth. Anemia and vitamin deficiencies may also occur as a result of celiac disease.

What are the risks?

Celiac disease is rare. A child with a relative who has celiac disease has a slightly higher than average risk of being born with it. In the very rare cases when a mild form of celiac disease is not detected in infancy, the child's growth may be affected.

What should be done?

If your child has the symptoms described, see your physician. Your child will probably have tests performed on his or her blood and stools. If these tests show evidence of the disease, a biopsy of the lining of the small intestine is performed. In a biopsy, a small amount of tissue is removed and examined. This test will confirm whether or not your child has celiac disease.

What is the treatment?

Wheat, rye, and other grains that contain gluten must be excluded from your baby's diet. Your physician may recommend that you discuss this with a dietitian. Rice and corn are safe for your child to eat, but he or she will need special bread and crackers, and you can make cakes or cookies with a special gluten-free flour. Within a few weeks of starting the diet, a child's symptoms usually clear up and he or she begins to thrive again. It is vital that your child continues with the diet. He or she may also need to take iron or vitamin supplements.

Your child needs to know the importance of avoiding certain foods, especially at school or friends' homes.

What is the long-term outlook?

A child with celiac disease can look forward to a full life, although he or she will have to stick to the special diet. The diet is restrictive, but many interesting and tasty foods can be prepared within its limits.

Recurrent stomachaches and headaches

Some children who are generally healthy have sudden stomachaches or headaches every few days, weeks, or months. They may look pale and often want to lie down. Generally the pain lasts a few hours, but it can last all day. When asked to locate the stomach pain, children usually point to the navel.

Many children stop having these problems by puberty. Others continue to have them in adult life.

Very few children who have recurrent stomachaches have an underlying disease. Food allergies such as lactose intolerance (see p.733) may cause the pains in some children. But in the majority of cases, the cause of the stomachaches is unknown, but may be psychological.

Headaches, too, are seldom a symptom of a serious underlying disorder. Most recurrent headaches in children are the result of emotional stress at home or at school. Stress can be caused by events such as the birth of a new brother or sister, or by the approach of exams at school.

In some cases, one or both parents may have frequent headaches, and may have had recurrent stomachaches as children. It is not known whether the tendency is inherited or whether it is the result of parental influence.

What should you do?

If your child has recurrent stomachaches, recurrent headaches, or a headache that lasts for more than one day, take him or her to a physician. If there is no underlying disease, your physician may recommend that you note whether the pains occur consistently after your child has eaten a particular food. For a severe headache, your physician may recommend that you give your child a pain-reducing medication such as acetaminophen. Do not give aspirin to children or adolescents who are ill with a fever because Reye's syndrome (see p.713), a potentially fatal condition, has been linked with aspirin.

If the stomachaches or headaches persist, they may result from psychological or emotional problems. Discuss the matter again with your physician, who may refer you to a child psychiatrist.

Cystic fibrosis

In this uncommon hereditary disease, the pancreas, a gland below and behind the stomach, fails to produce any digestive enzymes that are necessary to break down food into its component parts for digestion. The result is that a child's food is only minimally broken down by a small number of enzymes that are produced by the stomach, the intestinal wall, and the salivary glands. As a result, food retains its fats and most of its nutrients as it passes through the body (see Malabsorption, p.511).

In cystic fibrosis, the glands in the lining of the bronchial tubes in the lungs also malfunction. Instead of producing the normal thin mucus that traps germs and is then coughed up, they produce a thick, sticky mucus that tends to stagnate in the bronchial tubes. Germs multiply in this mucus and then cause respiratory infections, including pneumonia (see p.726).

What are the symptoms?

Symptoms sometimes occur immediately after birth. Mucous secretions in the baby's intestines make the first bowel movement too thick and sticky for the baby to pass, which can cause intestinal obstruction (see p.503). In all cases of cystic fibrosis, the child gains little weight right from birth, because failure of the pancreas to produce its enzymes means that hardly any nutrients are absorbed by the child. The child's stools are large, pale, foul-smelling, and greasy.

A child with cystic fibrosis may have recurrent respiratory infections, accompanied by a cough and fever, that are more severe and persistent than is normal. This is the result of the thick, sticky mucus that is typical of the disease. The mucus tends to trap and hold bacteria in the bronchial tubes. Children with cystic fibrosis often have large appetites and eat a great deal of food. Despite their malnutrition, they are not in pain and do not generally feel ill, unless they have acute bronchitis (see p.379).

What are the risks?

Repeated bouts of pneumonia are common in children with cystic fibrosis, and these repeated bouts usually lead to bronchiectasis (see p.389), which, in turn, makes the lungs even more susceptible to further pneumonia. Eventually this cycle may be fatal. However, treatment with antibiotic medications is enabling more children who have cystic fibrosis to survive the disease into early adulthood. Because cystic fibrosis is a hereditary disorder, it may affect several children in the same family (see Genetics, p.752).

What should be done?

The gene that is abnormal in cystic fibrosis has been identified, and this means that families with affected members can consult a genetic counselor (see p.664). In many cases, it is possible to perform blood tests on the prospective parents and chorionic villus sampling or amniocentesis on the fetus early in pregnancy (see p.684) to determine the chances of having a child with cystic fibrosis. If the diagnosis is made early, immediate treatment can lessen respiratory infections and lung damage and will also increase the child's life expectancy. In other cases, when symptoms occur soon after birth, the physician will be aware of a possible problem and check for the disease. But in some cases, respiratory infections are the main symptom, and these infections may not develop until some weeks after birth. If you are the first to discover the problem, you should see your physician as soon as possible. Diagnostic tests will then be performed on your child.

Although your child will be small for his or her age and will tend to miss school frequently, you should not overprotect him or her. Encourage your child to be positive and active and to live as full a life as possible. You may want to join a support group for families coping with cystic fibrosis.

What is the treatment?

Extracts of animal pancreas, in tablet, capsule, or granular form, are prescribed to replace the missing enzymes from the child's pancreas, and the amount of fat in the child's diet is reduced. With this treatment, the child begins to put on weight and the stools become much more normal. To keep the lungs as free of mucus as possible, your child may need to have daily respiratory physical therapy, which will include postural drainage (see Bronchiectasis, p.389). This program can be performed at home. Your physician or the physical therapist will show you and your child what to do.

Any respiratory infections are treated with large doses of antibiotics. The child may need to increase his or her salt intake, especially in hot weather or after exertion, to replace sodium lost in sweat. Some children with cystic fibrosis become increasingly disabled as they grow older because of damage to their lungs. In such cases, treatment may be a heart-and-lung transplant (see Transplants, p.433). This treatment has proved successful, but the supply of donor organs is limited.

Genetic engineering has produced the missing protein that loosens mucus, and has led to new methods of treatment.

Lactose intolerance

(lactase deficiency)

Enzymes are important substances in the body's chemical reactions. One enzyme, lactase, which is produced in the lining of the small intestine, breaks down lactose, the sugar found in milk. Most adult blacks, Asians, American Indians, and some whites produce little or no lactase and have difficulty digesting milk. This disorder is called lactose intolerance.

A severe episode of gastroenteritis (see p.491) in an infant can sometimes cause temporary damage to the intestinal lining, which then produces little or no lactase. The result of this is a temporary form of lactose intolerance. The baby may have no symptoms at first, because when diarrhea and vomiting associated with the gastroenteritis appear, your physician advises you to take the baby off milk and give him or her water instead. It is only when milk is reintroduced to the infant's diet that a reaction occurs and diarrhea reappears. The stools are often bubbly, and may cause diaper rash (see p.696) and may also be accompanied by vomiting. If lactose intolerance is present at birth, it causes bloating and persistent diarrhea immediately, and the affected child does not gain weight.

Teething problems

A baby's first teeth, the incisors, or front teeth, usually appear during the first year and seldom cause problems. The gum may be a little inflamed, there may be more drooling than usual, and the baby will probably chew a lot on his or her fingers or a teething ring. There may be a change in your baby's feeding, sleeping, and bowel habits, but he or she usually has very little discomfort.

The first and second molars, which usually appear between ages 1 and 3, are much more likely to cause problems. The gum may be tender and make eating painful. The cheek on the affected side of the mouth may be hot and flushed, and your child will probably be miserable for a few days. Parents would like to relieve their child's discomfort, but little can be done. Rubbing the gum gently, giving the child a cool drink from a cup, or giving the child a teething ring or a bagel to chew may ease the pain a little.

It is possible to overlook a disease or disorder in a child by attributing all symptoms to teething. If a child of teething age shows signs of distress, see your physician. Clutching one side of the face, for example, may be a sign that the child has an ear infection (see p.722).

Average ages for teeth to appear

Age	Baby teeth
6 months	First incisors
7 months	Second incisors
12 months	First molars
18 months	Canines
2–3 years	Second molars
	Full set: 20 teeth

Age	Permanent teeth
6–8 years	First incisors
6–7 years	First molars
7–9 years	Second incisors
9–12 years	Canines
10–12 years	First and second premolars
11–13 years	Second molars
17–20 years (or never)	Third molars (wisdom teeth)
	Full set: 32 teeth

Baby teeth

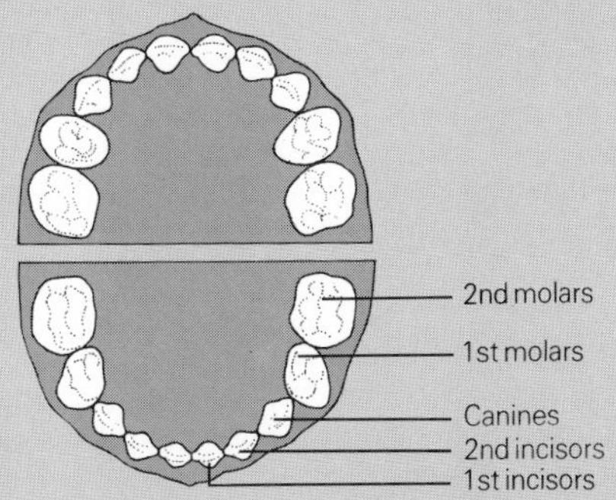

Permanent teeth

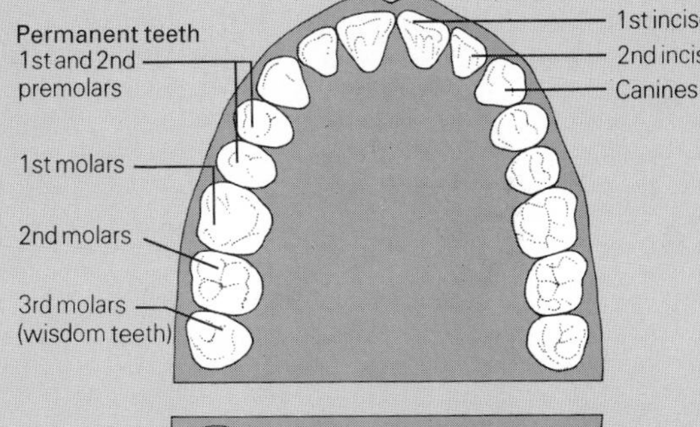

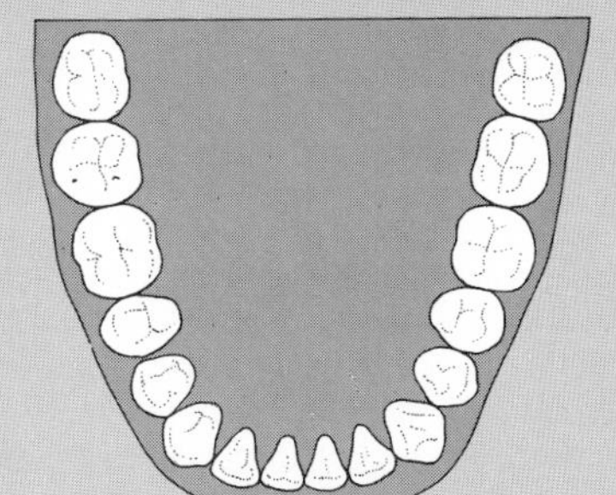

There are considerable variations in the ages at which teeth appear, and the ages listed above are just averages. Some children have one tooth or more at birth. Others have none at a year. Early or late teething has no effect on a child's general health or development.

What is the treatment?

If a physician who is treating a baby for recurrent diarrhea suspects temporary lactose intolerance, he or she will probably put the baby on a formula that has little or no lactose. Soybean-based formulas are often used because they supply protein without lactose. If the baby's condition improves, this formula is continued. The small intestine will eventually return to normal and milk can usually be reintroduced to the child's diet later.

If lactose intolerance is present at birth, or if there is a history of lactose intolerance in your family, ask your physician about nondairy formulas. Anyone who has had lactose intolerance from birth should realize that the condition is probably permanent and should continue to avoid milk and other dairy products. However, there are specially treated milk and nonprescription tablets available to help people with lactose intolerance to digest dairy products.

Hepatitis in children

Hepatitis is inflammation of the liver. In children, it is usually caused by a virus that enters through the mouth and is carried to the liver in the bloodstream. Of the various forms of hepatitis, the one that is most likely to affect children is acute hepatitis A (see p.523). The disease, which develops between 2 and 6 weeks after the virus enters the body, is milder in children than in adults. It frequently occurs in crowded, unsanitary living situations because closer contact with affected persons allows the disease to spread more easily.

What should be done?

A child who develops the symptoms of hepatitis (see p.523) should see a physician, who will usually advise bed rest as the only treatment necessary. One symptom of the disease is loss of appetite, so give your child small feedings of whatever he or she wants to eat. Encourage him or her to drink fluids that are high in calories, such as milk shakes. After about 2 weeks in bed, the child usually feels well enough to get up, and after 2 more weeks he or she can return to school.

Hepatitis is a contagious disease, so the child who has hepatitis, along with other members of the family, should be scrupulous about washing hands after using the toilet and before meals. And the toilet bowl, the bathroom sink, and any potty-chairs should be cleaned with antiseptic each time they are used by the affected child.

What are the long-term prospects?

The outlook after recovery from hepatitis is excellent. In children, there are usually no aftereffects of the disease except for immunity from further episodes of hepatitis.

Growth disorders

The charts on p.691 show that there is a wide range of height and weight in children. Usually it is only if a child's size falls well outside the total average range for his or her age that one of the following growth disorders may be responsible.

Nutritional disorders

The most common nutritional problem among American children today is being overweight, or obesity (see p.530), which means that a child weighs 20 percent more than the desirable weight for his or her height, build, and age. Obesity should be treated not because it is immediately harmful to the child's health, but because it often persists into adult life. In adults, obesity increases the risks that are related to many diseases. Malnutrition may result from inadequate intake of necessary nutrients or from illness.

Constipation in children

A child is constipated if he or she does not have a bowel movement for 4 days or more and if the stools are hard and dry and difficult to pass .

A diet deficient in fiber often causes constipation. Be sure to include fruit, vegetables, and whole grains in your child's diet (see Your diet and health, p.26). Babies 6 months old or older can be given whole-wheat cereals.

Another common cause of constipation is an anal fissure (see p.521), a small tear in the anus that makes bowel movements so painful that the child avoids having them. A child may also become constipated during an acute infection, by drinking less or sweating more. To prevent this, give your child as much liquid as possible.

Severe constipation that lasts 2 weeks or more may be a symptom of Hirschsprung's disease (see p.709) or of hypothyroidism (see next page).

If your child is severely constipated, see your physician. Do not give your child laxatives.

Among the disorders of the digestive tract that can limit growth are celiac disease (see p.731) and cystic fibrosis (see p.732).

Delayed puberty

Puberty usually starts in girls at about age 11½ and in boys a year or two later. If you are concerned about a delayed start of puberty in your child, see your physician.

Hormonal disorders

These disorders are usually caused by inadequate or excessive hormone production by the pituitary gland (see p.554) or the thyroid gland (see p.565). They are the least common of the growth disorders. They include gigantism (see p.555), short stature (see p.555), and hypothyroidism (see below).

Other causes of growth problems

Impairment of growth may also occur as a result of certain chronic diseases, including congenital heart disorders (see p.702), sickle-cell anemia (see p.453), thalassemia (see p.454), chronic kidney failure (see p.551), and rheumatoid arthritis (see p.589).

What should be done?

If you have looked at the charts (see p.691), and you are still concerned about your child's size, or if your child's pattern of growth has changed, take him or her to your physician. After examining your child, your physician may reassure you that your child does not have a growth disorder, may prescribe treatment for an obvious problem such as obesity, or may arrange for diagnostic tests.

Phenylketonuria

To develop and function, the body needs protein, which is made up of chemicals called amino acids. Normally, excess amounts of any amino acid in the food you eat are broken down or excreted, but in phenylketonuria (PKU), the body, because of an inherited defect, lacks the means to break down one of these amino acids, phenylalanine. The build-up of phenylalanine damages the brain.

How genetic defects such as the one that causes PKU are inherited is described elsewhere (see Genetics, p.752).

Phenylketonuria is extremely rare, but it is becoming slightly more common as more people with the disorder reach adulthood and have children.

What should be done?

A test for PKU is given to all babies shortly after birth. If the test shows that the baby has PKU, a special diet will be prescribed immediately to help prevent brain damage.

What is the treatment?

The baby is immediately put on a special formula that is low in phenylalanine. (Some phenylalanine must be in the diet because a certain amount of the amino acid is essential to the body.) Breast-feeding is not possible because breast milk contains phenylalanine. When the baby begins to eat specially selected solid foods, the special formula is continued as the child's protein source. Essentially the same diet must be followed at least until the child's nervous system has become mature at around the age of 10 to 12 years, but some children continue the diet beyond these ages because their nervous systems are not yet resistant to the damage that high levels of phenylalanine can cause.

A woman who has been treated for phenylketonuria and who has returned to a regular diet should return to the special low-phenylalanine diet before becoming pregnant to try to protect the health of the fetus.

Hypothyroidism

About one in every 4,000 white babies born in the US has a developmental defect of the thyroid gland that causes it to produce no hormones. The incidence of this disorder is lower in black infants. Without treatment, severe mental and physical disability result.

What should be done?

All newborns should have a blood test performed to check that the level of thyroid hormones in the blood is normal. If the test result is abnormal, further tests, such as a blood test to check for an excess of the pituitary hormone that stimulates the thyroid, will be performed. In most cases of hypothyroidism in newborns, however, the thyroid gland is absent at birth. Treatment with replacement thyroid hormone (in the form of thyroxine) must be given orally, every day for life, with periodic blood tests to adjust the dose as needed.

What are the long-term prospects?

When hypothyroidism is detected in the first few days of life, the outlook is excellent. Children treated with replacement thyroid hormone from birth develop normally, both physically and mentally.

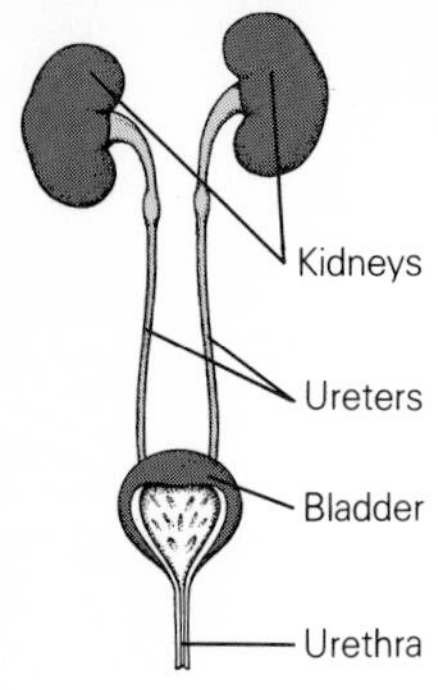

Urinary tract and sex organs

The urinary tract consists of the two kidneys, the two tubes called ureters that lead from the kidneys to the bladder, the bladder, and the tube that leads from the bladder to the outside, which is called the urethra (see p.540 for a detailed description of the urinary tract). Closely linked to the the urinary tract are the sex organs (see Men's health, p.611, and Women's health, p.623).

If your child has unusual urinary patterns, crying with urination, or blood in the urine, see your physician promptly so that he or she can provide treatment to prevent kidney failure (see p.550).

Bed-wetting

(enuresis)

By the age of 3½, about three fourths of all children stay dry at night. The other fourth continue to wet the bed, and in a few cases also wet themselves during the day. The medical term for this problem is enuresis, and it is sometimes called incontinence. If the child starts to wet the bed again after a long period of dryness following successful toilet training, it is called secondary enuresis.

The cause of enuresis, and especially secondary enuresis, may be psychological. It may be caused by stress from, for example, the arrival of a new baby or separation of the child from his or her mother. In a small minority of cases, there is an underlying illness, such as spina bifida (see p.700), or unrecognized or untreated diabetes (see p.558), which is usually marked by constant thirst. But in most cases, the cause of bed-wetting is unknown.

The problem can continue for several years. It is slightly more common in boys than in girls, and it often runs in families.

What should be done?

Have your child urinate before he or she goes to bed. Then, just before you go to bed, wake your child and have him or her urinate again. If your child is of school age, he or she may be able to deal with the problem by setting an alarm clock to go off in the middle of the night. Also, try to make clean pajamas and bed sheets available so your child does not have to wake you for assistance. If, after a few weeks, this approach does not have any effect on the problem, consult your physician to make sure there is nothing physically wrong with your child. Your physician may take a sample of urine for analysis, and, in rare cases, your child may need to have tests to evaluate functioning of the bladder.

The same principles that apply to toilet training should also be used to deal with bed-wetting. Praise your child for any dry nights and encourage him or her to keep a record of them, but never scold or punish your child for wet nights, and never make a record of them. This can deeply hurt the child's feelings, and it may also make the bed-wetting worse.

If your child is 7 or older, your physician may recommend the use of an alarm that rings loudly as soon as the first drop of urine touches the bed. Within a few days, most children find they are waking up before the alarm sounds and getting out of bed to go to the toilet. A few weeks of treatment is usually all that is required; if your child starts to wet the bed again, the alarm can be reintroduced.

Medical myths

1. Children who wet the bed sleep more deeply, and generally pass more urine, than other children.

Wrong. Children who wet the bed sleep as deeply and pass as much urine as other children.

2. Cutting down on the amount of liquid a child drinks before bedtime helps prevent bed-wetting.

Wrong. The amount of liquid the child drinks has no effect on the problem.

Urinary infections in children

In a urinary tract infection, infectious agents, usually bacteria, enter and multiply in the urinary tract. The process of infection and the symptoms produced are much the same in children as in adults. Girls are especially prone to infections because their urethra (the tube leading from the bladder to the outside) is relatively short. This makes it easier for bacteria to move into the bladder.

What are the risks?

Infections of the urinary tract are common during childhood. There are few risks from one or two bouts with such infections. However, if the problem recurs, it may be a sign that the child has some underlying abnormality of the urinary tract (see Chronic pyelonephritis, p.542). It is essential that any such abnormality be detected and corrected as soon as possible in order to help prevent the development of chronic pyelonephritis or even chronic kidney failure (see p.551). Take your child to your physician if you suspect he or she has a urinary infection. Always report bloody or very cloudy urine to your physician as soon as possible.

What should be done?

Your physician will have a sample of your child's urine tested. Next, if the infection recurs, your physician will arrange for further tests, including an ultrasound or CT scan of the abdomen, a radionuclide renal scan, and a voiding cystogram. The ultrasound or CT scan shows the shape of the kidneys, ureters, and bladder. The renal scan shows how well your child's kidneys work and shows any infections inside the kidney tissue. The voiding cystogram allows your physician to examine the bladder during urination.

Remember that even young children can be very sensitive about their genital organs and afraid of being in a hospital. If your child is embarrassed and afraid of the examination and tests, tell him or her that you understand and sympathize. Since the child's feelings are normal, it is a good idea to tell him or her that it is okay to feel this way, but that these procedures will help your physician to find out what is causing his or her problem.

What is the treatment?

Self-help: Be sure that your child follows your physician's instructions about drinking extra liquids. Encourage your child to empty his or her bladder completely when going to the toilet. Going again a few minutes later will help. Although symptoms subside a few days after the child begins to take the prescribed medication, all the medication must be taken to complete treatment.

Professional help: The infection is treated with antibiotics in tablet or, for younger children, in liquid form.

If the test results reveal any underlying abnormality of the urinary tract, corrective surgery may be necessary. Prospects are better for children whose urinary tract problems are diagnosed and treated early.

Glomerulonephritis in children

There are several forms of the kidney disease called glomerulonephritis (see p.543 for a general description, and also Nephrotic syndrome, next article). Poststreptococcal glomerulonephritis, or nephritis, is an acute form that develops in a child who has had a streptococcal (bacterial) infection, usually a sore throat, 2 to 3 weeks earlier. The body produces substances called antibodies to fight the bacteria, but because of some problem in the body's immune system, the antibodies continue to act after the bacteria have been destroyed, and they begin to harm the kidneys. The kidneys become inflamed and reduce urine production, and blood leaks from the glomeruli (filtering units of the kidney) into the urine.

What are the symptoms?

Symptoms appear over a few days. The main symptom is a reduced amount of urine. The urine that is produced looks smoky or reddish-brown because it is bloody. Another important symptom is accumulation of fluid throughout the body because of the reduced urine output. The excess fluid (edema) appears as swelling around the eyes and face, or over the entire body. In addition, some children have a headache and fever.

What are the risks?

Poststreptococcal glomerulonephritis is rare; the problem follows only a small fraction of streptococcal infections. Most children will recover completely from acute glomerulonephritis. During the illness, the buildup of fluid in the body may cause heart failure (see p.408). Also, the child's blood pressure may rise dramatically, and this produces a severe headache, vomiting, and sometimes seizures (see p.713). See your physician immediately if these symptoms appear.

In a few children, kidney problems persist. After many years, the result could be chronic kidney failure (see p.551).

What should be done?

Acute glomerulonephritis is a problem that requires medical attention. Always report abnormal-looking urine or abnormal amounts of urine to your physician. If after a physical examination your physician suspects acute glomerulonephritis, blood and urine samples will be taken. Laboratory analysis of the samples helps him or her make a diagnosis.

What is the treatment?

Your physician may recommend that your child rest in bed if he or she is very ill. In addition, your physician will recommend that your child be put on a diet to restrict the intake of sodium, liquids, and, sometimes, protein (meat, fish, eggs). The diet is designed to ease strain on the kidneys and to prevent accumulation of fluid in the body.

Your physician may prescribe antibiotics to eliminate any remaining infection. A diuretic drug may be given to increase the amount of urine, thereby eliminating excess fluids from the body.

If the child's condition worsens, he or she will be admitted to the hospital where any complications such as kidney failure and heart failure can be treated immediately. Your child's blood pressure will be checked regularly. If it rises to a very high level, your physician will prescribe antihypertensive medications (see High blood pressure, p.411). With most forms of glomerulonephritis, the prospects for a full recovery within a few months are excellent, even if there are complications.

Nephrotic syndrome

Nephrotic syndrome is a disorder of the kidney that mainly affects children. The filtering units of the kidneys, the glomeruli, are damaged, and proteins leak out of the blood into the urine. A second result is that the volume of urine is much reduced, so fluid that should be passed out of the body accumulates in the tissues. It is this fluid that produces the symptoms of the disorder.

What are the symptoms?

There are two main symptoms of nephrotic syndrome. One is the gradual appearance, over several weeks, of swelling throughout the child's body. This is due to accumulation of fluid and is called edema.

Another main symptom is a seriously reduced amount of urine, perhaps as little as one fifth of the normal amount. The urine usually looks normal.

What are the risks?

Nephrotic syndrome is uncommon. About 80 percent of the cases occur in children who are between ages 1 and 6, and most occur in children between ages 2 and 3. Boys are more likely than girls to get nephrotic syndrome.

A child with the syndrome is vulnerable to a variety of infections, including peritonitis (see p.503). But the main risk is that in a few cases, nephrotic syndrome persists despite intensive treatment and develops into chronic glomerulonephritis (see p.543), which can lead to kidney failure (see p.550).

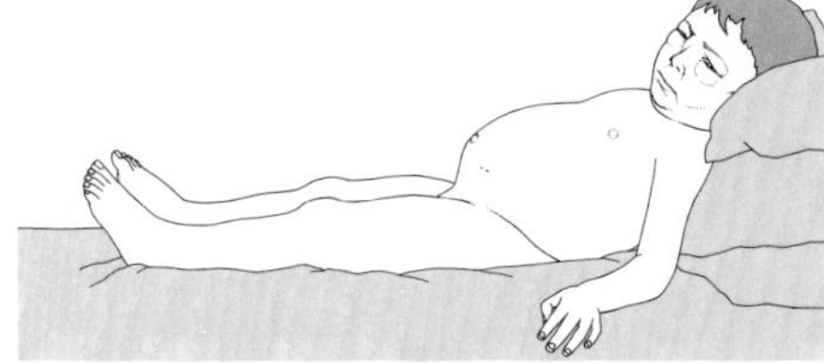

Edema in children
Edema, a condition characterized by a puffy face and swollen abdomen and ankles, may develop in a child with a kidney disorder.

What should be done?

See your physician if your child appears to have edema. He or she will examine your child and have samples of urine and blood taken for laboratory analysis. If results of the analysis suggest that your child has nephrotic syndrome, additional tests on samples of blood and urine, and possibly a biopsy of the kidney, will be needed to confirm the diagnosis. In a biopsy, a small amount of tissue is removed and examined.

What is the treatment?

Self-help: Although nephrotic syndrome often requires hospitalization, you can help your child by making sure that he or she sticks to the prescribed special diet and takes any medication exactly as instructed by your physician. Food should be cooked and served without salt, and the food should contain plenty of protein—fish, meat, eggs, and low-salt cheese. Your physician may also instruct you to restrict your child's liquid intake.

Professional help: Usually the child will be hospitalized so that treatment by diet and medication can be more easily supervised. The medications often used are diuretics, to promote fluid loss, and corticosteroids, to reduce inflammation and fluid accumulation. The corticosteroids are prescribed in high doses at first, but the amount is gradually reduced. The symptoms usually clear up by the end of the second week, and the child is allowed to go home to recover further.

In some cases, there is complete recovery with no aftereffects. In others, the child will have another episode of nephrotic syndrome after several weeks or months. Treatment as described will again relieve the symptoms. In a small number of cases, episodes continue to recur, and prolonged treatment with corticosteroid medications may eventually eliminate the condition.

Wilm's tumor

In Wilm's tumor, which almost exclusively affects children under 5 years of age, a malignant (likely to spread) tumor forms in one of the kidneys. Wilm's tumor may be an inherited disorder; there is a tendency for the disorder to run in some families.

What are the symptoms?

The main symptom of Wilm's tumor is a hard lump in the abdomen along with loss of weight and appetite. Anemia, causing weakness and paleness, and high blood pressure also occur.

What are the risks?

The disorder is very rare. However, the risks are those of any cancer. Without successful treatment, the malignant cells may spread to other parts of the body and start secondary tumors that are also life-threatening. However, advances in treatment have greatly improved chances of recovery.

What should be done?

If your child has any of the symptoms described above, see your physician, who will examine him or her. If your physician suspects a tumor, your child probably will be given an intravenous pyelogram (special X rays of the urinary tract) and a CT scan and/or an MRI scan. If Wilm's tumor is diagnosed, the affected kidney will be removed surgically to prevent the spread of the cancer. The remaining kidney will be able to take over the work of the one that is removed. The child will also be given anticancer medication and possibly also radiation therapy to destroy any remaining cancer cells.

Undescended testicles

(cryptorchidism)

In boys, the testicles (male sex glands) develop inside the abdomen from the same embryonic tissue that becomes the ovaries in girls. Normally, by a month before birth, both testicles have descended through the abdominal wall into the scrotum (a pouch of skin that surrounds the testicles).

In a very small number of boys, one testicle or both testicles do not descend by birth, for reasons that are not known. The condition does not cause any pain or problems with urinating, but there may be an associated inguinal hernia (see p.507).

What are the risks?

Usually the testicle or testicles descend during the boy's first few years, and regular medical checkups reveal when this has happened. Undescended testicles after age 5 may eventually cause a boy to become infertile if the problem is not corrected.

What is the treatment?

If either or both testicles have not descended by age 5, an operation known as an orchidopexy is performed to lower the testicle or testicles into the scrotum. Any inguinal hernia that is present is repaired at the same time. Once the testicles are descended, there usually are no further problems. However, in some cases it has been learned that some boys who were born with an undescended testicle or testicles have grown into men who have had decreased fertility.

Vulvovaginitis

Vulvovaginitis is redness, itching, and soreness of the vulva, the moist, normally pink fold that surrounds the opening to the vagina. It affects only a small number of girls, usually those whose vulva is already particularly sensitive to irritation. In many cases, no cause can be found for the condition. In other cases, it is caused by infectious agents (microorganisms) in stools or by a skin allergy to wool, nylon, fabric softeners, or detergents. Bed-wetting (see p.736) or pinworms (see p.751) are also possible causes of vulvovaginitis. Very rarely, the discomfort is caused by the child inserting a foreign object into her vagina. In such cases, there is usually a foul-smelling discharge. Vulvovaginitis may occur at any age. In some cases, vulvovaginitis can be a sign of child sexual abuse. The symptoms may result from someone inserting an object, a finger, or his penis into the child's vagina.

The soreness in the vulva can result in a frequent urge to urinate, and it can sometimes be very painful when the girl urinates. This frequent urge to urinate may sometimes lead you or your physician to the mistaken conclusion that the child has a bladder infection.

What should be done?

See your physician, who will examine your daughter's vagina. If a foreign object is in the vagina, the object will be removed. If you or your physician suspect that your daughter is being sexually abused, contact your local social services department at once.

In most cases, careful hygiene solves the problem. After a bowel movement, girls should wipe themselves from front to back. This assures that the soiled toilet paper will not touch the vaginal area. A girl with this disorder should take a bath every day, and the vulva should also be washed after each bowel movement. After bathing, the area should be dried thoroughly but gently and covered with zinc oxide paste or another protective ointment, also called "barrier creams."

The child should change her underwear daily. The underwear should be made of cotton or have a cotton insert or panel, and be loose fitting.

Muscles, bones, and joints

The most common cause of muscle, bone, and joint problems in children is injury (see p.573). Most childhood injuries heal quickly and completely. However, in addition to injuries, there are a few muscle, bone, and joint disorders that are especially risky in children. Rheumatic fever is very rare now, but severe or recurrent episodes can lead to valvular heart disease (see p.421). However, rheumatic fever does not cause permanent joint problems. Osteomyelitis, an infection of bone, can also have serious complications, but is usually treated successfully. Juvenile rheumatoid arthritis, a rare autoimmune disorder, usually runs its course by the time a child reaches puberty. However, some children will have permanent stiffness and deformity of the affected joints. Muscular dystrophy is an inherited disease that causes progressive wasting of the muscles. Intensive research is being conducted to find a cure for this crippling disease.

Rheumatic fever in children

Rheumatic fever is a disease that most commonly affects children of school age, particularly those 6 to 8 years old. It is usually, but not always, characterized by painful swelling in certain joints. Rheumatic fever originates, 1 to 6 weeks before its characteristic symptoms begin, in a throat infection caused by a certain strain of *Streptococcus* bacteria. The body produces antibodies to destroy the bacteria, but in some children these antibodies combine with antigens (see Glossary) and attack the tissues of their joints. Less commonly, the antibodies attack the tissues of the heart, or the tissues of both the heart and joints. Inflammation of the joints has no long-lasting aftereffects, but inflammation of the heart occasionally causes permanent damage to the heart valves.

Few children infected by the *Streptococcus* bacteria develop rheumatic fever. Those who do have some hereditary susceptibility, which is intensified if their living conditions and medical care are poor.

What are the symptoms?

The affected pair of joints becomes red, swollen, hot, and painful to move. The child also has a fever, loses his or her appetite, feels ill, and may be pale and sweaty. Inflammation of the joints usually disappears after about 24 hours, but if not treated, other joints may also become temporarily inflamed. The wrists, elbows, knees, and ankles are the most commonly affected joints. The hips, shoulders, fingers, and toes are also occasionally affected, but rarely without the condition first affecting other joints.

If only the heart has been affected and the disorder is mild, there are often no obvious symptoms, only vague symptoms such as tiredness, paleness, and general illness. This is why in many cases a child is not taken to his or her physician and the condition remains undiagnosed. But in severe cases of rheumatic fever, there are more obvious symptoms. The main symptom of the disease is breathlessness, especially during exertion or when the child is lying flat. Also, fluid accumulates under the skin of the legs and back, often causing swelling.

In some cases of rheumatic fever, a rash appears, usually on the chest, back, and abdomen. The rash consists of reddish circles with pale centers. The circles are 1 to 2 inches (2.5 to 5 cm) across and keep changing in shape. The rash does not itch.

Nodules, or small swellings, may appear (particularly when the heart is affected) just below the skin over bony areas such as the elbows, knees, knuckles, and the back of the head. The nodules are round, about ¼ to ½ in (5 to 10 mm) across, firm, and painless.

What are the risks?

In the 1960s and 1970s, the number of children in the US who had rheumatic fever gradually fell until the disease virtually disappeared, although it remained common in other parts of the world. This change was attributed partly to the treatment of infections with antibiotics and partly to improved nutrition. In the 1980s, however, a few small outbreaks of rheumatic fever occurred, indicating that the disease has not yet been eliminated. This is why it is vital for a child with a sore throat to have a test for the presence of *Streptococcus* ("strep") bacteria. Antibiotic treatment after a positive test result (meaning there is an infection) will prevent rheumatic fever.

Unless it is severe, a single episode of rheumatic fever is unlikely to lead to valvular heart disease (see Mitral stenosis, p.423, and Aortic incompetence, p.428). The risk of heart disease increases with one or more additional episodes of rheumatic fever. At one time, a child who had rheumatic fever once was more likely than other children to have an episode in the future, but today, lifelong treatment with antibiotics for a child who has had an episode usually protects against further streptococcal throat infections. A child still has a risk of developing heart disease if his or her episode of rheumatic fever has not been detected and treated.

In very severe cases that affect the heart, there is a risk of heart failure (see p.408).

What should be done?

If your child has any of the symptoms described, put him or her to bed and talk to your physician. If he or she suspects rheumatic fever, a throat culture and a sample of the child's blood may be taken for laboratory analysis. Your physician will also examine your child to determine whether his or her heart has been affected.

What is the treatment?

If an episode of rheumatic fever is mild, your child can rest in bed at home until tests show that the episode is over.

In more severe cases, a child is hospitalized. In the hospital, once the child's fever has subsided, the pain and swelling of inflamed joints may be treated with high doses of aspirin. When the heart is also affected, medication may be continued in smaller doses even after joint inflammation has disappeared. (But always consult a physician before you give aspirin to a child or adolescent who is ill with a fever because aspirin has been linked with Reye's syndrome (see p.713), a potentially fatal condition.)

In very severe cases of rheumatic fever, especially when the heart is seriously affected, your physician may prescribe more powerful anti-inflammatory medications such as corticosteroids.

In the rare event of heart failure, medications that strengthen the heart's pumping action may be prescribed by your physician. A diuretic may also be prescribed for heart failure. Diuretics rid the body of excess fluid that accumulates because of heart failure by stimulating urination. Whenever the heart is affected, a child will be more comfortable propped up in bed with pillows. This eases any breathlessness that might occur. In all cases of rheumatic fever, an antibiotic is prescribed to fight any bacteria that remain from the original throat infection and to prevent further infection.

What are the long-term prospects?

Today the long-term prospects are good. After any episode of rheumatic fever, mild or severe, physicians usually prescribe a low dose of an antibiotic to be taken daily to prevent another episode. Even when valvular heart disease does develop, either because of undetected episodes of rheumatic fever, or because the child did not take the prescribed medication regularly, current treatment allows most children who have had rheumatic fever to grow up and lead a full life.

Muscular dystrophy

(Duchenne muscular dystrophy)

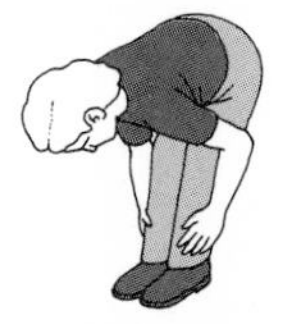

A distinctive sign of muscular dystrophy is that the child has difficulty moving into an upright position.

Muscular dystrophy is a progressive wasting and weakening of the muscles. There are several forms of the disease, but all of them are very rare. The most common and well-known type, which this article discusses, is Duchenne muscular dystrophy. This disease affects only boys, starts during early childhood, usually before a child reaches age 5, and first affects the muscles of the shoulders, hips, thighs, and calves. Gradually the disease spreads to all muscles and causes progressive disability and immobility. Because the weakened muscles interfere with respiration, the boy becomes susceptible to serious respiratory tract infections.

Although Duchenne muscular dystrophy affects only boys, it is usually inherited through female carriers, although 30 to 50 percent of cases occur in families that have no history of muscular dystrophy.

What are the symptoms?

Around age 3, a boy who has Duchenne muscular dystrophy first walks with his feet wide apart. He has trouble climbing stairs, falls easily, and finds it difficult to get up. He can barely lift his arms above his head. The affected muscles sometimes seem larger than normal, because fat replaces wasted muscle. The arms, legs, and spine usually become deformed. By the time he reaches adolescence the boy is confined to a wheelchair. If your son shows any of these signs, see your physician right away. Special tests, which may include a muscle biopsy, will show whether he has the disease. In biopsy, a small amount of muscle tissue is removed for examination under a microscope.

Any woman from a family with Duchenne muscular dystrophy should see her physician or a genetic counselor before deciding to get pregnant. Blood tests can be performed to find out whether female relatives of boys with the disorder are carriers of the gene (see Genetic counseling, p.664). If a female carrier has a son, there is a 50 percent chance that he will have the disorder. Chorionic villus sampling and amniocentesis can be performed during pregnancy (see p.684). These tests can indicate whether the fetus is affected. Your physician may refer you to a genetic counselor, who can explain the risks related to the disorder.

What is the treatment?

The gene responsible for some forms of muscular dystrophy has recently been identified and the basis for the disease is better understood. No cure is currently available. Treatment is physical therapy aimed at minimizing deformities.

Osteomyelitis in children

Osteomyelitis is an infection of bone and bone marrow. Although bone appears to be inactive, it is living tissue, honeycombed with blood vessels that deliver oxygen and nutrients that bone needs to stay alive.

Bacteria, from a contaminated wound for example, can get into the bloodstream and start an infection in the bone. The area of infection becomes inflamed and pus forms. Why the bone infection develops is unknown. Usually a single area near a joint in one of the arm or leg bones is affected. Rarely, more than one bone becomes infected.

What are the symptoms?

Symptoms usually develop over 2 or 3 days. The main symptoms are pain and tenderness in the affected area, particularly when the joint near it is flexed, along with high fever. An infant or young child won't want to move an affected arm or leg, and will probably scream if that arm or leg is touched or moved. If a leg bone is infected, a child is very reluctant to walk and, if forced to do so, has an obvious limp. If the condition is not treated within a day or two, the skin over the infection becomes red, swollen, and tender.

What are the risks?

In children, osteomyelitis seems to occur most frequently between ages 5 and 14, and more often in boys than in girls.

In the rare circumstance that osteomyelitis is not treated, the bacteria can spread and multiply in the bloodstream and cause blood poisoning (see p.452). A much more likely,

Flat feet, bow legs, and knock knees

From the time most children begin to learn to walk until the start of puberty, the bones of their legs and feet gradually change shape. Flat feet, bow legs, and knock knees are variations that may occur in almost all children, and they are usually no cause for concern.

At birth, all babies have flat feet. Arches develop slowly over the first 6 years. Until age 2, a child usually has bow legs—that is, when the ankles touch each other, the knees do not. As a child learns to walk, this is gradually reversed until, at age 3 or 4, he or she is usually knock-kneed. When a child stands with the knees together, the ankles do not meet. With continued growth, the knees and ankles become normally aligned.

In the majority of children with flat feet, bow legs, or knock knees, no treatment is necessary. Be sure that your child's shoes fit well, and that there is plenty of opportunity for your child to exercise his or her growing feet and legs. In some children, one or more of these variations in posture may last into adolescence and adulthood. Usually they are inherited, and only rarely are they caused by a disease. If your child's feet and/or legs seem to be developing abnormally, or your child's progress in learning to walk seems slow (see Milestones, p.691), talk to your physician.

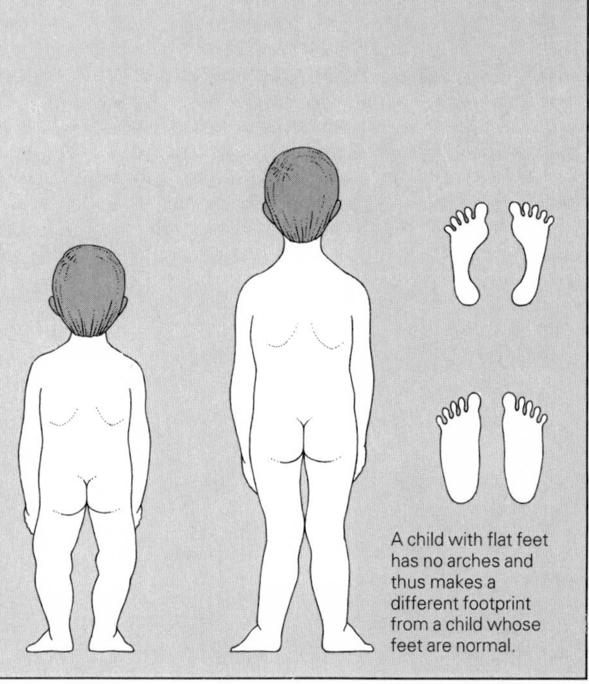

A child with flat feet has no arches and thus makes a different footprint from a child whose feet are normal.

although rare, risk is that the infection will destroy a large area of bone and may even spread into a neighboring joint. If this happens, the result is likely to be permanent stiffness or deformity of the infected joint.

Another risk is that the infection will spread and break through the surface of the skin. This takes the form of an abscess, which discharges pus and will not heal until the underlying bone infection is treated.

What should be done?

If your infant or child has symptoms of osteomyelitis, see your physician as soon as possible. If your physician's examination confirms that your child has osteomyelitis, he or she may be hospitalized immediately. To confirm the diagnosis, blood tests and X rays of the infected area will be performed.

Although osteomyelitis is rare, it is a good idea to take steps to prevent it. Clean any wounds your child receives thoroughly, and cover them with a clean bandage until they are completely healed.

What is the treatment?

The main treatment for osteomyelitis is an antibiotic given orally (or intravenously at first) for about 6 weeks.

If necessary, minor surgery is performed to drain and clean out the abscess. In some cases, your physician may immobilize your child's affected arm or leg in splints or in a cast. Once the infection is healing, the child will be sent home. It is important to follow your physician's instructions very carefully regarding antibiotics and exercise until your child is cured of the infection.

Juvenile rheumatoid arthritis

(Still's disease)

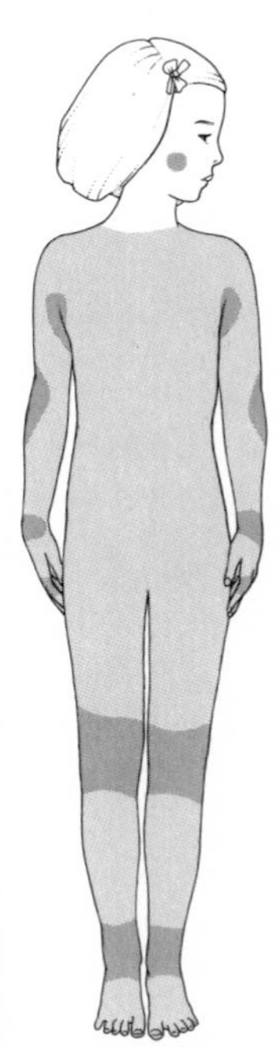

Sites of rash (gray) and other possible visible symptoms (dark gray) associated with juvenile rheumatoid arthritis.

Juvenile rheumatoid arthritis is an autoimmune disorder, which is an intermittent (coming and going) malfunctioning of the body's immune system (natural defense mechanism). Antibodies, which are produced to destroy invading infectious agents, combine with antigens (see Glossary) and attack the body's own tissues. These antibodies cause inflammation of organs, joints, and other parts of the body, resulting in variable amounts of damage and destruction. Juvenile rheumatoid arthritis usually starts between ages 2 and 5 and comes and goes over a number of years, usually disappearing by puberty. The episodes last for an average of a few weeks and tend to lessen in severity as they recur.

What are the symptoms?

Your child usually has a fluctuating temperature, which often swings from normal 98.6°F (37°C) in the morning to about 103°F (39.4°C) in the evening. The child has a poor appetite and loses weight. A blotchy, red rash may break out over the trunk, arms, and legs. Anemia often develops.

Sites of inflammation vary considerably from child to child. The area around one or both eyes may become red and painful, the lymph glands in the neck and armpits may swell, or the outer membrane of the heart may be inflamed and cause chest pain (see Acute pericarditis, p.430). The joints, usually the knees, ankles, elbows, and joints of the neck, may become swollen, stiff, and painful. The symptoms usually appear gradually, but sometimes they begin suddenly. In a few cases, the joints become deformed over time.

What are the risks?

Juvenile rheumatoid arthritis is uncommon, and girls are affected about 4 times as often as boys. In a few cases, inflammation of the joints leads to partial or disabling deformity, and inflammation of the eyes leads to partial or complete blindness.

What should be done?

If your child has any of the symptoms described, see your physician. A physical examination and blood tests are usually enough to make a diagnosis. If only the joints are swollen and there are doubts about the cause, a biopsy of the membrane that encloses one of the joints may be performed. In a biopsy, a small amount of tissue is removed for examination.

What is the treatment?

Self-help: Your child should get plenty of rest but should be allowed to get up when he or she feels like it. Encourage your child to eat, and provide a nutritious, balanced diet (see p.26) that contains plenty of protein. For children who have inflammation of the hand joints, special cutlery may help. If your child is not well enough to go to school but could study at home, ask your local school district to arrange a home-study program.

Professional help: Treatment is the same as for adult rheumatoid arthritis (see p.589). Your physician may recommend that you give your child acetaminophen to reduce fever, or he or she may prescribe a nonsteroidal anti-inflammatory medication to reduce swelling. In addition, physical therapy is prescribed when the joints are affected.

These are exercises both for the parents to perform on the joints and for the child to do alone. It is important that you make sure your child does the exercises, because they are crucial to minimizing the pain and the disabling effects of rheumatoid arthritis.

What are the long-term prospects?
With treatment, most children and young adults who have rheumatoid arthritis recover and function normally. However, in a few cases a child may be severely disabled by the disease, and a few will die.

Cancer in children

Regular visits to your child's physician and watching your child carefully for the warning signs of cancer (see p.16) will provide the best chances for early detection. With early diagnosis and treatment, some childhood cancers can go into remission (disappearance of symptoms) or be cured.

If your child is one of the few who does have some form of cancer, your physician should discuss with you the nature of the disease, the course of treatment, and the outlook for your child. No one knows exactly what causes cancer, but it is not contagious, and it is usually not hereditary. Ask your physician to recommend some support groups of parents whose children have had cancer. Learning how other parents have coped may help you and your child come to terms with cancer.

Most children with malignant (likely to spread) diseases are treated in a hospital that can provide the latest treatment. If your child needs to stay in the hospital for some time, he or she will require a lot of your time, care, and love. Being in a hospital may frighten your child. To make the hospital room less impersonal, bring your child a favorite toy or picture. After some time, your child may be allowed to go home, and probably return to school. Try to maintain as normal a home life as possible, and, within reason, do not lower your expectations of your child, either at school or at home.

Because you know your child better than anyone who may be involved in providing his or her treatment, you are probably the best person to judge how much to tell your child about the illness. If you are not sure how to explain the illness, discuss the problem with your physician or a nurse. He or she can help you decide on the most helpful way to talk to your child about his or her illness. Once you feel ready to talk to your child, do not hesitate. It is better for your child to learn about the cancer from you and your physician than to be told by someone who is less concerned about him or her, or to allow your child to imagine something worse than the truth.

In most cases, the chances are greater than 50 percent that your child will recover. If there is a strong possibility that the cancer cannot be cured, read the section Dying and death (see p.800), paying particular attention to the article Children and death (see p.807). But whatever the outlook, the months ahead will undoubtedly be difficult ones for your whole family. Do not keep your feelings bottled up inside. Discuss your feelings with physicians and nurses who are treating your child. Talking things over with friends and relatives may also be helpful. For information on support groups for parents and families of children with cancer, call the Cancer Information Service of the National Cancer Institute: 1-800-4 CANCER (1-800-422-6237).

Childhood infectious diseases

An infectious disease is a disease caused by infectious agents (microorganisms) that enter the body and multiply. Once you recover from certain infectious diseases of childhood, you are usually immune to reinfection. Measles, rubella (German measles), chickenpox, mumps, whooping cough, scarlet fever, and diphtheria are described in the following articles. Most of these diseases can be prevented by a program of immunization. (For other infectious respiratory diseases of childhood, see p.723.)

The childhood infectious diseases that are described in this section are contagious; that is, they spread from one person to another. The infectious agents that cause these diseases can live outside the body for only a few hours and are usually spread in tiny droplets coughed or sneezed into the air and by direct contact. Such diseases often spread through a school as a minor epidemic.

Infectious agents enter the body through the thin lining of the respiratory or digestive tract. Once inside, there is an "incubation period" during which infectious agents are not sufficiently numerous to cause symptoms.

The infectious agents increase in number and spread through the bloodstream and lymphatic system (see p.463); the disease becomes contagious and symptoms appear.

Meanwhile, the body is fighting off the infection in various ways. One way is to produce antibodies, special substances that neutralize or destroy the infectious agents. Each disease initiates the production of a particular kind of antibody. Gradually the body's immune system overcomes the infectious agents.

Once you have had certain childhood infectious diseases, your body can recognize any reinfection immediately, and antibodies destroy the infectious agents before they can cause symptoms. Once you have had the disease, you become immune, which means you cannot have measles, German measles, mumps, or chickenpox more than once. This is called natural immunity. Sometimes, although he or she did not have the disease before, a child's immune system is able to destroy infectious agents before they cause symptoms. Such children are immune afterward, although they were not actually ill. Also, the body can be stimulated to produce antibodies that will work against a particular disease by injecting a specially prepared, harmless version of the infectious agent (see Immunization, p.748). A small number of children have side effects such as pain and tenderness at the site of the injection, mild fever, swollen glands, headache, muscle ache, and joint ache, but these are far outweighed by the benefits of immunization.

Measles

(rubeola)

See p.247, **Visual aids to diagnosis, 26.**

Measles is a highly contagious disease caused by a virus that spreads throughout the body but chiefly affects the skin and respiratory tract. The incubation period (see introduction, previous page) is 7 to 14 days.

Measles is less common than it was at one time. This largely results from an immunization program that was introduced in the late 1960s. The Public Health Service continues its efforts to eliminate measles completely in the US, because it is the most serious of the preventable childhood infectious diseases. Measles has a high rate of complications, including pneumonia (see p.384) and encephalitis (see p.291).

What are the symptoms?

Typically, on days 1 and 2, the child has a fever, runny nose, red watering eyes, dry cough, swollen glands, and sometimes diarrhea. By day 3, the temperature falls and tiny white spots, like grains of salt, appear on the lining of the mouth. On days 4 to 5, the temperature rises again and a rash appears. The rash starts on the forehead and behind the ears as small (about 1/10 in, or 2 to 3 mm), dull red, slightly raised spots. As the spots gradually spread to the rest of the head and body, they get bigger and join together. By day 6, the rash begins to fade quickly, and usually by day 7 all the symptoms are gone.

When your child has an infectious disease

Here are some risks of childhood infections and tips to parents on caring for a sick child.

General risks of childhood infectious diseases

One rare, although possible, result of an infectious disease is encephalitis, which is inflammation of the brain (see p.291). Its symptoms are drowsiness or sleepiness so pronounced that it is difficult to wake the child completely; headache; sensitivity to bright light; and sometimes unconsciousness. It usually appears a week or so after the original disease has cleared up. Encephalitis is a medical emergency. If your child has symptoms of encephalitis, take him or her to a hospital emergency department quickly.

Other risks include febrile seizures (see p.713), acute infections of the middle ear (see p.359), and pneumonia (see p.384). If the symptoms of these complications occur, see your physician.

Children at special risk

Any child who develops an infectious disease can have complications, but certain children are at special risk. They include infants under 1 year old, children who are taking corticosteroid medication, and children who already have a long-term disease, such as diabetes mellitus or asthma.

If your child is at risk, talk to your physician as soon as symptoms of an infectious disease appear, or if you know that your child has been exposed to an infectious disease. For some diseases, such as measles and chickenpox, your physician may give your child an injection of antibodies called gamma-globulin. This injection may prevent the symptoms from developing or—if they develop—may make them much less severe.

How to take care of your child

To avoid spreading the infection and to help your child rest and recuperate, keep your child at home until your physician recommends that he or she return to school.

If your child has a fever, ask your physician to recommend a nonprescription antifever medication such as acetaminophen. Do not give aspirin to children or adolescents who are ill with a fever, because aspirin has been linked with Reye's syndrome (see p.713), a potentially fatal condition.

Do not force your child to eat or stay in bed. Encourage rest, but light activities such as reading, coloring, or watching television can help your child pass the time. Also see Caregiving at home, p.786.

Encourage your child to drink plenty of liquids.

Some children with measles complain that light hurts their eyes. Usually this symptom is no cause for concern, but let your physician know about it. In rare cases, it can indicate meningitis (see p.290).

What should be done?

Steps toward preventing measles are vital. Have your physician or the public health department in your area immunize your child against measles when he or she is 15 months old. (see Box, Immunization, p.748). Because the initial vaccination may not take, physicians recommend that you have your child revaccinated when he or she goes to school. Call your physician if you suspect your child has measles. If there is a local epidemic, your physician will know about it, and a telephone description of your child's symptoms may be enough for a diagnosis. Otherwise, your physician may want to examine your child. At the first sign of any complications, see your physician immediately.

Medical myths

If your child has measles, keep him or her in a darkened room because light can damage his or her eyes.

Wrong. While light may irritate the eyes of a child who has measles, it will not damage them. Darken your child's room if he or she complains that light is bothering his or her eyes.

What is the treatment?

Self-help: Make your child more comfortable and protect him or her against possible complications (see Box, When your child has an infectious disease, previous page) such as a type of encephalitis (see p.291). Because measles is so contagious, it is difficult to prevent other members of the family who are not immune from developing it.

Professional help: Prevention by immunization is vital. There is a combined vaccine for measles, mumps, and rubella (see Box, Immunization, p.748). However, if you or members of your family have not yet had measles or been immunized, and have been exposed to the disease, your physician may try to prevent it or lessen its effects. This is done by giving you an injection of antibodies called gamma-globulin. Your physician may prescribe antibiotic medications if complications caused by bacteria develop.

In most children, measles disappears within 7 to 10 days.

Rubella

(German measles)

See p.247, **Visual aids to diagnosis, 27.**

Rubella is a very mild contagious disease that is caused by a virus. In most children who catch it, rubella causes no more problems than a common cold (see p.368). Once inside the body, the virus has an incubation period (see the introduction to this section, p.744) of 14 to 21 days.

What are the symptoms?

For the first 2 days, the child has a slight fever, and sometimes swollen glands behind the ears, down the side of the neck, and on the back of the neck. A rash appears on the second or third day, consisting of flat, reddish-pink spots about 1/10 in (2 to 3 mm) across, on the head and/or body. The rash does not itch, and lasts for a day or so. By the fourth or fifth day, the symptoms are gone.

What are the risks?

Rubella is slightly less common than measles (see previous article), and it is not as contagious, so it does not spread from child to child at school as readily. Because rubella is such a mild disease, little treatment is required (see When your child has an infectious disease, previous page). Although the affected child is at very little risk, the disease can damage a growing fetus. It is therefore vital that any pregnant woman who has been exposed to rubella see her physician immediately. There is a combined vaccine for measles, mumps, and rubella available (see Box, Immunization, p.748) that may help prevent infection of the fetus.

All children should be immunized. Women who might become pregnant and have not been vaccinated for rubella should be immunized to prevent birth defects. Because the vaccination can cause problems for the fetus, it is essential that a woman not get pregnant before, during, or up to 3 months after vaccination (see also Rubella and pregnancy, p.661).

Roseola infantum

Roseola infantum is a common infectious disease caused by a virus (herpes simplex virus, type 6). The disease mainly affects children between ages 6 months and 3 years.

What are the symptoms?

Roseola infantum starts with a sudden fever and irritability. During the first few days of the infection, the child's temperature may rise as high as 104°F (40°C). About the fourth or fifth day, the child's temperature suddenly drops back to normal 98.6°F (37°C), and a rash appears on his or her trunk. The rash may quickly spread to the child's neck, face, arms, and legs, and usually lasts for no more than a couple of days. Other symptoms and signs are a sore throat and swollen lymph glands in the child's neck.

Sometimes a child may have febrile seizures (see p.713) during the course of the disease, but there are usually no serious aftereffects or complications.

What is the treatment?
Keep your child cool using a sponge or washcloth soaked in lukewarm water, and give him or her a nonprescription fever-reducing medication recommended by your physician, such as acetaminophen. Do not give aspirin to children or adolescents who are ill with a fever, because aspirin has been linked with Reye's syndrome (see p.713), a potentially fatal condition. No other treatment is necessary.

Fifth disease

(parvovirus infection)

Fifth disease gets its name because it is the fifth of the common childhood infections that cause fever and a rash—the others are measles, roseola, rubella, and scarlet fever. Sometimes chickenpox is included too. Fifth disease is less serious than the other four infectious childhood diseases. The cause of fifth disease is one of a group of viruses known as parvoviruses, which infect both humans and animals. Most parvoviruses do not seem to cause illness.

What are the symptoms?
The rash that indicates fifth disease is sometimes described as looking like a "slapped cheek"—the sides of the face are bright red—but the rash may also appear on the arms and legs, although rarely on the trunk. The rash may take the form of flat red spots, rings, or larger patches of reddish skin. Exercise or bathing often makes the rash worse. The child's temperature is usually slightly raised, and he or she may also have a sore throat or headache. Outbreaks of fifth disease occur most often in spring and early summer and usually affect children ages 5 to 14. Complications of fifth disease may include acute bone marrow failure (the marrow stops producing red and white blood cells and platelets) and joint pain.

What should be done?
The rash of fifth disease may persist for a couple of weeks but does not require any treatment. The child is not contagious when the rash is present. A soothing cream or lotion may be applied to the rash if it itches. Your physician may recommend that the child take acetaminophen to reduce any fever. Do not give aspirin to children or adolescents who are ill with a fever; aspirin has been linked to Reye's syndrome (see p.713), a potentially fatal condition. With bed rest and plenty of fluids, recovery takes about 10 days.

Chickenpox

(varicella)

See p.247, **Visual aids to diagnosis, 28.**

Chickenpox is a mild infectious disease that is caused by the varicella zoster virus. This is the same virus that, after years of dormancy, can cause shingles in adults (see p.602). The virus mainly affects the skin and the lining of the mouth and throat. After the virus enters the body, there is an incubation period (see the introduction to this section, p.744) of from 7 to 21 days.

What are the symptoms?
The main, and often the first, symptom of chickenpox is a rash. Groups of small, red, fluid-filled spots appear on many parts of the body. After a few days the spots burst or dry out, and then crust over. They are very itchy, and it is difficult to resist scratching them. Spots in the mouth, around the eyes, or in the vagina, may be very painful.

A child may also have a slight fever, but in general does not appear to be ill. However, adults who have the disease often have flulike symptoms (see Influenza, p.597) for 2 or 3 days before the rash appears. Children recover very quickly, within 7 to 10 days, but adults are more likely to develop complications, and they take longer to recover.

What are the risks?
Chickenpox is a fairly common and very contagious childhood disease. It occurs only rarely in adults.

If the rash is scratched excessively, it may become infected and produce pus. Your physician may prescribe antibiotic ointment or medication if the rash becomes infected.

What is the treatment?
Calamine lotion applied to the rash will help relieve itching. If the rash in the mouth or around the eyes is painful, your physician may recommend acetaminophen to relieve the pain. Read When your child has an infectious disease (p.745) for general treatment. Do not give aspirin to a child or adolescent who has (or may have) chickenpox, since using aspirin may lead to a potentially fatal disorder called Reye's syndrome (see p.713).

Immunization

Immunization is the process by which people are made immune, or resistant, to specific disease-causing microorganisms. There are two ways to become immune to a disease. If you catch an infectious disease such as measles, your body produces antibodies that neutralize or destroy the measles-causing organisms. Your symptoms disappear, and you recover from the disease. If you are exposed to measles-causing organisms again, the antibodies you have already produced will destroy them before they can cause any symptoms. Therefore, you will not have measles a second time. This is called natural immunity.

You can also become artificially immune to a disease without ever having it. Artificial immunity can be temporary or permanent. If you need temporary immunity—for example, if corticosteroid treatment makes you more prone to infection—your physician may treat you with antibody injections. This passive, or temporary, immunity can last up to several months. To ensure active, or permanent, immunity, your physician will give you a vaccine, which is made with dead or harmless versions of the infectious agent, by injection or by mouth. Your body will produce antibodies to fend off these agents, and while you do not have the symptoms of the disease (except, in some cases, a slight fever), you become immune to it. This is called vaccination or immunization.

Today, largely because of advances in immunization, many childhood infectious diseases that once caused serious illness and death are now extremely rare. One disease, smallpox (see p.605), has been completely eradicated. The chart here shows how a child's immunizations are usually scheduled, to offer maximum protection against serious infectious disease. These recommendations may change as new vaccines are developed and other medical discoveries are made, so ask your physician for the most current schedule.

Immunization schedule (American Academy of Pediatrics recommendations)

Age	Vaccine	Method
Birth	Hepatitis B	Injection
1–2 months	Hepatitis B	Injection
2 months	DPT* Polio Hib**	Injection By mouth Injection
4 months	DPT Polio Hib	Injection By mouth Injection
6 months	DPT	Injection
6–18 months	Hepatitis B	Injection
15 months	Measles Mumps Rubella	Injection
15–18 months	DPT Polio	Injection By mouth
4–6 years	DPT Polio	Injection By mouth
11–12 years	Measles Mumps Rubella	Injection
14–16 years	DT***	Injection

KEY: * Diphtheria, pertussis (whooping cough), and tetanus
** *Haemophilus influenzae* type b
*** Diphtheria and tetanus

If your child has ever had seizures (see p.713), be sure to tell your physician before your child is immunized. You should also tell your physician if your child is ill at the time scheduled for an immunization. If the illness is just a cold, your physician may go ahead with the immunization or may postpone it for a short time.

Mumps

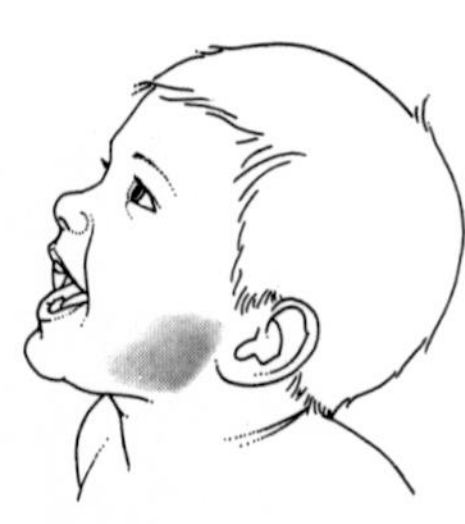

A child who has mumps usually feels generally sick and then develops swollen glands between the ear and the angle of the jaw.

Mumps is a common infectious disease that is caused by a virus. After an incubation period (see the introduction to this section, p.744) of from 14 to 28 days, the salivary glands (see p.486) begin to swell. The parotid glands, the largest pair of salivary glands, which are located at the angle of the jaw, are particularly affected.

What are the symptoms?

The parotid gland on one side of the face under the ear begins to swell. After another day, the parotid gland on the other side may also swell. This swelling is usually accompanied by a fever, diarrhea, and a general feeling of being sick. Occasionally the salivary glands under the jaw also swell, and it may be painful for the child to open his or her mouth or to swallow.

What are the risks?

Mumps is not very contagious, so it is uncommon for more than one member of a family to have the disease at the same time. There is a combined vaccine for measles, mumps, and rubella (see Box, Immunization, above) that is now in widespread use.

A fairly common risk of mumps is swelling and inflammation of the testicles in a boy or of the ovaries in a girl. Swelling and inflammation occur 3 to 4 days after the neck glands swell and are more common when the disease occurs in adults. A boy will definitely notice the swelling and it can be very painful for a day or two. A girl may have some discomfort in her lower abdomen. The swelling goes down after a few days and usually leaves no aftereffects. In rare cases, the swelling causes sterility.

In some cases, mumps is complicated by meningitis (see p.290). Another risk is acute pancreatitis (see p.528), which causes a stomachache that usually passes within 2 to 3 days. Other risks of mumps, and general treatment for the disease, are described in When your child has an infectious disease (see p.745). Mumps is generally mild. Contact your physician if your child has pain in his or her salivary glands or if your son has pain in his testicles. You can help relieve the pain in the swollen area by applying an ice pack wrapped in a towel. Complete recovery within about 10 days is usual.

Whooping cough

(pertussis)

Whooping cough is a contagious disease that affects the respiratory system. Bacteria called *Bordetella pertussis* infect the lungs and cause the air passages to become clogged with thick mucus. The extremely severe bouts of coughing characteristic of this disease are the body's attempts to clear the lungs of mucus. Symptoms develop after an incubation period of 7 to 14 days.

What are the symptoms?

The early symptoms are like those of an ordinary cold (see p.368): runny nose, dry cough, and slight fever. But unlike an ordinary cold, the symptoms do not improve after a few days. Instead, the symptoms get worse. The nasal discharge thickens, and the coughing becomes more severe until it occurs continuously in episodes up to a minute long. Because a child cannot breathe in during a bout of coughing, his or her face turns deep red, or even blue, from the lack of oxygen. At the end of each episode of coughing, as the child gasps for breath, he or she makes a "whooping" noise that gives the disease its name. Babies tend to whoop more quietly than older children.

Vomiting often occurs after a bout of coughing. The severe coughing phase of the disease can last from 2 to 10 weeks. Gradually the coughing and the vomiting become less severe and less frequent, although the cough may persist in a more ordinary form for several months.

What are the risks?

There is a combined vaccine for diphtheria, whooping cough, and tetanus (see Box, Immunization, previous page) available, so the disease is not common. But, as is true of all childhood diseases, if the number of children protected against whooping cough ever decreases, the disease will become more common again.

Symptoms of childhood infectious diseases

	Incubation period (days)	Fever	Rash	Swollen glands	Cough
Measles	7–14	Days 1 to 5	Day 4, dull red blotches	Neck	Day 1
Rubella (German measles)	14–21	Days 1 and 2	Day 2 or 3, flat, light red spots	Neck (including back of the neck)	None
Chickenpox	7–21	Variable	Day 1, groups of itchy, red spots that become blisters	None	None
Mumps	14–28	Day 1	None	One or both sides of the face	None
Whooping cough	7–14	Week 1	None	None	Week 1, becoming worse; week 2, severe bouts and characteristic whoop

There are serious risks associated with whooping cough. Rarely, bursting of blood vessels in the brain during a bout of coughing or asphyxia (lack of oxygen) can cause death. These risks can also produce permanent brain damage. Another risk is pneumonia (see p.726), which can produce permanent lung damage (see Bronchiectasis, p.389).

What should be done?

A child immunized against whooping cough (see Immunization, p.748) may still get a mild case but is not usually seriously ill with the disease. Immunization should be performed on young children because the risks associated with immunization are minor compared with the risks of whooping cough.

If your child is not protected by immunization, and he or she has a cough that does not clear up within a few days and seems to get worse, see your physician.

What is the treatment?

Self-help: Most children who become infected with whooping cough can be cared for at home if you carefully follow instructions you receive from your physician (see When your child has an infectious disease, p.745). Get medical help immediately if you notice that your child turns blue during a bout of coughing.

Do not give your child cough-suppressant medications to treat whooping cough unless prescribed by your physician, because the cough, although distressing, prevents mucus from clogging the lungs. You can counteract the tendency to vomit after coughing by feeding your child smaller, more frequent meals, and by not giving any food just after a period of coughing.

During an episode of coughing, it is best to lay a baby facedown with the foot of his or her crib raised. Be sure to turn the baby over after the coughing stops. Children usually prefer to sit up and lean forward. There is little else you can do except to comfort and reassure your child.

Professional help: Antibiotics sometimes reduce the severity of the coughing phase. If the cough is severe, infants are usually admitted to the hospital, where oxygen is provided with a face mask or a ventilator. Children who panic during coughing bouts should see a physician.

Scarlet fever

In scarlet fever, a type of *Streptococcus* bacteria enters the body through the throat and causes tonsillitis (see p.723). Without antibiotic treatment, the bacteria multiply and produce a toxin, or poison, that circulates in the blood and causes an infection. After an incubation period of 1 to 7 days, the amounts of toxin are sufficient to cause the symptoms of scarlet fever.

What are the symptoms?

Symptoms of scarlet fever vary from person to person. On day 1, a child develops a high temperature (as high as 104°F, or 40°C), a red, sore throat and tonsils, and a furred tongue (see p.487). A whitish coating may cover the tonsils and the child may vomit.

On day 2, a bright red (scarlet) rash appears on the child's face, except for just around the mouth. By day 3, this rash, which may itch, has spread to cover the rest of the body and the arms and legs. Meanwhile, the child's temperature starts to fall and the tongue becomes bright red.

By day 6, the rash has faded. Both skin and tongue may begin to peel, leaving a red, raw surface underneath. Peeling can last another 10 to 14 days.

The two main risks, both very rare and occurring about 2 to 3 weeks after the rash, are rheumatic fever (see p.740) and a form of glomerulonephritis (see p.737).

See your physician if you suspect your child may have scarlet fever. Follow the recommendations in When your child has an infectious disease (see p.745). Also, your physician may prescribe an antibiotic. Make sure that your child takes the entire prescription, as directed. Most children will recover completely with no aftereffects.

Diphtheria

Diphtheria is a serious disease that is uncommon in the US because of extensive immunization with a combined vaccine for diphtheria, whooping cough, and tetanus (see Box, Immunization, p.748). It is vital that your infant is immunized against diphtheria (see Immunization, p.748).

Symptoms of diphtheria include fever, rapid pulse, enlarged lymph glands in the neck, and, occasionally, a thick, yellow discharge from the nose. But the main symptom of diphtheria is a grayish membrane on the throat and tonsils. This membrane may become large enough to cause croup (see p.725) or prevent breathing. Talk to your physician immediately if these symptoms appear in your child. If diphtheria is diagnosed, the affected child's family, playmates, and classmates will be tested for immunity to the disease.

Treatment will require hospitalization. It involves injections of powerful antibiotics and antitoxins, and, if breathing is blocked, a temporary tracheotomy (an airway cut into the windpipe) may be necessary to prevent suffocation. Damage to the heart, kidneys, and nervous system, which can be caused by a toxin (poison) produced by the bacteria that causes diphtheria, may cause permanent disability or death, even with treatment.

Tuberculosis in children

Tuberculosis (TB) is an infectious disease caused by *Mycobacterium tuberculosis* bacteria. A skin test (tuberculin test) for tuberculosis should be performed at ages 12 months, 4 to 6 years, and 14 to 16 years on all children. Specially treated tuberculosis bacteria, or a protein derived from the bacteria, are injected into the skin of the forearm. If there is no change after 48 hours in the appearance of the skin at the site of injection, the reaction is negative. If a dime-sized or larger area of the skin becomes red, hard, and raised, the reaction is positive (indicating tuberculosis). Tuberculosis occurs in two stages. At one time, the first stage mainly affected children, but today it also develops in adults. The second stage occurs most commonly in older people who have suppressed immune systems or who are malnourished. Because the two stages of the disease are connected, they are described in full in the article on p.602.

While tuberculosis was uncommon for a period of years, it is now steadily increasing in the US. If your child has a cough, fever, fatigue, poor appetite, and weight loss, or chest pain and shortness of breath, see your physician. Also, if your child has been in contact with someone who has active tuberculosis, take your child to your physician, who will perform a skin test, since the child has been exposed to TB. If the skin test is positive, chest X rays may be needed to confirm the diagnosis, and antituberculosis medications will be prescribed for a prolonged period to prevent the disease from progressing to the second stage. The child will need to rest and follow a well-balanced diet.

Pinworms

Pinworms are tiny white worms, less than ½ in (about 3 cm) long, that are much more common in children, especially school-age children, than they are in adults. The worms' eggs can enter the body when swallowed by the child in contaminated food, or from clothing, toys, or a sandbox. The eggs hatch in the intestines, and young worms quickly begin to grow into adults. About 2 weeks later, a mature female worm lays eggs around the child's anus during the night. This may cause irritation, and if the child scratches the anus, he or she picks up some eggs on his or her fingers. Sucking the fingers or eating without washing thoroughly then causes reinfection. By contaminating food, drinking glasses, sheets, and towels, the child may pass on pinworms to other family members.

Scratching the anus may make it more inflamed. The small, white, threadlike worms can sometimes be seen in stools or around the child's anus at night.

If you see pinworms, or if your child's anus constantly itches, the entire family should see your physician. You can confirm the presence of pinworms by placing a strip of transparent tape across your child's anus in the early morning, preferably just before a bowel movement. Eggs in the area stick to the tape, which you can give to your physician, who will then confirm the diagnosis.

What is the treatment?

Self-help: The entire family should maintain strict hygiene. Wash your hands after going to the toilet, after handling a pet, which may also be infected, and before touching any food. Clip your fingernails short to lessen the chance of eggs being trapped under them. Change your sheets, pillowcases, and underwear daily. Wash these items in very hot water, or boil and iron them, to kill worms or eggs. If you have a pet, see a veterinarian about ridding the animal of the worms.

Professional help: The entire household needs to be treated, even those who have no symptoms. Your physician may prescribe medications used to treat worm infestations (antihelmintics) for a short time. Treatment is often repeated after 2 weeks. Anal inflammation may be relieved by using a nonprescription ointment, which may also contain a substance that kills the eggs. These treatments usually clear up the problem.

Genetics

Genetics is the study of the process of biological inheritance. It explains how and why certain characteristics such as hair color or blood types run in families.

Every human being develops from a single cell, the fertilized egg, which contains the genetic information necessary for the development of inherited mental and physical characteristics. This information is carried on 23 pairs of chromosomes. Every pair of chromosomes includes one contributed by the mother (in the egg) and one contributed by the father (in the sperm), and each chromosome contains thousands of genes. The genes determine specific physical features of a child such as eye color. What those features will be depends on how the chromosomes from each parent were shuffled as the fertilized egg developed, and how the genes from one parent combine with those from the other parent. To understand how certain disorders are caused by genetic transmission rather than by outside factors such as infection with a microorganism, or alcohol or drug use, it is essential first to understand the distinction between two types of genes: dominant and recessive.

Dominant means that the characteristic a gene determines will appear regardless of the character of the corresponding gene in the other chromosome of the pair. Characteristics determined by recessive genes will not appear in a child unless both parents contribute chromosomes that contain a recessive gene for that characteristic. For example, blue eyes are recessive and brown eyes are dominant, so a child will inherit blue eyes only if both parents contribute a gene for blue eyes. If one parent contributes blue and the other contributes brown, a child will have brown eyes. If both you and your partner have blue eyes, there are no genes for brown in either of you, since a gene for brown is dominant and would have given you brown eyes. Therefore, your children will have blue eyes. On the other hand, if both of you have brown eyes, there may be genes for blue eyes in the pair of chromosomes you each have that are related to eye color, so you could have children with blue eyes.

Single-gene disorders

Most serious genetic disorders are caused by a single defective gene, which is usually recessive. In other words, the disorder will not occur in a child unless both parents contribute the defective gene to the fertilized egg. An example of a single-gene disorder is cystic fibrosis (see p.732). About 1 in every 20 persons carries a gene for cystic fibrosis, usually without being aware of it. If two carriers have a child (a chance of 1 in 400), the disease can occur in their offspring, but the next generation may also include healthy carriers of the gene that causes the disease and children without the disease or the gene that causes it (see the accompanying diagram for more information).

The pattern is somewhat different when, as in hemophilia (see p.455), the defective gene is carried in one of the chromosomes that also determines the sex of the child. Females have two identical sex chromosomes, which are known as X chromosomes. Males have one X chromosome and one chromosome that is differently structured, which is known as a Y chromosome. If the sperm that fertilizes an egg carries an X chromosome, a baby will be female. If the sperm carries a Y chromosome, a baby will be male. Hemophilia is a sex-linked disease because the gene that governs the clotting ability of blood is carried in the X chromosome. Today, boys who have hemophilia are more likely to survive to become fathers, so it is theoretically possible for both parents to contribute a defective X gene to the fertilized egg. This means that there is an increased possibility of having a female child who has hemophilia. Most often, however, the mother (the carrier) contributes an X chromosome that contains the defective gene, and the father contributes a Y chromosome. There are some inevitable results of this combination:

1. The child will be male, because there is one X and one Y chromosome.
2. Although the defective gene is recessive, it cannot be overcome by a dominant gene since there is no gene for blood clotting on the Y chromosome. Therefore, a male child will be unable to produce the protein needed in blood clotting and will have hemophilia.

It also follows that:

1. All daughters of a man who has hemophilia will have received a defective X chromosome from him and will be carriers of the gene that causes the disease.
2. Only *some* of the daughters of a woman who is a carrier may be carriers, since they can inherit the normal X chromosome rather than the one with the defective gene.
3. A man with hemophilia cannot pass the defective gene on to his sons because they will inherit his Y chromosome, on which there is no gene for blood clotting.

In a few single-gene diseases, the defective gene is dominant instead of recessive. Anyone who inherits such a gene from either parent will have the condition. For example, read the article on Huntington's chorea (see p.313). Because symptoms of Huntington's chorea usually do not appear until middle age, many people who will develop the disease are not aware of it until after they have had children and possibly passed the abnormal gene to them. Alternatively, knowing that Huntington's chorea runs on one side of their family, some people decide not to have children and then discover that they have not inherited the disease and could not have passed it on. Tests are now available, however, that can identify many of the carriers of the Huntington's chorea gene at any age. If you think that you may be a carrier of the gene, see a genetic counselor (see p.664).

One might expect that abnormal genes that cause serious disorders would eventually disappear, because families with the gene would have fewer surviving children. In practice, this does not happen for two reasons. First, the carrier may have some survival advantage; for example, carriers of the gene for sickle-cell anemia are naturally resistant to malaria. Second, some genetic defects seem to develop in the process of cell division; for example, about one third of people with hemophilia are "new" cases who have no relatives with the disorder.

Genetic research has allowed scientists to map the location of many of the 50,000 genes in the body. It is now known where, on specific chromosomes, genes that determine physical characteristics such as tissue type, and genes for many of the single-gene disorders, are located.

Finding the location of the genes responsible for disorders such as cystic fibrosis, thalassemia (see p.454), and sickle-cell anemia (see p.453) has led to two important benefits. First, genetic counseling (see p.664) has been made more effective and accurate; adults can be tested to find out whether they are carriers, and these disorders can now be reliably diagnosed early in pregnancy (see Chorionic villus sampling, p.684). Second, in many conditions chemical changes caused by the defective gene have also been identified, and this presents the possibility of developing new and effective treatment methods—possibly by repairing the defective gene or by replacing the defective gene with a healthy gene.

Multiple-gene disorders

Many disorders are inherited through more than one gene. It is often said that these disorders tend to run in families (see, for instance, Coronary artery disease, p.400 and Asthma, p.381). What this means is that there is probably a genetic element present in susceptibility to the disorder, but that the genetic aspect is difficult to isolate and define.

In the case of coronary heart disease, however, some families are at a much higher risk than average because they have an inherited disorder that affects the amount of cholesterol in the blood. In such families, fatal heart attacks may occur in males or females in their teens or early twenties. If the disorder is recognized in childhood, however, treatment with diet and medication can reduce the risks.

If you or your partner have any relatives who have had illnesses or died in their teens or early adult life of unknown causes, you should consider the possibility of a genetic disorder and see a genetic counselor (see p.664) before becoming pregnant.

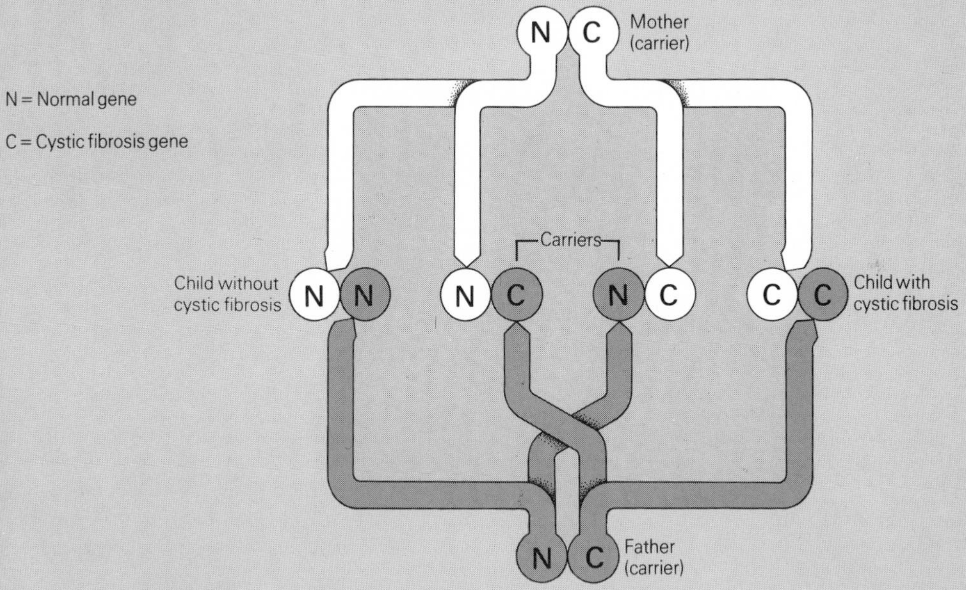

Cystic fibrosis is caused by an inherited genetic abnormality involving a single defective gene. The defective gene is recessive; a child inherits it only if both parents contribute a gene for cystic fibrosis. Most people have two normal genes (NN), one on each of the chromosomes, but a person with cystic fibrosis always has two cystic fibrosis genes (CC). In people with one C gene and one N gene, the N dominates the recessive C. Such people are free of the disease themselves but are "carriers" and can transmit the disease to their children.

If two carriers have a child, the child may inherit two normal genes (NN) and not have the disease, or he or she may inherit one normal gene and one cystic fibrosis gene (NC) and be a carrier. However, if the child inherits genes for the disease from both parents (CC), he or she will have cystic fibrosis. The diagram here shows all the possible combinations.

Allergies

An allergy is a disorder caused by hypersensitivity (abnormal or excessive sensitivity) to substances that are eaten, inhaled, injected, or brought into contact with the skin. Hypersensitivity results from a misdirected response by the body's immune system. Your immune system is designed to protect you from infection by infectious microorganisms such as bacteria or viruses (see General infections, p.596). It does this by producing antibodies that kill or neutralize these microorganisms. In people with allergies, antibodies attack normally harmless substances, which are called allergens.

The symptoms that an allergy produces depend on both the type of antibody and the part of the body in which the reaction between antibody and allergen takes place. In food allergies, for example, the allergen may cause symptoms that affect the intestines (as in celiac disease, see p.509), or the allergen may be absorbed into the bloodstream and react with antibodies in the blood vessels to produce certain kinds of headaches or skin rashes. In the type of allergic rhinitis known as hay fever, airborne pollens cause a reaction in the nose. In asthma, inhaled dust or pollen causes a reaction in the lungs.

In an allergic reaction, the cells of the immune system release irritant chemicals that cause symptoms characteristic of allergy attacks, including headaches, excessive production of mucus, constriction of bronchioles (small air passages in the lungs), and skin conditions such as redness, swelling, and itching.

Testing for allergy
It may be possible to identify an allergen by scratch testing. The skin is pierced or scratched, and a drop of solution containing a potential allergen is applied. Several scratches may be made, and a different suspected allergen put on each. If you are allergic to one of the substances, the area that has been in contact with it will produce a lump, and will be red and inflamed.

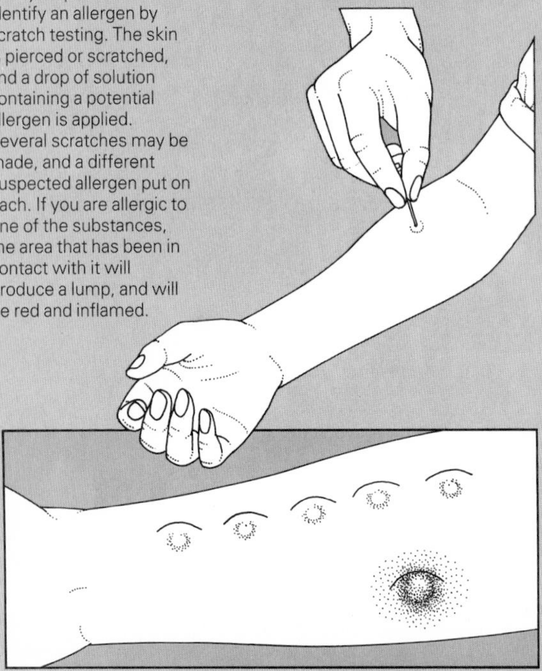

Who is susceptible?

Allergies are common—as many as one in ten children may have symptoms of asthma (see p.381) or eczema (see p.269). In recent years, however, allergies have been blamed for many common behavioral problems or recurrent physical disorders. This is especially true of allergies to food, food additives, food colorings, and toxic chemicals in the environment. It is possible that some children with destructive or hyperactive behavior (see p.719) have allergies of this kind, but research has shown that in most cases an allergy is not the cause of the symptoms. Nevertheless, some parents think that they or their children have an allergy, and in some cases they have gone on strict diets in an attempt to exclude the "allergen."

What is the treatment?

Self-diagnosis of allergy is risky, and people should also be suspicious of the many "allergy-testing" laboratories that advertise. If you suspect that your child's illness may be due to an allergy, consult your physician for a referral to an allergist or a pediatrician who specializes in allergies. Laboratory tests are available to determine whether a child has an allergy, and which substance is causing the allergy. If one or more foods (or food additives) are suspected, your child may be given an exclusion diet that eliminates the food or foods in question. The effects of this diet are then monitored. It is a good idea to start an exclusion diet with a physician's supervision. A change in diet that is expected to relieve symptoms of a condition such as asthma is likely to improve the condition temporarily. However, careful monitoring of the effects that the reintroduction of the suspected foods has on the child is essential. When these foods are reintroduced, they are given to the child without his or her knowledge, to ensure accurate monitoring.

Once an allergen has been identified, the best treatment is total avoidance of the allergen. This can be done only when it is possible to determine that you are allergic to a specific food or medication. Often an allergen is difficult to identify or to avoid. Pollen and animal dander (tiny particles from the feathers, fur, hair, or skin of an animal) are examples of this type of allergen. When an allergen has been identified, it is sometimes possible to make you less sensitive to the allergen (desensitization) with a series of injections that cause the body to get used to increasing doses of the substance. Desensitization is not used as often as it once was, however, because it occasionally causes serious reactions, and the results are often disappointing.

Current treatment for allergies is medications such as antihistamines that reduce or counteract allergic reactions. For further information read the articles dealing with allergy-based disorders, which include asthma (see p.381). allergic rhinitis (see p.370), eczema and dermatitis (see p.269), farmer's lung (see p.391), hives (see p.272), celiac disease (see p.509), and some forms of conjunctivitis (see p.343).

Adolescent health

Introduction

Adolescence, the period of transition from childhood to adulthood, is generally considered to last from about the beginning of puberty to age 18 or 20. Puberty is the period of life when a person becomes able to reproduce. Although there are individual variations in when adolescence begins and ends, it is practical to use the words "adolescent" and "teenager" interchangeably.

Many of the characteristic problems of adolescence stem from changes in the type and pattern of hormones present in the body (see Hormonal disorders, p.553, for more detailed information about hormones). These changes normally begin soon after age 10 or 11 in girls, and soon after age 12 or 13 in boys. Growth toward physical maturity tends to level off soon after age 17 or 18 in both sexes. During these developmental years, there are physical, mental, and emotional changes that make adolescence a particularly difficult time.

Some of the problems discussed in this section are physical, and others are psychological. In many cases, physical problems can have psychological effects, and psychological problems can have physical effects. For example, an adolescent who has acne, a very common physical problem, may react in a very emotional way.

It is hard to say whether teenagers or their parents are most affected by concerns such as sexual experimentation, and the use of cigarettes, alcohol, and other drugs. Therefore, teenagers and their parents alike may find it useful to read these articles. The key to a healthy adolescence is usually open and honest communication between adolescents and their parents.

Early or late sexual development

Although the hormonal changes that signal the beginning of puberty usually begin at about age 10 or 11 in girls and about 12 or 13 in boys, there are wide variations in adolescent growth patterns.

An important factor in sexual development is heredity (biological inheritance). For example, a girl whose mother started her periods late is also likely to begin late. Similarly, a boy's development is likely to follow the same pattern as his father's. Most teens are preoccupied with their changing bodies and concerned about being "normal." For example, many boys worry about the size of their penis. But, although soft penises differ widely in size, there is only a small difference in size among erect penises.

Whether an adolescent develops early or late is also affected by his or her general health. Poor nutrition or illness during childhood may delay the onset of puberty. In addition, a child who is smaller or thinner than average is likely to develop relatively late.

Children who develop early or late may be teased by their peers, but parents should be understanding and reassuring. Remind him or her that "differences" are not good or bad, they are just differences and usually are only temporary.

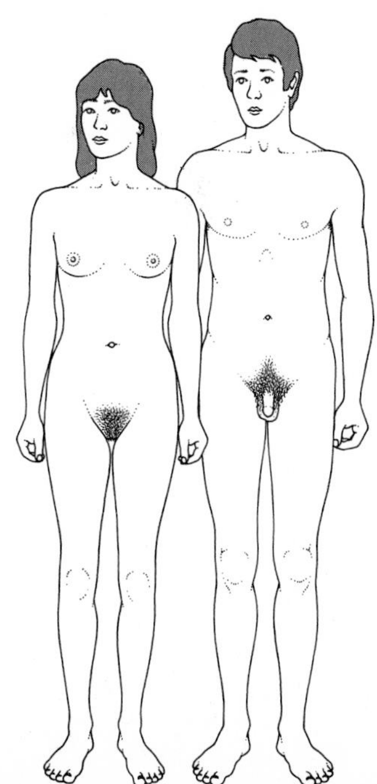

Reaching physical maturity
Many girls reach sexual maturity by the time they are 16. Their breasts have developed and the pelvis has broadened, underarm and pubic hair has grown, and fat has been laid down to create an adult female shape.

Most boys are sexually mature by the age of 17 or 18. Their genitals have grown, facial and body hair have appeared, the voice has deepened, and there have been important changes in the bones and muscles.

Normal adolescent development

Physical development in adolescent girls

	Age when noticeable change usually begins	Age when noticeable change usually stops	Remarks
Increase in rate of growth	10 to 11	15 to 16	If noticeable growth fails to begin by 15, see your physician.
Breast development	10 to 11	13 to 14	Noticeable development of breasts (one of which may begin to grow before the other) is usually the first sign of puberty. If change does not begin by 16, check with your physician.
Emergence of body hair	Pubic hair: 10 to 11 Underarm hair: 12 to 13	Pubic hair: 13 to 14 Underarm hair: 15 to 16	Development of body hair is extremely variable and largely dependent on heredity. Pubic hair usually darkens and thickens as puberty progresses.
Development of sweat glands under the arms and in the groin	12 to 13	15 to 16	Sweat glands are responsible for increased sweating, which causes underarm odor, a type of body odor not present in younger children.
Menstruation	11 to 14	15 to 17	Menstruation often begins with extremely irregular periods, but by 17 a regular cycle (3 to 7 days every 28 days) usually becomes evident. If menstruation begins before 10 or has not begun by 17, talk to your physician (see also Absence of periods, p.624).

Physical development in adolescent boys

Increase in rate of growth	12 to 13	17 to 18	If noticeable growth fails to begin by 15, see your physician.
Enlargement of genitals	Testicles and scrotum: 11 to 12 Penis: 12 to 13	Testicles and scrotum: 16 to 17 Penis: 15 to 16	As testicles grow, the skin of the scrotum darkens. The penis usually lengthens before it broadens. Ability to ejaculate seminal fluid usually begins about a year after the penis starts to lengthen.
Emergence of body hair	Pubic hair: 11 to 12 Underarm hair: 13 to 15	Pubic hair: 15 to 16 Underarm hair: 16 to 18	Development of body hair is extremely variable and largely dependent on heredity. Development of hair on the abdomen and chest usually continues into adulthood.
Development of sweat glands under the arms and in the groin	13 to 15	17 to 18	See the above table for girls.
Voice change	Enlargement of the larynx, or voicebox, begins at 13 to 14, and the voice deepens at 14 to 15	16 to 17	Growth of the larynx may make the "Adam's apple" more prominent. The voice may change rapidly or gradually. If childlike voice persists after 16, see your physician.

Medical disorders

Although adolescent boys and girls are susceptible to most of the general illnesses described in this book, the four disorders discussed in this section are far more common in adolescents. Other disorders that seem to be more common in teenagers or young adults are discussed in the sections that cover those problems. Some examples are Hodgkin's disease (see p.464), leukemia (see p.457 and p.458), and infectious mononucleosis (see p.601).

Teenagers and parents who are concerned about physical development should read the tables on the previous pages. Note the broad range of ages within which changes such as growth of body hair or beginning of menstruation occur. Many boys and girls begin to develop a bit earlier or later than the ages that are shown. Early development toward physical maturity is usually not a cause for concern. If development is unusually late, however, see your physician.

Acne

(acne vulgaris, common acne)

See p.248, **Visual aids to diagnosis, 30.**

Acne is a common skin disorder that is caused by inflammation of the hair follicles and sebaceous glands. Almost every part of your body is covered with hairs, most of them virtually invisible. Each hair grows from a follicle, which is a tiny pit in the skin. Inside each follicle is a sebaceous gland that produces an oily substance called sebum that lubricates the skin. If your body produces too much of this oily substance and some of it becomes trapped in a follicle, bacteria can multiply in the blocked follicle and cause it to become inflamed. This causes a pimple, which may be a small white plug (whitehead), a dark closed pore (blackhead), or a red lump that sometimes fills with pus. A pimple or two is nothing to worry about. You may be said to have acne only if you have a number of pimples on your body.

Certain medications, such as corticosteroids or antiepilepsy drugs, can also cause acne. Usually, however, acne is a problem that occurs during adolescence. It begins at puberty (when reproduction becomes possible) and usually clears up in the late teens or early twenties.

Many adolescents have acne because the level of male hormones in the body rises when a boy or girl reaches puberty, and this stimulates the sebaceous glands to increase their production of sebum.

What are the symptoms?

Pimples are usually concentrated on the face, but may appear on the back of the neck, the back, the chest, the buttocks, and in some cases the upper arms and thighs. An inflamed pimple may develop into a tender red lump with a white, pus-filled center. This tends to occur if you squeeze or pick the pimples. As individual acne pimples heal, other pimples appear. Each healed pimple leaves a purplish mark on the skin, but the mark usually fades. Severely inflamed pimples may take many weeks to clear up and may leave scars.

One psychological effect of adolescent acne may persist for years. Because many young people are extremely embarrassed and self-conscious about the appearance of their skin, they may be offended by comments made by their parents or other people, no matter how well-meaning they may be. This often places more stress on the teenager and increases the tension within his or her family.

What are the risks?

Most male adolescents aged 14 to 18 have some acne. Acne is slightly less common in adolescent girls, who usually develop pimples when they get their periods each month. With today's treatment, severe acne that leads to scarring occurs less frequently.

Acne can be distressing, but it is not a risk to your general health. Adolescent acne is not a disease or something shameful. It is a normal part of puberty.

What should be done?

If you have mild acne, the self-help measures suggested below should keep it under control. If it becomes severe, see your physician. Scrubbing your skin too hard is likely to do more damage than just leaving it alone. Even the dark part of blackheads is pigment (coloring) and not dirt and should not be scrubbed vigorously or squeezed.

What is the treatment?

Self-help: Keep your skin clean. Wash it with unscented soap twice a day, but not more often unless it becomes very dirty or oily. Ask your physician to recommend a

How an acne pimple forms

1. Sebaceous glands are usually found in or near a hair follicle through which they secrete sebum, an oily substance that lubricates the skin and hair.
2. A follicle may become blocked, usually by a mixture of excess sebum and dead skin cells. Then a white plug forms over the pore, or opening. Sebum, unable to escape, builds up in the blocked follicle.
3. Bacteria normally present on the skin may infect the sebum, causing inflammation, pus, and swelling, which is visible as an acne pimple.

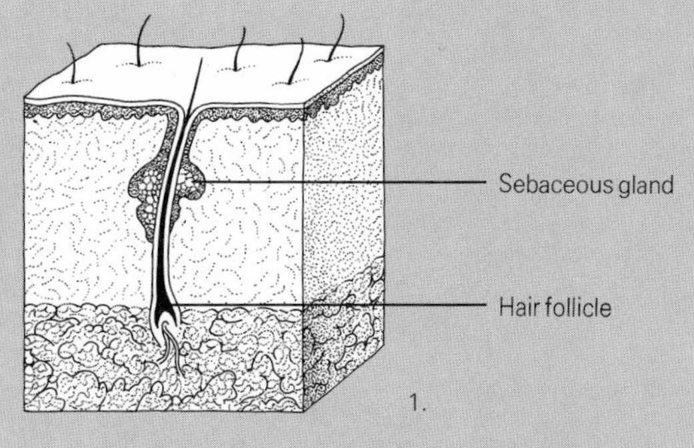

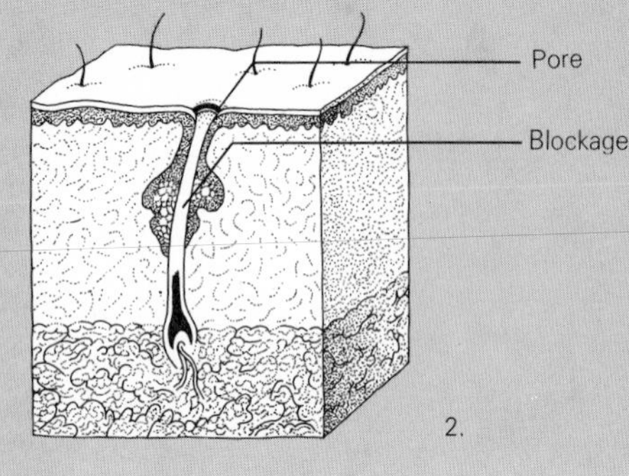

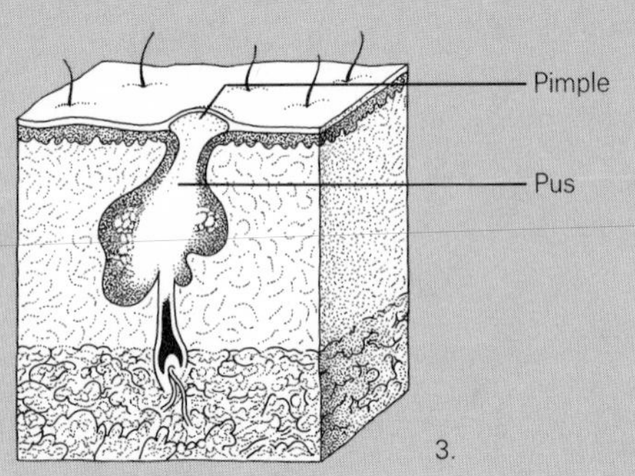

nonprescription cream or lotion that is often effective in treating acne. Girls should avoid wearing foundation makeup. If you feel you must wear it, use a water-based makeup, and be sure to clean your face thoroughly after removing your makeup. Also, remember that squeezing and picking pimples is likely to make your problem worse.

Professional help: If your acne is severe enough to require professional help, your physician may prescribe a special ointment that makes your skin peel and may also prevent new pimples from forming. If this treatment does not work, your physician may prescribe small, daily doses of oral antibiotics. If antibiotic treatment is unsuccessful, or if your acne is severe, your physician may recommend treatment with medications called retinoins. These medications are highly effective but can cause side effects, such as hair loss, joint pain, and sore eyes. Also, retinoins should not be taken during pregnancy because there is a significant risk of severe damage to the fetus.

Anorexia nervosa and bulimia nervosa

Anorexia nervosa is refusal to eat and can lead to extreme loss of weight, hormonal disturbances, and death. Bulimia nervosa is binge eating that is followed by self-induced vomiting. Both are primarily illnesses of adolescent girls and the causes are unknown. Girls with anorexia nervosa tend to come from families that frequently think and talk about the "right" amounts or kinds of things to eat and girls may use their refusal to eat as a tool to manipulate their parents, turning each mealtime into a battle.

Most teens diet to conform to strong social pressures that declare thin as ideal and indicate popularity. But in some cases, dieting becomes an illness that arises from a subconscious desire to retreat from sexual maturity. In anorexia nervosa, the adolescent girl diets to retain her preadolescent shape. This arrests the body's normal sexual development; occasionally, an early sexual experience has led to serious feelings of guilt. Sometimes an emotionally insecure girl will overhear a casual comment that she is too fat and decide she must lose weight to be popular. Even if she becomes emaciated, she still sees herself as overweight. Also, she often exercises excessively.

What are the symptoms?

Anorexia nervosa usually starts with normal dieting to lose weight, but the girl then eats less and less every day. She gives excuses for doing so, insisting, for example, that her legs or arms are still too fat. The less she eats, the less she wants to eat. Sometimes, however, she may go on binges, in which she consumes large quantities of a particular food and then makes herself vomit. She may also use large quantities of laxatives on a regular basis. If this binge-purge pattern is dominant, the condition is called bulimia nervosa. To counter family pressure, she may take food and throw it away, claiming she has eaten it. When her weight drops to about 26 lb (about 12 kg) below normal, she may stop having periods (see Absence of periods, p.624) and her body may become more hairy.

A girl who has anorexia nervosa is often abnormally energetic. She may cook large meals for others while starving herself, and she will insist that she feels fine. But her skin may begin to look sallow, waxy, and thin and she will eventually become very obviously ill. In later stages of anorexia nervosa, she may lapse into severe depressive illness (see Depression, p.321).

What are the risks?

Anorexia nervosa and bulimia nervosa are rare, but the number of cases of anorexia nervosa and bulimia nervosa seem to have risen in the past 20 years. They affect adolescent girls almost exclusively. Many teenagers go through a temporary phase of excessive dieting, but only a minority develop anorexia nervosa. Of those who develop the disease, up to 15 percent die; death results from starvation, from infections caused by poor nutrition, from dehydration caused by overuse of laxatives, or from suicide because of depression.

In bulimia nervosa, stomach acid from repeated vomiting usually causes severe damage to the teeth, making them sharp and rough. Bulimia nervosa also carries a risk of severe dehydration.

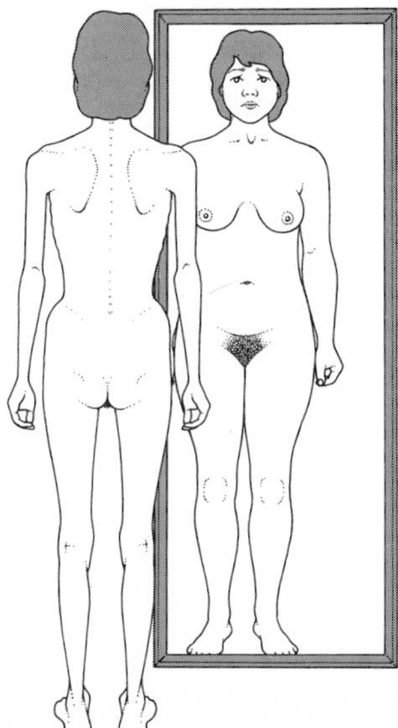

A distorted self-image
Even after dieting to the point where she is extremely thin or emaciated, a girl with anorexia nervosa still sees herself as overweight.

What should be done?

If your adolescent daughter has an unrealistic image of herself as being too fat and seems to be dieting excessively, take her to see your physician immediately. Effective treatment of these conditions becomes increasingly difficult as they progress. After examining your daughter, your physician may decide that she does not have either condition and may simply give you and her some advice on how to avoid problems with excessive weight loss. If her condition is diagnosed as anorexia nervosa or bulimia nervosa, your physician may arrange for immediate hospitalization and evaluation by a psychiatrist.

What is the treatment?

Even in the early stages, anorexia nervosa or bulimia nervosa is best treated in a hospital by a team of physicians, nurses, social workers, and dietitians who are experienced in treating these conditions. Your physician can discuss the illness with you and your daughter and help her to accept a suitable weight. Your physician and your daughter will then agree on the type of diet she should eat in order to gain weight at a healthy rate. While in the hospital, she will participate in individual and group psychotherapy. The more that is learned about personal and family problems, the better the chance of solving them. When the patient has made progress in treatment and no longer seems reluctant to accept physical and emotional maturity, she is permitted to return home. Before she leaves the hospital, however, the hospital staff usually advises the girl's family on how to interact with her and how to recognize recurrence of the disorder.

What are the long-term prospects?

A girl who has had anorexia nervosa or bulimia needs to visit her family physician and her psychiatrist frequently and regularly for some time, even after she appears to be eating normally. Many girls who seem to have recovered from these illnesses continue to have emotional problems.

Abnormal curvature of the spine

(scoliosis)

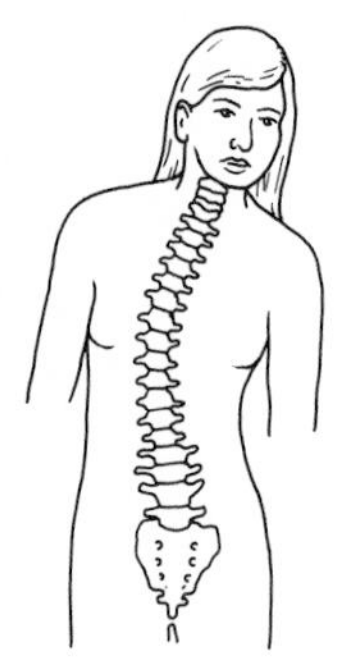

Sideways curvature of the spine that causes the rib cage to become tilted is called scoliosis. The curvature may be due to a congenital (present from birth) abnormality of the spinal column, to paralysis or weakness of the spinal muscles, or to abnormal growth of the spine associated with short stature (see p.555). Abnormal curvature of the spine runs in families. However, in most cases the cause of the curvature is not known.

Scoliosis becomes a noticeable problem mainly in the adolescent years and is much more common in girls than it is in boys.

What should be done?

If you think that your child may have an abnormal spinal curvature, see your physician. Early treatment can help to prevent the problem from getting worse. Without treatment, the lungs may be affected. In severe cases, the adolescent may also have recurrent chest infections. Once scoliosis has been diagnosed, your physician will examine your child's spine periodically to monitor the curvature. He or she may refer your child to an orthopedic surgeon (a physician who specializes in treating disorders of bones and joints).

What is the treatment?

If scoliosis is caused by spinal abnormality, your physician can diagnose and treat the underlying problem. Sometimes the only treatment that is needed is physical therapy, which concentrates on improving posture and toning spinal muscles. If physical therapy does not correct the curvature, your child may have to wear a spinal brace to help correct the curvature by immobilizing the spine. Spinal braces are fitted by an orthopedic surgeon and are worn for at least a year. Your child may need surgery, in which a steel rod is inserted to straighten the spine.

Phimosis

(tight foreskin)

Phimosis is the medical term for a tightness of the foreskin that prevents it from being comfortably drawn back over the glans at the tip of the penis. The problem cannot usually be detected before an uncircumcised boy reaches age 5, because the foreskin is usually small and tight until then. Most commonly, phimosis is discovered in adolescence, when it may become extremely painful or make it impossible for the boy to have an erection.

What should be done?

A boy can gradually stretch the foreskin over several weeks by retracting it with the aid of soap suds in the shower. Never use force, which can damage the tissues. If self-retraction is not possible, see your physician, who may recommend that your son be circumcised. This is a relatively minor operation in which the foreskin is removed (see Box, Should I have my son circumcised? p.698).

Psychological and behavioral disorders

The physical changes that occur during a child's adolescence are usually accompanied by emotional conflict. Teenagers must deal with changing social and sexual attitudes and also with the availability of illegal drugs. The demands of friends, family, and society place additional stress on teenagers. Although there are no easy answers to an adolescent's complex problems, open and honest communication between parents and teenagers is essential in dealing with this difficult period in a child's development. The following articles present some basic facts about the psychological and behavioral problems that can occur during adolescence and offer some suggestions for coping with these problems.

Rebelliousness

Most adolescents are self-conscious, self-aware, and self-centered. Also, adolescents have a stubborn determination to assert independence that conflicts with a continuing need to rely on adults for emotional and financial support. Most adolescents demand the right to question and criticize parental behavior and standards, and resent parental efforts to shape and control their behavior.

Although adolescents do not completely accept their parents' values, they will not completely reject their values either. Quiet, cooperative teenagers often have as much inner conflict as teenagers who are outwardly rebellious. Clashes between parents and teenagers are common, especially when the adolescents are between 13 and 16.

What are the signs?

Teenagers are often moody and sullen. They may act as if they know everything, reject advice from adults, and see situations only from their point of view. Inside, however, teenagers are not as confident as they seem. For example, teenagers usually attach extreme importance to their outward appearance. Wearing trendy clothing or hair styles may seem rebellious and unconventional to adults. However, this behavior usually indicates conformity resulting from peer pressure. Because they lack the self-confidence to be themselves, most teenagers, like many adults, need the security of dressing and behaving like the rest of their peer group.

Self-consciousness may also make some teenagers acutely aware of any real or imagined physical flaws, which they may blow out of proportion. Parents whose teenagers are convinced that their life is ruined because they have acne or curly hair may find it difficult to persuade their children that clear skin or straight hair is not very important in the long run. During adolescence, preoccupation with real or imagined physical imperfections can sometimes lead to serious disorders such as anorexia nervosa or bulimia nervosa (see p.758), anxiety (see p.324), or severe depression (see p.321).

Toward the end of adolescence, between ages 16 and 18, rebelliousness usually fades. A teenager may still often be critical, but criticism gradually becomes more constructive and less self-centered. Some intolerance of adults may continue, but the unpredictable irritability and moodiness of early adolescence is usually replaced by a willingness to compromise and accept differences as an adolescent nears age 20.

What should parents do?

Successful relationships between parents and adolescents depend on communication, and this is not always easy. Parents should try to be patient and tolerant and keep the lines of communication open.

Many parents aren't sure if they should continue to enforce their standards of behavior and discipline, or if they should relax the rules, after discussing them with their adolescent son or daughter. Too much parental concern can irritate a teenager, but too little concern may be interpreted as a lack of interest. Therefore, parents should base their decisions on standards of behavior and discipline that are suited to their particular family situation.

Both parents should agree on the ground rules for behavior and discipline. Begin by agreeing on the issues in two areas. First, decide what you both consider vital for your teenager's health and safety, which may include wanting to know where he or she is at a given time, or insisting that he or she not get into a car driven by someone who has been drinking alcohol. Second, agree on other issues that you both feel strongly about, such as how to discuss sexuality with your child. Once you have agreed on the ground rules, try to be flexible in other areas such as dress or use of slang, which are not as important.

Teenagers' anxieties about their appearance usually focus on hair, skin, or weight. Provide any practical help that you can. If your son is overweight, for example, help him modify his diet. Whatever the problem and however trivial it may seem to you, do not dismiss it. It is not until late adolescence that teenagers will have the confidence to accept themselves as they really are, and to believe that others can do the same.

What is abnormal behavior?

Adolescent rebelliousness sometimes reaches a point where professional help is needed. For example, some adolescents refuse to go to school. An established pattern of truancy can be very difficult to reverse, so parents should speak with their child's teacher or guidance counselor as soon as the problem begins. Similarly, if your child's behavior becomes violent or threatening, or if he or she is breaking the law, contact a counselor, a social worker, your family physician, or local juvenile authorities as soon as possible.

Occasionally the stresses of adolescence may lead to mental illness. Short periods of depression are common, but if a teenager's mood remains gloomy for more than a few days, and if symptoms of depression such as insomnia, loss of appetite, and/or withdrawal from friends and family appear, see your physician as soon as possible. Occasionally adolescent mood swings become so extreme that medical help is needed (see Manic-depression, p.323). Finally, a small number of adolescents are unable to cope with difficult emotional situations, such as the breakup of a relationship, and may take drastic action to escape reality. They might turn to alcohol or other drugs, or they may become physically violent or attempt suicide (see Box, Adolescent suicide, p.763). Medical help is vital for any teenager who threatens or resorts to such severe actions.

Drug abuse and adolescents

One of the major problems in the US is the availability of illegal drugs, which has made teenage drug abuse widespread. Marijuana and cocaine (including crack, the smokable form of cocaine) can be purchased easily in many rural, suburban, and urban schools. Nicotine and alcohol, which may be the most addictive drugs, are even more readily available. Many teenagers and younger children try drugs, making drug abuse an extremely important issue for every family (see Alcohol abuse, p.329, Drug abuse, p.332, and The dangers of tobacco, p.48).

Teenagers are particularly vulnerable to the risks of drug abuse because they tend to be attracted to behaviors that they associate with maturity and sophistication. Persistent feelings of rebelliousness (see p.760) may be expressed by drug use. Adolescents are also susceptible to peer pressure. They need to feel part of a group. And if their friends and classmates use drugs, including alcohol and/or nicotine, it is extremely difficult for teenagers to resist pressures to conform. Because teenagers generally think they will live forever, they mistakenly think that the risks of drug abuse do not apply to them. Trying a substance once may lead to repeated use; what begins as experimentation can result in dependence. Cigarette smoking is a good example. Research suggests that adolescents who do not smoke before age 20 are not likely to start, while those who smoke as teenagers often become addicted.

A national survey found that 10.6 million of 20.7 million adolescents between ages 12 and 17—more than half—drink alcohol. Eight million of them drink once a week, and 450,000 have 5 or more drinks per sitting.

Teenagers associate alcohol with good times and parties. Because of this, they need to know the risks of drinking alcohol. It is an illegal drug for teenagers in most states, and it is easy to develop dependence on it. Also, researchers have found evidence that some teenagers use alcohol in a misguided attempt to escape from their problems. Drunken driving kills or maims not only the driver, but also many innocent people.

What should parents do?

Talk to your children about drugs. Be honest and direct. Discuss the risks involved in using drugs, including alcohol and nicotine. (For additional suggestions on dealing with teenage drug abuse, see Box on this page.)

If you think that your teenager is using drugs, express your concern, offer help, and be supportive. Avoid hostile confrontations. Ask your family physician to recommend drug treatment programs such as inpatient or residential care, outpatient care, or self-help and peer counseling groups in your community, or call the National Institute on Drug Abuse Hotline at 1-800-662-HELP (1-800-662-4357) for information and referral.

Efforts to discourage teenagers from smoking cigarettes are more successful if you emphasize consequences such as bad breath and the smell of tobacco in hair and on clothing. It is hard to compete effectively with peer pressure and constant exposure to advertising, which gives smoking a positive image. Whether adolescents start to smoke depends mostly on the influence of friends and family and on how easy it is to get cigarettes. Friends who smoke are the main influence, but family environment is also important when an adolescent decides whether to smoke. Teenagers often resent double standards. Encourage your children not to smoke by not smoking.

What parents can do about teenage drug abuse

- Set an example; do not abuse drugs.
- Learn about drugs and the risks and signs of drug abuse.
- Talk to your children about drugs and the potential risks of drug abuse (see Alcohol abuse, p.329, Drug abuse, p.332, and The dangers of tobacco, p.48).
- Know where your children are and who their friends are.
- Actively encourage your child to participate in sports, school clubs, arts and crafts classes, or volunteer activities that will keep him or her busy and active.
- Watch your children for any signs of drug abuse, including changes in behavior, secretiveness, and declining grades at school.
- If you think your child has a drug problem, provide help and support.
- Call the National Institute on Drug Abuse Hotline at 1-800-662-HELP (1-800-662-4357) for information and referral.
- Get involved in (or start) a drug abuse education and prevention program at your child's school.
- Involve other members of your community in drug abuse prevention.
- Work with your local police department to help prevent drug abuse in your community.

Adolescent suicide

Suicide is the third leading cause of death among adolescents in the US. In fact, the adolescent suicide rate has tripled during the past 20 years, and it continues to increase. Girls attempt suicide more frequently than boys, usually by taking an overdose of drugs, which provides a much greater chance of survival and which in part may represent a cry for help. Boys are more often successful at killing themselves, because they tend to use such methods as guns or hanging.

In a recent year, there were 21.7 suicides for every 100,000 males between ages 15 and 24. There were 4.4 suicides for every 100,000 females in the same age group. These figures do not, however, reflect the large number of unsuccessful suicide attempts or the number of suicides that were incorrectly reported as accidental deaths. One study estimated that there are as many as 50 to 200 unsuccessful attempts for every completed suicide. In view of that estimate, the teenage suicide rate is probably much higher than it appears.

There have been reported cases of several suicides occurring over a short time in a limited geographic area. This has been called "cluster suicide." One possible cause of cluster suicide may be imitative behavior related to the suicide of a friend or classmate.

Although there is no "typical" suicidal person, someone who is suicidal may display one or more warning signs. These signs are not exclusively related to an increased risk of suicide, but, instead, indicate the presence of severe emotional disturbance or mental illness, which should never be overlooked or ignored. Parents should watch their teenagers for evidence of:

Withdrawal and isolation The child is uncommunicative and wants to be alone. He or she is no longer interested in his or her family, friends, or favorite activities. Poor grades in school may be a sign of withdrawal.

Depression A depressed adolescent does not function as he or she usually does and may express feelings of despair. He or she will be unable to sleep at night and will then have difficulty getting up in the morning. The teenager will lose interest in his or her surroundings, will have little or no appetite, and will begin to feel that no one cares. Teens can be overwhelmed by their problems and worry that a painful, distressing situation will never improve. A dangerous period for suicide is when a teen begins to regain energy and seems to be coming out of the depression. A teen who has recurrent, long periods of depression needs psychiatric treatment (see Depression, p.321).

Mood swings Although moodiness is a common feature of adolescence, drastic mood changes should be seen as significant. Note that a calm mood that follows an episode of profound anxiety and depression can be a sign that the child has chosen suicide as a means of escape from his or her problems.

Threats of suicide Never dismiss any talk of suicide. Statements like "I might as well be dead" should be taken seriously. It is a myth that people who talk about suicide never follow through.

Change in personality The teenager departs from his or her usual patterns of behavior. Watch for changes in attitude, demeanor, and appearance.

Giving away personal possessions The teenager may give his or her property to family or friends or say that they may have it when he or she is "gone."

Significant life events Death of a friend (especially by suicide), classmate, or relative, a parents' divorce, the breakup of an important relationship, or an accident can put unbearable stress on an adolescent.

Substance abuse Use of alcohol and other drugs, although frequently a part of adolescent experimentation, can indicate that a teenager is no longer concerned about his or her well-being. Use of hallucinogenic drugs can lead to accidental suicide when they cause a teenager to become confused and disoriented.

Risk-taking behavior Although teenagers may often take risks, participating in dangerous activities such as drinking and driving can be a sign that a teenager does not value his or her own life.

Preoccupation with death Constant talk about death and dying shows that an adolescent is preoccupied with thoughts about death and dying.

If your teenager exhibits one or more of these warning signs, take him or her to see your physician immediately. Even if your child's behavior does not signal a possible suicide attempt, it does indicate the presence of a problem that needs treatment. A child who is abusing alcohol and other drugs may need to enter a drug treatment program. Your physician may refer your son or daughter to a child psychiatrist or psychologist for psychotherapy. If there are problems at home, your physician may recommend family therapy. If your teenager is severely depressed, your physician may prescribe antidepressant medication or he or she may recommend treatment in a hospital psychiatric unit. If your teenager tells you he or she is contemplating suicide, consider it an emergency and take him or her to a hospital emergency department.

Not every teenager shows warning signs of suicide, and the expression of a warning sign varies from person to person, according to his or her usual patterns of behavior. It is important, however, that parents communicate with their adolescent sons and daughters. Talk to your children, and become familiar with their feelings and attitudes. Let your teenagers know that you care about their problems and are available whenever they need you. Then follow through. Adolescents need a great deal of love, support, and understanding from their parents.

Self-help or support groups can provide comfort for parents, family, and friends in the event of adolescent suicide. For information and referral to a group in your area, contact the American Association of Suicidology at 303-692-0985, or Compassionate Friends at 708-990-0010.

Adolescent sexuality

In early adolescence (about ages 12 to 15) a child's closest friendships are often made with people of the same sex. However, a teenager usually begins to seek relationships with people of the opposite sex. An increasing number of teenagers in the US have sexual intercourse. One study showed that 30 percent of 16-year-old girls and 70 percent of 18-year-old girls have had sexual intercourse. About 10 percent of teenagers who have had intercourse have had it often, and with different partners. A same-sex encounter may simply be sexual experimentation, and does not necessarily indicate homosexual orientation. However, as many as 10 percent of adolescents may be homosexual (attracted to people of the same sex).

Parents and children often have unrealistic views of each other's sexuality. Adolescents may find it difficult to believe that their parents are still interested (or were ever interested) in sex. Parents often feel that although their teenagers may be physically able to have sexual relationships, they are not emotionally prepared. Most adolescents, however, experiment with relationships and sex. If your children seem to be sensible and responsible in other ways, they may be responsible sexually as well, but it is likely that they will have had some type of sexual experience by the time they finish high school. Therefore, it is important that parents talk to their young teenagers about relationships, sex, and love, and explain that sex and love are not the same thing.

What should parents do?

Accept your child's sexuality and provide help and advice. Although parents may worry about masturbation, it does not involve any risk to health. It is normal. Say so to prevent your child from having guilt feelings. Explain the risks of sexual intercourse, including pregnancy and sexually transmitted diseases (STDs) including AIDS (see p.465).

If your child tells you that he or she is homosexual, or if you think this may be true, you can get further information and support from an organization such as Parents and Friends of Lesbians and Gays (PFLAG).

You have a responsibility to make sure that your children are well informed about your own beliefs about love, sex, contraception, and the health risks of sexual activity. If you find it difficult to talk to your children about sex, you can ask your physician to talk with them, or you can give your children a book on the subject and discuss any questions they may have. Adolescents should be informed about all available contraceptive techniques and should be told where they can go for sound contraceptive advice. Teenagers need to know that condoms help prevent conception and protect against sexually transmitted diseases. Teenagers also need to know where they can be treated for STDs. Emphasize the importance of reporting an STD to their physician so that their sexual contacts can be located and treated. Because many adolescents, like many adults, may be reluctant to reveal the names of their sexual partners, it may be helpful to stress that such reports are kept confidential.

Encourage self-confidence in your teenagers; that, along with an understanding of the complexities of sexual relationships, will help them to make responsible decisions regarding STDs, contraception, and pregnancy.

Adolescent pregnancy: a responsibility for both partners

Information about various methods of contraception appears in another section of this book (see Infertility and contraception, p.649). It is important for adolescents to know about contraception and the risks of sexual activity. Information about contraception can be obtained from your family physician or a family planning clinic.

Pregnancy is possible even if a girl's menstrual periods have not yet started. The first egg is released before the first period. The timing of her menstrual cycle may not be the same each month, and sperm can remain alive for up to 7 days after intercourse, so it is not a good idea to rely on timing intercourse with her menstrual cycle to try to prevent pregnancy.

Unplanned pregnancy can result in many kinds of difficult problems for teenagers. These include serious health risks for a pregnant adolescent and her fetus. Teens who are sexually active should always use a contraceptive to help prevent an unplanned pregnancy.

A boy is equally responsible for using contraception and supporting any child that is born.

If you become pregnant, or if you get someone pregnant, it is important to talk to your parents as soon as possible. The girl should see her family physician immediately if she plans to have the baby. The earlier help is sought, the more options are open to you. Continuing the pregnancy and either raising the child or arranging for adoption are possible choices. Abortion is another option. If you decide to have an abortion, it is safer and easier to do so as early as possible in the pregnancy. Legal restrictions on availability of abortion for pregnant minors varies from state to state. Talk to your physician or look in the phone book for the number of your local chapter of Planned Parenthood.

Older people's health

Introduction

Like all aging machines, a human body that has been functioning for a number of years tends to work less efficiently than it did when it was "new." This is mainly a reflection of normal aging-related changes in the body and does not mean that illness is an inevitable part of old age. However, aging is a process that affects individuals differently. Life-style habits such as smoking, drinking, diet, and exercise all influence your general health and your rate of aging. Aging should not be equated with unavoidable breakdown of body systems. You should neither expect nor accept illness as a necessary part of growing old.

The problems discussed in this section are those that affect only older people, or affect them primarily. If you have symptoms, check the self-diagnosis charts that start on p.74. Two of the charts deal specifically with problems of aging (see Chart 98, Incontinence in older people, and Chart 99, Confusion in older people). Two current and important concerns, the increasing number of older people with Alzheimer's disease and the growing need for special care arrangements for older people, are discussed in boxes on p.774.

How old is an "old" person? There is some truth in the saying that "you're as old as you feel." Many people of 75 or 80 years and over are as alert and active as they were at 60, but some 60-year-olds have bodies or minds that are much older. All of us can benefit from the advances being made in medicine and health care, and preventive medicine is important for all ages. Americans are living longer, on the average, and more attention is being given to providing social and psychological support for the older population.

The physical and mental disorders that mainly affect older people usually involve families too. For this reason, most of the following articles include suggestions for concerned family members along with direct information for older people. Also, if you have family members who are over 65, you should find out about government agencies or private organizations in your community that specialize in providing assistance and advice for older people and their families.

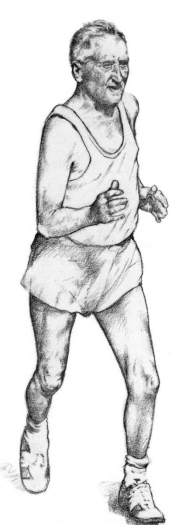

Aging and the body
The effect of age on different tissues and organs varies, but all become more vulnerable to disease.

Over the years, a gradual loss of elastic tissues causes everyone's skin to wrinkle and sag.

Aging in itself does not interfere with the functioning of your heart. But we become more susceptible to the effects of degenerative diseases, including atherosclerosis, which reduces blood flow to the heart and the brain. Damage to the heart and memory loss may occur.

In your eighties, bones become lighter and more brittle. They break more easily. Your vision and your hearing become less efficient as you age, and eyeglasses or a hearing aid may be recommended. Because of changes in body metabolism, the effects of drugs, including alcohol, may be exaggerated.

Planning for retirement

Now that many people retire earlier and live longer, more people spend a major part of their adult life in retirement while remaining physically and mentally active for much of this time. Yet some people approach this major period of their lives with no idea of how they can manage on their retirement income or of how they will fill their new free time.

Financial planning for retirement is essential. Seek professional advice, perhaps from your lawyer, accountant, or banker, about how to plan and manage any savings or investments as well as your social security and other retirement income. Be sure that you arrange for adequate and reliable medical and hospital insurance to supplement any available Medicare coverage. By planning in this way, you can help ease any worries that you may have about coping financially in retirement.

When planning for retirement, you will naturally seek advice from friends who have already retired.

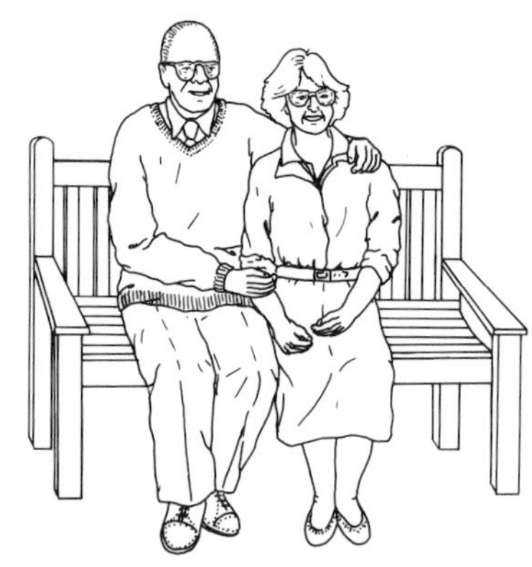

Relationships

Friends, relatives, and neighbors are one of the best insurance policies for a happy old age. Think of this before moving to another area when you retire, if you might find it difficult to give up old friends and meet people in a new community. If you decide to move to a new area, you should make a concerted effort to make new friends—by pursuing an activity or joining some social groups. Retirement communities are an increasingly popular option.

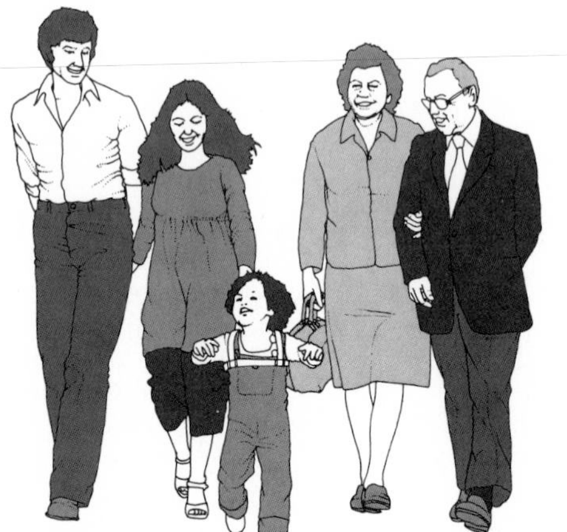

Recreation

Keep active and physically fit when you retire to help maintain your good health and to prevent illness. The trend toward a more sedentary life-style is being reversed, as people realize that lack of exercise contributes to the growing incidence of diseases linked with immobility, notably coronary artery disease (see p.400). It is good to have an established exercise program and stick with it; sudden changes in exercise habits that produce extra demands on the heart (such as shoveling snow) are harmful. Walking to the store and climbing stairs rather than using an elevator are both good forms of exercise. It is best to find a fitness activity that you enjoy participating in regularly.

Activities

Retirement will give you the opportunity to devote more time to interests such as hobbies. For example, you may enjoy traveling, swimming, or gardening. Being retired also gives you some time to develop new interests. Watch your newspapers, and contact any nearby schools that give adult education classes if you plan to explore new interests. Some communities offer senior citizen programs that may interest you. You may wish to work part-time to keep up your skills or to earn some extra money. Speak to a tax accountant about how this will affect the taxes on your pension or retirement income. You may want to do volunteer work instead.

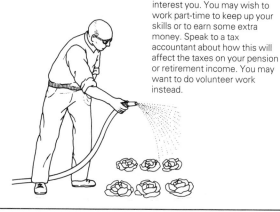

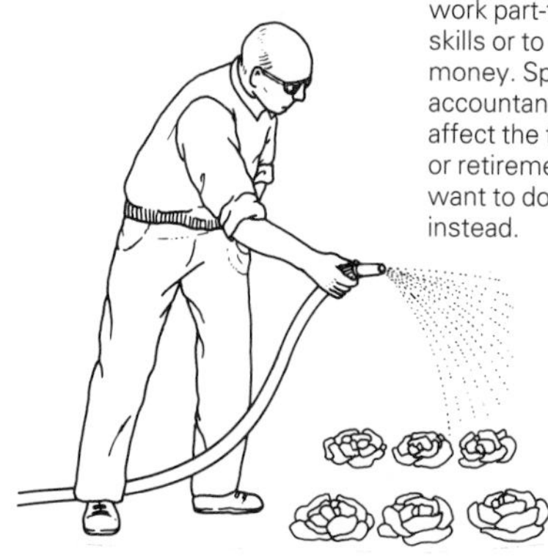

Incontinence

Incontinence is the term for uncontrollable, involuntary discharge of urine, stools, or both. Incontinence in older people, like incontinence in the young, is usually caused by an underlying condition, such as a urinary tract disorder or a problem with the nerves that control the bladder or the intestines. Incontinence is not an inevitable part of growing old and should not be accepted as such. It does, however, occur much more commonly in older people than in younger people. This is because the efficiency of muscle sphincters and the tone of other muscles connected with the urinary and digestive tracts diminish with age (see Prolapse of the uterus and vagina, p.640).

Incontinence will usually disappear after successful treatment of any underlying condition. For example, a urinary tract infection (see Infections, inflammation, and injury, p.541) or problems with the prostate gland (see p.615) may cause urinary incontinence. Similarly, certain gastrointestinal diseases or too little fiber in the diet are often responsible for loss of bowel control.

A few people who are incontinent have a more severe disorder such as stroke (see p.285), spinal cord injury (see p.296), or dementia in aging (see p.772). In at least some of these cases, the disorder causing the incontinence may not respond to treatment. The accompanying incontinence is then dealt with as a problem in itself.

The great majority of the older people who are incontinent have urinary incontinence only. Some can no longer suppress the urge to urinate on those occasions when going to the bathroom seems inconvenient. If their bladders are full, they may have stress incontinence, in which they may dribble urine when they cough or sneeze. Others have urge incontinence, in which they feel an uncontrollably powerful urge to urinate even though there may be hardly any urine to pass.

Most bowel incontinence is related to nerve-muscle control. An exception occurs in those who have fecal impaction, which is the accumulation of a hard mass of stools somewhere in the intestine. The partial blockage of the rectum by an oversize mass of hard stool prevents bowel movements, but it is not complete enough to prevent the more liquid portion of bowel contents from leaking out around the mass. If the blockage becomes big enough it can press on the bladder and cause urinary incontinence also.

What should be done?

Regardless of your age, you should consult your physician if you cannot control your bladder or bowels. Your physician may want you to have diagnostic tests. If the condition is reversible, you will be treated for it. If the cause turns out to be irreversible, much can be done to reduce the unpleasant effects of incontinence.

What is the treatment?

Self-help: You may be able to reestablish some control over your bladder by going to the bathroom at frequent, regular intervals (every 2 to 3 hours). Make sure your living and sleeping quarters are close to a bathroom, and keep a bedpan within reach of your bed. Make sure your garments are easy to remove. All bathroom facilities should be made as easy as possible to use. Handrails alongside the toilet may help if needed.

You can use memory aids or even an alarm clock to remind you to make regular visits to the bathroom. For urinary incontinence, drink sparingly if at all from the evening meal to bedtime. For bowel incontinence, eat plenty of high-fiber foods and drink plenty of fluids. If you do not move your bowels after breakfast, try a glycerin suppository. If nothing happens, try again the next morning.

As women age, muscles of the pelvic floor (which supports the bladder, intestines, and uterus) may weaken. If you have urinary incontinence, your physician may recommend that you do exercises at home to strengthen the pelvic-floor muscles. Tighten the muscles as you would to stop the flow of urine or stools. Relax and repeat this exercise 20 to 25 times in a series, several times a day. This may help curb the loss of urine by tightening the bladder opening.

Professional help: Your physician may prescribe a drug that stabilizes activity of the bladder so that urination times are further apart. But effective bowel-stabilizing drugs have not yet been developed. If you have a fecal impaction or chronic constipation (see p.510), consult your physician.

There are a number of incontinence aids that you can wear. Your physician or his or her nurse can tell you about them.

A typical example is specially designed disposable underwear that soaks urine into a porous outer layer and neutralizes the odor, leaving the inner layer (next to the skin) relatively dry. Another aid, which is for men, is a condom catheter, which is worn over the penis and is connected by a tube to a bag that can be emptied periodically. In some difficult cases of urinary incontinence, an indwelling catheter is used. A plastic tube is inserted into the bladder and drains urine into a bag. The bag can be emptied and cleaned regularly. The catheter must be changed periodically by your physician or a trained professional.

Falls

Everyone has an occasional fall, but falls among adults are common and especially serious in people over 65. Many such older people neglect the precautions listed in How to prevent falls (see p.769) and live in a home full of potential booby traps including slippery floors and stairs. Some older people have poor vision and poor general health, and some slowing of the reflexes is inevitable with age. Your bones also become more brittle as you age, making a fall a potentially serious injury. As you age, you become increasingly susceptible to disorders such as Parkinson's disease (see p.312) and various circulatory disorders (see Disorders of the heart and circulation, p.396) and arthritic conditions (see Bone diseases, p.581 and Joint disorders, p.588) that may affect your ability to maintain your coordination and balance. Finally, some prescribed drugs, especially sleeping pills and tranquilizers, may result in increased risk of falls.

What are the risks?

Falls are by far the most common type of injury in people over 65, because of the factors described above. Deaths from falls, or from complications directly related to falls, account for more than half of all accidental deaths of older people. In a typical orthopedic section of a hospital, about half the patients are likely to be older women with broken bones. The corresponding proportion of older men is lower, probably because women's bones tend to become more brittle somewhat earlier than men's and because there are more women than men in the older age groups.

Many falls, even for people over 65, cause nothing worse than a bruise. However, fragile skin and small blood vessels make bruising more serious and extensive in older people after even a minor fall. There is always a risk, moreover, of falling against or on something that is itself dangerous. Half of all deaths from burns in the US, for instance, occur among older people, who tend to have accidents such as stumbling against a stove or grabbing for support at the handles of pots of boiling liquid. And if you hit your head, the seemingly minor impact may cause dangerous delayed bleeding within the skull (see Subdural hemorrhage and hematoma, p.289).

One common result of an older person's fall is a fractured bone or bones, and those most frequently broken are much the same as the ones mentioned for the general population (see Fractures, p.575). So-called broken hips, which are in fact thighbones (femurs) that are broken near the top, are particularly common in older people. The chances of a hip fracture resulting from a fall increase significantly after age 50.

Apart from the injuries of the fall itself, there may be several indirect consequences of a fall. If, as sometimes happens, the person lies alone immobilized and undiscovered for hours or days, the result may be hypothermia (see p.772), pneumonia (see p.384), or even death. If the person with a broken bone must be hospitalized, the resultant possible long period of immobility may further deplete minerals from the bones, weaken aging bones and muscles, and permit deep vein thrombosis (see p.445) in the legs and pelvis.

Some older people who have had serious falls become permanently frightened and lose confidence in their ability to get around. They therefore become less and less active, and less and less confident. This vicious cycle can lead to becoming prematurely bedridden or, at least, confined indoors.

What should be done?

Protect yourself against falls by following the recommendations in the box on the next page. If you live alone, establish some way of alerting others quickly in case you have a problem. Some older people always carry an attention-getting device such as a whistle. Some have agreements with neighbors who check on them based on certain regular habits, such as a daily hour for raising a shade, opening a drape, or taking a stroll. The neighbor then checks for possible trouble whenever the habitual act is omitted. A word of warning, however—be careful not to develop a routine or set of signals that can be useful to burglars. If possible, it is useful to have a regular schedule of telephone calls or visits to and from friends and family, who then are alerted if the schedule is disrupted.

Remember that even a few days in bed may cause weakness and stiffness of your muscles and joints, and make your balance less steady. So stay active. If you think that you are not as steady on your feet as you should be, consult your physician. Since there are several possible causes of unsteadiness, your physician may order a series of tests to determine whether your problem is caused by a treatable disorder. Always see your physician, too, after you have had a bad fall, even if there seem to be no ill effects.

If you are with someone who falls, or if you find someone who is apparently immobilized by a fall, use appropriate first-aid measures (see Injuries and emergencies, p.842). However, don't move the person if you suspect an injury to the back. An older person who is in pain should be seen by a physician promptly. If you find anyone unconscious, you should call 911 if available in your area or summon emergency medical help at once. If a physician or someone who is trained in first aid is not available, call for an ambulance and stay with the unconscious person until help arrives.

What is the treatment?

Prevention is one of the best strategies for reducing the serious consequences of falls. If you need glasses, have them prescribed and

How to prevent falls

Because anyone can have a bad fall, the following suggestions are worth considering regardless of your age. However, older people are most likely to fall or to experience major problems as a result of a fall. If you are over 65 or if you are in any way responsible for the well-being of an older person, try to follow as many of these recommendations as are applicable in your situation.

1. If you need glasses, wear them, but never walk around wearing glasses that are meant only for reading. Take them off before moving around.

2. If you are even slightly unsteady on your feet, use a cane. Do not hesitate to use a walker outdoors as well as in the house if you feel safer with one or your physician recommends one.

3. Wear shoes with low heels that fit well or slippers with nonslip soles. Avoid long shoelaces, which can easily come untied and trip you.

4. Make sure that rugs and other floor coverings are secured around the edges, and tack down worn spots. Never use loose mats and rugs on shiny, polished floors.

5. Make sure that all potentially hazardous areas such as stairs and doorway entrances are brightly lit. White paint on either side of a flight of stairs can help.

6. A strong banister running along all indoor and outdoor steps is essential. Install one wherever such a support is not already in place.

7. Have a bedside lamp or low-wattage night-light in your bedroom so that you never have to grope around in the dark to go to the bathroom at night.

8. Install secure handrails in convenient places near the bathtub and toilet, and use nonslip mats both inside and alongside every bath or shower.

9. Do everything possible to minimize clutter in rooms, especially if there are several generations of people living together. Children's toys, especially those on wheels, are particularly hazardous.

10. Do not allow cords from electrical appliances to run loosely along the floor. Wherever possible, wires should be attached to walls or moldings.

11. Store frequently used dishes, clothes, and other items in places where you can reach them easily without standing on a stool or chair. If you must climb up to get something from a high shelf, use a stable stepladder or sturdy chair.

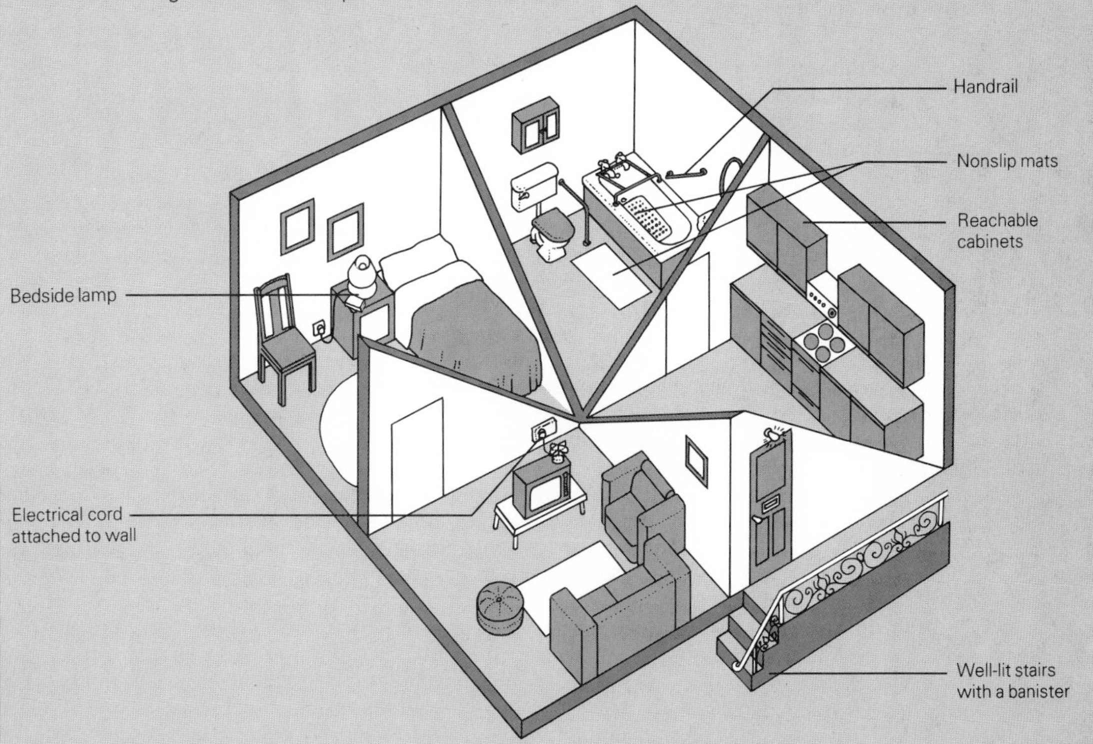

fitted; then wear them. Report to your physician any changes that you believe are related to the effects of any new medication. Also, a regular exercise program will help strengthen your legs; if necessary, use walking aids such as a cane.

The pain and discomfort of a fall, even if no bones have been broken, may be considerable. (If there is any possibility of broken bones, go to an emergency department where X rays can be taken.) It is important to relieve the pain with the use of aspirin or acetaminophen. Once you are sure there are no serious injuries, get the person moving again. Bed may seem to be a comfortable place, but it is too easy for an older person who is already stiff and sore after a fall to become bedbound and immobile. Cold compresses for the first 24 hours, and warm compresses thereafter, can reduce the pain and swelling of bruises. Applying heat with a hot water bottle or a heating pad can help relieve muscle stiffness. See also Injuries and emergencies, p.847.

For treatment of fractures, see p.575. Older people who have been treated in the hospital for broken bones (or any disabling disorder) should inquire about home health care services and housekeeping help during their recovery period.

Skin problems of older people

(including degenerative purpura)

Aging skin becomes increasingly thinner, more wrinkled, and less flexible, in part because there is a gradual change in the nature of the fibrous and elastic elements that keep your skin supple and smooth. This and other physical changes are irreversible, and as the aging process continues, the skin may also become more susceptible to some skin disorders (see Skin, hair, and nail disorders, p.266). Smoking increases wrinkling. In addition, many blotches and pigmented patches tend to appear in old age. Often called age spots, they may come and go and usually are not a problem.

Degenerative purpura

Reddish-brown or purplish areas, sometimes as large as 2 in (about 5 cm) across, may appear anywhere on the body. They are usually most noticeable on the legs, the forearms, or the back of the hands. These markings are caused by bleeding under the skin. Blood seeps slowly from tiny vessels that have become damaged by loss of elasticity in the skin. Although the blood is gradually reabsorbed, the underlying defect is irreversible, and the spots may recur.

Most such spots are harmless, but you should see a physician about any spot that concerns you, because there is a possibility of skin cancer. For more information, read the articles on basal cell carcinoma (see p.274), malignant melanoma (see p.275), and squamous cell carcinoma (see p.275). Most skin cancers can be cured if treated early.

Itching

As you age you may develop extremely dry, itchy skin. If you are bothered by constant itching, see your physician, who will examine you for a possible underlying condition such as jaundice (see p.522). If there is no cause other than age, your physician may recommend an ointment or lotion, sometimes along with superfatted soap and advice not to wash your skin with soap and water too often.

Trigeminal neuralgia

(tic douloureux)

This kind of neuralgia ("neuralgia" means pain from a damaged nerve) is more common in people over 70 and almost never affects anyone under 50 except in cases of multiple sclerosis (see p.316). The trigeminal nerve is a major nerve in the face. If it is damaged, the result is severe pain, which usually occurs on only one side of the face. It is not known what causes the nerve damage or why the condition occurs mainly in older people. Although it is not life threatening, trigeminal neuralgia can be agonizing and disabling.

What are the symptoms?

The pain of trigeminal neuralgia shoots through one side of the face along the length of the nerve. An episode may last for a few seconds or as long as a minute or more, and while it lasts it can be excruciating. The pain may be triggered just by touching a sensitive place somewhere on the face or even by sitting in a draft or inhaling cold air through the nose. Sometimes these physically disabling and emotionally exhausting episodes occur for no apparent reason every few minutes over a period of several days or weeks. They may then fade, but stabbing pains usually return at shorter intervals, and bouts of trigeminal neuralgia may eventually become almost continuous. In some cases, occasional muscular spasms accompany the pain and cause a facial tic, or twitching.

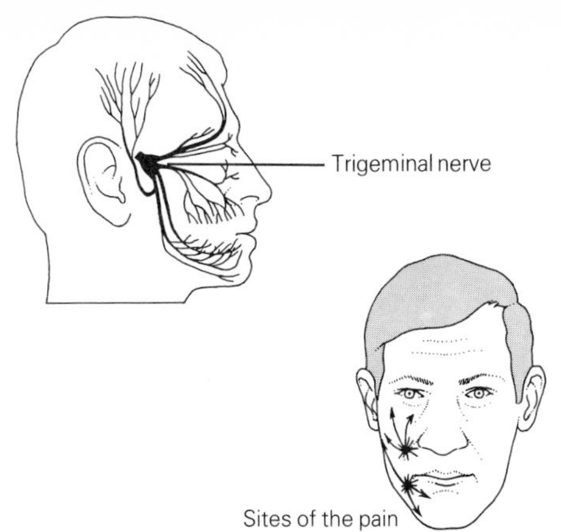

The trigeminal nerve
This nerve supplies sensation to the face, teeth, mouth, and nasal cavity and stimulates the group of muscles that move the jaw.

What should be done?

If you have what seems to be trigeminal neuralgia, consult your physician, who may refer you to a neurologist or neurosurgeon. If you have trigeminal neuralgia, your physician may prescribe a drug that can help prevent episodes. The medication should be taken exactly as prescribed. If drugs are not effective, you may be advised to have an operation to destroy the trigeminal nerve, by using high-frequency radio waves to cut it, severing it with a surgical knife, or injecting alcohol around it. But because destruction of the nerve leaves part of the face permanently numb, surgery is not usually recommended except in cases of extreme, persistent pain.

Aging and the senses

The senses, most notably sight and hearing, are likely to deteriorate with age. Often, however, declining sensitivity turns out to be at least partly caused by factors other than aging. Such cases can be treated. Even when the problem cannot be reversed, medical devices such as hearing aids and glasses can significantly improve your ability to see and hear, so consult your physician about how you can take advantage of them.

Vision

By age 50, most people rely on glasses to read, walk, or drive. Most people over 65 have presbyopia (see p.337), in which the lens of the eye focuses less easily on nearby objects. There is no cure for such changes, but you should visit an ophthalmologist regularly (see Box, p.338) for a checkup. A new pair of glasses may help you or, even more important, an examination may reveal an underlying disorder such as a cataract (see p.345) or glaucoma (see p.346). If you have diabetes, you should pay especially close attention to any changes in your vision (see Diabetic retinopathy, p.349).

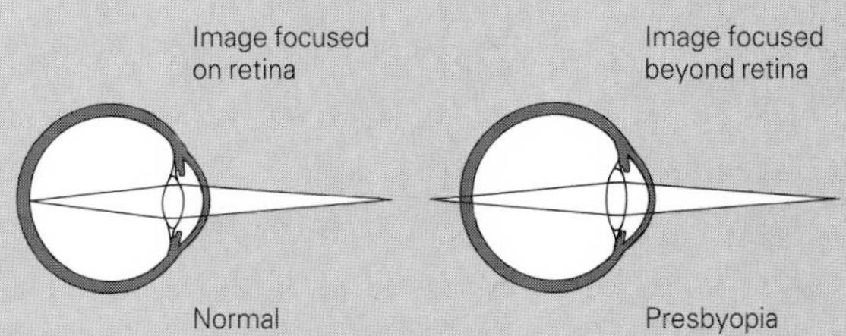

Hearing

Many people have difficulty hearing but have not consulted a physician about the problem. This is unfortunate because hearing loss may result from an easily treated underlying cause such as an accumulation of wax in the ear. Wax accumulates faster as you get older (see Wax blockage, p.356), so ask your physician about the possibility of flushing out your ears and the use of ear wax softeners whenever you notice that your hearing seems to be impaired. Another possible cause of hearing loss that can be treated is otosclerosis (see p.358).

There is no magic cure for the gradual impairment of hearing due to natural deterioration of the hearing mechanisms in the ear. Do not hesitate, however, to ask your physician whether you would benefit from a hearing aid; then get and learn how to adjust it so that you can make the most of it. Do not buy a hearing aid without first consulting your physician, since there are some untrained and unscrupulous sales people who may sell you a hearing aid that will not help your particular problem. For information on types of hearing aids, read the Box on page 361.

Other senses

Among other senses that often become less sharp as you grow older are taste, smell, and balance. Do not worry if food tastes and smells less appetizing than it used to. Continue to eat a sensible and varied diet and try increasing the amount of spices you use when cooking. Balance is a more serious matter, since unsteadiness can lead to falls (see p.767).

There is one other kind of sense perception, sensitivity to changes in temperature, that can be life threatening if it deteriorates. The skin of healthy young adults can detect a temperature drop of only 1°F (about ½°C) in the surrounding air. As you age, this sensitivity to temperature can diminish, and you may fail to notice a drop of up to 9°F (about 5°C). This is one reason why older people tend to be susceptible to hypothermia (see p.772).

Altered sensitivity to temperature can also be caused by disorders of the thyroid gland (see Thyroid and parathyroid glands, p.565). If you are warm when others are cold, or cold when they are warm, talk to your physician.

Hypothermia

In hypothermia, body temperature falls more than 4°F (about 2°C) below the healthy norm of 98.6°F (37°C). Death is a real possibility if hypothermia persists for more than a few hours. Anyone can acquire hypothermia and freeze to death if exposed to extreme cold for some time without adequate protection. So hypothermia is a risk for anyone who lives in a cold climate or spends a lot of time outdoors in winter weather.

However, older people are susceptible to hypothermia in less extreme temperatures. There are two main reasons for this. First, as we age, the body becomes progressively less able to maintain an even temperature when subjected to external cold. Second, the body mechanism that normally would detect a drop in its own temperature gradually loses its sensitivity as you age. The older person's reaction to cold is slower and incomplete. As a result, some older people do not realize that they are dangerously cold in a chilly environment (see Box, Aging and the senses, p.771) and may even die.

If you are over 60, be sure your residence is well heated and that you are well clothed. If you are cold and also sleepy or slightly confused, call your physician.

What are the symptoms?

If you find an older person sitting listlessly in a cold room or outdoors in cold weather, suspect hypothermia even if he or she is covered by several blankets or layers of clothing. Early symptoms of hypothermia may include drowsiness, mental confusion, and pallor. Loss of consciousness follows. The hands and feet of a person with hypothermia may feel cold to the touch, but a much more telling indication of hypothermia is cold skin over the abdomen.

The best way to determine whether someone's body temperature is dangerously low is to use a thermometer.

What should be done?

If you have older relatives or neighbors, visit them as often as you can in cold weather, encourage other friends to do so too, and make sure that they have plenty of warm clothes and blankets, that they eat well, and that their house or apartment is kept at a temperature at which they are comfortable.

There are many organizations such as local aging groups, home health services, visiting nurse associations, some hospitals, and community food programs (sometimes called "meals on wheels") that are prepared to assist older people in a variety of ways. Consult your physician or clergy for advice.

If you find an older person in what appears to be an early stage of hypothermia, take him or her to the nearest hospital emergency department or call for medical help. If the person is unconscious, the unconsciousness may result from some other condition such as a stroke or heart attack; emergency treatment is necessary in any case. While waiting for help to arrive, do what you can to warm the person slowly. Additional blankets and warm, nonalcoholic drinks may help if the person is still conscious. Do not give the person alcohol to drink, because it reduces body heat. Do not pile very heavy blankets or quilts on the person, and do not try to force him or her to eat or drink. Do not rub the person's hands or feet roughly in an attempt to restore warmth. Be gentle, calm, patient, and understanding.

The key to treatment of hypothermia is gentle, gradual rewarming of the person, and this should be done by a physician. The treatment must be gradual because too rapid an application of heat can cause sudden enlargement of blood vessels to the skin and just under the skin. If this happens, a rush of blood into the swollen vessels may rob vital inner organs of the blood they need in order to continue functioning.

Dementia and aging

Dementia is a brain disorder that results in the progressive loss of certain intellectual functions, particularly the memory. The disorder can develop at any age.

What are the causes?

A common cause of dementia in older people is Alzheimer's disease. In this disease, degeneration takes place in the brain, and many cells are lost. The underlying cause of the disease is unknown. Stroke is another common cause of dementia. A form of dementia more common among those over 75 is known as multi-infarct dementia. It is due to many blockages of cerebral blood vessels. Usually with multi-infarct dementia, the person does not become paralyzed, does not have other major symptoms, but ultimately will have dementia. Alcohol use is another major cause of dementia in older people. For other conditions that may lead to mental confusion, see Dementia, p.314.

What are the symptoms?

The symptoms of dementia usually begin with loss of memory, particularly for recent

Drugs and older people

Even minor disorders are often treated, at least in part, with tablets, pills, or liquid medication. As a result, many older people take several different drugs at one time, prescription and nonprescription drugs alike, often in different forms and on different schedules. It is very easy to forget whether a pill has been taken, to become confused about which medications to take when, or to forget whether the correct dose of a given drug is one, two, or three pills. Research has shown that about four in every ten people who are under a physician's care do not take their medication as prescribed by the physician. This is a remarkable figure when you consider the total number of people who are involved and the potential danger of skipping doses or taking too much or too little of some drugs.

The following list of DOs and DON'Ts should help you to avoid making serious mistakes. The list has been compiled primarily for the use of people who are over 65, but it contains good advice for anyone who takes medication. If you use medication regularly, keep this list available and review it every now and then.

Do

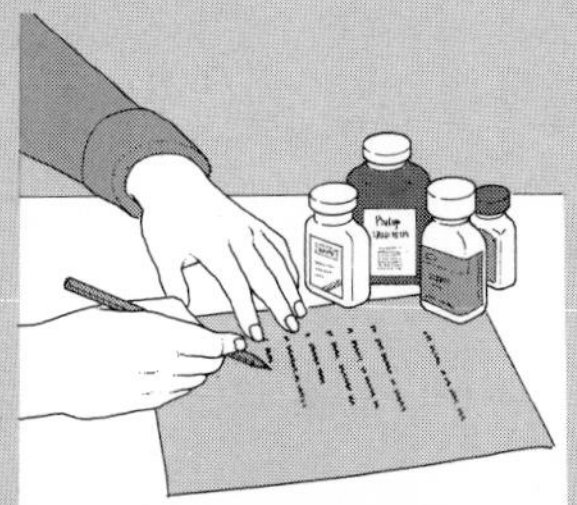

Use memory aids to help you remember dose times. For example, a once-a-day drug might always be taken at bedtime, and a three-times-a-day drug after each meal. Write down a checklist of all the drugs you are taking, and update the list whenever there are changes. It may also help to prepare your list in the form of a calendar so that you can mark off each dose of each drug as you take it. Another aid is to use an egg carton or plastic container with a place for up to four doses of drugs for each day of the week; put each required dose of medication in a separate section.

Make sure that all containers are clearly labeled with their contents and when they should be taken. If you have trouble reading a label, ask your pharmacist how often to take the drug and whether it should be taken with food. Also, request easy-to-open containers if child-proof containers are difficult for you to open.

Ask your physician to give you a drug in the easiest possible form to take. For instance, if you find it difficult to pour a liquid medication into a measuring spoon without spilling some, it may be possible to get the same drug in tablet form. Sometimes a change is not possible, however, because different forms of drugs are absorbed in different ways into your body.

Be sure to inform all physicians who treat you about all the drugs you are taking. Show them your checklist or take in the containers for the drugs you are taking. This will help prevent excessive doses or dangerous interactions of drugs.

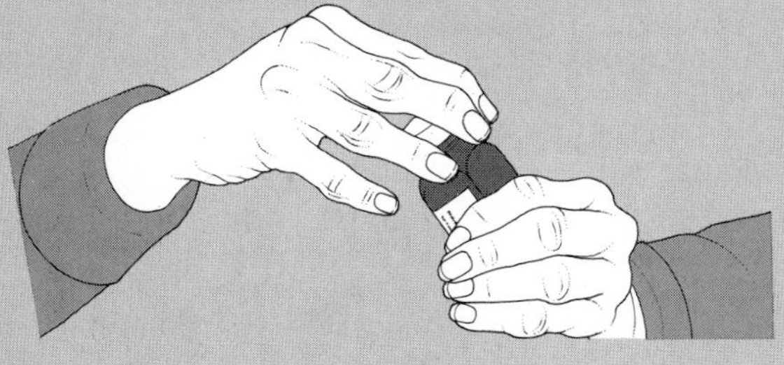

Don't

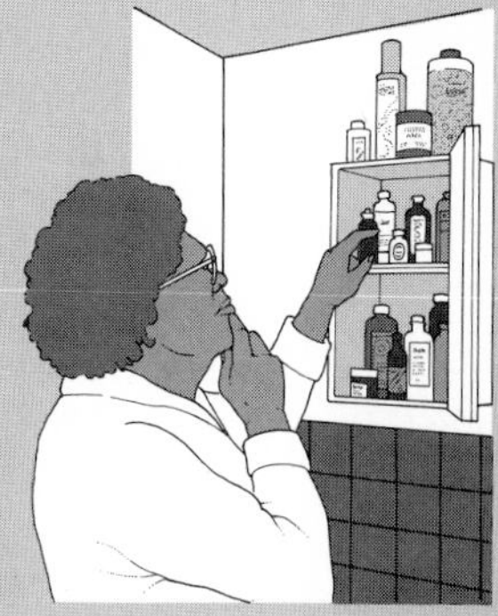

Don't be a drug hoarder, or keep unused medication in your medicine cabinet. Keep drugs that you are currently using, and those you use occasionally such as antihistamines or aspirin, and throw away (or flush down the toilet) partially used supplies of all others. Never give your prescription drugs to others or take medication prescribed for someone else.

Don't start taking a medication again after a long interval without consulting your physician. Your present symptoms may result from a different disorder from the one for which last year's drug was prescribed. Moreover, another drug that you may now be taking could interact dangerously with the old one. Also, many drugs have a limited period of effectiveness.

Do not discontinue a drug unless you talk to your physician about it first; this is especially important if you are taking beta-blockers, anticoagulants, or ulcer medications. You should not transfer drugs from one container to another without making absolutely sure that the new container is correctly and clearly labeled.

Don't keep medication containers on your bedside table unless it is absolutely necessary. There is a great risk of taking either the wrong medicine or an overdose of the right one when you are sleepy. This can happen especially if, instead of switching on a light, you trust your sense of touch in the dark.

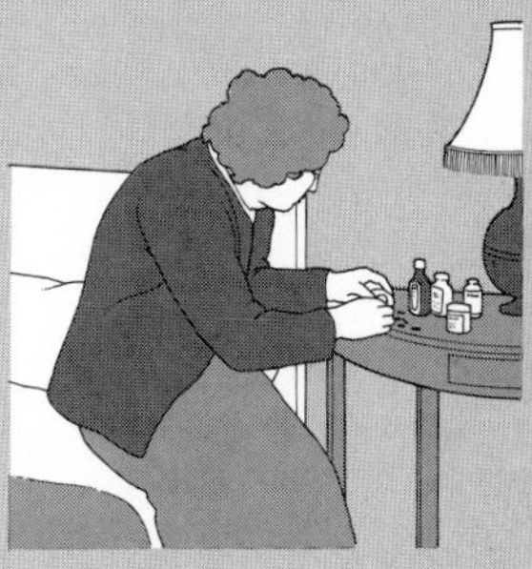

events. Gradually other intellectual functions, such as the ability to reason and understand, become increasingly impaired, and the affected individual may lose interest in his or her surroundings and even in simple, basic activities. Often, a total disintegration of personality may occur. In advanced stages, movement becomes increasingly difficult due to generalized stiffness of the arms and legs. Mental and physical deterioration resulting from dementia may gradually progress over 10 or more years.

What should be done?

Many people who appear to have dementia may actually have symptoms of an underlying disorder that can be treated. It is important that any older person with any loss of memory that interferes with daily life (such as losing important items) have a thorough evaluation by a physician.

Drugs such as sleeping pills, tranquilizers, and some pain medications can cause the symptoms of dementia. Depression, too, can be an important treatable cause of the disorder. Bronchitis and other infections tax your circulatory system, diverting blood from the brain; this can lead to the sudden onset of reversible dementia. Today, most forms of dementia in older people are irreversible, but research continues. For advice on caring for a person with dementia, see Dementia, p.314.

Alzheimer's disease

The death rate from Alzheimer's disease in the US increased from 857 in 1979 to 11,311 in 1987. Public health experts were uncertain whether the number of cases of Alzheimer's was growing or whether the dramatic increase represented an increased awareness of the disease on the part of physicians. Men had a slightly higher rate than women; whites, a higher rate than blacks. Alzheimer's disease is a leading cause of dementia (see Dementia and aging, p.772), and it is not known exactly what produces it (see also Dementia, p.314). For more information on how to cope with a family member who has Alzheimer's disease, or any condition causing progressive dementia, contact the Alzheimer's Association in Chicago, or ask your physician about an Alzheimer's Family Support Group in your area.

Special care for older people

The combined effects of disease and increasing age can lead to an inability to cope, either mentally or physically, with everyday tasks. Many older people are highly independent and may try to hide any disability because they are afraid of being put into a nursing facility. However, only about 5 percent of older people are in residential care—either public or private. The other 95 percent are largely independent, dependent on friends or relatives, or being supported in some way with the help of community social services.

Most older people feel more secure with an arrangement where they are cared for by relatives who live with or near them. However, this is often a tremendous challenge for the families involved (see Caregiving at home, p.786) and is practical only as long as the person can get around and is able to take care of himself or herself. The family physician or local social agencies may be able to make arrangements for day care or short-term care to relieve the caregiver. In such an arrangement, the older person may go to a special center or residential home for a week every few months, or for 1 or more days every week.

Full-time residential care, usually supported privately, is recommended only for older people for whom the alternatives are impractical. Many older people adapt well to life in a nursing facility after an initial upheaval, but it is important for the family to monitor the quality of care. Adult day care centers are now being provided in some communities and may be the answer for the many older people who need daily professional care but want to retain a measure of independence; they prefer to spend the night with family or friends in familiar surroundings at home.

The decision to send a relative away from home is very difficult for the whole family. It is best to discuss such a decision with your physician and all family members. Then, if you must send the person to a nursing facility, you can be certain that the move is best for everybody concerned.

PART FOUR

Caring for the sick

The American health care system

Introduction

Like many of our institutions, the US health care system relies on a wide variety of public and private resources. Health care is provided in several ways: by physicians in private practice; by prepaid plans; by municipal, county, state, and federal institutions, such as the Veterans Administration; and by hospitals, which may be owned by religious groups or profit-making corporations, or which may be financed through charitable or community efforts. The US has more than a half million physicians, who practice medicine in a variety of settings: in solo, partnership, or group practice; in prepaid clinics and health maintenance organizations (HMOs); as hospital or governmental employees; and in ambulatory surgical centers, immediate care facilities, and emergency departments. Health care may be financed by the individual, by private or employer-employee insurance plans, through Medicare and Medicaid, or through other governmental programs.

The American health care system is large, employing more than 6 million people, handling more than 3.5 million patients a day, and absorbing more than 12 percent of our annual gross national product. For more than a quarter of a century, the number of physicians per 100,000 population has been increasing and many common measurements of health—such as life expectancy at birth—have been improving. As a result, the US is today one of the healthiest large nations with heterogeneous populations. Scientifically, American medicine is often regarded as the best in the world. In recent years, however, access to care and costs have become major issues. According to some estimates, at least 38 million people have no health insurance coverage.

Using the health care system

With all the well-trained people and with thousands of health care facilities in the US, it is important to learn how best to make use of them. How do you choose a physician, or, for that matter, change physicians? What are the differences in the different kinds of medical practices? What are skilled nursing facilities like and what is home health care? What happens during an operation? What happens in an intensive care unit? What is "alternative medicine"?

This section contains answers to these questions and many more that you might ask. Reading it will help you understand how to use the American health care system.

Voluntary health organizations

Voluntary health organizations are usually formed by citizens who have an interest in a specific disease or disorder. Such associations bring the energy and interest of the general public to the ongoing needs of patients with serious and/or chronic diseases. Physicians and other health workers often join these organizations also. Many voluntary health organizations exist to assist people with various diseases and conditions, including alcohol and other drug abuse, Alzheimer's disease, heart disease, bleeding disorders, blindness, cancer, arthritis, autism, diabetes, kidney disease, mental and emotional illness, muscular dystrophy, over- or undereating, occupational diseases, cystic fibrosis, facial deformities, hearing and speech disorders, Parkinson's disease, epilepsy, respiratory diseases, cerebral palsy, mental retardation, multiple sclerosis, and spinal cord injuries and other diseases and injuries that cause paralysis.

These voluntary associations are usually nationwide, statewide, or regional, with local chapters in cities and large towns. The activities of these groups include services such as providing patients, their families, and the public with information about various medical conditions, working toward related legislation, and supporting research and health care programs.

Choosing and using physicians

Everyone wants his or her physician to be well trained, competent, and accessible. Compassion and high ethical standards are also important. These are the basic features of good health care. But there are other factors that you should consider when you are choosing or evaluating a physician. When selecting a physician, you should be sure to consider your own preferences and needs. For example, would you prefer a physician who is older than you are, or one who is close to your own age? Do you want a physician who is the same sex as you are? Would you prefer a physician who appears warm and personally concerned about you, or are you more interested in a physician's technical knowledge? In general, both patient and physician are most satisfied and the care is most successful when each participant feels comfortable with the other.

Local and state medical societies usually can provide the names of physicians accepting new patients in your area. In addition, many hospitals offer physician referral services at no charge.

It is difficult to define a "good" physician. That may be mostly a matter of personal preference. But here are some criteria to consider: Does your prospective physician have a good reputation among other physicians in your area? What do his or her patients say? Does he or she have privileges at a good hospital? How many years of residency training has he or she completed? Is he or she certified by a medical specialty board (indicating special training)?

Evaluating your physician

Once you have a physician, how can you assess the quality of the care you are receiving? Medicine and the human body are far too complex to base such an assessment only on outcomes. Some conditions are more difficult to diagnose and cure than others, and some diseases cannot be cured.

What follows are three areas that you can try to evaluate as rough indicators of your physician's performance.

First, you can look at how well your physician's practice is organized. This is important because a well-organized practice should allow for effective follow-up, accurate recordkeeping, a minimum of waiting time before appointments, and adequate time for your physician to spend with you. It is also important that your physician has an effective system for after-hours and weekend care in emergencies, and that the practice manages to take care of patients who do not have appointments but who need care urgently.

Second, think about how your physician treats you personally. Does he or she spend enough time with you to assess a problem? Does he or she explain what is wrong with you and what the treatment is in such a way that you can understand it? If you do not understand, do you feel that you can ask questions? Does your physician give you a chance to explain your symptoms before asking a lot of questions? Does he or she communicate the reasons for any diagnostic tests that are ordered? Do you find out what you can expect from treatment, and do you feel free to call to ask about drug side effects, changes in your condition, or questions that you thought of after you left the office? Finally, do you feel that your physician is really listening to what you have to say?

A good physician should be willing to discuss any questions you have about your treatment, especially in cases where a disease has been under treatment for a long time and no apparent progress is being made. Your physician should also discuss alternative treatments with you when there are choices, and be able to tell you the advantages and disadvantages of each, so that you are in a position to make informed choices.

A third area that you can evaluate is your physician's willingness to consult with other physicians if your problem is outside his or her area of expertise, if it appears to be especially complex, or if it requires a particular procedure performed by that consultant. Your physician should explain to you why the consultation is needed, and he or she should provide adequate information for the second physician to evaluate your condition. Your physician should also try to send you to the most appropriate specialist available, and should be concerned to learn what the second physician found. If your physician is concerned, he or she can also act as an advocate for you or a coordinator of care if you have problems that may require the attention of various medical specialists.

Second opinions and changing physicians

If you have chosen a physician on the basis of your general preferences and his or her qualifications, give the relationship a chance. If you have one unsatisfactory appointment, it may have been just a bad day for one or both of you. But if communication is poor after several attempts and your condition is not improving, it may be in your best interest either to seek the opinion of another physician or to change physicians. Although this is a wise and rational decision, many people are reluctant to make it, often fearing that their physician's feelings may be hurt. This should not be a consideration, however; most physicians understand such changes. Your first concern must be your health and the best way to protect and maintain it.

In general, it is better to let your regular physician know about any consultation with another doctor so that the second physician can get a copy of your medical records and the results of any tests that have already been performed. This can save you much time and money. Do not worry that your physician will talk the second physician into believing his or her diagnosis; physicians are trained to reach their own, independent conclusions.

There are good reasons not to change physicians under certain circumstances. For example, if your health problem is unusual or rare and you are receiving care from a specialist, there may not be another specialist available to treat your problem. Changing physicians in this situation could be risky.

If you are unhappy with the care you are receiving, talk to your physician. If you cannot work out the problems you are having, both you and your physician may welcome a change. However, you may belong to a health maintenance organization (HMO) or other health plan that requires you to visit its own physicians. If you have problems relating to your HMO physician, call your plan coordinator to request a change.

Second opinions on surgery

Since most operations are not emergencies, you usually have enough time to get a second opinion, if your health insurance policy requires one, or if you or your physician feel that it is necessary. Getting second opinions for a minor problem can be costly and confusing. Help from your family physician in arranging your referral to a surgeon may be your best and easiest route to good surgical care. Many health insurers or employers now require a second opinion before they will pay for some elective operations; find out what your insurance policy requires.

Your need for a second opinion on surgery is also crucial when the problem you have can be treated without an operation, is particularly complex or rare, or is especially dangerous. In addition to providing information about whether surgery is necessary, a second surgical opinion in these situations provides an opportunity for you to obtain the names of and ask about several surgeons. Then, if the second physician agrees that surgery is necessary, you can, with the help of your physician, decide who should perform the operation.

Office and clinic care

People in the US average almost five visits to a physician per year. Much of this care is provided in ambulatory care settings, that is, walk-in care that does not involve spending a night in a hospital or other health care facility. Examples include the care that you receive in your physician's office, in the outpatient department of a hospital, including an emergency department, in a free clinic, or in a health center. Also included are the many home care services that may be available. In recent years, private home care services have provided an increasing number of home care visits by various therapists or nurses, offering more complex treatment, such as intravenous drugs, at home.

Office-based practice

There are three ways in which physicians usually organize their office practices: solo practices, partnerships, and group practices.

Solo practices: A solo practice is one in which a physician works alone, although sometimes a solo physician shares some office expenses with other physicians in what is called an association. Solo practice is becoming much less popular with physicians, partly because of costs and because of the problems inherent in trying to be available 24 hours a day, 365 days a year.

Partnerships: A partnership involves a specific legal agreement between two or more physicians to share income, office space, and equipment. The major advantages of a partnership over solo practice are that physicians in a partnership can help each other provide after-hours care, consult each other with difficult cases, and share some responsibility for care when appropriate.

Group practices: A group practice is an association of three or more physicians who use common facilities and share income and expenses. Such a practice has many of the same advantages as a partnership.

Health maintenance organizations (HMOs) are group practices that are organized to provide complete care for patients on a prepaid basis. Each patient (and/or his or her employer) pays a set amount each month, and the group provides medical care and preventive services, including checkups and, in some cases, medication. Hospitalization and referral for services that the group cannot supply directly are also covered by the monthly fee. Your physician's group practice may decide to join another prepaid plan, including an independent practice association (IPA) or a preferred provider organization (PPO). Prepaid plans vary greatly, depending on the contract with patients.

Hospital clinics

Some physicians have practices that are located in hospitals. They see patients in the outpatient departments, in clinics, or in the emergency department.

In large cities, hospital outpatient clinics have been a major source of medical care for the poor. However, university teaching hospitals may serve all income groups in their clinics. Depending on the hospital, patients may receive care from resident physicians who are supervised by senior specialists, or they may receive care directly from the specialist physicians.

Hospital clinic care is usually of high quality because of the availability of many qualified specialist physicians.

Ambulatory care centers

These centers may be "walk-in" centers for basic medical care or surgical centers for procedures that do not require an overnight hospital stay. Ambulatory care centers may be either independent facilities or part of a hospital. Surgical centers do not require the same equipment necessary in an operating room where complex surgical procedures can be performed, nor do they need as many beds, staff, and services. As a result, surgical centers can sometimes provide surgery at a reduced cost.

Public health

Public health, sometimes called community health, services are provided by county health departments, city health departments, or other publicly supported agencies.

Preventive medicine plays a very important role in maintaining good health and is therefore often considered to be a part of public health. In most states, health departments are organized to deliver services to a city, town, county, or region.

Organization and function of state health agencies vary, but state health departments usually are responsible for coordinating and planning public health activities. Local and county health departments often deliver more direct services. These may include school health services, health screening, immunization programs, pest control, nutrition programs, prenatal maternal and child health services, and other similar programs.

School health

In many communities, nurses and other health professionals are assigned to schools. A variety of services may be provided, including consultation with administrators, teachers, and parents in matters of physical and emotional health; home visitation to assist parents in planning follow-up treatment for their children; educational support for teachers, students, and parents in health-related subjects; screening programs to detect dental, vision, and hearing problems; and checking immunization records. A school nurse may also plan and/or participate in health conferences and classes.

Health screening

In health screening, large numbers of people with no symptoms are tested for disease, so that early detection can lead to treatment of the disease. Local public health departments can usually provide information on voluntary health screening agencies and may also offer such services. Screening may include testing for infectious diseases, or illnesses such as high blood pressure, diabetes, and some types of cancer. Such programs may also help with diet or medication problems. For children, there are case-finding programs available for early diagnosis of many diseases. These programs may include a health history, vision and hearing tests, a dental examination, and a blood test for anemia.

Maternal and child care

Maternal and child care programs are available in many city neighborhoods and communities. These federally funded programs are aimed at upgrading prenatal, and maternal and child health.

The WIC (women, infants, and children) program seeks to help pregnant women, new mothers, infants, and children up to age 5 whose weight is low for their age or who are anemic or near-anemic. You must have income below a certain level to qualify.

Local health departments may offer instruction in prenatal care, infant care, nutrition, family planning, and other topics.

Disease prevention and control

Immunization programs are available in many communities. Immunization protects people against diphtheria, pertussis (whooping cough), tetanus, polio, measles, rubella (German measles), and mumps.

In some communities, health departments screen people for chronic diseases such as tuberculosis. Testing and counseling programs for HIV (human immunodeficiency virus), which causes AIDS (acquired immune deficiency syndrome), are offered by many public health departments, and in many urban areas, voluntary groups provide a large share of health care and social services for people with HIV-related conditions and AIDS. Sexually transmitted disease control may also be handled by the local health department.

Communicable diseases that threaten the general population are called "reportable diseases," because all public health workers are required to report such cases to their local health department.

Medicare and Medicaid

Medicare finances medical care for older people and other selected beneficiaries. All Medicare beneficiaries are covered under Part A, which pays for many hospital services. Medicare beneficiaries may choose to subscribe to Part B, which helps pay for physicians' fees and home care services.

Medicare pays for hospital services using a system of reimbursement called diagnostic related groups (DRGs), which determines how much Medicare will pay the hospital, independent of how long you stay. For each episode of illness, you pay one deductible established by the federal government.

Physician fees are reimbursed by Medicare under a different system, called the Resource-Based Relative Value Scale (RBRVS). The RBRVS system is part of an effort to stabilize the mounting costs of medical care.

Many private insurance companies sell policies that supplement Medicare coverage (so-called Medigap insurance). A Medicare beneficiary needs only one Medigap policy.

Medicaid provides federal subsidies for state programs that finance health care for eligible people. The federal government regulates the use of Medicaid funds, but each state has rules and eligibility criteria within the limits of federal regulations.

All states must provide coverage for the following groups: people receiving Supplemental Security Income, people receiving Aid to Families with Dependent Children, and any children under age 5 in other low-income families. Reimbursement for nursing facility charges has become a large portion of Medicaid spending. Again, state regulations vary on eligibility.

Mental health

Community mental health programs attempt to prevent, detect, and treat mental illness. Trained mental health workers on staff provide such services as consultation for detention centers and departments of social service, educational support for civic and fraternal groups and schools, alcohol and drug abuse rehabilitation programs, and emergency care for the mentally ill.

In recent years, however, the mental health system has had problems coping with an increasing number of homeless mentally ill people living on the street in urban areas. Many homeless people were or would have been hospitalized in psychiatric hospitals before budget cuts and the advent of major antipsychotic drugs.

The term developmental disability is used to describe the problems of people whose mental and/or physical development is impaired. State institutions for the severely developmentally disabled provide a wide range of services. Churches and other voluntary organizations have a tradition of building and administrating institutions for the severely mentally or physically disabled.

The hospital

There has been a major shift of emphasis away from hospital care and toward care in the outpatient department, the physician's office, and at home. Nevertheless, sooner or later most of us must go to a hospital—to the outpatient department for tests requiring sophisticated equipment, for surgery as an outpatient or inpatient, or for other specialized medical care.

Hospitals can be classified on the basis of ownership, type of services provided, length of stay, and as teaching or nonteaching facilities. However, the variety within these types is so great that any classification has exceptions. The two most important groups by size and volume of care provided are voluntary, short-stay, general community hospitals and nonfederal, long-term hospitals.

Emergency care

Although every hospital does not have an emergency department, those that do provide a great deal of a community's trauma and emergency care. They have also been used by people for routine treatment. Care received in emergency departments is substantially more expensive than care received in a clinic or physician's office. Also, emergency department treatment usually does not provide for continuity of care by a single physician, and the most seriously ill or injured patients must be cared for first, no matter when they arrived. For these reasons, it is best to go to an emergency department only for truly urgent problems. Specialized centers for emergency care in some hospitals deal with burns, accidents, heart attacks, and other life-threatening conditions.

Quality of health care

Hospitals are subject to regular reviews to help maintain the quality of care that they provide. The hospital regulations that are designed to assure quality care are complex. Some reviews are required by government regulations, and some are voluntary.

The major voluntary mechanism for reviewing a hospital and its performance is the formal accreditation process of the Joint Commission on Accreditation of Healthcare Organizations. Hospitals are accredited, or approved, by the commission for no more than 3 years at a time.

All hospitals have medical staff bylaws. These rules and regulations are developed by the medical staff to assure the high quality of their work. In addition, a credentials committee reviews all physicians on the medical staff on a regular basis and determines which physicians are qualified to perform various types of surgery and complex diagnostic procedures.

Hospital review mechanisms also include committees that are responsible for quality assurance, utilization review (evaluating whether the facilities are overused or underused), written reports on surgical specimens, patient complaints, the quality of medical records, frequency and control of infections, and the use of prescription drugs. These committees meet regularly to discuss their findings and make recommendations.

Having an operation

Before any operation, you will be told what the surgeon plans to do and be given information about the possible risks and outcomes of the operation. You will then be asked to sign a consent form, which may be long and detailed. Before signing it, you should read it carefully and ask your physician about anything you do not understand.

On the morning of the operation, it is important not to eat or drink; if your stomach is not empty, the anesthetic may cause you to vomit while you are unconscious, which could be very dangerous. Any shaving to remove hair from the area to be operated on may be done at this time or earlier. You are then dressed in a clean gown to minimize the risk of infection. Thirty minutes or so before the operation is scheduled, you receive an injection that makes you sleepy. The anesthetic is administered in the operating room.

Except when blood vessels are being stitched, internal and membranous areas that have been cut or injured are closed with dissolving stitches. Small skin incisions are usually closed with thin synthetic fiber thread or clips. Larger incisions may be held together by stronger supporting stitches.

After any surgery, the patient goes immediately to a recovery room for about half an hour to two hours, to be watched closely until the staff approves a transfer to the patient's hospital room. If the patient is very ill or the surgery extensive, he or she may be sent to an intensive care unit (see next page).

After some types of surgery, particularly abdominal surgery, you may have to be fed or given fluids through an intravenous drip (a tube inserted into a vein) for a day or two. Other tubes (drainage tubes) may also be used to drain fluids and pus.

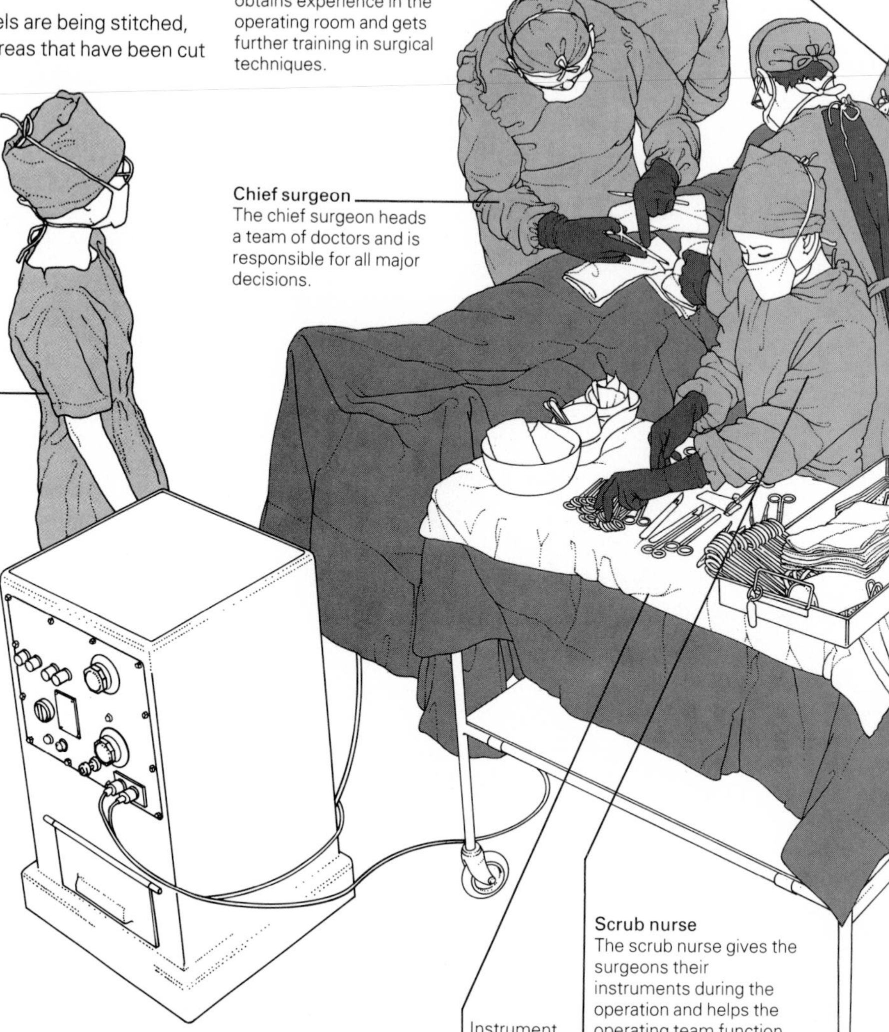

Anesthesiologist
The anesthesiologist administers anesthetics and is an expert in treatment of surgical shock, maintenance of lif support, and relief of the pain that follows the operation.
Surgical resident
The surgical resident obtains experience in the operating room and gets further training in surgical techniques.
Chief surgeon
The chief surgeon heads a team of doctors and is responsible for all major decisions.
Circulating nurse
One nurse helps the surgeons and the entire surgical team.
Instrument table
Scrub nurse
The scrub nurse gives the surgeons their instruments during the operation and helps the operating team function smoothly.

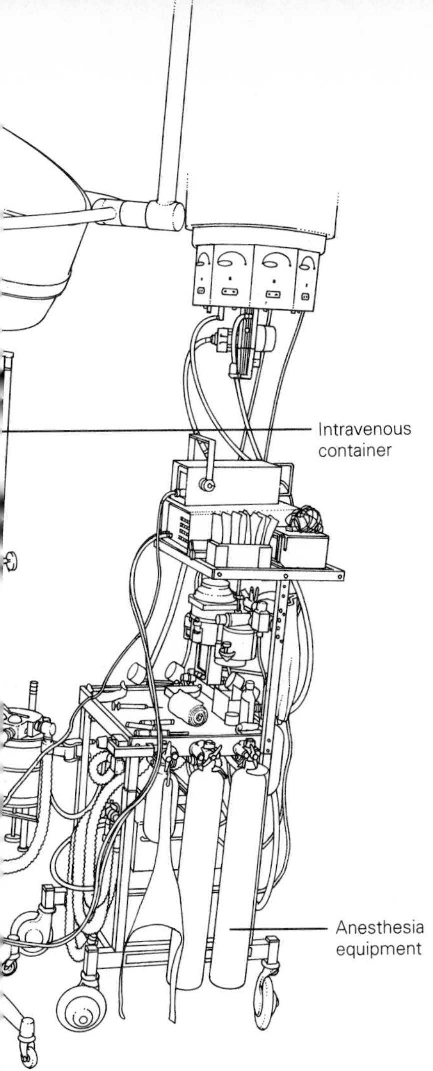

Assisting surgeon
The assisting surgeon is the chief surgeon's assistant and also may perform much of the surgery.

Intensive care

After some major operations and during some serious illnesses, a patient may need an artificial ventilator or extra oxygen in order to breathe. Continuous electronic monitoring of blood pressure, heart rate, and other vital body functions may also be required. The equipment necessary to provide intensive care after an operation is usually concentrated in a unit where patients are cared for by specialized medical and nursing staff. Most patients remain in an intensive care unit, under close supervision (with a ratio of one nurse for every one or two patients), for only a few days. They are then transferred to a less intensive hospital unit to continue their recovery.

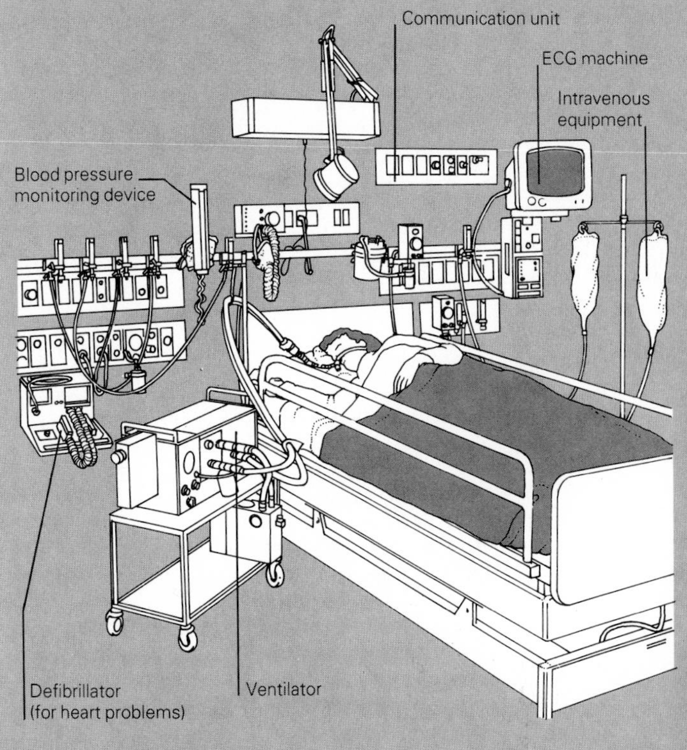

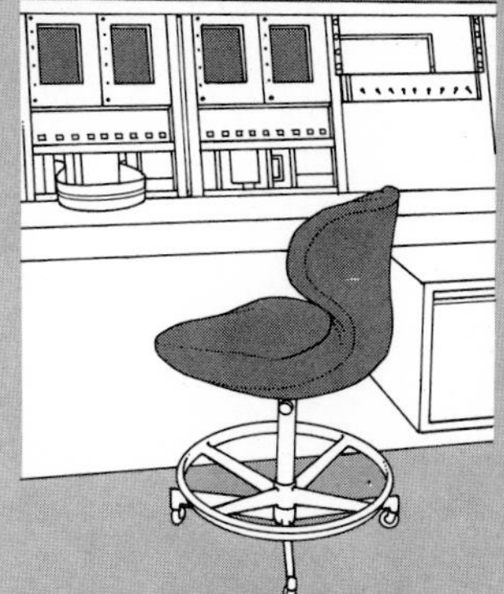

Central nursing station

An intensive care unit often has a central console, which allows the nursing staff to monitor the condition of all the patients in the unit. The recordings made of each patient's vital functions are shown on the console, and the instruments have automatic alarms to indicate any emergency.

Nursing facilities

Families are still the major caretakers of older, dependent, or disabled persons in the US. However, the number of people over 65 in nursing facilities (formerly called nursing homes) is rising, because the population in that age group is increasing. Many people now live longer, healthier lives, and this longevity has increased the need for nursing facilities and other long-term care facilities.

A "long-term care" facility is designed for people who need care for a longer period of time than is usually possible in an acute care hospital. Thus, a nursing facility is only one type of long-term care facility. Long-term care may also be given in rehabilitation and psychiatric hospitals, hospitals for people with chronic diseases, and hospitals for people who are mentally disabled. Nursing facilities accommodate patients of all ages and with a variety of conditions but are primarily populated by older people.

Choosing a nursing facility, like choosing any new place to live, is an important decision. It is difficult to decide quickly, but disabling illness can occur suddenly. So it may be wise to learn about the available facilities and their costs.

Nursing facility accommodations are in short supply in some areas, and the person may have to be placed on a waiting list. The cost of the nursing facility is also important, and early exploration allows a greater chance of finding one within your family budget.

Older people often dread moving into a nursing facility. They may feel they are going away to wait to die. They may fear not only abandonment by family and friends, but also having to adapt to a totally new environment and new people. Family members should be positive and reassure such a person. In practice, many older and disabled people adjust extremely well to nursing facilities.

Types of nursing facilities

There are many types of nursing facilities. It may help you choose a facility if you are familiar with the types and terminology.

A residential care facility (RCF) provides meals and sheltered living (with little or no housekeeping responsibilities for the resident) and some medical monitoring. This type of facility is appropriate for someone who needs to give up household chores, but does not need continuous medical attention. Many RCFs have exercise, social, and recreational programs.

An intermediate care facility (ICF) provides room and board and regular nursing care (not around-the-clock) for patients who cannot live independently. Physical, social, and recreational activities may be provided and some ICFs have rehabilitation programs. The cost of care in an ICF may be covered in part by some government programs.

A skilled nursing facility (SNF) provides physician coverage and full 24-hour nursing care by registered nurses, licensed practical nurses, and nurse's aides. An SNF is the right place for someone who requires intensive nursing care and rehabilitation services. An SNF may be paid for by a private insurance company or by either Medicare or Medicaid programs (see p.780). Medicare and Medicaid have certain eligibility conditions that usually include a prior hospitalization. Up-to-date information can be obtained from your nearest Social Security Administration office.

A hospice provides a caring environment in which efforts of the staff are concentrated on relieving pain, so that terminally ill patients can spend as much of their remaining time as possible with relatives and friends. For further information about hospices, see Terminal illness, p.801.

Determining the quality of care

Quality of care is of vital importance in choosing a nursing facility and there is no substitute for "shopping around." Talk to residents and their families and to health workers who have worked in a long-term care center, read brochures, speak with the administrators, and visit the facilities on more than one occasion.

State regulation of nursing facilities varies widely. Official certification as a skilled nursing facility or as an intermediate care facility is important and signifies that the facility has met all state standards. Although certification is not a guarantee of high-quality care, lack of certification is a signal that the facility could have serious problems.

Alternative medicine

In recent years, interest in alternative medicine, or those treatments generally not considered to be standard medical practice, has increased. Such treatments appeal to many people, particularly those who are deeply dissatisfied with modern medicine, its cost, and its emphasis on the scientific rather than the spiritual or personal approach.

The following are a few examples of alternative medicine that are available in the US today. The list and descriptions are intended purely as a source of information, not as an endorsement.

Holistic health care

This approach to health care attempts to focus on the whole person. This is not really radical, since health workers traditionally put a high priority on a person's total welfare. Also, all trained health professionals are aware that physical conditions do not exist in isolation. However, the number of medical specialists who concentrate on a single organ system—as cardiologists do—also has increased as the amount of medical knowledge has expanded. It is not surprising, therefore, that a renewed interest in the "whole patient" has developed. Holistic health care is an attempt to combine scientific treatment of medical problems with treatment of psychological, social, and spiritual problems.

Herbalism

In herbalism, plants are used in prevention (rosemary as an insect repellent), cures (garlic as a germ killer), and relief of pain and discomfort (aloe vera for arthritis pain).

Centuries ago, herbs and their extracts were the only available medications for many diseases. Today, however, pharmacies stock many medications that have been derived from natural sources to treat specific diseases, as well as purified herbs in the form of pills, pastes, or liquids.

In herbalism, the number of plants that are used medically is diverse and further complicated by the differing effects of barks, leaves, stalks, roots, flowers, and seeds.

Chiropractic

Chiropractic is a theory of healing founded on the belief that disease results from interference with nerve function. Chiropractic does not use drugs or surgery, nor is it intended to treat diseases as such. Instead, it attempts to maintain the structural and functional integrity of the nervous system. According to the theory of chiropractic, this is accomplished by massage and manipulation of the spine, joints, and soft tissues.

Acupuncture

Acupuncture is used in the US mostly to treat pain. There is no scientific explanation of how it works, but ancient Chinese theories are of interest to today's physicians. The theory of acupuncture is that a cycle of energy flows through the body along meridians, or channels. If energy is blocked at any point along a meridian, according to the theory, illness results that may be corrected with acupuncture.

The effect of treatment is unpredictable, but it may provide relief. Acupuncturists insert thin needles at key locations in the body, and may apply a herbal preparation to the points of insertion (moxibustion) or apply pressure with their fingers (acupressure).

Naturopathy

Naturopathy attempts to use natural forces to maintain health and treat disease. Typical remedies include sunbathing, diet regimens, steam bathing, exercise, and manipulation. High vegetable consumption is encouraged, as is abstinence from salt and stimulants.

Spiritual healing

Spiritual healing refers to the restoration of physical, mental, emotional, or spiritual health through prayer, meditation, and other practices. Through the ages, most religions have practiced some form of spiritual healing. Some other semispiritual groups that use spiritual healing border on the magical or occult. Be very cautious if a spiritual healer asks you to suspend your own religious values or give up large amounts of money or property to participate in a form of therapy.

Homeopathy

Homeopathy is a form of medical practice in which the practitioner administers remedies in minute quantities that cause reactions in a patient that are similar to symptoms of the illness being treated. Homeopathic theory contrasts with standard medical practice, which uses medications to counteract symptoms. An example of homeopathy is treating diarrhea with a very small dose of a laxative.

Caregiving at home

Introduction

Today, it is recognized that people who are ill or injured should be cared for in their own homes whenever possible. Besides keeping the costs of care down, caregiving at home keeps hospital beds and services more available to people who really need them. In addition, home care can be more reassuring and pleasant for the person, which can make it conducive to a speedy recovery. At some time or another, almost every family will need to provide home care for a family member who is ill. You may have to care for a person who is severely disabled and bedridden. Such a person may need full-time care and attention. More often, however, the illness will be simpler and more temporary, like episodes of "flu" and childhood infectious diseases.

Caregiver skills and priorities

Do not feel intimidated by the role of caregiver, even if you have had no previous experience caring for someone who is ill. Caregiving calls for a combination of common sense and a caring approach that virtually anyone can provide. Difficult procedures and sophisticated equipment are rarely necessary. However, when necessary, caregivers can often be trained to perform more difficult tasks effectively. Basic caregiving skills such as taking a temperature, making a bed, preventing bedsores, and knowing the best way to move an immobile person are all procedures that are easily learned. In many cases, these skills are all that is required. Many routine caregiving procedures are illustrated in this section.

Your main goal is to keep the person comfortable, optimistic, and clean. When someone is confined to bed, small problems tend to be magnified. However ill the person feels, he or she will probably feel better when you provide fresh, cool sheets. If you are caring for someone who is likely to be in bed for some time, one or two pairs of cotton sheets will make your task of laundering bed linen much easier. Special diets are seldom necessary. Your physician will tell you if there are any foods the person should eat or avoid.

If you are caring for a member of your family, do not try to do everything. If more complex care is needed than you are able to give, your physician can often arrange for professional assistance through a home health care agency or a visiting nurse association. These organizations can provide someone to perform special procedures such as giving injections or changing dressings, or simply offer you guidance and teach you procedures you can do yourself.

Long-term illness or disability

Long-term illness or disability can be a tremendous strain on the entire family. An exhausted caregiver is not likely to be efficient, so the burden of care should not fall on one person. Every member of the family can do errands, help with bed-making, and provide company. Home health agencies should be used if their help is needed. Ask your physician about such services (see Home services, p.799). Financial assistance may be available for people who are caring for someone who is ill or disabled. Equipment such as portable commodes, bedpans, urinals, and other caregiving aids can be rented from medical supply companies.

Children and older people

Children and older people can pose special caregiving problems because they are sometimes more demanding patients, both emotionally and physically. Information in this section and elsewhere in the book may help you cope with the possible difficulties involved in caring for both children and older people.

Convalescence

Convalescence, or the process of recovery, can be an even more difficult time than illness for the person who is ill and his or her caregivers. The better the person feels, the more impatient for recovery he or she is likely to become. Sometimes, however, someone who has been well cared for may be reluctant to abandon the comfort involved in receiving loving attention for his or her illness. So it is vital that you encourage the person to be active in whatever way that he or she can manage throughout the course of the illness.

Home health care

The following pages include many practical suggestions on caregiving at home. Give some thought to the day's routine and the arrangement of furniture and equipment, so that potential problems are minimized. Your physician or a visiting nurse can provide you with additional help and guidance.

Planning the person's room

If you are caring for someone who is likely to be ill for some time, plan the person's room carefully. In a two-story house, it may be better for the person to be in the living room on the first floor rather than in an upstairs bedroom, so that he or she will not feel isolated, and you will not have to make as many trips up and down the stairs.

Your main goal in arranging the room is to make things comfortable and convenient for the person who is ill and his or her caregivers. A single bed is easier to make. If possible, the bed should be accessible on both sides. This will make it easier to reach and move the person while he or she is in bed. If you can, place the bed so that the person can see out of the window. The changing views provide welcome distraction and a feeling of being connected with the outside world. Have a bedside table to hold medications, water, tissues, a whistle (so that you can be called if you are needed), and other items. If the person is allowed out of bed but cannot easily get to a bathroom, a commode (a chair with a bedpan in it) is essential. You can rent or buy one from a medical supply store. Also, local community health agencies or volunteer organizations may have such equipment available to lend to those in need.

As long as there is air circulation in the room, a person does not need fresh air, but he or she may feel more comfortable if a window is left slightly open. This is a matter of individual preference. Whether the room is ventilated or not, it should be kept free from drafts and comfortable.

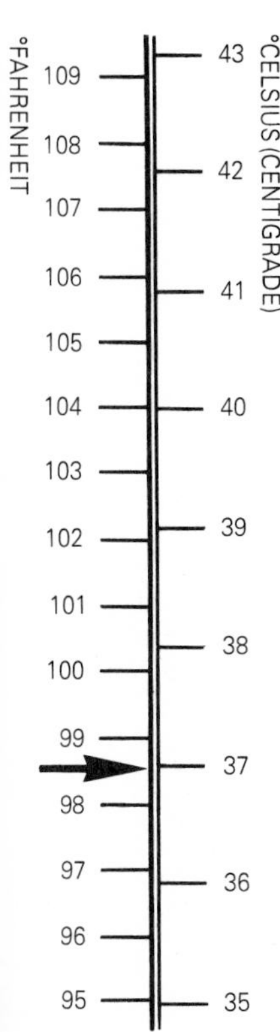

Temperature conversion scale

Taking medication

It is essential for medications to be taken exactly as prescribed by your physician. Make a point of finding out and writing down a schedule of doses per day for each drug; check off the drugs when you give them. Do not stop giving a person medication without the approval of your physician just because he or she appears to be getting better.

If a medication is prescribed four times a day, ask your physician if the doses can be taken at meal times and bedtime. Measure the dose of a liquid medication, using a special spoon if it is provided, to ensure accuracy. When you pour the medication, hold the bottle with the label facing up so that any overflow does not make it illegible. If the person finds it difficult to swallow tablets or capsules, a glass of water or a small dish of applesauce, ice cream, or frozen yogurt usually helps make swallowing easier.

Most drugs have predictable side effects, and your physician should discuss them with you. Occasionally a person experiences an unexpected allergic response to medication. Penicillin and related antibiotics are among the most common drugs to cause an allergic reaction, and the most usual reactions are a rash, hives (see p.272), itching, or wheezing. If, after taking medication, a person develops symptoms that seem unrelated to his or her illness, call your physician to find out if you should stop giving the drug (see also Drugs and older people, p.773).

Taking a temperature

Normal body temperature is about 98.6°F (37°C), but it may vary by 1° to 2°F (0.5° to 1°C) during the day. Body temperature is usually at its lowest in the early hours of the morning. A rise in temperature (a fever) is not dangerous in itself unless it exceeds 106°F (41.1°C). If the person's temperature exceeds 104°F (40°C) and he or she is uncomfortable, sponge him or her with lukewarm water, which may provide relief.

You can take a person's temperature with a thermometer in the mouth, under the arm, or in the rectum. Oral thermometers (also used under the arm) have a long, narrow bulb at the end, and rectal thermometers have a short, stubby bulb.

The thermometer: There are a variety of thermometers available today. The traditional glass tube thermometer has a mercury-filled bulb at one end and is marked with a temperature scale. Normal body temperature is marked with an arrow. As the mercury is heated in the person's mouth, armpit, or rectum, it expands and rises up the tube to a point on the scale that indicates the body temperature. A small kink in the tube prevents the mercury from sinking back into the bulb when the thermometer is removed from the mouth or armpit. Before you buy a thermometer, examine it carefully to be sure that the mercury column and the markings on the scale are easy to read.

A thermometer in the mouth gives an accurate reading of body temperature. But it may be both easier and safer to take the temperature of a young child by putting the thermometer in the armpit. In this case, add about 1°F (0.5°C) to the reading you get, to determine the equivalent temperature you would have gotten with an oral thermometer.

Another method is to use a rectal thermometer. Insert the bulb end of the thermometer just a short way into the child's rectum while gently holding the child down, if necessary, with your forearm. A rectal temperature reading will be approximately 1°F (0.5°C) higher than an oral reading.

Never leave a young child alone with a glass thermometer, since both the glass and the mercury can be harmful to the child if the thermometer is broken.

In addition to glass thermometers, there are electronic thermometers, temperature strip thermometers, and disposable thermometers. All of these types of thermometers, however, have disposable elements that increase their cost, and their reliability and accuracy have been questioned. In general, it is best to purchase a glass thermometer.

Whether you use a glass thermometer or another type, do not take a temperature immediately after the person has had a bath, a meal, a hot or cold drink, or a cigarette, since you may then get a false reading.

If a person has a fever, do not try to "sweat it out" by turning up the heat or putting on extra blankets. This may make the person's temperature rise even further. Check with your physician before giving aspirin or an aspirin substitute to help bring the temperature down. Do not give aspirin to a child or adolescent who is ill with a fever; aspirin has been linked with Reye's syndrome (see p.713), a potentially fatal condition.

While the person's temperature is falling, he or she may sweat a lot. To replace body fluids and salt lost through sweating, give the person plenty of water, soup, and fruit juice.

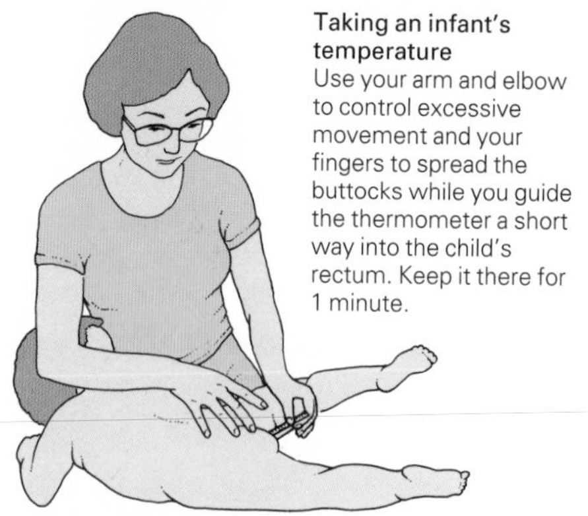

Taking an infant's temperature
Use your arm and elbow to control excessive movement and your fingers to spread the buttocks while you guide the thermometer a short way into the child's rectum. Keep it there for 1 minute.

Bed-making

Sheets for the person's bed should be made of cotton, which will absorb sweat, not of synthetic fabrics.

How to take a temperature

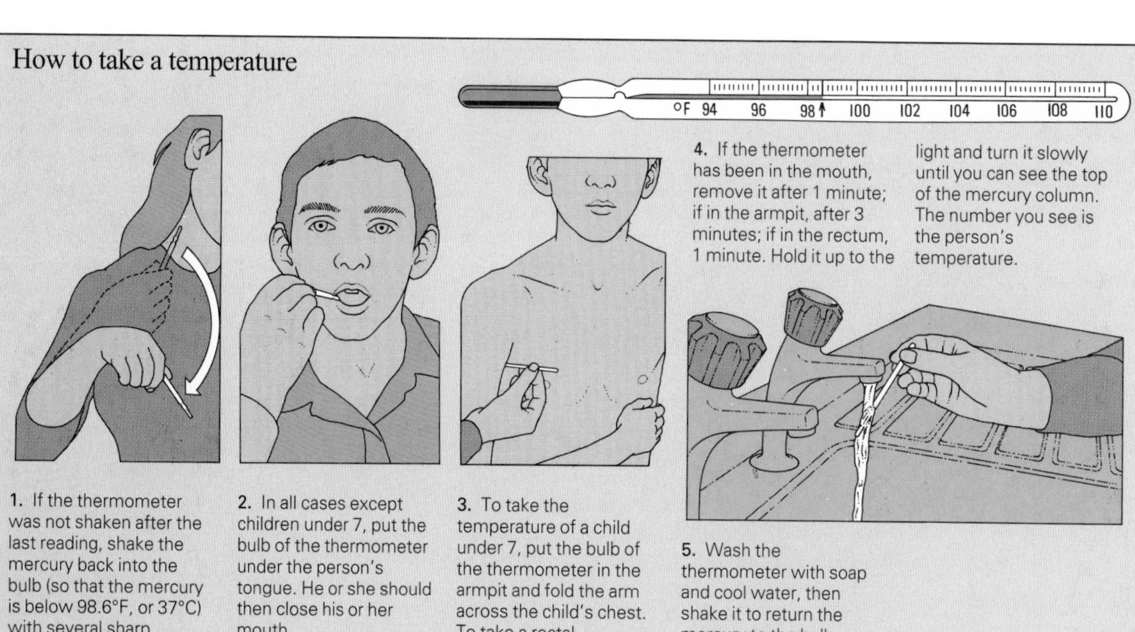

1. If the thermometer was not shaken after the last reading, shake the mercury back into the bulb (so that the mercury is below 98.6°F, or 37°C) with several sharp, downward flicks of the wrist. Wash the thermometer with soap and cool water.

2. In all cases except children under 7, put the bulb of the thermometer under the person's tongue. He or she should then close his or her mouth.

3. To take the temperature of a child under 7, put the bulb of the thermometer in the armpit and fold the arm across the child's chest. To take a rectal temperature, see above.

4. If the thermometer has been in the mouth, remove it after 1 minute; if in the armpit, after 3 minutes; if in the rectum, 1 minute. Hold it up to the light and turn it slowly until you can see the top of the mercury column. The number you see is the person's temperature.

5. Wash the thermometer with soap and cool water, then shake it to return the mercury to the bulb.

Changing a bottom sheet

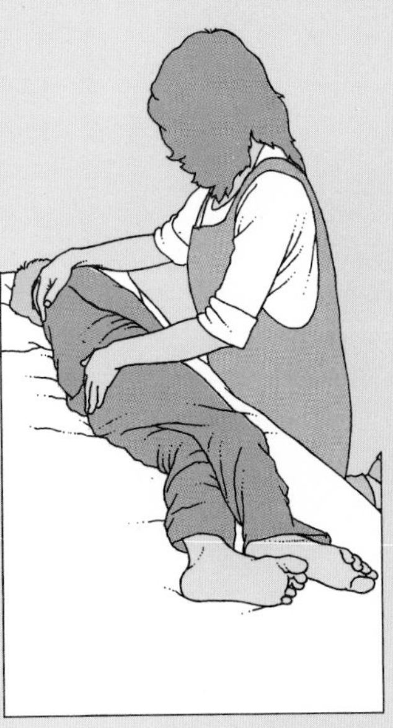

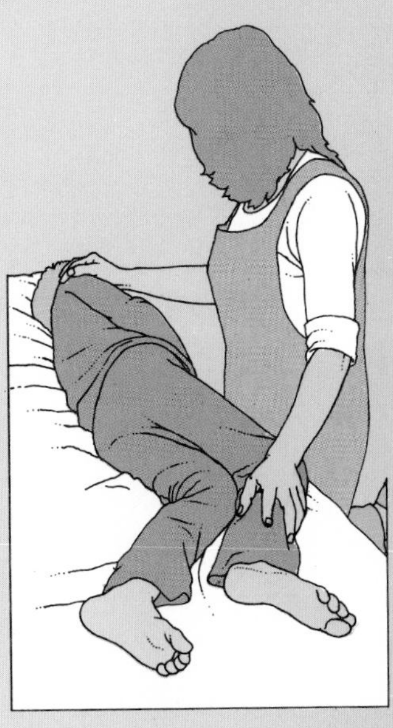

1. If the person cannot get out of bed at all, there is still an easy way of changing the bottom sheet. First, turn the person on one side.

2. Move the person to the edge of the bed, making sure that he or she is lying in a stable position.

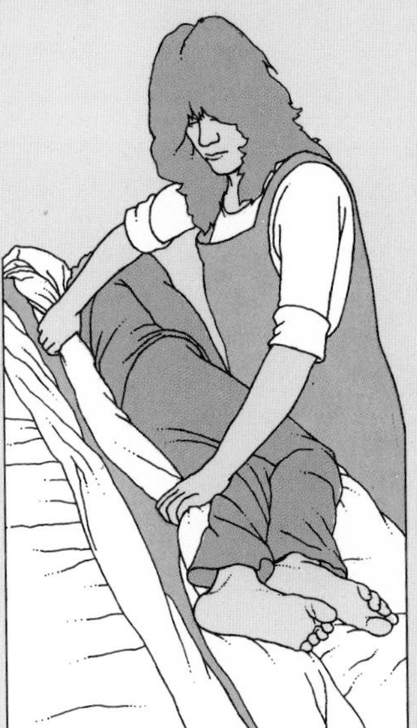

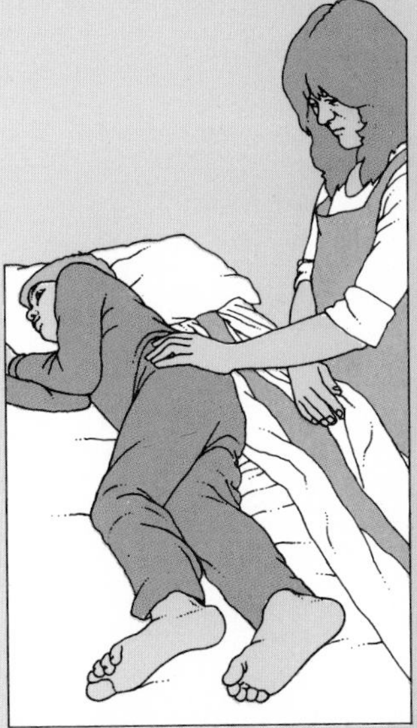

3. Roll one half of the soiled sheet lengthwise up against the person, then roll one half of the clean sheet lengthwise and put it on the bed with the rolled-up half of the sheet in the center of the bed.

4. Roll the person onto the clean half and take off the soiled sheet. Finally, unroll the rest of the clean sheet, stretch it tight, and tuck it in.

A bedridden person needs his or her bed made twice a day (morning and evening) and straightened up in between. Change the sheets every 4 to 5 days, and more often if the sheets become soiled. Always pull the bottom sheet tightly so that there are no wrinkles, and tuck it in well. Arrange the pillows so that they support the person's shoulders as well as his or her head. The most comfortable arrangement for someone who must lie on his or her back is two pillows placed side by side vertically against the headboard, with a third lying across their base. If the person prefers only one pillow, pull it well down so that the neck and shoulders as well as the head are supported and kept comfortable.

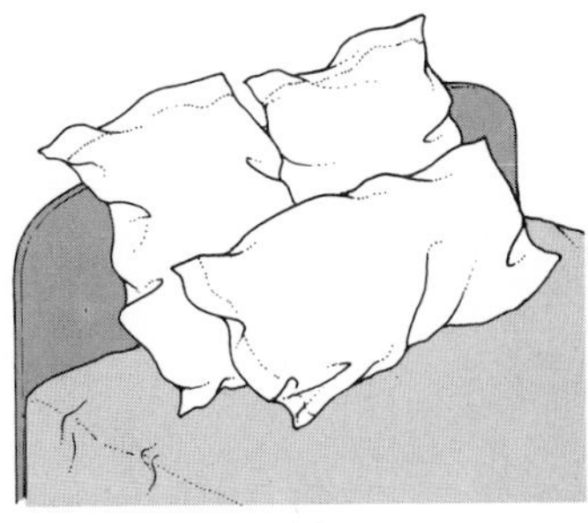

Once the person can sit up, he or she will need greater support for the back. This can be accomplished by adding more pillows or by using a lounging pillow with arms. Also, provide something to brace the feet against to prevent a shorter person from sliding down toward the foot of the bed.

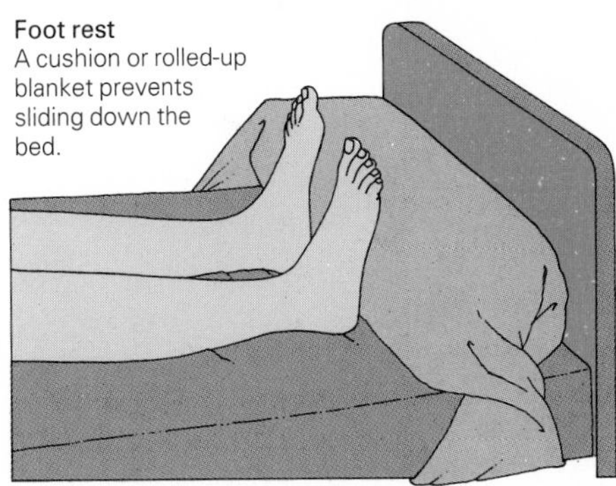

Foot rest
A cushion or rolled-up blanket prevents sliding down the bed.

If the person cannot get out of bed at all, you can still change the bottom sheet. First, turn the person on one side and roll one half of the soiled sheet lengthwise up against his or her back. Then roll one half of the clean sheet lengthwise and put it on the bed with the rolled half in the center. Roll the person onto the clean half, and remove the soiled sheet. Finally, unroll the rest of the clean sheet, stretch it tight, and tuck it in.

Drawsheets

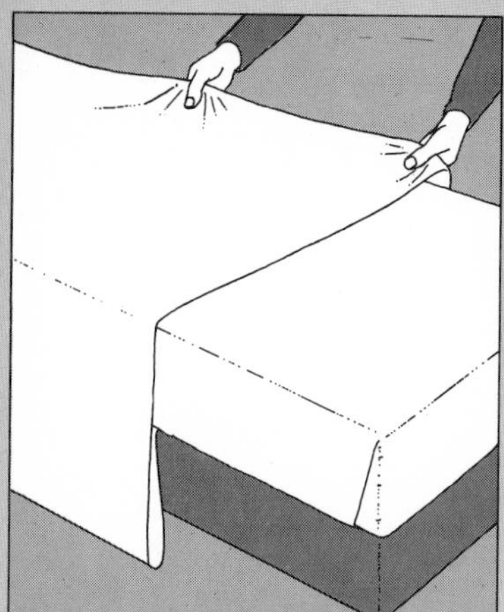

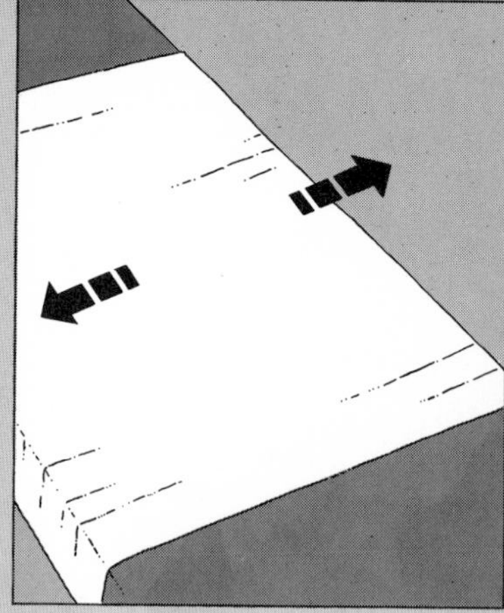

A drawsheet is an ordinary sheet folded and positioned so that it can provide a clean, unwrinkled sheet to lie on without having to remake the bed. Fold the sheet in half lengthwise and put it over the bed crosswise, so that it extends from the person's head to his or her knees, and overlaps the bed more on one side than the other. Tuck one end in, pull the sheet tight, and tuck in the other end. When you want to provide a clean surface, untuck both ends of the sheet, pull a clean area into position, and tuck in both ends tightly again. For the person's comfort, make sure the drawsheet is kept tight.

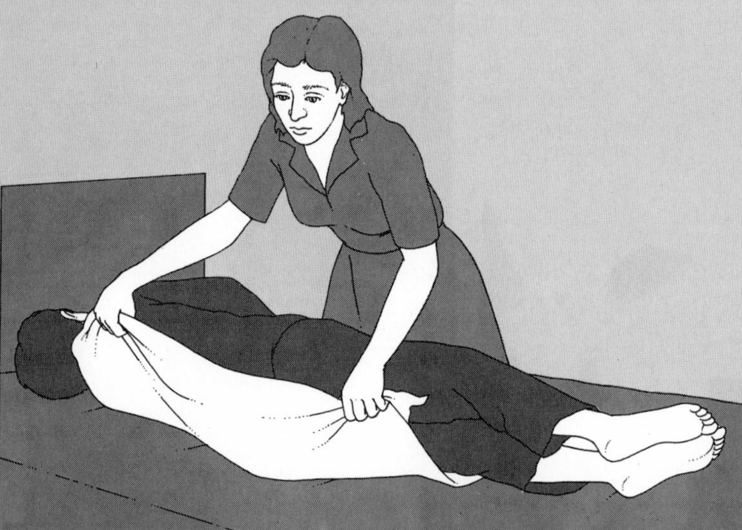

A drawsheet can also be used as an aid in moving an immobile or very weak person. If you want to move the person sideways, first untuck the end of the drawsheet opposite to the side of the bed to which you want the person to move. Then cross to that side of the bed, lean across the bed, and hold onto the untucked end of the drawsheet. Use that end to roll the person toward you. To move the person up the bed, you need another person's help. Both ends of the drawsheet are untucked, each of you holds one end, and the person is lifted on the drawsheet to the desired position.

Hospital corners

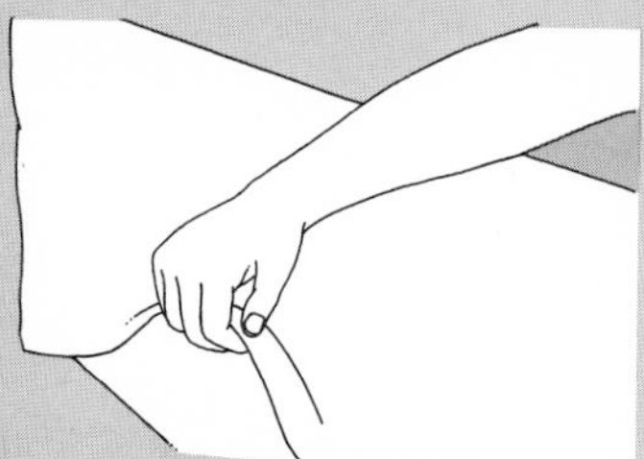

1. Hospital ("mitered") corners make a neat and comfortable finish to the bed. After you have put on the bottom sheet, place the top sheet in position and tuck it in at the end. With one hand, lift the side of the sheet about 16 in (40 cm) from the foot of the bed.

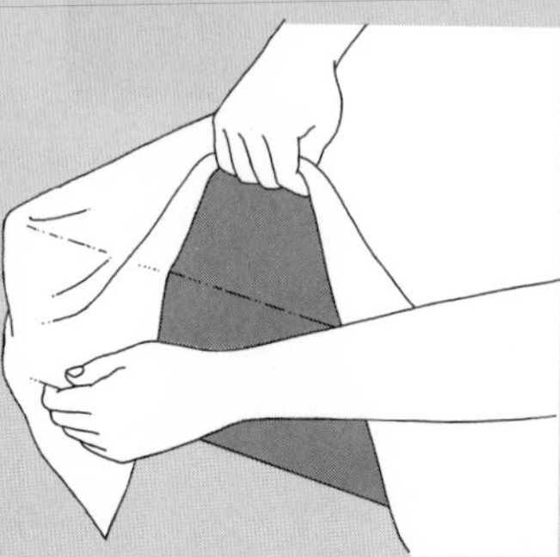

2. Tuck the flap of sheet that hangs between the side of the bed and your hand under the mattress with your other hand. Then let the side of the sheet fall to form a fold at the side of the bed.

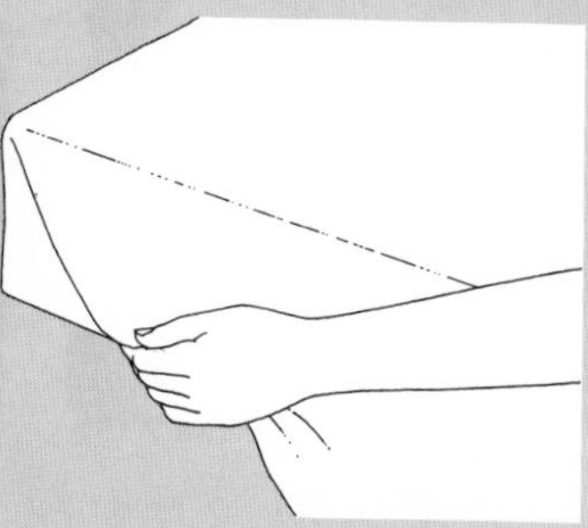

3. Tuck the fold smoothly beneath the mattress. Repeat on the other side of the bed. Once you learn how to make corners, you can make them for sheets and blankets too.

Giving food, drink, and special diets

Mealtime is a sociable activity and is often a highlight of the day for a person who is confined to bed. Unless your physician recommends a special diet, you can safely give the person a normal, balanced diet. Many snack foods such as potato chips and peanuts are high in sodium and fat, so check to be sure the person is not on a low-sodium or calorie-restricted diet before offering these foods. The person will probably most enjoy small helpings of simple foods that are easy to eat until his or her appetite returns. Make sure the person gets plenty of liquids.

If your physician has prescribed a special diet, and if you will have to provide it for a long time, you may want to get a special cookbook on the subject. Your physician may recommend a good one, or may refer you to a nurse or dietitian who is knowledgeable about that type of diet.

Low-sodium diet: Your physician may recommend a low-sodium diet for someone who has heart disease (see p.399), liver disease (see Liver, gallbladder, and pancreas, p.522), kidney disease (see Disorders of the urinary tract, p.539), or high blood pressure (see p.411). In the US almost everyone eats more salt than the body requires. Sodium usually can be reduced substantially simply by adding no extra salt at the table, and by making certain that no salt is added to food during preparation. Also, avoid foods with high sodium content such as cured or tenderized meat, smoked fish, cheese, canned food other than fruit, food made with baking powder, and butter or margarine. Another possible source of extra salt in the diet is a water softener on the cold water line. This can be eliminated, if necessary, or bottled water can be used for cooking and drinking.

If your physician considers it necessary to restrict the salt intake even further, he or she will advise you on how to cut down on food items that contain even moderate amounts of sodium. The flavor that a salt-free diet lacks can be provided by using a salt substitute, other spices, or lemon juice. Also, after several weeks on a low-sodium diet, many people find they do not miss the salt flavor. If the person has kidney disease, check with your physician to see if you should choose a salt substitute that is also free of potassium.

Low-protein diets: A low-protein diet may be recommended for some kidney disorders. Such a diet will involve reducing the intake of meat, fish, eggs, dairy products, and other protein-rich foods. Because protein provides a part of the body's energy needs, extra sugar and fat are needed to make up for this loss.

Spoon-feeding: A person who is aging or very ill may need to be spoon-fed. If this is the case, feed the person with foods that are well cut, minced, or pureed, since these are the easiest to serve and to swallow. Make sure the person is in a comfortable position before you start, and tuck a napkin under his or her chin. Taste the food yourself to be sure it is not too hot. Spoon-feeding often takes a long time, and you may find that the food stays hot longer if you use a special dish with a hollow base that you fill with hot water, or a similar type of dish that is warmed electrically. When giving fluids, always elevate the person's head slightly to prevent choking. It's easiest for the person to drink from a cup through a flexible straw.

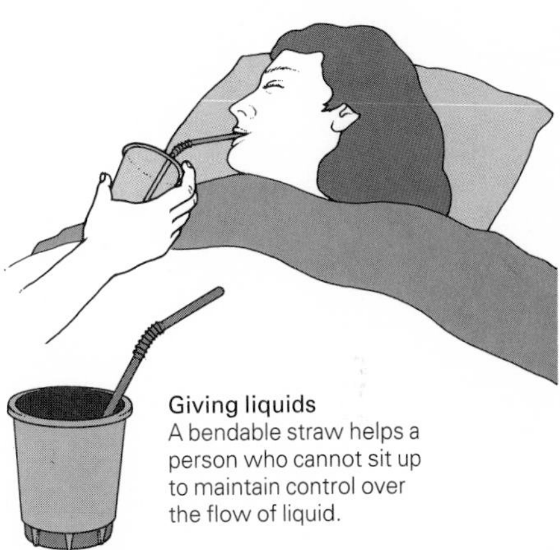

Giving liquids
A bendable straw helps a person who cannot sit up to maintain control over the flow of liquid.

Someone who is seriously ill may be able to take only liquid foods. Your physician may advise you to consult a dietitian to make sure that the diet will provide adequate nutrition. There are many commercial liquid products that contain nutritional supplements. Your physician can also suggest some alternatives if you are having problems with feeding. Check with your physician also if the person appears to be losing any weight.

If a stroke has paralyzed one side of a person's body, food may tend to collect in the paralyzed cheek. If the food accumulates in the person's mouth, knead the cheek with your finger to help move the food along.

Managing a bedpan

A toilet or commode (a chair with a bedpan in it) is the easiest way for people who are ill to eliminate because it allows for a sitting position. But if a person is too ill or disabled to get out of bed, a bedpan, and for a male a bed urinal, will be needed. Most people who are not used to a bedpan find it inconvenient and inhibiting, especially if someone else is present, so make sure that the person has complete privacy, and give him or her enough time to let the bowel and bladder relax. Keeping the person's sensitivity in mind is part of good care. Such thoughtfulness often can contribute to a more rapid recovery and helps avoid fecal impaction.

Before you give a bedpan, warm it in hot water, dry it well, and sprinkle the rim with talcum powder to make it easier for the pan to be slipped under the buttocks. If the person cannot lift himself or herself up in the bed, help the person use the pan lying down. Lift the person's hips while another person maneuvers the pan beneath the buttocks, with the open end toward the feet. The easiest way to give a bedpan to a totally immobile person is to turn the person on his or her side, put the pan against the buttocks, press the pan down into the bed as much as possible, and roll the person back on top of it. When the pan has been used, hold it firmly and roll the person off, away from you.

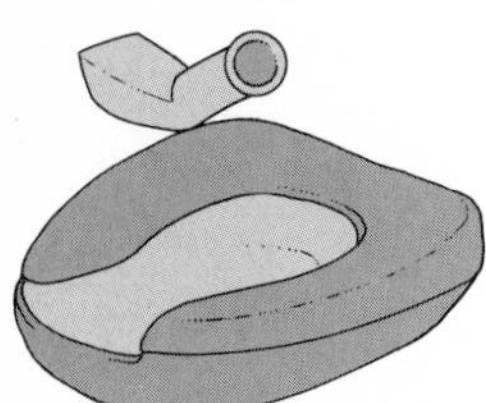

Bedpan and urinal
These items are essential for anyone who is likely to be confined to bed for a long time.

After use, bedpans and urinals should be washed thoroughly in a disinfectant diluted with water. Always put them back in the same place so that they can be found in a hurry. A urinal should be left within easy reach of the bed so that the person has no need to call for it. Keep it in a plastic bowl or bucket to lessen the possibility of spills.

Preventing bedsores
Anyone who is confined to bed for a long time risks developing bedsores, especially if movement is restricted or if sensation is impaired. Bedsores occur on those parts of the body that bear the weight of the body or rub constantly against the bedclothes. The most common sites are the elbows, knees, shoulder blades, spine, and buttocks.

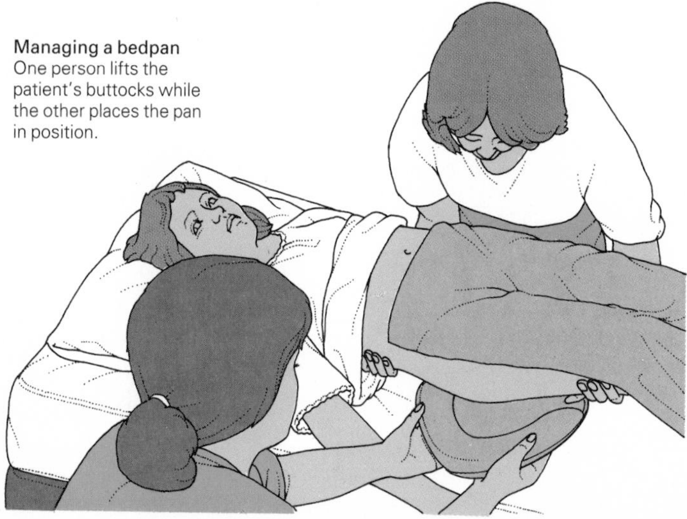

Managing a bedpan
One person lifts the patient's buttocks while the other places the pan in position.

A bedsore begins as a patch of tender, reddened, inflamed skin. Later, the skin can become purple. Then it breaks down and an ulcer or sore develops. If any skin redness or inflammation occurs, consult your physician immediately. The ulcers generally take a long time to heal, are painful, and are harmful to the person's health.

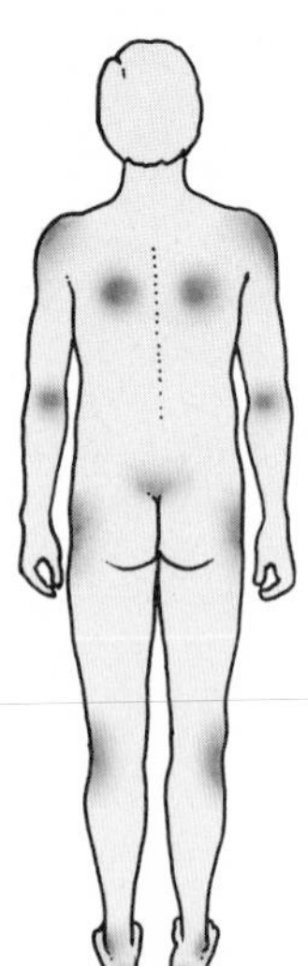

Common sites for bedsores include the shoulders, elbows, lower back, hips, buttocks, knees, ankles, and heels.

Bedsores can and must be prevented. Unless immobile, someone confined to bed can still exercise. Every hour or so, a period of wriggling the toes, rotating the ankles, flexing the arms and legs, tightening and relaxing muscles, and stretching the whole body will both stimulate circulation and prevent joint contracture, or stiffening. If the person cannot move or is very weak, the caregiver can offer passive exercise by gently bending and straightening the person's joints manually several times a day. Also, change his or her position as often as you can—at least every 2 to 3 hours, but more often if possible—so that the pressure of the body on any particular area is relieved. This is most easily accomplished, especially if the person is a great deal heavier than you, by using a drawsheet (see p.790) or by rolling the person from side to side. Otherwise, lift the person into a new position (with help from someone else, if necessary). Dragging the person may damage his or her skin and increase the chance of bedsores.

Many people use a so-called egg carton foam mattress cover, which allows air to circulate around the person's skin. Also, use a bed- or foot-cradle (frames that raise the covers) to keep the weight of the bedclothes off the person's legs and feet. You can rent one from a medical supply company, or you can improvise by using a stool or a wooden box with two opposite sides cut out. If the person is lying permanently on his or her side, support the upper arms and thighs with soft pillows to keep the elbows and knees apart, and put a pillow between the ankles to keep them from rubbing together. However, you will still need to turn the person frequently to prevent bedsores.

Relieving pressure
Use plenty of soft pillows or cushions to relieve pressure that leads to bedsores.

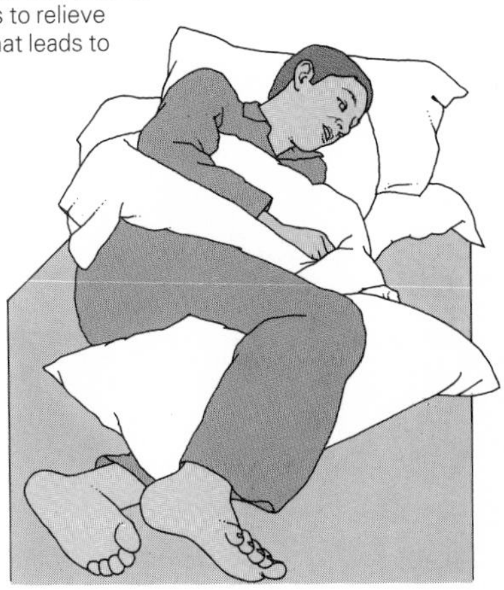

If the person will be bedridden for a long time, you may want to get a fluffy sheepskin (preferably a synthetic, washable one) for the person to lie on, to decrease friction from sheets and to help cushion the body. Special air mattresses are also available. Sheepskin booties protect the heels and ankles.

Make sure that the sheets are always clean, dry, crumb-free, and pulled as tightly as possible to prevent wrinkling. Also, wash the person frequently and keep his or her skin particularly clean and dry on places that are vulnerable to bedsores. Check every day for reddening; if you see any, keep pressure off the area and let your physician know that a bedsore is beginning to form.

In addition to adequate turning, movement, exercise, and cleanliness, a balanced diet can help prevent bedsores.

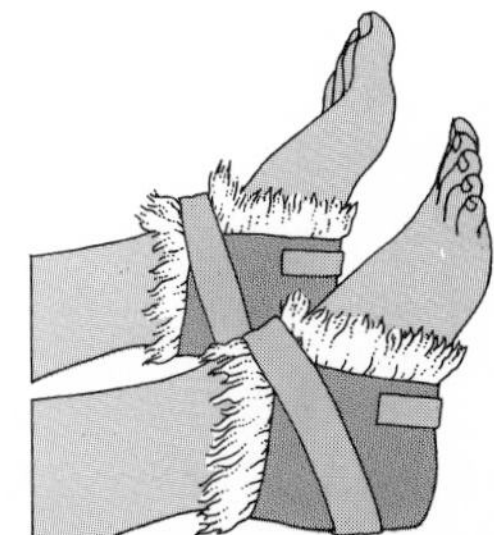

Sheepskin booties
These help protect the skin of the heels and ankles from bedsores.

Moving an immobile person

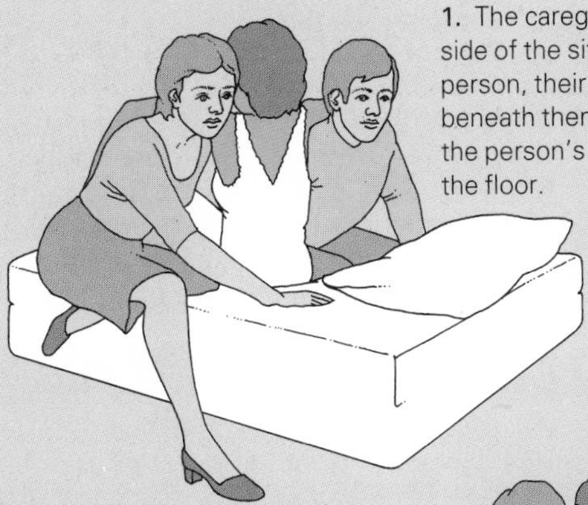

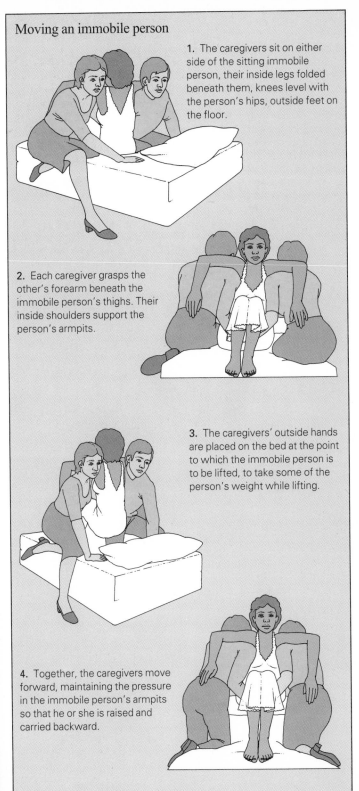

1. The caregivers sit on either side of the sitting immobile person, their inside legs folded beneath them, knees level with the person's hips, outside feet on the floor.

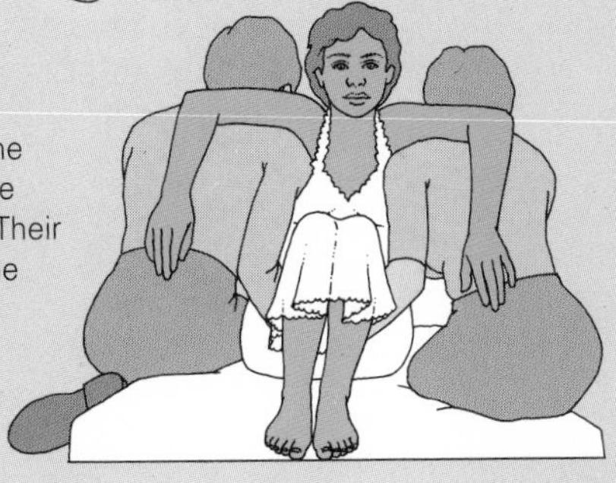

2. Each caregiver grasps the other's forearm beneath the immobile person's thighs. Their inside shoulders support the person's armpits.

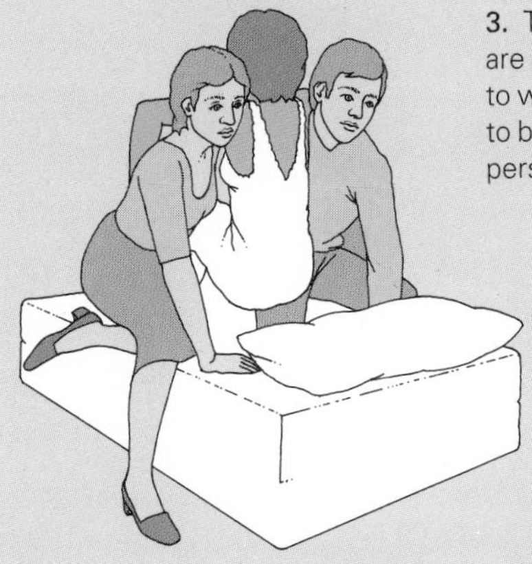

3. The caregivers' outside hands are placed on the bed at the point to which the immobile person is to be lifted, to take some of the person's weight while lifting.

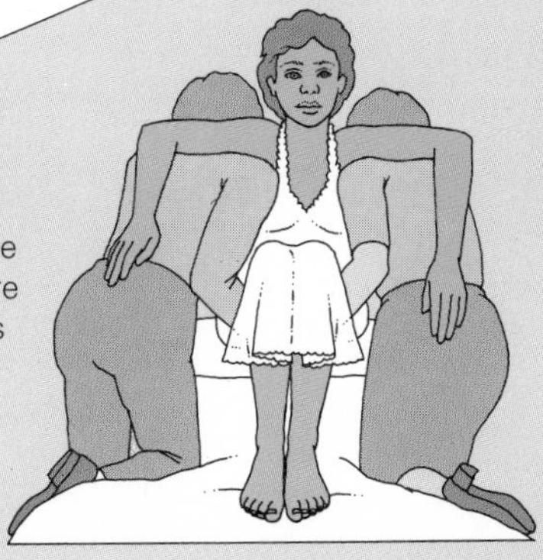

4. Together, the caregivers move forward, maintaining the pressure in the immobile person's armpits so that he or she is raised and carried backward.

Dealing with vomiting

Most people prefer to be left alone while they are vomiting, but others find it comforting to have you hold their forehead for support. After comforting someone in this way, offer him or her some water to rinse out the mouth and then gently sponge his or her face with cool or lukewarm water.

After an episode of vomiting, do not give the person solid food for several hours, but once the nausea subsides do give sips of water, tea, broth, or fruit drinks to replace the lost body fluids. If the person continues to vomit repeatedly, call your physician for any additional treatment. Your physician may recommend that you observe the person for signs of dehydration after vomiting; these include dry lips, loss of skin elasticity, and reduced output of urine. When the nausea subsides, let the person's own inclinations determine the amount and type of liquid he or she drinks. Soft foods (custards, puddings, oatmeal, gelatin dessert) may then be easier to eat than regular food.

Coping with incontinence

Some loss of bladder control is common in older people or in those who are paralyzed below the waist. For a full description of the problem and how to cope with it, see Incontinence in older people, p.766.

Relieving congestion

While a stuffy nose can be relieved by giving a nasal spray, overuse of these medications can lead to more nasal congestion. Consult your physician if the nasal spray does not seem to be working. Your physician may recommend that you make sure that the humidity is appropriate in the person's room.

Giving a bath in bed

If the person is unable to give himself or herself a bath, you can give one. Be sure that the room is warm before you remove the person's pajamas. Cover his or her body with a large towel and place another one beneath the body to protect the bedclothes. If the person is immobile or heavy, you can get the second towel into position in the same way that you change the bottom sheet (see p.789).

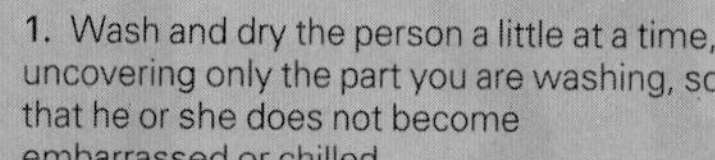

1. Wash and dry the person a little at a time, uncovering only the part you are washing, so that he or she does not become embarrassed or chilled.

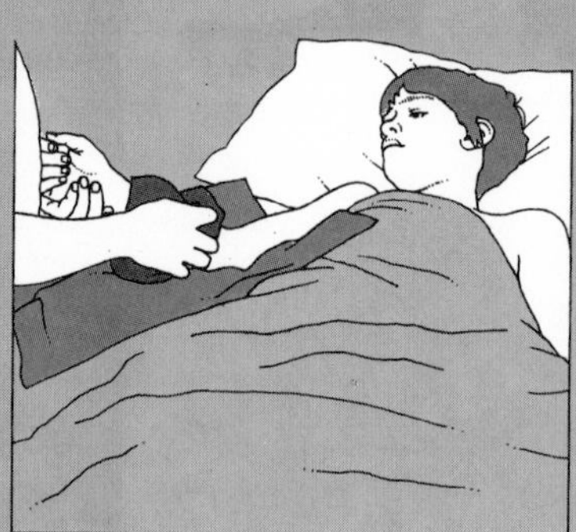

2. Soap is needed only for sweaty areas such as the armpits, groin, and buttocks.

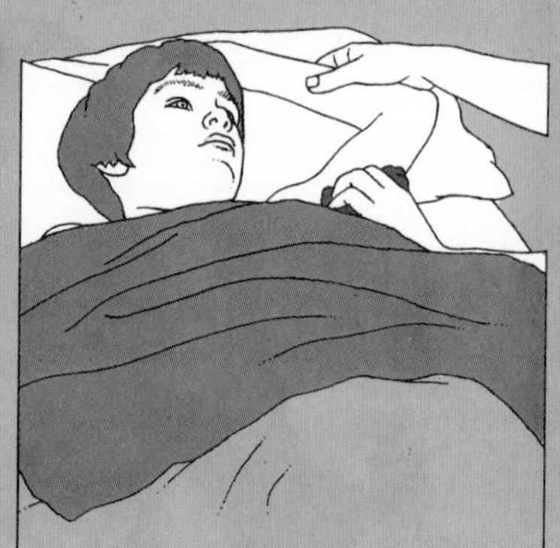

3. Pat the person dry gently—do not rub. Work from head to feet.

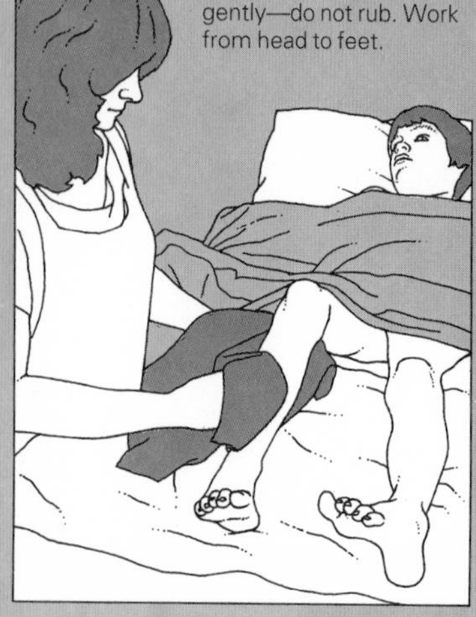

4. Roll the person onto one side so you can wash and dry his or her back (for how to move an immobile or heavy person, see p.793).

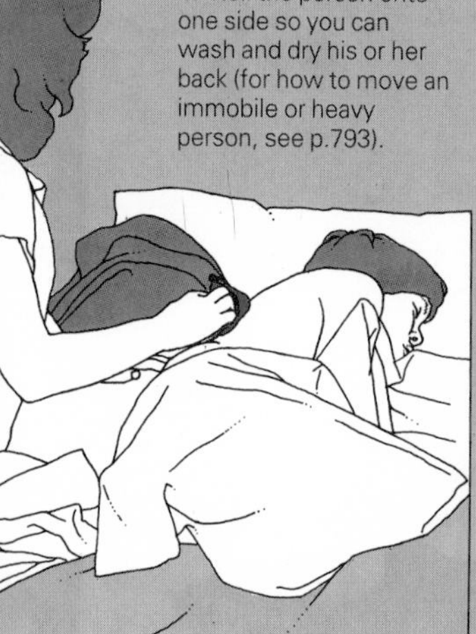

5. Help the person dip his or her own hands in the bowl of water you are using. He or she will find this much more refreshing than simply having the hands wiped with a sponge or cloth.

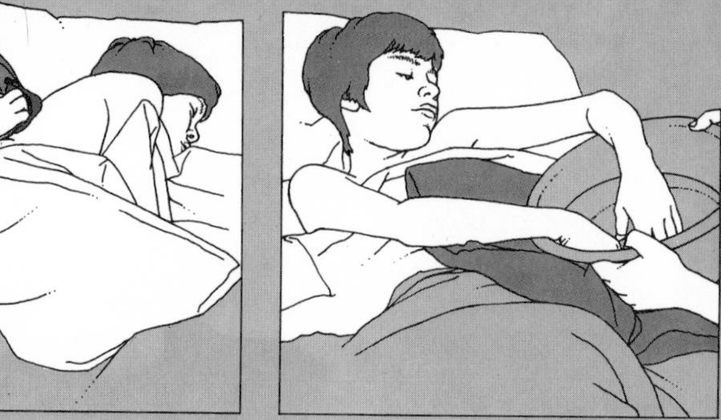

Bathing a person who is ill

Whether ill or well, everyone should be encouraged to keep clean. The face and hands should be washed and the teeth brushed twice a day, and the body should be washed once a day. This is not only a matter of hygiene. Feeling clean and fresh boosts the person's morale and may play a part in speeding recovery. Even bedridden people, unless they are extremely ill, can usually manage to keep themselves clean. Before giving a bedridden person a basin of water and toiletries, place a large towel beneath him or her to protect the bedclothes. If the person is going to have a sponge bath, make sure the room is warm, and provide a second large towel to be draped over the parts of the body that are not being washed, so that the person does not become embarrassed or chilled.

Washing hair

Having clean hair will also boost a person's morale. If the person cannot get up, it is possible to wash his or her hair in bed.

First, protect the bottom sheet by placing a plastic cover underneath a towel. Move the person down the bed, raise his or her shoulders on a pillow, and place a bowl or a dishpan under the head. To wet the person's hair before shampooing and to rinse it, pour several cups of water over it. If the person has long hair, it may be easier to wash if the person rests his or her head on the edge of the bed so that the hair hangs over a bowl or dishpan placed on the floor. Place one end of a large tray under the person's head and the other end in the bowl or dishpan. Wet and rinse the hair as for short hair. The water will run down the tray into the bowl or dishpan.

After washing the person's hair, rub it thoroughly with a warm towel and finish drying it with a blow-dryer.

Washing hair
Wet and rinse the hair over a bowl or dishpan placed near the bed.

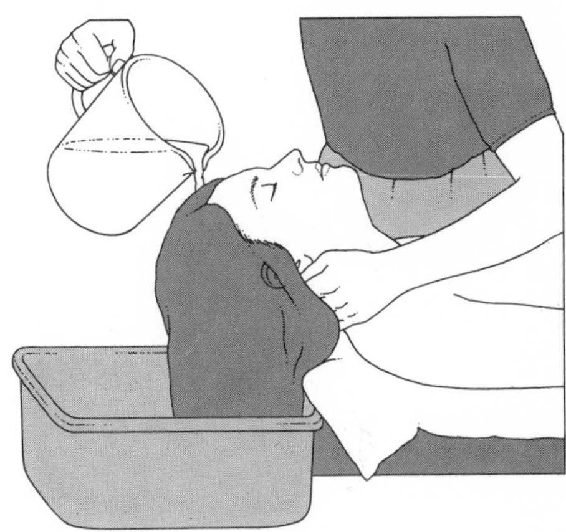

Caring for children who are ill

In general, children do not become as seriously ill as adults and older people. However, when they are ill they require almost constant attention to prevent boredom. You should make sure that you are prepared for this or you may find yourself resenting the time and effort involved in caring for your child. A child who is ill needs at least one caregiver, preferably one of his or her parents, on hand almost constantly in order to raise morale and promote a speedy recovery. For specific information on various childhood illnesses, read the section entitled Children's health (see p.690).

Should you keep your child in bed?

Unless your physician has told you to keep your child in bed, your child can decide whether he or she feels well enough to get up.

A child who is ill but close to recovery will make the most demands on your time. In these circumstances, it may be helpful to make up a bed in the living room or on the first floor (in a two-story house), so that you do not have to keep climbing the stairs and so that your child has your household activities as a distraction. You also may want to put a television near your child's bed.

Medications and children

It is important that a child who is ill takes all the medication prescribed by your physician. Because small children often cannot swallow pills easily, their medications are usually prescribed in liquid form. Be sure to measure out the exact dose as prescribed. It can be difficult to get a child to take an unpleasant-tasting medication. It may help if you sit your child on your knee and give him or her a pleasant drink to hold, ready to be swallowed after the medication. Also, because most of the taste buds lie at the front of the tongue, tip the medication into your child's mouth as far back as you can. Show by your manner that you assume he or she will take the medication. If your child senses that you expect trouble, he or she may provide it for you. Sometimes encouragement helps in the form of a favorite treat, promised as soon as your child actually has taken the medication.

If your child refuses to take the medication, try mixing it with a spoonful of something he

Entertaining a child who is ill

Adults usually like to be left alone when they are ill, but children, unless they are very ill, usually want company or entertainment. The younger the child, the greater the demands on your time, because the child will be more dependent on you for amusement.

Generally a child will not feel like concentrating on one thing for very long, and will not want to do anything intellectually demanding. He or she will probably want to play with familiar toys and games or read a favorite book rather than learn something new. Children tend to regress a little when they are ill and may prefer toys and activities meant for slightly younger children.

or she likes, such as applesauce or pudding. If your child refuses, ask your physician if the medication can be given in tablet or capsule form. A child of 3 or older may be able to swallow a tablet or capsule whole with the help of a drink. If the child cannot do this, you may be able to get him or her to take a tablet by crushing it (this cannot be done with a capsule) and again mixing it with a food the child likes, in a spoon. With luck, the spoonful will slip down and the child will not even taste the medication.

Dealing with a fever

A fever is not always dangerous and rarely has any harmful effects. In a few susceptible children, however, a high temperature may cause febrile seizures (see p.713).

Unless a child's temperature is higher than 102°F (38.9°C), all you need to do is make sure that he or she drinks plenty of liquids and keep him or her lightly clothed or covered. Forget anything you may have heard about sweating out a fever by covering the child with lots of heavy blankets.

Above 102°F, you can, if your child seems miserable or uncomfortable, give him or her a child's acetaminophen, but check with your physician first. When it is time for another dose, first take your child's temperature again. If it has started to fall, do not give the medication. If your child is asleep, do not wake him or her; sleep will do your child good. Do not give aspirin to children or adolescents who are ill with a fever because Reye's syndrome, a potentially fatal condition, has been linked with this drug.

If your child's temperature continues to rise in spite of the medication, and reaches 104°F (40°C) or higher, call your physician. In the meantime, relieve the discomfort of the fever by sponging his or her face, neck, arms, and legs with water and leaving them to dry naturally. Evaporation cools the skin.

If your child has had a previous febrile seizure make sure your physician knows this. Your physician may recommend that you try to lower your child's temperature at an early stage by giving medications at the first sign of a fever and sponging the child as soon as he or she feels hot.

Feeding a child who is ill

Unless your physician has recommended a special diet, let the child eat what he or she wants, within reason, rather than offering what you think is good. Provide smaller helpings than usual, and do not worry if the child does not eat much. In cases of fever or diarrhea, it is important to give the child plenty of liquids to drink. The same is true for vomiting, once the nausea subsides. The amount of liquid the child drinks is what matters, not the content.

Dealing with vomiting

Children vomit much more easily than most adults. Often they vomit without warning, at the beginning of an illness. Support your child's head with one hand pressed against his or her forehead and, with your other hand, hold a bowl in which to catch the vomit. If your child can hold the bowl, put your other hand firmly on his or her stomach to support it. Afterward, give your child a glass of water to rinse out his or her mouth and a bowl to spit in, and then wash your child's face.

Caring for a convalescent

After a long illness, it takes time for a person to recover and return to routine activities. During this convalescent period, all activities, including physical and mental exercise as well as work, must be resumed gradually. This gradual return to everyday life is essential to genuine recovery.

General care

People who are convalescing from an illness often become bored and frustrated by their enforced inactivity, especially if they were very active before their illness. Radio, television, newspapers, books, puzzles, and the company of other people will help to occupy such a person's mind and lessen the frustration the person feels. If work can be done at home, it may be helpful for him or her to ease back into this activity.

However, there is another side to this. The person may feel that he or she is more fully recovered than is actually the case, and may consequently take on too much too soon. This may overtax his or her strength. The person may become depressed and have a setback in his or her convalescence. It is important to try to prevent this. Ask your physician what the individual can reasonably do, and if the person shows any signs of going beyond this limit, gently but firmly persuade him or her to stop. Your physician will also tell you if the person needs a special diet and, if necessary, can suggest sources of help for you in caring for the person.

The risks of inactivity

It is possible for people (especially older people) who are convalescing from an illness to become unnecessarily immobile. With this kind of inactivity comes a rapid physical deterioration. Unused muscles become weak, joints stiffen, and constipation, bedsores, and weak bladder and bowel control may develop. The inactive older person is also more prone to thrombosis (see p.445) or embolism (see p.446) and is more likely to develop severe respiratory infections such as pneumonia (see p.384). Mental confusion also seems to occur more easily when an older person is confined to bed. Therefore, encourage the convalescing older person to get up as soon as possible and to stay active, within the limits recommended by your physician.

Getting out of bed

Anyone who has been ill and bedridden for a long time will feel weak and probably dizzy when getting out of bed for the first time. Have the person first sit on the edge of the bed for a few minutes before attempting to stand. Put a chair covered with a blanket beside the bed. When the person feels steady, stand in front of him or her so that the person can use your body as a support while standing up, and provide extra support by holding the person under the arms. Then help to lower the person onto the chair and wrap the blanket around him or her if necessary. Once he or she feels stronger, a few steps can be tried, using your arms for support.

Professional services

Anyone who recently has had a long illness or a lengthy stay in the hospital may benefit from the extended services of home nursing, physical therapy, occupational therapy, or a visiting social worker. Nursing services are only necessary when specific medical activities need to be performed, such as managing catheters. Physical therapy is appropriate when a convalescing individual continues to show progress in regaining muscle strength, flexibility, and mobility following a stroke, orthopedic surgery, or injury. Occupational therapists are sometimes called on to suggest ways of accomplishing a daily task or making adaptations in the home environment that will help conserve the person's energy.

A social worker can be helpful in exploring possible sources of financial aid for getting equipment and home modifications for a homebound or disabled person. A speech therapist can help a person who has had a stroke or another type of brain injury to learn how to swallow without choking, relearn how to speak, or learn to communicate in other ways. Your physician can help arrange for these allied health professionals to work with you, in order to restore the person to as much independence as is possible.

Caring for older people

The increasing likelihood of illness in old age means that older people tend to spend more and more time at home, perhaps in bed. Many families with aging relatives can obtain practical advice and assistance from local community health agencies. Ask your own physician about health services that may be available in your community (see also Home services, p.799). For details on some of the specific illnesses that affect older people, see Older people's health, p.765.

Food

The appetite of an older person who is ill will probably be small. It is therefore important that the food that is served be nutritious. Each day give at least one meal that includes high-protein foods such as meat, cheese, fish, or eggs, about half a pint of milk, and some high-fiber foods such as fruit, vegetables, or bran cereal. Unless there is a medical reason not to, encourage the person to drink plenty of liquids to avoid dehydration.

Modifying the home environment

With more people over age 80, and more people with Alzheimer's disease and other kinds of senile dementia (see p.774), families may need to modify their home or that of an older friend or relative living alone nearby.

First, make changes to help prevent falls (see p.769). To prevent fires, make sure that electrical cords are not frayed and sockets are not overloaded. Also, a large sign in the kitchen with a reminder to turn off the stove is often helpful.

For someone who has memory problems or is disoriented, consider a wrist bracelet with the person's name, address, and telephone number so that someone can help him or her get home again if he or she wanders away. Designate a special place to keep items that are frequently misplaced, including keys, pill bottles, and eyeglasses.

A large calendar with large numbers can be used to keep track of days of the week, and the older person can check off each day as a means of orientation. If the older person is living in a home with many doors on a hallway, and this seems confusing, you can paint his or her door a special color—or perhaps the bathroom door, if that becomes hard to locate at night. It's also important to provide a night-light in the bathroom and any hall the person might use at night.

An electronic monitoring system can summon help in an emergency via a telephone connection. These systems are voice-activated so that the older person can call for emergency assistance even if he or she has become immobilized.

To keep your aging family member comfortable at home, make sure that he or she takes all necessary medications on schedule. A large pillbox divided by day of the week can help the person keep track of when to take which medications. Adequate nutrition is also vital; many seniors living alone subsist on "junk food" to the detriment of their general health. Family members should also monitor personal hygiene, making sure that the older person takes a bath regularly; also, check on bladder and bowel control and provide adult-type diapers if necessary. You may need to visit someone with dementia who lives alone each day to help him or her with meals, baths, and medications. (Or you may be able to hire a home health aide to visit and care for the person each day.)

Your local chapter of the Alzheimer's Association can offer additional suggestions about the long-term care of a person with dementia. It is vital for the health of both caregiver and patient that caregivers with major responsibilities for an older person find ways to take a break from their duties.

Preventing arms and legs from stiffening

A period of bed rest is often necessary after a major illness or operation. Although most people prefer to stay in a position they find comfortable, they should be encouraged to move around in bed as much as possible to prevent the joint stiffness and loss of muscle tone that may follow prolonged inactivity. You can help to prevent joint stiffness, first by carefully placing and supporting the person's arms and legs in the most comfortable, natural, and strain-free positions and resting them on pillows, cushions, or foam-rubber rolls. Encourage the person to exercise each joint through its whole range of motion several times each day. If he or she is immobile, you can help him or her do this. Gently bend and straighten each elbow and wrist, and the fingers and thumb of each hand. Raise each leg in turn, bending and straightening the hip, knee, and ankle.

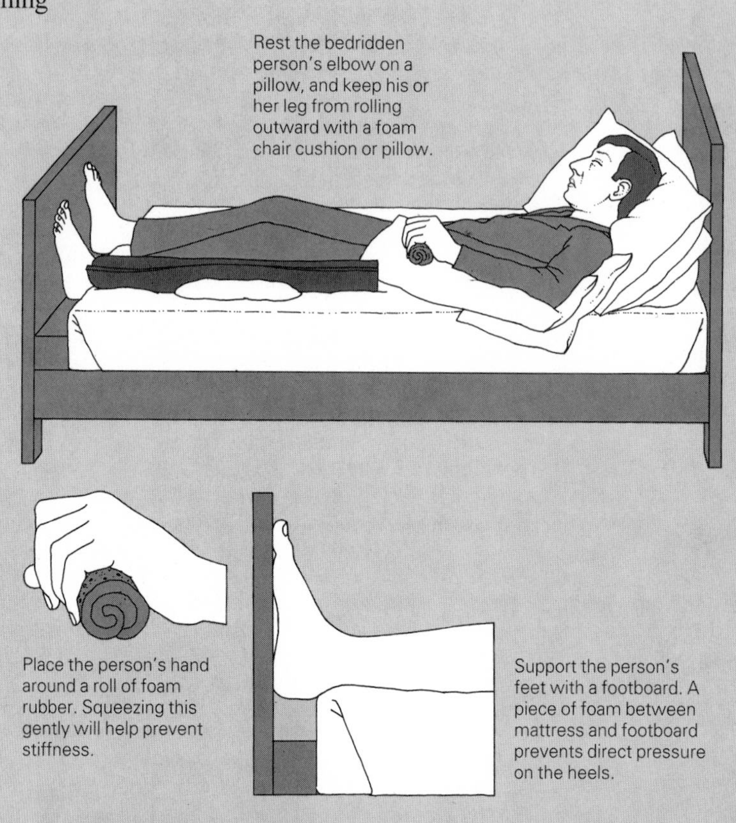

Rest the bedridden person's elbow on a pillow, and keep his or her leg from rolling outward with a foam chair cushion or pillow.
Place the person's hand around a roll of foam rubber. Squeezing this gently will help prevent stiffness.
Support the person's feet with a footboard. A piece of foam between mattress and footboard prevents direct pressure on the heels.

Home services

The following services help provide care at home for people who are ill or disabled:

Home health services are medical services that are provided in a person's home under a physician's direction. A visiting nurse association or a county or city health department, for example, may provide a variety of types of physician-directed care. These might include home visits by nurses to give injections, give medications, and teach family members how to give such care.

In many areas, one or more home health agencies may provide physical therapy, occupational therapy, speech therapy, general health assessment, social work services, counseling, and nutrition programs. If an agency has home health aides or homemakers on staff, a person can receive help with personal and household tasks. Charges for these services may or may not be paid by Medicare, Medicaid, or private insurance companies. Check with your physician's office or insurer to make sure you are eligible.

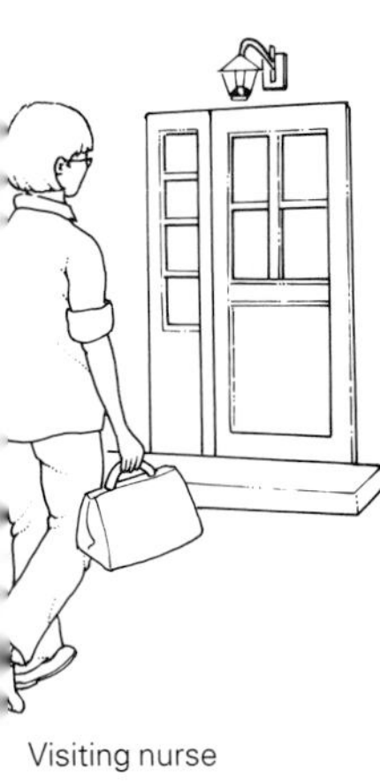

Visiting nurse

Friends and relatives can be of great help in caring for someone at home. When they ask what they can do, think of what needs to be done this week and next (errands, phone calls, letters, meals, and day care relief) and then offer a couple of suggestions from which they can choose. Do not feel you are imposing on them. They are probably very concerned and eager to help.

Organizations to which you belong, such as a church or a social group, may ask to help. Accept the offers, because such relationships can be important in the future.

Physicians and other health workers, especially social workers, will be familiar with public and private agencies that can provide specialized services. A social worker will often spend time with both the patient and the family while he or she is still in the hospital, to gather information and make suggestions about how problems might be solved. In addition, the social worker can help you identify and contact the agencies that provide the specific services you need.

Drugstores and medical supply companies stock home care equipment and supplies. Try to rent, rather than buy, the items you need, such as a walker (left). Renting may be economical if there is only a temporary need for expensive equipment. Renting also allows a person who is ill to try out several types of equipment before purchasing.

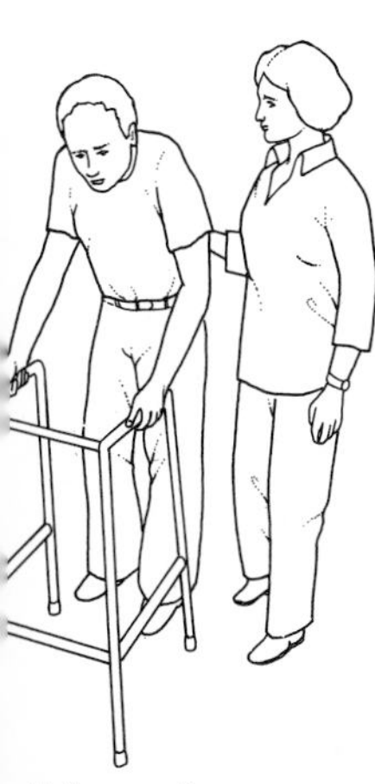

Using a walker

Hospice is the name for programs that are specially designed for the terminally ill and emphasize relief of pain and the security of a caring environment. The goal is to have the dying person spend time with family and friends, while still involved in activities of his or her choice. This may be accomplished at a specified facility or might be arranged in your home. At either site, several dedicated professional personnel will closely follow a family and their dying loved one throughout the remainder of his or her life.

Adult day care programs may provide either supervised medical and rehabilitative services or recreational and social activities. These programs are primarily for older people who want to remain at home instead of living in a nursing facility. Adult day care may be available for just 1 day a week, or for as many as 5 days a week, depending on the program. Community services or church-related groups may offer this service.

Door-to-door transportation for older and disabled people provided at minimal cost is available in some cities and can be very useful. Ask the visiting nurse, a social worker at the hospital, or your physician if such a program exists in your area.

Homemaker services are available in some areas. This program provides trained people to do difficult home chores for older or disabled people. Such services are sometimes available through church-related groups.

Special meals Home delivery of meals, often called "meals-on-wheels," is available from many religious and social agencies. Check with your physician or a social worker at the hospital whether this service is available in your area. Preference may be given to low-income older people.

Senior citizen centers in many areas of the US offer communal lunch or supper activities. The older person who can travel to the center has the benefit of a hot meal and companionship with his or her peers.

Local voluntary health organizations such as the American Cancer Society and the Easter Seal Society may be able to lend specialized equipment and provide you with information. These organizations often have programs that benefit the ill or disabled.

Vocational rehabilitation programs provide guidance, training, and employment placement assistance with the goal of enabling a person to perform within the limits of his or her current abilities. People who have had a stroke or serious head injury may be good candidates for such a program.

Recorded audio messages are available by telephone through some hospitals and medical societies that subscribe to libraries of recorded medical information. You can dial a message from the hospital or from your home on a variety of topics such as how to care for a person with diabetes.

Dying and death

Introduction

Most people hope for a long life and a quick death, but only a few people have this wish fulfilled. Most of us will die slowly over a period of weeks or months. Although a slow death may seem like a burden to the dying person and his or her family and friends, it can provide everyone concerned with the opportunity to come to terms with death and prepare for it.

People who are close to a dying person have to bear the emotional, and sometimes physical, stress of caring for him or her. Also, after someone has died, there are various practical and legal matters that must be dealt with. The articles that follow discuss these matters and also provide information about helping a bereaved person cope with his or her grief.

Life expectancy and death rates in the US

The first table below shows life expectancy—the average number of years of life left—at different ages for white and black men and women. On average, women live longer than men and, in the US, whites have greater life expectancies than blacks. The second table lists major causes of death; for each cause the figures show the total number of deaths for every 100,000 people, the number of male deaths (per 100,000 males), and the number of female deaths (per 100,000 females). Thus heart disease, the most common cause of death, accounted for 156 deaths per 100,000 people, and the death rate in men was almost twice the death rate in women. (The figures in both tables are based on 1989 data from the US Census Bureau.)

However, the pattern of causes of death changes over time as a result of such factors as medical research and new methods of treatment. The total death rate due to heart disease, for instance, declined from 286 deaths per 100,000 people in 1960 to 156 deaths per 100,000 people in 1989. In contrast, the death rate from cancer has shown an increase over the same period, from 126 deaths per 100,000 people in 1960 to 133 deaths per 100,000 people in 1989.

Life expectancy in the US in 1989 (by age, sex, and race)

Age (in years)	Male life expectancy (in years)		Female life expectancy (in years)	
	White	Black	White	Black
0 (Birth)	73	65	79	74
20	54	47	60	55
40	36	30	41	37
60	19	16	23	20
80	7	7	9	9

Major causes of death in the US in 1989

Cause of death	Death rate (per 100,000 people)	Male deaths (per 100,000 males)	Female deaths (per 100,000 females)
Heart disease	156	210	112
Cancer	133	162	112
Accidents	34	50	19
Stroke and related disorders	28	30	26
Chronic lung disorders	19	26	15
Pneumonia and influenza	14	18	11
Suicide	11	19	5
Cirrhosis of the liver	9	13	6
Diabetes mellitus	12	12	11
Homicide	9	15	4

Terminal illness

Some terminally ill people want to know the facts regarding their condition while others may deny the terminal nature of their illness in order to carry on. A dying person's physician, family, and friends should be gentle when talking about death. Although it is important for the dying person to organize his or her affairs, hope should never be compromised by insensitive talk about death.

When and what to tell a dying person

Let a terminally ill person decide the timing and extent of any discussion of death. If a dying person asks questions about dying, this indicates that he or she has been thinking about death and has, to some extent, already come to terms with it. If no questions are asked, do not force information on the dying person. This does not mean, however, that you should encourage false hopes of recovery. Someone who is misled in this way may be unable to understand why he or she is growing weaker instead of stronger and may lose confidence in medical treatment. He or she may also miss the chance to put his or her affairs in order. Also, if the patient suspects the truth he or she will be prevented from discussing fears and seeking reassurance.

A dying person will usually make it clear how much he or she wants to know. Someone who is terminally ill usually seeks some reassurance, however, and you should give an honest, comforting answer.

Physicians are commonly asked how much time the dying patient has left to live. Usually only an approximate answer is possible, such as "anything from a couple of weeks to several months." It is impossible to give a more precise answer than this.

A person who is terminally ill may find it easier to talk about his or her death with someone who is not a relative, such as a member of the hospital staff. This usually does not indicate any lack of affection or trust, but may indicate a desire to spare others pain. The closer the relationship, the more each person may want to protect the other, and the more difficult it may be to talk freely. This may cause problems for the terminally ill patient. Members of the hospital staff are often too busy to spend much time comforting the dying person. They may find it difficult to talk about dying since they may see themselves primarily in a healing role. Some hospitals have tried to help cope with this problem by training professional staff members to work with terminally ill patients and their families. A psychiatrist or the clergy may be consulted to help the family deal with their feelings about dying and death. Counseling programs both in the hospital and outside may be helpful.

The patient may find that his or her family physician is the best person to help with this problem. A physician who knows the family can sometimes help the dying person and his or her relatives come to terms with death.

Care at home or in the hospital

It is rarely true that nothing can be done for a dying person when curative treatment is no longer appropriate. The dying person still needs relief from symptoms and pain, along with understanding and comfort. Sometimes this kind of care is best provided in the dying person's own home rather than in a hospital. At home, the person can remain more independent, feel more like an individual, participate in his or her family life, and avoid some feelings of loneliness and isolation. Hospitals are more geared to treating acutely ill patients than to caring for terminally ill patients. Among home, nursing facility, and hospital care, home care may be the best choice. It is not necessarily physically demanding, pain relief does not always require an injection, and many cases of terminal illness do not require complicated caregiving. Even for cases that do require such care, it is usually needed for only a few weeks.

If you do plan to care for a terminally ill relative at home, regular visits from your family physician, along with support from family and friends, will be essential. Visiting nurse services should be used if available. Many hospitals have home care services to provide support for families that want to care for a dying relative at home.

Hospices

Hospices are small facilities (often associated with general hospitals) that have been set up especially to care for people who are dying and to help their families. These facilities are becoming increasingly widespread.

In a hospice, a dying person may not be bothered with the usual hospital routine such as temperature-taking. The efforts of the staff are concentrated on relieving pain and comforting the dying person and his or her family. One might think that seeing others dying would be depressing for terminally ill people, but many are reassured because the deaths are peaceful. Hospice-related services can also be provided for patients choosing to stay at home.

Physical pain

Pain is often the most feared problem associated with terminal illness. Continuous pain over a long period usually wears down a terminally ill person and sometimes blocks thoughts of anything else.

Today, such suffering, even with some of the most painful forms of cancer, is usually avoidable. Analgesics (painkilling drugs), can be used before the person needs to ask for medication. When painkillers are used in this way, the dose can usually be kept low, so that the dying person remains virtually pain-free and alert.

In terminally ill people, severe pain is usually controlled by an opiumlike drug. Risk of addiction to the drug is outweighed by the pain relief that the drug provides.

Emotional pain

A terminally ill person also has emotional pain at the thought of dying. Anger and depression are common reactions to the prospect of death. Some terminally ill people may have feelings of guilt or dissatisfaction when they look back on their lives and their achievements. In the end, given loving support from people around them, most terminally ill people come to terms with death, in their own way and in their own time.

Dying people often resent their growing helplessness and fear a loss of dignity. For this reason, someone who is dying should be given every opportunity to manage his or her own affairs for as long as possible and should be encouraged to do as much as possible for himself or herself. A terminally ill person should be consulted on family matters and should help his or her family plan the future.

Many dying people fear that the moment of death will be unpleasant and violent, and many are afraid of dying alone. Although fear sometimes makes a dying person seem demanding, caregivers should always try to be understanding and reassuring. You can decrease fear of an unpleasant or violent death by telling the person, if he or she asks, that in nearly all cases a dying person will feel overwhelming drowsiness just before the end of life and will lapse into unconsciousness before death occurs.

The approach of death

Toward the end of life the dying person may become restless, or his or her breathing may become labored, because the lungs may become congested as the heart fails. If you are at home with the person and these symptoms occur while he or she is still conscious, call your physician. He or she can prescribe medications to help make the person more comfortable. If the person is still alert, you can make breathing easier either by propping him or her up in a sitting position with pillows, or by laying the person on his or her side, with the top arm and leg pulled out a little for support and a single pillow beneath the person's head.

You should assume that the dying person can hear what you say up until the time of death. You may feel helpless in the presence of a person near death, but your presence is important. Often nothing more is necessary than holding the person's hand so that he or she does not feel alone.

Death

Death occurs when both breathing and heartbeat have stopped. It usually is easy for a physician to determine that this has happened if the patient is not on a life-support system. In such cases, the physician performs a specific series of tests to determine if the brain is actually dead or if the patient is simply unconscious. If the brain is dead, physical death is established and any life-support equipment is disconnected.

Delaying death

In order to prolong their lives, people with diseases such as cancer may choose to undergo treatment that is both unpleasant and uncomfortable. However, as the periods of relative health between these treatments shorten, treatments may simply prolong the dying process. At this stage, with clear prior instructions from the patient, treatment may be stopped and only painkillers and sedatives may be prescribed. In this way, a terminally ill person may be allowed to die more peacefully and with dignity.

People in a coma who are unable to breathe or maintain a heartbeat can be kept alive with intravenous or tube feedings, ventilators, and pacemakers. With legal preparation by the patient, the medical staff may be asked not to perform lifesaving measures. In these circumstances, it may be best to withhold heroic efforts and to refrain from interfering with the natural process of death. Quality of life should also be a consideration.

In 1990, the US Supreme Court ruled that a state could require clear and convincing evidence of the wishes of a patient concerning the withdrawal of life-support treatment and did not have to accept the substituted judgment of family members. Most states have passed "living will" laws, which provide that the dying person's written advance instructions will be honored regarding the use of artificial life support. A living will must be drawn up while you are still competent to make decisions (although the will becomes effective only after you are incompetent to make decisions). Some states have also enacted laws to provide for a durable power of attorney for health care, which permits you to name someone (usually a spouse or other close family member) who will have the right to make medical decisions if you become incompetent.

Criteria of death

Death occurs if both breathing and heartbeat have stopped. In the case of serious injury (from a traffic accident, for example, when life-support equipment is not immediately available), it may be possible to maintain breathing and heartbeat for a short time with emergency first-aid procedures. Eventually, however, if the heart and lungs do not begin to function on their own, first-aid measures will not be effective.

In a hospital, equipment is available to maintain breathing and heartbeat functions, which can make the diagnosis of death by loss of breathing and heartbeat uncertain. This has led to the concept of brain death. Brain death involves an irreversible state of brain damage; in fact, the areas of the brain (primarily the brain stem) necessary to maintain life have stopped functioning. Brain death can be diagnosed after a physician has performed a neurological examination and has ruled out causes of temporary brain dysfunction such as drug overdose or chemical imbalances inside the body. An electroencephalogram (a recording of the electrical impulses of the brain) is sometimes used to confirm the diagnosis but is not required and may even be misleading. Brain death is the medical, legal, and ethical equivalent of death diagnosed by the criteria of loss of breathing and heartbeat. It should not be confused with rare reports of deep coma from which people awaken after months or years. When a diagnosis of brain death is made, life-support systems are disconnected. An exception occurs if organ donation is planned, in which case life support is maintained until the organs are removed.

Practicalities of death

When someone dies, there are several legal matters to take care of before the funeral: obtaining a medical certificate of the cause of death (death certificate), registering the death, and contacting an undertaker to organize funeral and burial arrangements. There are other formalities if the death has to be reported to the medical examiner or coroner, if the body is to be cremated, or if the body is to be used for research or organ donation.

In the information that follows, it is assumed that you are either the next of kin of the dead person or his or her executor—that is, someone appointed by the dead person to carry out his or her will.

Death certificate

Only a licensed physician can certify that someone is dead and state the cause of death. The first thing to do if someone dies at home is call your family physician or the police. In most cases, your physician will have been caring for the person during his or her illness and will usually have no difficulty identifying the cause of death. If your physician has seen the person within an amount of time specified by state law, he or she is not legally obligated to examine the body before signing a death certificate that states the cause of death. However, if they are present at the time of death, most family physicians examine the body before filling out the certificate. If your physician has not seen the dead person within the time specified by law, the case may be referred to the coroner or medical examiner. Also, your physician must examine the body if it is to be cremated; if a cremation is planned, tell your physician. You should also tell your physician if the dead person's body is to be used for medical research or organ donation (see Medical use of the body, p.805). Arrangements for organ donation must be made before the person is removed from life-support systems.

If the person has died in the hospital, one of the physicians who has taken care of the person will complete the death certificate. A member of the hospital staff will tell relatives of the death and arrange for them to claim the dead person's possessions. He or she will also request permission for an autopsy so that your physician can learn more precise details regarding the cause of death and any medical conditions that may be important for the family to know. There is no charge for an autopsy. If a person has died of an injury and been brought to a hospital, the police will ask the relatives to identify the body. If the dead person has donated certain organs for transplant, or if you wish to donate any organs, the organs usually can be removed for transplantation only after the person has died in a hospital, since removal should be carried out promptly after death, before life-support systems are disconnected. If organs are to be donated, tell the hospital physician.

After the physician has completed the death certificate, the funeral director picks it up and files it with the authorities.

Referral to the medical examiner or to the coroner

Depending on where you live, one of two offices is authorized to investigate deaths—the medical examiner or the coroner. A coroner may be appointed or elected. A medical examiner usually holds office as part of the civil service system.

Mention of the coroner or medical examiner often worries people because of the implication that foul play is suspected. In fact, most of the circumstances in which the coroner must be informed of a death are innocent ones. In most states, a death is reported to the coroner or medical examiner by a physician or the police if no physician cared for the person during his or her final illness. Other circumstances in which a report to the coroner or medical examiner is required vary from state to state. Your physician, a lawyer, or the police department will be able to tell you if such a report is necessary. In general, investigation of a death is required when the cause of death is not known or when a death is known or suspected to have been caused by violence.

The medical examiner or coroner may require that an autopsy be performed to establish the cause of death (see Autopsies, next article). If the results of the autopsy are satisfactory, a death certificate is issued.

Inquests

If the autopsy does not reveal the cause of death and the death was violent, unnatural, or resulted from an injury, there may be an inquest, or public court hearing. Procedures for inquests and investigations of deaths vary depending on state and local laws. In some cases, a jury is convened. If there is a public hearing, some people may be ordered to attend as witnesses. Anyone can attend and may be represented by an attorney. This is probably a good idea if compensation claims are being considered or if there is a possibility of a criminal charge.

Once a verdict has been announced and the inquest is over, the medical examiner or coroner issues a death certificate. Permission for burial or cremation may be granted. This usually occurs as soon as the body has been identified. If the investigation is going to take a long time, the inquest may be formally opened and then adjourned. You may then be able to get a letter confirming the fact of death, which will serve in place of the death certificate as proof of death for social security and insurance claims.

The funeral

It is sensible to contact a funeral director soon after your physician has signed the death certificate. Even though you may not feel like it, it is wise to obtain price quotations from more than one funeral director. It is also a good idea to have someone who was not as personally involved with the dead person as you were, such as a member of the clergy or a lawyer, accompany you to the funeral home to help you decide on the arrangements. You are likely to be very distressed and vulnerable at this time, so another person may be able to help you make arrangements and choices that are most appropriate for your needs and your financial circumstances.

Most funeral directors offer funerals ranging from simple to elaborate. Often there is a flat fee that includes the coffin, preparation of the body for burial, and procedures such as filing the death certificate and putting notices in the newspaper. Be sure to find out what is included in the price, which costs are extra, and what other details you must take care of yourself. You will have to make decisions about the type of casket, the type and location of the burial service and who is to conduct it, whether the body is to be embalmed, whether you want to have an open casket and viewing of the body, and whether the body is to be buried or cremated.

It is possible to make arrangements for your own funeral before your death. There are consumer organizations called memorial societies that can help you make such plans. These usually nonprofit organizations are not affiliated with any particular undertaker. However, they can provide information such as which undertakers will allow payment in advance for a funeral and which ones will provide the simplest funeral. In some cases, this can save money and can spare your relatives from making these arrangements after your death when they are bereaved.

A funeral is usually held 2 to 4 days after the death. Many funeral ceremonies are performed either at a church or at a funeral home and have two parts—the ceremony at the church or funeral home and the ceremony at the graveside. Those who want a nonreligious ceremony can arrange for it with the funeral director. A memorial service is another possibility. The body is not present at a memorial service, which may change the emphasis of the ceremony so that the focus is on the person's life rather than on death. A memorial service can be held at any time and in a variety of places.

Burial and cremation

If the body is to be buried, you will need to find out whether the dead person had bought a cemetery plot or if there is a family plot. If he or she has not made arrangements for a grave site, you will have to purchase a plot.

Any instructions left by the dead person that he or she should or should not be cremated are not necessarily legally binding on the next of kin.

If the body is to be cremated instead of buried, additional arrangements are involved. This is to prevent destruction of the body before the possibility of a crime has been eliminated. The funeral director will explain what forms you need to fill out. After the cremation, you can collect the ashes to keep, bury or scatter them yourself, or ask the crematorium to dispose of them.

Paying for the funeral

The funeral expenses are the first claim on a dead person's estate. However, the person responsible for the funeral cannot obtain the money from the estate until he or she has obtained a grant of probate or letters of administration from the local probate court. Procedures vary depending on state law. Some people have life insurance policies that are intended to cover funeral expenses. Also, some trade unions, credit unions, and fraternal organizations have death benefits that can be used to help pay for a funeral. Be sure to find out if such benefits are available and how to apply for them. If the dead person was eligible for social security benefits, he or she will be eligible for a small death benefit from that source.

In some states, local government is required to arrange a funeral if no one else will. A hospital, too, may arrange a funeral for anyone who dies in the hospital and whose relatives cannot be traced.

Medical use of the body

If a person has (either in writing or verbally before two witnesses) forbidden that his or her body be used for medical research or organ donation, those instructions must be followed when the person dies. However, under the Uniform Anatomical Gift Act, it is possible to leave instructions for your body or your organs (or both) to be donated after your death. One way to accomplish this is to complete a Uniform Donor Card, which you can carry with you so that your wishes are known in the event of accidental death. The card should be signed by two witnesses in the spaces provided. It is considered a legal document in most states. These cards are available from the AMA and several other sources. Some states print a legal donor card on the back of drivers' licenses.

In most states, however, a surviving spouse or next of kin can refuse to allow your instructions to be carried out, so it is important to discuss your intention to be an organ donor with your family, and ask them to honor your wishes. If you have not left specific instructions, your spouse or next of kin is allowed to donate your body or organs for medical use (see also Autopsies, next article). If the death has been reported to the medical examiner or to the coroner, permission is needed before the body or organs can be donated.

If a body is to be donated for research, contact the appropriate medical school or organization as soon as possible after death.

Acting as an executor

If the dead person has left a will, the person appointed as executor (who is often a spouse or other close relative) is required to pay any claims against the estate (including funeral costs) and distribute other assets to the named beneficiaries.

If the dead person does not have a will, the local probate court will appoint an administrator for the estate. The spouse, if any, has the primary right to nominate an administrator. The estate is then distributed according to the laws of your state.

Autopsies

An autopsy is a detailed examination of a body after death. It is also referred to as a postmortem examination. There are two different kinds of autopsies. A "medicolegal" autopsy is ordered by the legal authorities. Its purpose is to establish the cause of death and to gather information about the death to be used as evidence in any legal proceedings that may follow. This is done to be sure that crimes that involve death are detected. It may also be done to investigate possible industrial hazards or contagious diseases that may endanger the public health, or to establish the cause of death for insurance purposes.

The second type of autopsy is performed for medical or educational reasons, usually in the hospital where the person died, and may be requested by the attending physician or the next of kin. Medical and educational autopsies cannot be performed unless the next of kin gives his or her permission. Procedures for granting such permission vary from state to state. The general purposes of this type of autopsy are to increase medical knowledge and to provide the family with a more exact cause of death, and with information concerning any diseases that might be contagious or inherited.

Both types of autopsies are usually performed before the body is embalmed. Afterward, the body is given to the funeral director so that the funeral can be held.

Medicolegal autopsies

When the coroner, the medical examiner, or a judge orders an autopsy, the family has no choice. If there is any question about the order, consult an attorney.

Medicolegal autopsy can range from a simple examination of the appearance of the body and the situation in which it was found, to a study of the entire body and all its parts, including the structure of the individual cells. The thoroughness of the autopsy depends on what is being investigated. A pathologist (a physician who performs autopsies and studies tissues and organs) must always make extremely detailed records of everything that is done, in case the information is needed as evidence for legal proceedings.

Disorders discovered by autopsies
Listed below are a few of the diseases and disorders that have been discovered as a result of autopsy studies:

Connective tissue diseases
Effects of potassium deficiency on kidneys and heart
Hyperparathyroidism
Viral hepatitis
Industrial hazards
Effects of toxic chemicals

Medical and educational autopsies

Until about the 13th century, very few autopsies were performed for any reason. However, during the 13th and 14th centuries, physicians began to perform autopsies to learn about the structure and function of the human body. Much of today's basic medical knowledge was discovered and confirmed through autopsies. Since that time, more and more medical students have learned about human anatomy by dissecting a human body.

New discoveries continue to be made from autopsies (see list at left). In diseases such as cancer and heart disease, an autopsy study of diseased organs or systems provides information that can be used to help improve treatment of the disease and to increase medical knowledge.

Autopsies are also occasionally performed to check on the accuracy of diagnosis and the appropriateness of treatment. If the patient died unexpectedly or if the symptoms were puzzling, the physician involved with the case may want an autopsy to find out exactly what happened. The family may also want to know. In some cases, the family may want information about possible inherited diseases (see Genetics, p.752); this information can sometimes be obtained from an autopsy.

If you are asked to approve an autopsy, remember that you can allow a limited autopsy; that is, you can specify which parts of the body can be studied. The pathologist is legally obligated to follow the next of kin's instructions. Also, it does not have to be evident (at the funeral, for instance) that an autopsy was performed because, in most cases, any obvious marks can be covered by clothing. Autopsies are performed with respect in a carefully regulated and confidential setting. Much can be learned from an autopsy, both for the benefit of medical science and for the benefit of the family.

Bereavement

Immediately after the death of someone close, many people feel mainly numb and empty. For a while they may move through life almost as if nothing has happened, until they are eventually stricken with intense grief. During the period immediately after a loss, delusions of seeing the dead person are common and not abnormal. There is a tendency to forget that the person is dead and act as though he or she were still alive. Idealization of the dead person and feelings of guilt for not doing more when the person was alive are also common. Guilt and intense grief are much more common in cases when the person died unexpectedly; by contrast, when death occurred after a long illness, the bereaved person was usually able to provide care and anticipate his or her loss.

If someone close to you dies, try to acknowledge your loss rather than attempt to remove it from your consciousness. Talk about the dead person to relatives and friends and sort out his or her possessions to help you come to terms with your loss.

The intensity of grief usually starts to lessen after about 6 weeks and is sometimes replaced by a more general state of depression and apathy. Grief will usually become minimal by 1 year. During this year, your feelings of grief may reappear unpredictably, and will probably recur occasionally in the years that follow. By the end of a year, most bereaved people have recovered from their loss and have started building a new life.

Occasionally, however, grief is prolonged or intense and cannot be relieved without help from a professional such as a psychiatrist. Support groups are available for people who may find comfort in sharing their feelings with others who have had similar experiences. Ask your physician about support groups in your area. Bereaved people most likely to need help are those who are particularly susceptible to grief, those whose relationship with the dead person has left them with strong feelings of guilt or anger, and those who tend to be socially isolated.

In recovering from the death of someone close to you, it is important to meet new people and to interest yourself in new activities. Give yourself time to accept your loss, allow your feelings of grief to flow, and then begin to rebuild a life that allows you to forget the loss most of the time through positive activities and new relationships. Ask for help if you need it.

Helping the bereaved

A bereaved person will need practical help at first to continue day-to-day existence and, in some cases, to make decisions. Besides that, it may seem that there is little real comfort you can offer, but this is not true. By allowing the person to talk about his or her loss, you encourage an outlet for the expression of grief that can be highly beneficial.

Take any threat of suicide seriously. Call a physician or a suicide hot line, or take the person to a hospital emergency department to get immediate assistance.

Do not limit your help only to the first few difficult days. The bereaved person will need support throughout the lonely months that follow. The first anniversary of a death, or the first holiday spent alone, can be a particularly difficult time, and a visit or an offer of hospitality from you may be very welcome.

Children and death

Until about age 3, children have no concept of death. By age 9, most children are at least partially able to understand that death is the end of life and is inevitable.

The bereaved child

Children should be allowed to grieve in their own way and not forced to conform to adult ideas about grieving. Young children often appear to recover from bereavement very quickly, especially if they can become attached to a substitute for the dead person.

Adults should not try to suppress their own grief in front of a child. Children can often sense unexpressed feelings, and this might make a child feel even more uneasy. Give the child every opportunity to ask questions about the death. Some children feel that the death may somehow be their fault, and they may need to be reassured that this is not true.

Even if a child appears to show minimal signs of grief after the death of a close relative, it is best to try to avoid any major changes in the child's life for about 6 months, if possible. Stability and a feeling of security are important to a bereaved child.

The dying child

A child may be able to face the prospect of his or her own death better than his or her parents can. A child may fear pain and, if admission to the hospital is necessary, separation from his or her parents more than he or she fears death. It will usually help a child come to terms with death if he or she is told about his or her illness. Death should not be treated as a forbidden subject. The most important thing that parents can give to a child is security—physical security by their presence and emotional security by their loving support.

It is important that a terminally ill child lead as normal a life as possible for as long as possible. Avoid treating him or her in any special way that will make your child feel different from his or her friends. School work, seeing friends, and normal family activities and discipline should be continued for as long as possible.

If possible, it is much more comforting for a terminally ill child to be cared for at home rather than in a hospital. However, it is necessary for parents who take on home care to have a family physician who can be called on in any circumstance. The family physician will try to arrange hospital admission if the parents can no longer cope with a difficult situation or if the child needs more sophisticated medical care.

Death of a child

Death of a child can cause more grief than death of an adult because we frequently experience distress and perhaps even anger about the fact that a young life has been cut off before it has really begun. Sudden death is often more difficult to bear than a death that occurs after a long illness. Professional counseling may be important for the parents and, in some cases, siblings. Support groups or group therapy with other parents who have had similar experiences can provide great comfort. Ask your physician about organizations in your area.

Drug glossary

This glossary briefly describes more than 700 prescription and over-the-counter drugs that are available in the US. The listings give (1) the generic name of the drug (brand names of drugs are not included) and, in many cases, (2) the drug group to which the drug belongs (set in italics) and/or (3) a brief explanation of the drug or its primary uses (for drugs with several actions, only the most important use or uses are given). If your physician has prescribed or you have purchased a brand-name product, you can find the generic name of the drug by asking your physician or pharmacist or by reading the label. The drug that has been prescribed or that you have purchased may or may not be discussed elsewhere in this book; please see the Index. If the drug is not listed in the Index, you can look it up in this section to determine the drug group to which it belongs, and then use the Index to learn more about that group.

A

ACE inhibitors these drugs interfere with the action of a substance called angiotensin-converting enzyme and thereby block one of the stages in a chain of biochemical reactions controlling blood pressure. They are used to treat high blood pressure and certain forms of heart failure.

acebutolol a *beta blocker* primarily used to treat high blood pressure and angina.

acetaminophen a nonnarcotic *analgesic* (painkiller).

acetazolamide a weak *diuretic*; also used to treat glaucoma.

acetohexamide a drug used to treat diabetes mellitus.

acetophenazine an *antipsychotic* used to treat acute psychosis.

acetylcysteine a mucolytic (mucus thinner); also used as an antidote for acetaminophen poisoning.

acyclovir an *antiviral* used to treat herpes virus and cytomegalovirus infections.

adenosine an *antiarrhythmic* used to treat irregular heartbeat.

albuterol a *bronchodilator* primarily used to treat asthma.

alclometasone dipropionate a *corticosteroid* used to treat inflammation and itching of the skin.

allopurinol a drug used to prevent attacks of gout.

alprazolam an *antianxiety drug* primarily used to treat panic disorders and anxiety.

alprostadil a drug used to treat congenital heart disease in infants and Raynaud's disease (disorder of the blood vessels).

alteplase a *thrombolytic* used to dissolve blood clots in the heart and the lungs.

aluminum hydroxide an *antacid.*

amantadine an *antiviral*; also used to treat parkinsonism.

ambenonium a drug used to treat myasthenia gravis (muscle disorder).

amcinonide a topical *corticosteroid* used to treat skin disorders.

amikacin an aminoglycoside *antibiotic.*

amiloride a weak *diuretic* primarily used to treat high blood pressure.

aminocaproic acid a drug used to prevent abnormal bleeding.

aminoglutethimide an *anticancer drug.*

aminophylline a *bronchodilator* used to treat narrowing of the airways in the lung caused by muscle spasm.

amiodarone an *antiarrhythmic* used to treat life-threatening irregular heartbeat.

amitriptyline a tricyclic *antidepressant.*

amlodipine a *calcium channel blocker.*

amobarbital a *barbiturate* primarily used as a *sedative.*

amoxapine a tricyclic *antidepressant.*

amoxicillin a penicillin *antibiotic.*

amphetamine a drug that stimulates the central nervous system; used to treat narcolepsy (sleep disorder) and attention deficit disorder.

amphotericin B an *antifungal.*

ampicillin a penicillin *antibiotic.*

amsacrine an investigational *anticancer drug* used to treat leukemia.

analgesics drugs that relieve pain. There are two main types of analgesics: non-narcotic analgesics for treating mild to moderate pain, and narcotic analgesics (based on opium) for treating severe pain. Most nonnarcotic analgesics contain aspirin or acetaminophen, and are also *antipyretics.* Many analgesics that are related to aspirin are *anti-inflammatories* also. Many brand name products are a combination of nonnarcotic analgesics, sometimes with codeine, a weak narcotic analgesic. Although these are more costly, they are rarely more effective than single-ingredient preparations. Narcotic analgesics may be taken as tablets or by injection. Possible side effects: nausea, constipation, dizziness, inability to urinate. All narcotic analgesics cause gradual development of some degree of tolerance and are habit-forming. The risk of becoming addicted to weaker narcotics such as codeine is lower than it is with powerful morphine derivatives. Narcotic analgesics are not prescribed for anyone who has chronic pain not caused by cancer, who is taking monoamine oxidase inhibitors (a type of *antidepressant*), or who has low blood pressure, asthma, liver damage, or head injury.

anisindione an *anticoagulant* used to prevent blood clots.

anistreplase a *thrombolytic* primarily used to dissolve blood clots.

antacids drugs that relieve indigestion and heartburn by neutralizing the effects of stomach acid. Antacids are taken in tablet or liquid form or as a powder mixed with water. Liquid preparations or powders are most effective. Possible side effects: constipation (from aluminum compounds), diarrhea (from magnesium compounds). In preparations made by combining different antacids, the side effects may neutralize each other. Antacids may be combined with an *anti-spasmodic* to treat peptic ulcers. Anyone who has kidney problems should not take preparations that contain magnesium or sodium bicarbonate. Antacids are taken between meals, and because they interfere with absorption of many drugs, they should not be taken with other medications.

anthralin a drug used to treat psoriasis (skin disease).

antianxiety drugs drugs (sometimes called anxiolytics, sedatives, or minor tranquilizers) that suppress anxiety and relax muscles. Some are also used as *sleeping drugs* or for relief of premenstrual tension. Possible side effects: drowsiness, dizziness, confusion, unsteadiness (especially in older people). Because they can become habit-forming and users develop tolerance, antianxiety drugs are usually prescribed for periods of no more than 4 months of continuous use. To avoid withdrawal symptoms, decrease the dosage gradually, not abruptly. Effects last for several hours, and driving or working with potentially dangerous machinery is not recommended during that time. The effects of alcohol may be dangerously increased by the drugs.

antiarrhythmics drugs used to control irregularities of heartbeat. The oldest antiarrhythmics are digitalis and quinidine, both of which are plant extracts. More recently introduced antiarrhythmics include *beta blockers*, such as propranolol.

antibacterials drugs used to treat infections. See *antibiotics*.

antibiotics drugs made from naturally occurring and synthetic substances that combat bacterial infection. Some antibiotics are effective only against limited types of bacteria. Possible side effects: nausea, vomiting, diarrhea, and, especially from the use of broad-spectrum antibiotics, secondary infections such as yeast infections that result from an upset in the balance of natural bacteria within the body. Allergic reactions, particularly to penicillin and its many derivatives, may occur. Among the reactions are rashes, fever, painful joints, body swelling, wheezing, and some blood disorders. If you are diagnosed as allergic to a particular antibiotic, remember to tell this to any new physicians you see. Once treatment begins, the prescribed course should be completed even if the infection seems to have been cured. Failure to take the entire prescription may allow relapse of the infection and may increase the chances of bacterial resistance to further treatment with the drug.

anticancer drugs anticancer drugs are often cytotoxic; that is, they kill or damage cells. Anticancer drugs include *antineoplastics* and *immunosuppressants*. They are taken as tablets or given by injection, and several anticancer drugs with different types of action may be used in combination. Possible side effects: nausea, vomiting, loss of hair. Because anticancer drug action can affect healthy as well as cancerous cells, these medications may also have a more dangerous side effect. For example, they can damage bone marrow and affect the production of blood cells, causing anemia, increased susceptibility to infection, and hemorrhage. Therefore, frequent blood tests are recommended for anyone who is having such a treatment.

anticoagulants drugs that prevent blood from clotting. Possible side effects: bleeding from nose or gums, bruising, smoky or pink urine, bleeding into the intestinal tract. Because anticoagulants interact adversely with many other drugs including aspirin, users should carry a warning card and take other medicine only under a physician's direction. *Thrombolytics* increase levels of a clot-dissolving blood enzyme; they are used to treat thrombosis and embolism.

anticonvulsants drugs that prevent epileptic seizures. In certain types of epilepsy, once the patient has remained free of seizures for 2 or 3 years, the dose may be gradually reduced, and in some cases may eventually be stopped altogether. However, in many types of epilepsy, medication must be continued for life. Possible side effects: drowsiness, rashes, dizziness, headache, nausea. Abrupt withdrawal can precipitate a seizure. Drinking alcohol, taking *antihistamines,* or operating potentially dangerous machinery are not recommended while taking anticonvulsants.

antidepressants there are several groups of mood-lifting antidepressants, including tricyclics and monoamine oxidase inhibitors (MAOIs). Beneficial effects may take 3 to 4 weeks to develop, so patients may need encouragement from relatives and friends to continue the treatment. Possible side effects of tricyclics: drowsiness, dry mouth, blurred vision, constipation, difficulty urinating, faintness on standing, sweating, trembling, rashes, palpitations. Possible side effects of MAOIs: dizziness, faintness on standing, headache, trembling, constipation, dry mouth, blurred vision, difficulty urinating, rashes. The MAOIs interact adversely with other drugs and several foods and are usually prescribed only if depression fails to respond to tricyclics. Individuals taking MAOIs are advised to carry a warning card. Drinking alcohol, driving, or using complex machinery are not recommended after taking any antidepressant.

antidiarrheals drugs used for the relief of diarrhea. Two main types of antidiarrheal preparations are simple absorbent substances (for instance, kaolin, chalk, or charcoal mixtures) and drugs that slow down the contractions of the intestinal muscle so that the contents are propelled more slowly. Antidiarrheals are available in tablet and liquid form. Because treatment of diarrhea can lead to constipation, using antidiarrheals for prolonged periods is not recommended.

antiemetics drugs used to treat nausea and vomiting. Certain *antihistamines* and *antispasmodics* are also commonly used as antiemetics for prevention of motion sickness. Antiemetics are usually taken as tablets, but may be taken in liquid or suppository form or by injection. For possible side effects see *antihistamines, antispasmodics*, and *antipsychotics*. Driving, using potentially dangerous machinery, or drinking alcohol are not recommended after taking an antiemetic. Antiemetics are not recommended in cases where the cause of vomiting is not known and should not be taken by pregnant women without a physician's advice.

antifungals drugs used to treat fungal infections, the most common of which affect the hair, skin, nails, or mucous membranes. Antifungals may be taken in tablet form or applied locally as creams, ointments, or suppositories. Internal fungal infections are treated by antifungal drugs given by injection.

antihemophilic factor a substance used to promote clotting of blood in hemophiliacs.

antihistamines drugs used primarily to counteract the effects of histamine, one of the chemicals involved in allergic reactions. They are used with variable success to treat hay fever. Many antihistamines are also beneficial for relief of stuffy or runny nose, nausea, and vertigo (dizziness). They are therefore common ingredients of *cold remedies* and are used to prevent motion sickness. Possible side effects: drowsiness, blurred vision, dry mouth. Driving, operating potentially dangerous machinery, or drinking alcohol are not recommended after taking an antihistamine.

antihypertensives drugs that lower blood pressure. The two groups that are most commonly used are *beta blockers* and *diuretics*, but other categories also are prescribed and these agents are referred to in this glossary simply as antihypertensives. Antihypertensives are usually taken as tablets or capsules, but may be given by injection for rapid effect.

anti-inflammatories drugs used to reduce inflammation, the redness, heat, swelling, and increased blood flow found in infections and in many chronic noninfective diseases such as rheumatoid arthritis and gout. Three main types of drugs are used as anti-inflammatories: *analgesics* such as aspirin, *corticosteroids*, and nonsteroidal anti-inflammatory drugs (NSAIDs) such as indomethacin. The analgesics that are especially effective for treating rheumatic conditions also reduce the fever and inflammation of the joints, and may help correct some of the blood abnormalities found in those disorders. Nonsteroidal drugs similar to indomethacin have little effect on pains such as those from a toothache or a bruise, but are very effective in relieving the inflammation and the pain of diseases such as gout. *Corticosteroids* may be applied locally as cream or eye drops for inflammation of the skin or eyes, but they are not generally prescribed for rheumatic conditions unless such disorders have failed to respond to treatment with nonsteroidal drugs.

antineoplastics drugs used to treat cancer. See *anticancer drugs*.

antipsychotics drugs used to treat symptoms of severe psychiatric disorders. These drugs are sometimes called major tranquilizers. Some antipsychotics also may be useful in treating migraine headaches. They may be taken in tablet, liquid, or suppository form, or given by injection. Possible side effects: faintness on standing, dry mouth, constipation, abnormal face and body movements.

antipyretics drugs that reduce fever. Those most commonly used are aspirin and acetaminophen, which are both also *analgesics*. This double action makes them particularly effective for relieving the symptoms of illnesses such as flu.

antirheumatics see *anti-inflammatories* and *analgesics*.

antispasmodics drugs for reducing spasm of the intestine to relieve the pain of conditions such as irritable colon or diverticular disease. Some antispasmodics are used to treat asthma. A few are also used as *antiemetics*. Antispasmodics may be taken in tablet or liquid form or by injection. Possible side effects: dry mouth, palpitations, difficulty urinating, constipation, blurred vision.

antivirals drugs used to treat viral infections or to provide temporary protection against infections such as influenza. Few viral disorders respond to drugs, and those that do respond, such as cold sores and shingles, will do so only if treatment is started early.

aprobarbital a barbiturate used as a *sedative*.

aspirin an NSAID *analgesic* used to treat pain, stiffness, and inflammation (especially arthritis).

astemizole a nonsedating *antihistamine* used to prevent symptoms of allergies.

atenolol a *beta blocker* primarily used to treat angina, irregular heartbeat, heart attack, and high blood pressure.

atropine an antiarrhythmic; also used as an antidote for some types of pesticide poisonings.

auranofin an oral *antirheumatic* gold compound used to treat arthritis.

aurothioglucose an intramuscular *antirheumatic* gold compound used to treat arthritis.

azathioprine an *immunosuppressant* used to treat immune disorders and prevent rejection of transplanted organs.

azithromycin a macrolide *antibiotic*.

azlocillin a penicillin *antibiotic*.

aztreonam an *antibiotic*.

B

bacampicillin a penicillin *antibiotic*.

bacitracin a topical *antibiotic*.

baclofen a *muscle relaxant* primarily used in the treatment of spastic conditions.

barbiturates see *sleeping drugs*.

beclomethasone a *corticosteroid* used as an inhalant to treat inflammation due to asthma and rhinitis and topically to treat allergic skin disorders.

belladonna a drug primarily used to reduce cramping of the intestines.

bendroflumethiazide a *diuretic* primarily used to treat high blood pressure.

benzalkonium chloride a topical antiseptic (prevents infection).

benzocaine a topical anesthetic (causes loss of sensation).

benzonatate a *cough suppressant*.

benzoyl peroxide a topical *antibacterial* used to treat acne.

benzquinamide an *antiemetic* used to treat nausea and vomiting.

benztropine a drug used to treat parkinsonism.

benzyl alcohol a topical anesthetic (causes loss of sensation).

benzyl benzoate a topical drug used to treat scabies (skin infestation).

beta blockers beta adrenergic blocking agents, or beta blockers for short, reduce the oxygen needs of the heart by reducing heartbeat rate. They are used as *antihypertensives* and *antiarrhythmics* to treat angina due to exertion, and to ease symptoms such as palpitations and tremors in people with anxiety. They are used occasionally for migraine headaches. Beta blockers may be taken as tablets or given by injection. Possible side effects: nausea, insomnia, physical weariness, diarrhea. Overdose can cause dizziness and fainting spells. Discontinuation of treatment with these drugs should be gradual, not abrupt. Beta blockers are not prescribed for people who are known to have either asthma or heart failure.

betamethasone a topical *corticosteroid* used to treat inflammation and allergic skin disorders.

betaxolol a *beta blocker* used to treat glaucoma.

bethanechol a drug used to treat retention of urine after an operation.

bichloracetic acid a corrosive substance used topically for removal of warts, corns, and calluses.

biperiden a drug used to treat parkinsonism.

bismuth a substance primarily used in the treatment of peptic ulcers and diarrhea.

bitolterol a *bronchodilator* used to treat asthma.

bleomycin an *anticancer drug*.

botulinum A toxin a substance used to treat spasmodic muscle disorders.

bretylium an *antiarrhythmic* used to treat irregular heartbeat.

bromocriptine a drug used to treat parkinsonism and infertility and to regulate ovarian function and breast milk secretion.

bromodiphenhydramine an *antihistamine* primarily used in cold preparations.

brompheniramine an *antihistamine* primarily used in cold preparations.

bronchodilators drugs that open up the bronchial tubes within the lungs when the tubes have become narrowed by muscle spasm. Bronchodilators ease breathing in diseases such as asthma. They are most often taken as aerosol sprays, but they are also available in tablet, liquid, or suppository form. In emergencies such as severe asthma attacks, they may be given by injection. The effects of these drugs usually last for 3 to 5 hours. Possible side effects: rapid heartbeat, palpitations, tremor, headache, dizziness. Because of the possible effects of bronchodilator drugs on the heart, prescribed doses should never be exceeded. When asthma does not respond to the prescribed doses of these drugs, emergency medical treatment is needed.

buclizine an *antiemetic* used to treat nausea and vomiting and motion sickness.

bumetanide a *diuretic* used to treat high blood pressure.

buprenorphine a narcotic *analgesic* (painkiller).

buspirone hydrochloride an *antianxiety drug.*

busulfan an *anticancer drug.*

butabarbital a *barbiturate* primarily used as a sedative.

butamben a topical anesthetic (causes loss of sensation).

butoconazole nitrate an *antifungal* used to treat fungal infections of the vagina.

butorphanol a narcotic *analgesic* (painkiller).

C

calamine a lotion used to soothe irritated skin.

calcitonin a *hormone* drug used to treat bone loss.

calcitriol a *vitamin D* preparation used to elevate levels of calcium in the blood.

calcium channel blockers these drugs slow down calcium movement through cell membranes, dilate blood vessels, and reduce the heart's workload. They are used to treat hypertension, angina, and arrhythmias (abnormal heart rhythms).

cantharidin a blistering agent used to remove warts.

capreomycin an *antibacterial* used to treat tuberculosis.

captopril an *ACE inhibitor* used to treat high blood pressure and congestive heart failure.

carbachol a drug used to treat glaucoma.

carbamazepine an *anticonvulsant* used to treat epilepsy; also used to reduce pain in neuralgias.

carbamide peroxide a topical drug used to soften earwax and as a mouthwash.

carbenicillin a penicillin *antibiotic.*

carbidopa a drug used to treat parkinsonism.

carbinoxamine an *antihistamine* primarily used to treat allergies.

carbonic anhydrase inhibitors drugs used to decrease pressure within the eye in the treatment of glaucoma. Possible side effects: loss of appetite, weight loss, nausea, vomiting, diarrhea, weakness, depression, dizziness.

carboplatin an *anticancer drug.*

carboprost a drug used to stimulate contractions of the uterus.

carisoprodol a *sedative* used to promote muscle relaxation.

carmustine an *anticancer drug.*

carteolol a *beta blocker* used to treat high blood pressure.

cefaclor a cephalosporin *antibiotic.*

cefadroxil a cephalosporin *antibiotic.*

cefazolin a cephalosporin *antibiotic.*

cefixime a cephalosporin *antibiotic.*

cefoxitin a cephalosporin *antibiotic.*

ceftriaxone a cephalosporin *antibiotic.*

cefuroxime a cephalosporin *antibiotic.*

cephalexin a cephalosporin *antibiotic.*

charcoal, activated used to absorb poisons and to treat drug overdoses.

chenodiol a drug used to dissolve gallstones.

chloral hydrate a *sleeping drug.*

chlorambucil an *anticancer drug.*

chloramphenicol an *antibiotic.*

chlordiazepoxide an *antianxiety drug;* also used to treat symptoms of alcohol withdrawal.

chlorhexidine a topical antiseptic (prevents infection).

chlormezanone an *antianxiety drug.*

chloroquine a drug used to treat malaria; also used to treat liver abscess caused by a parasite and rheumatoid arthritis.

chlorotrianisene a *hormone* drug primarily used to treat cancer of the prostate gland.

chlorphenesin a *sedative* primarily used to promote muscle relaxation.

chlorpheniramine an *antihistamine* primarily used to treat allergies and cold symptoms.

chlorpromazine an *antiemetic* used to treat nausea and vomiting; an *antipsychotic* used to treat psychosis.

chlorpropamide a drug used to treat diabetes mellitus.

chlorprothixene an *antipsychotic* used to treat acute psychosis.

chlortetracycline a tetracycline *antibiotic.*

chlorthalidone a *diuretic* primarily used to treat high blood pressure.

chlorzoxazone a *sedative* primarily used to promote muscle relaxation.

cholestyramine a *lipid-lowering drug* used to reduce levels of cholesterol in the blood.

choline salicylate a non-narcotic *analgesic* (painkiller).

ciclopirox an *antifungal.*

cilastatin/imipenem a combination *antibiotic* given by injection.

cimetidine a drug used primarily to treat peptic ulcers.

cinnamates a group of sunscreens.

cinoxacin an *antibacterial* primarily used to treat urinary tract infections.

ciprofloxacin an *antibacterial.*

cisplatin an *anticancer drug.*

clarithromycin an oral macrolide *antibiotic.*

clavulanic acid a drug used to inactivate bacterial enzymes that destroy some penicillin antibiotics.

clemastine an *antihistamine* primarily used to treat allergies.

clidinium bromide a drug primarily used to treat irritable bowel syndrome.

clindamycin a lincosamide *antibiotic.*

clioquinol a topical *antibacterial* and *antifungal.*

clobetasol a topical *corticosteroid* used to treat inflammation and allergic skin disorders.

clocortolone a topical *corticosteroid* used to treat inflammation and allergic skin disorders.

clofazimine an *antibacterial* used in the treatment of leprosy.

clofibrate a *lipid-lowering drug* used to reduce levels of fatty substances in the blood.

clomiphene a drug used to treat infertility.

clomipramine a tricyclic *antidepressant* used to treat obsessive-compulsive disorders.

clonazepam an *anticonvulsant* primarily used to treat epilepsy.

clonidine a drug primarily used to treat high blood pressure.

clorazepate an *antianxiety drug;* also used to treat symptoms of alcohol withdrawal.

clotrimazole an *antifungal.*

cloxacillin a penicillin *antibiotic.*

clozapine an *antipsychotic* primarily used to treat schizophrenia.

coal tar a substance used topically to treat psoriasis (skin disease) and dandruff.

cocaine a drug that stimulates the central nervous system; also used as a local anesthetic (causes loss of sensation).

codeine a narcotic *analgesic* (painkiller).

colchicine a drug used to treat and prevent attacks of gout.

cold remedies although there is no drug that can cure a cold, the aches, pains, and fever that accompany a cold can be relieved by aspirin or acetaminophen taken with plenty of liquid. Cold remedies are often available in fizzy or fruit-flavored preparations. Many preparations also contain *antihistamines* and *decongestants,* for dealing with nasal symptoms. However, taken by mouth, these drugs are unlikely to be effective unless swallowed in doses high enough to produce side effects that outweigh the benefits. Possible side effects: drowsiness, giddiness, headache, nausea, vomiting, sweating, thirst, palpitations, difficulty urinating, weakness, trembling, anxiety, insomnia. Cold remedies should be avoided by people who have angina, high blood pressure, diabetes, or thyroid disorders and by anyone who is taking monoamine oxidase inhibitors, a type of *antidepressant.* Driving or using potentially dangerous machinery is not recommended after taking a remedy that contains an *antihistamine.*

colestipol a *lipid-lowering drug* used to reduce levels of fatty substances in the blood.

colistin an *antibiotic.*

corticosteroids these hormonal preparations are used primarily as *anti-inflammatories* in arthritis or asthma or as *immunosuppressants,* but they are also useful for treating malignancies or compensating for a deficiency of natural hormones in disorders such as Addison's disease. They are effective for many types of dermatitis when applied to the skin. Corticosteroids may be taken as tablets, applied locally as cream or eyedrops, or given by injection. Possible side effects of overuse: swollen ankles, raised blood pressure, fat deposits on face, shoulders, and abdomen, hairiness, flushing, acne, disturbance of menstrual patterns, muscle weakness, mood changes, peptic ulcers, cataracts. Corticosteroid tablets also reduce the body's resistance to infection, and they may suppress growth in children. Given as eye drops, they may cause glaucoma; as creams they may cause rashes, acne, and other skin problems. In all forms, these drugs should be used sparingly and for limited periods only. Discontinuation of treatment should be gradual, not abrupt.

corticotropin a *hormone* drug used to stimulate the adrenal glands to produce more hydrocortisone.

cortisone a *corticosteroid* used to treat inflammation.

cough suppressants simple cough medicines, which contain substances such as honey, glycerine, or menthol, soothe throat irritation but do not actually suppress coughing. They are most soothing when used as lozenges and dissolved in the mouth. As liquids they are probably swallowed too quickly to be effective. A few drugs, notably dextromethorphan and codeine, are actually cough suppressants; that is, they can help to control a dry, unproductive (nothing coughed up) cough.

cresol a disinfectant.

cromolyn sodium a drug used in the preventive treatment of asthma and hay fever.

crotamiton a topical drug used to treat scabies (skin infestation) and itching.

cyclacillin a penicillin *antibiotic.*

cyclizine an *antiemetic* used to treat nausea and vomiting.

cyclobenzaprine a *muscle relaxant* used to treat muscle spasms.

cyclophosphamide an *anticancer drug.*

cycloserine an *antibiotic* used to treat tuberculosis.

cyclosporine an *immunosuppressant* primarily used to prevent rejection of transplanted organs.

cyclothiazide a *diuretic* used to treat high blood pressure and edema.

cyproheptadine an *antihistamine* primarily used to treat itching and hives.

cytarabine an *anticancer drug.*

cytomegalovirus immune globulin an intravenous solution that delivers human antibodies against cytomegalovirus, given to kidney transplant recipients and other people with suppressed immune systems.

D

dacarbazine an *anticancer drug.*

dactinomycin an *anticancer drug.*

danazol a drug with hormone-like action used to treat endometriosis (fragments of the lining of the uterus present in the abdominal cavity) and cystic breast disease.

dantrolene a *muscle relaxant* primarily used to treat muscle spasticity caused by stroke and malignant hyperthermia (life-threatening drug reactions with high fever and muscle spasms).

dapsone an *antibacterial* used to treat leprosy.

decongestants drugs that reduce swelling of the mucous membranes that line the nose by constricting blood vessels, thus relieving nasal stuffiness. Decongestants are most effective in the form of a nasal spray or drops. Overuse can lead to increased stuffiness. They can also be taken by mouth as one ingredient of *cold remedies,* but they are less effective in this form. Large doses taken by mouth may adversely affect heart rate.

deferoxamine a drug used to treat iron poisoning.

dehydrating agents See *diuretics.*

demecarium a drug used to treat glaucoma.

demeclocycline a tetracycline *antibiotic.*

desipramine a tricyclic *antidepressant.*

desmopressin a drug used to prevent excess water loss from the kidney.

desonide a topical *corticosteroid* used to treat inflammation and allergic skin disorders.

desoximetasone a topical *corticosteroid* used to treat inflammation and allergic skin disorders.

dexamethasone a *corticosteroid* used to treat inflammation.

dexchlorpheniramine an *antihistamine* used to treat symptoms of allergies.

dextroamphetamine a drug that stimulates the central nervous system; primarily used to treat narcolepsy and attention deficit disorder.

dextromethorphan a *cough suppressant.*

dextrothyroxine a *lipid-lowering drug* used to reduce levels of fatty substances in the blood.

diazepam an *antianxiety drug;* also used as an *anticonvulsant.*

diazoxide an *antihypertensive* used to treat high blood pressure; also used to treat hypoglycemia (low blood sugar level) and hyperinsulinemia (excessive secretion of insulin).

dichlorphenamide a weak *diuretic* primarily used to treat glaucoma.

diclofenac an NSAID *analgesic* used to treat pain, stiffness, and inflammation (especially arthritis).

dicloxacillin a penicillin *antibiotic.*

dicumarol an *anticoagulant* used to prevent blood clots.

dicyclomine a drug used to treat irritable bowel syndrome.

dienestrol a *hormone* drug primarily used to treat atrophic vaginitis (dry, irritated mucosal lining of the vagina).

diethylpropion a drug that stimulates the central nervous system; used to suppress appetite.

diethylstilbestrol a *hormone* drug used to treat advanced prostate cancer and as a form of contraceptive.

diflorasone a topical *corticosteroid* primarily used to treat inflammation and allergic skin disorders.

diflunisal an NSAID *analgesic* used to treat pain, stiffness, and inflammation (especially arthritis).

digoxin a drug primarily used to treat congestive heart failure and irregular heartbeat.

dihydrocodeine a narcotic *analgesic* primarily used as a cough suppressant.

dihydroergotamine a drug used to treat migraine headache.

dihydroxyaluminum an *antacid.*

diltiazem a *calcium channel blocker* primarily used to treat angina and high blood pressure.

dimenhydrinate an *antiemetic* used to treat nausea and vomiting.

dimercaprol a drug used as an antidote for metal poisoning.

dimethicone a water repellent used in barrier creams.

dinoprostone a drug used to stimulate contractions of the uterus.

diphenhydramine an *antihistamine* used to treat allergies and in cold preparations; an *antiemetic* used to treat nausea and vomiting; also used to treat insomnia.

diphenidol an *antiemetic* used to treat Meniere's disease, nausea, and vertigo.

dipivefrin a drug used to treat glaucoma.

dipyridamole a drug used to prevent blood clots.

disopyramide an *antiarrhythmic* used to treat irregular heartbeat.

disulfiram an alcohol abuse deterrent.

diuretics drugs that increase the quantity of urine produced by the kidneys and passed out of the body, thus ridding the body of excess fluid. Diuretics reduce waterlogging of the tissues caused by fluid retention in disorders of the heart, kidneys, and liver. They are useful in treating mild cases of high blood pressure. They are usually taken as tablets. Possible side effects: rashes, dizziness, weakness, numbness, tingling in the hands and feet.

dobutamine a drug used to treat severe heart failure.

dopamine a naturally occurring neurotransmitter (chemical messenger) used to treat shock syndrome and heart failure.

doxapram a drug used to stimulate respiration after anesthesia or drug overdose.

doxepin a tricyclic *antidepressant.*

doxorubicin an *anticancer drug.*

doxycycline a tetracycline *antibiotic.*

doxylamine an *antihistamine* primarily used to induce sleep.

dronabinol an *antiemetic* used to treat nausea and vomiting induced by *anticancer drugs.*

droperidol a drug used as a preanesthetic medication.

dyclonine a topical anesthetic (causes loss of sensation).

dyphylline a *bronchodilator* used to treat narrowing of airways in the lungs.

E

echothiophate a drug used in the treatment of glaucoma.

econazole an *antifungal.*

edetate calcium disodium a drug used to treat lead poisoning.

edetate disodium a drug used to reduce calcium levels in the blood.

edrophonium a drug used in the diagnosis of myasthenia gravis.

emetine a drug used to treat disease caused by protozoa (single-celled organisms).

enalapril an *ACE inhibitor* used to treat high blood pressure and heart failure.

encainide an *antiarrhythmic* used to treat life-threatening irregular heartbeat.

ephedrine a drug primarily used to treat asthma; also used as a *decongestant.*

epinephrine a drug primarily used in emergency treatment of cardiac arrest, anaphylactic shock (life-threatening allergic reaction), and acute asthma attacks; also used to treat glaucoma and cataracts.

epoetin alfa a drug used to stimulate production of red blood cells in the treatment of anemia associated with chronic renal failure (inability of kidneys to filter waste products from blood) and cancer.

ergocalciferol a *vitamin D* preparation used to treat parathyroid and vitamin D deficiencies.

ergonovine a drug used to stop bleeding after childbirth.

ergotamine a drug used to treat migraine headache.

erythrityl a drug used to treat angina.

erythromycin an *antibiotic.*

esmolol a *beta blocker* used to treat irregular heartbeat.

estradiol a *sex hormone* used to treat estrogen deficiency in menopausal women and to treat some types of prostate and breast cancer.

estramustine an *anticancer drug.*

estrogens see *sex hormones (female).*

estrogens, conjugated *sex hormones* used as hormone replacement therapy in postmenopausal women.

estrogens, esterified *sex hormones* used in hormone replacement therapy.

estrone a *sex hormone* used to treat symptoms of menopause, underactivity of ovaries or testes, and prostate cancer.

estropipate a *sex hormone* used to treat symptoms of underactivity of ovaries.

ethacrynate sodium a *diuretic* used to treat edema.

ethacrynic acid a *diuretic* used to treat edema.

ethambutol an *antibacterial* used to treat tuberculosis.

ethchlorvynol a *sleeping drug.*

ethinamate a *sleeping drug.*

ethinyl estradiol a *sex hormone* (estrogen) used in oral contraceptives.

ethionamide an *antibacterial* used to treat tuberculosis and leprosy.

ethopropazine a drug used to treat parkinsonism.

ethosuximide an *anticonvulsant* primarily used to treat epilepsy.

ethotoin an *anticonvulsant* used to treat epilepsy.

etidronate a drug used to treat Paget's disease (bone formation disorder) and osteoporosis (decreased bone density).

etodolac an NSAID *analgesic* used to treat osteoarthritis.

etoposide an *anticancer drug.*

etretinate a vitamin A derivative used to treat psoriasis (skin disorder).

expectorant a drug that stimulates the flow of saliva and promotes coughing to eliminate phlegm from the respiratory tract.

F

factor VII a preparation containing human antihemophilic factor derived from blood plasma, used to treat hemophilia A.

factor IX complex a preparation containing blood

coagulation factors and other blood proteins, used to treat hemophilia B and Christmas disease.

famotidine a drug used to treat peptic ulcers.

fenfluramine a drug that stimulates the central nervous system; used to suppress appetite.

fenoprofen an NSAID *analgesic* used to treat pain, stiffness, and inflammation (especially arthritis).

ferrous sulfate a mineral used to treat iron deficiency anemia.

fibrinolytic drugs these dissolve recently formed blood clots in arteries and veins and are used to treat coronary thrombosis and venous thromboembolism.

filgrastim a preparation containing human blood proteins, used to treat side effects of *anticancer drugs.*

finasteride an enzyme inhibitor used to treat enlarged prostate.

flecainide an *antiarrhythmic* used to treat life-threatening irregular heartbeat.

floxuridine an *anticancer drug.*

fluconazole an *antifungal.*

flucytosine an *antifungal.*

fludrocortisone a *cortico-steroid* used in the treatment of Addison's disease.

flunisolide a *corticosteroid* primarily used to treat asthma and hay fever.

fluocinolone a topical *corticosteroid* used to treat inflammation and allergic skin disorders.

fluocinonide a topical *corticosteroid* used to treat inflammation and allergic skin disorders.

fluorometholone a topical *corticosteroid* used to treat eye disorders.

fluorouracil an *anticancer drug.*

fluoxetine an *antidepressant.*

fluoxymesterone a *sex hormone* used to treat underactive testes and delayed puberty in men.

fluphenazine an *antipsychotic* used to treat mental disorders.

flurandrenolide a topical *corticosteroid* used to treat inflammation and allergic skin disorders.

flurazepam a drug primarily used to induce sleep.

flurbiprofen an NSAID *analgesic* used to treat pain, stiffness, and inflammation (especially arthritis).

flutamide a *hormone* drug used to treat prostate cancer.

foscarnet an *antiviral* used to treat cytomegalovirus retinitis in AIDS patients.

fungicides see *antifungals.*

furosemide a *diuretic* used to treat high blood pressure and edema.

G

ganciclovir an *antiviral* used to treat cytomegalovirus retinitis in AIDS patients and others with suppressed immune systems.

gemfibrozil a *lipid-lowering drug* used to reduce levels of fatty substances in the blood.

gentamicin an aminoglycoside *antibiotic.*

gentian violet an antiseptic skin preparation.

glipizide a *hypoglycemic* drug used to treat diabetes mellitus.

glucagon a *hormone* drug used in emergency treatment of very low blood sugar levels in people with diabetes mellitus.

glutethimide a *sedative* used to induce sleep.

glyburide an oral *hypoglycemic* drug used to treat diabetes.

glycerin ingredient in cough mixtures, skin preparations, laxative suppositories, and earwax-softening drops.

gold sodium thiomalate an *antirheumatic* gold compound used in the treatment of arthritis.

gonadotropin, human chorionic a *hormone* drug used to treat infertility.

goserelin acetate a *hormone* drug used to treat prostate cancer and fibroids (non-cancerous growths in the uterus).

gramicidin an *antibiotic* used topically to treat eye infections.

griseofulvin an *antifungal.*

growth hormone a *hormone* drug used to treat short stature in children due to a disorder of the pituitary gland.

guanabenz a drug used to treat high blood pressure.

guanadrel a drug used to treat high blood pressure.

guanethidine a drug used to treat high blood pressure.

guanfacine a drug used to treat high blood pressure.

H

halazepam an *antianxiety drug.*

halcinonide a topical *corticosteroid* used to treat inflammation and allergic skin disorders.

haloperidol an *antipsychotic* used to treat agitated dementia; also used to treat Tourette's syndrome.

haloprogin a topical *antifungal.*

heparin an *anticoagulant* used to prevent blood clots.

hormones chemicals produced naturally by the endocrine glands (thyroid, adrenal, ovary, testis, pancreas, parathyroid). In some disorders, for example, diabetes mellitus, in which too little of a particular hormone is produced, synthetic equivalents or natural hormone extracts are prescribed to restore the deficiency. Such treatment is known as hormone replacement therapy. For other uses of hormones, in particular the *corticosteroids* and *sex hormones,* and for side effects, see appropriate entries in this glossary.

hydralazine a *vasodilator* used to treat high blood pressure.

hydrochlorothiazide a *diuretic* used to treat high blood pressure and edema.

hydrocodone a narcotic *cough suppressant.*

hydrocortisone a *hormone* drug used to treat Addison's disease (underactive adrenal glands) and to treat inflammation.

hydroflumethiazide a *diuretic* used to treat high blood pressure and edema.

hydromorphone a narcotic *analgesic* (painkiller).

hydroquinone a topical drug used to bleach the skin in people with pigmentation disorders.

hydroxychloroquine a drug used to treat malaria; an *antirheumatic* used to treat arthritis.

hydroxyprogesterone a *hormone* drug used to treat a variety of menstrual disorders.

hydroxyurea an *anticancer drug.*

hydroxyzine an *antihistamine* used to treat allergic skin conditions; also used as a *sedative* to induce sleep and occasionally to treat anxiety.

hyoscyamine a drug used to treat irritable bowel syndrome.

hypnotics see *sleeping drugs.*

hypoglycemics (oral) drugs that lower the level of glucose in the blood; used to treat diabetes mellitus. Oral hypoglycemic drugs are used if the diabetes cannot be controlled by diet alone, but does not require treatment with injections of insulin. Possible side effects: loss of appetite, nausea, indigestion, numbness or tingling in the skin, fever, rashes, jaundice. If the glucose level falls too low, weakness, giddiness, pallor, sweating, increased saliva flow, palpitations, irritability, and trembling may result. If such symptoms occur several hours after eating, this indicates that the dose of the medication is too high and the symptoms should be reported to the physician.

I

ibuprofen an NSAID *analgesic* used to treat pain, stiffness, and inflammation (especially arthritis).

idoxuridine an *antiviral* used topically to treat herpes simplex infections of the eye.

ifosfamide an *anticancer drug.*

imipramine a tricyclic *antidepressant;* also used in treatment of bed-wetting in children.

immunosuppressants drugs that prevent or reduce the body's usual reaction to invasion by disease or by foreign tissues. Immunosuppressants are used to treat autoimmune diseases (in which the body's defenses work abnormally, and attack its own cells and tissues) and to help prevent the body from rejecting organ transplants. Most drugs used in this way are *anticancer drugs* or *corticosteroids.*

indapamide a *diuretic* used to treat high blood pressure and edema.

indomethacin an NSAID *analgesic* used to treat pain, stiffness, and inflammation (especially arthritis).

insulin a *hormone* drug used to treat diabetes.

interferons a group of drugs, prepared from blood proteins, that are *antiviral* and *anticancer.*

interleukins a group of drugs, prepared from blood proteins, that alter the immune response and act as *anticancer drugs.*

iodoquinol a drug used to treat disease caused by protozoa (single-celled organisms).

ipecac a drug used to induce vomiting in cases of drug poisoning.

ipratropium a *bronchodilator* primarily used to treat narrowing of airways of the lungs.

isocarboxazid an MAOI *antidepressant.*

isoetharine a *bronchodilator* primarily used as an inhalant to treat narrowing of airways of the lungs.

isoflurophate a drug used to treat glaucoma.

isoniazid an *antibacterial* used to treat tuberculosis.

isopropyl alcohol a topical antiseptic (prevents infection).

isoproterenol a *bronchodilator* primarily used to treat irregular heartbeat and narrowing of airways of the lungs.

isosorbide dinitrate a *vasodilator* used to treat angina.

isotretinoin a derivative of vitamin A used topically to treat severe acne.

K

kanamycin an aminoglycoside *antibiotic.*

kaolin a substance that can adsorb (attract and retain) bacteria, viruses, and poisons; used as an ingredient of some antidiarrheal drugs.

ketoconazole an *antifungal.*

ketoprofen an NSAID *analgesic* used to treat pain, stiffness, and inflammation (especially arthritis).

ketorolac an NSAID *analgesic* used to treat pain, stiffness, and inflammation (especially arthritis).

L

labetalol a *beta blocker* used to treat high blood pressure.

lactulose a *laxative*; also used to treat dementia caused by cirrhosis.

lanolin a preparation used in the treatment of dry skin.

laxatives drugs that increase the frequency and ease of bowel movements, either by stimulating the bowel wall (stimulant laxative), by increasing the bulk of colon contents (bulk laxative), or by lubricating them (stool softeners). Laxatives may be taken by mouth or directly into the lower bowel as suppositories or enemas. Bulk laxatives must be taken with plenty of water. If laxatives are taken regularly, the bowels may ultimately become unable to work properly without them.

leucovorin a substance used to counteract adverse effects of some *anticancer drugs.*

leuprolide a *hormone* drug used to treat prostate cancer and endometriosis.

levamisole an *anticancer drug*; also used to treat parasitic infestations.

levobunolol a *beta blocker* used to treat glaucoma.

levodopa a drug used to treat parkinsonism.

levorphanol a narcotic *analgesic* (painkiller).

levothyroxine a *hormone* drug used to treat hypothyroidism (underactivity of the thyroid gland).

lidocaine a local anesthetic and *antiarrhythmic* used to treat irregular heartbeat.

lincomycin an *antibiotic.*

lindane a topical drug used to treat scabies and lice infestations.

liothyronine a *hormone* drug used to treat hypothyroidism (underactivity of thyroid gland).

liotrix a *hormone* drug used to treat hypothyroidism (underactivity of thyroid gland).

lipid-lowering drugs these drugs control the level of fatty substances in the blood. People with atherosclerosis (a condition in which fatty plaque clogs the arteries) take these drugs, preferably in combination with a low-fat diet. Lipid-lowering drugs are taken orally and often are prescribed for indefinite periods of time. Side effects may include cramps, changed sense of taste, change in bowel movements, gas, heartburn, indigestion, and nausea. Lipid-lowering drugs taken in combination with selected other drugs can cause serious interactions; ask your physician about this.

lisinopril an *ACE inhibitor* used to treat high blood pressure and heart failure.

lithium a drug used to treat the manic phase of manic-depressive illness.

lomustine an *anticancer drug.*

loperamide an *antidiarrheal.*

lorazepam an *antianxiety drug*; also used to treat insomnia.

lovastatin a *lipid-lowering drug* used to reduce the level of cholesterol in the blood.

loxapine an *antipsychotic* used to treat mental disorders.

lymphocyte immune globulin an *immunosuppressant* used to prevent tissue rejection in kidney transplant patients.

lypressin a *hormone* drug used as an antidiuretic.

M

mafenide an *antibacterial* used topically to treat serious burns.

magnesium hydroxide an *antacid* and a *laxative.*

magnesium oxide an *antacid.*

magnesium salicylate an *anti-inflammatory* used to treat arthritis.

magnesium sulfate an *anticonvulsant* primarily used to treat or prevent convulsions associated with some conditions in pregnancy; also used as a *laxative.*

mannitol a *diuretic* used to treat glaucoma and swelling of the brain.

maprotiline a tetracyclic *antidepressant.*

mazindol a drug that stimulates the central nervous system; used to suppress appetite.

mebendazole a drug primarily used to treat worm infestations.

mecamylamine a drug used to treat severe high blood pressure.

mechlorethamine an *anticancer drug.*

meclizine an *antiemetic.*

meclocycline a tetracycline *antibiotic* used topically to treat acne.

meclofenamate an NSAID *analgesic* used to treat pain, stiffness, and inflammation (especially arthritis).

medroxyprogesterone a *hormone* drug used to treat a variety of menstrual disorders and in the treatment of cancers of the kidney and endometrium (lining of the uterus); also used as a long-acting contraceptive.

medrysone a topical *corticosteroid* used to treat inflammatory conditions of the eye.

mefenamic acid an NSAID *analgesic* used to treat pain, stiffness, and inflammation (especially arthritis).

mefloquine a drug used to treat malaria.

megestrol a *hormone* drug used to treat cancers of the breast and endometrium (lining of the uterus).

melphalan an *anticancer drug.*

menotropins a *hormone* drug used to treat infertility.

meperidine a narcotic *analgesic* (painkiller).

mephenytoin an *anticonvulsant* used to treat epilepsy.

mephobarbital a *barbiturate* used as a *sedative* and to control epileptic seizures.

mepivacaine a local anesthetic (causes lack of sensation).

meprobamate a *sedative* used to treat anxiety.

mercaptopurine an *anticancer drug.*

mesalamine an aspirin derivative used to treat ulcerative colitis.

mesoridazine an *antipsychotic* used to treat mental disorders.

metaproterenol a *bronchodilator* used to treat narrowing of airways in the lungs caused by muscle spasm.

metaraminol a drug used to treat shock.

methacycline a tetracycline *antibiotic.*

methadone a narcotic *analgesic* used to treat heroin addiction and withdrawal symptoms.

methamphetamine a drug that stimulates the central nervous system; used to treat attention deficit disorder and to suppress appetite.

methandrostenolone an anabolic steroid used to treat osteoporosis.

metharbital a *barbiturate* used to treat epilepsy.

methazolamide a weak *diuretic* used to treat glaucoma.

methdilazine an *antihistamine* primarily used to treat allergies.

methenamine an *antibacterial* used to treat urinary tract infections.

methicillin a penicillin *antibiotic.*

methimazole a drug used to treat hyperthyroidism (overactivity of the thyroid).

methocarbamol a *muscle relaxant.*

methotrexate an *anticancer drug*; also used to treat psoriasis (skin disease) and arthritis.

methoxsalen a drug used to treat psoriasis (skin disease) and vitiligo (disorder of skin pigmentation).

methsuximide an *anticonvulsant* used in the treatment of epilepsy.

methyldopa a drug used primarily to treat high blood pressure and Raynaud's disease (disorder of the blood vessels).

methylene blue a substance used as an antidote for cyanide poisoning.

methylergonovine a drug used to stimulate contractions of the uterus during labor.

methylformamide an *anticancer drug.*

methylphenidate a drug that stimulates the central nervous system; used to treat narcolepsy (sleep disorder) and sometimes used to treat attention deficit disorder.

methylprednisolone a *corticosteroid* used to treat inflammation.

methyltestosterone a *hormone* drug used to treat hypogonadism (underactivity of the testes) and impotence caused by hypogonadism.

methyprylon a *sedative* used to induce sleep.

methysergide a drug used to prevent migraine headache.

metoclopramide a drug used to stimulate stomach emptying into the small intestine; also used as an *antiemetic* to treat nausea and vomiting associated with *anticancer drugs.*

metolazone a weak *diuretic* used to treat glaucoma.

metoprolol a *beta blocker* primarily used to treat angina and high blood pressure.

metronidazole an *antibacterial*; also used to treat disease caused by protozoa (single-cell organisms).

metyrosine a drug primarily used to treat pheochromocytoma (tumor causing excess hormone secretion).

mexiletine an *antiarrhythmic* used to treat irregular heartbeat.

mezlocillin a penicillin *antibiotic.*

miconazole an *antifungal.*

minor tranquilizers see *antianxiety drugs.*

minoxidil an *antihypertensive*; also used to stimulate hair growth.

mitomycin an *anticancer drug.*

mitotane an *anticancer drug.*

mitoxantrone an *anticancer drug.*

molindone an *antipsychotic* used to treat acute psychosis.

mometasone furoate a topical *corticosteroid* used to treat inflammation and allergic skin disorders.

monobenzone a depigmenting agent used to treat severe vitiligo (disorder of skin pigmentation).

moricizine an *antiarrhythmic* used to treat life-threatening irregular heartbeat.

morphine a narcotic *analgesic* (painkiller).

moxalactam a cephalosporin *antibiotic.*

muscle relaxants drugs that relieve muscle spasm in disorders such as backache. *Antianxiety drugs*, which also have a muscle-relaxant action, are used most commonly. This term is applied also to drugs such as curare that are used only during surgery.

N

nabilone an *antiemetic* used to treat nausea and vomiting.

nabumetone an NSAID *analgesic* used to treat osteoarthritis and rheumatoid arthritis.

nadolol a *beta blocker* primarily used to treat angina and high blood pressure.

nafarelin a *hormone drug* used to treat endometriosis.

nafcillin a penicillin *antibiotic.*

naftifine an *antifungal.*

nalbuphine a narcotic *analgesic* (painkiller).

nalidixic acid an *antibacterial* used to treat urinary tract infections.

naloxone used as an antidote for narcotic drug poisoning.

naltrexone a drug used to treat narcotic drug addiction.

nandrolone an anabolic steroid used to treat some types of anemias.

naphazoline a *decongestant.*

naproxen an NSAID *analgesic* used to treat pain, stiffness, and inflammation (especially arthritis).

natamycin an *antifungal.*

neomycin an aminoglycoside *antibiotic.*

neostigmine a drug used to treat myasthenia gravis (muscle disorder).

netilmicin an aminoglycoside *antibiotic.*

niacin a *lipid-lowering drug* used to reduce the level of fatty substances in the blood.

niacinamide a *lipid-lowering drug* used to reduce the level of fatty substances in the blood.

nicardipine a *calcium channel blocker* primarily used to treat high blood pressure and angina.

niclosamide a drug used to treat worm infestations.

nicotine polacrilex a gum used to help the symptoms of nicotine withdrawal.

nifedipine a *calcium channel blocker* primarily used to treat angina; in the sustained-release form, used to treat high blood pressure.

nifurtimox a drug used to treat diseases caused by protozoa (single-cell organisms).

nimodipine a *calcium channel blocker* used to treat spasm after bleeding from an aneurysm (ballooning of an artery) in the brain, and for migraine headache; also used investigationally in the treatment of stroke.

nitrofurantoin an *antibacterial* used to treat urinary tract infections.

nitrofurazone an *antibacterial* used topically in the treatment of burns.

nitroglycerin a drug used to relieve pain caused by angina and congestive heart failure.

nizatidine a drug used to treat peptic ulcers.

nonoxynol 9 a spermicide used as a contraceptive.

norepinephrine a chemical messenger produced in the body and *hormone* used to treat shock.

norethindrone a *hormone* drug used in oral contraceptives.

norfloxacin an *antibacterial* used to treat urinary tract infections.

norgestrel a *hormone* drug used in oral contraceptives.

nortriptyline a tricyclic *antidepressant.*

nystatin an *antifungal.*

O

octoxynol a spermicide used as a contraceptive.

octreotide acetate a derivative of a *hormone* drug used to treat the diarrhea associated with some types of tumors.

ofloxacin an *antibacterial* used to treat urinary tract infection.

olsalazine a drug used to treat inflammatory bowel disease.

omeprazole a drug used to treat peptic ulcers.

ondansetron an *antiemetic* injection used to prevent chemotherapy-induced nausea and vomiting.

oral contraceptives see *sex hormones (female).*

orphenadrine an anticholinergic (blocks muscle contractions) *antispasmodic* used to treat muscle spasm and nocturnal leg cramps.

oxacillin a penicillin *antibiotic.*

oxaprozin an NSAID *analgesic* used to treat osteoarthritis and rheumatoid arthritis.

oxazepam an *antianxiety drug*; also used to treat insomnia.

oxiconazole nitrate an *antifungal.*

oxtriphylline a *bronchodilator* primarily used to treat asthma.

oxybutynin a drug used to treat urinary incontinence.

oxycodone a narcotic *analgesic* (painkiller).

oxymetazoline a *decongestant.*

oxymetholone an anabolic steroid used to treat some types of anemia.

oxymorphone a narcotic *analgesic* (painkiller).

oxyphencyclimine a drug used to treat peptic ulcers.

oxytetracycline a tetracycline *antibiotic.*

oxytocin a *hormone* drug used to induce labor and to control bleeding after childbirth.

P

paclitaxel an *anticancer drug* derived from yew trees, used to treat ovarian cancer.

painkillers see *analgesics.*

pamidronate a drug used to treat Paget's disease, hypercalcemia, and other bone-loss conditions.

pancreatin a preparation containing pancreatic enzymes; used in pancreatic deficiency.

pancrelipase a preparation containing pancreatic enzymes; used in pancreatic deficiency.

papaverine a *vasodilator* primarily used to treat circulatory problems.

para-aminobenzoic acid a sunscreen.

paramethadione an *anticonvulsant* used to treat epilepsy.

paramethasone a *corticosteroid* used to treat inflammatory or allergic conditions.

paregoric a narcotic *antidiarrheal.*

paromomycin an aminoglycoside *antibiotic*; a drug used to treat worm infestation or protozoal diseases.

pemoline a drug that stimulates the central nervous system; sometimes used to treat attention deficit disorder.

penbutolol a *beta blocker* used to treat high blood pressure.

penicillamine an *antirheumatic* used to treat rheumatoid arthritis; also used to treat metal poisoning and a form of cirrhosis.

penicillin G a penicillin *antibiotic.*

penicillin G benzathine a penicillin *antibiotic.*

penicillin V a penicillin *antibiotic.*

pentaerythritol tetranitrate a *vasodilator* used to treat angina.

pentamidine a drug used to treat pneumonia caused by *Pneumocystis carinii.*

pentazocine a narcotic *analgesic* (painkiller).

pentobarbital a *barbiturate* used to treat insomnia.

pentostatin an *anticancer drug* used to treat hairy-cell leukemia.

pentoxyfylline a drug used to treat intermittent claudication and sometimes transient ischemic attacks.

pergolide a dopamine-boosting drug used to treat parkinsonism and to regulate ovarian function and breast milk secretion.

permethrin a drug used to treat head-lice infestation.

perphenazine an *antipsychotic*; also used as an *antiemetic.*

phenazopyridine an *analgesic* used to treat pain caused by urinary tract infection.

phendimetrazine a drug that stimulates the central nervous system; used to suppress appetite.

phenelzine an MAOI *antidepressant.*

phenindamine an *antihistamine* primarily used to treat allergies.

phenobarbital a *barbiturate* used to treat epilepsy and anxiety.

phenoxybenzamine a drug used to treat pheochromocytoma.

phentermine a drug that stimulates the central nervous system; used to suppress appetite.

phentolamine a drug used to treat pheochromocytoma.

phenylbutazone an NSAID *analgesic* used to treat pain,

stiffness, and inflammation (especially arthritis).

phenylephrine a *decongestant.*

phenylpropanolamine a *decongestant*; also used to suppress appetite.

phenytoin an *anticonvulsant* used to treat epilepsy.

physostigmine a drug used to treat glaucoma.

the pill oral contraceptives; see *sex hormones (female).*

pilocarpine a drug used to treat glaucoma.

pindolol a *beta blocker* used to treat high blood pressure.

piperacillin a penicillin *antibiotic.*

piperazine a drug used to treat worm infestations.

pirbuterol acetate a *broncho-dilator* used to treat narrowing of airways of the lungs.

piroxicam an NSAID *analgesic* used to treat pain, stiffness, and inflammation (especially arthritis).

plicamycin an *anticancer drug*; also used to treat high levels of calcium in the blood.

podophyllin a topical drug used to treat genital warts.

polycarbophil a bulk-forming *laxative.*

polymyxin B an *antibacterial* used to treat skin infections.

polythiazide a *diuretic* used to treat high blood pressure.

potassium iodide an *expecto-rant* (promotes coughing up of mucus); also used to treat hyperthyroidism (overactivity of the thyroid gland).

povidone-iodine a topical antiseptic (prevents infection).

pralidoxime an antidote to poisoning by some pesticides.

pramoxine a topical anesthetic (causes loss of sensation).

pravastatin a *lipid-lowering drug.*

prazepam an *antianxiety drug.*

praziquantel a drug used to treat worm infestation.

prazosin a drug used to treat high blood pressure and prostate problems.

prednisolone a *corticosteroid* used to treat inflammation and symptoms of a variety of disorders (including skin disorders, eye irritations, and ulceration of the colon).

prednisone a *corticosteroid* primarily used to treat inflammatory bowel disease and rheumatoid arthritis (inflammatory disorders).

primaquine a drug used to treat malaria.

probenecid a drug used to reduce uric acid levels that occur with gout; also used to enhance levels of penicillin and cephalosporin antibiotics.

probucol a *lipid-lowering drug* used to reduce the level of fatty substances in the blood.

procainamide an *antiarrhythmic* used to treat irregular heartbeat.

procarbazine an *anticancer drug.*

prochlorperazine an *antiemetic* used to treat nausea and vomiting; an *antipsychotic* used to treat mental disorders.

procyclidine a drug used to treat parkinsonism.

promazine an *antipsychotic* used to treat psychosis.

promethazine an *antihistamine* primarily used to treat allergy; an *antiemetic* used to treat nausea and vomiting.

propafenone an *antiarrhythmic* used to treat irregular heartbeat.

propantheline an *antispasmodic* used to treat peptic ulcers.

propoxyphene a narcotic *analgesic* (painkiller).

propranolol a *beta blocker* used to treat angina, heart attack, and high blood pressure; used to prevent migraine headache.

propylhexedrine a *decongestant.*

propylthiouracil a drug used to treat hyperthyroidism (overactive thyroid gland).

protriptyline a tricyclic *antidepressant.*

pseudoephedrine a *decongestant.*

psyllium a bulk-forming *laxative.*

pyrantel a drug used to treat worm infestations.

pyrazinamide an *antibacterial* used to treat tuberculosis.

pyrethrin a drug used to treat lice infestation.

pyridostigmine a drug used to treat myasthenia gravis.

pyrilamine an *antihistamine* primarily used to treat allergies.

pyrimethamine a drug used to treat malaria (combined with sulfadoxine).

Q

quazepam an *antianxiety drug* used to treat insomnia.

quinacrine a drug used to treat giardiasis.

quinapril an *antihypertensive.*

quinestrol a *hormone* drug used to treat symptoms of menopause.

quinethazone a *diuretic* primarily used to treat high blood pressure.

quinidine an *antiarrhythmic* used to treat irregular heartbeat.

quinine a drug used to treat malaria; also used to treat nighttime cramping of the legs.

R

ramipril an *antihypertensive.*

ranitidine a drug used to treat peptic ulcers.

ribavirin an *antiviral* used to treat viral infections of the respiratory tract in high-risk infants.

rifampin an *antibacterial* used to treat tuberculosis.

S

salicylic acid a drug used to treat acne, warts, and other skin disorders.

salsalate an NSAID *analgesic* used to treat pain, stiffness, and inflammation (especially arthritis).

scopolamine an *antispasmodic* used to prevent motion sickness.

secobarbital a *barbiturate* primarily used to induce sleep.

sedatives see *antianxiety drugs.*

selegiline a drug used to treat parkinsonism.

selenium sulfide an agent included in dandruff shampoos.

semustine an *anticancer drug.*

sertraline an *antidepressant.*

sex hormones (female) there are two groups of these hormones (estrogens and progesterone), which are responsible for development of female secondary sexual characteristics. Small amounts are produced in males. As drugs, female sex hormones are used to treat menstrual and menopausal disorders and are also used as oral contra-ceptives. Estrogens may be used to treat cancer of the breast or prostate, progestins (synthetic forms of proges-terone) to treat endometriosis. Sex hormones may be taken orally, given by injections, implanted in muscle tissue, or worn in a skin patch. Possible side effects: nausea, weight gain, headache, depression, breast enlargement and tenderness, skin problems, changes in sexual drive, and abnormal blood clotting, which can cause heart attack, stroke, or venous thrombosis. Estrogen treatment is usually not prescribed for anyone who has circulatory or liver disorders, and must be carefully controlled for people who have had jaundice, diabetes, epilepsy, or heart or kidney disease. The risk of clotting disorders and strokes is greater in patients who smoke and also increases with age. Progestin is usually not prescribed for people with liver disorders and must be carefully controlled for anyone who has asthma, epilepsy, or heart or kidney disease.

sex hormones (male) androgenic hormones, of

which the most powerful is testosterone, are responsible for development of male secondary sexual characteristics. Small quantities are also produced in females. As drugs, male sex hormones are given to compensate for hormone deficiency in hypopituitarism or disorders of the testes. They may be used to treat breast cancer in women, but either synthetic derivatives (anabolic steroids), which have less marked side effects, or specific antiestrogens are often preferred. Anabolic steroids also have a "body building" effect that has led to their (usually nonsanctioned) use in competitive sports, for both men and women. Male sex hormones (androgens) and anabolic steroids can be taken as tablets, given by injection, or implanted in muscle tissue. Possible side effects: edema, weight gain, weakness, loss of appetite, drowsiness, nausea. High doses in women may cause increased libido, cessation of menstruation, enlargement of the clitoris, deepening of the voice, shrinking of the breasts, hairiness, or male-pattern baldness. These hormones are usually not prescribed for people with kidney or liver problems and must be carefully controlled for anyone who has epilepsy or migraine headaches.

silver nitrate a chemical used topically to prevent gonorrheal eye infections in newborns; also used to cauterize tissue.

silver sulfadiazine an *antibacterial* used to treat burns.

simvastatin a *lipid-lowering drug* used to reduce the level of fatty substances in the blood.

sleeping drugs the two main groups of drugs that are used to induce sleep are *antianxiety drugs* and barbiturates. All such drugs have a sedative effect in low doses and are effective sleeping medications in higher doses. *Antianxiety drugs* are used more widely than barbiturates because they are safer, the side effects are less marked, and there is less risk of eventual physical dependence. Possible side effects of all types: "hangover," dizziness, dry mouth, and (especially in the elderly) clumsiness and confusion. Sleeping drugs are habit-forming, should be taken for short periods only, and should be discontinued gradually. Broken, restless sleep and vivid dreams may follow withdrawal and may persist for weeks. Driving, operating dangerous machinery, and drinking alcohol are not recommended until the effects of a sleeping drug have completely worn off.

sodium bicarbonate an *antacid.*

sodium iodide a drug used to treat hypothyroidism (underactive thyroid gland) and some cancers of the thyroid gland.

sodium nitroprusside a *vasodilator* used to treat extremely high blood pressure in emergencies.

sodium salicylate an NSAID *analgesic* used to treat pain, stiffness, and inflammation (especially arthritis).

sodium thiosulfate an antidote for cyanide poisoning.

somatropin a *hormone* drug used to treat growth hormone deficiency in children.

spectinomycin an *antibiotic* used to treat penicillin-resistant gonorrhea.

spironolactone a *diuretic* used to treat overproduction of the hormone aldosterone and in combination with a thiazide *diuretic* to treat high blood pressure or edema.

stanozolol an anabolic steroid used to reduce the frequency and severity of angioedema (an allergic reaction).

stibocaptate a drug used to treat worm infestations.

stibogluconate a drug used to treat disease caused by protozoa (single-cell organisms).

streptokinase a *thrombolytic* used to dissolve blood clots.

streptomycin an *antibiotic.*

streptozocin an *anticancer drug.*

sucralfate a drug used to treat peptic ulcers.

sulconazole nitrate an *antifungal* primarily used to treat superficial skin infections.

sulfacetamide an *antibacterial* used to treat vaginal infections and superficial eye infections.

sulfadiazine an *antibacterial.*

sulfadoxine a drug used with pyrimethamine to treat drug-resistant malaria.

sulfamethizole an *antibacterial.*

sulfamethoxazole an *antibacterial* used to treat urinary tract infections.

sulfamethoxazole/ trimethoprim a combination *antibacterial* commonly used to treat urinary tract infections.

sulfasalazine an *anti-inflammatory* used in the treatment of inflammatory bowel disease.

sulfinpyrazone a drug that promotes urinary excretion of uric acid in order to prevent gout attacks.

sulfisoxazole an *antibacterial* used to treat eye infections.

sulindac an NSAID *analgesic* used to treat pain, stiffness, and inflammation (especially arthritis).

sumatriptan a drug used to treat acute migraine headache attacks.

suramin a drug used to treat sleeping sickness.

T

tamoxifen an *anticancer drug.*

temazepam an *antianxiety drug.*

terazosin a drug used to treat high blood pressure, female urethral syndrome, and enlarged prostate.

terbutaline a *bronchodilator* used to treat narrowing of airways in the lungs.

terconazole an *antifungal.*

terfenadine a nonsedating *antihistamine.*

testolactone an *anticancer drug.*

testosterone a *hormone* drug used to promote male sexual characteristics when testicular function is deficient or absent.

tetracaine a local and topical anesthetic (causes loss of sensation).

tetracycline a tetracycline *antibiotic.*

theophylline a *bronchodilator* used to treat narrowing of airways in the lungs.

thiethylperazine an *antiemetic* used to treat nausea and vomiting.

thioguanine an *anticancer drug.*

thioridazine an *antipsychotic* primarily used to treat schizophrenia.

thiotepa an *anticancer drug.*

thiothixene an *antipsychotic* used to treat psychosis.

thrombolytics drugs that help dissolve and disperse blood clots and may be prescribed for people with recent arterial or venous thrombosis.

ticarcillin a penicillin *antibiotic.*

ticlopidine a drug used to prevent recurrence of stroke.

timolol a *beta blocker* used to treat heart attacks and high blood pressure; also used to treat glaucoma.

tioconozole an *antifungal* used to treat yeast infection (candidiasis).

tobramycin an aminoglycoside *antibiotic.*

tocainide an *antiarrhythmic* used to treat life-threatening irregular heartbeat.

tolazamide a *hypoglycemic* drug used to treat diabetes mellitus.

tolbutamide a *hypoglycemic* drug used to treat diabetes mellitus.

tolmetin an NSAID *analgesic* used to treat pain, stiffness, and inflammation (especially arthritis).

tolnaftate an *antifungal.*

tranquilizer this is a term commonly used to describe any drug that has a calming or sedative effect. However, the drugs that are sometimes called minor tranquilizers should be called *antianxiety drugs*, and the drugs that are sometimes called major tranquilizers should be called *antipsychotics*.

trazodone an *antidepressant*.

tretinoin a derivative of vitamin A used to treat acne.

triacetin an *antifungal*.

triamcinolone a *corticosteroid* used to treat inflammatory disorders.

triamterene a *diuretic* primarily used in combination with a thiazide diuretic to treat high blood pressure and edema.

triazolam an *antianxiety drug*; also used to treat insomnia.

trichlormethiazide a *diuretic* used to treat high blood pressure and edema and to prevent some types of kidney stones.

trientine a drug that removes excess copper in the treatment of Wilson's disease.

trifluoperazine an *antipsychotic* used to treat mental disorders.

triflupromazine an *antipsychotic* used to treat mental disorders; an *antiemetic* used to treat nausea and vomiting.

trifluridine an *antiviral* used to treat herpes virus infections of the eye.

trihexyphenidyl a drug used to treat parkinsonism.

trilostane a drug used in the treatment of Cushing's syndrome.

trimeprazine an *antihistamine* used to treat itching.

trimethadione an *anticonvulsant* used to treat epilepsy.

trimethaphan a drug used to reduce blood pressure in emergencies.

trimethobenzamide an *antiemetic* used to treat nausea and vomiting.

trimethoprim an *antibacterial* used to treat urinary tract infections.

trimipramine a tricyclic *antidepressant*.

trioxsalen a drug used to treat vitiligo (disorder of skin pigmentation).

tripelennamine an *antihistamine* primarily used to treat seasonal allergies.

triprolidine an *antihistamine* primarily used to treat allergies.

tropicamide a drug used to dilate the pupil.

trypsin a naturally occurring enzyme used to treat malabsorption.

U

urea a natural substance included in remedies for dry skin.

urofollitropin a *hormone* drug used to induce ovulation (to treat infertility).

urokinase a *thrombolytic* used to dissolve blood clots.

ursodiol a drug used to dissolve gallstones.

V

valproic acid an *anticonvulsant* primarily used to treat epilepsy.

vancomycin an *antibiotic*.

vasodilators drugs that dilate blood vessels. These medications are used to prevent and treat angina, but they are also useful for treating heart failure and certain circulatory disorders. Vasodilators are taken as tablets, often dissolved beneath the tongue for rapid action. Possible side effects: headache, palpitations, faintness, nausea, vomiting, diarrhea, nasal stuffiness.

vasopressin a *hormone* drug used to treat diabetes insipidus.

verapamil a *calcium channel blocker* used to treat angina, irregular heartbeat, and high blood pressure; also used to prevent migraine headache.

vidarabine an *antiviral* used to treat herpes virus infections.

vinblastine an *anticancer drug*.

vincristine an *anticancer drug*.

vindesine an *anticancer drug*

vitamins chemicals essential for good health. Some vitamins are not manufactured by the body, but adequate quantities are present in a normal diet. People whose diets are inadequate or who have digestive tract or liver disorders may need to take supplementary vitamins. These are generally available without a prescription; see tables of vitamins and minerals, p.534.

warfarin an *anticoagulant* primarily used to prevent blood clots.

witch hazel a soothing astringent.

X

xylometazoline a *decongestant*.

Z

zidovudine an *antiviral* used in the treatment of AIDS.

zinc oxide a soothing agent used in skin preparations and sunscreens.

zinc sulfate an astringent.

Glossary

A

abortion a medical term describing either premature spontaneous loss of a fetus during pregnancy (see also *miscarriage* in this glossary) or elective termination of pregnancy (see Box, p.671).

abscess a collection of pus, caused by a local infection, that builds up and may spread into the bloodstream.

acupuncture a system of treatment in which needles are inserted into the skin and either left or manipulated for several minutes. The treatment is used most widely in China. Acupuncturists are not usually medical doctors.

acute a term used to describe an illness in which symptoms develop over only a few hours or, at most, a few days. A person with an acute illness recovers quickly; if the disease becomes long-lasting, it is chronic.

adhesion fibrous scars that form when tissues heal and cause adjacent organs to stick together. Adhesions in the abdomen may be painful when pulled or stretched, because fibrous tissue is not elastic.

AIDS acquired immune deficiency syndrome, a disorder of the body's immune system caused by infection with HIV (human immunodeficiency virus). People with AIDS have a significantly lowered resistance to various infections and diseases that are rarely found in people who are not infected with HIV. See AIDS, p.465.

allergen a substance, such as animal fur, pollen grains, or dust, that is normally harmless but causes an allergic reaction in susceptible people.

Alzheimer's disease an incurable, progressive, degenerative brain disorder of unknown cause that produces personality changes and gradual loss of memory and other intellectual functions. It is the most common cause of dementia in older people. See Dementia, p.314, and Dementia and aging, p.772.

amniocentesis a procedure in which a sample of fluid that surrounds the developing fetus in the uterus is removed through a needle. An examination of the cells, proteins, and other chemicals in the fluid enables physicians to diagnose, and in some cases monitor, certain fetal disorders.

anaphylactic shock an intense allergic reaction to a substance such as a drug or venom that quickly leads to difficulty in breathing and speaking, low blood pressure, rapid pulse, paleness, sweating, and collapse.

androgen the term applied to several male sex hormones that promote the development of male sexual characteristics. Androgens are produced by the testes and the adrenal glands. For further information see Sex hormones (male) in Drug glossary. See also *estrogen* in this glossary.

angiogram see *angiography.*

angiography a technique for examining blood vessels by injecting into them a solution visible on X rays. The passage of the solution can be followed on a monitor at the same time a recording is made on film of the appearance of the vessel. This record is called an angiogram.

angioplasty a procedure in which a catheter (see *catheter* in this glossary) with an attached inflatable balloon, boring tool, or laser is used to open a section of an artery that has become narrowed.

anoxia lack of oxygen. Anoxic tissues cannot function properly. If tissues are completely deprived of oxygen for more than a few minutes, they will die. See also *cyanosis* in this glossary.

antibodies complex substances formed to neutralize or destroy foreign substances or organisms (antigens) in the blood. Each individual type of antibody recognizes only the substance or organism that provokes its formation. Antibody activity normally fights infection but can be damaging in allergies and a group of diseases that are called autoimmune diseases.

antigen any substance, such as an infectious agent or a poison produced by it, that can be detected by the body's immune system. The immune system usually produces antibodies to combat the antigen.

appendectomy removal of the appendix, a small organ located at the point where the large and small intestines join. An inflamed appendix may rupture, spread pus through the abdomen, and eventually cause peritonitis.

arrhythmia variation in the regular rhythm of the heartbeat. Arrhythmias may cause serious conditions such as shock and congestive heart failure, or even death. They may be treated with drugs or electrical current. A pacemaker may be implanted to correct certain altered rhythms.

arteriogram see *arteriography.*

arteriography angiography of an artery. See *angiography* in this glossary. The resultant pictures are known as arteriograms.

arthroscopy examination of the inside of a joint with a viewing instrument.

ascites an abnormal collection of fluid inside the abdominal cavity resulting from cancer, infection, or disease of the heart, liver, or kidney.

aspiration a procedure in which fluid is sucked from a body cavity with an instrument such as a needle and syringe. The cavity may be a natural one (the abdominal cavity, for example), one made by disease (a liver abscess, for example), or one present from birth (a kidney cyst, for example).

ataxia lack of coordination in body movements due to some form of nerve or brain damage.

atheroma cholesterol that accumulates in an arterial wall and forms a build-up that narrows the artery.

atrophy shrinkage or wasting of one or more muscles from lack of use or of an organ such as the liver as a result of disease.

autoimmune a term used to describe a condition in which the body manufactures antibodies against its own tissues, and damages itself. Such a defect in the immune system produces symptoms of autoimmune disease (for instance, rheumatoid arthritis).

autopsy examination of a dead body in order to discover and document the cause of death.

B

bacteremia the presence of bacteria in the blood. This sometimes occurs after minor surgery, such as tooth extraction, is performed or when contaminated needles and syringes are shared by people who use intravenous drugs. Toxins produced by some of these bacteria can cause toxemia (see *toxemia* in this glossary) or septicemia (see Blood poisoning, p.452).

bacteria single-celled microorganisms with no nucleus that multiply by division and are visible under a conventional light microscope. Bacteria are classified according to their shape, such as cocci (round cells) or bacilli (rod- or cylinder-shaped cells).

balloon angioplasty see *angioplasty*.

barium enema an enema containing the chemical barium sulfate, which is visible on X-ray film. A series of pictures taken while the enema is retained in the large intestine, often while air is pumped into the large intestine, reveals the lining of the colon and rectum. See also *gastrointestinal (GI) series* in this glossary.

barium meal or swallow a liquid containing the chemical barium sulfate, which is visible on X-ray film. After you drink the liquid, its progress down the digestive tract is recorded on a series of X-ray pictures. The procedure is used to detect diseases of the digestive tract, including the esophagus, stomach, and duodenum. When necessary, the barium is also tracked into the small intestine via X ray. See also *gastro-intestinal (GI) series* in this glossary.

bedsores skin ulcers caused by prolonged pressure on parts of the body when a person is confined to bed or immobile. Bedsores occur most commonly on areas of the body where the person's weight presses against the mattress and blocks the normal flow of blood. See Preventing bedsores, p.792.

benign a term used to describe an abnormal growth that will neither spread to surrounding tissues nor recur after surgical removal. See also *malignant* in this glossary.

biopsy removal of a small piece of tissue for microscopic analysis from any area of the body that seems abnormal. Biopsies are usually performed in order to determine whether an abnormal growth is malignant or benign.

bisexuality see *sexuality*.

blood clot a clump of coagulated blood. The medical term for blood clot is thrombus (see *thrombus* in this glossary). When a blood clot breaks off and travels through the bloodstream it is called an embolus (see *embolus* in this glossary). An embolus may block an artery and cut off blood flow to the lungs, causing pulmonary embolism (see p.446), or to the brain, causing a stroke (see p.285).

blood poisoning (septicemia) invasion of the bloodstream by bacteria or fungi that may also form poisons. Blood poisoning was usually fatal before sulfa drugs and antibiotics became available.

blood pressure the pressure of the blood on the walls of the arteries, which varies with the demand placed on the circulatory system. Maximum (systolic) pressure occurs when the heart muscle contracts and blood surges through the aorta. Minimum (diastolic) pressure occurs when the ventricles and aorta relax between heartbeats. See Testing blood pressure, p.412.

blood test analysis of blood samples taken by puncturing an ear or finger or by putting a needle into a vein. A blood sample can be tested for counts of red blood cells, white blood cells, and platelets; antibodies to HIV or other infections; and hemoglobin concentrations. Levels of cholesterol, sugar, and triglycerides (fatlike substances) in the blood can also be measured. The process of blood clotting can also be tested.

botulism a rare type of food poisoning caused by poisons formed by a bacterium usually found in improperly canned or preserved foods. Early symptoms—vomiting, abdominal pains, and double vision—begin hours after you eat a contaminated substance. Severe breathing difficulties may develop later and risk of death is high.

brachytherapy a method of treating a malignant (likely to grow or spread) tumor in which a radioactive substance is inserted directly into the tumor or surrounding tissue. This procedure is performed in an attempt to keep a cancer from spreading by destroying or slowing the growth of abnormal cells.

bronchoscopy a diagnostic procedure in which a flexible endoscope (a viewing tube) with a lighting system is passed down the throat to examine the air passages (bronchi) of the lungs.

bronchospasm temporary narrowing of the bronchi (the airways into the lungs) caused by contraction of the muscles in the walls of the bronchi. Bronchospasm occurs in people who have asthma (see p.381) and it can also occur in people who have chronic lung disease such as emphysema (see p.383) and chronic bronchitis (see p.380). It can also result from shock (see p.414) or an allergic reaction.

C

calculus **1.** a hard white, creamy, or brown deposit that forms on tooth surfaces. Also known as tartar when dental plaque hardens. **2.** a gallstone or kidney or bladder stone.

calorie a measurement of energy used in nutrition that represents the amount of energy contained in foods.

capsule **1.** an oval or cylindrical pill containing a liquid, granular, or powdered drug inside a soluble plastic-like coating. **2.** the tough fibrous tissue that encloses an organ or surrounds a joint.

carcinogen any substance that can cause cancer.

carcinoma a malignant growth composed of abnormally multiplying surface tissues such as those of the skin, linings of internal organs (such as the bladder or intestines), or linings of glands (such as the breast or prostate).

Carcinomas, the most common type of cancer, can often be treated successfully if discovered early.

cardiac catheterization a diagnostic procedure in which a catheter, or tube, is passed along a blood vessel into the heart in order to investigate the heart at work. The procedure is performed with a local anesthetic where the catheter is inserted. It is usually virtually painless.

caries tooth decay or "cavities." Bacteria act on food trapped between teeth and produce acid. This progressively attacks the enamel, dentin, and pulp of the tooth, and can eventually destroy it.

carotid arteriograms X-ray pictures of the blood vessels in the neck that go to the brain; used as a diagnostic aid in a transient ischemic attack or a stroke. An opaque dye is injected into the carotid artery in the neck. The dye moves through the artery and a rapid series of X rays shows how the blood is moving through the vessels of the brain.

CAT scan see *CT scan*.

catheter a flexible tube used to withdraw liquid (or air) from, or to squirt fluid into, a part of the body such as the bladder or a blood vessel.

cauterization destruction of tissue by burning it away with a caustic chemical, heat, or electricity. Cauterization is most often used to remove growths, such as warts, on the skin or mucous membrane.

cerebral angiography angiography of blood vessels inside the skull that supply the brain. The resultant pictures (cerebral angiograms) can indicate the presence of disorders such as tumors and aneurysms.

chemotherapy treatment or control of cancer by the use of drugs that kill cells (cytotoxic drugs). These drugs are either injected into the bloodstream or taken by mouth.

chiropractic a theory of healing based on the belief that health and disease are related to the function of the nervous system. Therapy involves physical manipulation and adjustment of the spinal column, joints, and soft tissues, and does not include surgery or medication.

chlamydia a type of microorganism that causes a wide variety of diseases in humans and animals, including a sexually transmitted disease.

cholecystectomy surgical removal of the gallbladder, performed either as traditional surgery or by passing surgical instruments through a type of endoscope (a viewing tube) that has been inserted through a small incision. The gallbladder is then removed through the tube in small pieces. See Gallbladder removal by laparoscopy, p.527.

cholesterol a steroidlike chemical present in some foods, notably animal fats, eggs, and dairy products. An excessively high level of cholesterol in the blood is associated with atherosclerosis, and excess cholesterol in the bile may cause gallstones. However, some cholesterol in the body is necessary for healthy functioning.

chorionic villus sampling removal and examination of a small piece of one of the membranes (the chorion) that surround the developing embryo in the uterus. This procedure makes possible the diagnosis of many genetic disorders early in pregnancy.

chromosomes threadlike structures in a living cell that contain the cell's genetic information. Each chromosome is composed of thousands of genes. All cells in complex organisms, except reproductive cells, contain paired sets of chromosomes (one from each parent). Chromosomes in reproductive cells are not paired.

chronic a term used to describe a disorder or symptom that lasts a long time—weeks, months, or even years.

chronic fatigue syndrome a disorder of unknown cause that lasts for prolonged and variable periods of time and causes a person to feel weak and exhausted. A person who has chronic fatigue syndrome may have fever, headache, muscle ache, and joint pain.

clubbing a condition in which fingertips become thickened and nails unnaturally curved. Clubbing itself is harmless and requires no treatment, but it is a common symptom of disorders such as bronchiectasis and congenital heart disease.

colic **1.** abdominal pain that comes in waves separated by relatively pain-free intervals. The precise site of pain depends upon the cause. Biliary colic, for example, affects the upper right area of the abdomen, near the gallbladder. **2.** in infants, episodes of crying and irritability that are distressing to parents but that do not involve any underlying disease.

colonoscopy examination of the colon (large intestine) by means of a fiberoptic endoscope containing a miniature TV camera. A long, flexible tube on the instrument transmits images. This allows the physician to make a direct visual examination of the colon to diagnose disorders.

colposcopy visual examination of the vagina and cervix by inserting a special microscope that has various lenses for magnification. Colposcopy is performed to look for any precancerous conditions or cancer in its early stages. See also Cervical dysplasia, p.640.

coma a state of unconsciousness from which the victim cannot be easily aroused (by speech or touch, for instance). In a light coma the victim may move his or her limbs to avoid painful sensations, but in a deep coma all limb movements cease.

cone biopsy a surgical procedure in which a cone-shaped portion of the cervix is removed for laboratory examination.

cones nerve endings in the retina that detect color and are responsible for vision in normal light and fine details. See also *rods* in this glossary.

congenital a term describing a disease or condition that is present at birth.

congestive a term applied to heart failure when both left and right sides of the heart are affected.

contagious a term applied to diseases that can spread from person to person, usually by personal contact or by respiratory droplets.

contracture abnormal shortening of a muscle, a tendon, or scar tissue that produces deformity or distortion. Joint contracture often affects the hips, knees, and shoulders of elderly people because of lack of use of the joint.

coronary arteriography angiography of the coronary arteries performed during cardiac catheterization. The resultant pictures (coronary arteriograms) can show the location of patches of atheroma, blockage due to thrombosis, and other problems in the arteries of the heart.

critical care unit (CCU) see *intensive care unit*.

cryosurgery use of extreme cold to destroy tissues. Cryosurgery is used to freeze excessive or abnormal tissue. It is used experimentally to destroy cancer in the prostate, brain, and liver. It is an effective treatment in some cases of hemorrhoids, cervical erosion, and some brain disorders.

cryotherapy see *cryosurgery*.

CT scan an abbreviation for computed tomography, a painless diagnostic procedure in which hundreds of X-ray pictures are taken as a camera revolves around the area being examined. The pictures are fed into a computer, which integrates them to reveal extremely detailed cross-sectional views of structures inside the body.

curettage a procedure involving the removal of a thin layer of skin or internal lining (for example, from the uterus). The purpose of curettage is either to remove tissue or to obtain a sample of tissue for microscopic analysis.

cyanosis blueness of skin and lips caused by a lack of oxygen in the blood. This condition can be caused by respiratory or heart problems, and is often a sign of serious illness.

cyclothymic an inborn tendency to experience repeated swings of mood from elation to depression not directly related to external events. People with cyclothymic temperaments are not necessarily mentally ill.

cystogram see *cystography.*

cystography a diagnostic procedure in which an X ray (cystogram) of the bladder is obtained by injecting a solution visible on X-ray film into the bladder.

cystography, voiding an X-ray examination of the bladder that starts with injecting a dye that is visible on X-ray film. A film of the bladder is then made while the person urinates. This test is performed to evaluate the emptying of the bladder.

cystoscopy examination of the bladder using a type of *endoscope* (a viewing tube) passed through the urethra. The procedure is usually performed under a general anesthetic and requires an overnight stay in the hospital.

D

D and C abbreviation for dilatation and curettage, a procedure in which the lining of the uterus is scraped away. D and C is used in the diagnosis and treatment of heavy menstrual bleeding, cancer, and various other disorders of the uterus, as a means of terminating pregnancy, and sometimes after a miscarriage to ensure complete removal of fetal tissue from the uterus. See also D and C, p.637.

decibel a unit (abbreviated dB) for expressing the loudness of sounds. Ten decibels represents the faintest audible sound, and 120 decibels is the average pain threshold.

defibrillation a procedure in which medical professionals administer an electric shock to the heart through electrodes placed directly on the surface of the heart muscle or on the chest wall. It is used as treatment to restore an extremely rapid or uncoordinated heartbeat to its normal pattern.

dehydration a physical condition caused by the loss of an excessive amount of water from the body, often resulting from severe vomiting or diarrhea. Easily recognized signs of dehydration are sunken eyes, wrinkled skin, dry mouth, and, in babies, a sunken fontanelle (area at the top of the head).

delirium tremens a group of symptoms that may occur if an alcoholic abstains from drinking for a day or so. Symptoms range in severity from shaking limbs to hallucinations, often of insects crawling over the person's body. The condition is occasionally fatal.

dementia a progressive loss of intellectual function that includes personality changes and impairment of memory, judgment, and thought processes. Alzheimer's disease is a common cause of dementia. See Dementia, p.314, and Dementia and aging, p.772.

dialysis a technique for artificial removal of waste products from the bloodstream either by a machine (hemodialysis) or by using the abdominal cavity (peritoneal dialysis). Dialysis is a way to compensate for the inadequate functioning of diseased kidneys. All artificial kidney machines use some form of dialysis.

diastolic the blood pressure reading obtained when the ventricles (lower chambers of the heart) have completely relaxed. Diastolic refers to diastole, the part of the heart's cycle when the ventricles are refilling with blood. See also *systolic* in this glossary.

diathermy use of a high-frequency electric current to heat body tissues. A current passed through a small electrode can burn away the tissues it touches and may be used as a form of bloodless surgery because the intense heat immediately seals any cut vessels.

dilation or dilatation widening of a passageway or body opening either intentionally, as with an instrument or drug, or by involuntary relaxation of constricting walls or encircling tissue.

DNA deoxyribonucleic acid, the large molecule that is the main carrier of genetic information in cells. DNA is found mainly in the chromosomes (see *chromosomes* in this glossary) of cells. See also Genetics, p.752.

Doppler ultrasound scan a diagnostic technique that uses the changes in reflected sound wave frequencies in ultrasound scanning to evaluate blood flow or narrowing of a blood vessel. See also *ultrasound* in this glossary.

DPT vaccination a series of injections given at specific ages throughout childhood that makes a person resistant to diphtheria, pertussis (whooping cough), and tetanus. See also Immunization, p.748.

dyspepsia a medical term for indigestion, which is a group of symptoms that may include nausea, heartburn, upper abdominal pain, gas, belching, or a feeling of extreme fullness after a meal.

dysplasia a term that describes abnormal development. It is used to refer to abnormal formation of body structures such as the skull (cranial dysplasia) and to abnormal growth of cells (cellular dysplasia), which sometimes precedes cancerous changes in the cells.

dysuria painful or difficult urination.

E

echocardiogram see *echocardiography.*

echocardiography use of ultrasound waves to examine the structure of the heart, thickness of the heart walls, the health of the valves, and the way in which the walls move when you are at rest or are exercising. Findings are recorded graphically on an echocardiogram.

echography a diagnostic procedure that uses ultrasound wave echoes to detect possible abnormalities. The ultrasound pattern can help identify types of tumors (for example, whether it is a fluid-filled cyst or a solid tumor). The recording is called an echogram.

ectopic a term used to describe something that is in a false or abnormal position, such as in ectopic pregnancy (implantation of the fertilized egg in a fallopian tube rather than in the uterus).

edema swelling of body tissue due to excess water content. The swollen tissue may "pit," or remain indented, when you press it with your finger.

effusion a collection of fluid in space between neighboring body tissues that are normally in contact (for instance, between the lung and pleura or where bones meet within a joint).

electrocardiogram (ECG) see *electrocardiography.*

electrocardiography a painless procedure for making a graphic recording (electrocardiogram, abbreviated ECG) of the electrical impulses that start in and pass through the heart to initiate and control its activity. Electrocardiography is done by placing metal plates called electrodes on body surfaces. These plates are attached to a voltage measuring and recording device, and they pick up the electrical impulses that begin just before the heart beats, which are altered by heart disease.

electroencephalogram (EEG) see *electroencephalography.*

electroencephalography a painless procedure for recording electrical impulses of the brain. A variety of patterns normally produced by nerve cells are altered in recognizable ways by abnormal conditions (such as epilepsy). Electroencephalography is done by placing metal electrodes on the head. The electrodes are attached to a recording device that reproduces the activity graphically. The recording is called an electroencephalogram (EEG).

electromyogram (EMG) see *electromyography.*

electromyography a test to analyze the electrical activity in muscle tissue to help diagnose various muscular or neuromuscular disorders. Electrodes are attached to needles that are inserted directly into the muscle, and the electrical impulses are recorded. The recording is called an electromyogram (EMG).

electroshock therapy (EST) a treatment for depression in which an electric current is passed through the brain while the patient is under a general anesthetic. Drowsiness and some loss of recent memories are possible side effects of this treatment.

embolectomy emergency surgery to remove an embolus that has caused an embolism, or blockage, in a blood vessel. A successful embolectomy restores the flow of blood to deprived tissues.

embolism sudden blockage of a vessel caused by an embolus.

embolus a blood clot or other material (such as a fragment of fat or a piece of tumor tissue) that is carried along in the bloodstream. See also *thrombus* in this glossary.

endoscope an instrument that enables a physician to look into a hollow organ or body cavity, photograph or videotape the interior, and (if necessary) take a sample of tissue or remove a small growth. The basic instrument is a tube equipped with a miniature TV camera. A clawlike attachment can be passed through the tube for cutting. Endoscopes designed for use in different parts of the body have special names such as cystoscope (used to examine the bladder) or bronchoscope (used to examine the bronchi, the airways to the lungs).

endoscopy any procedure involving the use of an endoscope. Special names are usually given to endoscopic procedures involving different parts of the body.

enema a liquid instilled into the rectum through a tube or syringe and held for a set time before release by defecation or by being drained away. Enemas are used for treatment (as in relief of constipation) or for diagnostic purposes (as in a barium enema).

enzymes substances in the body necessary for accomplishing chemical changes such as burning sugar to produce energy or breaking down food in the intestinal tract. Many of the enzymes in the body are found in digestive juices.

estrogen one of the main sex hormones responsible for female sexual characteristics. In women, estrogen is produced mainly in the ovaries. In men, small amounts are produced in the testes and adrenal glands. For further information see Sex hormones (female) in the Drug glossary. See also *androgen* in this glossary.

exchange blood transfusion repetitive withdrawal of small amounts of blood and addition of donated blood, until most of the blood in the patient's body has been replaced.

exclusion diet a diet from which all foods likely to cause an allergic reaction have been excluded. If symptoms disappear, food allergy may be suspected. Confirmation is sometimes obtained by offering the suspected food in small quantities without the person's knowledge, to avoid the power of suggestion.

extracorporeal shock wave lithotripsy (ESWL) see *lithotripsy.*

F

failure to thrive a condition in which an infant lags in normal growth and development because of some physical problem or simply a shortage of comfort and attention.

fecal impaction hard masses of stool that block the rectum.

fiber **1.** any body tissue composed mainly of threadlike structures (for example, nerve fibers, muscle fibers, and connective tissue). **2.** indigestible components (mostly cellulose) of plant cell walls. Eating fibrous fruit and vegetables can help relieve constipation and may also reduce the risk of cancer of the colon.

fibrillation rapid "quivering" of the heart muscle instead of normal regular rhythmical heart muscle contractions. Fibrillation may affect either the atria (the smaller heart chambers) or the ventricles (the larger heart chambers). Ventricular fibrillation is fatal unless normal rhythm is restored quickly by electric shock.

fibrin an insoluble protein formed in blood as it clots. Fibrin is the substance that unites the blood cells to close any damage to blood vessel walls.

fluorescein angiography a procedure for the study of disorders of the eye. A fluorescent dye is rapidly injected into an arm vein. As the dye reaches the blood vessels in the retina, a series of pictures reveals the passage of the dye through the retinal arteries, veins, and capillaries.

gamma globulin a type of blood protein that includes antibodies. Gamma globulins can be extracted from the blood of many donors, combined, and used to prevent or treat infections such as hepatitis.

gastrectomy surgical removal of all or part of the stomach.

gastrointestinal (GI) series diagnostic examinations performed to detect or monitor various diseases of the gastrointestinal tract (esophagus, stomach, and intestines) by using barium sulfate, a chemical that will appear on a special monitor or on an X ray. To prepare for an upper GI series, the person drinks a special mixture (see *barium meal or swallow* in this glossary) that reveals an image of the esophagus, stomach, and small intestine. To prepare for a lower GI series, barium is introduced into the patient's rectum (see *barium enema* in this glossary). This provides an image of the large intestine and rectum. These examinations are usually performed on an outpatient basis, and no anesthetic is needed.

gene this segment of a DNA (deoxyribonucleic acid) molecule is the basic unit of biological inheritance. There are about 100,000 genes in each human cell, and each one plays a part in determining various characteristics (such as eye color or hair texture) that are passed from one generation to the next. See also Genetics, p.752.

genetics the study of biological inheritance; how characteristics are passed from one generation to the next. See also Genetics, p.752.

German measles see *rubella.*

gingivectomy a dental procedure that involves removal of diseased areas of the gums. The resultant wound may be covered with a protective dressing, which is left in place for several days while the gum heals.

H

HDL cholesterol high-density lipoprotein cholesterol (often called good cholesterol) is one type of cholesterol (see *cholesterol* in this glossary) that is made by the liver and transported in the blood. If the blood level of this type of cholesterol is high, there is a lower risk of developing atherosclerosis (see p.398). See also *LDL cholesterol* and *VLDL cholesterol* in this glossary.

hematoma a swelling that contains blood, usually clotted, in an organ, space, or tissue. A hematoma is caused by a break in the wall of a blood vessel.

hematuria the medical term for blood in the urine.

hemolysis a disorder in which red blood cells are destroyed prematurely. Hemolysis may be caused by defects in the blood cells, and by certain infections (for example, malaria). It may also occur as a side effect of drugs such as methyldopa (see Methyldopa in the Drug glossary). Severe hemolysis causes anemia and jaundice (see *jaundice* in this glossary).

hemorrhage a medical term for excessive bleeding. A hemorrhage may be internal (inside a body cavity) or external (from the skin or an opening).

heredity transmission of biological characteristics from one generation to the next through genetic inheritance. See also Genetics, p.752.

herpes, genital a sexually transmitted disease caused by a herpes simplex virus. The virus, which produces a sometimes painful rash on the genitals, is transmitted by sexual contact with an infected person. See Genital herpes, p.656.

herpes simplex a virus that causes cold sores around the lips and mouth, and that also causes painful blisters on the genitals and in the pubic area, thighs, and buttocks.

herpes zoster a painful viral disease of the nerves commonly known as shingles.

Hib vaccination a series of injections given at specific intervals to make a child resistant to infection from the bacteria called Hib (*Haemophilus influenzae* type b; see Immunization, p.748). These infections commonly involve epiglottitis (see also Croup and stridor, p.725) or childhood pneumonia (see Pneumonia in children, p.726).

histamine a chemical that is released into the body when an allergic reaction occurs and causes various symptoms, such as itching. Another common symptom caused by a histamine is dilation and leakage of small blood vessels; as a result, surrounding tissues become swollen.

HIV human immunodeficiency virus, the cause of AIDS (acquired immune deficiency syndrome). HIV is transmitted through contact with the blood, semen, or vaginal fluids of an infected person. See also *AIDS* in this glossary.

Holter monitor a portable device used to keep track of the heart rhythm, or to show the result of inadequate blood flow through the heart muscle (see *electrocardiography* in this glossary) over a 24-hour period. It is worn over the patient's shoulder, and electrodes are attached to the surface of the chest. While the patient follows his or her usual daily routine, the electrodes transmit the heartbeat to a cassette tape inside the monitor, where it is recorded for analysis by the physician. See also Tests for coronary artery disease, p.402.

hormone replacement therapy use of hormones, in drug form, to replace those that the body no longer makes naturally. Hormone replacements may be given in the form of an injection, tablet, or patch; they must be taken regularly, often for life. The most familiar example of hormone replacement therapy is the treatment of diabetes with insulin.

hypertension high blood pressure that does not go down to normal levels. Although blood pressure normally rises in response to exertion or stress, people with hypertension have high blood pressure at all times, even when they are resting. See also High blood pressure, p.411.

hysterectomy surgical removal of the uterus (see Box, p.638). This procedure can be performed either through an incision in the lower abdomen or through an incision in the vagina. Hysterectomy is usually performed to treat fibroid tumors of the uterus (which are noncancerous) or cancer of the uterus or cervix. The ovaries and fallopian tubes may also be removed during this procedure.

hysterosalpingography a process in which an X ray is taken of the uterus and fallopian tubes after injection of an opaque liquid.

hysteroscopy examination of the inside of the uterus with a type of endoscope (a viewing tube) to look for infection or tumors or to enable treatment of any excessive vaginal bleeding that occurs when a woman is near menopause.

I

immobilization placing fractured bones or damaged joints in their correct position and holding them in place so that they will heal properly. The procedure usually involves the use of splints or casts, but it sometimes requires an operation in which fractures are repaired with metal splints attached directly to the bones. See also *traction* in this glossary.

immunity resistance to disease through the body's immune system, its own mechanism for recognizing and destroying foreign material or infectious agents by producing antibodies. Immunity can be present at birth, can develop as a result of having the disease, or can be induced through vaccination with small doses of a specific infectious agent altered to avoid active infection. See also *immunization* in this glossary.

immunization the process by which people are made resistant to specific infectious diseases. Immunization may be active or passive. In active immunization, a person is given small doses of a vaccine, which is a specific infectious agent that has been killed or altered. This usually does not cause disease, but stimulates the body's defense mechanism (immune system) to produce antibodies (substances that recognize and destroy foreign material or infectious agents) to that infectious agent. Resistance to that disease is permanent. In passive immunization, a person is injected with antibodies taken from the blood of another person who was previously ill with a disease, thereby providing temporary resistance to that disease. Such resistance will last for only a few weeks at most. See Immunization, p.748.

incubation period time lag between the moment of infection and the appearance of symptoms. During this period infectious agents are multiplying but are insufficient in number to cause symptoms or infect other people. Incubation periods range from a few days (for example, in influenza) to months (for example, certain types of hepatitis).

intensive care unit (ICU) a section in most hospitals in which intense surgical and medical care is given to injury victims, premature babies, burn patients, people who are recovering from major surgery, and others who are seriously ill. ICUs are equipped with monitoring devices, respirators, defibrillators, and other lifesaving equipment.

intravenous drip a term used for a liquid substance introduced into the body by letting it drip from an elevated sterile container, through a tube inserted into a vein. The rate of flow is measured by counting the rate at which the liquid drips through a transparent chamber.

intravenous fluid such essentials as salt, water, sugar, protein, minerals, and vitamins, which are given to a patient intravenously in liquid form, often after surgery.

intravenous infusion see *intravenous drip.*

intravenous pyelography (IVP) a diagnostic procedure involving the injection into a vein of a solution visible on X rays. The test is used to examine the urinary system. The result is a series of pictures known as pyelograms. An IVP is painless, but patients often feel faint and experience a warm flush for a few minutes after the injection. In rare cases, a serious allergic reaction occurs.

involuntary a term applied generally to any physical activity not subject to conscious control. In particular, muscles that are not under your conscious control, such as those that propel food through the digestive tract, are known as involuntary muscles.

irreducible a term applied to a hernia, fractured bone, or dislocated joint that cannot be returned to its natural position.

J

jaundice yellow discoloration of the skin and whites of the eyes as a result of an excess of the pigment bilirubin in the bloodstream. Bilirubin is a breakdown product of the blood pigment hemoglobin, and jaundice may be due to either excessive destruction of red blood cells (see also *hemolysis* in this glossary), or to a liver disorder that impairs the normal excretion of bilirubin in the bile.

K

keratin a hard substance present in skin, hair, and nails.

L

laparoscopy examination of the inside of the abdomen by means of a type of endoscope (a viewing tube). Laparoscopy is also used for some surgical prodecures.

laparotomy, exploratory a surgical procedure in which the surgeon makes an incision in the abdominal wall to enable him or her to examine the inside of the abdomen. Exploratory laparotomy is performed to help arrive at a diagnosis after other tests have failed to reveal the cause of an illness. See also Laparotomy and acute abdomen, p.513.

laser a device that produces a highly concentrated, powerful beam of light of a single specific wavelength (or a narrow band of wavelengths) that can be used as a surgical cutting tool.

LDL cholesterol low-density lipoprotein cholesterol is one type of cholesterol (see *cholesterol* in this glossary) that is made by the liver and transported in the blood. Eating animal fat increases LDL cholesterol levels and in turn increases the risk of atherosclerosis (see p.398). See also *HDL cholesterol* and *VLDL cholesterol* in this glossary.

leukemia any of the various types of cancer in which there is excessive production of abnormal white blood cells (leukocytes) or, more rarely, red blood cells (erythrocytes) in the bone marrow, thereby interfering with the production of normal white blood cells, platelets, and red blood cells. See Leukemia, p.457, and Leukemia in children, p.729.

lithotripsy a term that describes destruction of a stone. Ultrasonic or hydraulic shock waves are used to break stones in the kidneys or upper urinary tract into tiny pieces. In extracorporeal shock wave lithotripsy (ESWL), a device produces external shock waves to break up the stones, which are then passed in urine. In percutaneous lithotripsy, a small incision is made and a type of endoscope (a viewing tube) is inserted directly into the kidney. A probe that produces ultrasonic waves is passed through the tube to break up the stones, which are then removed through the tube. See also Kidney stones, p.548.

lobectomy surgical removal of a lobe, or section, of an organ, such as the thyroid, liver, brain, or lung.

lumbar puncture a procedure for investigating or treating diseases of the nervous system by inserting a needle between the vertebrae in the lower spine to remove cerebrospinal fluid and, occasionally, inject drugs. Lumbar puncture is done under local anesthetic and takes about 20 minutes.

lumpectomy a surgical procedure for breast cancer in which only the tumor and a small surrounding area of normal tissue are removed. See also Surgery for breast cancer, p.633.

Lyme disease a disease caused by bacteria transmitted by tick bites, it is named for the Connecticut town in which it was first observed. Characteristics of the disease include skin rash, arthritis, and heart problems. See Lyme disease, p.605.

lymphadenectomy surgical removal of a lymph node.

lymphoma any of the types of cancer in which there is excessive production of abnormal lymphoid tissue cells. Hodgkin's lymphomas are distinguished by the presence of a certain type of abnormal cell. All other lymphomas are called non-Hodgkin's lymphomas. See Lymphoma, p.463. Chances for recovery from this kind of tumor are good.

M

magnetic resonance imaging (MRI) an imaging technique based on a computer analysis of the response of atoms of hydrogen, phosphorus, or other elements to a generated magnetic field and radio signal.

malignant a term applied to cancers, or to a growth that is likely to penetrate the tissues in which it originated to spread further (metastasize), and eventually cause death. Because of their pervasive qualities, malignant growths sometimes recur after apparent removal, and complete eradication may be impossible. See also *benign* in this glossary.

mammography a procedure for detecting breast cancer by means of X rays. The photographic result is known as a mammogram. Mammography takes about half an hour in an office or clinic.

measles see *rubeola.*

melanoma a life-threatening type of skin cancer that occurs in the cells (melanocytes) that produce melanin, the pigment found in skin, hair, and the iris of the eyes. Melanoma usually develops from an existing mole, which may increase in size, become lumpy, change color, bleed, develop an irregular border, or begin to itch. Melanoma frequently spreads to other parts of the body. See Malignant melanoma, p.275.

meninges membranes that cover the brain and spinal cord. When they are inflamed (meningitis), stiff neck, persistent headache, vomiting, and fever result.

menopause technically, the end of a woman's final menstrual period. As commonly used, the word denotes the time of a woman's life usually between the ages of 40 and 54 when menopause occurs. The medical term for what is sometimes called "change of life" is climacteric.

metastasis a term applied to a malignant growth that develops in one part of the body as a result of the spread of abnormal cells from another part. Cancer that has spread from one tissue to another is said to have metastasized.

metastasize spreading of malignant tissue from one part of the body to another.

miscarriage loss of a fetus before the beginning of the 20th week of pregnancy, before it is able to survive outside the uterus without artificial support. This is also known as a spontaneous abortion. See Miscarriage, p.674.

monounsaturated see *unsaturated.*

myelogram see *myelography.*

myelography a diagnostic procedure for X raying the fluid-filled space around the spinal cord in order to detect disorders such as prolapsed disks or growths on the cord, or compression of the cord. The basic method involves a lumbar puncture, removal of some cerebrospinal fluid, and injection of a solution visible on X-ray film into the space; then the patient is tilted in various ways so that the movement of the solution can be recorded on a series of pictures known as myelograms.

myringotomy a surgical procedure in which a small cut is made in the eardrum to release fluid trapped in the middle ear.

N

nasogastric tube a term describing a thin, flexible tube that can be passed through a nostril into the stomach via the throat. Nasogastric tubes are used either for passing nourishment into the digestive tract or for draining away digestive fluids. This may be helpful when the intestines are not working properly.

nebulizer a device that mixes a drug with water vapor to produce a medicated mist suitable for inhalation. Nebulizers are used to help treat asthma.

neonatal a term that refers to newborn infants, particularly during the first 4 weeks of life.

nuclear medicine see *radioactive isotope.*

O

obstructed blocked. This term is usually used when a passageway from one part of the body to another is blocked. A common example is blockage of part of the intestine. Another example is obstructed labor, in which the fetus cannot pass out of the uterus because it is too large for the woman's birth canal.

occlusion **1.** a term that dentists apply to a person's "bite," the way in which upper and lower teeth come together as the mouth closes. **2.** blockage of a passageway such as a blood vessel by a clot or bubble.

ophthalmoscopy examination of the inside of the eye with an ophthalmoscope (a viewing instrument).

orifice the entrance or outlet of a body cavity; an opening.

osteoma a benign growth of hard, bony tissue, which needs to be removed only if it causes problems.

osteomyelitis an infection of bone and bone marrow, usually by bacteria, that is more common in children. Osteomyelitis most often affects a single area near a joint in one of the long bones of the arms and legs. In rare instances more than one bone becomes infected. See also Osteomyelitis in children, p.742.

osteopathy a system of medicine based on the interrelationships between all of the various body systems, with emphasis on the musculoskeletal systems (bones, muscles, tendons, tissues, nerves, and spine). A Doctor of Osteopathy (DO) is a fully licensed physician who uses manipulation techniques along with traditional methods of diagnosis and treatment. Doctors of Osteopathy prescribe medications and perform surgery.

osteotomy a surgical procedure involving the cutting and repositioning of bones in order to treat diseased or deformed joints or the bones themselves.

otoscopy examination of the internal parts of the ear from the outer ear canal through the slightly transparent eardrum using an otoscope (a viewing instrument).

P

papilloma a wartlike tumor that can occur in the colon, bladder, or cervix, or on the skin. Most are benign but some may become malignant (cancerous) or may induce the growth of a cancer. Some papillomas are caused by viral infections, but others (such as bladder papillomas) may be caused by toxic chemicals.

paracentesis a diagnostic procedure or treatment for draining fluid from part of the body (especially the abdomen). Paracentesis involves puncturing the affected area with a needle and in some cases requires a local anesthetic, but the procedure is usually painless.

paranoid see Behavioral and emotional problems, p.318.

patch test a test performed to identify substances that cause allergic reactions in the individual. Small amounts of substances that may cause a reaction (redness and swelling) are applied to small patches of the skin to determine whether or not the person is allergic to them.

peak-flow meter an instrument used to determine lung efficiency by measuring how swiftly a person can expel air from the lungs. Peak-flow meters are used to diagnose respiratory tract diseases or to evaluate recovery rate.

perforation a hole formed in the wall of an organ or the digestive tract from penetration by a duodenal ulcer or appendicitis, or a stone through the wall of the ureter or gallbladder.

peristalsis rhythmic, wavelike contractions of digestive tract muscles that move food along the tract and mix it with digestive substances. Peristaltic action occurs from the moment of swallowing to the expulsion of waste matter from the rectum.

peritonitis inflammation of the peritoneum (the membrane that lines the abdominal wall and covers the abdominal organs). Peritonitis is a life-threatening condition that is almost always caused by bacterial infection. See Peritonitis, p.503.

pertussis the medical term for whooping cough. See p.749.

PET see *positron emission tomography.*

photophobia the sensation that light is painful to the eyes. Photophobia is a significant symptom of certain nervous system diseases.

phototherapy treatment of disease by exposure to ultraviolet rays. Phototherapy is used on the skin or on blood elements that are removed, exposed, and returned to the body. Severe jaundice in newborns, psoriasis in adults, and certain diseases of the

T cells (lymphocytes) are sometimes treated by phototherapy.

placenta the bowl-shaped organ that nourishes a fetus while it is in the uterus and that also produces hormones responsible for many of the changes in a woman's body during pregnancy. When the baby is born, the placenta is expelled and is known as the afterbirth.

plaque (arterial) a patch of atheroma (fatty tissue) on the inside lining of an artery.

plaque (dental) coating on the teeth made up of mucus, food particles, and bacteria. Without regular, effective brushing and flossing, plaque builds up rapidly, leading to tooth and gum diseases.

plasmapheresis a procedure in which blood is removed from a vein and spun in a centrifuge to separate plasma or to remove certain proteins or blood cells. The remaining cells, along with replacement fluids, are then reinjected into the patient's vein. Plasmapheresis takes about 2 hours and is virtually painless.

pneumonectomy surgical removal of an entire lung or of one or more lobes of a lung. See also *lobectomy* in this glossary.

polyp an outgrowth of tissue from the skin or a mucous membrane that appears in the form of a short stalk with a knob on the end (like a grape on a stem).

polyunsaturated see *unsaturated.*

positron emission tomography (PET) a diagnostic scanning procedure in which short-lived radioactive isotopes (see *radioactive isotope* in this glossary) are injected or inhaled to help produce a graphic image of the structure or metabolic activity of an organ. PET scanning is as yet mainly used for research. See also Brain-imaging techniques, p.295.

postmortem another name for autopsy. See *autopsy.*

proctoscopy examination of the anus and rectum with an endoscope (viewing tube); often the examination is extended into the sigmoid colon (large intestine). The procedure may be uncomfortable, but it is usually not particularly painful.

prolapse partial or full slipping of a body organ or structure (the uterus, or a segment of the rectum) from its normal position. Prolapse is usually caused by a weakening of surrounding supportive tissues.

prophylactic a substance or procedure that helps to prevent disease (for example, an antimalarial drug, an immunization, or a condom).

prostatectomy surgical removal of all or part of the prostate gland.

prosthesis an artificial appliance used to replace lost natural structures. Common prostheses are dental bridges and plates, artificial arms and legs, breast implants, and glass eyes.

psychosis see Behavioral and emotional problems, p.318.

psychotherapy see Behavioral and emotional problems, p.323.

psychotic see Behavioral and emotional problems, p.319.

puberty the age when children begin to develop adult sexual characteristics, capabilities, and feelings. Puberty usually occurs sometime between the ages of 10 and 15.

R

radial keratotomy an operation to correct nearsightedness in which a series of spokelike cuts is made in the cornea, causing it to flatten, thereby improving the ability of the eye to focus on distant objects. Radial keratotomy may cause complications and the surgery may not produce predictable results.

radiation therapy treatment of disease by radioactivity or X rays. It is mainly used to destroy malignant or cancerous growths and prevent their spread.

radioactive implant a pellet of radioactive material such as radium that is inserted into a cancerous tumor as a treatment. The pellet, usually implanted under general anesthetic, is left in place for several days and then removed.

radioactive isotope a substance (such as radioactive iodine) that gives off beta or gamma rays (similar to X rays). Radioactive isotopes are used in some diagnostic scanning procedures to check the structure and function of an organ. For example, in thyroid scanning, a radioactive isotope is either swallowed or injected into the bloodstream; it then collects in the thyroid, where it helps to produce a graphic image. In radiation therapy, some types of cancer are treated with a radioactive isotope (for example, radioactive phosphorus) that is swallowed, injected, or inserted into the body, or cobalt that is aimed at a particular part of the body in an attempt to keep the disease from spreading by destroying abnormal cells.

radioimmunoassay a technique used to measure very small amounts of substances such as hormones in the circulation. It involves the use of laboratory-produced antibodies labeled with radioactive chemical elements.

radioisotope scan a diagnostic procedure that uses a radioactive isotope to view a body organ and examine some aspect of its structure or function. The isotope can be detected and followed with specialized equipment. Findings of radioisotope scans are recorded either in still photographs or on a moving picture.

rape sexual intercourse by the use or threat of force or violence and against the victim's will or without the victim's consent. Rape is a felony in every state, although the exact definition varies by state. Rape has been viewed traditionally as a violent crime committed by a man against a woman, but some states now use the broader term aggravated sexual assault instead of rape. Some state laws now recognize as crimes some forms of marital rape, homosexual rape, incest, and other sexual offenses. Rape is not a crime of passion; it results from the offender's urge to dominate and humiliate the victim.

reducible a term applied to a hernia, fractured bone, or dislocated joint that can be successfully treated by restoration to its normal position.

reduction **1.** manipulation into correct position of a dislocated joint or a fractured bone. **2.** pushing of a hernia back into its proper place.

refraction the process by which light and images entering the eye are bent (refracted) by the cornea and the lens to bring the image into sharp focus on the retina.

rehabilitation **1.** restoration of movement and strength to a limb in which a bone or joint has been immobilized after an injury. **2.** preparation or education of a patient recovering from an injury or serious illness for a return to working and domestic life. This type of treatment is largely carried out by occupational and physical therapists and vocational rehabilitation counselors, under the direction of a physician.

rejection an attack by the body's immune defense system on a transplanted organ or a skin graft. Rejection may be prevented by treatment with immunosuppressive drugs. For further information see the Drug glossary.

remission disappearance of the symptoms of a chronic disease, especially of cancer. If remission lasts for more than 5 years, the condition is usually regarded as having been cured.

respirator see *ventilator.*

respiratory failure failure of the lungs, which may be either acute or chronic. In either case insufficient oxygen is extracted from the air for the body's needs.

RNA ribonucleic acid, a type of genetic material that carries out the instructions of a cell's DNA. See also Genetics, p.752.

rods nerve endings in the retina that contribute to night vision, recognition of general shapes, and movements seen from the "corner of the eye." See also *cones* in this glossary.

rubella (German measles) a non-life-threatening infectious viral disease, usually occurring during childhood, that causes a fever, rash, and swollen lymph glands. If a pregnant woman becomes infected with the virus in the early stages of pregnancy, fetal deformities may develop. The disease is preventable by vaccination.

rubeola (measles) a potentially dangerous infectious disease of childhood that causes a fever, rash, red eyes, and a runny nose. Complications include inflammation of the ears, lungs, and brain. The disease is preventable by vaccination.

S

Salmonella a type of bacteria that causes food poisoning, gastrointestinal inflammation, or disease of the genital tract.

sarcoma a malignant tumor that starts in bones, cartilage, or fibrous or muscular tissues. All types of sarcoma are rare and tend to be difficult to treat successfully.

saturated a type of fat that is readily converted to LDL cholesterol and is thought to encourage production of arterial disease. Saturated fats tend to be hard at room temperature. Among saturated fats are animal fats, dairy products, and such vegetable oils as coconut and palm oils. See also *cholesterol* and *unsaturated* in this glossary.

sclerosant an irritant substance sometimes used to treat hemorrhoids and varicose veins. Sclerosants form thick scar tissue in the vein, blocking the channel.

sensory a term describing nerves or body organs that relay information about the senses to the brain. The areas of the brain that receive this information are known as sensory centers; they provide your consciousness with knowledge of your environment.

sepsis infection of blood or tissues with bacteria. Sometimes the body's immune system can eliminate the bacteria or prevent them from multiplying. However, if an excessive amount of rapidly multiplying bacteria are present in the blood, the toxins (poisons) they produce can spread and cause toxemia (see *toxemia* in this glossary) and septicemia (see Blood poisoning, p.452).

septicemia see *blood poisoning.*

sexuality in biology, sex refers to the anatomical differences that distinguish male from female. Sexuality refers to an individual's attitudes, behaviors, and responses with regard to sexual attraction. The term is also used in reference to the sex organs and reproduction. Heterosexuality refers to sexual attraction toward people of the opposite sex (male/female), and homosexuality refers to sexual attraction toward people of the same sex (female/female; male/male). Bisexuality refers to sexual attraction toward people of both sexes. See also Homosexuality, p.660, and Adolescent sexuality, p.764.

sexually transmitted diseases (STDs) any of the various infections (also called venereal diseases) that are usually spread through sexual intercourse with an infected person, but that can also be spread through other forms of sexual contact, through sharing of contaminated needles and syringes by people who use intravenous drugs, and through contact with infected blood. People who have many sexual partners are at greatest risk for contracting STDs. However, the risks are reduced if a latex condom is always used during sexual intercourse.

shock life-threatening collapse in blood circulation that causes reduction in the flow of blood throughout the body, leading to an inadequate supply of oxygen to the vital organs. Shock can result from any severe injury or disease in which there is dehydration, loss of blood, or loss of central nervous system control. Symptoms include sweating; rapid, shallow breathing; nausea; cold, clammy skin; rapid, weak pulse; dizziness; confusion; and fainting. Shock may lead to coma and death. See Shock, p.414.

sialogram see *sialography.*

sialography a diagnostic procedure for examining the ducts in a salivary gland. A solution that is visible on X rays is injected into the gland, and pictures (sialograms) are taken while the solution is in place. The procedure is usually painless.

sigmoidoscopy, flexible examination of the rectum and the last portion of the large intestine with a type of endoscope (a viewing tube) that bends so it can move easily through the intestine. Sigmoidoscopy is performed to check for benign (not likely to spread) growths, ulcers, or cancer. A small cutting instrument can be passed through the viewing tube to perform biopsy (removal of a small tissue sample for analysis).

spasm uncontrollable contraction of one or more muscles.

SPF (sun protection factor) rating system for sunscreen lotions. The higher the number, the more protection you get from the sun's ultraviolet rays.

sphincter a ring of muscle that narrows or closes off a passageway by contracting. Sphincters are found at the anus and at the opening from the bladder to the urethra.

sphygmomanometer an instrument for measuring blood pressure in the arteries. Its components include an inflatable cuff that is wrapped around the upper arm, a rubber bulb that is squeezed to inflate the cuff, and a mechanism that displays a reading of the blood pressure. A new electronic version does not involve a bulb. See also Testing blood pressure, p.412.

splenectomy surgical removal of the spleen. Emergency splenectomy is necessary if the spleen is torn or severely bruised. A splenectomy is performed usually as partial treatment for diseases of the blood.

sprain the injury or tearing of supporting structures around a joint, such as ligaments.

stapedectomy a surgical procedure for restoring hearing by removing a diseased stirrup bone (stapes) from the middle ear and replacing it with an artificial substitute.

status asthmaticus sudden, intense, and continuous aggravation of a state of asthma, marked by shortness of breath to the point of exhaustion and collapse. This condition does not respond to the usual treatments for asthma.

stenosis a term used to describe the narrowing of any channel in the body, but in particular a narrowing of arteries or of the openings of the heart valves.

stethoscope an instrument for monitoring the activity of various organs, especially the lungs, heart, and bowel sounds. Internal sounds are picked up by the bell-shaped end (or flat end covered by thin plastic), which rests on the body surface while the physician listens through the ear-pieces for unusual or abnormal sounds that may indicate disease.

strain to exercise to an extreme or harmful degree—for example, overstretching or overexerting a particular muscle or group of muscles.

strangulation **1.** prevention of respiration by compression of the trachea. **2.** prevention of circulation by compression of the blood vessels. This type of strangulation occurs if a swollen hernia blocks the flow of blood through the muscular gap through which the hernia protrudes. Such hernias are called strangulated hernias. A strangulated intestine occurs when the intestine twists on itself enough to shut off the blood supply.

Streptococcus a group of bacteria responsible for diseases such as pneumonia, scarlet fever, rheumatic fever, and glomerulonephritis. They also cause "strep" throat.

stress test sometimes called exercise stress test. A test to determine how the heart responds to physical activity. Blood pressure, pulse rate, electrical activity of the heart, and any symptoms of inadequate blood flow through the heart muscle (for example, chest pain or fainting) are monitored while the person performs some type of standardized physical activity, such as walking on a treadmill. Exercise stress tests are used to check the adequacy of blood flow through the coronary arteries. A modified exercise stress test is used to evaluate function of the lungs.

stridor noisy breathing, usually due to inflammation of the epiglottis or larynx (voice box).

stroke damage to part of the brain caused by interruption of blood flow due to blockage (as by a blood clot) or rupture of the cerebral blood vessels. Symptoms such as paralysis, loss of consciousness, loss of sensation, or loss of speech depend on the extent of damage, and on the side and area of the brain that has been damaged. See Stroke, p.285, and *transient ischemic attack* in this glossary.

sunscreen a substance that protects skin from the harmful effects of excessive exposure to ultraviolet radiation found in sunlight. Sunscreens are used in many suntanning products to help prevent sunburn.

suppository a soluble cylindrical medication that can be inserted into the rectum or vagina to act directly on the surrounding area or to be absorbed into the body.

suture **1.** thread for stitching wounds or surgical incisions. Stitches fashioned from the thread are also called sutures. The stitching process is called suturing. **2.** interlocking joints that unite the bones of the skull, holding them firmly in place.

synovectomy surgical removal of a diseased synovium. Synovectomy relieves pain but is not practical if several joints or tendons are affected. The operation is done under general anesthetic.

synovium a membrane that lines the tough layers surrounding a joint or tendon. Synovial membranes normally produce small amounts of fluid to lubricate adjoining surfaces.

syringe a device for injecting fluid into or withdrawing fluid from a blood vessel, tissue, or body cavity. One common type of syringe consists of a hollow tube with a plunger at one end, and a nozzle for attaching a hollow needle at the other. Most syringes available today are presterilized and made of disposable plastic.

systolic the higher of the two readings obtained when blood pressure is measured. Systolic refers to systole, the period when the ventricles of the heart contract and blood is pumped into the arteries. See also *diastolic* in this glossary.

T

testosterone a male sex hormone. For further information see Sex hormones (male) in the Drug glossary.

tetany muscle twitchings, cramps, and spasm caused by a lack of calcium in the blood. Tetany is especially apt to affect the hands, feet, and/or throat muscles. It should not be confused with tetanus, a disease that causes similar symptoms for different reasons.

throat culture laboratory examination of a sample of mucus taken from the throat, performed in order to detect the possible presence of infectious agents. The sample, or specimen, is used to start a colony (or culture) of the infectious organism in a laboratory dish under sterile conditions.

thrombosis formation of a blood clot (thrombus) on the lining of a blood vessel or the heart. A thrombus that breaks away and is carried along in the bloodstream is one type of embolus. See also *embolus* in this glossary.

thrombus a blood clot that forms inside the heart or a blood vessel and remains attached to its point of origin. See also *embolus* in this glossary.

thyroid scan see *radioisotope scan.*

TIA see *transient ischemic attack.*

tonometry measurement of the fluid pressure inside the eyeball. Elevated pressures inside the eye often indicate glaucoma.

tonsillectomy surgical removal of the tonsils.

toxemia the presence of toxins (poisons) in the bloodstream. Toxemia may be related to septicemia, a life-threatening condition in which bacteria in the blood multiply and spread their toxins (see Blood poisoning, p.452). If untreated, septicemia can lead to a dangerous condition called septic shock (see also Shock, p.414). Toxemia of pregnancy is a disorder in which the woman has high blood pressure, tissue swelling, and protein in the urine. Severe toxemia of pregnancy is a serious condition that can lead to seizures and coma; treat this condition as an emergency. See also Preeclampsia and eclampsia, p.676.

toxic poisonous.

toxin a poisonous substance produced by bacteria, other infectious agents, and some plants and animals.

traction a treatment for broken legs, broken vertebrae, and other bone disorders in which damaged parts that have become compressed or broken are pulled apart and held in place long enough for healing to occur. See also *immobilization* in this glossary.

transfusion provision of blood collected from another person (the donor) or from oneself into the bloodstream. Before donor blood is used for transfusion, it is screened for infections, such as syphilis, HIV, and hepatitis, and then matched to test that it is compatible with the recipient's blood type.

transient ischemic attack temporary deficiency of blood flow to the brain caused by narrowing or blockage of an artery. Symptoms include headache, dizziness, tingling, numbness, blurred or double vision, confusion, or loss of the use of part of one side of the body. Although the symptoms last for less than 24 hours, transient ischemic attacks may signal an impending stroke. An episode that lasts for more than 24 hours is called a stroke. See Transient ischemic attack, p. 287, and Stroke, p.285.

transplant surgery a procedure in which a diseased or damaged organ or tissue is replaced with a healthy organ or tissue. The replacement can be provided by a donor, as in kidney or heart transplants, or it can come from the recipient of the transplant, as in skin or bone marrow transplants. See Transplants, p.432.

trauma any wound or injury, whether physical or mental.

tremor involuntary trembling or quivering. Tremors may be inherited or caused by a disease such as Parkinson's or multiple sclerosis, the effects of alcohol or other drugs on the nervous system, or emotional disorders.

tuberculin skin test a test performed to determine whether a person has been previously exposed to the bacteria that cause tuberculosis. A substance derived from tuberculosis bacteria is injected into the skin of the arm. After 48 hours, the site of the injection is examined for a skin reaction. No change in the appearance of the skin means that the reaction to the test is negative; that is, the person has not been exposed to tuberculosis. However, if a dime-sized or larger area of the skin becomes red, hard, and raised, the reaction to the test is positive; that is, the person has been exposed to tuberculosis. See Tuberculosis, p.602, and Tuberculosis in children, p.751.

U

ulcer an open sore on any external or internal surface of the body.

ulceration the formation or development of an ulcer.

ultrasound high-frequency sound waves, which are absorbed and reflected to different degrees by various body tissues. Ultrasound is useful for both diagnosis and treatment. The reflections may be recorded pictorially to reveal the inside of such organs as the gallbladder or uterus. Also, doses of ultrasound can be used to destroy abnormalities such as bladder stones.

ultrasound scan see *ultrasound.*

unsaturated a type of fat that is thought to lower the risk of cardiovascular disease. Eating polyunsaturated fats instead of saturated fats reduces LDL cholesterol (see *LDL cholesterol* in this glossary) levels, but may also lower HDL cholesterol (the good cholesterol; see *HDL cholesterol* in this glossary) levels. Monounsaturated fats reduce LDL cholesterol levels. Unsaturated, polyunsaturated, and monounsaturated fats tend to be soft or fluid at room temperature and to come from fish or vegetable sources.

V

vaccine a preparation containing killed or altered versions or a portion of a specific infectious agent. Vaccines are given to make people immune (resistant) to the infectious agents of specific diseases. See also Immunization, p.748.

valvuloplasty a surgical procedure, performed as open-heart surgery, to repair, reconstruct, or replace a defective heart valve. When the defect is a narrowed heart valve, however, a special technique called balloon valvuloplasty can be performed. Balloon valvuloplasty does not require open-heart surgery. In this technique, a catheter with a balloon at the tip is inserted into a blood vessel and passed through the blood vessel to the heart, where the balloon is inflated to separate the flaps of the heart valve that have fused together.

venography a technique for viewing the inside of a vein by injecting a solution visible on X-ray film. Passage of the solution through the vein is recorded on a series of pictures (venograms). Venography is used to detect deep-vein thrombosis.

ventilator a machine that regularly pumps air in and out of the lungs to compensate for the loss of natural breathing.

virus any of a group of simple microorganisms that are too small to be visible under a light microscope (although they can be seen under an electron microscope). Viruses are smaller than bacteria and can multiply only by utilizing the DNA inside living cells. They are responsible for most coughs, colds, and childhood fevers and are unaffected by the common antibiotics (see Drug glossary).

VLDL cholesterol very low-density lipoprotein cholesterol is one of the types of cholesterol (see *cholesterol* in this glossary) that is made by the liver and transported in the blood. If the blood level of this type of cholesterol is high, there is an increased risk of developing atherosclerosis (see also Atherosclerosis, p.398).

X

X rays electromagnetic rays with a short wavelength that pass through body tissues. An exposed X-ray film resembles a negative of an ordinary photograph, with dense tissues such as bones showing up as white shapes. X rays with very short wavelengths, which can penetrate tissues deeply enough to destroy them, are used in radiation therapy.

Injuries and emergencies

First aid

The goals of first aid are to help someone who is injured or ill to recover, or at least to prevent the injury or illness from getting worse; to provide reassurance; to organize help; and to make the person as comfortable as possible until professional help arrives.

For many minor injuries, first aid may be all that is needed. More serious injuries may require professional medical attention and further treatment. Sometimes first aid is needed to deal with life-threatening injuries and may involve quickly stopping the bleeding from a severe wound or resuscitating someone whose breathing has stopped. Correct and rapid assessment of what needs to be done is crucial, and this assessment often requires a healthy dose of common sense. There is little point in diving in to save a drowning person unless you know how to swim. It is just as important to know what you should do first in an emergency, so a priority checklist for life-threatening emergencies is provided below.

The more knowledge you have before an injury or emergency occurs, the more useful you can be. It is a good idea to review this section and familiarize yourself with first-aid techniques and procedures now. The following pages will supply you with valuable information, but please be aware that information is no substitute for the practical experience you get if you attend first-aid classes. This book does not include instruction in cardiopulmonary resuscitation (CPR). CPR should be used only by a person trained in this procedure.

First-aid index

Priority checklist for life-threatening emergencies

If you have to handle an emergency on your own, first call 911 or the number for emergency services in your area. If possible, send someone for help while you check this list.

1. Check breathing. If person is choking (see p.835), clear airway. If breathing has stopped (see p.834), perform resuscitation.
2. If breathing is still absent, check heartbeat. If heart has stopped (see p.836), perform cardiopulmonary resuscitation (CPR) if you have been trained to do it.
3. Attempt to control any severe bleeding (see p.838).
4. If person is unconscious but breathing, place in recovery position (see p.837).
5. Deal with any severe burns (see p.840) or fractures (see p.842).
6. Prevent shock (see p.839).

Absence of breathing

If a person's breathing has stopped, artificial respiration is needed immediately. If the brain is deprived of oxygen for more than 4 or 5 minutes, permanent brain damage or death can occur.

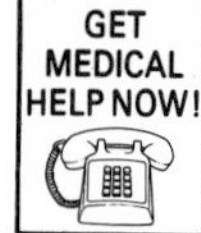

When someone has stopped breathing, there is no rise-and-fall movement of the chest or abdomen, his or her face becomes bluish gray in color, and you can feel no exhaled breath. First call 911 or your emergency number. As soon as someone stops breathing, start artificial respiration. Continue to give artificial respiration about 12 to 14 times per minute until the person resumes normal breathing.

How to resuscitate infants and children

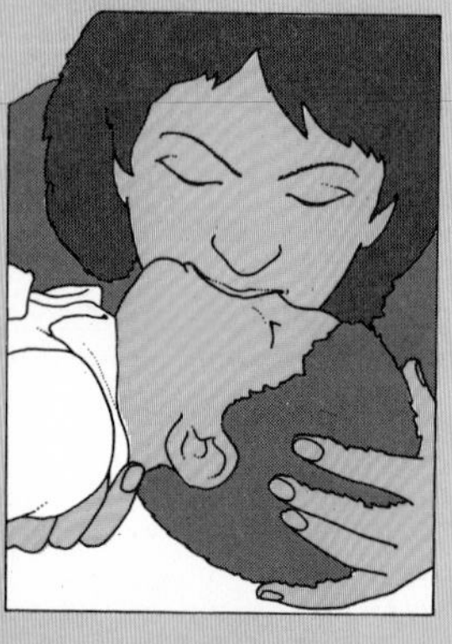

Resuscitating an infant or small child is the same as resuscitating an adult, except you will find it easier to seal your mouth over both the mouth and nose of the child. Do not tip the child's head back very far; this can cut off the airway. Blow gentle breaths, one every 4 seconds (15 per minute) for a child, one every 3 seconds (20 per minute) for an infant. Stop each breath when the child's chest starts to rise. Remove your mouth to get a fresh breath before every attempt.

Mouth-to-nose resuscitation

A facial injury may prevent you from breathing easily into the person's mouth. In such cases, follow steps 1 and 2 at right, then take a deep breath and seal your mouth around the person's nose. Close the mouth by lifting his or her chin. Blow strongly into the person's nose. Remove your mouth and hold the person's mouth open with your fingertips, so that air can escape. Repeat as for mouth-to-mouth resuscitation, every 5 seconds.

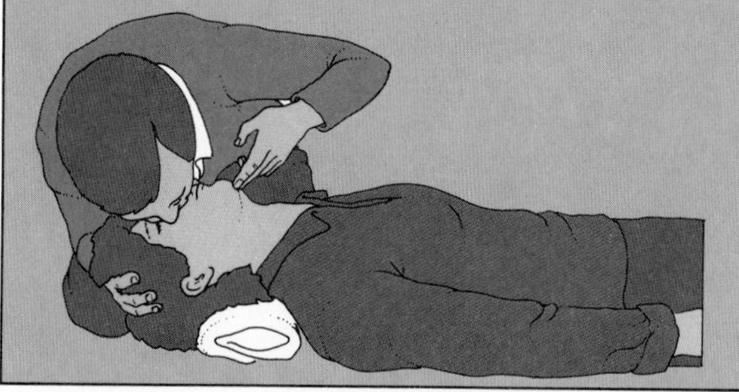

Mouth-to-mouth resuscitation

The simplest and most effective method of artificial respiration is to vigorously exhale your breath into the person's lungs. Mouth-to-mouth resuscitation can safely be used on a person whose breathing, while regular, is very weak, shallow, or labored. Time your exhalations with the person's inhalations.

1 After you call 911 or your emergency number, start first aid immediately. Lay the person down on his or her back on a firm, rigid surface.

2 Tilt the person's head backward by placing one hand beneath his or her chin and lifting upward. Place the heel of your other hand on his or her forehead and press downward as the chin is elevated.

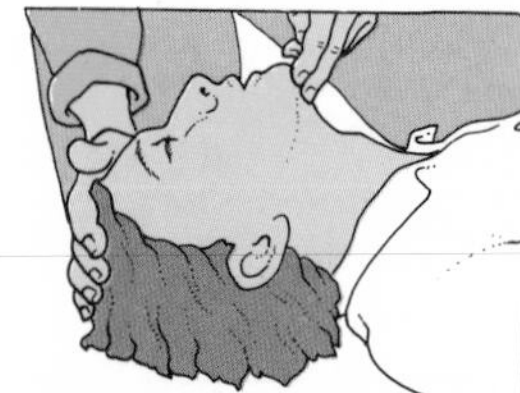

3 With the hand on the person's forehead, pinch his or her nostrils closed using your thumb and index finger. Take a deep breath. Place your mouth tightly over the person's mouth and give 2 full breaths. Then give about 12 breaths per minute (1 breath every 5 seconds). Each breath should cause the person's chest to rise.

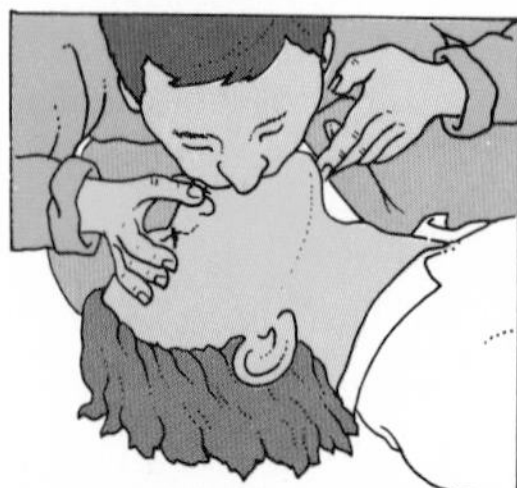

4 Stop blowing when the person's chest is expanded. Remove your mouth and turn your head toward the person's chest so that your ear is over his or her mouth. Listen for air leaving his or her lungs and watch the chest fall. Repeat breathing procedure.

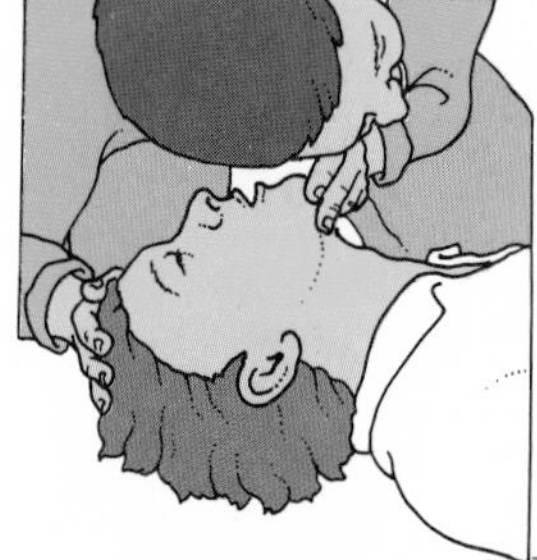

5 Check the person's wrist or neck artery for a pulse. If no pulse is present, begin cardiac compressions if you are trained in cardiopulmonary resuscitation (CPR). This must be done in conjunction with artificial respiration. Continue until medical help arrives or until the person begins breathing on his or her own.

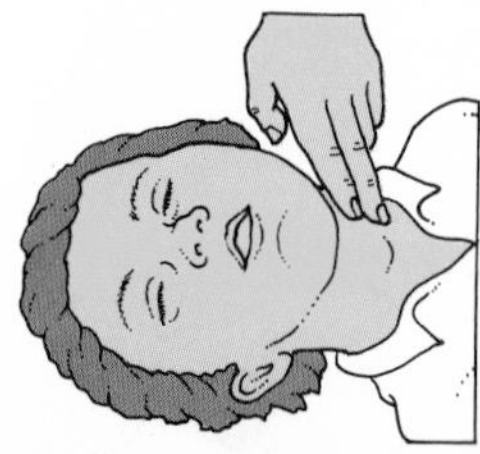

Choking

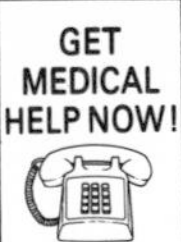
GET
MEDICAL
HELP NOW!

Obstruction of the airway by a piece of food or any object is an emergency. The airway may be only partly blocked; as long as the person is coughing and has good color (not bluish), do not interfere. However, if the person is coughing weakly and is having difficulty breathing, immediate first aid is needed. Call 911 or your emergency number. A person whose airway is totally blocked will be unable to speak, cough, or breathe. He or she may look blue in color or clutch at his or her throat and will soon become unconscious. Sweeping a finger deep inside the person's mouth and dislodging the object may clear the obstruction. Look to see if an object is visible at the top of the throat; if so, try to remove it, being careful not to force it deeper into the throat. If the object cannot be removed, start the Heimlich maneuver (see below).

1 To begin the Heimlich maneuver, hold the person up in a standing position from behind, with one fist against his or her waist area, keeping your thumb inside. Hold your other hand over the fist and quickly thrust hard, in and up, above the person's belt line, forcibly, 6 to 10 times.

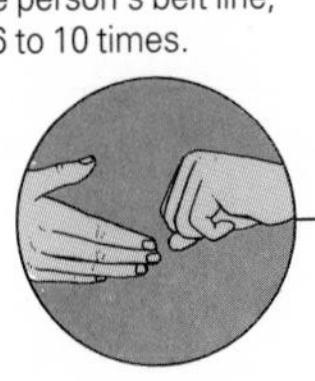

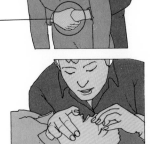

2 These abdominal thrusts should dislodge the obstruction. If they do not, repeat 3 times. Then, if the obstruction is still there and the person has lost consciousness, help him or her to the floor; open the airway with your finger; try mouth-to-mouth resuscitation (see previous page). If this is unsuccessful, begin the Heimlich maneuver by placing the heel of one hand above the person's navel. Put your other hand over the first hand. Give 4 quick, forceful thrusts forward and downward toward the person's head. If the obstruction is dislodged, give mouth-to-mouth resuscitation.

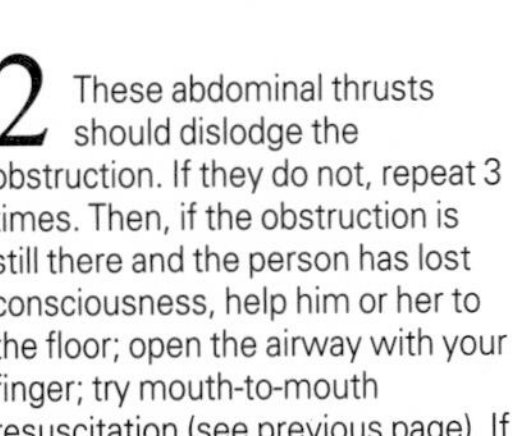

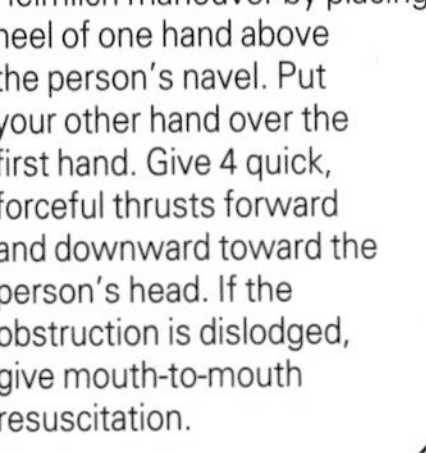

Drowning

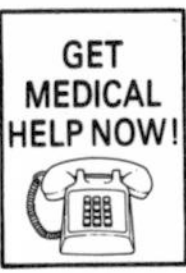
GET
MEDICAL
HELP NOW!

In almost all cases of drowning, speed in starting artificial respiration is essential. First call 911 or your emergency number. Open the airway; attempt to breathe into the person's mouth. You may need to blow fairly hard, but the air you breathe into the person's lungs will pass through any water in them.

If you are alone and the person is in shallow water, start resuscitation (see previous page) immediately in the water. If helpers are available, start resuscitation while they carry the person out of the water and make him or her comfortable. Do not stop respirations even while moving the person.

1 Start mouth-to-mouth resuscitation (see previous page). Do not stop until the person breathes on his or her own again or medical help arrives.

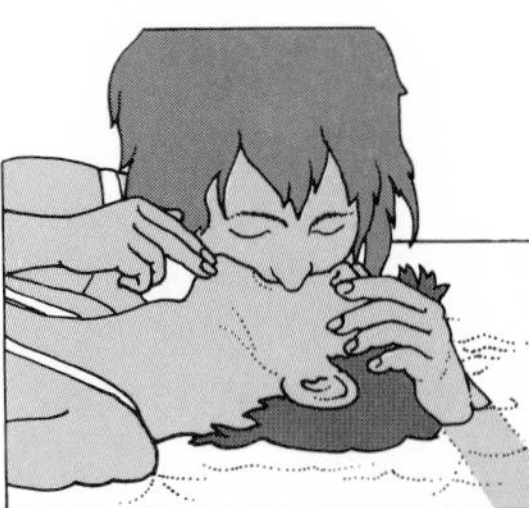

2 Once the person is breathing on his or her own, place in the recovery position (see p.837), and keep warm.

How to revive a choking baby or child

Sit down and lay the child facedown across your knee. Give several thumps with the heel of your hand between the child's shoulder blades, more gently than you would on an adult. A baby can be held face down, supported by one hand under the chest, while being thumped with the other hand.

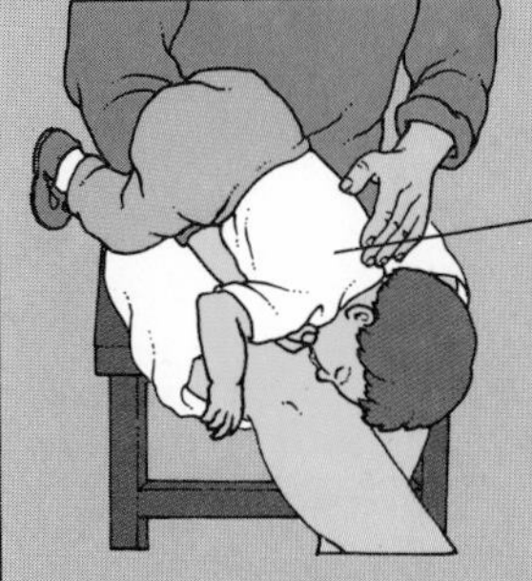

Thump gently between the shoulder blades with the heel of your hand.

Heart attack

A heart attack is a life-threatening emergency. It occurs when there is not enough blood and oxygen reaching a portion of the heart due to a narrowing or obstruction of one of the coronary arteries that supply the heart muscle. If this lack of blood and oxygen is prolonged, a part of the heart muscle will die (see also p.406).

The symptoms of heart attack may include some or all of the following: pain in the central chest that comes on suddenly and feels like a crushing (not sharp) pressure, is constant, and often lasts for 20 minutes or longer; chest pain that spreads through the chest to either arm, shoulder, neck, jaw, mid-back, or pit of the stomach; heavy sweating; nausea and vomiting; extreme weakness; anxiety and fear; pale or bluish gray skin color, and blue fingernails; and/or shortness of breath (mild to severe). The pain of a heart attack may be mistaken for indigestion. If you are not sure about the cause of your pain, treat it as a heart attack to be safe. Call 911 or your emergency number immediately, and follow the first-aid directions given below.

Treatment of a heart attack differs depending on whether the person is conscious or unconscious (see below).

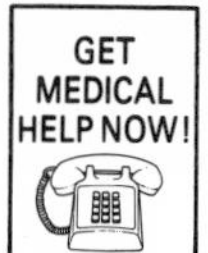

Unconscious person who is not breathing

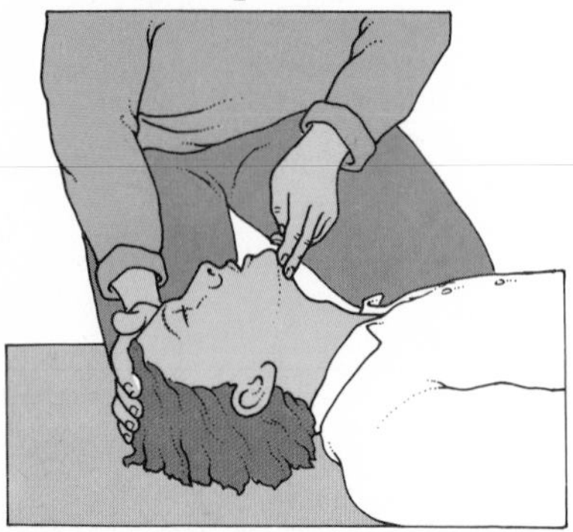

1 First, call 911 or your emergency number; then start first aid. Lay the person on his or her back on a firm, rigid surface. Tilt the person's head backward by placing one hand beneath the chin and lifting upward. Place the heel of your other hand on the person's forehead and press downward as the chin is elevated.

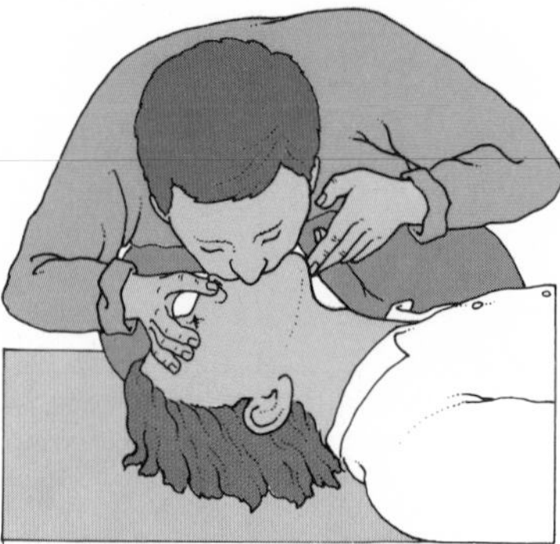

2 With the hand on the person's forehead, pinch his or her nostrils closed using your thumb and index finger. Take a deep breath. Place your mouth tightly over the person's mouth and give 2 slow, full breaths, taking a fresh breath between them so you have air to breathe into the person. Blow air in until you see the chest rise.

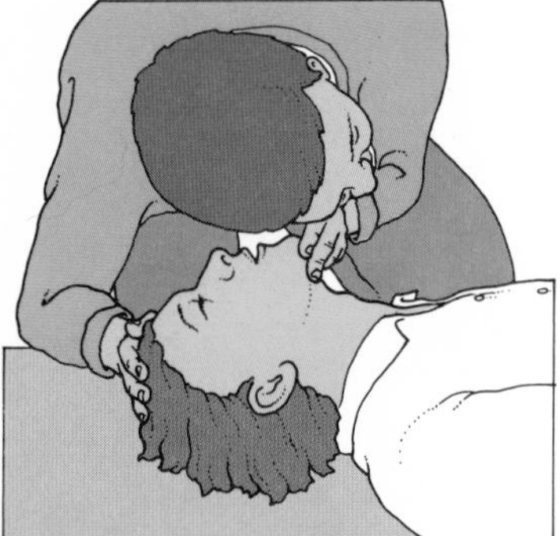

3 Stop blowing when the person's chest is expanded. Remove your mouth and turn your head toward the person's chest so that your ear is over the person's mouth. Feel and listen for air leaving his or her lungs and watch the chest fall. Repeat the breathing procedure, giving one breath every 5 seconds.

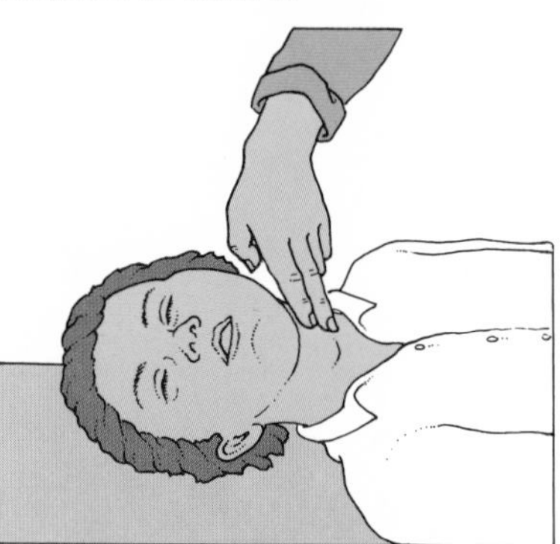

4 Check the person's wrist or neck artery for pulse for 5 to 10 seconds. If no pulse is present, begin cardiac compressions if you are trained in cardiopulmonary resuscitation (CPR). Artificial breathing must be continued during CPR. Continue until medical help arrives or the person begins breathing on his or her own.

Conscious person

1 Gently place the person in a comfortable position, either sitting up or partially sitting. Lying down makes breathing feel more difficult.

2 Loosen tight clothing, particularly around the neck, and keep the person warm with a blanket or coat.

3 Calm and reassure the person, but do not offer anything to eat or drink.

4 Call 911 or your emergency number and inform the operator of a possible heart attack and need for oxygen. If no ambulance is available, take the person to the nearest hospital emergency department.

5 Follow these steps also if an unconscious person regains consciousness and resumes breathing. The same basic instructions apply if you have a heart attack when you are alone.

Unconsciousness

Unconsciousness refers not only to a coma but also to a state in which a person is drowsy, confused, and unable to respond to your presence. It may result from brain damage (head injury or stroke), loss of blood, lack of oxygen in the blood (drowning), or chemical changes caused by disease (diabetic coma) or drugs. First, call 911 or your emergency number; then start first aid.

Note: If you suspect a possible spinal injury, do not move the person into the recovery position (right) unless he or she is vomiting. Then move him or her without flexing the spine by turning the head and body simultaneously, keeping them in exact alignment.

How to treat unconsciousness

When a person is unconscious, the body's normal reflexes disappear and the muscles may lose their tone and become floppy. The main danger is obstruction of the airway, either because the lower jaw and tongue have fallen backward, blocking the airway, or because the person can no longer cough to clear vomit or other matter from the back of the throat. Even after you open the airway and restore breathing to the unconscious person, never leave him or her unattended. A person who goes into a coma may stop breathing and his or her heart may stop as a result.

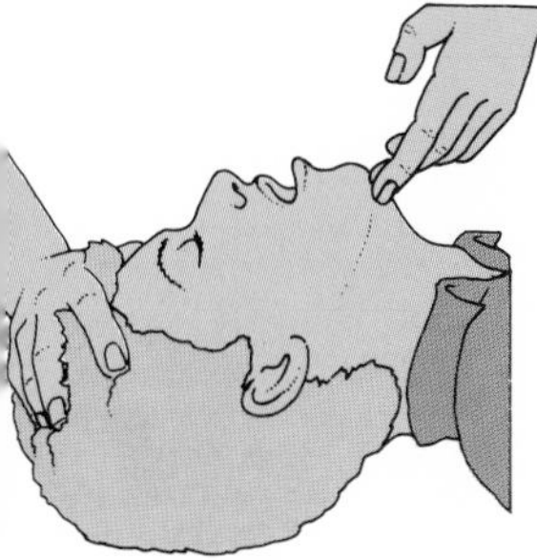

1 After you call 911 or your emergency number, bend the person's head well back. If the person is not breathing, start artificial respiration (see previous page).

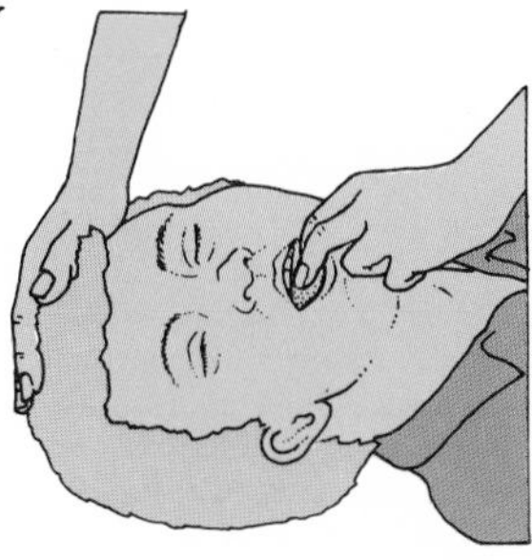

2 If the person's breathing sounds noisy or gurgling, sweep a finger around deep inside the person's mouth. Remove any loose or false teeth.

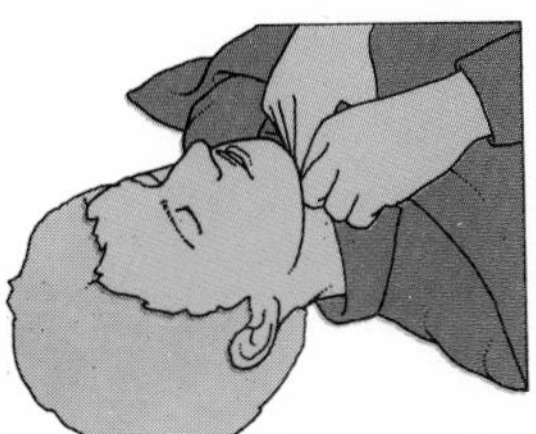

3 Loosen any tight clothing around the person's neck and chest once normal breathing is reestablished.

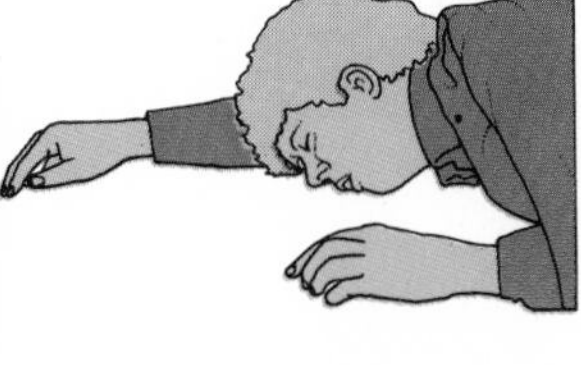

4 Place the person in the recovery position (right), on a blanket, if possible, to minimize heat loss. Cover with a coat or blanket and stay close by.

Recovery position

Note: Do not use the recovery position if you suspect a spinal injury, unless the person is vomiting.

When you have done everything you can to alleviate the person's condition (see priority checklist, p.833), place him or her in the recovery position while waiting for emergency medical help to arrive.

In the recovery position, the head hangs forward so that the person can breathe freely and liquids can drain easily from the mouth. The placement of the arms and legs supports the body in a stable and comfortable position, with the person's body weight evenly distributed.

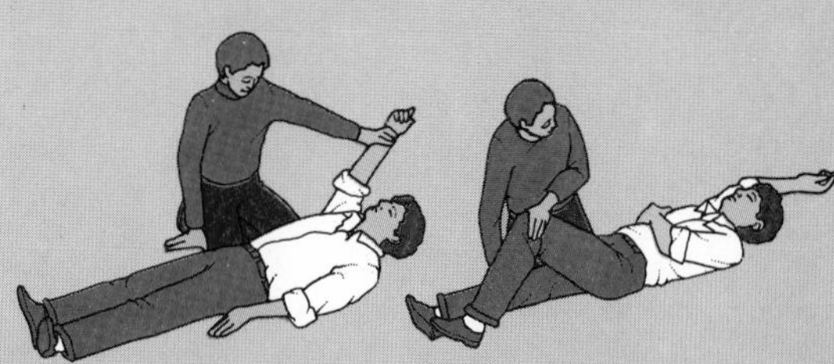

1 Kneeling at the person's side, straighten the arm and hand nearest to you and place it behind his or her head.

2 Cross the far arm over the chest, and the far leg over the near one at the knee.

3 Grasping clothing at the hip, pull the person gently over toward you with one hand, rotating the head with the body and protecting his or her face with the other hand.

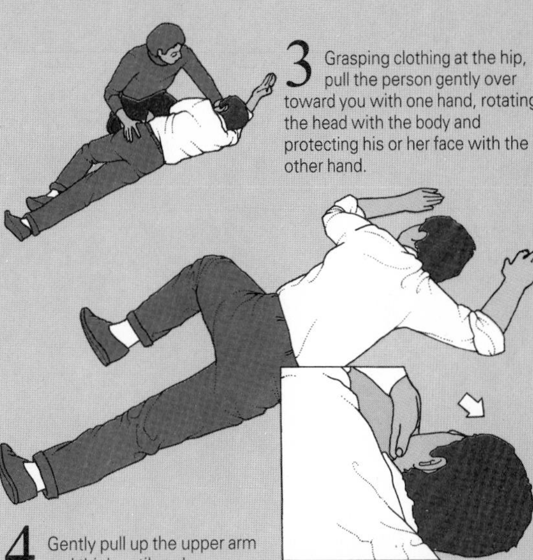

4 Gently pull up the upper arm and thigh until each one forms a right angle with the body, bent at the elbow and knee.

5 Tilt the person's head back so that the chin juts forward, enough so that he or she can breathe. But keep the chin lower than the body. Keep the person warm, and stay close by.

Severe bleeding and wounds

Large quantities of blood can be lost very rapidly from a severed or torn artery. Severe blood loss can lead to shock and unconsciousness, and if the bleeding is not stopped it is fatal. If an adult loses more than 1½ pints of blood or a child loses one-half pint, the blood loss is considered severe.

The muscles in the wall of a damaged artery will contract, which combines with formation of a blood clot to seal the wound (see Bleeding, p.455). If the blood does not clot for any reason, such as hemophilia (see p.455), or because of anticoagulant or antithrombotic medication, bleeding will be more difficult to control. First, call 911 or your emergency number; then start first aid.

GET MEDICAL HELP NOW!

Arterial pressure points

If direct pressure on the wound is not effective, or if a wound is too extensive for direct pressure, there is another way to stop bleeding. Apply pressure to a major artery, at a point between the wound and the heart where the artery can be compressed against a bone.

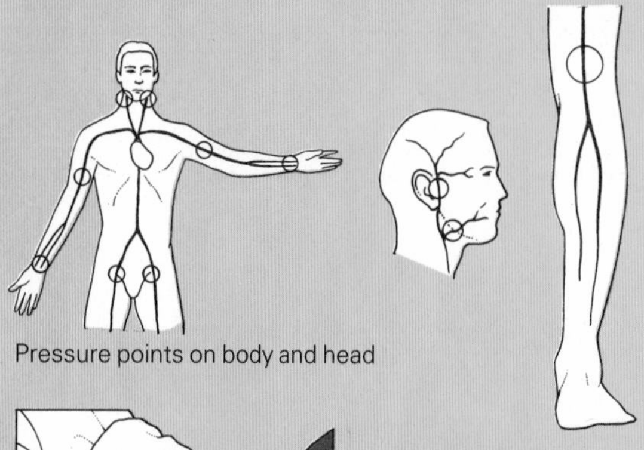

Pressure points on body and head

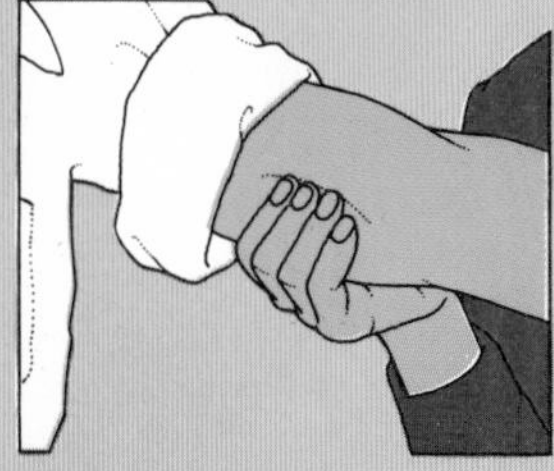

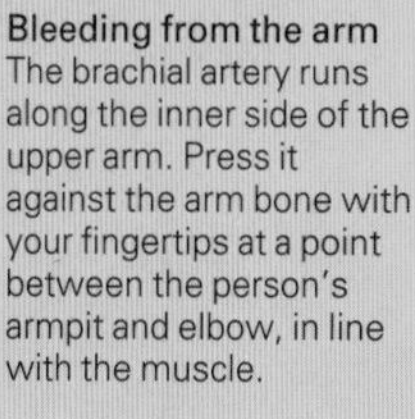

Bleeding from the arm
The brachial artery runs along the inner side of the upper arm. Press it against the arm bone with your fingertips at a point between the person's armpit and elbow, in line with the muscle.

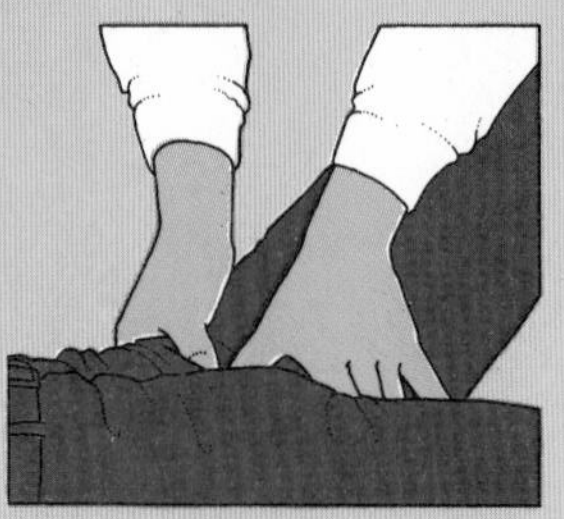

Bleeding from the leg
The femoral artery runs across the groin before going down the leg. Hold the person's upper thigh with both hands and press hard in the center of the groin with both thumbs, one on top of the other.

Stopping severe bleeding

In a minor wound, bleeding usually stops by itself after a short time. In a severe wound, blood may flow so freely that there is no chance for a clot to form. The goal of first aid is to stop the flow of blood as quickly as possible.

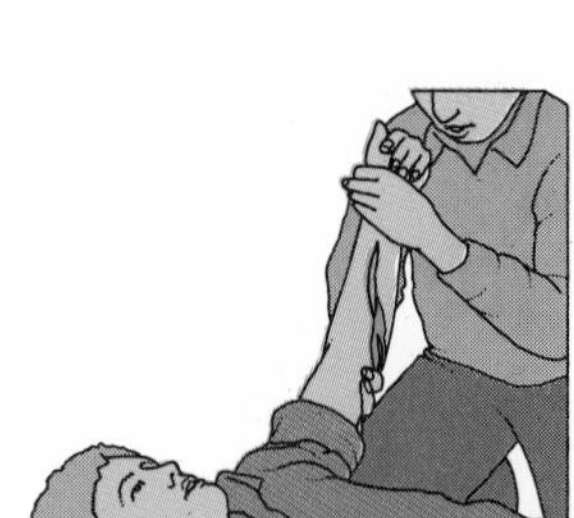

1 Lay the person down and, if possible, raise the injured part. This will reduce the flow of blood from the wound.

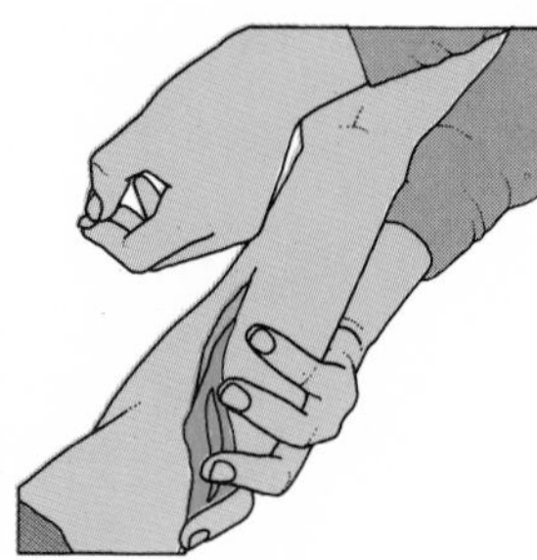

2 Pick out any visible and easily removable objects not deeply embedded, such as glass or metal, but do not probe for anything embedded in the wound.

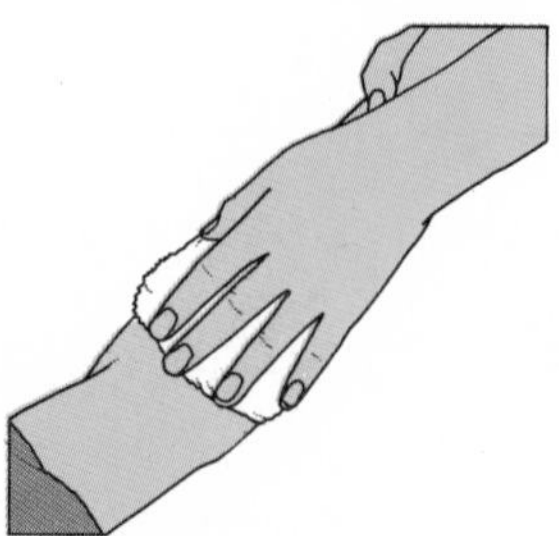

3 Press hard directly on the wound for 5 to 10 minutes, until visible bleeding stops, with a pad that is as clean as possible. If the wound is gaping, hold its edges firmly together. If there is anything in the wound, exert pressure around it, not over it.

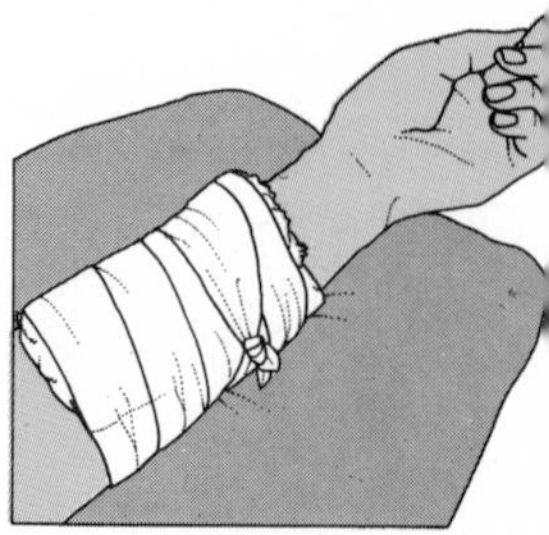

4 Take a firm pad and bind it tightly over the whole wound so that pressure is maintained. If no bandage is available, use an item of clean clothing. Do not use a tourniquet. Check for a pulse below the bandage (that is, on an artery farther away from the heart).

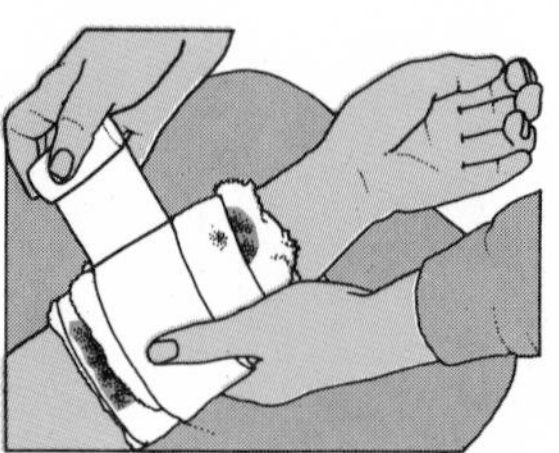

5 If blood oozes through the bandage, do not remove it. Instead, put more padding over the wound and bandage it tightly.

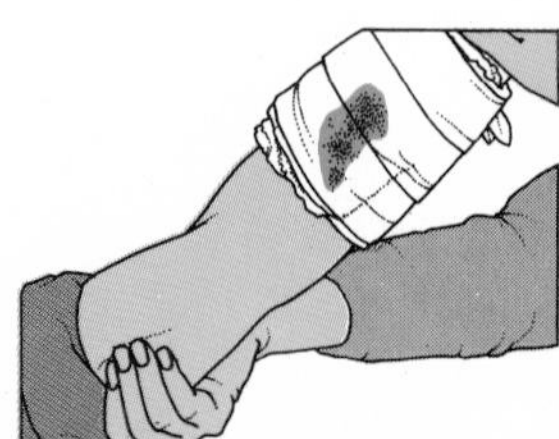

6 If direct pressure fails to slow or stop the bleeding, you may be able to control it more effectively by pressing on an arterial pressure point (see Box).

Shock

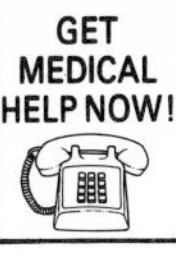

A person in shock usually looks very pale, feels faint and sweaty, and has a weak, rapid pulse and cold, moist skin. He or she is drowsy and confused, and will eventually become unconscious. A person who is in shock requires immediate first aid and medical treatment. (For general information, see Shock, p.414.) First, call 911 or your emergency number; then start first aid.

How to prevent shock

Shock can follow any severe injury, particularly if there are severe burns or blood loss. Blood loss can be internal, so you may not see any blood. First-aid treatment after all severe injuries should include measures to prevent—or at least minimize—shock.

1 Lay the person down, head low, face up, and with legs raised about 1 ft (30 cm), so blood will flow from the legs to the upper body. If the person is unconscious, place in the recovery position (see p.837).

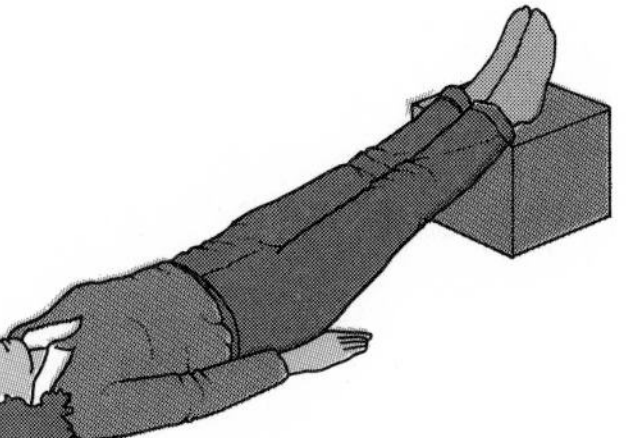

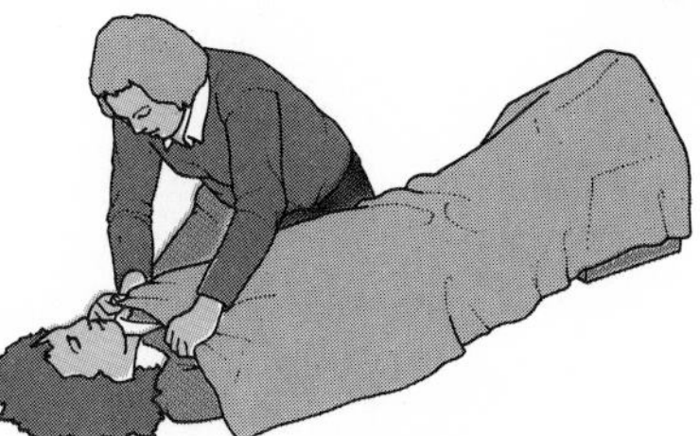

2 Loosen any tight clothing, and prevent heat loss by wrapping the person in a coat or blanket. Do not use a hot-water bottle or electric blanket.

3 Do not offer anything to eat or drink unless medical help is several hours away. Then you can give a conscious person water or a weak solution of water and salt or baking soda. Mix 1 level teaspoon of salt or a level half-teaspoon of baking soda in 1 quart (about 1 liter) of water. Give the adult victim 4 oz (120 mL), a child 2 oz (60 mL), and an infant 1 oz (30 mL); have the person sip that amount slowly over 15 minutes. Offer reassurance and make the person as comfortable as you can.

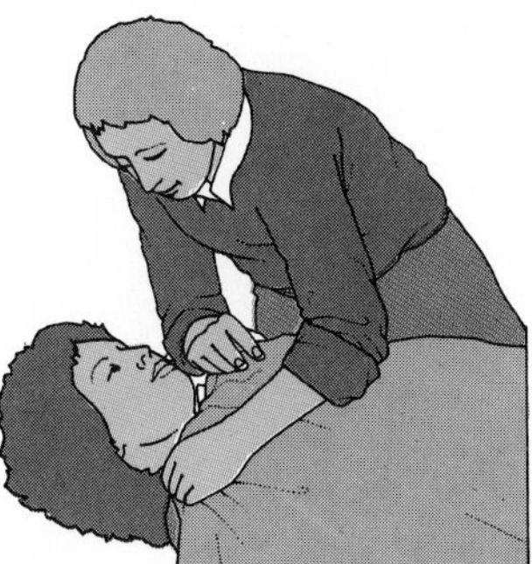

Head injuries

Scalp injuries usually bleed profusely because of the scalp's rich blood supply. If you are treating a superficial head wound, apply a clean pad or handkerchief to the wound with steady pressure.

If the person has a severe head injury, tie a clean pad loosely over the wound. If you apply pressure on the wounded area to stop the bleeding, you may press broken fragments of skull bone or other foreign material into the brain. So press very carefully around the edges of the wounded area, especially if a fracture is visible or suspected.

If a clear, watery fluid (known as cerebrospinal fluid) comes out of an injured person's ear, place a clean pad loosely over the ear, but do not try to prevent the fluid from draining.

Treating a severed arm, leg, finger, or toe

If a part of the body is cut off, it is vital to get both the person and the severed part to an emergency department immediately. The greater the time lapse, the less chance there is of successfully rejoining the severed part to the body. It is important to keep the part clean and cool. If possible put it in a plastic bag and then inside another plastic bag with ice in it. If this is impossible, place the part inside any clean container. Take the person to the hospital immediately with the severed part. Make sure that emergency department personnel understand the situation.

Chest injuries

If the chest wall is penetrated in an injury, air can enter the chest cavity, displacing and collapsing a lung. This reduces the amount of air entering the lungs. You will be able to hear the noise of air being sucked in as the person inhales, and see blood-stained bubbles around the wound as he or she exhales. Do not remove any object that is embedded in the wound, and do not offer anything to eat or drink.

1 Press firmly with a clean pad held in the palm of your hand over the site of the wound, to make an airtight seal.

2 Lay the person down, with head and shoulders raised and the body leaning slightly toward the injured side.

3 Cover the entire wound with a large dressing. A cloth or sheet of foil will do if no sterile dressing is available.

4 Cover the dressing with a thick pad of cotton and tie or tape it firmly on, so that the seal remains airtight.

5 Call (or have someone call) 911 or your local emergency medical services system, or take the person to a hospital as soon as possible.

Electric shock

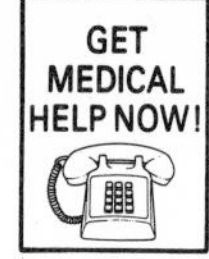

The shock of an electric current entering and leaving the body can knock someone down, cause unconsciousness, or stop breathing and heartbeat. The current fans out through the underlying tissues and may cause deep and widespread damage, even though a small mark is all that is visible on the skin where the current entered and exited the body.

First aid for electric shock

First, turn off the current, if possible, or safely separate the person from the source of the current with a nonconducting material such as wood or a dry rope. Until this has been done, the person may be conducting electricity; anyone trying to offer first aid will also receive a shock. This does not apply to someone who has been struck by lightning; he or she is not conducting electricity and can be given first aid immediately.

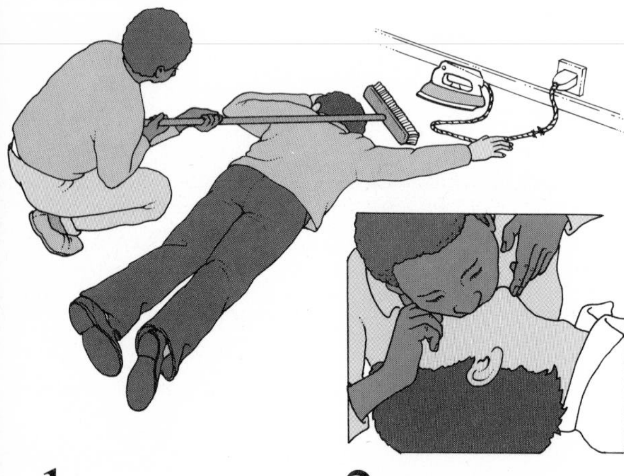

1 Turn off the current, or push the person away from the source of electricity with a dry, nonconducting object such as a wooden chair or a broom handle.

2 Check breathing and heartbeat. If the person is not breathing, start mouth-to-mouth resuscitation (see p.834).

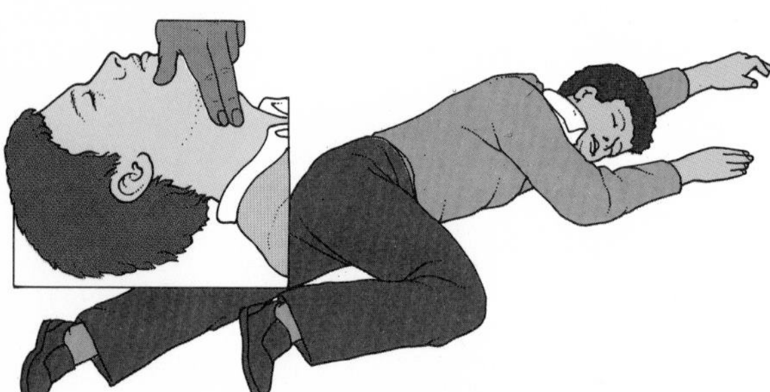

3 If the person's heart is not beating, start cardiopulmonary resuscitation (CPR) if you are trained in the procedure.

4 If the person is breathing but unconscious, place in the recovery position (see p.837). Treat any burns (right), and call 911 or your emergency number.

Severe burns

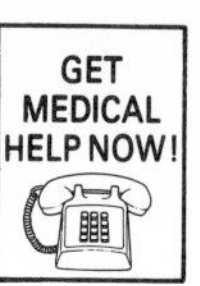

Burns may be caused by dry heat, moist heat (steam, hot liquids), electricity, friction, or corrosive chemicals. First, call 911 or your emergency number; then start first aid as discussed below. A severe (third-degree) burn will destroy all the layers of the skin, leaving a relatively painless area that may look white or charred.

First aid for severe burns

If someone's clothing is on fire, quickly help the person to the ground with the burning side face-up. Smother the flames with a blanket or whatever is at hand, directing the flames away from the head toward the feet. Cool the burned area with cold water as soon as possible.

Do not prick or burst blisters, and do not breathe or cough over the burned area. Quickly remove anything constricting (shoes, rings, bracelets) from the burned part, because later it will swell and make it difficult to remove the items. Do not cover the burn with anything fluffy such as cotton, and *do not apply any lotions or ointments to it.*

Note: Nothing but cold water should be put on the burn. If the skin has been burned by a corrosive chemical, it is vital to put the entire area under a steady flow of running water immediately to dilute and wash off the chemical.

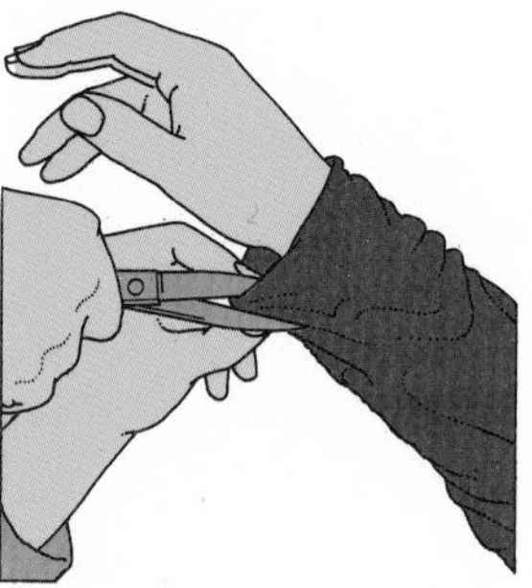

1 Remove clothing that has been soaked in hot grease or oil or boiling water immediately. Do not remove dry, burned clothing or any clothing that is stuck to the burn.

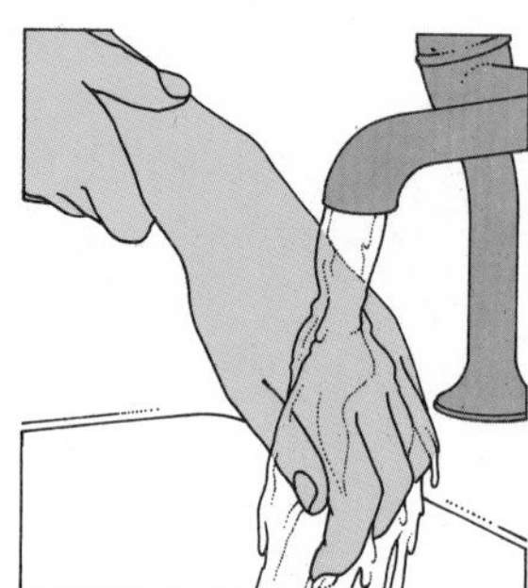

2 Immerse the burned part in cold water for at least 10 minutes, if possible. If the burned area is extensive, cover it with a folded sheet or towel soaked in cold water. Do not apply ointments or lotions.

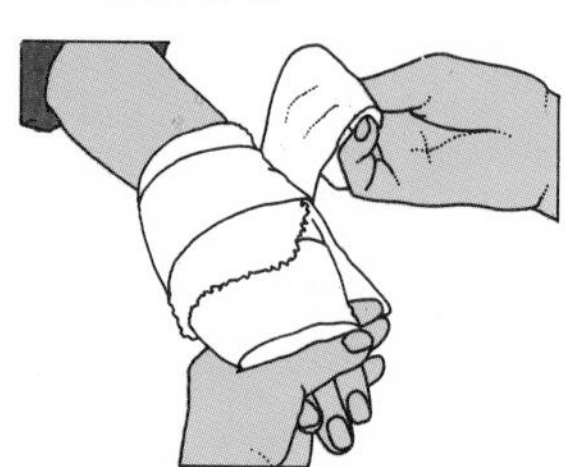

3 Lightly cover the entire burned area with a clean, dry dressing. If fluid oozes through, cover with another layer. An arm or leg can be protected inside a clean plastic bag.

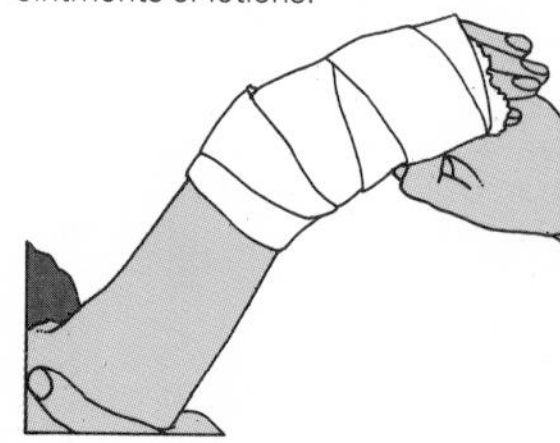

4 Raise a burned arm or leg to reduce swelling, and give the person frequent small sips of cool water to combat fluid loss, as long as he or she is conscious and not vomiting.

Hypothermia

Body temperature is normally constant at 98.6°F (about 37°C). During prolonged exposure to cold, more body heat may be lost than can be replaced, so body temperature may drop. Hypothermia occurs when the body temperature falls.

In young, healthy people, hypothermia occurs only after prolonged physical exertion in cold, windy conditions. In older people (see p.772) and young children, it can occur more easily. Once the stores of energy that produce body heat have been used up, the fall in body temperature causes a gradual physical and mental slowing that may not be noticed. The affected person becomes increasingly clumsy, unreasonable, irritable, and sleepy. The person's speech becomes slurred. He or she becomes confused and drowsy, and eventually goes into a coma, with slow, weak breathing and a slow, weak heart rate. First, call 911 or your emergency number; then start first aid.

GET MEDICAL HELP NOW!

1 If the person is unconscious, check breathing. If he or she has stopped breathing regularly, artificial respiration (see p.834) may be necessary.

2 Once breathing is regular, shelter the person from the cold. If you have to remain outdoors until help arrives, cover the person's head and insulate him or her from the ground to prevent further heat loss.

3 If possible, dress the person in warm, dry clothes and give warm drinks if he or she does not cough or vomit. Do not offer the person alcohol.

4 A healthy adult can be rewarmed gradually in a well-heated room, or more rapidly in a warm (not hot) bath.

Frostbite

Frostbite is the freezing of parts of the body, which results in blockage of blood flow and damage, usually to the fingers, toes, ears, and nose. Frostbite (see p.440) requires immediate medical attention. Get the person indoors as soon as possible and send for help. Meanwhile, shelter the person from the wind, give warm nonalcoholic drinks, and cover the frozen part with extra clothing or blankets, or warm it against your body. Do not use direct heat and do not rub the area. As frostbitten parts warm up, encourage the person to move them gently, but do not let the person walk if his or her feet are frostbitten or frozen.

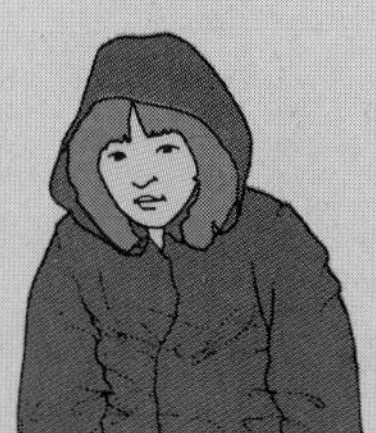

If the hands are frostbitten, tuck them into the person's armpits under his or her coat or put the hands in warm water (101°–104°F, about 38°–39°C).

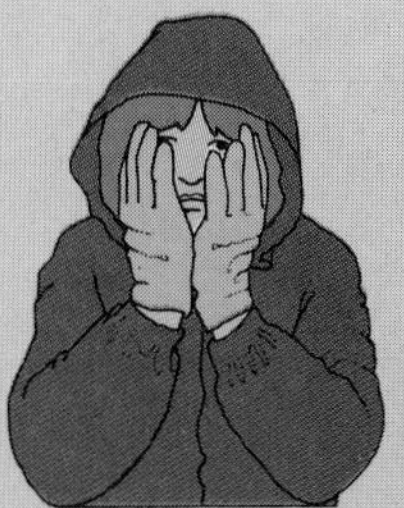

If the face is affected, cover it with dry, gloved hands until normal color returns.

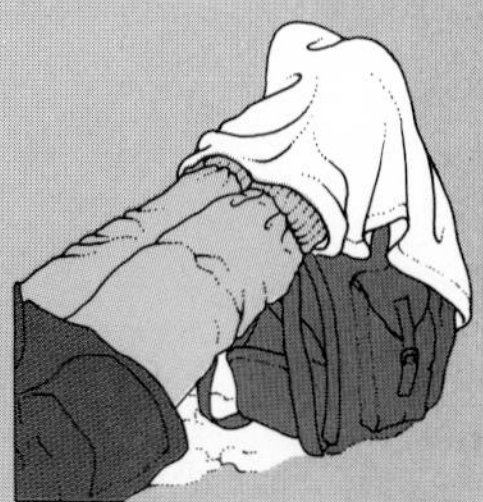

If toes or feet are affected, keep them elevated and covered, or immerse them in warm water (101°–104°F, about 38°–39°C).

Heat exhaustion

Heat exhaustion occurs when someone is exposed to very hot weather, and does not take in adequate salt and water; as a result, the body cannot get rid of the heat load placed on it. Water and salt loss is caused by excessive sweating as the body unsuccessfully attempts to cool off. The skin becomes pale and clammy. The person may feel sick, dizzy, and faint. His or her pulse rate and breathing become rapid and a headache or muscle cramps may develop. Heatstroke may follow.

1 Lay the person down in a cool, quiet place, with feet raised a little.

2 Loosen any tight clothing and give water to drink. Add one level teaspoonful of salt to each quart (liter).

Heatstroke (sunstroke)

Heatstroke usually occurs because of prolonged exposure to very hot conditions. The mechanism in the brain that normally regulates body temperature stops functioning, and the temperature rises to 104°F (40°C) or higher. The person is confused or unconscious, and is flushed, with hot, dry skin and strong, rapid pulse. Heatstroke is a medical emergency. First move the person to the coolest available place and call 911 or your emergency number.

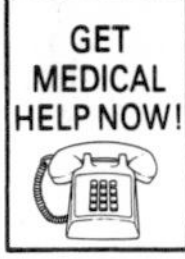

1 Remove clothing and sponge the person with cool or tepid water.

2 Fan the person, either by hand or with an electric fan or blow-dryer set on cold.

3 When body temperature drops to about 101°F (38°C), place the person in the recovery position (see p.837).

4 Continue to fan. If body temperature starts to rise again, repeat the process.

Fractures and dislocations

Without an X ray, it is not always possible to tell if a bone is fractured, or broken, so if you are not sure, treat an injury as if a fracture has occurred. Suspect a dislocation or fracture if the person cannot move or put weight on the injured part, or if it feels very painful or looks misshapen (see Fractures, p.575).

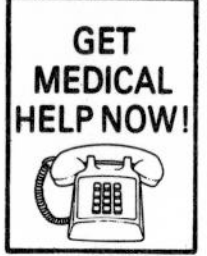

How to treat a broken or dislocated bone

Do not try to force back a dislocated bone yourself. This should be done only by a physician. Splint the arm or leg in the position in which you found it, and take the person to a hospital, unless the injury makes it hard to walk. In such cases, call 911 or your emergency number and wait for help.

1 Treat any bleeding (see p.838). Move the person as little as possible. Movement may further displace broken bones and damage organs. Cover an open wound with a clean dressing and secure in place.

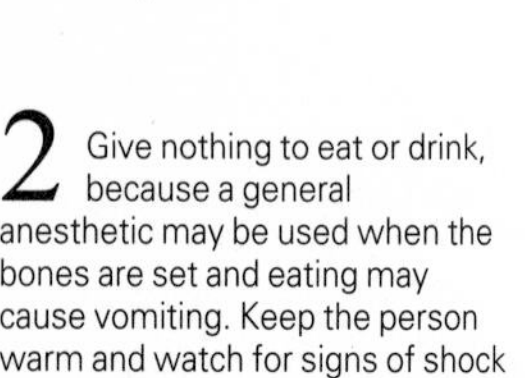

2 Give nothing to eat or drink, because a general anesthetic may be used when the bones are set and eating may cause vomiting. Keep the person warm and watch for signs of shock (see p.839).

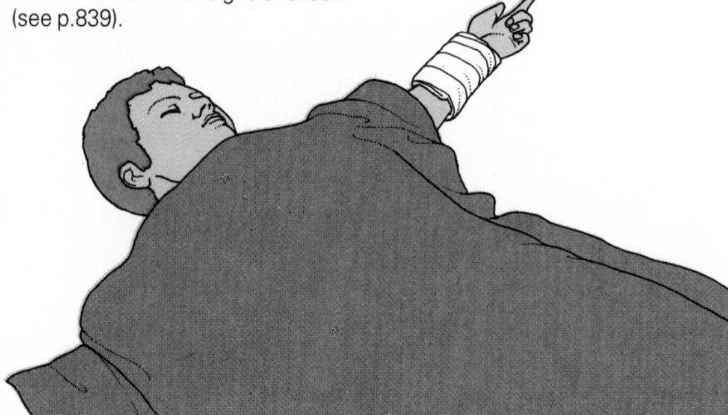

Applying a splint

Splinting is usually necessary. By preventing movement, you avoid provoking pain and keep the break from getting worse. This is especially valuable if you have to move the injured person or if there will be a long delay before help arrives. A splint should be rigid and, if possible, long enough to immobilize the joints above and below the injury. Splints can be made with padded pieces of wood, magazines, or even pillows if necessary.

For a broken upper arm or a broken leg, be sure to put some padding between the arm and the torso or between the legs, before splinting the injured limb. Use cloth (bandages, ties, or scarves) to tie the splint in place.

Broken lower arm
Place lower arm at a right angle across the person's chest, with palm facing toward the chest and thumb pointing upward. Put padded splint around lower arm. Splint should reach from the elbow to beyond the wrist.

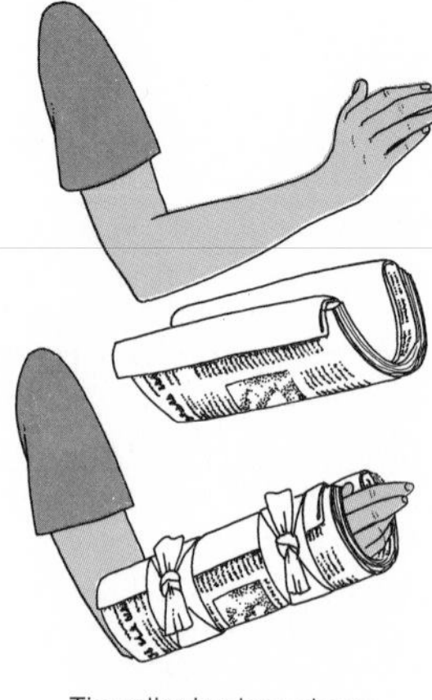

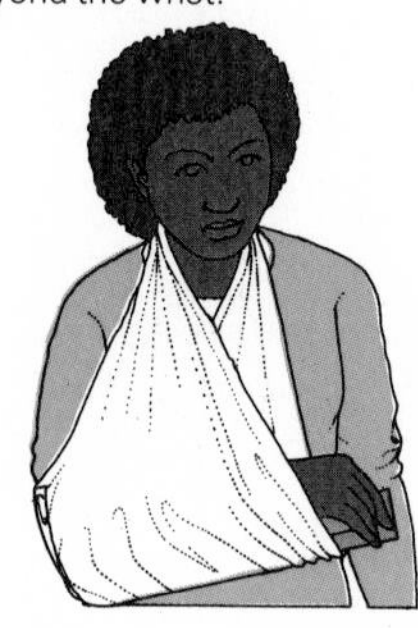

Tie splint in place above and below the break. Support lower arm with a wide sling tied around the neck, so the fingers are slightly higher than the elbow.

Splinting injured leg to uninjured leg
Gently straighten the knee of the injured leg. Place some padding between the person's legs. Tie the injured leg to the other leg in several places, but not directly over the break.

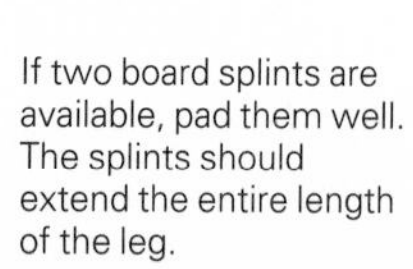

If two board splints are available, pad them well. The splints should extend the entire length of the leg.

Spinal injuries

If the person has severe pain in the neck or spine, any tingling or loss of feeling or control in his or her arms or legs, or any loss of bladder or bowel control, the spinal column may be fractured or dislocated. In such cases, do not move the person unless his or her life is in immediate danger or he or she is choking on vomit. If the person must be moved, keep his or her body straight, do not bend the back or neck, and do not twist the body. Move the person's body in a straight line, preferably placing him or her on a rigid surface such as a door, a table, an ironing board, or a wide plank.

Poisoning

Swallowing is the most common way in which a poison enters the body (including food poisoning and accidental or deliberate self-poisoning). Other forms include bites, stings (see p.844), drugs injected through the skin, inhaled gases such as exhaust fumes (right), and chemicals absorbed through the lungs or skin.

GET MEDICAL HELP NOW!

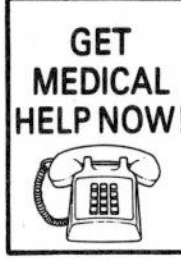

How to deal with a poisoning emergency

First contact a poison control center, 911 or your emergency number, or a physician for instructions. Tell them the person's age, the name of the poison, how much was taken and when, whether the person has vomited, whether he or she is conscious, and how far you are from medical help. Follow the instructions you are given exactly. If the person is conscious, you may be told the following: If the poison was swallowed, give the person water or milk to dilute the poison; then induce vomiting to eliminate the poison.

However, do not induce vomiting if you do not know what the person has swallowed, or if he or she has taken an acid, an alkali, or a petroleum product, unless the poison control center specifically tells you to do so. Water, not milk, is used if the person has swallowed a petroleum product. Keep syrup of ipecac and activated charcoal in your first-aid kit at home; use only as directed by your poison control center.

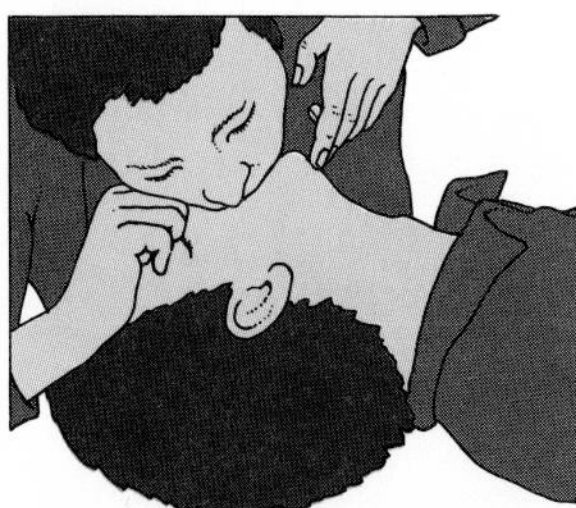

1 If the person is unconscious, check breathing. If he or she is not breathing, start mouth-to-mouth resuscitation (see p.834).

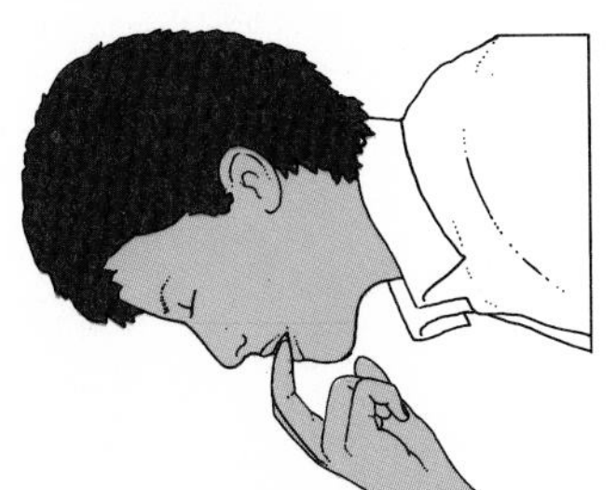

2 If the person is conscious, and the poison is not acid, alkali, or a petroleum product, put the person sitting or lying face down (so he or she does not breathe in vomit) and stick your finger down his or her throat to induce vomiting.

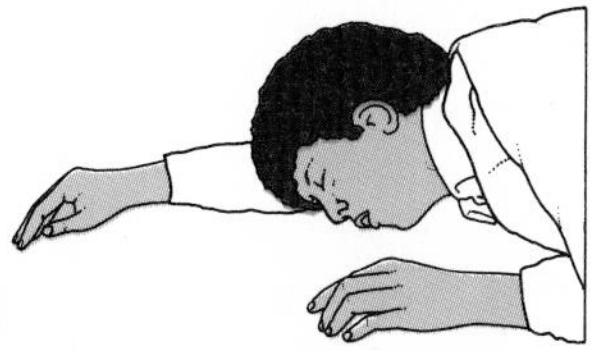

3 If the person is unconscious but breathing or conscious but drowsy, place in the recovery position (see p.837).

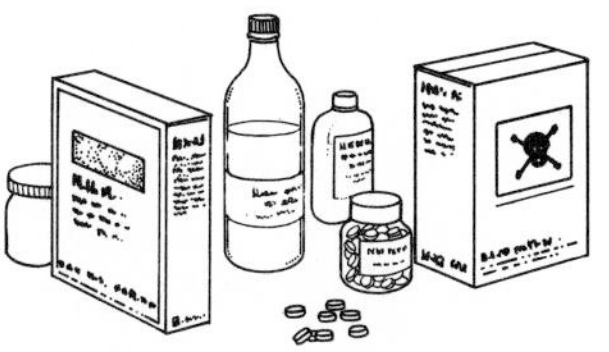

4 Keep any containers that may have held the poison, and a sample of any vomit, for the hospital to analyze. Get medical help as soon as possible.

Poisoning from smoke, chemical, or gas fumes

Be extremely careful when rescuing a person from an area filled with fumes or smoke. If possible, avoid making the rescue attempt alone. Breathe deeply and rapidly two or three times, then take a deep breath and hold it before entering the area. Remain close to the ground to avoid inhaling hot air and fumes (hot air rises toward the ceiling). If the area is very hot or the fumes are very heavy, you should have an independent source of air (an air tank and mask). Do not try to do anything except move the person into the fresh air.

Once you have moved the person away from the smoke or fumes, check to see if he or she is breathing. If the person is not breathing, start mouth-to-mouth resuscitation (see p.834).

Loosen tight clothing. Get medical help immediately for the person even if he or she appears to recover completely.

Common household poisons

Keep the telephone number for your local poison control center by every telephone in your home. The following substances are found in most homes. If they are swallowed or get into your eyes, they are extremely harmful and possibly fatal. All such substances should be stored out of reach of young children and kept in childproof containers. Also, be sure these items are always labeled correctly.

Alcohol
Aspirin
Bleach
Cigarettes and tobacco
Cosmetics
Dishwasher detergent
Dishwashing detergent
Drain cleaner
Drugs of any kind
Furniture polish
Glass cleaner
Grease remover
Insecticide
Laundry detergent
Nail polish and nail polish remover
Oven cleaner
Paint and paint thinner
Scouring pads
Scouring powder
Toilet cleaner
Weedkiller

Bites and stings

The injuries that come under this heading are varied, and they range from mild to extremely serious and possibly fatal. Each geographical area of the US has its own risks, so make sure that you and your children know about local poisonous plants and insects and dangerous animals found in your area.

Insect bites and stings

Allergic reactions to insect stings

Some people are allergic to stings from certain insects such as honey bees. An allergic reaction to a sting may be life-threatening. The extreme case of a total body allergic reaction is called anaphylactic shock. Symptoms may include severe swelling in parts of the body other than the area of the sting, such as the eyes, lips, and tongue; weakness; coughing or wheezing; severe itching; stomach cramps; nausea and vomiting; anxiety; difficulty breathing; bluish color of skin; dizziness; collapse; unconsciousness; and/or hives. Many people know that they have such an allergy, and have an emergency kit available. If this is not the case, remove the stinger by scraping it out with a knife or fingernail (do not use tweezers, as you may squeeze more venom out) and apply a light constricting band 2 in to 4 in (5 cm to 10 cm) above the sting (below right). Make the person as comfortable as possible, and get medical help immediately.

Minor bites and stings

Symptoms of a minor insect bite or sting may include pain, swelling at the site, redness, itching, and/or burning. Multiple stings may cause a toxic reaction with headache, muscle cramps, fever, drowsiness, or even unconsciousness. A severe toxic reaction may require medical treatment. Remove any stinger without using tweezers. Wash the area with soap and water. Apply an ice pack or cold compresses to the area.

Bees, wasps, and hornets Only the honey bee leaves a stinger in the skin. Remove it without using tweezers, to avoid squeezing more venom into the area.

Spiders Bites from poisonous spiders are especially dangerous for young children, older people, or people who are ill. Two kinds of poisonous spiders are found in the US: black widows and brown recluse, or fiddleback, spiders. If you have severe pain or other symptoms after being bitten by a spider, put ice or cold compresses on the bite and get medical help immediately. Take the spider with you, if possible, if you can do so safely.

Scorpions The venom of some scorpions is more poisonous than the venom of others. Treat a scorpion sting like a spider bite, and get immediate medical help.

Snakebites

If you are bitten by a snake, it is important to know whether or not the snake is poisonous. There are four major kinds of poisonous snakes in the US: rattlesnakes, copperheads, cottonmouths, and coral snakes. You should become familiar with the appearance of these snakes. Try to capture and kill the snake that bit you, without damaging the head, or at least be able to describe the snake.

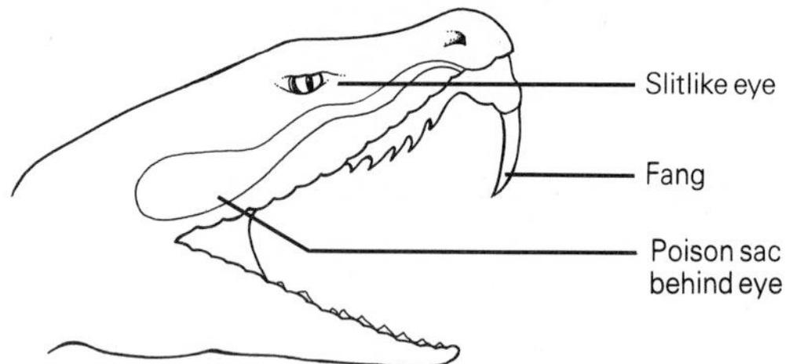

Poisonous snakes
The rattlesnake, copperhead, and cottonmouth all have slitlike eyes with poison sacs behind them. They also have long fangs. The coral snake has rounded eyes, but has fangs and poison sacs like the other poisonous snakes.

Rattlesnakes have a characteristic rattle on the end of their tails. Cottonmouths, also called water moccasins, have a white lining in their mouths, for which they are named. A coral snake has red, yellow, and black rings and a black nose.

Treating snakebites
The instructions below do not apply if the person is bitten by a coral snake. In such cases, the person should be immobilized and medical help obtained immediately. In the case of any snakebite, keep the bitten area below the person's heart, if possible.

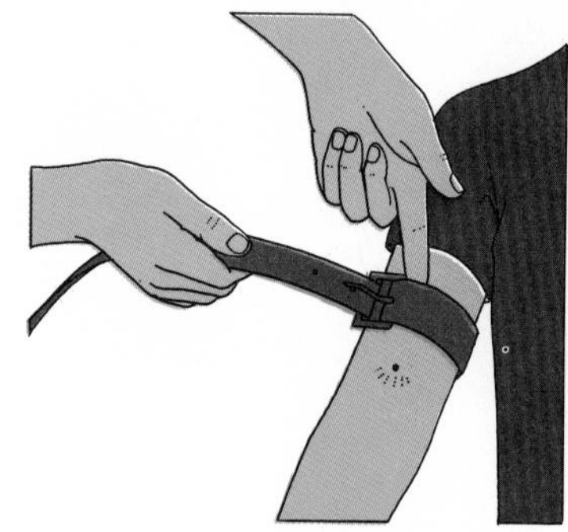

1 First call 911 or your emergency number. If the bite is on an arm or leg, place a light constricting band 2 in to 4 in (5 cm to 10 cm) above the bite toward the body. Do not cut off circulation. Leave the band on until medical help arrives. Wash the bite area with soap and water. Immobilize the area. Do not use ice or cold compresses.

2 Keep the person as quiet as possible. This will help to slow the circulation, which will, in turn, help stop the venom from spreading. Do not let the person walk unless absolutely necessary and, if so, then very slowly. Do not attempt to suck out the venom.

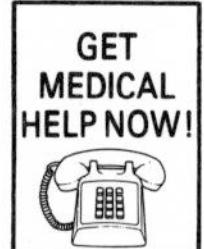

Animal (mammal) bites

Treat superficial bites and scratches the same way as cuts and scrapes (see p.846). Get immediate medical help for human bites or any deep bites, especially the puncture wounds of any animal, since such bites can easily become infected. A tetanus injection may be needed. If you are bitten by any animal, domestic or wild, the animal should be caught and impounded so it can be immediately checked for rabies. If the animal is dead, it should still be checked. The person may need treatment with antirabies serum and vaccine (see Rabies, p.603).

Jellyfish stings

Jellyfish stings are seldom dangerous, although they may cause painful burning and swelling. Relieve the symptoms with calamine lotion. The Portuguese man-of-war may cause a more serious reaction, with shortness of breath and fainting. Scrape off the stingers, which stick to the skin, with dry sand, if possible, and get medical help immediately. Place the person in the recovery position (see p.837) and keep him or her warm while waiting for help to arrive.

Foreign object in the ear or nose

Children often put small objects such as beans or beads into their ears or noses. Do not try to remove them; take your child to a physician.

Insect in the ear

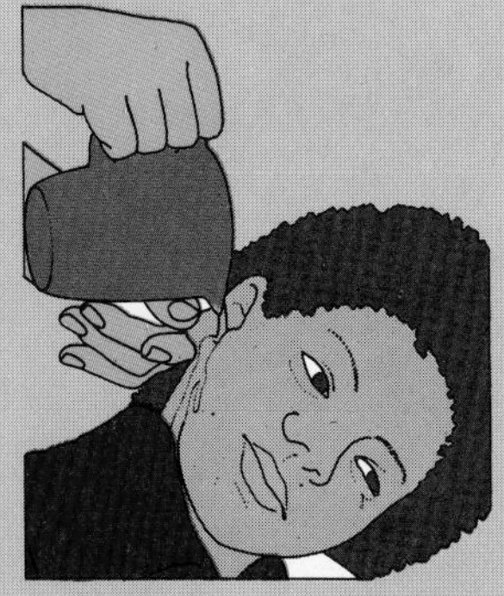

If an insect becomes lodged in the ear, ask the person to tilt his or her head with the affected ear up. Then float out the insect by pouring warm (not hot) mineral, olive, or baby oil into the ear. Pull the ear lobe gently backward and upward to straighten the ear canal while you do this. If the insect does not come out, take the person to a physician.

Poisonous plants

Some plants can cause an allergic reaction or direct chemical reaction (burn or blister) on the skin of some people. Poison ivy, poison oak, and poison sumac are three of the most common of these plants. They may grow anywhere, but are often found in woods and uncultivated fields. If you touch the plant, an oily substance on the leaves gets on your skin and causes an itchy, oozing rash. You may unintentionally spread the rash all over your body and cause considerable discomfort if you don't wash off the oily plant substance.

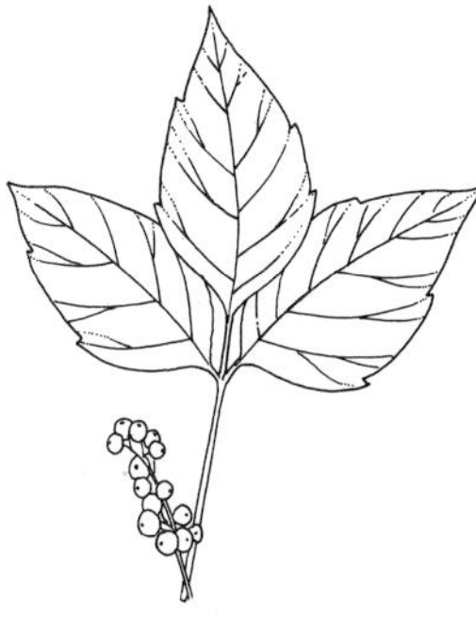

Poison ivy may grow as a plant, bush, or vine. It has three shiny leaflets on a stem.

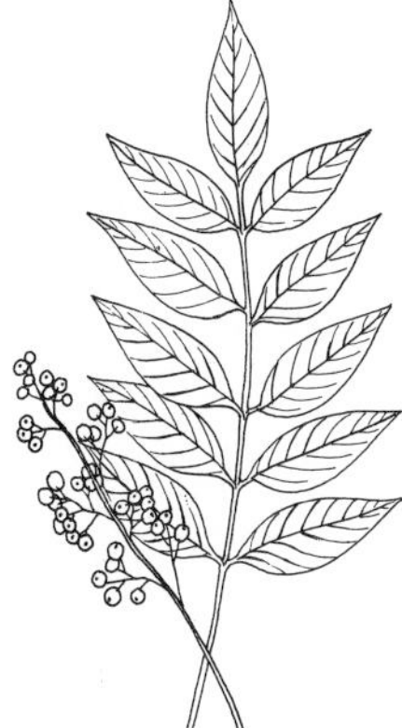

Poison sumac may be a bush or a tree. It has two rows of leaflets opposite each other and a leaflet at the tip.

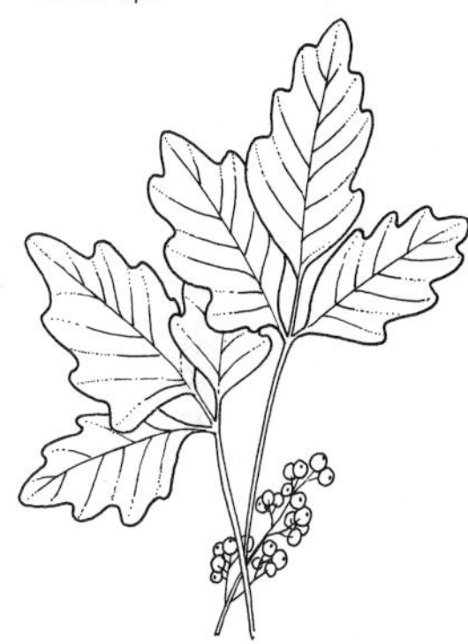

Poison oak is similar to poison ivy except for the shape of the three leaflets, which resemble oak leaves.

After exposure, remove your clothes and wash the exposed area with soap and water to remove the oily plant substance. Then sponge off with rubbing alcohol, except in the genital area. Wash the clothes also. If you scratch the rash, it may spread and get worse. See a physician if the reaction is severe or if the rash appears on your face or genitals.

Other plants such as nettles can cause temporary irritation and/or rashes or swelling that occur in a limited area. The symptoms usually disappear within a few hours (see also Eczema and dermatitis, p.269).

Cuts and scrapes

If blood spurts from a wound or flows so heavily that it cannot be stopped after a few minutes of pressure, this is severe bleeding (see p.838) and is a medical emergency.

Slight bleeding from a cut or a scrape usually stops on its own within a few minutes. If it does not stop, press a gauze pad firmly over the wound for about 5 to 10 minutes. Any wound that later becomes tender or inflamed or appears to contain pus should be examined by a physician.

If the cut is deep (you can see yellow fatty tissue), irregular, or on the face, or if the edges gape so badly that they cannot easily be pulled together with surgical tape, seek medical help. Such cuts probably need stitching to aid healing and to reduce scarring. A scrape with dirt or grit embedded under the skin should be properly cleaned and bandaged by a physician.

If bleeding or a clear, watery fluid comes from the ear or nose after a severe blow to the head, the base of the skull may be fractured. Keep the person's neck and back aligned and firmly supported and do not bend them. Call 911 or your emergency number immediately. Do not move the person unless absolutely necessary (see Head injuries, p.839).

Puncture wound A deep wound caused by something dirty such as a nail or an animal's tooth is more likely than other wounds to become infected; dirt and bacteria are carried deep into the tissues and the wound bleeds very little. Numbness, tingling, or weakness in an arm or leg can follow a deep cut or puncture wound, indicating that nerves or tendons may be damaged. Antibiotics and a tetanus injection may be necessary after a deep wound, to prevent infection.

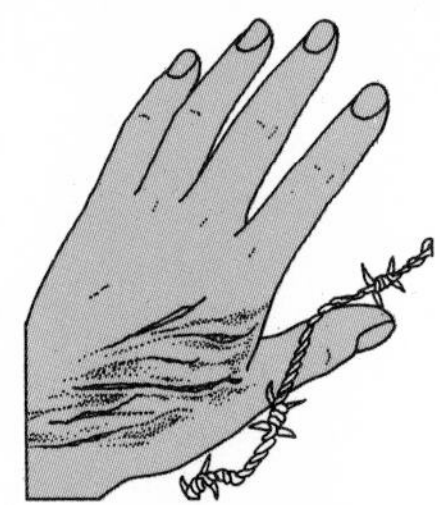
Lacerated wound

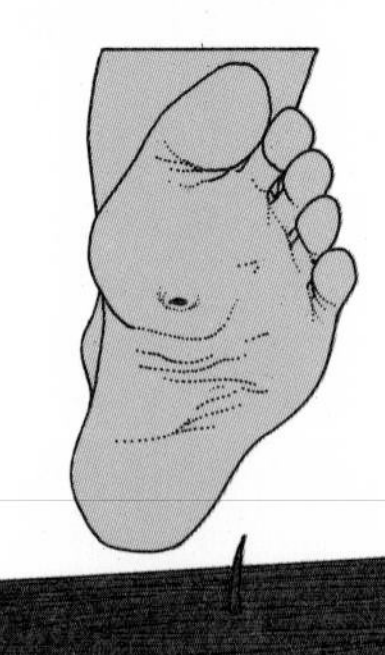
Puncture wound

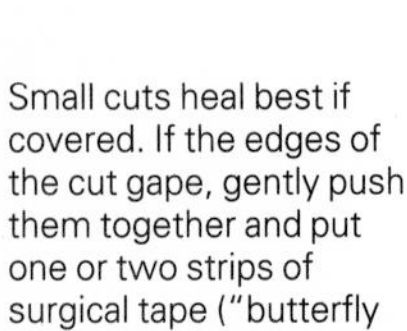
Bleeding carries some dirt out of most wounds, so you only need to clean around a cut. Wipe from the edges of the wound outward, using a clean gauze or cotton pad for each stroke.

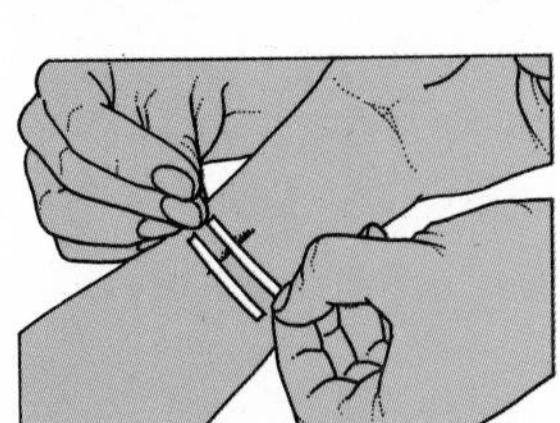
Small cuts heal best if covered. If the edges of the cut gape, gently push them together and put one or two strips of surgical tape ("butterfly strips") across the cut.

Minor burns and scalds

If a burn or scald damages only the outer layer of skin over a fairly small area, causing reddening and perhaps blistering, it can be treated at home. Severe burns (see p.840) are a medical emergency. Sunburn is usually only a minor burn.

Superficial burns are very painful, so the goal of first aid is to relieve the pain. If blisters form over a burn, do not break them. If they are on a part of the skin normally rubbed by clothing, cover them with a light dressing (see Blisters, next page). Do not put any cream, grease, or ointment on a burn, except for a large area of mild sunburn, which can be soothed with calamine lotion. The pain of sunburn can also be relieved by applying cool compresses to the skin at intervals, taking cool baths, or taking aspirin or an aspirin substitute.

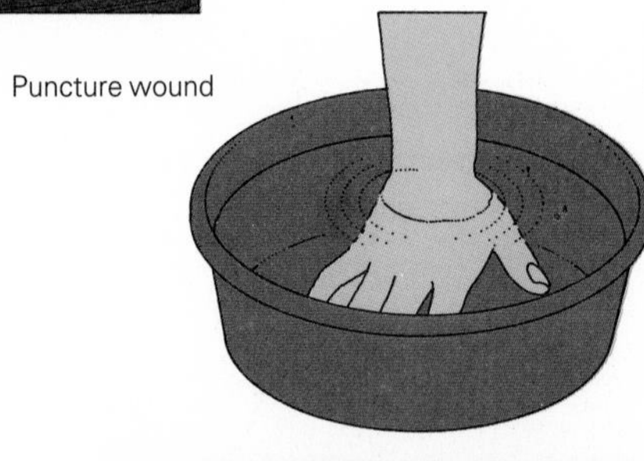
Plunge the burned area into cold water, or hold it under a cold running tap for 10 minutes or until the pain stops or lessens. Do not put ice on a burn because it may injure the tissue. Also, do not apply creams or ointments.

Fishhook in the skin

If the barb of a fishhook becomes embedded in the skin, get a physician to remove it. Try to remove it yourself only if medical help is not available, and consult a physician afterward because of the high risk of infection.

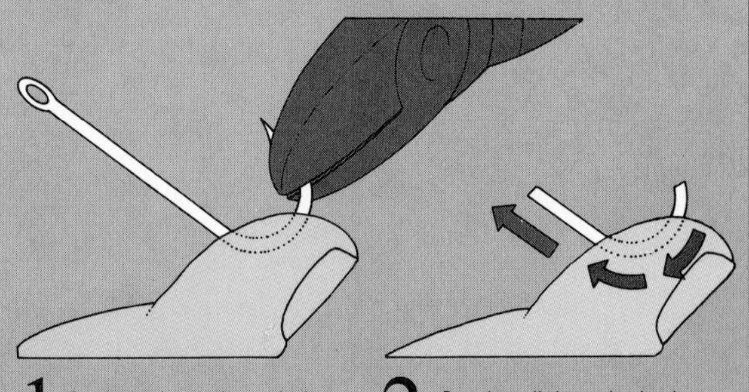

1 Push the hook through the skin until the barb protrudes. Then cut off either the barb or the shank, close to the skin.

2 Gently pull the unbarbed portion through the skin at the same angle as the curve in the hook. Clean the wound and cover it with a bandage.

Splinters

A small splinter projecting from the skin can usually be removed by a gentle pull with tweezers. To remove a splinter embedded just under the skin, slit the skin over one end of the splinter with the tip of a needle or point of a razor blade that has been sterilized in a flame and allowed to cool for a moment, and lift up the end of the splinter with the needle tip or razor blade. You should then be able to remove the splinter with tweezers. If it does not come out easily, do not probe further. Go to a physician.

Bruises

Bruises occur when a fall or blow causes bleeding into the tissues beneath the skin. Bruises normally fade slowly, change color as they fade, and disappear without any treatment after 10 to 14 days. If any bruise does not fade or disappear, or if you notice bruises appearing for no obvious reason, see your physician.

Bruises on the head or the shin, where the bone is just beneath the skin, may swell significantly. To reduce pain and swelling, apply an ice pack or wring out a cloth in cold water and lay it over the bruise for about 10 minutes with moderate pressure.

Bruising around the eye, known as a "black eye," may swell significantly. Apply a cool or cold wet cloth to the area for 10 minutes. If any disturbance of vision follows a blow to the eye, seek medical help.

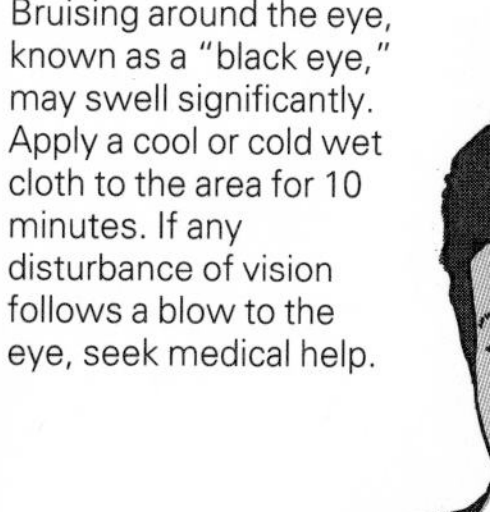

Blisters

Blisters form on the skin because of allergic reactions, or when the skin is damaged by friction, burns, or chemicals. New skin forms under the blister, and the fluid in the blister is gradually absorbed. Eventually the outer layer of skin comes off. No first-aid treatment is needed unless the blister breaks or is likely to be damaged by further friction. In such cases, wash the area with soap and water, and protect it with an adhesive bandage.

Do not prick the blister or try to remove it. This will leave the raw skin under it painful and open to infection.

Sprains and strains

A tear in a muscle or tendon is called a strain, and a tear in a ligament or joint capsule is called a sprain (see p.573). Both sprains and strains result from overstretching the tissues, and the symptoms for both injuries are the same: pain, swelling, and bruising. A severe sprain may be indistinguishable from a fracture and should be treated as if it were a fracture (see p.575).

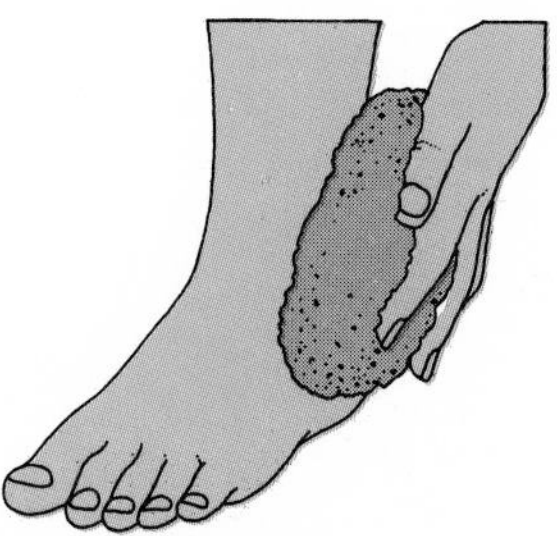

1 Sponge a mild strain or sprain with cold water or apply ice wrapped in a cloth to reduce pain and swelling.

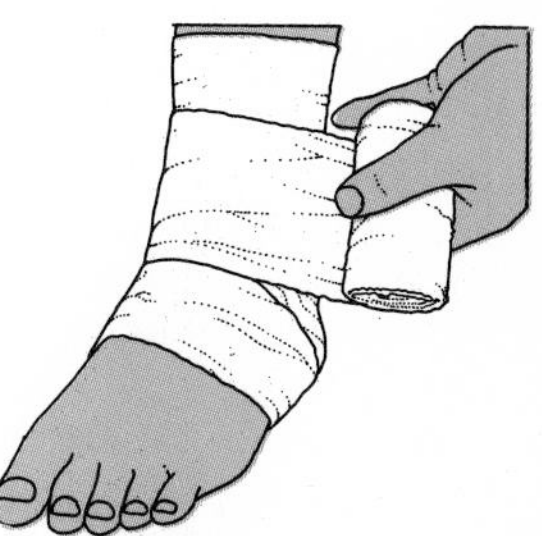

2 Support the joint or muscle with an elastic, figure-eight bandage, and do not put any weight on it for a day or two.

Applying a figure-eight bandage

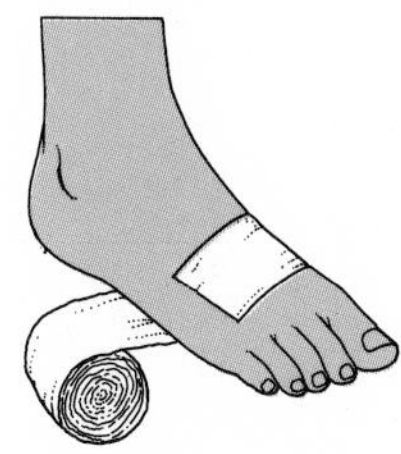

1 Anchor the bandage by making one or two circular turns around the foot.

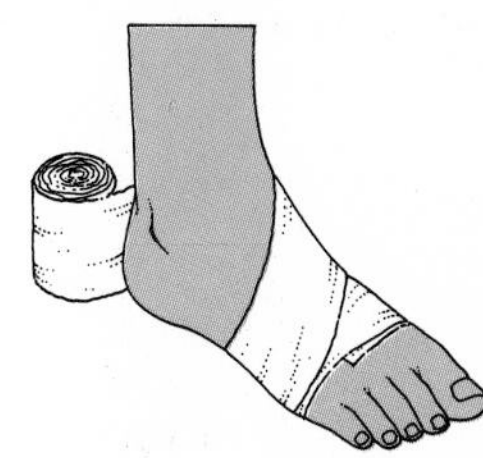

2 Bring the bandage diagonally across the top of the foot and around the ankle. Continue to bring the bandage down across the top of the foot and under the arch of the foot.

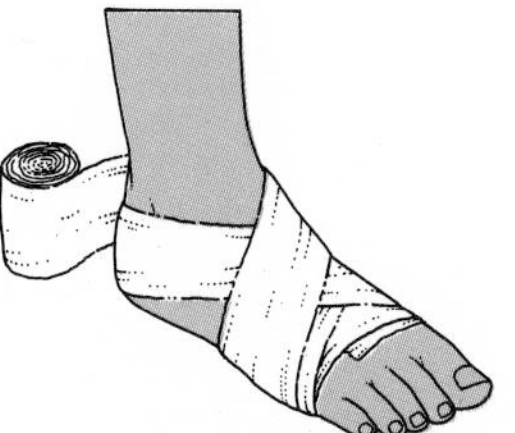

3 Continue figure-eight turns, with each turn overlapping the last one by about three-fourths of the width of the bandage.

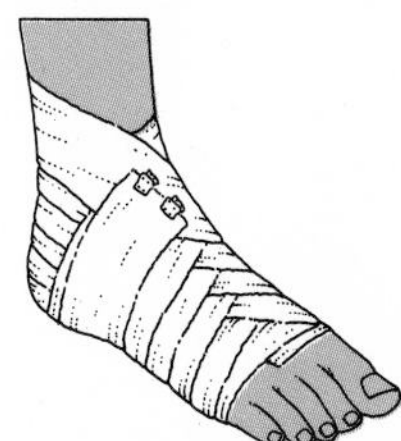

4 Bandage until the foot (not toes), ankle, and lower leg are covered. Secure bandage with tape or clips.

Foreign object in the eye

Never try to remove anything that is on the pupil of the eye, or that seems to be stuck or embedded in the white of the eye. In such circumstances, do not let the injured person rub the eye, but cover both eyes with a soft pad to help stop eye movements, and get medical help.

If the foreign object is floating on the white of the eye or on the inside of the eyelid, try to remove it with the corner of a clean cloth, handkerchief, or tissue, or with a cotton-tipped swab, as described below. Do not let the person rub the eye.

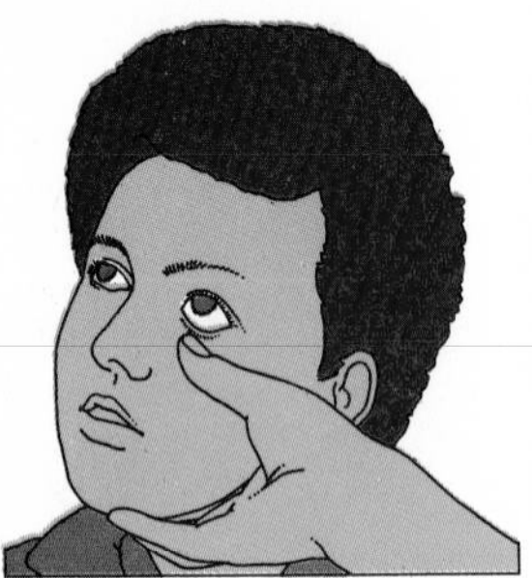

1 Seat the person in good light. Get the person to look up while you gently pull the lower lid down. If you can see the object, pick it off gently with the corner of the cloth.

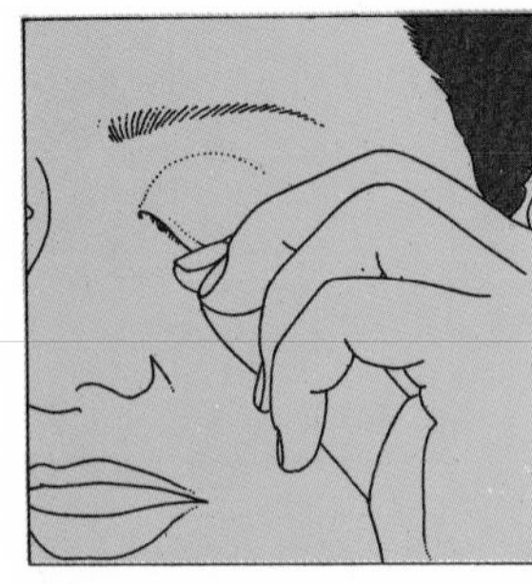

2 If you cannot see the object, pull the upper lid down and out over the lower lid and let it slide back. This may be enough to dislodge the object.

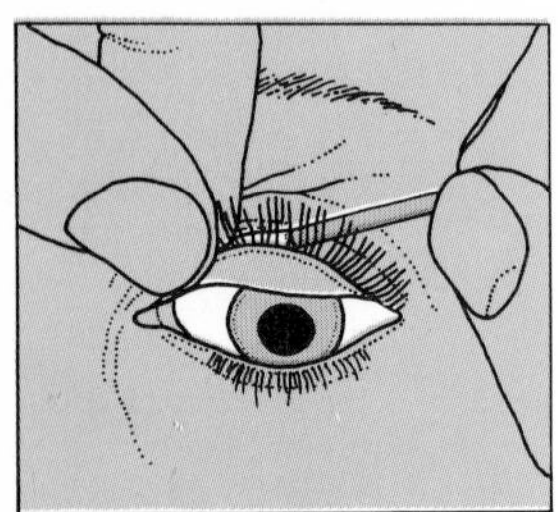

3 If nothing happens, ask the person to look down while you place a swab or toothpick above the upper lid and fold the lid up over it.

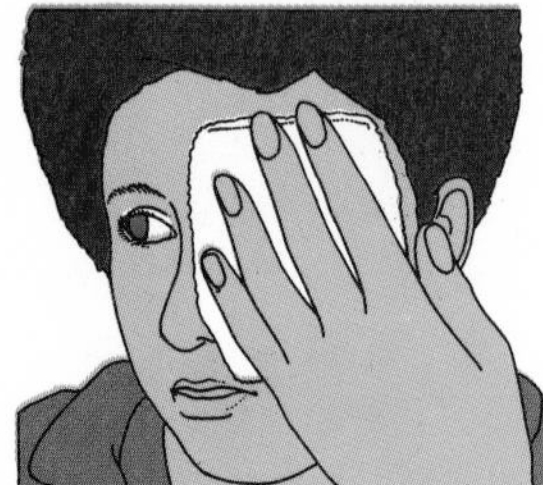

4 If you can see the object, pick it off with the cloth. If not, cover the eye with a soft pad and get medical help.

Chemicals in the eye

Chemicals or corrosive fluids splashed in the eye must be washed out quickly by holding the person's opened eye under gently running water. Tilt the head toward the injured side so that the chemical is not washed into the uninjured eye. Keep the eyelids apart with your fingers. After 10 to 20 minutes, cover the eye with a pad and take the person to a hospital emergency department immediately.

Emergency childbirth

Sometimes a pregnant woman's labor proceeds so fast that there is not enough time to reach a hospital or get medical help before the baby is born. If you are the only person present at such a birth, remember that it is a natural process: interfere as little as possible. Most births do not have complications.

GET MEDICAL HELP NOW!

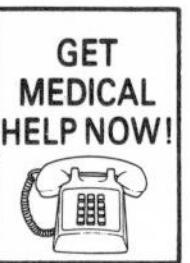

Preparing for birth

Try to make the site warm. Make the woman comfortable with pillows. Put a clean sheet or newspapers under her, if possible, with a plastic sheet under them. Wash your hands with soap and water. If you can, sterilize a pair of scissors and a length of string by boiling them.

If the woman seems distressed or in a lot of pain, be calm and reassuring. As the birth proceeds, there may be a lot of blood-stained fluid. This is normal during birth.

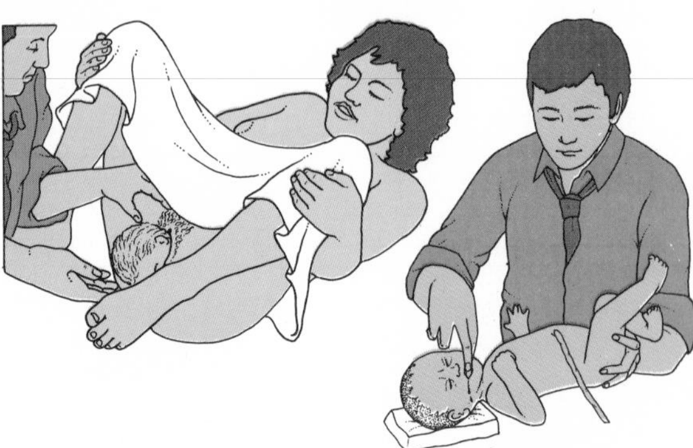

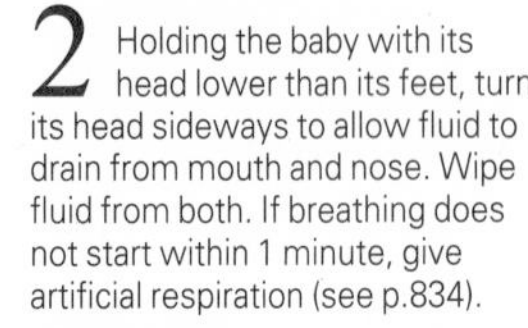

1 When the baby's head is visible in the vagina, birth is imminent. Once its head and shoulders emerge, support the baby by holding its head up. Do not pull. The rest of the baby's body will slide out.

2 Holding the baby with its head lower than its feet, turn its head sideways to allow fluid to drain from mouth and nose. Wipe fluid from both. If breathing does not start within 1 minute, give artificial respiration (see p.834).

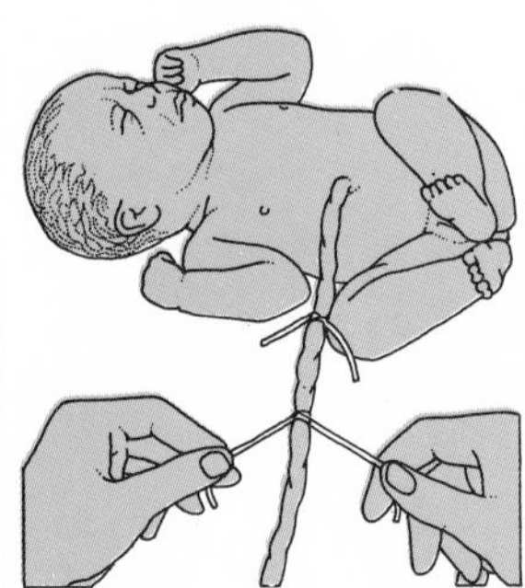

3 Wait until the umbilical cord stops pulsating before cutting it. Tie a tight knot with sterilized string at least 4 in (10 cm) from the baby's navel and another knot 2 in to 4 in (5 cm to 10 cm) away. Cut the cord between the two knots.

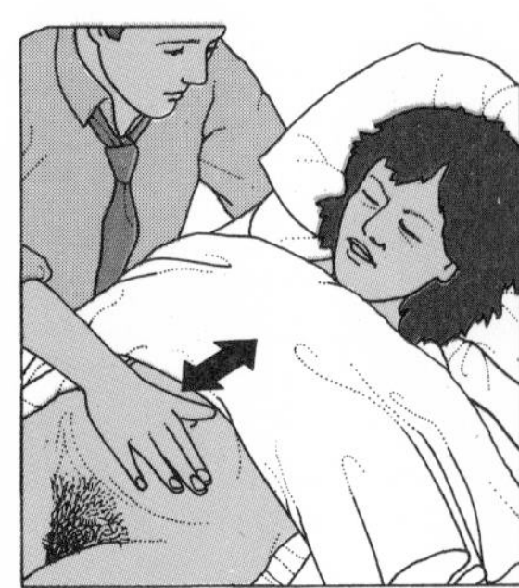

4 Within 20 minutes after the baby is born, the placenta (afterbirth) will usually emerge. Do not pull on the cord; it may tear off. If bleeding seems heavy, massage the woman's lower abdomen gently every few minutes until medical help arrives.

Index

A

B

C

D

F

G

H

J

M

N

O

P

Q

R

S

T

W

Acknowledgments

DORLING KINDERSLEY WOULD LIKE TO THANK THE FOLLOWING INDIVIDUALS, DEPARTMENTS, AND COMPANIES FOR THEIR HELP:

Commissioned photography
Andy Crawford, Steve Gorton

Illustrators
Simone End, Guy Smith, John Temperton, Debra Woodward

Retouching/Airbrushing
Roy Flooks, Selwyn Hutchinson

Design assistance
Anne Renel, Alastair Wardle

Editorial assistance
Joanna Chisholm, Howard Farrell, Stephanie Jackson, Mary Lindsay, Margaret Little, Martyn Page, Teresa Pritlove

Models
Tina Brazil, Fiona Courtenay-Thompson, Amy Evans, Carole Evans, Leigh Evans, Karen Good, John Goodwin, Emily Gorton, Kashi Gorton, Ian Henderson, Iris Henderson, Mary Lindsay, Phil Ormerod, Susan St Louis, Amy-Beth Walton-Evans, Ellen Woodward

Picture research
Kathy Lockley

Index
Sue Bosanko

Typesetting
Tradespools Ltd.

Reproduction
International Graphic Studios Ltd.

Film outputting
Graphical Innovations

PHOTOGRAPHIC CREDITS:

American Academy of Dermatology: 251 (below)
Audio-Visual Services: 260 (top left)
Biophoto Associates: 258 (top left), 258 (top right)
Children's Memorial Hospital, Chicago: 693 (below)
Image Bank/Ted Russell: 46
Images Colour Library: 17 (below)
National Medical Slide Bank: 49 (right center), 49 (below right)
Papworth Hospital Nuclear Medicine Department: 263 (top right), 263 (below right)
Science Photo Library: /Chris Priest & Mary Clarke: 17 (top); /Prof. P. Motta/Dept. of Anatomy, University "La Sapienza," Rome: 24 (left), 24 (right); /Peter Ryan: 48; /Biophoto Associates: 49 (top right); /Alexander Tsiaras: 49 (right above center), 264 (below left); /John McFarland: 49 (right below center); /James Stevenson: 49 (below left), 49 (below center); /Mehau Kulyk: 257 (center right); /Omikron: 257 (left); /CNRI: 257 (center left), 257 (right), 259 (top center), 259 (top right), 259 (below left), 259 (below right); /King's College School of Medicine, Dept. of Surgery: 258 (below right); /J.C.Revy: 259 (top left); 260 (below right); /Custom Medical Stock Photo: 260 (below left); /Clinique Ste. Catherine/CNRI: 261 (top right), 261 (below right); /Dr Raymond Damadian: 262 (top left), 262 (top right); /Simon Fraser/Medical Physics, RVI, Newcastle: 263 (top left), 263 (below left); /Petit Format/Nestle: 264 (top left), 264 (top right); /Manfred Kage: 264 (below right)
Tony Stone Images/Chris Harvey: 40; /Don Smetzer: 43
Dr Ian Williams: 258 (below left), 261 (top left), 261 (below left), 260 (top right), 262 (below left), 262 (below right)
ZEFA: 23 (center), 39, 54 (top), 54 (below), 55

Every effort has been made to trace the copyright holders and we apologize in advance for any unintentional omissions. We would be pleased to insert the appropriate acknowledgment in any subsequent edition of this publication.